Netter's Neurology

Netter's Neurology

Edited by
H. Royden Jones, Jr, MD
Jaime Ortiz-Patino Chair in Neurology
Lahey Clinic
Clinical Professor of Neurology
Harvard Medical School

Illustrations by Frank H. Netter, MD

Contributing Illustrators

John A. Craig, MD
Carlos A. G. Machado, MD
James A. Perkins, MS, MFA

Associate Editor for Neuroimaging

Richard A. Baker, MD
Emeritus Chair
Department of Radiology
Lahey Clinic

Icon Learning Systems · Teterboro, New Jersey

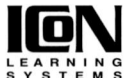

Published by Icon Learning Systems LLC, a subsidiary of MediMedia USA, Inc.
Copyright © 2005 MediMedia, Inc.

All rights reserved. No part of this book may be reproduced in any form or by any electronic or mechanical means, including information storage and retrieval systems, without permission in writing from the publisher.

Requests for permission should be addressed to Permissions Editor, Icon Learning Systems, 295 North Street, Teterboro, NJ 07608; or may be made at www.netterart.com/request.cfm.

ISBN 1-929007-06-X

Library of Congress Catalog No.: 2004114325

Printed in the U.S.A.

NOTICE

Every effort has been taken to confirm the accuracy of the information presented and to describe generally accepted practices. Neither the publisher nor the authors can be held responsible for errors or for any consequences arising from the use of the information contained herein, and make no warranty, expressed or implied, with respect to the contents of the publication.

Before prescribing pharmaceutical products, readers are advised to check the product information currently provided by the manufacturer of each drug to be administered to verify the recommended dose, the method and duration of administration, and the contraindications. It is the responsibility of the treating physician, relying on experience and knowledge of the patient, to determine dosages and the best treatment for the patient. Neither the publisher nor the editors assumes any responsibility for any injury and/or damage to persons or property.

Executive Editor: Paul Kelly
Editorial Director: Greg Otis
Managing Editor: Jennifer Surich
Production Manager: Stephanie Klein
Digital Asset Manager: Karen Oswald
Director of Manufacturing: Mary Ellen Curry

Binding and Printing by Quebecor World
Digital Separations by R.R. Donnelly and Page Imaging
Color Correction by Strine Printing

10 9 8 7 6 5 4 3 2 1

Dedication

To Mary Norman Jones, my beloved wife

Mary has been a steadfast and loyal supporter of my various academic pursuits. Their beginnings can be traced to my first major clinical research project during my neurology residency at Mayo. There are not enough words to begin to appropriately thank Mary for her love, dedicated parenting of our four wonderful children, companionship, and encouragement in these various projects, particularly including my two Netter volumes. Mary also became a friend and admirer of Frank Netter's many talents during our frequent sojourns to Palm Beach from 1982 to 1985 while Frank and I were composing the Nervous System Part II.

ABOUT THE EDITOR

H. Royden Jones, Jr, MD, the Jaime Ortiz-Patino Chair of Neurology at the Lahey Clinic, was born in central New Jersey and grew up in North Plainfield and Point Pleasant Beach. He graduated from Tufts College with a Bachelor of Science degree and, on the advice of his dean at Tufts, "went west" to obtain his MD at Northwestern University. While there, he met and married Mary Elizabeth Norman. Dr Jones served as a rotating intern at the Philadelphia General Hospital. An internist at Northwestern encouraged him to take his internal medicine residency at Mayo. During this period, a neurology rotation rekindled his neuroscience interests, and Dr Jones transferred to Mayo's neurology program. This experience was interrupted by a commitment to the United States Army Medical Corps, where he became Chief of Neurology at the 5th General Hospital, Bad Cannstatt, Germany.

After Dr Jones completed his residency, he moved to Boston to join the Lahey Clinic, where he has been a member of the neurologic staff since 1972. He has served there in a variety of administrative roles, including chair of the departments of education and neurology, the personnel committee, and the divisions of medicine and medical specialties, as well as being a member of the board of governors.

Neurologic education has always been one of Dr Jones' major interests. After coming to Lahey, he was also appointed to the teaching staff of the neurologic unit at Boston City Hospital, led by a superb educator, Norman Geschwind, MD. Here he received his initial Harvard appointment, as a clinical instructor. In 1978, based on his training with Ed Lambert, MD, at Mayo, Dr Jones was asked to develop the pediatric electromyographic laboratory at Children's Hospital Boston, where he maintained his Harvard Medical School academic affiliation, leading to his later becoming a Clinical Professor of Neurology.

His initial clinical research interests were in cerebrovascular diseases. However, as his experience at Children's Hospital Boston increased, Dr Jones focused his attention on neuromuscular disorders of children and concomitantly on Lambert-Eaton myasthenic syndrome, stiff man syndrome, and variants of immune-mediated motor neuropathies in adults.

Dr Jones edited the original *Part II, Neurologic and Neuromuscular Disorders, of Netter's Nervous System*, Volume 1, as well as two other monographs as a primary editor, including *Clinical Pediatric Electromyography* with Drs Bolton and Harper and *Neurologic Disorders of Infants, Childhood, and Adolescence* with his child-neurology colleagues Drs De Vivo and Darras. He has served on the American Board of Psychiatry and Neurology in a number of capacities, most recently completing an 8-year term as an elected director, has been a member of the Residency Review Committee of the Accreditation Council of Graduate Medical Education and previously represented the American Academy of Neurology at the American Association of Medical Colleges.

At the conclusion of 2004, Dr Jones will have completed all of his local and national administrative responsibilities and plans to return to his primary neurologic interests, seeing patients in the clinic and electromyography laboratory, while hoping to do more teaching and clinical research once again. Equally importantly, he plans to spend more time with his family, including Mary; his four children, Roy, Kate, Fred, and David; and his grandchildren, Erik, Kristin, Kendall, and Sam.

H. Royden Jones, Jr, MD
Jaime Ortiz-Patino Chair in Neurology
Lahey Clinic
Burlington, Massachusetts

Preface

The spectacular developments within clinical neurology during my lifetime often have been beyond any reasonable prediction. Consider just a few: One of the most dramatic has been the successful introduction of new pharmacologic modalities as well as deep brain stimulation for Parkinson disease; truly miraculous changes occurred for some individuals as portrayed by Oliver Sachs, MD, in *Awakenings*. Another is the discovery of the role of autoimmune pathophysiology in various peripheral and central nervous system disorders, including myasthenia gravis, and the acquired demyelinating polyneuropathies. This has led to very successful novel therapeutic intervention that have literally put many patients back on their feet. More in-depth neurophysiologic techniques have provided for an increased role of surgery for patients with previously socially devastating seizure disorders, especially in those uncommon scenarios where the many new and usually effective anticonvulsants have failed to control these events. In the past decade, the multiple sclerosis enigma has finally been opened with some effective prophylactic therapies; however, we need more innovative measures that will be effective early in the disease. Our psychiatric colleagues now possess specific and effective new medications targeted for depression and the affective disorders as their neurochemistry is being refined.

In neuroradiology, the replacement of direct-puncture carotid angiography and/or pneumoencephalography first by computed tomography imaging and now by finely tuned magnetic resonance imaging has led to Nobel recognition for 2 different teams of basic physical scientists. New classes of fine catheters now provide access to the almost microscopic cerebral arteries, providing the potential for direct infusion of thrombolytic agents or placement of coils directly into a berry aneurysm. Positron emission tomography scanning now offers another adjunctive role in clinical research and particularly our understanding of various seizure and neurodegenerative disorders.

Although spongiform encephalopathy has been recognized for many years, Prusiner's novel concept that a prion is the responsible mechanism has led to yet another Nobel award to a neurologic colleague. However, many challenges remain as there are still no effective therapies for a number of devastating neurodegenerative and biochemical disorders of the nervous system, including these rare prion disorders as well as the much more prevalent dementing disorder of Alzheimer disease. Many eagerly await further pathophysiologic elucidation that will lead to effective therapy. The emergence of the human immunodeficiency virus (HIV) pandemic, with its potential to involve so much of the entire nervous system, has caught us all by surprise; not since syphilis was conquered by penicillin 60 years ago have we witnessed a neurologic disorder with such an overwhelming and devastating predilection for both the central and the peripheral nervous system. This terrible epidemic has also emphasized the vast capabilities of our bench researchers at various medical industrial complexes. They have developed novel therapies, some proving so effective that some of us have not evaluated a new case of neurologic acquired immunodeficiency syndrome (AIDS) in more than 10 years.

Lou Gehrig disease, ie, amyotrophic lateral sclerosis, remains one of our greatest challenges. This and other neurodegenerative disorders, such as the spinocerebellar ataxias, deprive patients of their strength and equilibrium, respectively. All neurologists eagerly await resolution of these complex problems; we hope that these means will be expedited in the near future. To be successful, our colleagues will undoubtedly be aided by the many discoveries accruing within the framework of the DNA revolution; these findings may provide great help for our many patients with genetic disorders, particularly within the framework of child neurology.

My own romance with neurology began as a result of 2 interrelated events during my first year of medical school at Northwestern University in Chicago. The first was a wonderful

Preface

teacher, Ray Snider, PhD, who was a very wise neuroanatomist. He had the pedagogic gift to make this complex subject intellectually stimulating and clinically relevant. My second was our introduction to the magnificent artwork of Frank H. Netter, MD, through his initial collection of Nervous System Illustrations. Dr Netter's skillful interpretations allowed me to more easily and clearly conceptualize this most complicated of body systems. Frank Netter soon became one of my first medical heroes. At that time, it would have never entered my imagination that I would one day have the opportunity to work closely with Dr Netter, let alone that this would eventuate in our becoming dear friends. His was a special career that few physicians have successfully emulated.

Colleagues have often asked how I came to work with Dr Netter. In 1978, at the American Medical Association meeting in San Francisco, I serendipitously visited the CIBA (now Novartis) pharmaceutical booth when I noted in passing that it was promoting Dr Netter's artwork. By this time, Frank was the world's most prestigious medical artist. I naively inquired of the CIBA representative whether Dr Netter had considered doing a *Clinical Symposia* on the mononeuropathies. A few months later, I received a letter from Frank Netter asking me to elaborate on my ideas, and soon after, I was sitting in Frank's Palm Beach studio smoking cigars with this icon of medical artistry. During these sessions, Frank would have me discuss the various clinical entities. Then he would ask for my suggestions as to how he might conceive plates for the subject. Dr Netter always demanded that he himself fully understand the specific medical issues appropriate to the subject at hand. Together we would decide on the most suitable venue to illustrate each entity. On an average day, we would get through 12 to 15 potential subjects, with Frank taking notes for his planned rough drafts that he would later send on to me. Even though I would have loved to watch him paint, I never asked to do so; from my own amateurish experience, I knew that this was a very private moment for an artist trying to conceptualize something.

On a return visit, Frank first mentioned to me that he was giving serious consideration to updating his original nervous system volume; he asked me to join with him in bringing this project to completion and asked that I propose a plan to complete this venture by utilizing his previously completed plates and helping him consider what new art was necessary. Thus was born the 2-volume Netter Nervous System published in 1986. We hoped to make the clinical volume relevant for a long time to come by illustrating the basic anatomy, pathophysiology, and clinical symptomatology of the most common of the many neurologic disorders. My subsequent long weekend visits with Dr Netter became a cherished time for both my wife Mary and me. Frank was a gentleman in the classic definition, a dedicated and passionate artist, and a superb golfer. It was on the links that he frequently took challenging projects to finalize their conceptualization.

We usually started our days together at about 7 AM. Although most of the original Netter plates were designed for ongoing relevance, sometimes new information made them obsolete. For example, in the mid 1950s, Frank had painted some 20 plates on the thoracic outlet syndrome. Then it was thought that this entity was the underlying mechanism for that most common of all neurologic complaints, ie, intermittent, usually nocturnal, numbness and tingling of the hands. When electromyography came into early use at the Mayo Clinic and Queens Square later in that decade, it was then recognized that the primary lesion related to median nerve entrapment at the wrist, ie, carpal tunnel syndrome; this had nothing to do with cervical ribs. Frank was very proud of his thoracic outlet syndrome plates and it took a lot of gentle per-

PREFACE

suasion to get him to agree not to publish even one of his artistically accomplished but now scientifically rarely relevant plates.

The resultant text, Nervous System Part II, *Neurologic and Neuromuscular Disorders*, became very dated over the past 10 years. This related to the tremendous surge in neuroscience advances particularly in the "decade of the brain." Some of these milestones are highlighted in an earlier paragraph. When Icon Learning Systems had the good judgment to gain publication access to the Netter plates and asked me to help with this neurology volume, I could not have been more thrilled.

As neurology is the finest tuned of the clinical sciences, I wished to infuse life within this volume by including clinical vignettes in each chapter; many were or are patients of mine and the remaining are from my Lahey coauthors. In so doing, my colleagues and I wanted to bring special relevance to the student of neurology, whether someone very early on in their medical education, or the resident or fellow, or even the practitioner. We think that this case method approach, with emphasis on the history and clinical examination, will enlighten the student as well as even stimulate the most experienced clinician's interest. Probably a number of the "patients" presented here will be old friends to our neurologically savvy readers.

Because neurology and neuroscience have been constantly advancing, we needed to update some of the original classic Netter illustrations as well as to develop a number of new ones. In this all-important task, my new artistic collaborators John A. Craig, MD, an ophthalmologist, and Carlos A. G. Machado, MD, a cardiologist, have been superb colleagues who have followed the pathway that Frank Netter, MD, so spectacularly blazed while still being true to their own artistic expressions. It has been an honor to get to know these wonderful and superbly talented artists and physicians.

My colleagues and I hope the readers of this volume will find in it a resource that will be useful to many neurologic "students" throughout all stages of their professional lives. Furthermore, we particularly feel that the artwork of Frank Netter will once again come full circle to inspire yet another generation of medical students to enter the forever stimulating fields of neuroscience.

H. Royden Jones, Jr, MD
Burlington and Boston, Massachusetts

Frank H. Netter, MD

Frank H. Netter was born in 1906 in New York City. He studied art at the Art Student's League and the National Academy of Design before entering medical school at New York University, where he received his MD degree in 1931. During his student years, Dr Netter's notebook sketches attracted the attention of the medical faculty and other physicians, allowing him to augment his income by illustrating articles and textbooks. He continued illustrating as a sideline after establishing a surgical practice in 1933, but he ultimately opted to give up his practice in favor of a full-time commitment to art. After service in the United States Army during World War II, Dr Netter began his long collaboration with the CIBA Pharmaceutical Company (now Novartis Pharmaceuticals). This 45-year partnership resulted in the production of the extraordinary collection of medical art so familiar to physicians and other medical professionals worldwide.

Icon Learning Systems acquired the Netter Collection in July 2000 and continues to update Dr Netter's original paintings and to add newly commissioned paintings by artists trained in the style of Dr Netter.

Dr Netter's works are among the finest examples of the use of illustration in the teaching of medical concepts. The 13-book Netter Collection of Medical Illustrations, which includes the greater part of the more than 20,000 paintings created by Dr Netter, became and remains one of the most famous medical works ever published. The Atlas of Human Anatomy, first published in 1989, presents the anatomical paintings from the Netter Collection. Now translated into 11 languages, it is the anatomy atlas of choice among medical and health professions students the world over.

The Netter illustrations are appreciated not only for their aesthetic qualities but, more importantly, for their intellectual content. As Dr Netter wrote in 1949, "... clarification of a subject is the aim and goal of illustration. No matter how beautifully painted, how delicately and subtly rendered a subject may be, it is of little value as a medical illustration if it does not serve to make clear some medical point." Dr Netter's planning, conception, point of view, and approach are what inform his paintings and what makes them so intellectually valuable.

Frank H. Netter, MD, physician and artist, died in 1991.

Acknowledgments

It is very important for me to be able to pay tribute to some of my teachers, first and foremost my loving Mom and Dad, who always encouraged my academic interests. In high school, I found that one special teacher, Albert A. Surina; it was his chemistry course that stimulated me to seek a career in science and not the law. My family internist Leonard Williams, MD, also took a special interest in my career when I entered Tufts as an undergraduate; "Doc Willie" gave me the necessary confidence to consider a career in medicine. Our organic chemistry professor at Tufts, "Pop" Dolman, turned this subject into the most intellectually stimulating of my college career; in a way, his approach to teaching, this most important of the premed courses, set the stage for the reasoning process so essential to the differential diagnosis a neurologist entertains each time she or he takes a history. Clifton Emery, PhD, Tufts' Dean, encouraged me to consider Northwestern. Instead of "becoming a provincial New Englander," he told me to expand my horizons.

At Northwestern University medical school, Ray Snider, PhD, our teacher of neuroanatomy, was the initial preclinical scientist to bring clinical medicine into the first-year classroom. His challenging and thoughtful lectures and examinations made the nervous system take a life of its own for me, and I began to consider a career in this field. Later, the opportunity to study with Martin Brandfonbrenner, MD, a brilliant young cardiologist with whom I was privileged to spend almost an entire year, introduced me to clinical research and didactic teaching rounds at their best. Neurology took a back seat in my career plans. Lastly, a clinical internist at Evanston Hospital, Dr Franklin Kiser, was the one who encouraged me to go to Mayo, and there my medical career became truly blessed.

Mayo was endowed with so many fine clinicians and clinical researchers I will certainly be remiss when I mention just a few. At the beginnings were Peter J. Dyck, MD, and Kendall Corbin, MD, PhD, who were my first neurology attendings, or visits, as they say here in Boston. In January 1965, having had almost 3 years of internal medicine, I was fully committed to becoming a cardiologist. However, a 6-week rotation on the hospital neurology service was so stimulating with Dr Corbin that he encouraged me to speak with Robert G. Siekert, MD, about a neurologic career. Thus, my initial medical school interests were vitally reactivated.

Once this decision was reached, I had the good fortune to work with many other masters of the neurology profession. Some of the foremost being Drs Donald Mulder, Norman Goldstein, and Bill Karnes as well as Don Klass and Ed Lambert in their renowned neurophysiologic laboratories. Most influential was Dr Bob Siekert, who has continued to be a dear friend as well as an early collaborator. Peter Dyck is still available for phone consultations in addition to reading all our sural nerve biopsies some 40 years later. One could never have dreamed of having such wonderful role models.

I wish to pay special thanks to my Lahey colleagues who have been so supportive over the years. This includes Steve Kott, MD, our chair for more than 2 decades; Steve Freidberg, MD, chair of neurosurgery; his predecessor, Charles Fager, MD; and Dick Baker, MD, Lahey's first neuroradiologist, who has been a major help as a contributor of all neuroradiographic images for both the Nervous System Part II and this volume. Our former chief executive officer Robert Wise, MD, supported an all-too-spirited young neurologist through thick and thin, in particular making it possible for me to found the electromyography laboratory at Children's Hospital Boston, when I was recruited there in 1979, while maintaining a full time appointment at Lahey. It has been a great pleasure to see our neuroscience efforts grow so strongly here over these 3-plus decades. The continued support and friendship of our outstanding current chief executive officer at Lahey, David Barrett, MD, is also greatly appreciated. Many others deserve

Acknowledgments

mention, but space is short, and so to those dear colleagues all I can say is many thanks, the trip has been a ball!

Very importantly, I will forever be indebted to my dear friend, Jaime Ortiz-Patino, who underwrote the Jaime Ortiz-Patino Chair in Neurology at Lahey for me. This Medici-like gift has made it possible for me to have time for this second venture with Frank Netter, albeit in absentia this time since Frank's death in 1991. No one could be more fortunate. I feel truly blessed to have had the tremendous collaboration of my many Lahey Clinic neuroscience colleagues to bring this latest Netter venue to fruition.

Additionally, I wish to acknowledge Susan Gay, Jennifer Surich, Carolyn Kruse, Tamara Myers, Jennifer Withers, and Greg Otis at Icon Learning Systems who have so faithfully worked on the nuts and bolts of this venture. It has been a pleasure to have the opportunity to be colleagues with my new artist heroes, John Craig, MD, and Carlos Machado, MD, to whom I owe many, many thanks. It has been an honor to work with them as well as much fun; I hope that we can collaborate in the future.

Lastly, I wish to thank Carol Spencer for her special help with this project, as well as her ongoing dedication to all of the physicians at Lahey. Carol has continually made it easier for us to accomplish our clinical research projects by creating a wonderfully accessible medical library for many years. In addition, I wish to acknowledge the many contributions of Joyce Royston, Carol's able assistant in our medical library.

H. Royden Jones, Jr, MD
Burlington and Boston, Massachusetts

CONTRIBUTORS

All of the contributors are associated with the Lahey Clinic Medical Center unless otherwise noted.

Editor

H. Royden Jones, Jr, MD
Emeritus Chairman, Department of Neurology and Division of Medical Specialties
Clinical Professor of Neurology, Harvard Medical School
Director EMG Lab, Children's Hospital Boston

Associate Editor

Richard A. Baker, MD
Diagnostic Radiologist
Lecturer on Radiology, Harvard Medical School
Associate Clinical Professor of Radiology, Tufts University School of Medicine

Assistant Editors

Gregory Allam, MD
Department of Neurology

Ted M. Burns, MD
Assistant Professor
Department of Neurology
University of Virginia

Ann Camac, MD
Department of Neurology

Claudia J. Chaves, MD
Director of Multiple Sclerosis Clinic
Department of Neurology

Stephen R. Freidberg, MD
Chair, Department of Neurosurgery

Kinan K. Hreib, MD, PhD
Director Stroke Service
Assistant Clinical Professor, Tufts University

James A. Russell, DO
Director of Muscular Dystrophy Association Clinic
Vice Chairman, Department of Neurology

Monique M. Ryan, MB BS, MMed, FRACP
Former Fellow in Clinical Neurophysiology/Electromyography and Neuromuscular Disorders
Senior Lecturer
Discipline of Pediatrics and Child Health
University of Sydney

Jayashri Srinivasan, MBBS, PhD, MRCP
Department of Neurology

Yuval Zabar, MD
Director, Center for Memory and Cognitive Disorders
Department of Neurology

Contributing Authors

Lloyd M. Alderson, MD, DSc
Department of Neurosurgery

Timothy D. Anderson, MD
Senior Staff
Department of Otolaryngology

Diana Apetauerova, MD
Department of Neurology

Jeffrey E. Arle, MD, PhD
Director, Functional Neurosurgery
Department of Neurosurgery

Peter J. Catalano, MD, FACS
Chairman, Department of Otolaryngology
Associate Professor of Otolaryngology, Boston University

Ellen Choi, BS
Senior Medical Student, Tufts University Medical School
Department of Otolaryngology, Head and Neck Surgery

Contributors

Donald E. Craven, MD
Chair, Department of Infectious Diseases
Professor of Medicine, Tufts University School of Medicine

Carlos A. David, MD
Director Cerebrovascular Surgery
Co-Director Skull Base Surgery
Department of Neurology
Clinical Assistant Professor, Tufts University School of Medicine

Peter K. Dempsey, MD
Department of Neurosurgery

Francesco G. De Rosa, MD
Assistant Clinical Professor
Infectious Diseases, University of Turin

Robert A. Duncan, MD, MPM
Senior Staff Physician
Center for Infections Diseases

Jennifer A. Grillo, MD
Former Fellow in Clinical Neurophysiology/Electromyography and Neuromuscular Disorders
Staff Neurologist, Holy Family Hospital

Paul T. Gross, MD
Chair, Department of Neurology
Clinical Professor of Neurology, Tufts University

Jose A. Gutrecht, MD, MSc
Department of Neurology

Aaron C. Heide, MD
Director of Stroke Services
Department of Neurology
Valley Medical Center

Alice A. Hunter, MD
Department of Orthopaedic Surgery

Allison Gudis Jackson, MS CCC-SLP
Speech-Language Pathologist
Department of Otolaryngology

Edward R. Jewell, MD
Chair, Department of Vascular Surgery

N. George Kasparyan, MD, PhD
Director of Hand Surgery
Assistant Professor of Orthopedics, Boston University, School of Medicine

Kenneth Lakritz, MD
Department of Psychiatry and Behavioral Medicine

Marie C. Lucey, BS, PT
Physical Therapist
Center for Balance and Mobility, Gordon College

Subu N. Magge, MD
Department of Neurosurgery

Steven W. Margles, MD
Department of Orthopaedic Surgery, Section of Hand Surgery
Assistant Clinical Professor, Department of Orthopaedic Surgery, Boston University

John Markman, MD
Department of Anesthesiology and Neurology

Ippolit C. A. Matjucha, MD
Neuro-ophthalmologist
Department of Ophthalmology

Daniel P. McQuillen, MD
Department of Infectious Disease
Assistant Professor, Tufts University School of Medicine

Michael P. McQuillen, MD, MA
Professor of Neurology and of the Medical Humanities
University of Rochester, School of Medicine and Dentistry

Eva M. Michalakis, MS CCC-SLP
Clinical Director of Speech, Voice, Swallowing
Department of Otolaryngology

Mary Anne Muriello, MD
Department of Neurology
Associate Professor of Clinical Neurology, Tufts University School of Medicine

Contributors

Winnie Ooi, MD, MPH, DMD
Travel and Tropical Medicine Clinic
Department of Infectious Diseases

Joel M. Oster, MD
Director of Epilepsy and EEG
Department of Neurology

E. Prather Palmer, MD
Staff Physician
Department of Neurology

Kevin B. Raftery, MD
Department of Vascular Surgery

Edward Tarlov, MD
Department of Neurosurgery

Eric T. Tolo, MD
Orthopaedic Surgeon
Division of Hand and Upper Extremity Surgery
Department of Orthopaedic Surgery

Robert J. Updaw II
Senior Medical Student, Medical School of Ohio

Michal Vytopil, MD
Fellow in Clinical Neurophysiology/Electromyography and Neuromuscular Disorders
Department of Neurology

Harold J. Welch, MD
Senior Vascular Surgeon
Department of Vascular Surgery

Judith White, MD, PhD
Head, Section of Vestibular and Balance Disorders
Head and Neck Institute, The Cleveland Clinic

Table of Contents

I. NEUROLOGIC EXAMINATION
Kinan K. Hreib, Associate Editor

Chapter 1. Clinical Neurologic Evaluation 2
Kinan K. Hreib and H. Royden Jones, Jr

Chapter 2. Cognitive and Language Evaluation 40
Kinan K. Hreib

II. NEURO-OPHTHALMOLOGY
H. Royden Jones, Jr, Associate Editor

Chapter 3. Retina and Optic Nerve 54
Ippolit C. A. Matjucha and Robert J. Updaw II

Chapter 4. Optic Chiasm, Optic Tract, Lateral Geniculate Nucleus, and Optic Radiations 64
Ippolit C. A. Matjucha and Robert J. Updaw II

Chapter 5. Primary Visual Cortex 72
Ippolit C. A. Matjucha and Robert J. Updaw II

Chapter 6. Cranial Nerve III: Oculomotor 77
Ippolit C. A. Matjucha

Chapter 7. Cranial Nerve IV: Trochlear 85
Ippolit C. A. Matjucha

Chapter 8. Cranial Nerve VI: Abducens 89
Ippolit C. A. Matjucha

III. CRANIAL NERVES
Kinan K. Hreib, Associate Editor

Chapter 9. Cranial Nerve I: Olfactory 96
Michal Vytopil and H. Royden Jones, Jr

Chapter 10. Cranial Nerve V: Trigeminal 101
Michal Vytopil and Edward Tarlov

Chapter 11. Cranial Nerve VII: Facial 112
Michal Vytopil, Peter J. Catalano, and H. Royden Jones, Jr

Chapter 12. Cranial Nerve VIII: Vestibular 126
Kinan K. Hreib, Judith White, and Marie C. Lucey

Chapter 13. Cranial Nerve VIII: Auditory 134
Ellen Choi and Peter J. Catalano

Table of Contents

Chapter 14. Cranial Nerve IX, Glossopharyngeal, and Cranial Nerve X, Vagus: Swallowing *143*
Eva M. Michalakis, Allison Gudis Jackson, and Peter J. Catalano

Chapter 15. Cranial Nerve X, Vagus: Voice Disorders *153*
Timothy D. Anderson

Chapter 16. Cranial Nerve XI: Spinal Accessory *157*
Michal Vytopil and H. Royden Jones, Jr

Chapter 17. Cranial Nerve XII: Hypoglossal *163*
Michal Vytopil and H. Royden Jones, Jr

IV. HEADACHE
Ann Camac, Associate Editor

Chapter 18. Primary and Secondary Headache *170*
Jose A. Gutrecht and Edward Tarlov

V. CEREBROVASCULAR DISORDERS
Claudia J. Chaves, Associate Editor

Chapter 19. Arterial Supply to the Brain and Meninges *188*
Aaron C. Heide and Claudia J. Chaves

Chapter 20. Ischemic Stroke *195*
Claudia J. Chaves and H. Royden Jones, Jr

Chapter 21. Endarterectomy for Extracranial Carotid Artery Atherosclerosis *218*
Edward R. Jewell, Harold J. Welch, and Kevin B. Raftery

Chapter 22. Cerebral Venous Thrombosis *223*
Gregory Allam

Chapter 23. Intracerebral Hemorrhage *234*
Kinan K. Hreib and H. Royden Jones, Jr

Chapter 24. Cerebral Aneurysms and Subarachnoid Hemorrhage *248*
Carlos A. David

VI. EPILEPSY AND SYNCOPE
Gregory Allam, Associate Editor

Chapter 25. Epilepsy and Syncope *264*
Joel M. Oster, Jose A. Gutrecht, and Paul T. Gross

Chapter 26. Surgical Treatments for Epilepsy *281*
Jeffrey E. Arle

TABLE OF CONTENTS

VII. SLEEP DISORDERS
Gregory Allam, Associate Editor

Chapter 27. Sleep Disorders *288*
Paul T. Gross

VIII. DISORDERS OF CONSCIOUSNESS
Gregory Allam, Associate Editor

Chapter 28. Coma *296*
Gregory Allam

Chapter 29. Increased Intracranial Pressure and Cerebral Herniation *307*
Gregory Allam

Chapter 30. Brain Death *316*
Gregory Allam

IX. MEMORY AND COGNITIVE DISORDERS
Yuval Zabar, Associate Editor

Chapter 31. Acute Cognitive and Behavioral Disorders *322*
Yuval Zabar

Chapter 32. Alzheimer Disease *327*
Yuval Zabar

Chapter 33. Dementia With Lewy Bodies *347*
Yuval Zabar

Chapter 34. Frontotemporal Dementia *351*
Yuval Zabar

Chapter 35. Vascular Dementia *356*
Yuval Zabar

Chapter 36. Transmissible Spongiform Encephalopathy *360*
Yuval Zabar

X. PSYCHIATRIC DISORDERS
Yuval Zabar and H. Royden Jones, Jr, Associate Editors

Chapter 37. Major Depression *366*
Kenneth Lakritz

Chapter 38. Bipolar Disorder *369*
Kenneth Lakritz

TABLE OF CONTENTS

Chapter 39. Schizophrenia *372*
Kenneth Lakritz

Chapter 40. Obsessive-Compulsive Disorder *375*
Kenneth Lakritz

Chapter 41. Panic Disorder *378*
Kenneth Lakritz

Chapter 42. Dysthymia *381*
Kenneth Lakritz

Chapter 43. Borderline Personality Disorder *384*
Kenneth Lakritz

Chapter 44. Attention Deficit Disorder *387*
Kenneth Lakritz

Chapter 45. Drug and Alcohol Abuse *390*
Kenneth Lakritz

Chapter 46. Delirium *399*
Kenneth Lakritz

XI. MOVEMENT DISORDERS
Ann Camac, Associate Editor

Chapter 47. Parkinson Disease *402*
Diana Apetauerova

Chapter 48. Atypical Parkinsonian Syndromes *414*
Diana Apetauerova

Chapter 49. Tremors *422*
E. Prather Palmer

Chapter 50. Medication-Induced Movement Disorders *432*
Diana Apetauerova

Chapter 51. Dystonia *438*
E. Prather Palmer

Chapter 52. Myoclonus *447*
Diana Apetauerova

Chapter 53. Chorea *453*
Diana Apetauerova

TABLE OF CONTENTS

Chapter 54. Tic Disorders 460
E. Prather Palmer

Chapter 55. Wilson Disease 466
E. Prather Palmer

Chapter 56. Psychogenic Movement Disorders 472
Diana Apetauerova

Chapter 57. Surgical Treatments for Movement Disorders 475
Jeffrey E. Arle

XII. GAIT DISORDERS AND DIZZINESS
Kinan K. Hreib, Associate Editor

Chapter 58. Gait Disorders 480
Kinan K. Hreib

XIII. MYELOPATHIES
Ann Camac, Associate Editor

Chapter 59. Anatomical Aspects of Myelopathies 492
Ann Camac and H. Royden Jones, Jr

Chapter 60. Acute Myelopathies 503
Ann Camac and H. Royden Jones, Jr

Chapter 61. Chronic Myelopathies 514
Ann Camac and H. Royden Jones, Jr

XIV. MULTIPLE SCLEROSIS AND OTHER DEMYELINATING DISORDERS
Ann Camac, Associate Editor

Chapter 62. Multiple Sclerosis and Acute Disseminated Encephalomyelitis ... 538
Mary Anne Muriello, H. Royden Jones, Jr, and Claudia J. Chaves

XV. INFECTIOUS DISEASE
Claudia J. Chaves, Associate Editor

Chapter 63. Bacterial Meningitis 560
Donald E. Craven, Francesco G. De Rosa, Daniel P. McQuillen, and Robert A. Duncan

Chapter 64. Parameningeal Infections 566
Donald E. Craven, Francesco G. De Rosa, and H. Royden Jones, Jr

Chapter 65. Neurosyphilis 570
Daniel P. McQuillen

TABLE OF CONTENTS

Chapter 66. Viral Infections of the Nervous System 574
Francesco G. De Rosa, Daniel P. McQuillen, Donald E. Craven, John Markman, and H. Royden Jones, Jr

Chapter 67. Tuberculosis of Brain and Spine 583
Daniel P. McQuillen

Chapter 68. Infections in Immunocompromised Hosts 586
Donald E. Craven, Francesco G. De Rosa, Daniel P. McQuillen, and H. Royden Jones, Jr

Chapter 69. Tetanus 594
H. Royden Jones, Jr

Chapter 70. Poliomyelitis 597
Daniel P. McQuillen and Michael P. McQuillen

XVI. NEURO-ONCOLOGY
H. Royden Jones, Jr, Associate Editor

Chapter 71. Neuro-oncology Differential Diagnosis 604
H. Royden Jones, Jr, Peter K. Dempsey, and Lloyd M. Alderson

Chapter 72. Malignant Brain Tumors 611
Peter K. Dempsey and Lloyd M. Alderson

Chapter 73. Benign Brain Tumors 622
Peter K. Dempsey and Lloyd M. Alderson

Chapter 74. Spinal Cord Tumors 635
Peter K. Dempsey, Lloyd M. Alderson, and H. Royden Jones, Jr

XVII. TRAUMA TO THE BRAIN AND SPINAL CORD
Stephen R. Freidberg, Associate Editor

Chapter 75. Brain Trauma 644
Carlos A. David

Chapter 76. Trauma of the Spine and Spinal Cord 658
Stephen R. Freidberg and Subu N. Magge

XVIII. RADICULOPATHIES
Stephen R. Freidberg, Associate Editor

Chapter 77. Cervical Radiculopathy 672
Subu N. Magge and Stephen R. Freidberg

Chapter 78. Lumbar Radiculopathy 679
Stephen R. Freidberg and Subu N. Magge

TABLE OF CONTENTS

Chapter 79. Lumbar Spinal Stenosis 691
H. Royden Jones, Jr, and Stephen R. Friedberg

Chapter 80. Rheumatologic, Functional, and Psychosomatic Back Pain 694
H. Royden Jones, Jr

XIX. PLEXOPATHIES
Ted M. Burns, Associate Editor

Chapter 81. Brachial Plexus and Brachial Plexopathies 700
Ted M. Burns and H. Royden Jones, Jr

Chapter 82. Lumbosacral Plexopathies 708
Ted M. Burns and Monique M. Ryan

XX. MONONEUROPATHIES
James A. Russell, Associate Editor

Chapter 83. Overview of Mononeuropathies 716
N. George Kasparyan and James A. Russell

Chapter 84. Mononeuropathies Presenting With Upper Extremity Symptoms 726
Steven W. Margles and James A. Russell

Chapter 85. Mononeuropathies Presenting With Shoulder Pain and Weakness 741
Alice A. Hunter and James A. Russell

Chapter 86. Mononeuropathies Presenting With Lower Extremity Weakness 746
Eric T. Tolo, James A. Russell, and H. Royden Jones, Jr

Chapter 87. Primary Sensory Neuropathies of the Lower Extremity 757
N. George Kasparyan and James A. Russell

XXI. MOTOR NEURON DISORDERS
James A. Russell, Associate Editor

Chapter 88. Overview of Motor Neuron Disease 764
James A. Russell and H. Royden Jones, Jr

Chapter 89. Motor Neuron Disease Presenting in the Limbs With Lower Motor Neuron Features 777
James A. Russell and H. Royden Jones, Jr

Chapter 90. Primary Lateral Sclerosis: Motor Neuron Disease Presenting With Upper Motor Neuron Features in the Limbs 783
James A. Russell

Table of Contents

Chapter 91. Motor Neuron Disease: Bulbar, Head Drop, and Ventilatory Presentations ..*789*
James A. Russell

Chapter 92. Stiff Person Syndrome *794*
Ted M. Burns and H. Royden Jones, Jr

XXII. POLYNEUROPATHIES AND AUTONOMIC DISORDERS
James A. Russell, Associate Editor

Chapter 93. Overview of Peripheral Nerve Disease *800*
Ted M. Burns and James A. Russell

Chapter 94. Length-Dependent Polyneuropathy *808*
Jennifer A. Grillo, James A. Russell, and H. Royden Jones, Jr

Chapter 95. Acquired Demyelinating Polyradiculoneuropathies: Guillain-Barré Syndrome and Chronic Inflammatory Demyelinating Polyradiculoneuropathy *818*
Ted M. Burns, James A. Russell, and H. Royden Jones, Jr

Chapter 96. Multifocal Neuropathies *827*
Monique M. Ryan, Ted M. Burns, James A. Russell, and H. Royden Jones, Jr

Chapter 97. Sensory Neuropathy and Neuronopathy *834*
Jennifer A. Grillo, James A. Russell, and H. Royden Jones, Jr

Chapter 98. Leprosy (Hansen Disease) *839*
Jayashri Srinivasan and Winnie Ooi

Chapter 99. Disorders of the Autonomic Nervous System *843*
Ted M. Burns, Jayashri Srinivasan, and James A. Russell

XXIII. NEUROMUSCULAR TRANSMISSION DISORDERS
Ted M. Burns, Associate Editor

Chapter 100. Neuromuscular Junction Anatomy and Physiology *850*
Monique M. Ryan

Chapter 101. Lambert-Eaton Myasthenic Syndrome *858*
Ted M. Burns and H. Royden Jones, Jr

Chapter 102. Myasthenia Gravis *864*
Ted M. Burns, Monique M. Ryan, and H. Royden Jones, Jr

TABLE OF CONTENTS

XXIV. MYOPATHIES
James A. Russell, Associate Editor

Chapter 103. Overview of Muscle Disease 872
James A. Russell and H. Royden Jones, Jr

Chapter 104. Acute or Subacute Proximally Predominant or Generalized Myopathies Presenting With Weakness 884
Jayashri Srinivasan, James A. Russell, and H. Royden Jones, Jr

Chapter 105. Myopathies: Chronic Proximally Predominant or Generalized Weakness ..892
Jayashri Srinivasan, James A. Russell, and H. Royden Jones, Jr

Chapter 106. Distal Predominant Myopathies 906
Monique M. Ryan and James A. Russell

Chapter 107. The Channelopathies: Myopathies Presenting With Episodic Weakness 909
Monique M. Ryan and James A. Russell

Chapter 108. Myopathies Presenting With Exercise Intolerance 914
Monique M. Ryan and James A. Russell

INDEX 923

Section I
NEUROLOGIC EXAMINATION

Chapter 1
Clinical Neurologic Evaluation 2

Chapter 2
Cognitive and Language Evaluation 40

Chapter 1
Clinical Neurologic Evaluation

Kinan K. Hreib and H. Royden Jones, Jr

Neurology is a rewarding, intellectually demanding clinical discipline involving careful history taking, detailed patient examination, formulation of diagnostic evaluations, and development of treatment and supportive plans for patients. The most important encounter with a patient is the initial examination, during which the physician should endeavor to build trust and encourage the patient to communicate openly. This chapter provides the information that forms the basis of the performance of detailed neurologic evaluations.

NEUROLOGIC HISTORY

An accurate history requires attention to detail, reading the patient's body language, and interviewing family members and, sometimes, witnesses to patient's difficulties. History taking is an art even more time consuming than a complete, careful neurologic examination. Some patients have seen one neurologist before they seek another's opinion. To prevent bias, a neurologist should not read others' notes or look at previous neuroimages before taking the history and performing the examination.

One of the most important attributes of a skillful neurologist is the ability to be a good listener so as not to miss crucial historic points. It is important to begin the initial meeting by asking patients why they have come; this offers them the opportunity to express concerns in their own words. If possible, the neurologist should not interrupt, so that the patient may provide the information they deem of greatest importance. Rarely, anxious or compulsive patients may speak of their concerns at great length; with experience, physicians learn to use interjections to maintain control of the evaluation and draw the patient back from tangents.

When the patient's primary concerns have been established, specific issues can be explored. Additionally, making careful observations during the history review allows better focus for subsequent questions. An accurate assessment of mental status and language can be obtained from listening to the patient and observing responses to questions. Although time-consuming, the history is the most important factor leading to accurate diagnoses.

Unfortunately, the economics of modern health care has forced primary care physicians to shorten encounters with patients and their families. Many physicians use tests as substitutes for careful clinical evaluation. The combination of the detailed medical information available on the Internet and the adversarial medical-legal environment have enhanced patients' knowledge bases, although not always in a balanced way. Patient expectations sometimes affect the diagnostic approach of physicians. In this environment, it is not surprising that imaging techniques such as MRI and CT have replaced or supplemented a significant portion of clinical judgment. However, even the most dramatic test findings may prove irrelevant without appropriate clinical correlation. To have patients unnecessarily undergo surgery because of MRI findings that have no relation to their complaints may lead to a tragic outcome. Therein lies the importance of gaining complete understanding of the clinical issues.

Although neurology may seem in danger of being subsumed by overreliance on highly sophisticated tests, these studies have improved diagnostic skills and choice of therapy. For example, much knowledge regarding the early recognition, progression, and response to treatment of multiple sclerosis (MS) depends on careful MRI imaging.

It is essential to make patients feel comfortable in the office, particularly by fostering a positive interpersonal relationship. Taking time to ask about patients' lives, education, and social habits often provides useful clues. A careful set of questions providing a general review of systems may lead to the key diagnostic clue that focuses the evaluation. When the patient develops a sense of confidence and rapport with an empathetic physician, he or she is more willing to return for follow-up, even if a diagnosis is not made at the initial evaluation. Sometimes a careful second or third examination reveals a crucial difference that leads to a specific diagnosis. If patients feel rushed on their first visit, they may not return for follow-up, thus denying the neurologist a chance at crucial diagnostic observations. The physician-patient relationship must always be carefully nourished and highly respected.

AN APPROACH TO THE NEUROLOGIC EVALUATION

Throughout training, examination skills are continually being amplified, based on ever-evolving clinical experience and observation of varied approaches of academic physicians to different types of patients. It is essential to interpretation of the neurologic examination to understand what is normal at different ages as well as learning how to elicit important, sometimes subtle clues to diagnosis.

One of the most intellectually challenging aspects of neurology relates to the multiple potential neuroanatomical sources for many complaints. Therefore, although carpal tunnel syndrome is the most common cause for a numb hand, be certain not to overlook other anatomical sites, such as at the level of the brachial plexus, cervical nerve root, spinal cord, or brain.

Essential to the practice of neurology is gaining as much information as possible in patients presenting with unusual or unfamiliar neurologic complaints. A carefully obtained history and examination is essential to discerning the eventual diagnosis and exploring treatment options. A hasty history and examination can be misleading. For example, a diagnosis of early MS may be missed by not asking about such things as previous problems with visual function, shooting electric paresthesiae when bending the neck (Lhermitte sign), or sphincter problems. Alternatively, failure to undress a patient with numb hands may deny the examining physician the opportunity to elicit an unexpected positive Babinski response or even a spinal cord level indicative of a myelopathy and not a peripheral neuropathy. This omission may delay recognition that the problem lies at the level of the CNS, in the spinal cord or brain.

As clinicians mature, they learn to eliminate or put into perspective information and findings irrelevant to current problems. Although a full neurologic examination may not be necessary in every patient, a thorough examination can be used to establish a future baseline for each patient. Noting a patient's slightly asymmetric smile, somewhat irregular pupils, or hint of ptosis is important. Even though these findings may have no bearing on the issue, their notation may prove helpful to the patient later. This is especially true if another neurologist calls for patient records for comparison or if the patient returns with another clinical concern.

Basic Tenets

The examination begins the moment the patient walks down the hall to enter the neurologist's office; it continues during the conversations requisite to history taking. By the end of the examination, the findings must be able to be categorized and organized for easy interpretation and, eventually, diagnostic formulation. Many of the patient's cognitive abilities are readily assessed during the history as well as the formal neurologic examination. Concurrently, the neurologist is always looking for abnormal clinical signs. Some are overt movements (tremors, restlessness, dystonia or dyskinesia); others are subtler, eg, vitiligo, implying a potential for a neurologic autoimmune disorder. Equally important may be the lack of normal movements, as seen in patients with Parkinson disease.

The examination is divided into several sections. Speech and language are assessed during the history taking. The cognitive part of the examination is the most time consuming and complicated (chapter 2). However, unless a cognitive or language dysfunction is suspected, the multisystem neurologic examination provides a careful basis for the essential clinical evaluation.

CLINICAL NEUROLOGIC EVALUATION

Neurologists in training and their colleagues in practice cannot expect to test all possible cognitive elements in each patient evaluated. Certain basic elements are required, most of which are readily observable or elicited during initial clinical evaluation. These include documentation of language function, affect, concentration, orientation and memory. When concerned about the patient's cognitive abilities, the neurologist must elicit evidence of an apraxia or agnosia and test organizational skills, constructional ability, calculation abilities, and any tendency to neglect anatomical structures, particularly nondominant limbs or visual fields.

When language and cognitive functions have been assessed, gait and equilibrium, visual fields, cranial nerves (CNs) (Figure 1-1), coordination, muscle strength, muscle stretch reflexes (MSRs), plantar stimulation, and sensory modalities should be examined in an organized fashion. The patient's general health, nutritional status, and cardiac function, including the presence or absence of significant arrhythmia, heart murmur, or signs of congestive failure, should be noted. If the patient is encephalopathic, it is important to search for subtle signs of infectious, hepatic, renal, or pulmonary disease.

THE CRANIAL NERVES: AN INTRODUCTION

The 12 CNs subserve multiple types of neurologic function (Figure 1-2). The special senses are represented by all or part of the function of 5 CNs: olfaction, the olfactory (I); vision, the optic (II); taste, the facial (VII) and the glossopharyngeal (IX); and hearing as well as vestibular function, the cochlear and vestibular (VIII). Another 3 CNs are directly responsible for the coordinated, synchronous, and complex movements of both eyes: III (oculomotor), IV (trochlear), and VI (abducens). The primary CN responsible for facial expression is CN-VII, which is important for setting the outward signs of immediate emotional bearing. Facial sensation is subserved primarily by the trigeminal nerve (V); however, it is a mixed nerve also having a primary motor contributions to mastication. The ability to eat and drink also depends on CNs IX, X (vagus), and XII (hypoglossal). The hypoglossal and recurrent laryngeal nerves are also important to the mechanical function of speech. Last, CN-XI, the accessory, contains both cranial and spinal nerve roots that provide motor innervation to the large muscles of the neck and shoulder.

Disorders of the CNs can be confined to a single nerve such as the **olfactory** (from a closed head injury or meningioma), **trigeminal** (tic douloureux), **facial** (Bell palsy), **acoustic** (schwannoma), and **hypoglossal** (carotid dissection). However, a single lesion, such as within the median longitudinal fasciculus, as seen with MS, or, less commonly, a small brainstem stroke can lead to involvement confined to the nerves supplying multiple extraocular muscles.

Additionally, a subset of systemic disorders has the potential to infiltrate or seed the base of the brain and the brainstem at the points of exit of the various CNs from their intraaxial origins. These processes lead to a clinical picture of multiple, sometimes disparate cranial neuropathies, including leptomeningeal seeding of metastatic malignancies, such as in the lung, breast, and stomach, as well as various lymphomas. In these instances, a stuttering onset of various symptoms related to each CN may develop within a short time. Common problems that bring patients to medical attention include diminished visual acuity (optic nerve), diplopia (oculomotor, abducens), facial pain (trigeminal), an evolving facial weakness (facial), difficulty swallowing (glossopharyngeal and vagus), and slurred speech (hypoglossal).

Similarly, some chronic granulomatous infections, such as tuberculosis and Lyme disease, or infectiouslike processes, including sarcoidosis, also require diagnostic consideration in patients with multiple or isolated cranial neuropathies. The latter is particularly relevant to patients presenting with Bell palsy because sarcoidosis and Lyme disease have a predilection for CN-VII. When a facial paresis has an atypical nonacute and progressive temporal profile, a search for focally invasive malignancies, particularly of the parotid gland, is essential.

CRANIAL NERVE TESTING
I: Olfactory Nerve

In a few specific circumstances, olfactory nerve function testing is relevant despite its only occasional clinical indications. Olfactory function may be impaired after head trauma and in individuals

CLINICAL NEUROLOGIC EVALUATION

Figure 1-1

Cranial Nerves: Distribution of Motor and Sensory Fibers

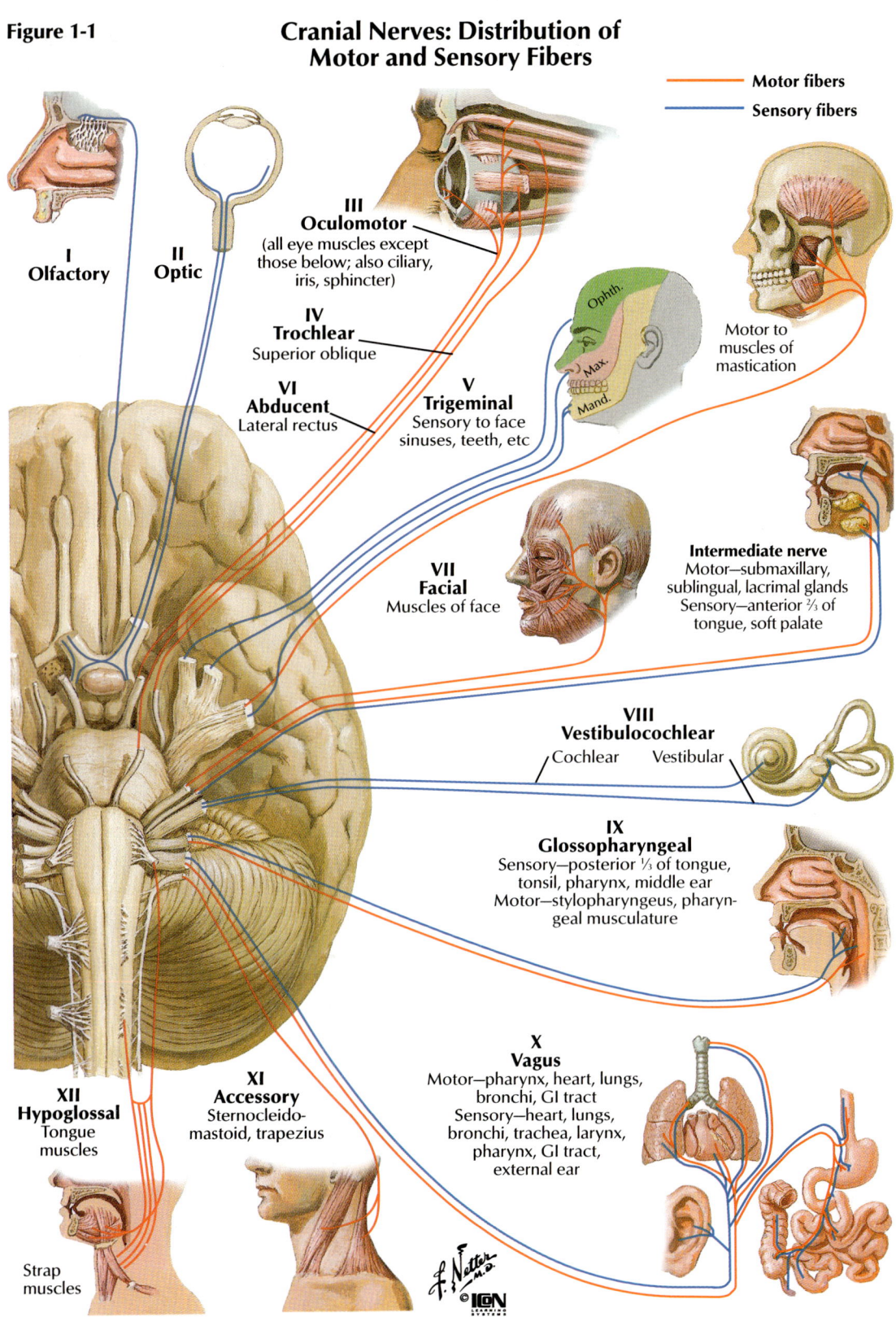

NEUROLOGIC EXAMINATION

CLINICAL NEUROLOGIC EVALUATION

Figure 1-2A   Cranial Nerves: Nerves and Nuclei Viewed in Phantom From Behind

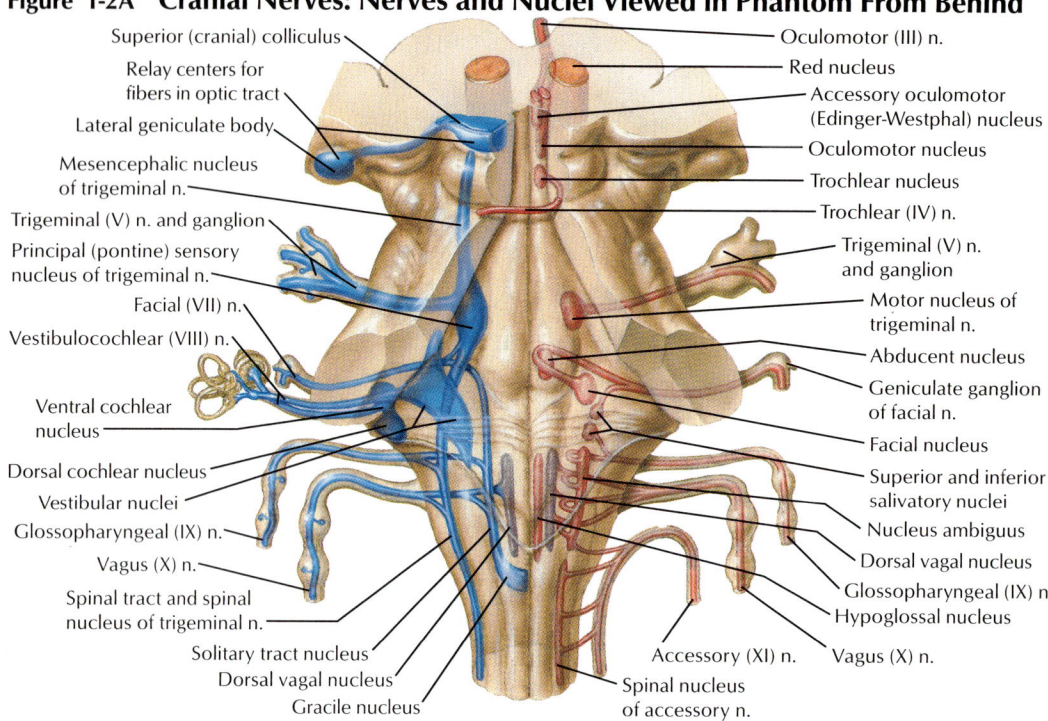

Figure 1-2B   Cranial Nerves: Schema of Nerves and Nuclei in Lateral Dissection

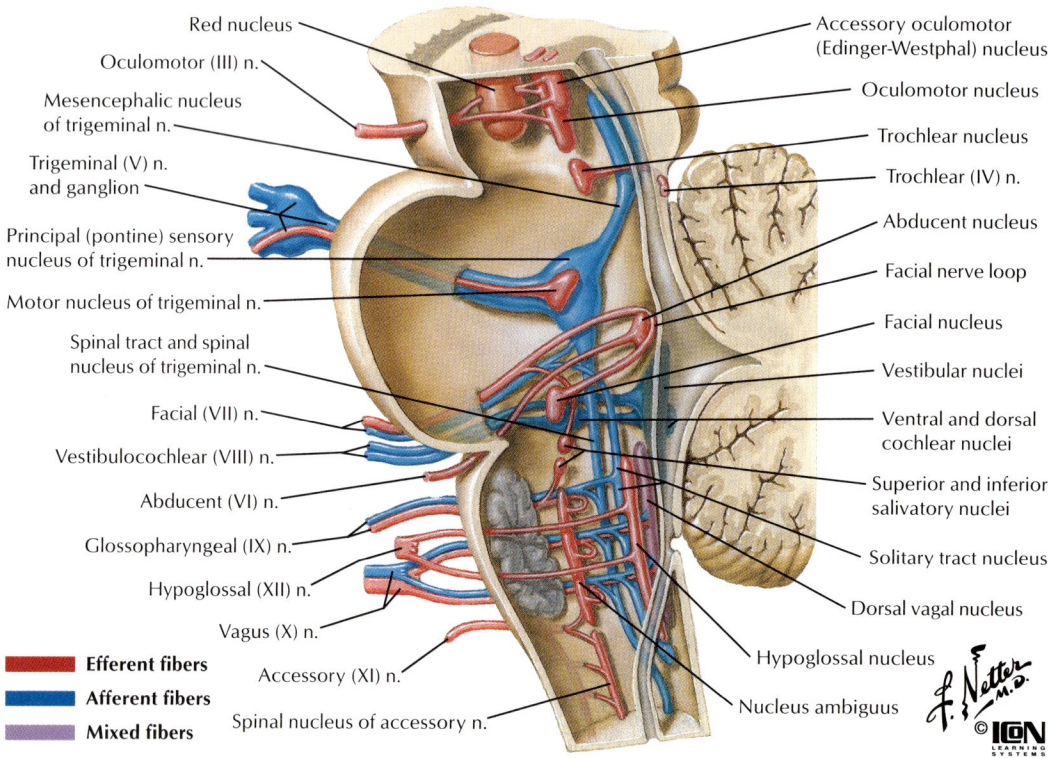

NEUROLOGIC EXAMINATION

with various causes of frontal lobe dysfunction, especially an olfactory groove meningioma.

Clinical evaluation of olfactory functions is straightforward. The examiner has patients sniff a substance of familiar odor (coffee beans, leaves of peppermint, lemon). Ideally, patients keep the eyes closed, and each nostril is tested separately while the other is occluded with a finger. Subsequently, patients are asked whether they detect an odor and, if so, to identify it. Important conclusions are drawn from this simple test: inability or reduced ability to detect an odor suggests **anosmia** or **hyposmia**, respectively; inability to identify an odor correctly implies **smell distortion** (**parosmia** or **dysosmia**); and whether an olfactory disturbance is bilateral or unilateral, ie, whether the patient has a total loss of smell or only loss on 1 side.

Olfactory nerve damage can have significant consequences. When individuals lose their sense of smell, their important ability to smell fires or burning food is compromised.

II: Optic Nerve

Blurred vision, a relatively nonspecific symptom, is the most common problem resulting from optic nerve dysfunction (Figure 1-3). When examining optic nerve function, one needs to look first for concomitant ocular abnormalities that may affect vision, including proptosis, ptosis, scleral injection (congestion), tenderness, bruits, and pupillary changes.

Visual acuity is screened using a standard Snellen vision chart held 14 inches from the eye. Screening must be performed in light to the patient's refractive advantage using corrective lenses or a pinhole when indicated.

A careful visual field evaluation is the other important means to assess visual function. These tests are complementary, one testing central resolution at the retinal level and the other an evaluation of peripheral visual field detection secondary to lesions at the levels of the optic chiasm, optic tracts, and occipital cortex. Visual fields are evaluated most simply by having the patient sit comfortably facing the examiner, who faces the patient at a similar height. First, each eye is tested independently. The patient is asked to look straight at the examiner's nose. The examiner extends an arm laterally, equidistance from the patient, and asks the patient to differentiate between 1 or 2 fingers. Most patients inadvertently look laterally at the fingers. The patient's attention must be refocused, and the test is repeated. Each quadrant of vision is tested separately. After individual testing, both eyes are tested simultaneously for visual neglect, as may occur with right hemispheric lesions (Figure 1-4).

Progressively complex perimetric devices can produce rich data on the health of the visual system. In **kinetic perimetry**, a stimulus is moved from a nonseeing area (far periphery or physiologic blind spot) to a seeing area, with patients indicating at what point the stimulus is first noticed. Testing is repeated from different directions until a curve can be drawn connecting the points at which a given stimulus is seen from all directions. This curve is the *isopter* for that stimulus for that eye. The isopter plot has been likened to a contour map, showing "the island of vision in a sea of darkness." The Goldmann perimeter, a halfsphere onto which spot stimuli are projected, is the premiere device for this mapping. The normal visual field extends approximately 90° temporally, 45° superiorly, 55° nasally, and 65° inferiorly, resembling the oblique teardrop shape of aviator-style sunglass lenses.

In **static perimetry**, the test point is not moved, but turned on in a specific location. Typically automated, computer testing preselects locations within the central 30° of field. Stimuli are dimmed until they are detected only intermittently on repetitive presentation—this intensity level is called the *threshold*. The computer then generates a map of numeric values of the illumination level required at every test spot, or the inverse of this level, often called a *sensitivity value*. Values may also be displayed as a grayscale map, and statistical calculations can be performed—by comparing to adjacent spots or precalculated normal values or noting sudden changes in sensitivity—to detect abnormal areas.

Most visual field changes have localizing value: specific location of the loss, its shape, border sharpness (ie, how quickly across the field the values change from abnormal to normal), and its concordance with the visual field of the other eye tend to implicate specific areas of the visual system. Localization is possible because details of anatomical organization at any level predispose to particular types of loss.

CLINICAL NEUROLOGIC EVALUATION

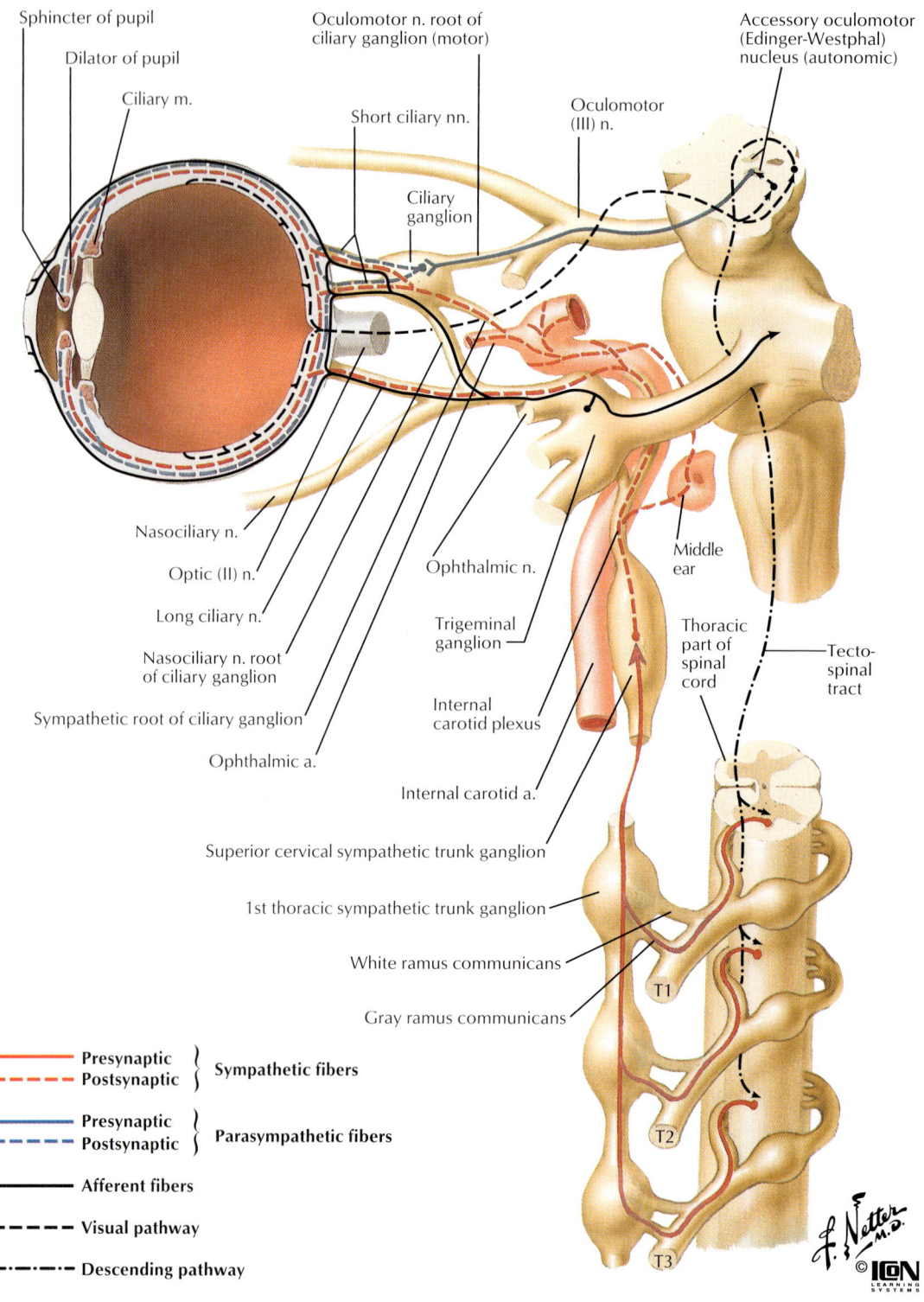

Figure 1-3 Autonomic Innervation of Eye

CLINICAL NEUROLOGIC EVALUATION

Figure 1-4 — Visual Pathways: Retina to Occipital Cortex

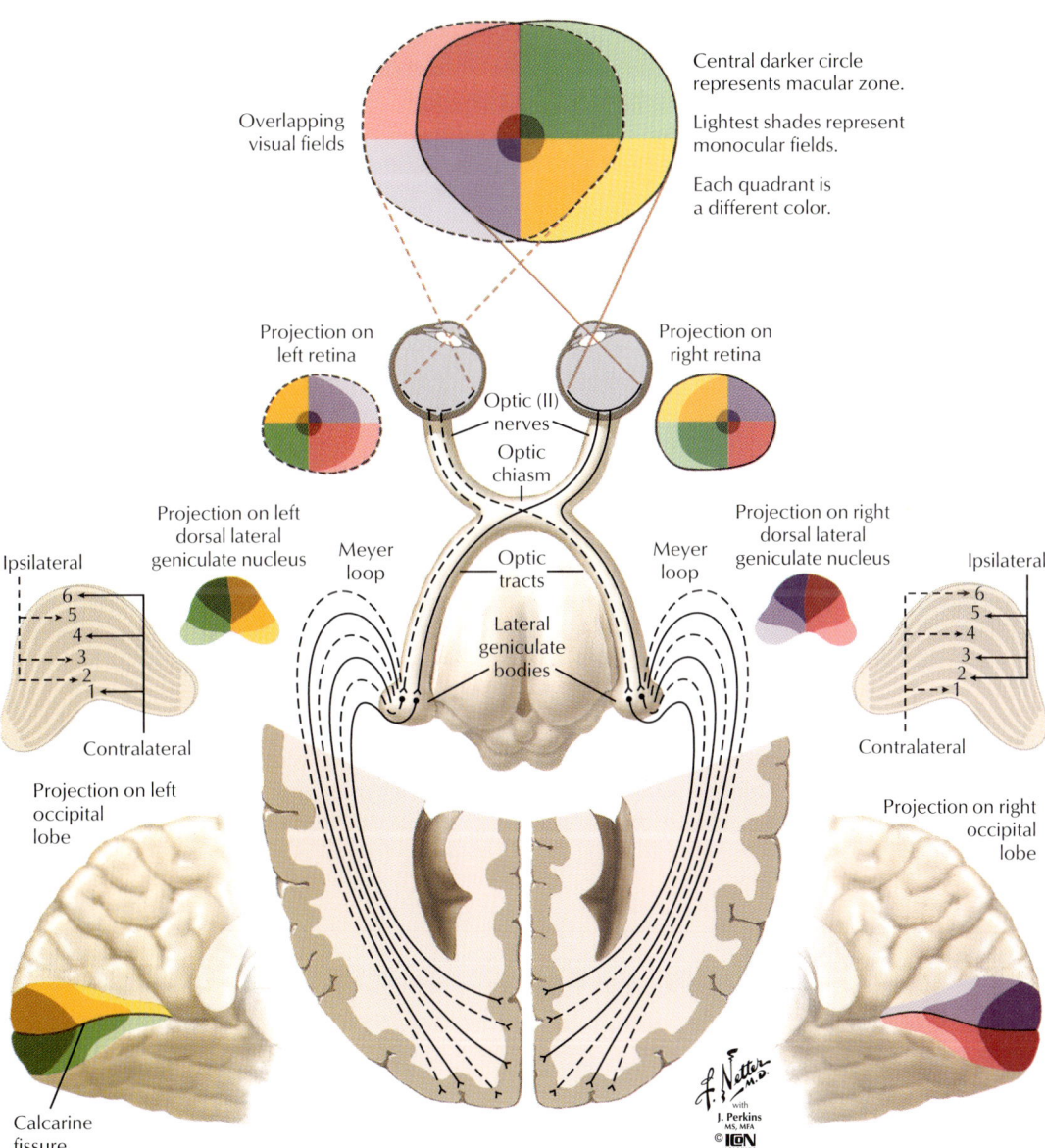

In examining the pupils, one should note the shape and size. A 1-mm size difference in otherwise round pupils is acceptable as a normal variant. Pupillary responses are tested with a bright flashlight. A normal pupil reacts to light by constricting. Normally, the contralateral pupil also constricts. These responses are called the **direct** and **consensual reactions**, respectively. The pupils also constrict when shifting focus from a far to a near object (**accommodation**) and during **convergence** of the eyes, as when patients are asked to look at their nose.

The **ciliospinal reflex** is useful for evaluating comatose patients. When the examiner pinches the neck, the ipsilateral pupil should transiently dilate. This provides a means to test the integrity of neuropathways to midbrain structures.

The short ciliary nerve, supplying parasympathetic inputs to the pupil, may be damaged by various forms of trauma. This results in a

CLINICAL NEUROLOGIC EVALUATION

unilateral dilated pupil with preservation of other third nerve function. Significant unilateral pupillary abnormalities are usually related to innervation changes in pupillary muscles.

A number of pathophysiologic mechanisms lead to **mydriasis** (pupillary dilatation) (Table 1-1). Atropinelike eye drops, often used for their ability to produce mydriasis, are important mechanisms that are occasionally overlooked as potential causes of otherwise asymptomatic, dilated, poorly reactive pupils. Other medications may cause certain atypical reactions to light. Bilaterally dilated pupils, in otherwise neurologically intact patients, likely do not reflect significant pathology and are probably related to medications. Parasympathomimetic drugs, such as those typically used to treat glaucoma, cause prominent pupillary constriction.

Horner Syndrome

In **Horner syndrome**, the affected pupil is typically constricted from interference with the sympathetic nerves at one of many levels. The sympathetic efferents originate within the hypothalamus and traverse the brainstem and cervical spinal cord to reach the superior cervical ganglia, where they subsequently accompany the carotid artery in the neck, proceeding intracranially to eventually innervate the pupilodilator musculature of the eye. Typically, patients with Horner syndrome have an ipsilateral loss of sweating in the face, a sympathetic paralysis with subsequent miosis (constricted pupil), and ptosis from loss of smooth muscle innervation. The levator palpebra, a striated muscle innervated by the oculomotor nerve CN-III, is not affected. (See Horner syndrome image in Figure 20-6B.)

Optic Fundus

A careful **optic funduscopic** examination is essential. This evaluation is best performed in a relatively dark environment to increase pupillary size and improve contrast of the posterior chamber structures. Findings that should be documented include margins of the optic nerve, venous pulsations, hemorrhages, exudates, any obvious obstruction to flow by embolic material (such as cholesterol plaque in patients complaining of transient visual obscuration), and pallor of retinal fields that may reflect ischemia.

Papilledema is characterized by elevation and blurring of the optic disk, absence of venous pulsations, and hemorrhages adjacent to and on the disk (Figure 1-5). The finding of papilledema may be consistent with anything from increased intracranial pressure, including brain tumors, subarachnoid hemorrhage, and metabolic processes, to pseudotumor cerebri.

Table 1-1
Pupillary Abnormalities*

	Argyll Robertson	Horner	Hutchinson	Holmes Adie
		Eponym		
Response to light	None	Yes	None	None
Other responses	Converge	Yes	NA	Accommodate
Margins	Irregular	Regular	Regular	Regular
Associated changes	Iris depigmented	Ptosis/anhydrosis	Ptosis	Loss of MSR
Causes	Tabes dorsalis	Carotid dissect Carotid aneurysm Pancoast tumor Syringomyelia	III nerve compression	Ciliary ganglion
Anatomy	Unknown	Loss of sympathetic	Loss of parasympathetic	Loss of parasympathetic

*MSR indicates muscle stretch reflex; NA, not applicable.

CLINICAL NEUROLOGIC EVALUATION

Figure 1-5   **Effects of Increased Intracranial Pressure on Optic Disk and Visual Fields**

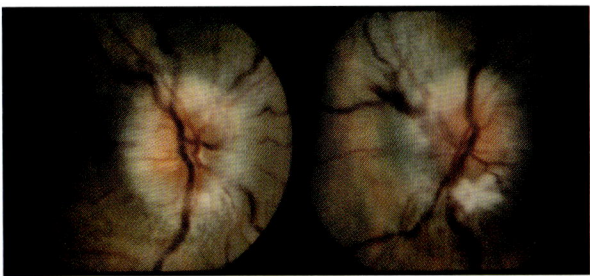

Optic fundus with papilledema

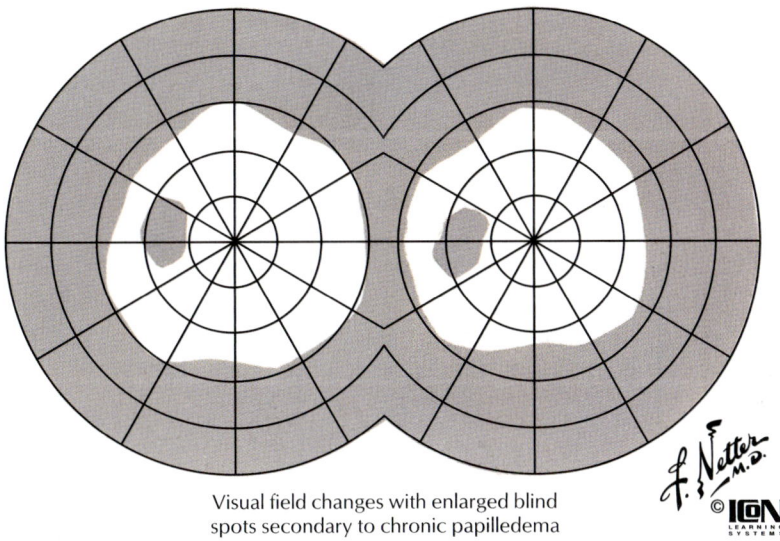

Visual field changes with enlarged blind spots secondary to chronic papilledema

III, IV, VI: Oculomotor, Trochlear, and Abducens Nerves

Testing each eye individually is less confusing and helps to identify isolated ocular dysfunction. It is best to describe the observed loss of specific function, ie, an abduction paresis as opposed to CN-VI palsy, because it is possible that the dysfunction is partial or is not related to CN abnormalities. In testing extraocular muscle function, the patient is instructed to follow the examiner's finger without allowing head movement. Gently touching the patient's forehead may remind the patient to keep the head still.

The medial longitudinal fasciculus is responsible for controlling extraocular muscle function because it provides a means to modify central horizontal conjugate gaze circuits. The medial longitudinal fasciculus connects CN-III on one side and CN-VI on the opposite side. Understanding the circuit of horizontal conjugate gaze helps clinicians to appreciate the relation between the frontal eye fields and the influence it exerts on horizontal conjugate gaze as well the reflex relation between the ocular and vestibular systems (Figure 1-6).

The connection of the vestibular system to the medial longitudinal fasciculus can be tested by cold-water calorics or by the doll's eye maneuver, wherein the head is rotated side to side while the examiner watches for rotation of the eyes. Rotation of the head to the left normally moves the eyes in the opposite direction, with

NEUROLOGIC EXAMINATION

CLINICAL NEUROLOGIC EVALUATION

Figure 1-6

Control of Eye Movements

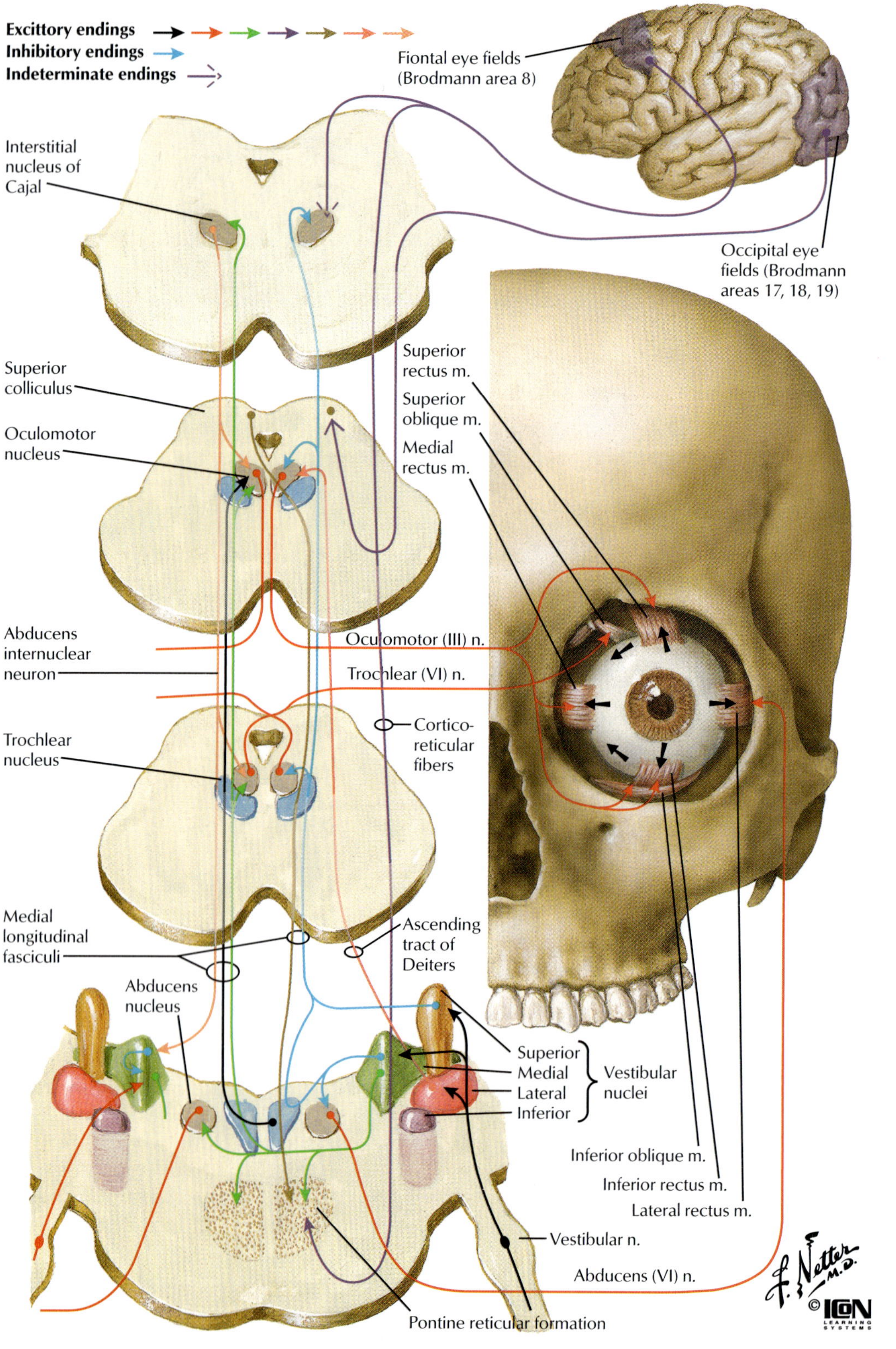

12

NEUROLOGIC EXAMINATION

CLINICAL NEUROLOGIC EVALUATION

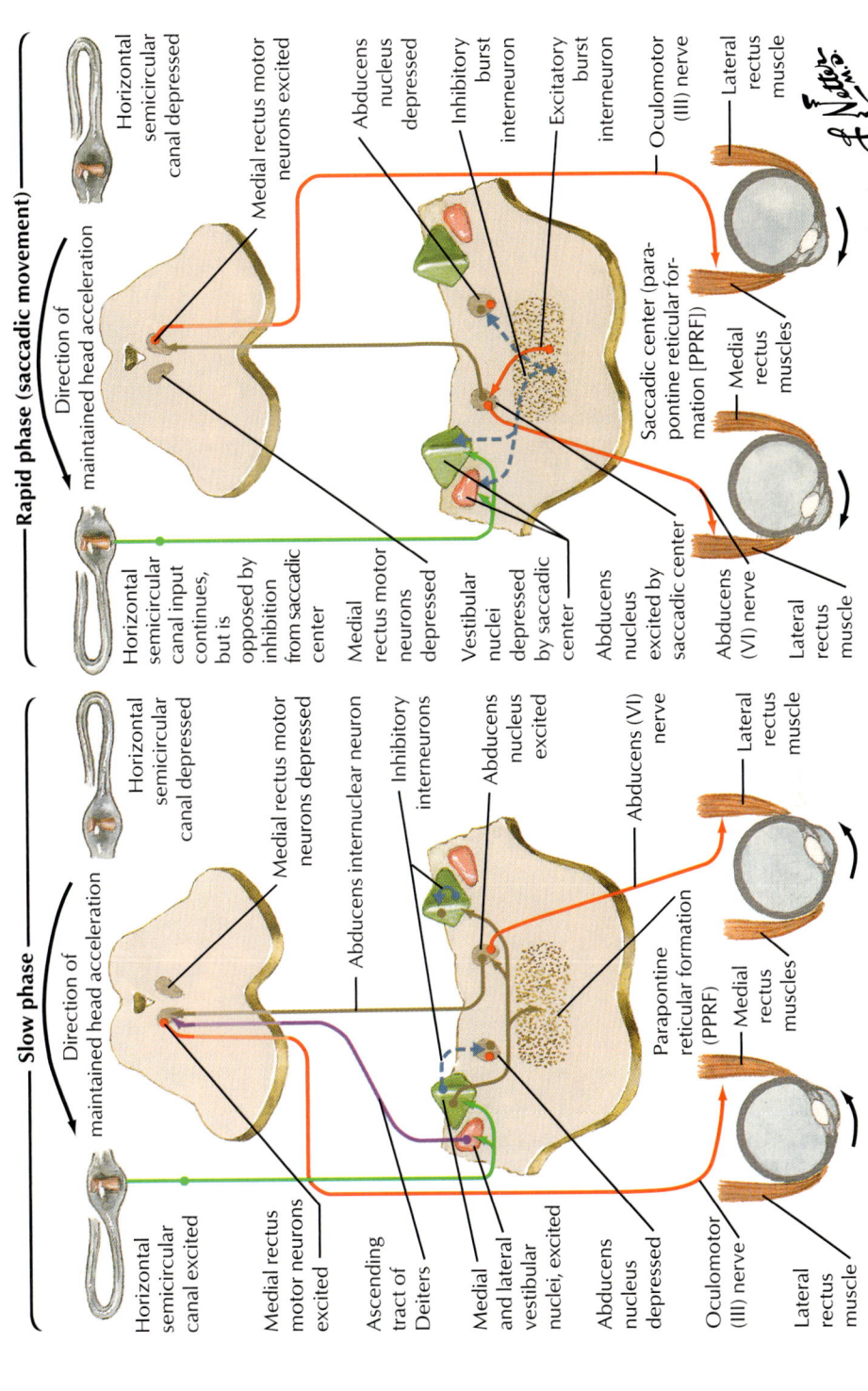

Figure 1-7

Nystagmus

NEUROLOGIC EXAMINATION

CLINICAL NEUROLOGIC EVALUATION

the left eye adducting and the right eye abducting. The opposite occurs when the head is rotated to the right. The cold caloric test evaluates the vestibular-ocular reflex function on each side. This test generally is used for the examination of comatose patients and will rouse a patient in a nonorganic or feigned coma. The study is performed by filling a 50-mL syringe with ice water. Patients are placed at an elevation of approximately 45°. The tympanic membranes are checked for intactness, and then the ice water is gradually infused into each ear. In a normal response, left ear stimulation in the awake patient leads to slow deviation of the eyes to the left followed by rapid movement to the right. Comatose patients who retain intact brainstems have a persistent ipsilateral deviation of the eyes to the site of stimulation; however, the rapid eye movement component is lost.

The center for vertical conjugate gaze and convergence is located in the midbrain, although the underlying circuit is not delineated (Figure 1-7). The vertical conjugate gaze centers can be tested by flexion of the neck while holding the eyelids open and watching the eye movements. In central processes affecting conjugate gaze, eg, MS, there is often prominent nystagmus. The nystagmus results from an attempt to maintain conjugate function of the eyes and minimize double images.

V: Trigeminal Nerve (Figure 1-8A)

The larger part of the nerve is classified into 3 sensory divisions, supplying the face and anterior aspects of the scalp. The angle of the jaw is spared within the trigeminal sensory territory, providing an important landmark to differentiate patients with conversion disorders or obvious secondary gain.

The clinical testing of nerve functions is generally performed by gently using a sharp object and a wisp of cotton. The **corneal reflex** depends on afferents from the first division of the trigeminal nerve and efferents from the facial nerve. This is tested using a wisp of cotton. The examiner approaches the patient from the side or has the patient look away when stimulating the cornea. When the cornea on one side is stimulated, both eyelids close because of multisynaptic pathways within the brainstem. To evaluate the broad spectrum of facial sensation, the examiner uses a cotton wisp and the tip of a new, previously unused safety pin, the cold handle of a tuning fork, or both. In a symmetric fashion, the physician asks whether the patient can perceive each stimulus in the 3 major divisions of trigeminal nerve supplying the face. Additionally, trigeminal motor function may be assessed by having the patient bite down and try to open the mouth against resistance.

VII: Facial Nerve (Figure 1-8B)

The motor functions of CN-VII are tested by asking patients to wrinkle their forehead, close their eyes, and smile. Whistling and puffing up the cheeks are other techniques to test for subtle weakness. When unilateral peripheral weakness affects the facial nerve after it leaves the brainstem, the face may look "ironed out," and when the patient smiles, the contralateral healthy facial muscle pulls up the opposite half of the mouth. Patients often cannot keep water in their mouths, and saliva may constantly drip from the paralyzed side. With peripheral CN-VII palsies, patients are also unable to close their ipsilateral eye or wrinkle their foreheads on the affected side. However, although the lid cannot close, the eyeball rolls up into the head, removing the pupil from observation. This is known as the **Bell phenomena**.

In addition, another motor branch of the facial nerve innervates the stapedius muscle. This helps to modulate vibration of the tympanic membrane and dampens sounds. When this part of the facial nerve is affected, the patient notes hyperacusis, an increased perception of sound, when primarily listening with the ipsilateral ear.

VIII: Cochlear and Vestibular Nerves (Figure 1-8C)

Clinical evaluation of CN-VIII dysfunction is often challenging. Bedside hearing tests sometimes help to demonstrate diagnostically useful asymmetries. Using a tuning fork, it is possible to differentiate between nerve deafness caused by cochlear damage and that caused by conduction deafness with 2 different applications of the standard tuning fork. With the **Rinne test**, a vibrating tuning fork is placed on the mastoid. As soon as the patient is unable to appreciate the sound, the

CLINICAL NEUROLOGIC EVALUATION

Figure 1-8A
Trigeminal Nerve Territories

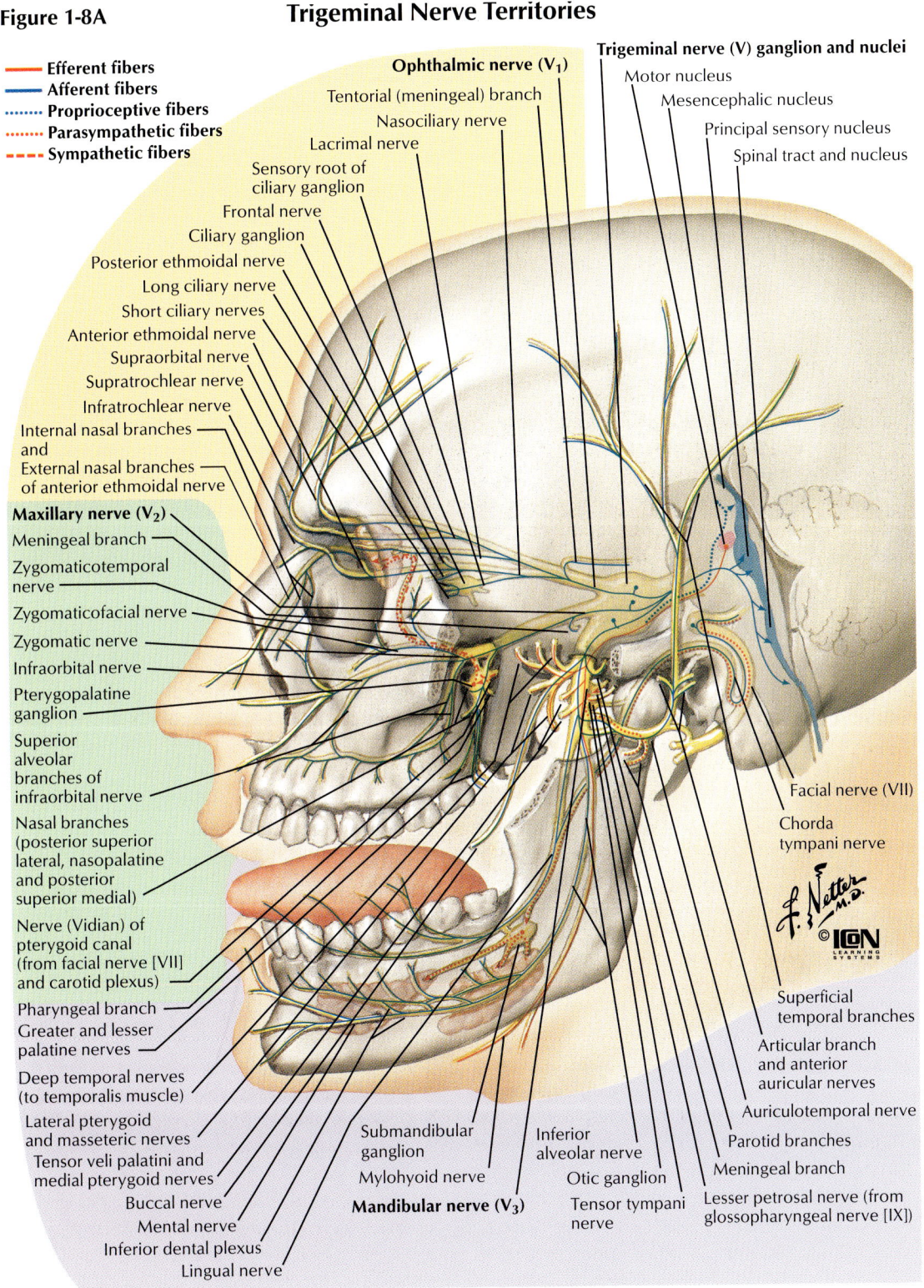

NEUROLOGIC EXAMINATION 15

CLINICAL NEUROLOGIC EVALUATION

Figure 1-8B
Facial Nerve Muscle Innervation

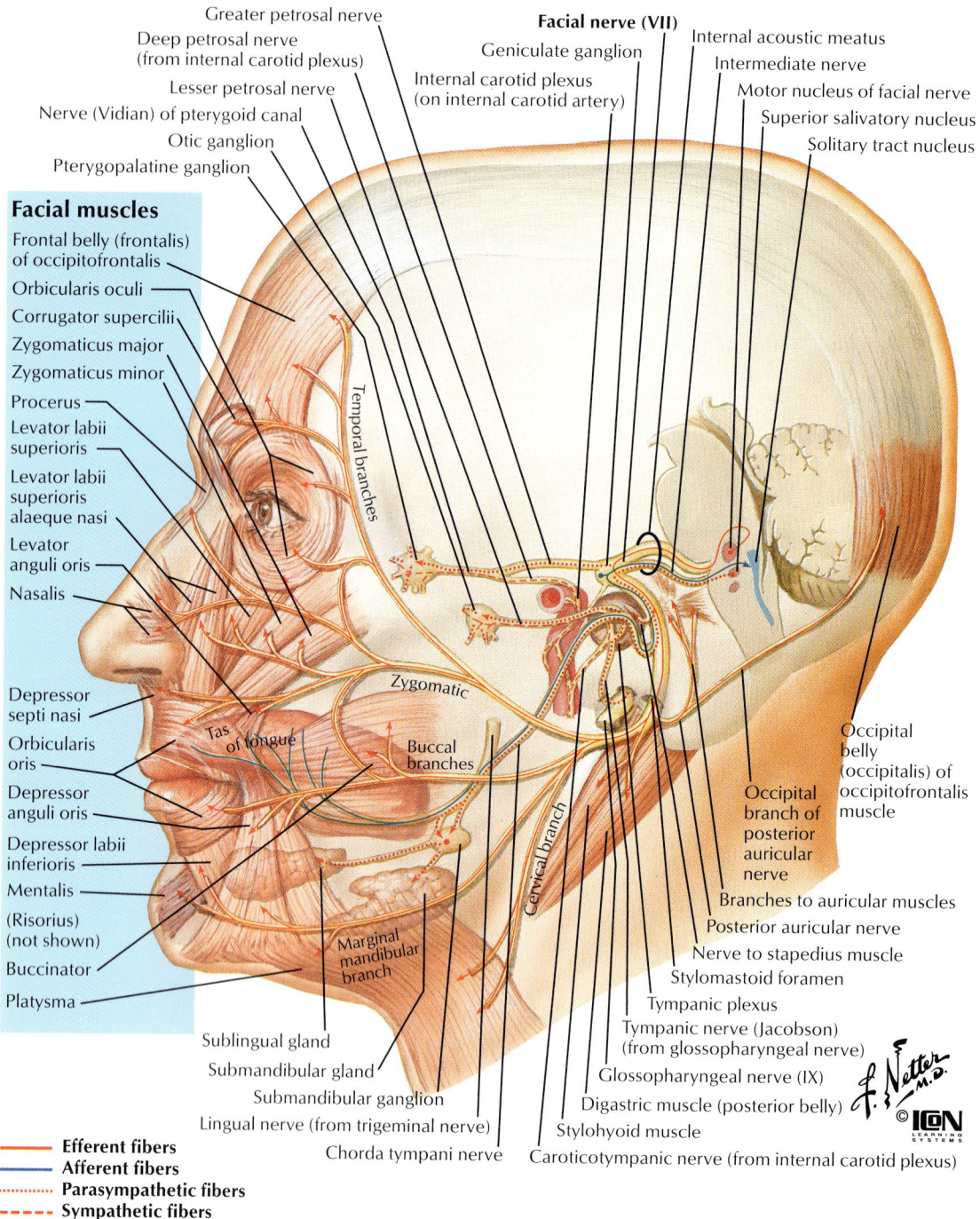

— Efferent fibers
— Afferent fibers
···· Parasympathetic fibers
--- Sympathetic fibers

NEUROLOGIC EXAMINATION

16

CLINICAL NEUROLOGIC EVALUATION

Figure 1-8C **Auditory Nerve Testing: Weber and Rinne Testing**

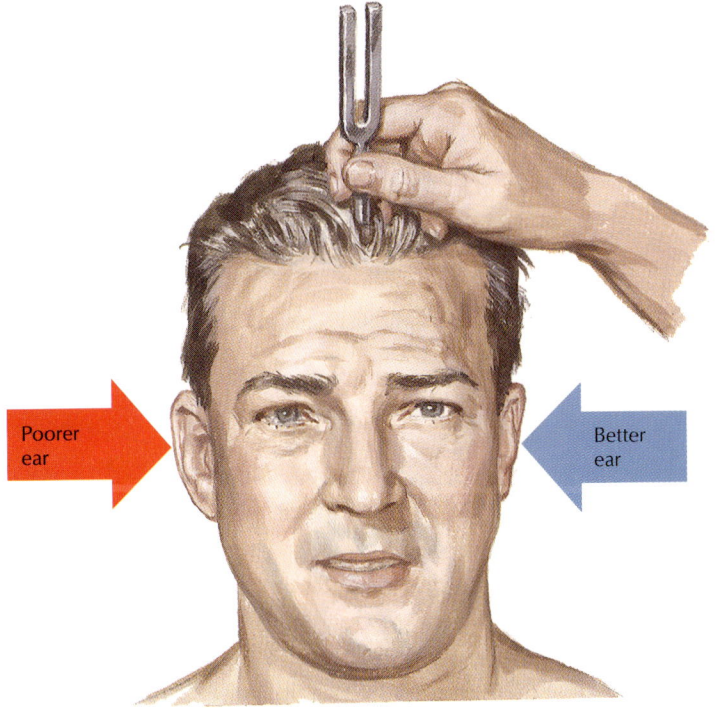

Tone referred to poorer ear indicates conductive impairment.

Tone referred to better ear indicated perceptive impairment.

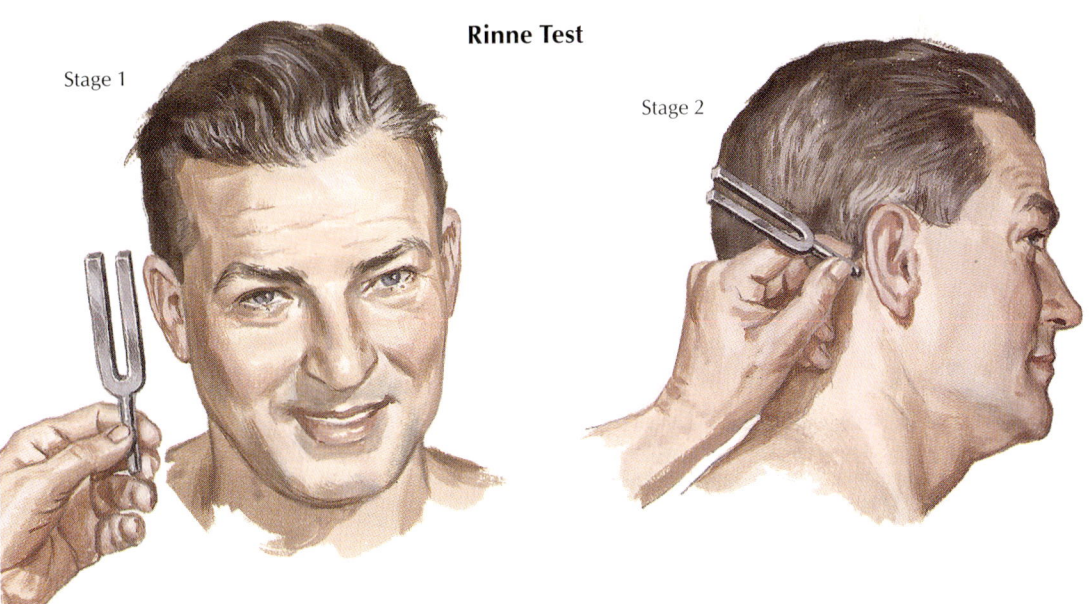

Tone heard longer by air conduction = Rinne positive: indicates perceptive loss
Tone heard longer by bone conduction = Rinne negative: indicates conductive loss

CLINICAL NEUROLOGIC EVALUATION

Figure 1-9   **Test for Positional Vertigo**

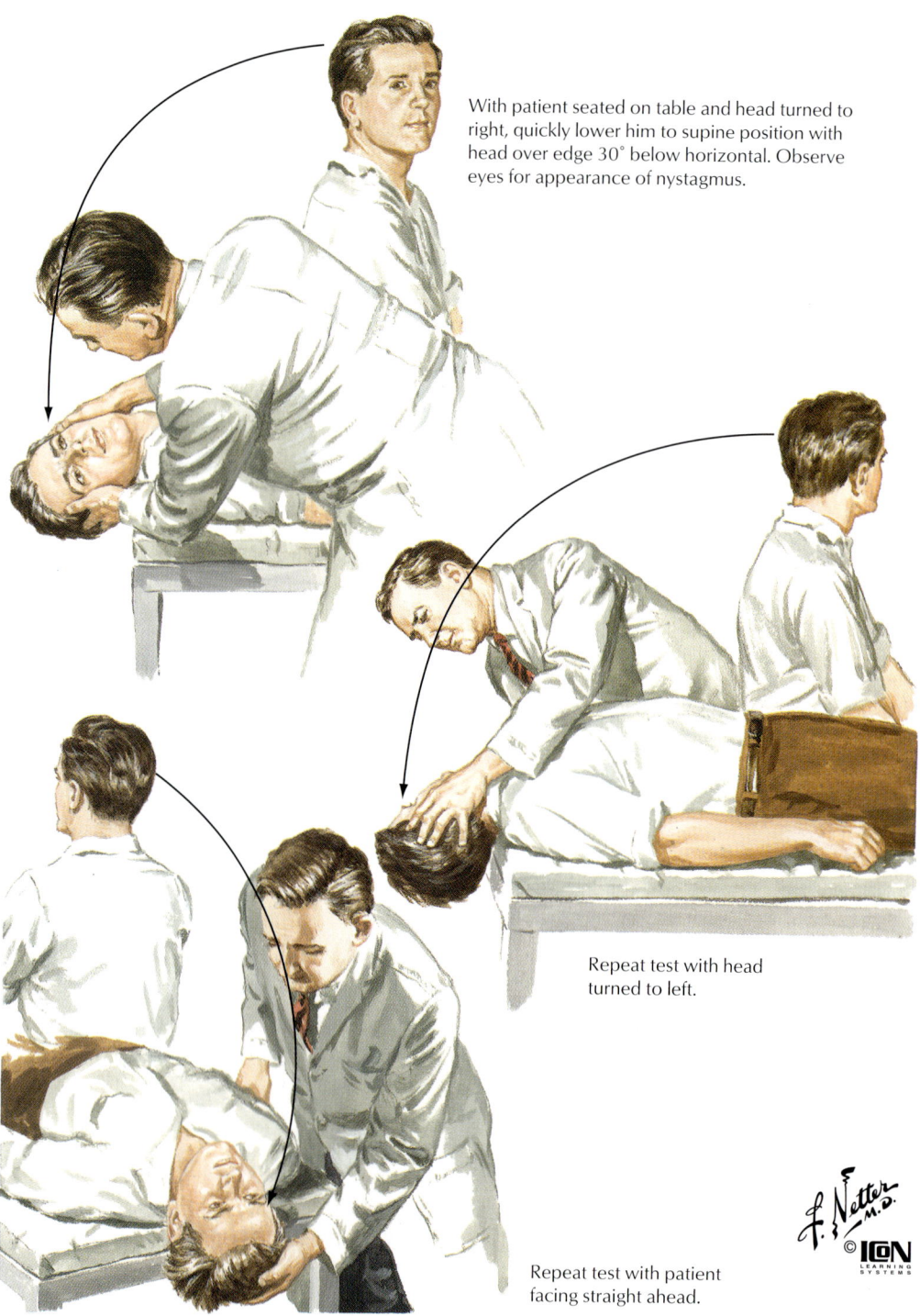

With patient seated on table and head turned to right, quickly lower him to supine position with head over edge 30° below horizontal. Observe eyes for appearance of nystagmus.

Repeat test with head turned to left.

Repeat test with patient facing straight ahead.

instrument is moved close to the opening of the external ear canal to evaluate air conduction. If the individual has **normal hearing**, air conduction is better than bone conduction. If the patient has **nerve deafness**, bone and air conductions are diminished, but air conduction is still better than bone conduction. In contrast, this finding is reversed in patients with middle ear pathology, ie, **conduction deafness**. Here, when the patient's bony conduction has ceased, air **conduction** is limited by the intrinsic disorder within the middle ear. Therefore, the sound can no longer be heard. In the **Weber test**, the tuning fork base is placed in the middle of the skull, and the patient is asked to decide whether one ear perceives the vibration better. In **conduction deafness**, the vibrations are better appreciated in the abnormal ear. In **nerve deafness**, the sound is best appreciated in the normal ear.

The vestibular system can be tested indirectly by evaluating for nystagmus during testing of ocular movements or by positional techniques, such as the Barany maneuver, that induce nystagmus. At the bedside, with the patient in a seated position, the examiner turns the head and lays the patient back, with the head slightly extended to provoke the characteristic rotary, delayed, fatiguing nystagmus (Figure 1-9).

Eye movements depend on 2 primary components, the induced **voluntary frontal eye field** and the **reflexive vestibular-ocular** movement controlled by the connections. The ability to maintain conjugate eye movements and a visual perspective on the surrounding world is an important brainstem function. It requires inputs from other receptors in muscles, joints, and the cupulae of the inner ear. Therefore, in vestibular-ocular or cerebellar dysfunction, the maintenance of basic visual orientation becomes more challenged. Nystagmus is a compensatory process that attempts to help maintain visual fixation.

Traditionally, when one describes nystagmus, the fast phase is described. For example, left semicircular canal stimulation produces a slow nystagmus to the left, with a fast component to the right. As a result, the nystagmus is referred to as *right beating nystagmus*. Direct stimulation of the semicircular canals or its direct connections, ie, the vestibular nuclei, often induces a **torsional nystagmus**. This is described as clockwise or counterclockwise, according to the fast phase.

In most individuals, a few beats of horizontal nystagmus occurring with extreme horizontal gaze is normal. The most common cause of bilateral horizontal nystagmus occurs secondary to toxic levels of alcohol ingestion or some medications, ie, phenytoin and barbiturates.

IX, X, XI: Glossopharyngeal, Vagus, and Accessory Nerves

Swallowing difficulties (**dysphagia**) and changes in voice (**dysphonia**) are the most common complaints related to the dysfunction of the vagal system. A patient with a glossopharyngeal nerve paresis presents with flattening of the palate on the affected side. When the patient is asked to produce a sound, the uvula is drawn to the unaffected side (Figure 1-10). Indirect mirror examination of the vocal cords may demonstrate paralysis of the ipsilateral cord. The traditional test for gag reflex, placing a tongue depressor on the posterior pharynx, is of equivocal significance at best, because the gag response varies significantly. Preservation of swallowing reflexes is best tested by giving the patient 30 mL fluid to drink through a straw while seated at 90°. Patients with compromised swallowing reflexes develop a "wet cough" and regurgitate fluids through their nose. Accessory nerve damage limits the ability to turn the head to the opposite side.

XII: Hypoglossal Nerve

Damage to the hypoglossal nucleus or its nerve produces tongue atrophy and fasciculations (Figure 1-10). The fasciculations usually are seen best on the lateral aspects of the tongue. If the nerve is affected on one side, the tongue often deviates to that side. Two means to test for subtle weakness include asking the patient to push against a tongue depressor held by the examiner and having the patient push the tongue into the cheek.

CRANIAL NEUROPATHIES AND SYSTEMIC DISEASE

In evaluating patients for any cranial neuropathy, other neurologic and systemic complaints

CLINICAL NEUROLOGIC EVALUATION

Figure 1-10

Evaluation

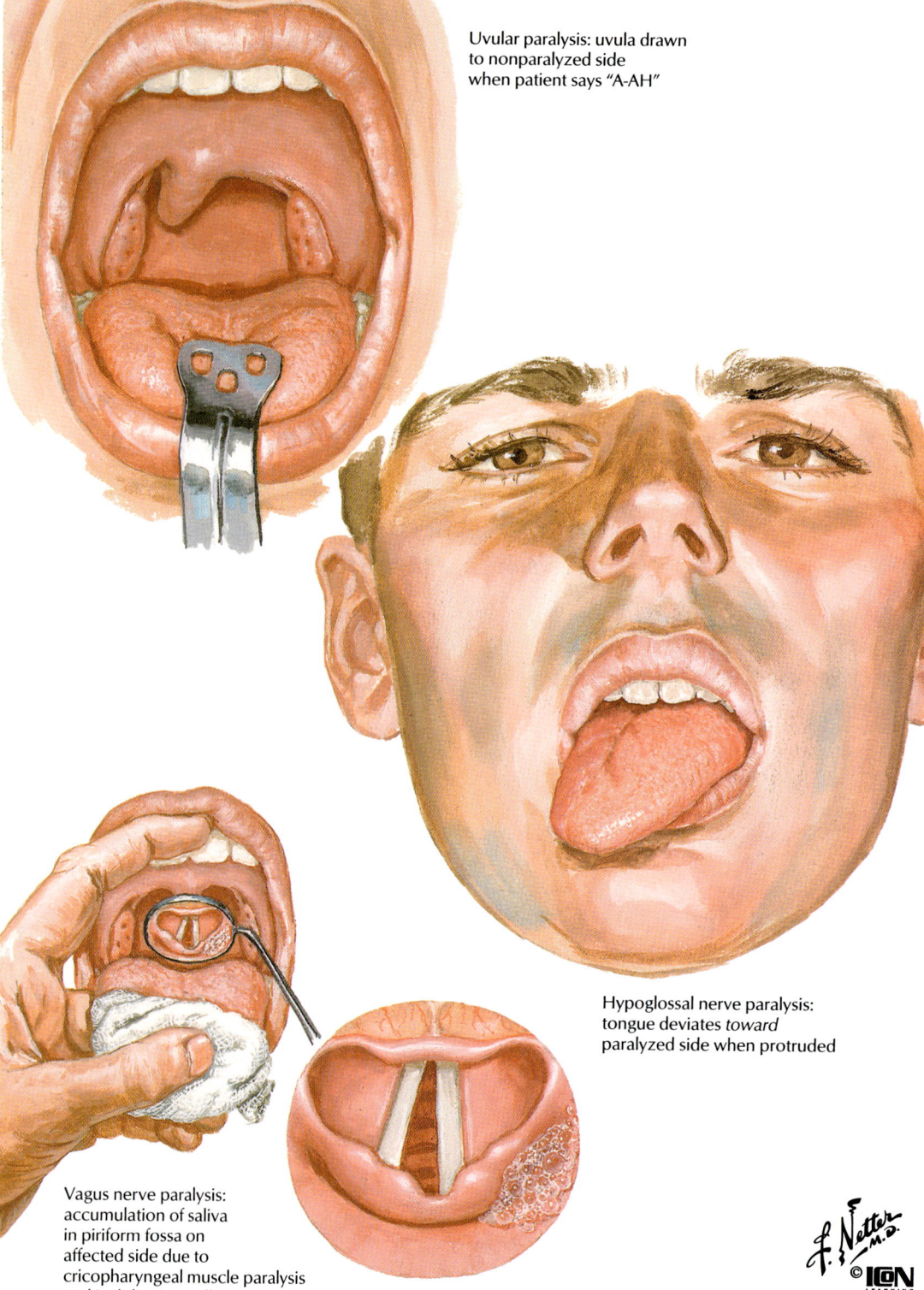

Uvular paralysis: uvula drawn to nonparalyzed side when patient says "A-AH"

Hypoglossal nerve paralysis: tongue deviates *toward* paralyzed side when protruded

Vagus nerve paralysis: accumulation of saliva in piriform fossa on affected side due to cricopharyngeal muscle paralysis and inability to swallow

NEUROLOGIC EXAMINATION

and findings must always be considered. This is especially true in unusual cranial neuropathies.

CEREBELLAR DYSFUNCTION

Evaluation of posture and gait provide the opportunity to observe the most dramatic clinical manifestations of cerebellar dysfunction. With midline cerebellar lesions affecting the vermis, the patient characteristically assumes a broad-based stance when walking, not unlike an inebriated individual. At the extreme, these individuals are unable to maintain a stance. In contrast, when there is a cerebellar hemisphere problem, the patient has a tendency to veer to the affected side. With midline lesions, gait is usually unchanged whether the eyes are open or closed, suggesting that this is not the result of disruption of proprioceptive inputs. Patients with unilateral lesions are often able to compensate with their eyes open but deteriorate when they loose visual inputs.

Loss of limb coordination is the result of cerebellar inability to calculate inputs from different joints and muscles and coordinate them into smooth movements. This abnormality is best observed by testing finger-to-nose and heel-to-shin movements and comparing the responses on both sides. When performing the finger-to-nose test, the examiner's finger is the target; it is sequentially moved to different locations. The patient in turn keeps the arm extended and tries to touch the examiner's finger at each location. When unilateral cerebellar dysfunction is present, the patient overshoots the target, so-called past pointing. In patients with focal motor or sensory cerebral cortex lesions leading to mild arm weakness or even more so with proprioceptive sensory loss affecting that limb, some dysmetric movements may occur that are difficult to distinguish from cerebellar dysfunction. However, in cerebellar dysfunction, the movement improves after a few trials, but with cortical dysmetria, the movement continues to deteriorate.

Dysdiadochokinesia is a sign of cerebellar dysfunction that occurs when the patient is asked to rapidly change hand or finger movements, ie, alternating between palms up and palm down. Patients with cerebellar dysfunction typically have difficulties switching and maintaining smooth, rapid, alternating movements.

Other important cerebellar signs include tremor, nystagmus, and hypotonia. Tremors may develop from any lesion that affects the cerebellar efferent fibers via the superior cerebellar peduncle. This is most obvious with coarse, irregular movement. Nystagmus may also occur with a cerebellar lesion. This is often seen with unilateral cerebellar disease; the nystagmus is most prominent on the affected side. Hypotonia may be present but difficult to document. Best observed when testing MSR, the most common finding is seen on the quadriceps knee jerk. Here, the normal "check" does not occur after the initial movement, so the leg on the affected side swings back and forth a few times after the initial patellar tendon percussion.

GAIT EVALUATION

When meeting the patient, the neurologist always observes the gait as the patient walks into the office. A smooth gait requires multiple inputs from the cerebellum and primary motor and sensory systems. Gait disorders may be caused by frontal lobe processes leading to apraxia or weakness (Figure 1-11E) and or spasticity, neurodegenerative conditions (particularly those affecting the basal ganglia), posterior column dysfunction within the spinal cord, peripheral neuropathies, myopathies, and changes in vision. These disorders are particularly common among the elderly. It is important to record the temporal profile of the gait decline and the circumstances or situations that lead to falls, such as catching the toe on a rug as one circumducts a spastic leg or having a leg give out going down stairs secondary to weakness of the quadriceps femoris muscle. Therefore, when testing gait function, one must assess all aspects of the neurologic examination.

Gait is tested under several circumstances, including walking straight, walking at least 10 yd in open space, making turns, and maneuvering through a tight corridor. The examiner should note arm swing and the ease of gait initiation. Patients with Parkinson disease have difficulty getting their feet started when they stand and tend to take small steps (Figure 1-11A). There is an innate, almost waxlike rigidity to their stooped body carriage, including the frozen posture of one or both arms, which lack the normal arm swing. The normal degree of foot separation (the

CLINICAL NEUROLOGIC EVALUATION

Figure 1-11   Various Gait Disorders

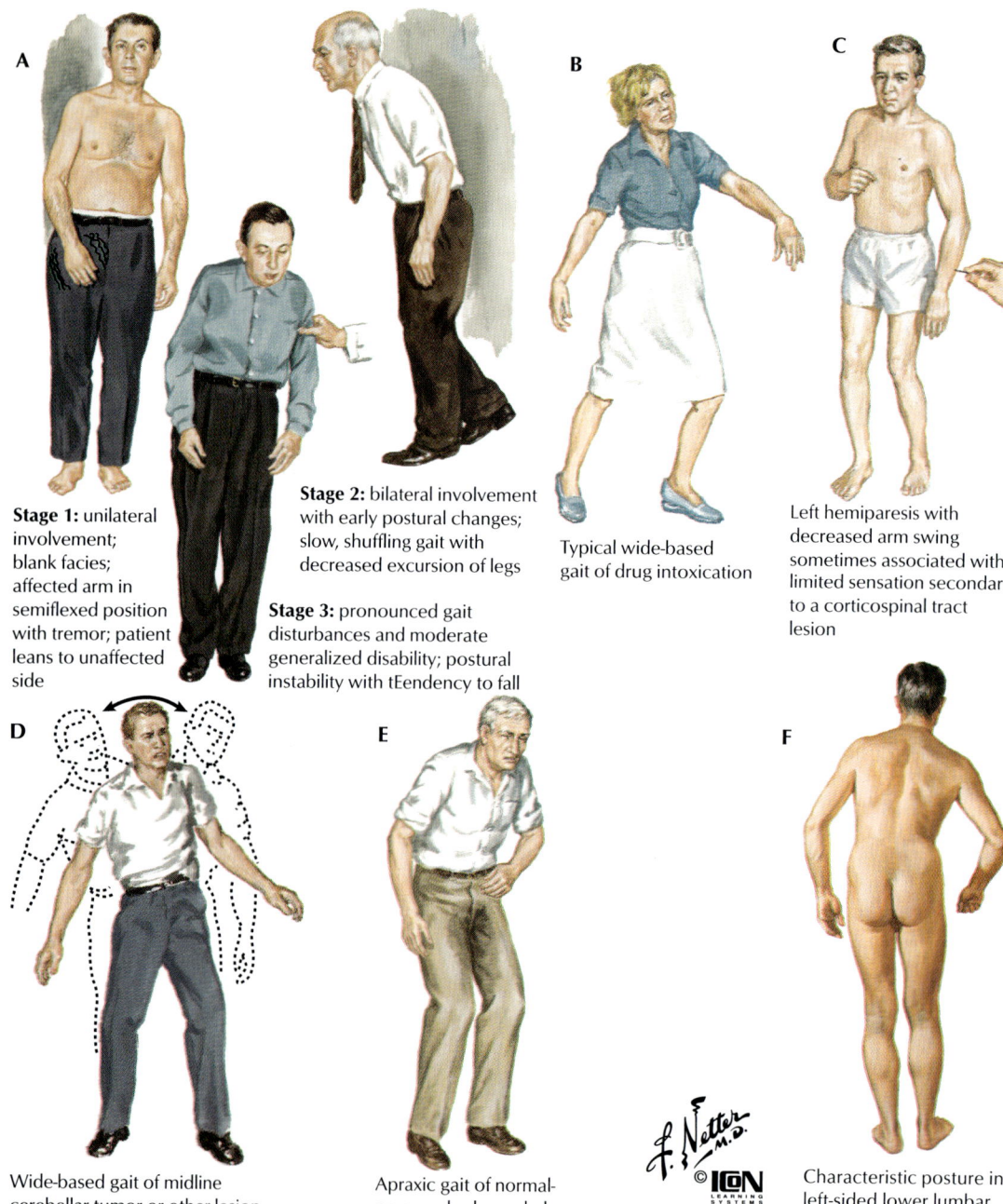

Stage 1: unilateral involvement; blank facies; affected arm in semiflexed position with tremor; patient leans to unaffected side

Stage 2: bilateral involvement with early postural changes; slow, shuffling gait with decreased excursion of legs

Stage 3: pronounced gait disturbances and moderate generalized disability; postural instability with tEendency to fall

Typical wide-based gait of drug intoxication

Left hemiparesis with decreased arm swing sometimes associated with limited sensation secondary to a corticospinal tract lesion

Wide-based gait of midline cerebellar tumor or other lesion

Apraxic gait of normal-pressure hydrocephalus

Characteristic posture in left-sided lower lumbar disc herniation

base) is widened when proprioception or midline cerebellar vermis function is compromised (Figures 1-11B and D). The examiner should note the ability to maintain a relatively straight line, any loss of balance when the patient turns, and any tendency of one side not to function as well as the opposite, ie, circumducting (Figure 1-11J) the leg, moving the leg through an arc that scuffs the toe instead of pursuing a normal straight course (Figure 1-11C). The patient is asked to walk in tandem, with one foot in front of the other. This is the well-known DWI (driving while

NEUROLOGIC EXAMINATION

CLINICAL NEUROLOGIC EVALUATION

Figure 1-11   Various Gait Disorders (continued)

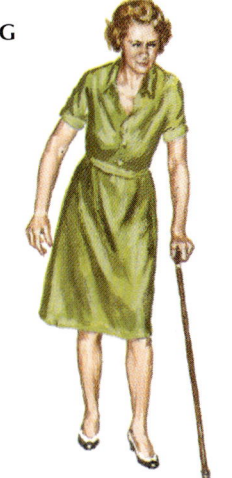
Patient walks gingerly due to loss of position sense and/or painful dysesthesia

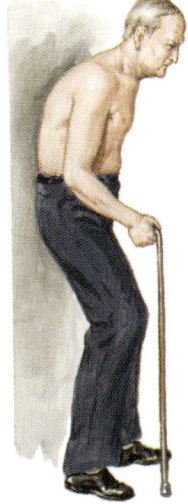
Patient with lumbar spinal stenosis with forward flexion gait

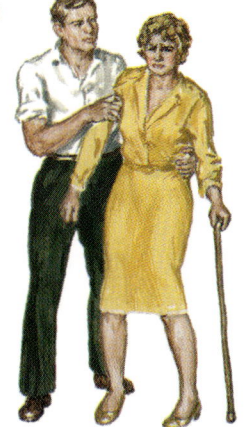
Patient with peripheral neuropathy and loss of proprioception

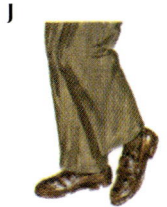
Typical spastic gait, scuffing toe of affected leg

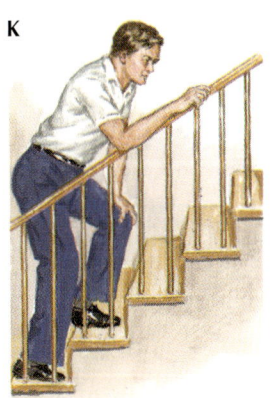
Severe myopathy or NMJ lesion with proximal weakness

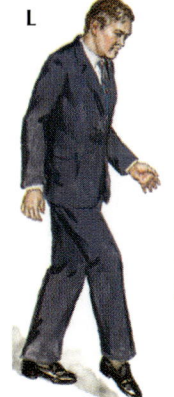
Sudden occurrence of foot drop while walking (peroneal nerve)

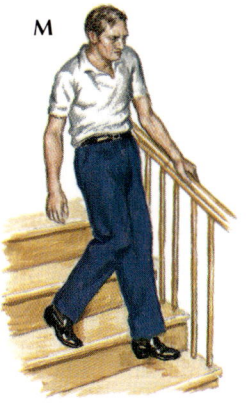
Sudden buckling of knee while going down stairs (femoral nerve)

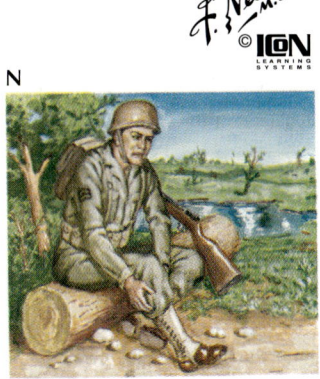
Muscle cramps from defection energy metabolism, ie, McArdle disease

intoxicated) test and is an effective means to elicit a subtle dysequilibrium often related to midline cerebellar dysfunction such as with simple entities including alcohol intoxication. Occasionally, having the patient climb stairs reveals a subtle degree of iliopsoas weakness as found in various peripheral motor unit disorders (particularly myopathies) (Figure 1-11K) and, less commonly, neuromuscular junction or proximal peripheral neuropathies. Finally, the appearance of spasticity may be enhanced by having the patient walk longer distances and even asking him or her to walk several blocks and return to the clinic. Rarely, this uncovers an unsuspected corticospinal tract lesion (Figures 1-11C and J; see Figure 12-1).

ABNORMAL MOVEMENTS

During the examination, the neurologist is always alert to any adventitious movements, including tremors, chorea, dyskinesias, and ballismus. The most common movement disorder encountered in the office is "essential tremor," a

CLINICAL NEUROLOGIC EVALUATION

Figure 1-12
Pyramidal System

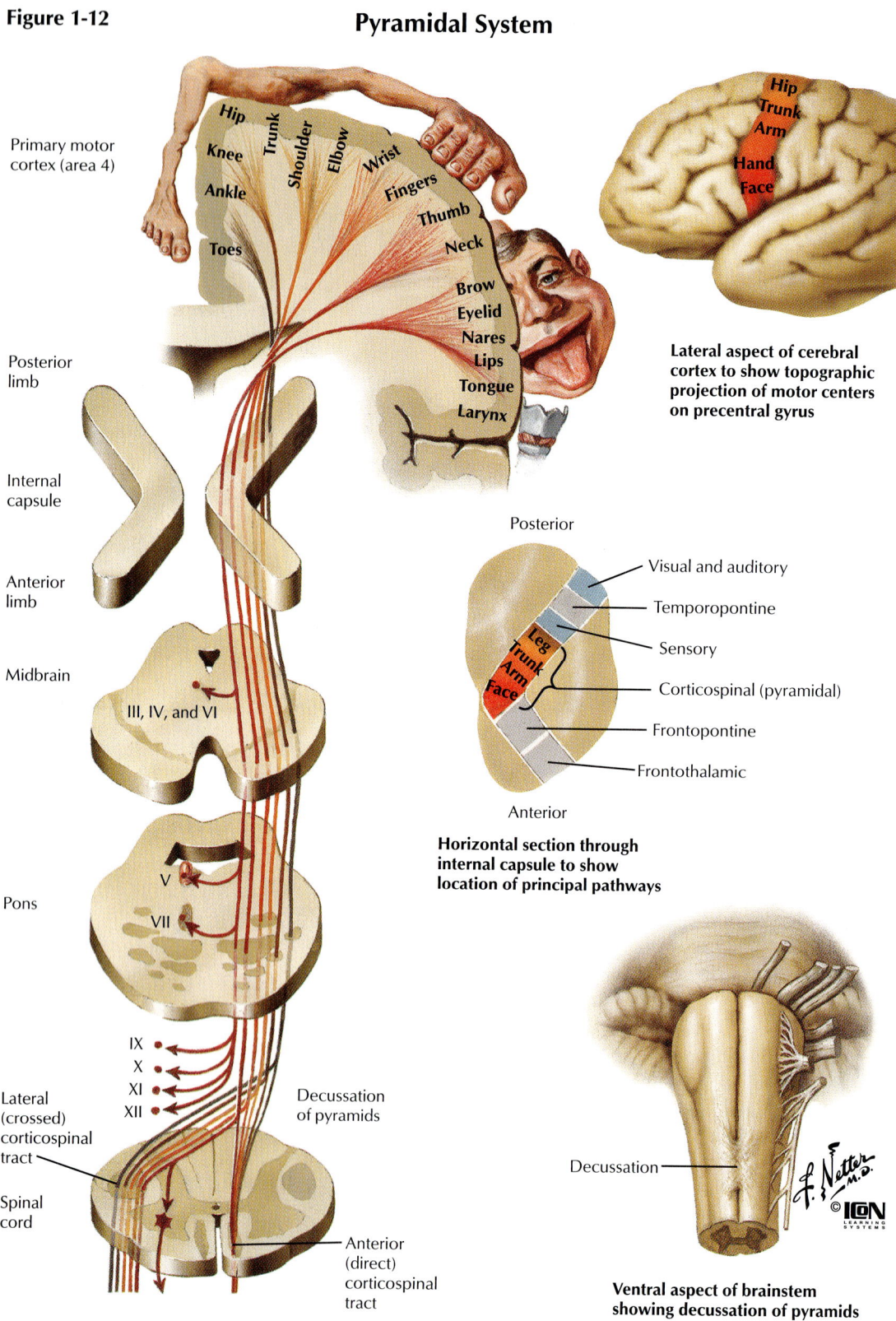

Lateral aspect of cerebral cortex to show topographic projection of motor centers on precentral gyrus

Horizontal section through internal capsule to show location of principal pathways

Ventral aspect of brainstem showing decussation of pyramids

NEUROLOGIC EXAMINATION

CLINICAL NEUROLOGIC EVALUATION

usually benign hereditary condition. These patients often seek medical attention because they are concerned that their tremors are a sign of Parkinson disease. Therefore, differentiating between different types of tremors is a common and important concern. An essential tremor characteristically occurs during certain voluntary actions, such as when bringing a cup of coffee to the mouth. In contrast, with classic Parkinson disease, the pill-rolling tremor is primarily evident at rest, when the patient is seated or walking, and disappears with use of the extremity.

MUSCLE STRENGTH EVALUATION

Weakness is one of the most common complaints of patients seeking neurologic care. The motor pathways encompass multiple anatomical areas within the CNS, including the cerebral cortex and important subcortical structures such as the basal ganglia, the brainstem, the cerebellum, and the spinal cord (Figure 1-12). Although generalized weakness, fatigue, or both often are not caused by a neurologic disorder, the possibility of a CNS disorder should always be considered, including MS in younger individuals and Parkinson disease in older patients. Less commonly, even sleep apnea may come into consideration when the patient is significantly overweight. Lesions of the peripheral motor unit warrant consideration in the evaluation of a patient with generalized weakness (Figure 1-13). These may include processes affecting the anterior horn cell (ie, amyotrophic lateral sclerosis), peripheral nerve (ie, Guillain-Barré syndrome), neuromuscular junction (including Lambert-Eaton myasthenic syndrome), or muscle cells (various myopathies).

Focal weakness often has a subtle character that frequently is not recognized by the patient as loss of motor strength. Dropping objects or clumsy handwriting may represent a single peripheral nerve lesion such as a radial neuropathy leading to a wrist drop, or tripping on rugs or steps may be the expression of a peroneal nerve lesion causing a foot drop (Figure 1-11L). In contrast, a dramatic whole limb weakness is obvious and of greater patient concern, often leading to immediate seeking of medical opinion. Bilateral motor loss is most commonly due to lesions affecting the spinal cord or peripheral motor unit.

Partial limb weakness is referred to as *monoparesis*. Total limb paralysis is referred to as *monoplegia*. Unilateral weakness of the limbs is referred to as *hemiparesis* or *hemiplegia*. *Paraparesis* is used when both legs are affected; if no motor function remains, this is considered *paraplegia*. Similarly, *quadriplegia* relates to total paralysis of all 4 extremities.

When analyzing the complaint of weakness, the physician must consider the presence or absence of associated neurologic complaints or difficulties, such as language, speech, and visual changes; gait dysfunction; difficulty with rising from chairs and associated movements; and alteration in sensation. The neurologist testing for strength must search for atrophy and fasciculations, note the degree of patient effort and cooperation, and consider associated problems that may compromise the testing, such as pain and skin or orthopedic lesions. Formal strength testing must be conducted in a systematic manner. Most neurologic physicians proceed from the CN to the neck, the upper extremities, and finally the lower extremities, usually proceeding proximal to distal. Initial focus is on the major muscle groups, such as the flexors and extensors, to seek out any areas of weakness. More specific muscle testing is particularly useful when distinguishing between lesions of the nerve root and plexus or mononeuropathies (Table 1-2).

When individual muscle testing does not demonstrate specific weakness, other techniques sometimes uncover more subtle function loss. If the patient is instructed to extend the arms with the palms up and the eyes closed, subtle arm weakness may manifest as downward or lateral drift of the affected extremity. Similarly, moving the fingers as if playing piano or rapidly tapping may demonstrate a subtle incoordination. Subtle proximal lower extremity weakness may not be appreciated with individual muscle testing. Watching the patient rise from a chair may demonstrate use of furniture arms to "push off" and is a good means to identify proximal leg weakness. Particularly effective means to uncover proximal strength loss include having the patient climb stairs or squat and attempt to rise without arm use. Also asking the patient to walk on the heels or the tips of the toes is helpful in uncovering distal leg weakness.

CLINICAL NEUROLOGIC EVALUATION

Figure 1-13 — Primary Sites of Motor Disorders

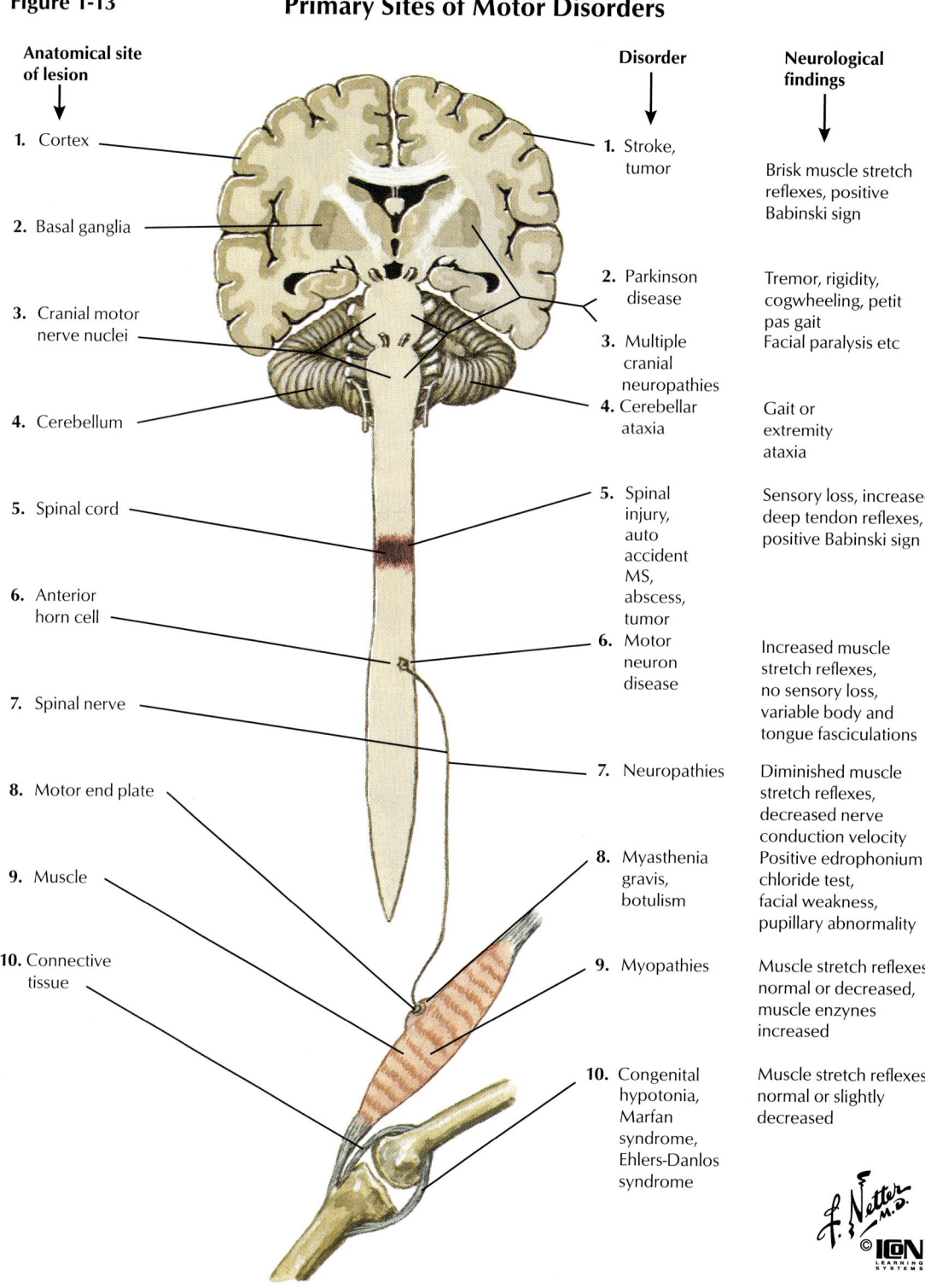

Anatomical site of lesion	Disorder	Neurological findings
1. Cortex	1. Stroke, tumor	Brisk muscle stretch reflexes, positive Babinski sign
2. Basal ganglia	2. Parkinson disease	Tremor, rigidity, cogwheeling, petit pas gait
3. Cranial motor nerve nuclei	3. Multiple cranial neuropathies	Facial paralysis etc
4. Cerebellum	4. Cerebellar ataxia	Gait or extremity ataxia
5. Spinal cord	5. Spinal injury, auto accident MS, abscess, tumor	Sensory loss, increased deep tendon reflexes, positive Babinski sign
6. Anterior horn cell	6. Motor neuron disease	Increased muscle stretch reflexes, no sensory loss, variable body and tongue fasciculations
7. Spinal nerve	7. Neuropathies	Diminished muscle stretch reflexes, decreased nerve conduction velocity
8. Motor end plate	8. Myasthenia gravis, botulism	Positive edrophonium chloride test, facial weakness, pupillary abnormality
9. Muscle	9. Myopathies	Muscle stretch reflexes normal or decreased, muscle enzymes increased
10. Connective tissue	10. Congenital hypotonia, Marfan syndrome, Ehlers-Danlos syndrome	Muscle stretch reflexes normal or slightly decreased

NEUROLOGIC EXAMINATION

CLINICAL NEUROLOGIC EVALUATION

Table 1-2
Muscles to Test in a Routine Neurologic Examination*

Muscle	Action	Nerve	Root
Infraspinatus	External rotation of arm	Suprascapular	C5
Biceps	Flexion of forearm	Musculocutaneous	C5-6
Deltoid	Abduction of arm	Axillary	C5
Triceps	Extension of forearm	Radial	C7
Extensor digitorum	Extension of fingers	Posterior interosseous of radial	C7
Flexor digitorum	Grip	Median	C7-8
APB/opponens pollicis	Abducting thumb and touching tip to fifth finger	Median	T1
Dorsal interossei	Spread fingers apart	Ulnar	C8
Iliopsoas	Flexion of thigh	Femoral	L2-3
Quadriceps	Extension of leg	Femoral	L3-4
Hamstring	Flexion of knee	Sciatic	S1
Gluteus medius	Abduction of thigh	Superior gluteal	L5
Gluteus maximus	Extension of thigh	Inferior gluteal	S1
Tibialis anterior	Dorsiflexion of foot	Deep peroneal	L5
Tibialis posterior	Inversion of foot	Tibial	L5
Peroneus longus	Eversion of foot	Superficial peroneal	L5, S1
Gastrocnemius	Plantar flexion of foot	Tibial	S1-2

*APB indicates abductor pollicis brevis.

Grading Weakness

The traditional, most widely used system for quantifying degrees of weakness is based on a scoring range of 0 to 5, with 5 being normal. The extremes of grading are easy to understand, although the subtle grading between 4 and 5 (ie, 4−, 4, 4+, 5−) may be slightly different depending on the examiner's own strength (Table 1-3). The examiner must recognize that this is not an athletic match but rather a determination of whether the patient has normal strength. There is a significant range of normal, and a sense of that latitude can only be gained by examining multiple individuals.

The examiner assesses the symmetry of function and coexisting changes in tone to formulate appropriate conclusions regarding the significance of subtle changes. The patient's degree of effort must be assessed to distinguish organic disorders from feigned weakness in those with somatoform disorders or individuals with potential for secondary gain, as may occur with workman's compensation or other litigation. This is an important and occasionally difficult differentiation. Always listen carefully to the patient, conduct reexaminations, and use available imaging and neurophysiologic modalities before reaching a diagnosis of a functional nonorganic disorder.

CLINICAL NEUROLOGIC EVALUATION

Table 1-3
Grading System for Clinical Documentation of Degree of Weakness*

Grade	Interpretation
0	No movement (complete paralysis)
1	Able to move a muscle but no movement of limb
2	Minor movement of limb but inability to overcome gravity
3	Moderate weakness; movement of limb against gravity
4	Mild weakness; some resistance against mild pressure
5	Normal; resistance against moderate pressure

*Adapted from Brain. Aids to the Examination of the Peripheral Nervous System. 4th ed. Philadelphia, Pa: WB Saunders; 2000.

When evaluating patients with focal weakness, one should document the evolution of symptoms and any associated changes in sensation or pain. Sudden onset of weakness, without preceding trauma or associated pain, suggests ischemic or hemorrhagic nervous system damage. Pain with localized weakness and sensory changes may imply nerve root involvement or peripheral nerve damage. Most myopathic processes cause symmetric proximal weakness, although such can occur with other motor unit disorders, particularly chronic inflammatory demyelinating polyneuropathy or rare neuromuscular transmission defects, such as Lambert-Eaton myasthenic syndrome. In contrast, CNS processes cause preferential weakness of the arm extensors and leg flexors. The strength of muscles that are not usually examined, such as neck flexors and extensors, must always be assessed when a myopathic process is suspected. Certain illnesses, particularly myasthenia gravis and inflammatory myopathies, may lead to weakness of these muscles. In the most extreme state, some patients may present with a floppy head.

Other lesions are often localized to specific parts of the nervous system by analyzing the pattern of weakness, the onset of symptoms, and the associated findings. For example, neglect of the affected arm or hand, in association with variable degrees of left-sided weakness, often occurs with pathologic processes in the right hemisphere.

Pure motor weakness of the arm and leg, with slurring of speech, is the hallmark of a stroke in posterior limb of the internal capsule. Deeper strokes involving the brainstem can often be associated with cranial nerve findings. Language deficits usually point to a left hemispheric processes. Visual field deficits may also develop, depending on whether there is concomitant involvement of the optic nerve, chiasm, tract, radiation, or optic cortex.

It is also important to differentiate weakness caused by brain processes from weakness caused by spinal cord or peripheral nerve processes. The most common lesions affecting the spinal cord are compressive lesions from progressive spondylosis (thickening of the bony spinal canal), metastases, trauma, and inflammatory processes, particularly MS or transverse myelitis. Depending on the location and temporal profile, spinal cord lesions often begin with subtle symptoms of gait disturbance, weakness, or both. Concomitantly, spinal cord lesions are usually associated with sensory findings and urinary bladder difficulties. A careful examination is important to elicit a sensory level; this is often best documented by using pin and temperature modalities even with uncooperative patients. Looking for a sweat level is also sometimes helpful because the skin below the level of a significant spinal cord lesion will be noticeably drier.

Pain is often an associated symptom when lesions of peripheral nerves, including nerve roots and plexuses, cause weakness. Sensory changes are frequently identified, but occasionally, they are subtle in character and not yet recognized by the patient. Because sensory examination is the most subjective part of the neurologic examination, its reliability sometimes must be called into question. Asking the patient to roughly outline the area in question using a finger can often be very useful, particularly when the pattern of loss

CLINICAL NEUROLOGIC EVALUATION

Figure 1-14 **Dermal Segmentation**

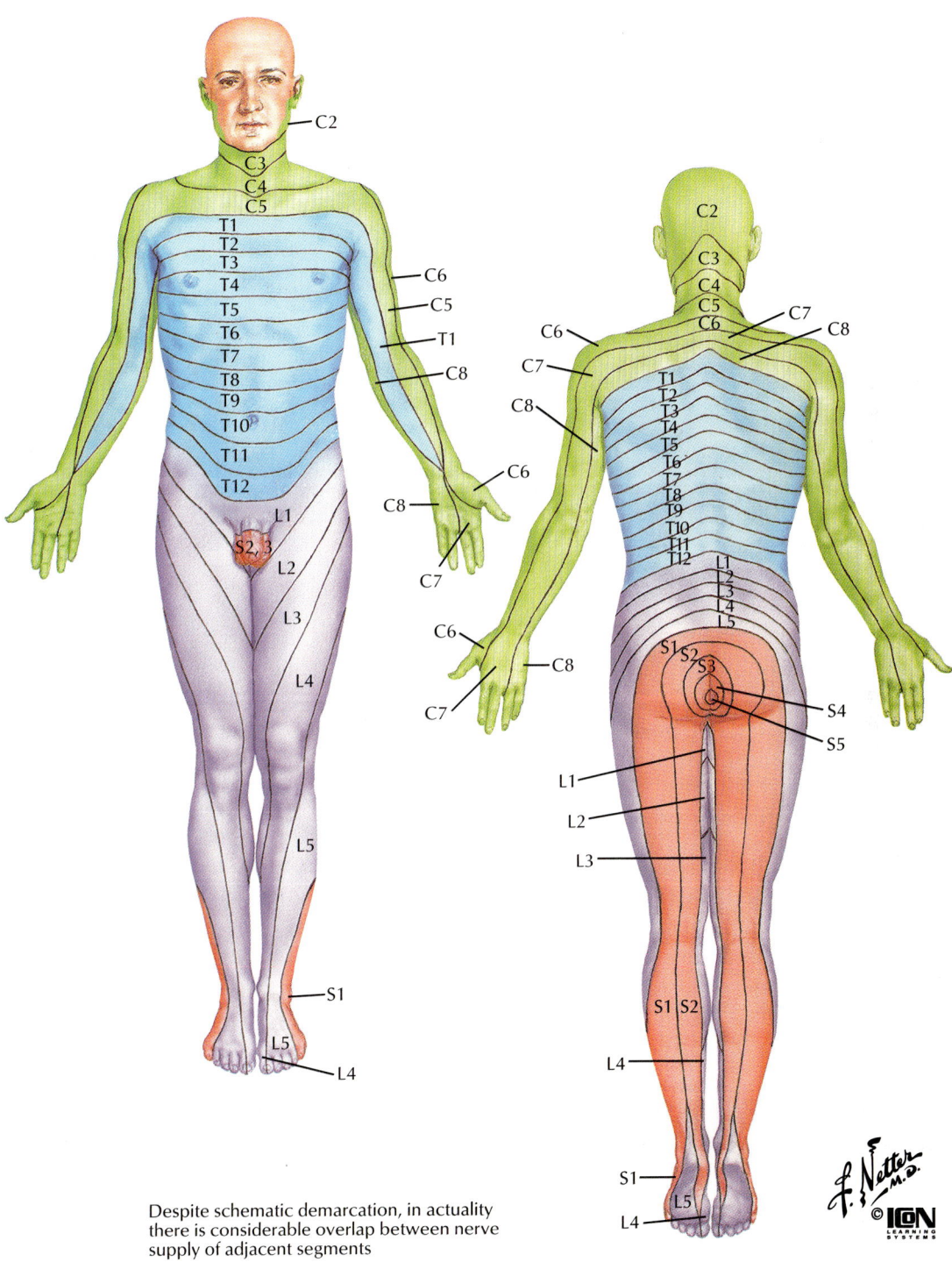

Despite schematic demarcation, in actuality there is considerable overlap between nerve supply of adjacent segments

CLINICAL NEUROLOGIC EVALUATION

fits the distribution of a particular peripheral nerve or nerve root dermatome. Detailed knowledge of the specific sensory territories of the nerve root dermatomes (Figure 1-14) and the specific peripheral nerves is essential to performing an accurate and useful clinical sensory examination.

Some peripheral mononeuropathies presenting with unilateral weakness, particularly the wrist drop of radial nerve lesions, are mistaken for processes above the foramen magnum, often mimicking a stroke. Understanding the motor distribution of the major peripheral nerves ultimately aids in the correct diagnosis. Although a peroneal nerve lesion similarly causes a foot drop, an L5 nerve root lesion also presents with a foot drop. However, the L5 lesion also produces weakness of the posterior tibial muscle, providing the means to make a clinical distinction from a common peroneal nerve lesion.

Typically, concomitant sensory involvement manifests as back pain. Interspinal disc herniation and spinal stenosis are the most common processes affecting individual nerve roots. The symptom onset and progression can help in the diagnosis.

Peripheral nervous system involvement often leads to atrophy of muscles innervated by the involved nerve. Measuring extremity circumference may document significant side-to-side asymmetries and, by inference, muscle atrophy secondary to anterior horn cell, nerve root, or peripheral nerve damage.

Fasciculations, spontaneous firing of small groups of muscle fibers, commonly accompany lower motor neuron weakness, particularly with lesions at the motor neuron or nerve root level. Although often perceived by the patient as twitching or jumping, they may not be easily seen with the naked eye. Sometimes it may be necessary to watch a specific muscle for several minutes to see these signs. Placing a hand on the muscle when the patient is at rest may allow fasciculations to be felt. Additionally, with lower motor nerve lesions, there is a concomitant diminution or absence of specific MSRs.

MOTOR TONE

In its most basic form, the motor system depends on inputs from the cerebrum, basal ganglia, cerebellum, brainstem, and spinal cord. Projections from the pontine reticular formation and reticulospinal tract also have direct connections with α and γ motor neurons in the proximal and axial musculature of the body. These fibers originate from the cerebrum and cerebellum and are inhibitory, functioning to decrease motor tone. Subsequent to damage of structures above the pontine reticular formation, this circuit loses its inhibitory input from the cerebrum and cerebellum, leading to excessive stimulation of a motor neurons, especially in the antigravity muscles, the arm flexors, and the leg extensors. This increase in tone is referred to as **spasticity**. Its most extreme clinical manifestation is found in severely ill patients who have decerebrate rigidity (Figure 1-15) or posturing, analogous to spasticity.

Three primary types of changes in tone are found in patients with primary CNS disease: **spasticity, flaccidity,** and **rigidity**. It is important to consider perceived changes in motor tone in the context of the complete neurologic examination rather than in isolation. The patient's body tone is best evaluated when the individual is fully relaxed. Sometimes it is useful to check tone more than once during the examination. *Tone* is described as the patient's primary level of muscular tension. To become comfortable with this part of the examination, students should perform this test as frequently as possible.

Hypotonia is occasionally demonstrable in patients with cerebellar hemispheric lesions. For example, the distal part of the ipsilateral extremity may not be able to perform rapid alternate movements (called *dysdiadochokinesia*) because of the inability to maintain a stable posture. Similarly, the smooth, straight pursuit seen when one elicits the knee MSR loses the out-and-back motion that typically has an inhibitory cerebellar check. Instead, on return, there is overshoot with no check, leading to a repetitive pendular response. This classic hypotonic cerebellar tone is a relatively uncommon finding. A more generalized loss of normal tone is most commonly seen among infants with either central or peripheral motor unit disorders, classically spinal muscular atrophy (Werdnig-Hoffmann disease). Although a similar example is not seen in adults, rarely, floppy head syndrome develops in an older patient.

CLINICAL NEUROLOGIC EVALUATION

Figure 1-15   **Motor Tone Abnormalities**

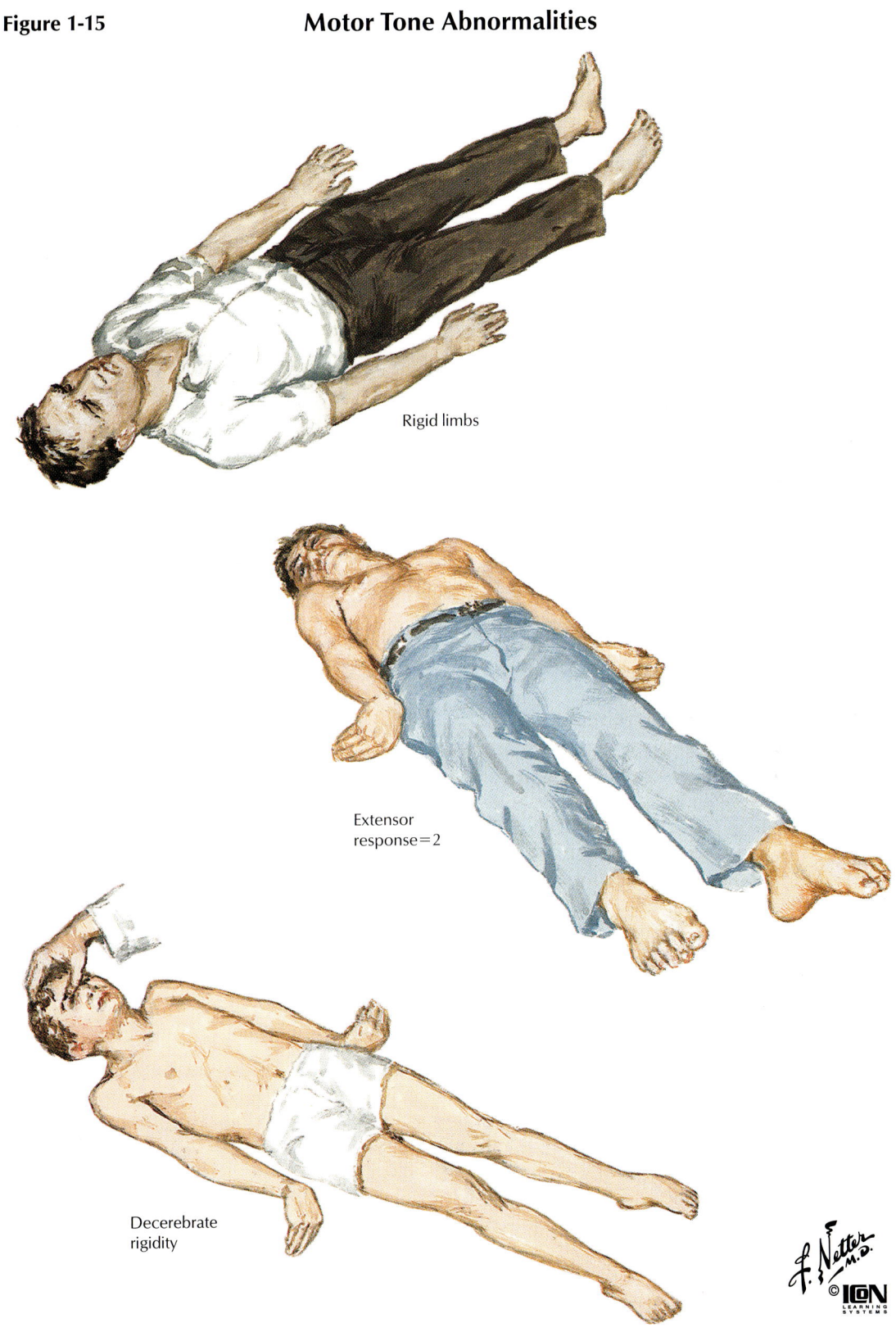

Rigid limbs

Extensor response=2

Decerebrate rigidity

NEUROLOGIC EXAMINATION

CLINICAL NEUROLOGIC EVALUATION

Flaccidity, a total loss of tone, is seen in various disease processes affecting the upper motor neurons. Most commonly, this occurs with a recent stroke or an acute spinal cord injury, ie, **spinal shock**. However, with both of these, the flaccidity is temporary, and tone increases later to present with significant **spasticity**.

Spasticity is defined by extreme muscle tone that is maximal at the initiation of the physician's attempt to move the limb and then suddenly releases partway through the movement (a clasp-knife, **spastic release**). Significant degrees of spasticity are easily elicited with any reasonable stimulation of muscles that induces the stretch reflex. More subtle spasticity may be obvious only with stretching the muscle in a specific direction and at a specific rate. Increased tone, such as may occur with stroke or spinal cord injury, evolves from flaccidity to spasticity over a matter of days to weeks subsequent to the initial neurologic injury.

When there is total loss of a motor neuron inhibition, as may occur with an upper brainstem injury, one sees the syndrome of **decerebrate rigidity**. Here, a simple noxious stimulus leads to bilateral extension in unison of all 4 extremities, with the arms rotated inward. Most commonly, one sees this in the setting of cardiac arrest or from shear injuries to the brain from automobile accidents. When such patients survive 1 to 3 months and are totally otherwise unresponsive, they are said to be in a ***persistent vegetative state***.

Increasing tone from basal ganglia disorders, as may occur with Parkinson disease, is known as ***rigidity***. Rigidity creates a continuous sense of tightness in the attempt to move the joint through a full excursion from extension to flexion.

MUSCLE STRETCH REFLEXES

The Ia and Ib afferents join the fibers of the spinal cord posterior columns, whose primary function is to convey information from touch and pressure receptors. Therefore, although the muscle spindles and Golgi tendon organs cannot be specifically tested, some of their spinal cord connections can be clinically evaluated by testing position and vibration sensory modalities. Additionally, the Ia and Ib afferents convey similar information to the cerebellum via the posterior spinocerebellar tract that travels into the cerebellum through the inferior cerebellar peduncle (Figure 1-16). In isolation, it is difficult to assess the contribution to motor control of each tract. Experimental posterior spinocerebellar tract lesions result in muscular movement incoordination or asynergia.

With simple passive stretching, such as occurs with tapping the patellar tendon at the knee, the intrafusal muscle spindle is activated, leading to a direct stimulus to the large a motor neurons. These in turn stimulate the extrafusal skeletal muscle fibers leading to the clinically observed muscle contraction (Figure 1-17). If the afferent sensory or efferent motor limb of this nerve supply is damaged, the MSR is affected and may be diminished or lost, as occurs with many peripheral neuropathies. These reflexes are sometimes inappropriately referred to as *deep tendon reflexes* when in fact their physiologic basis primarily depends on the intrafusal muscle spindle fibers, not the Golgi tendon organs. *MSR* is a more accurate term.

During the neurologic examination, MSRs (named for the muscle stretched) are usually readily elicited by tapping lightly over the muscle insertion tendon while palpating the tendon and then percussing the palpating digit. Occasionally, it is difficult to obtain MSRs in healthy individuals. It is sometimes useful to distract the patient or apply techniques that reinforce the reflex to potentiate MSRs. The most common method is the Jendrassik maneuver, wherein patients flex their fingers, interlocking one hand with the other and pulling on the count of 3 while the clinician percusses the appropriate tendon at the knee or ankle. For the upper extremities, the patient may be asked to clench the contralateral fist as the neurologist percusses over the arm tendons, activating the intrafusal muscle spindle.

When grading MSRs, the extremes are easy to appreciate and range from 0 to 4. A reflex grading of 0 is indicative of complete lack of MSR. A generalized loss of reflexes is pathologic and is known as **areflexia**; this typically occurs in Guillain-Barré syndrome. Briskly responding MSRs are graded as 4. In brisk MSRs, a single Achilles tendon percussion sometimes elicits a repetitive series of dorsi movements, plantar movements, or both in the foot. This is known as

CLINICAL NEUROLOGIC EVALUATION

Figure 1-16 **Cerebral Afferent Pathways**

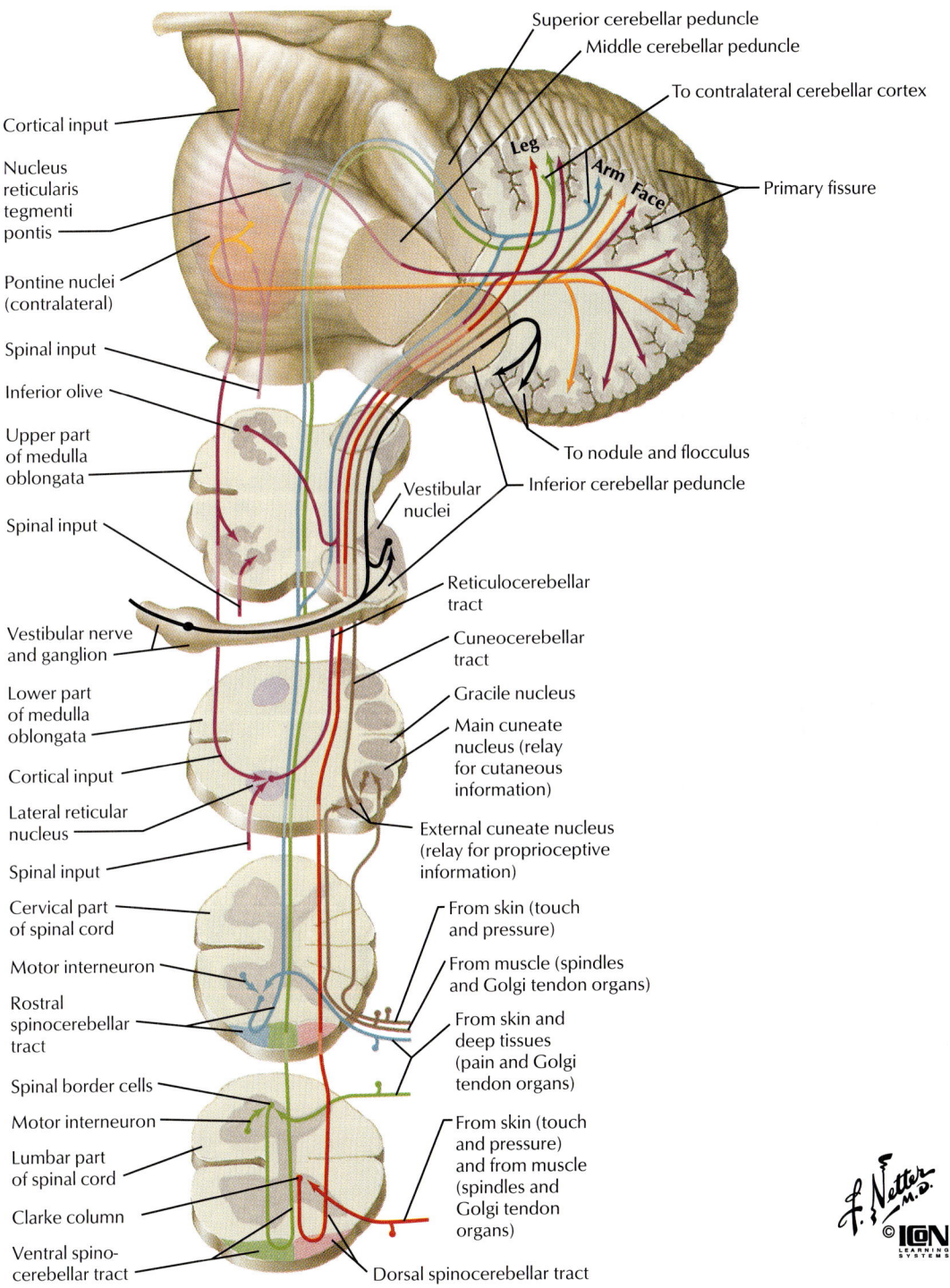

NEUROLOGIC EXAMINATION

33

CLINICAL NEUROLOGIC EVALUATION

Figure 1-17 Muscle and Joint Receptors and Muscle Spindles

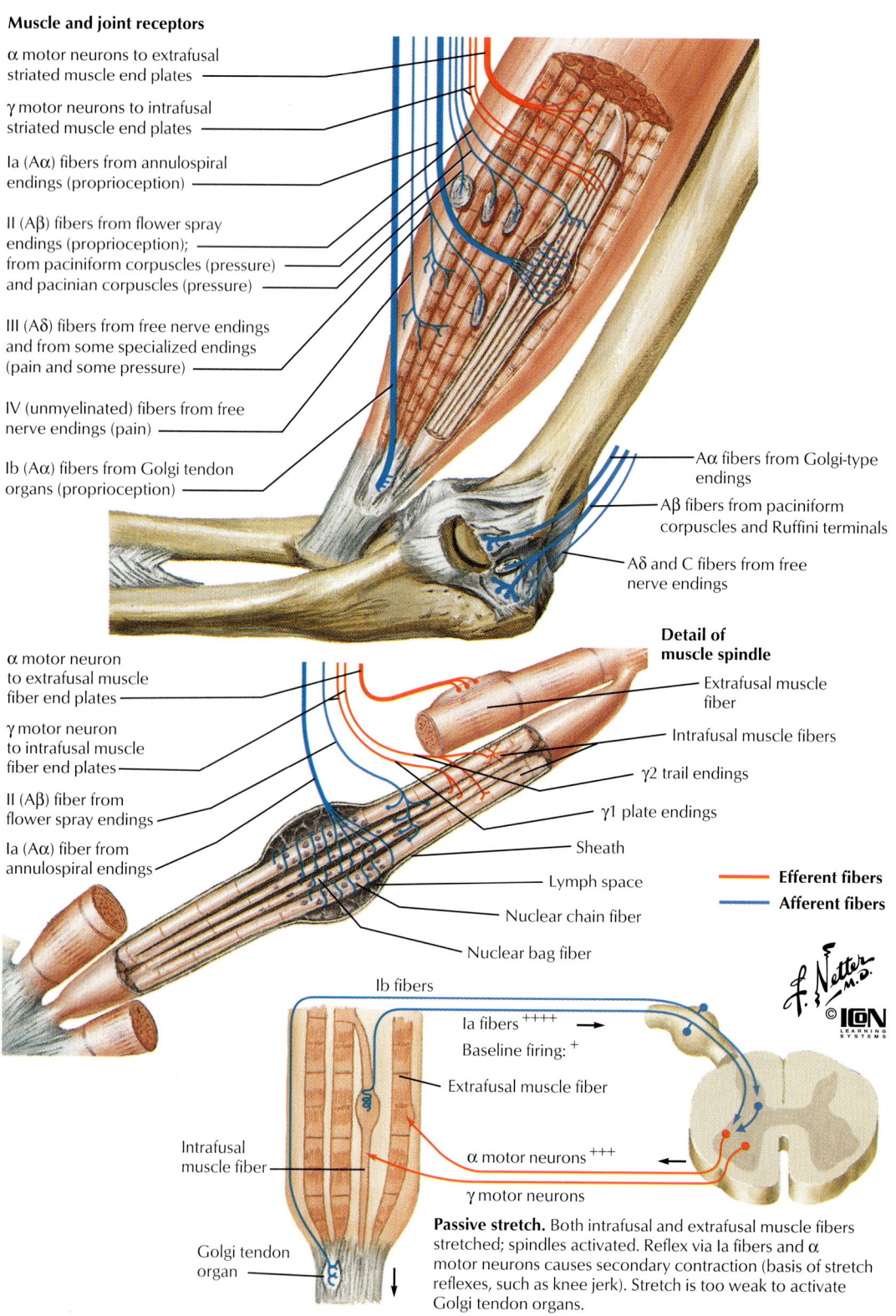

CLINICAL NEUROLOGIC EVALUATION

Figure 1-18   Elicitation of the Babinski Sign

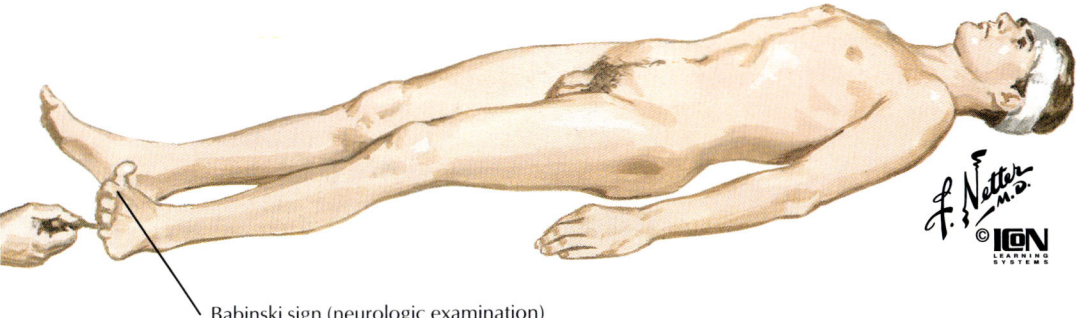

Babinski sign (neurologic examination)

clonus. This does not commonly occur spontaneously, but clonus may be elicited by giving a quick snap to the dorsiflexed foot as it is held in the palm of the hand. This also occurs, rarely, at the quadriceps tendon. The remainder of the grading is easier to understand. A reflex of 1 is a mere contraction of the muscle, a 2 is a contraction that leads to actual limb movement, and a 3 is a reflection of brisker and more forceful movement.

The **Babinski sign** is an important **pathologic reflex** that is elicited at the lateral, plantar surface of the foot using subtle, careful stroking with a tongue depressor or the base of a key. The great toe extends, and the remaining toes fan out (Figure 1-18). A more exaggerated response, known as **triple flexion**, includes flexion of the hip, knee, and foot, often with a Babinski response. Because this reflex primarily depends on sensory stimulation of the foot, a kind, gentle, nonirritating stimulus is best to obtain an accurate response. It absolutely does not require excessive or painful pressure. With sensitive or ticklish patients, appropriate responses can usually be obtained from a careful stimulation of the lateral outside foot surface. However, some patients have a **withdrawal response** wherein the foot and entire set of toes dorsiflex. This is often overcome by separately pulling down on the middle toe while carefully stimulating the sole in traditional fashion.

A clinical combination of brisk MSRs, clonus, and a Babinski sign indicates an **upper motor neuron lesion**. These abnormalities result from various pathophysiologic mechanisms originating in the brain or spinal cord. The many possibilities include destructive cerebral lesions, such as stroke, tumor, encephalitis, and spinal cord trauma, or demyelinating disorders affecting the spinal cord, the brain, or both. Additionally, these signs of upper motor neuron lesions are observed in patients during the postictal period after a seizure or in patients who have toxic or metabolic encephalopathies. Therefore, although brisk MSRs and a Babinski sign are nonspecific regarding the anatomical setting of the CNS abnormality, their presence provides unequivocal evidence of upper motor neuron pathology.

SENSORY EXAMINATION

A carefully designed sensory system evaluation serves to define the presence or absence of normal sensation and, if abnormal, to define specific anatomical patterns of loss for the affected modalities. Because part of the sensory examination is fairly subjective, the examiner should analyze the consistency of responses. Additionally, the relevance of sensory changes to the patient's complaints and other findings needs to be evaluated. Initially, the examination should focus on defining the presence or loss of sensation. One needs to avoid having the patient be overly cooperative, trying to define the subtlest differences in sensory appreciation. This often leads to an exhausted patient and a frustrated clinician. In most clinical settings, it is best to separate the sensory examination into 2 major categories derived from superficial skin receptors or deeper mechanoreceptors. The former are small, unmyelinated, slowly conducting type C fibers or larger, slightly-myelinated, somewhat more rapidly conducting type A-δ fibers. These small fibers primarily subserve pain (tested using

NEUROLOGIC EXAMINATION

CLINICAL NEUROLOGIC EVALUATION

Figure 1-19

Documentation of Various Types of Sensory Modalities in a Peripheral Neuropathy

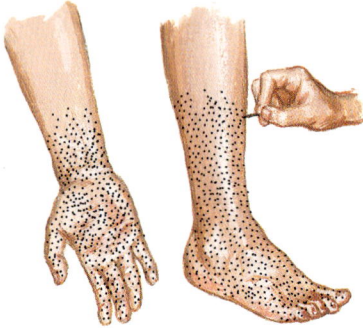

Graduated glove-and-stocking hypesthesia to pain and/or temperature

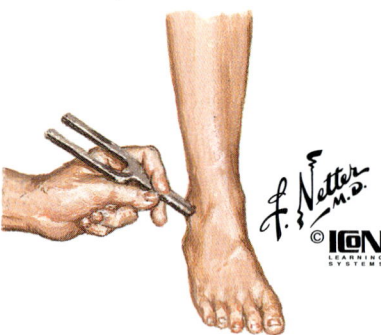

Impaired vibration sense

a pinpoint), temperature (tested using a cold object such as the handle of a tuning fork), deep pressure, and gross touch modalities. The large, well-myelinated type A-α and A-β fibers carry the kinesthetic modalities of position studied by the examiner's passively moving the digit in the vertical plane and asking the patient whether the movement was up or down. Additionally, fine tactile discrimination can be evaluated by using a pair of calipers to check their ability to recognize whether 1 or 2 points are applied to the digit. Some vibratory modalities are probably also subserved by type A-δ fibers.

Classic Syndromes of Sensory Dysfunction
Peripheral Nervous System

Generalized polyneuropathies typically present with symptoms of numbness and tingling at the tips of the toes and, later, fingers, ie, a stocking-glove distribution (Figure 1-19). These then spread proximally past the ankles and wrists into the legs and forearms. On examination with a cold object, a pin (for small fiber function), a tuning fork, and position sense (if large fibers are also involved), the examiner notes a distal loss that is maximal in the periphery and gradually reaches normal at a more proximal site.

Individual mononeuropathies are typified by symptoms and findings specific to a peripheral nerve. For example, the patient notes numbness in the thumb, index, middle fingers, and adjacent lateral aspect of the fourth finger if the median nerve is involved. In carpal tunnel syndrome with entrapment of the median nerve at the wrist, the examination results are often normal. However, using a reflex hammer to tap over the entrapment site commonly elicits brief paresthesiae in the classic distribution of the median sensory fibers. This maneuver is known as the ***Tinel sign***; the name applies to instances wherein a simple provocative test is used to define the lesion site with a mononeuropathy.

Plexopathies are usually unilateral in distribution, affecting the brachial or lumbosacral groups of nerves. Typically, they have combined sensory loss involving multiple peripheral nerves within the affected limbs. These have a broader distribution of motor and sensory loss than a single nerve root or mononeuropathy. Therefore, when the examination reveals findings not exclusively delegated to the defined distribution, the possibility of a plexus lesion must be considered.

Radiculopathies are frequently more subjective, with intermittent or persistent symptoms confined to the dermatomal patterns of one specific nerve root (Figure 1-14). Pain is the most common symptom, starting in the neck, shoulder, and low back, often radiating down the posterior thigh. The classic examples include the C7 nerve root in the neck with paresthesiae primarily in the index and middle fingers and the L5 nerve root in the low back, where the patient reports numbness in the first and second toes and the lateral calf. Concomitant MSR loss often occurs, ie, the triceps reflex with a C7 root and the Achilles reflex with an S1 root. If the lesion is severe, the examiner often notes concomitant weakness in a specific radicular distribution, such as the triceps muscle with a C7 radiculopa-

NEUROLOGIC EXAMINATION

CLINICAL NEUROLOGIC EVALUATION

Figure 1-20

Somesthetic System: Body

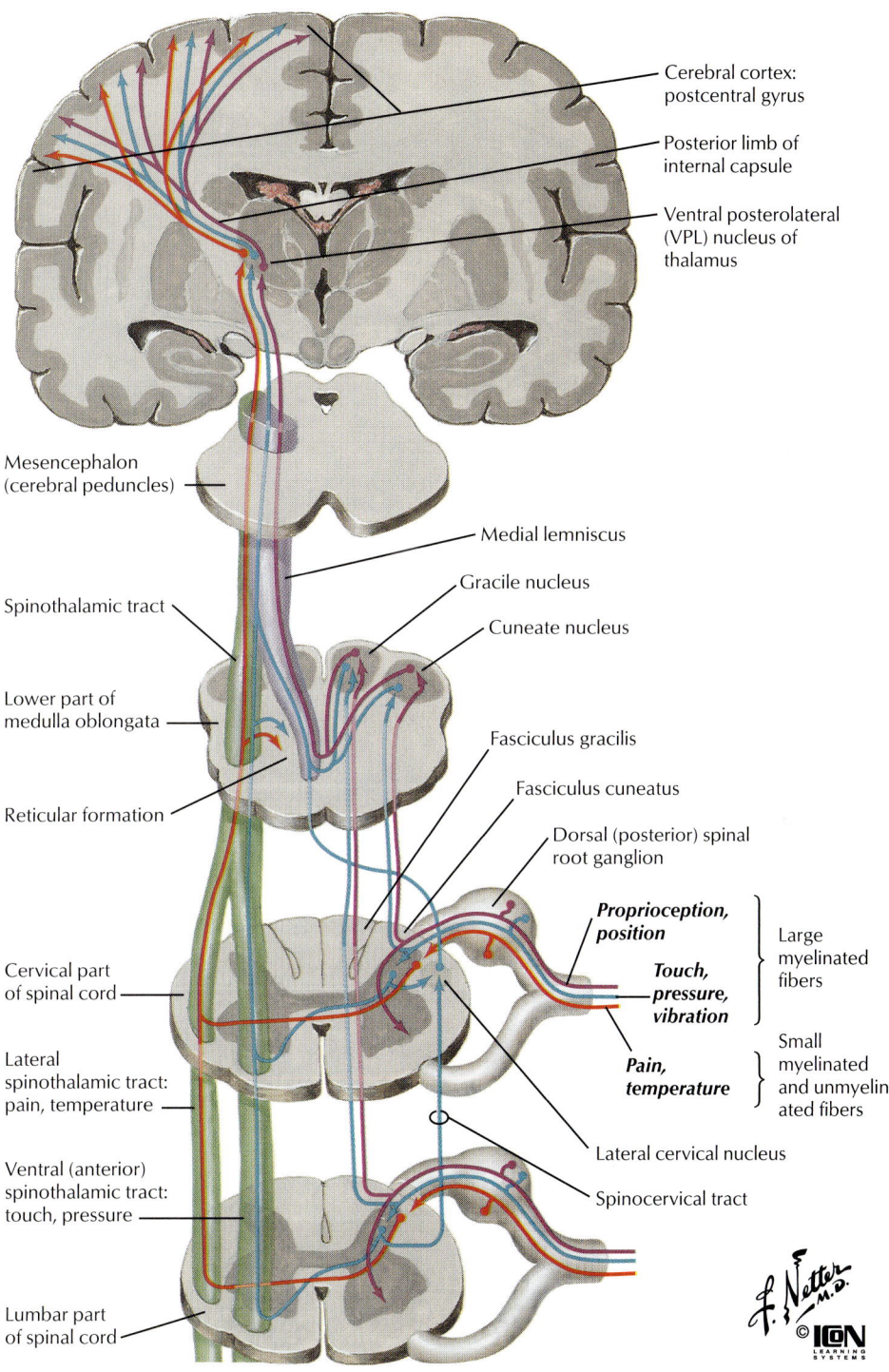

NEUROLOGIC EXAMINATION

CLINICAL NEUROLOGIC EVALUATION

thy and the tibialis anterior and tibialis posterior in the case of an L5 root involvement.

Spinal Cord Syndromes

The site of a spinal cord lesion is defined by identifying the exact distribution of specific motor and sensory deficits of various modalities (Figure 1-20). A complete lesion of the spinal cord leads to total loss of function distal to the site of the abnormality. A distinct level of sensory loss can be discerned with tests for loss of pain and/or temperature sensations, associated with loss of sweating below the lesion level. Concomitantly, all muscles subserved by anterior horn cells distal to the site of the lesion experience paralysis (Figure 60-3).

A lesion in the anterior lateral aspect of the spinal cord causes contralateral loss of pain and temperature sensation. If the lesion is more extensive, leading to damage of the anterior and posterior aspects of the cord on one side, **Brown-Séquard syndrome** occurs. This syndrome is characterized by contralateral loss of pain and temperature sensation, ipsilateral loss of position and vibration sensation, and ipsilateral upper motor neuron weakness.

Syringomyelia or a central hemorrhage leads to another anatomically specific spinal cord lesion. The pathology occurs at the center of the cord, destroying fibers carrying pain and temperature sensation from both sides as they cross in the anterior commissure. Because the fibers carrying vibration and position sense do not cross in the spinal cord and ascend posteriorly, a small lesion in the center of the cord spares those pathways. This causes a **dissociated sensory loss** with isolated loss of pain and temperature sensation, usually in a "cape" distribution, while concomitantly, position sense is preserved.

A patient with an **anterior spinal artery** infarction presents another classic sensory picture. Here, the bilateral damage to the spinothalamic

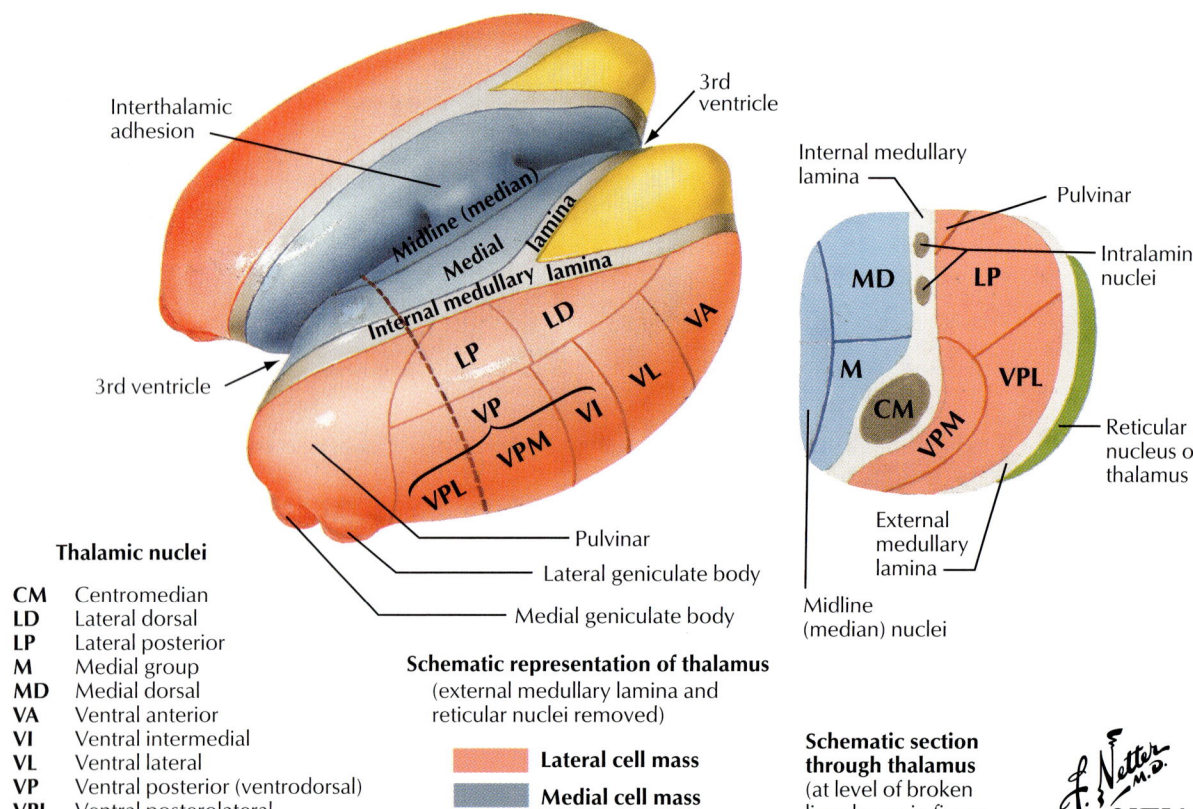

Figure 1-21 **Thalamus and Its Multiple Nuclei**

NEUROLOGIC EXAMINATION

and corticospinal tracts spares the posterior column function. The patient is paralyzed and has total loss of pain and temperature sensation, but position and often vibratory sensory modalities are preserved.

Thalamic Involvement

The ventral posterior lateral and ventral posterior medial thalamic nuclei are the 2 major sensory relay nuclei (Figure 1-21). Lesions in these areas can cause loss of sensation to all modalities involving the entire contralateral half of the body. This most commonly occurs in patients with bland or hemorrhagic infarcts. Initially presenting with a relatively tolerable numbness, eventually the damage incurred from the stroke may produce an unpleasant, sometimes disabling, hyperpathic sensory alteration known as the **thalamic pain syndrome**. Rarely, this loss of sensation can lead to limb sensory choreoathetosis. Lesions within the corona radiata, undercutting the parietal cortex, can cause similar, although often less extensive, findings.

Cortical Sensory Involvement

The parietal lobe receives topographically organized sensory inputs from the thalamic nuclei brainstem, spinal cord, plexi, and peripheral nerves (Figure 1-20). The important function of the parietal lobe is the integration of that information with other sensory and motor information to formulate body awareness. In the purest form of cortical sensory dysfunctions, patients are unable to differentiate the location of their toes or fingers in space, between 1 point and 2 points of contact, and points separated by 1 cm (**2-point discrimination**). They are unable to recognize numbers traced on the palm (**graphesthesia**).

Many other sensory abnormalities occur, including complete loss of sensation on the contralateral side of large strokes involving the parietal area and a neglect with right parietal lesions, wherein the patient is unaware of paralysis or sensory loss of the contralateral limbs. These are especially obvious with double simultaneous stimulation (extinction). One or two sides of the body are variably stimulated, and the patient is asked to identify the stimulus location. Individuals with a more subtle parietal sensory loss cannot identify the contralateral stimulus when bilateral stimuli are applied.

REFERENCES

Bates B. *A Guide to Physical Examination and History Taking*. 4th ed. Baltimore, Md: JB Lippincott Co; 1987.

Brain. *Aids to the Examination of the Peripheral Nervous System*. 4th ed. Philadelphia, Pa: WB Saunders; 2000.

Brazis P, Masdeau J, Biller J. *Localization in Clinical Neurology*. 3rd ed. Baltimore, Md: Lippincott Williams & Wilkins; 1996.

Carpenter MB, Sutin J. *Human Neuroanatomy*. 8th ed. Baltimore, Md: Williams & Wilkins; 1983.

Kandel, ER, Schwartz JH, Jessell TM. *Principles of Neural Science*. 4th ed. New York, NY: McGraw-Hill, Health Professions Division; 2000.

Luria AR. *Higher Cortical Functions in Man*. 2nd ed. Basic Books, Inc; 1980.

Mayo Clinic Department of Neurology. *Mayo Clinic Examinations in Neurology*. 7th ed. St. Louis, Mo: Mosby; 1998.

Miller N. Clinical signs and symptoms. In: *Walsh and Hoyt's Clinical Neuro-Ophthalmology*. 5th ed. Baltimore, Md: Lippincott Williams & Wilkins; 1998.

Peters A, Jones EG, eds. *Cerebral Cortex: Vol 4. Association and Auditory Cortices*. New York, NY: Plenum Press; 1985.

Chapter 2
Cognitive and Language Evaluation

Kinan K. Hreib

Clinical Vignette

A 70-year-old previously healthy man was referred for evaluation of an inability to ambulate. According to the family, during the past year, the patient had had difficulties standing up and getting out of the car and often sat in the car for hours until someone actively encouraged him by either gently pushing or pulling him out of the car. On further questioning, it became evident that he had similar problems under other circumstances. He tended to sit on the toilet seat for hours. His wife reported that often in public places, she had to ask security to get him out of the bathroom. In the morning, the patient stayed in bed until physically coaxed to get up.

The family commented that he had experienced a concomitant change in behavior. He might lie in urine while in bed, often seemingly unaware of the problem. On a regular basis, he was incontinent of stool, often while standing up. His wife would urge him to clean up, but to her amazement when she returned a few hours later, she found him still standing in the same spot.

He ate if reminded and shown the food but usually did not ask for or make his own meals. At dinner, he typically took a piece of bread, eating it slowly but often not proceeding to the rest of the food unless helped by the family. He read the newspaper regularly, usually comprehending and remembering its content. However, when he finished reading, he folded and unfolded the newspaper for hours. When the patient was asked about these issues, his answer was brief: "I do not know." His wife did not notice any problems with his memory but emphasized that his level of interaction with the family had significantly decreased.

During his neurologic examination, he often smiled and looked around the room as if searching for something. He was always pleasant but not conversational. When asked a question, his responses were brief and usually monosyllabic but appropriate, without speech or language dysfunction. He did not seem to have prominent memory difficulties, nor did he have cranial nerve involvement or motor or sensory deficits. His gait was normal. His reflexes were 1+ throughout, and his toes were down.

Subsequently, his symptoms have progressed. He is now less interactive and continues to be unable to participate in his own hygiene or to eat on regular basis. MRI demonstrated significant frontotemporal atrophy (Figure 2-1). This clinical picture is compatible with the diagnosis of frontal-type dementia. Pick disease may have a similar presentation but often with significant language difficulties (chapter 34).

The initial clinical evaluation affords the opportunity to assess whether a neurologic patient has overt cognitive or language difficulties. The ability to give a well-organized history provides the experienced neurologist with insight into the patient's general language and cognitive function. It is usually clear that intellect and speech are appropriate to the setting, so a more formal set of mental status tests is unnecessary. However, in instances of overt intellectual function changes, when the patient's demeanor suggests that possibility or the family suggests an additional problem to the primary complaint of the patient (as in the vignette in this chapter), a more detailed cognitive examination is needed in addition to the standard (chapter 1) neurologic examination.

This part of the neurologic evaluation strives to determine the precise level of various higher cortical functions. The human cerebral cortex, with its multiple gyri and network of many million interconnections, is the most complex part of the brain. Anatomically, the cortex is classified into 4 major functional areas: frontal, temporal, parietal, and occipital lobes (Figure 2-2). These anatomic substrates are carefully interconnected in a complex network. For the sake of discussion, these cortical areas are described in isolation, but in reality, interconnections with other

COGNITIVE AND LANGUAGE EVALUATION

Figure 2-1

Frontal Temporal Atrophy

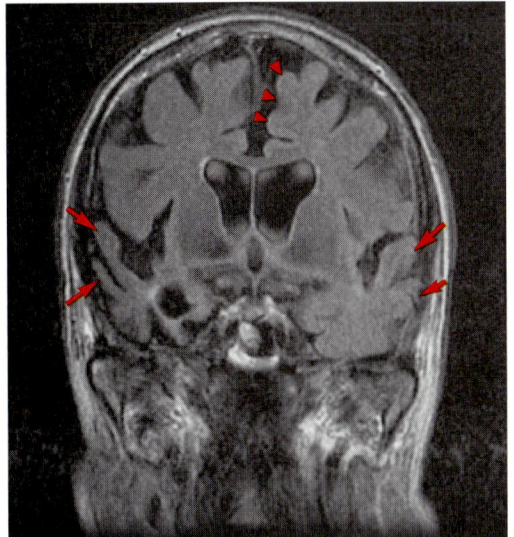

Coronal FLAIR MR image demonstrates ventricular enlargement especially of the right temporal horn, atrophy of superior and middle temporal gyri (arrow), and prominence of frontal sulci. Notice prominent widening of the interhemispheric fissure (arrowheads). Courtesy of Richard Caselli, MD.

cortical and subcortical areas are critical for brain function (Figure 2-3). Because some patients are not able to give a history or cooperate with the examiner, the history from reliable family and friends is the most important part of the evaluation. Interactions with the patient also help to determine the level of cognitive neurologic function. The patient's attitude, affect, level of cooperation, and distractibility are noteworthy. For example, patients with dementia may seem pleasant and jovial, often finding excuses for their inability to answer questions, rarely with any insight into their deficit. In contrast, patients with severe posterior aphasia may seem agitated and uncooperative, and often respond intermittently to certain commands but not to others.

Many fascinating and complex syndromes affect higher cortical function. Often they occur in association with other significant neurologic deficits, particularly with a stroke, the most frequent clinical cause for these lesions.

COGNITIVE TESTING

Factors to be documented in an elementary cognitive examination include level of alertness, orientation, concentration, constructional ability, apraxia, any language deficit, and recall (Figure 2-4). The Mini-Mental Status Examination, often used to quantitate cognitive function, is limited by its lack of a true language element and inability to test for most frontal lobe dysfunctions. Language deficits provide another major obstacle in a detailed cognitive examination. Similarly, the delirious patient with poor concentration, poor attention, or both has a limited capacity to respond to the examination.

APHASIA

Language dysfunction is manifested by impairment in oral or written communication or both. Deficits vary in quality and severity depending on the extent of anatomic involvement within the language areas. Aphasias result from involvement of the dominant hemisphere, which is the left hemisphere in all right-handed individuals and approximately 50% of native left-handed individuals. In the remaining left-handed population, the language center is located in the right hemisphere. The aphasia may not be accompanied by other neurologic deficits; therefore, such patients are often initially mistaken as being confused. A good history from the family regarding symptom onset or other important medical history often helps in the diagnosis.

In the acute clinical setting, the classification of aphasia is challenging. The different types of language deficits depend on the brain area involved (Table 2-1). The easiest to understand are those involving the cortex (Figure 2-5). Although aphasias are often part of a large hemispheric stroke, many devastating aphasias can result from small processes affecting the temporal or frontal lobes, or even some subcortical structures, such as the thalamus.

The degree of language fluency is the earliest manifestation of aphasia that can help to determine its specific characteristics. For example, a patient with a posterior temporal infarct of the dominant hemisphere presents with poor comprehension but fluent speech, ie, the patient is often talkative, albeit his or her language is not normal. In contrast, fluency is significantly diminished in patients with a frontal lobe lesion, particularly with Broca aphasia. Thalamic aphasias are often characterized by apathy, hypophonia, and

COGNITIVE AND LANGUAGE EVALUATION

Figure 2-2

Superolateral Surface of Brain

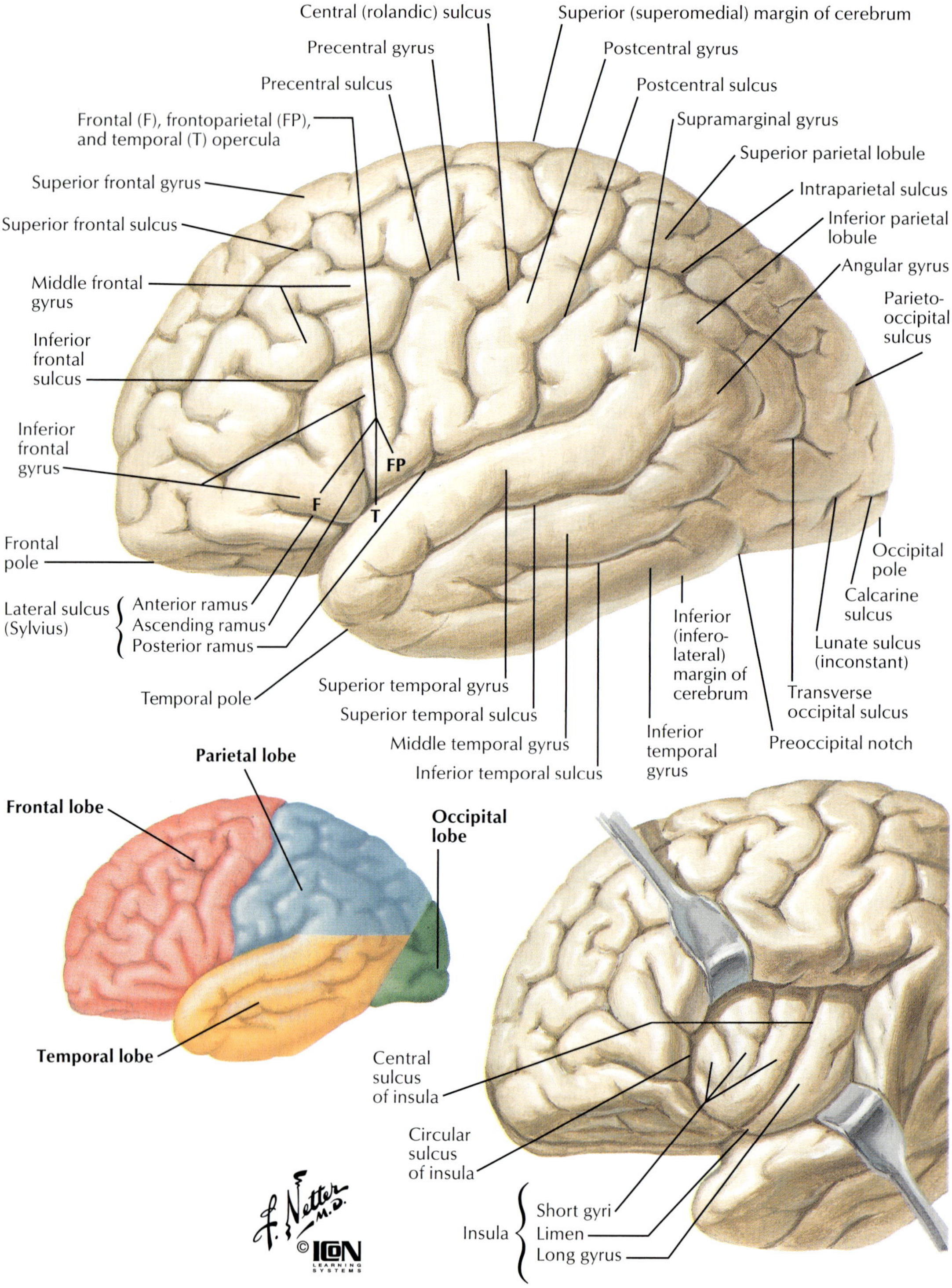

Labels: Central (rolandic) sulcus; Superior (superomedial) margin of cerebrum; Precentral gyrus; Postcentral gyrus; Precentral sulcus; Postcentral sulcus; Frontal (F), frontoparietal (FP), and temporal (T) opercula; Supramarginal gyrus; Superior frontal gyrus; Superior parietal lobule; Superior frontal sulcus; Intraparietal sulcus; Middle frontal gyrus; Inferior parietal lobule; Inferior frontal sulcus; Angular gyrus; Parieto-occipital sulcus; Inferior frontal gyrus; Frontal pole; Occipital pole; Calcarine sulcus; Lateral sulcus (Sylvius) { Anterior ramus, Ascending ramus, Posterior ramus }; Lunate sulcus (inconstant); Inferior (inferolateral) margin of cerebrum; Transverse occipital sulcus; Temporal pole; Preoccipital notch; Superior temporal gyrus; Superior temporal sulcus; Middle temporal gyrus; Inferior temporal sulcus; Inferior temporal gyrus

Frontal lobe — **Parietal lobe** — **Occipital lobe** — **Temporal lobe**

Central sulcus of insula; Circular sulcus of insula; Insula { Short gyri, Limen, Long gyrus }

NEUROLOGIC EXAMINATION

42

COGNITIVE AND LANGUAGE EVALUATION

Figure 2-3

Cerebral Cortex: Localization of Function and Association Pathways

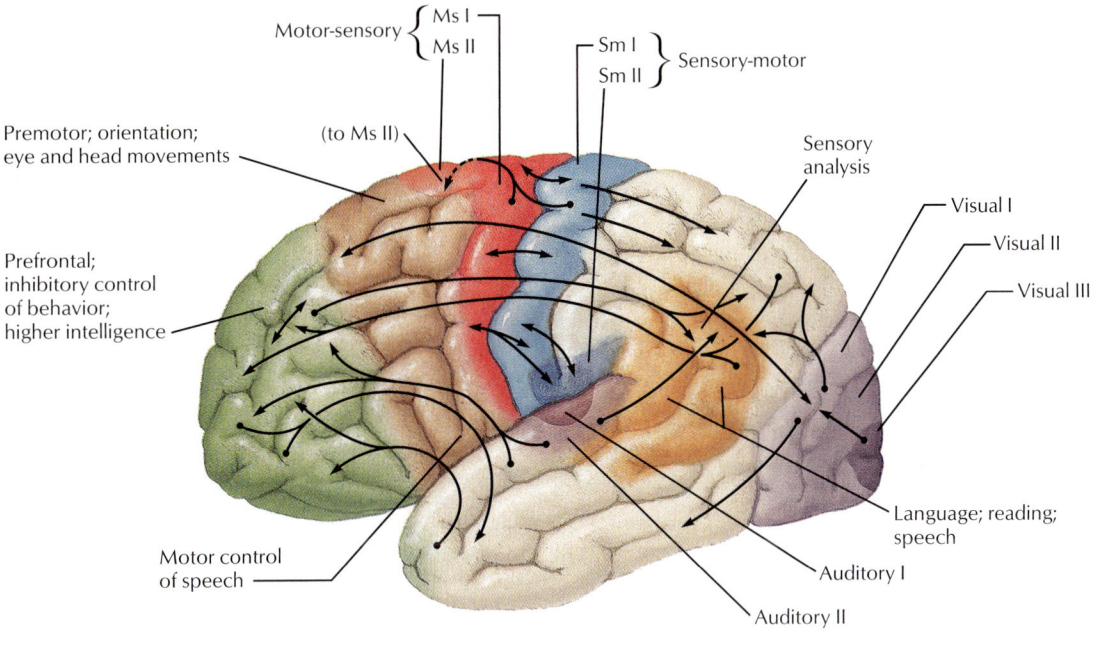

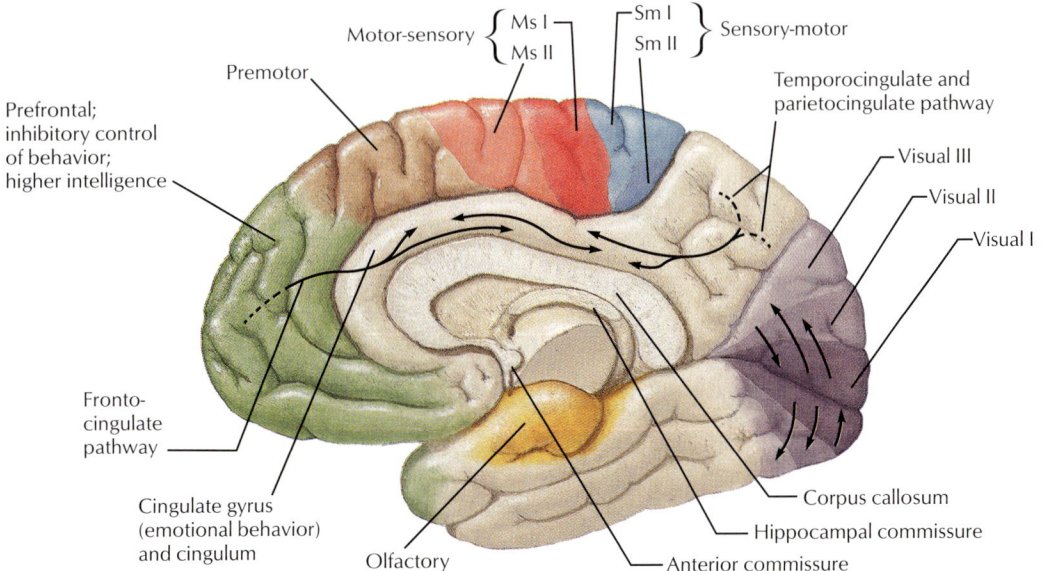

COGNITIVE AND LANGUAGE EVALUATION

Figure 2-4 **Testing for Defects of Higher Cortical Function**

A. Appearance and interpersonal behavior

Pleasant, neatly dressed, good spirits

Depressed, sloppily dressed, careless

Belligerent

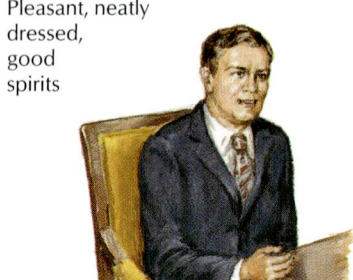
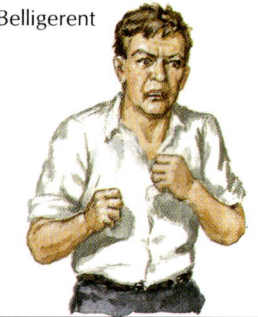

B. Language

Good   Defective

Doctor: "Write me a brief paragraph about your work."

C. Memory

Doctor: "Here are 3 objects: a pipe, a pen, and a picture of Abraham Lincoln. I want you to remember them and in 5 minutes, I will ask you what they were."

5 minutes later:
Patient: "I'm sorry, I can't remember. Did you show me something?"

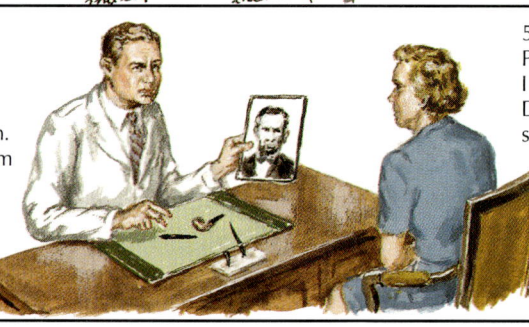

D. Constructional praxis and visual-spatial function

Doctor: "Draw me a simple picture of a house."

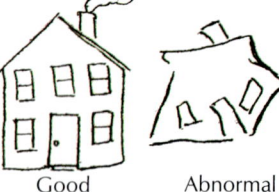
Good   Abnormal

"Draw a clock face for me."

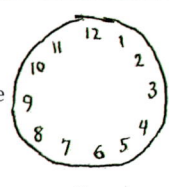
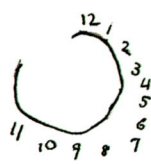
Good   Abnormal

E. Reverse counting

Doctor: "Count backward from 5 to 1 for me."
Patient: "5...3...4..., sorry, I can't do it."

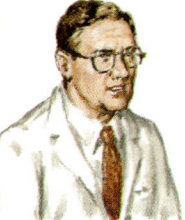
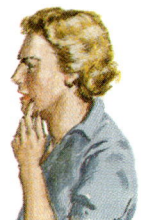

Doctor: "Spell the word *worlds* backward for me."
Patient: "W..L..R..D..S."

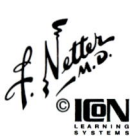

NEUROLOGIC EXAMINATION

Table 2-1
Characteristics of Aphasias

Parameter	Anterior	Posterior	Conduction	Subcortical	Transcortical		
Location	Frontal/Broca	Temporal/Wernicke	L.-inf.-parietal	Basalganglia/white matter	Thalamus/anterior-lateral	Motor	Sensory
Fluency	Poor	Good	Good	Variable	Poor	Poor	Good
Naming	Poor	Poor	Poor-fair	Variable	Poor	Poor	Good
Repetition	Poor	Poor	Poor	Good	Good	Good	Good
Paraphasia	Common	Common	Common	Variable	Variable	Common	Common
Comprehension	Good	Poor	Good	Good	Poor	Good	Poor

echolalia. Most often, lesions in the anterior-lateral thalamus cause the most profound aphasia.

Transcortical aphasia refers to aphasias near the classic language areas. These include the posterosuperior temporal lobe (Brodmann area 40, for Wernicke aphasia) and the posteroinferior frontal lobe (Brodmann area 44 for Broca aphasia). However, transcortical aphasia does not directly involve these areas. Most investigators agree that receptive transcortical aphasia involves the posterior-inferior temporal gyrus, ie, Brodmann area 37. Transcortical motor aphasia occurs with left frontal lobe lesions. Echolalia is common in these latter aphasias, whereas right visual deficits are common in the sensory transcortical aphasias.

Some patients with Wernicke aphasia are able to mimic certain movements, especially midline commands such as opening the mouth, closing the eyes, and standing up. Another common phenomenon, best described as a crowding effect, occurs when patients seem to be able to follow the first command and perhaps the second, but their performance deteriorates with subsequent testing. The cause may be partially intact language function becoming overwhelmed by persistent use. The aphasia also seems worse when patients are anxious or upset.

FRONTAL LOBE DYSFUNCTION

The frontal lobe comprises approximately 30% of brain mass occupying the motor area (Brodmann area 4), the premotor cortex (Brodmann areas 6 and 8), and significant prefrontal areas. Significant prefrontal areas are distinct from the adjacent motor and premotor areas, particularly in their connections with other cortical areas and the thalamus. Most thalamic connections are with the dorsal medial nucleus, a prime relay center for limbic projections originating from the amygdala and the basal forebrain. The reciprocal inputs are the most prominent cortical connections, originating from second-order sensory association and paralimbic association areas, including the cingulate cortex, temporal pole, and parahippocampal area. The frontal lobe is an integrator and analyzer of highly complex multimodal cortical areas, including limbically processed information.

Experimental animals demonstrated unusual behavior after ablation of both frontal lobes. Some of the most dramatic symptoms, including automatic nonpurposeful behaviors with a tendency to chew randomly on objects, led to the conclusion that the frontal lobe was important for the integration of goal-directed movement. Investigations in the 1950s began to define the importance of the frontal lobe in analyzing stimuli. Lesions in the frontal lobe resulted in loss of normal social interchange, personal internal reinforcement, and judgment. Therefore, patients are unable to modify behavior despite potentially harming or embarrassing effects of their actions. Furthermore, patients tend to repeat automatic behaviors that do not result in conclusive actions, as seen in perseveration testing.

In humans, one of the earliest descriptions of frontal lobe damage included significant personality changes and "release of animal instincts." Subsequent reports described patients with apa-

COGNITIVE AND LANGUAGE EVALUATION

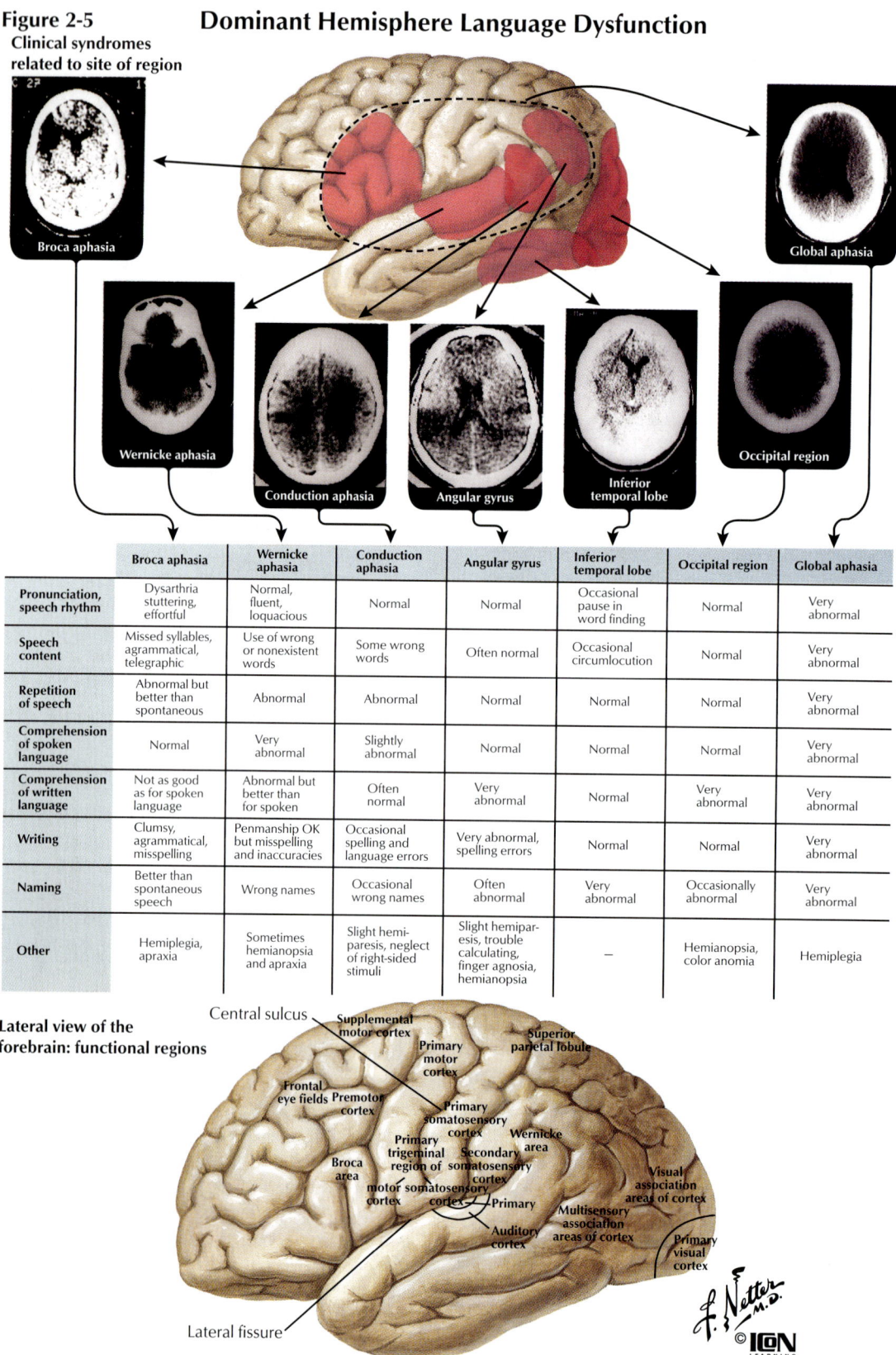

Figure 2-5 Clinical syndromes related to site of region

Dominant Hemisphere Language Dysfunction

	Broca aphasia	Wernicke aphasia	Conduction aphasia	Angular gyrus	Inferior temporal lobe	Occipital region	Global aphasia
Pronunciation, speech rhythm	Dysarthria stuttering, effortful	Normal, fluent, loquacious	Normal	Normal	Occasional pause in word finding	Normal	Very abnormal
Speech content	Missed syllables, agrammatical, telegraphic	Use of wrong or nonexistent words	Some wrong words	Often normal	Occasional circumlocution	Normal	Very abnormal
Repetition of speech	Abnormal but better than spontaneous	Abnormal	Abnormal	Normal	Normal	Normal	Very abnormal
Comprehension of spoken language	Normal	Very abnormal	Slightly abnormal	Normal	Normal	Normal	Very abnormal
Comprehension of written language	Not as good as for spoken language	Abnormal but better than for spoken	Often normal	Very abnormal	Normal	Very abnormal	Very abnormal
Writing	Clumsy, agrammatical, misspelling	Penmanship OK but misspelling and inaccuracies	Occasional spelling and language errors	Very abnormal, spelling errors	Normal	Normal	Very abnormal
Naming	Better than spontaneous speech	Wrong names	Occasional wrong names	Often abnormal	Very abnormal	Occasionally abnormal	Very abnormal
Other	Hemiplegia, apraxia	Sometimes hemianopsia and apraxia	Slight hemiparesis, neglect of right-sided stimuli	Slight hemiparesis, trouble calculating, finger agnosia, hemianopsia	—	Hemianopsia, color anomia	Hemiplegia

Lateral view of the forebrain: functional regions

NEUROLOGIC EXAMINATION

thy and disturbed emotions. Elucidation of the frontal lobe connections, particularly the medial-basal portion, shows that the limbic system provides significant input to that area. Autonomic centers originating in the brainstem and hypothalamus also have significant connections with the basal frontal lobe. When these connections are disrupted, aggressive, impulsive, and uncontrolled behavior results.

Frontal lobe syndromes are classified clinically, anatomically, and neuropsychologically into lateral and medial-basal groups. Patients with lateral frontal lesions experience significant difficulties in executing a purely motor function, with general slowing of speech, gait, or other previously learned motor action, and are sometimes described as behaving "like a bump on a log." Individuals with medial-basal lesions display prominent behavioral and emotional difficulties and disturbances of consciousness.

Broca aphasia is the classic form of frontal lobe language dysfunction, exhibited as a nonfluent stuttering, very effortful, agrammatic speech in association with poor naming but with normal comprehension. Often, these individuals have an associated apraxia and weakness of the right side of the face and right hand.

Testing

One of the simplest frontal lobe tests is sequencing movements, ie, rapid alternating movements. Although this test may serve several purposes during the neurologic examination, it is most useful in frontal lobe syndrome diagnosis. One set of 3 motor movements includes tapping with the hand on the thigh, forming the letter *O* with the index finger and the thumb, and forming the letter *T* by placing an open hand on top of the other. With the rapid alternating movement sequences, the patient is asked to place the hand in 3 different positions: flat, then sideways, and finally with the fist clenched. Many variations of these tests exist. Patients with frontal lobe dysfunction fail them, either by performing haphazard movements or by perseverating on the same movement. Other tests for eliciting frontal lobe dysfunction include copying certain randomly repeating shapes. Such patients suddenly start drawing the previous shape repeatedly even when instructed to draw a different shape. Similarly, when asked to draw a circle, they may draw many superimposed circles. The classic grasp response is also a form of perseveration. The exact pathophysiologic mechanisms underlying these dysfunctions are not well defined. However, it is thought that perseveration inertia is a form of disinhibition; the patient is unable to differentiate between activities because of an inability to appropriately process many sensory and motor inputs normally handled in the frontal lobes.

As the vignette in this chapter illustrates, patients with frontal lobe dysfunction typically have preserved memory and no obvious primary motor or sensory deficits. They may have visual fixation problems from frontal visual field involvement but do not experience severe visual disturbance. Sometimes, patients may lose the details of moving objects or misinterpret a complicated drawing; an individual shown a picture of an airplane may misinterpret it as a bird. Their limited visual scanning and fixation and their impulsive nature may produce erroneous interpretation of stimuli. This disturbance in frontal lobe function extends to a variety of tasks, including memory. A patient with severe frontal lobe dysfunction may recognize that his sister is a family member but then refer to her as his mother, because of resemblance in hair or height or other isolated features. When given a set of 3 words to memorize and then given another set of 3 words, these patients often repeat the first set. Even when told of the mistake, the patient is unable to correct it. These patients also have difficulties associating words with certain pictures and recalling them in a specific order. Patients with frontal lobe dysfunction become severely impaired as a result of disconnection of an important analyzer that processes sensory and motor inputs. Frontal lobe syndromes at the earliest stages may be difficult to diagnose. Sometimes, they are misinterpreted, and occasionally, a psychiatric illness is diagnosed. Traditional imaging studies often help to demonstrate a focal pathologic process, although even sophisticated modalities do not always demonstrate a specific lesion.

TEMPORAL LOBE DYSFUNCTION

Wernicke aphasia is the best-known neurologic presentation of a dominant posterior tem-

COGNITIVE AND LANGUAGE EVALUATION

poral lobe lesion. It is characterized by fluent, often nonsensical jargon, many neologisms, poor naming ability, and difficulty comprehending spoken language. More anterior portions of the superior temporal gyrus, the Heschl transverse gyrus, receive auditory inputs. Therefore, the most important connections of the superior temporal gyrus are those involving complex analyses of sound. Lesions in the dominant superior temporal gyrus can lead to word deafness. Unlike patients with typical Wernicke aphasia in many aspects, these patients are able to recognize written words. Linguistically, word deafness deficit is an inability to differentiate phonemes, sounds that allow differentiation of closely related words. In English, phonemic differentiation occurs between fricatives such as *F* and *V* or *Z* and *SH* and nonfricatives such as *zipper* and *tipper*. In other languages (eg, French), phonemes are vowels. Some patients with word deafness may also be unable to recognize music. Amusia can occur with unilateral lesions of the temporal lobe.

The inferior and medial temporal gyri are functionally less well understood. Connections of the inferior temporal gyrus include input from visual processing areas and connections with the parietal cortex. The meaning of these connections and their contributions to certain cognitive functions are not well understood. Prominent changes in monkey behavior follow the removal of both temporal lobes. More focal lesions involving the medial parts of the temporal lobes produce sudden outbursts of rage, fluctuating levels of consciousness, inability to acquire new skills, and disappearance of previously learned skills. Similar deficits occur in patients with temporal lobe tumors or temporal lobe epilepsy. Prominent deficits include a heightened anxiety level and short-term memory difficulties. Memory and learning are complex processes and require integration of information at multiple levels from multiple sources. The ability to retain information starts with registering, integrating, retaining, recalling, and reproducing the information. Memory may not become encoded if one of these steps fails.

Often, a neurodegenerative process presents with confusion and disturbed thinking and perception, compromising the processes that help to formulate memory. Memory seems to involve both hemispheres. Right temporal lesions result in disturbance of imprinting and storage of memory traces, whereas left temporal lesions produce disturbance of delayed recall. These types of memory mechanisms have also been called *involuntary* and *voluntary memory*, referring to right and left hemispheric functions, respectively. Separating testing for involuntary and voluntary memory is beyond the scope of this text.

Testing

Documenting long-term and short-term recall and new learning are the basic elements of memory testing. Remote memory testing can involve asking the patient about relevant past events such as birthdays or anniversaries. Short-term memory can be tested with a pure measure of attention and immediate memory, the Digit Span Forward test. It is administered by asking the patient to repeat a series of numbers with increasing length, from 3 digits up to 8 digits. The Digit Span Backward test, giving the patient a series of numbers to repeat in reverse order, tests the ability to manipulate information in memory. Naming 3 objects and then asking the patient to repeat the list 3 to 5 minutes later can easily test learning. These memory problems may be dramatic and accompanied by confabulations, similar to Korsakoff syndrome.

Word list testing is a nonspecific test of recall, learning, and executive function. The patient is asked to produce, over 1 minute, a list of words beginning with a specific letter or in a specific category. This task requires input from multiple cortical areas and tests several cognitive deficits.

PARIETAL LOBE DYSFUNCTION

Sensory alterations are typically characterized by a loss of cortical sensory modalities (chapter 1). One of the most dramatic changes with nondominant parietal lobe pathology is neglect syndrome, ie, asomatognosia. This mind-body dissociation manifests with curious behavioral changes, sometimes including a form of confabulation. For example, when an affected patient is asked about his paretic arm, he may state that it is not paretic and proceed to demonstrate the motor function of the normal arm. When his neglected and paretic arm is shown to him, he does not recognize it as his arm. In addition, many patients perceive distortion of the size and shape of their limb. The neglect, often associated with a relatively blunted affect, may be difficult to differentiate from visual field deficits, especially in the early stages of the disease. However, neglect seems to be more prominent with exposure to multiple stimuli, ie, double simultaneous stimulation. Smaller parietal lobe lesions may manifest as geographic disorientation. For example, patients may not be able to find their way around their home.

Apraxia, a form of movement construction failure, is defined as an inability to perform purposeful movement in the absence of elementary sensory or motor disturbance. Ideational apraxia is characterized by patients who cannot create the image of the required movement. The responsible lesion is located near the parieto-occipital junction, although some frontal lobe lesions may mimic it. Motor apraxia causes disturbances of coordination of previously learned motor movements and results from lesions just anterior to the parieto-occipital sulcus. The evaluation of patients with possible apraxia involves asking them to perform certain tasks: pretending to hold a toothbrush and brushing the teeth or pretending to hold a comb and combing the hair. In patients, oral apraxia develops as a manifestation of inferior post–central gyrus lesion, testable by asking the patient to perform or mimic certain movements, such as chewing, smiling, or kissing. Dominant hemispheric lesions account for most of these apraxias. Dressing apraxia, another common symptomatic apraxia, is a combination of apraxia and a topographical disorientation usually seen in nondominant parietal lesions. An extension of spatial dysfunctions is the inability to copy three-dimensional figures, such as a cube.

Testing

There are multiple tests for nondominant hemispheric dysfunction (Figure 2-6). These include asking the patient to mark the numbers of a clock on a large circle covering an entire sheet of paper, followed by drawing the hands of a clock to indicate 10:10, or asking the patient to draw transecting lines that fill an entire sheet. Alternatives include showing patients the classic "boy and the cookie jar" drawing and asking them to describe what they see. Gerstmann syndrome, found in dominant posteroinferior parietal lobe dysfunction, results in right and left confusion, finger agnosia, and acalculia. These problems are easily tested by asking the patient to raise his or her right or left hand or identify the examiner's crossed right or left hand. Similarly, asking the patient to show his thumb or index finger and perform several levels of calculation help to diagnose left parietal lesions.

Some patients with dominant hemispheric lesions may have alexia or other language difficulties. Although it is uncommon and difficult to recognize as a language problem, alexia is confirmed when patients are able to write but cannot read their writing (alexia without agraphia). Reading numbers is usually more preserved than reading letters or words. Some patients also have difficulties identifying colors. Occasionally, the adjacent occipital lobe is involved; most patients have a contralateral visual field deficit. Alexia is related to inability to relay visual information to the angular gyrus. Therefore, a lesion in the splenium of the corpus callosum or underlying white matter may interrupt this topographic information to the language areas in the dominant hemisphere.

OCCIPITAL LOBE DYSFUNCTION

At the most elementary level, occipital lobe lesions cause visual field defects (Figure 2-7). Rudimentary visual information is processed in the striate cortex, or Brodmann visual area 17. Complex visual information is processed more anteriorly, relying on inputs from multiple cortical areas. The complex nature of visual processing and integration of visual information in memory and orientation suggest that a vision disturbance may lead to several neuropsychological abnormalities. The primary visual areas project to midtemporal areas, temporal polar regions, and the parahippocampal gyrus. These regions receive extensive input from other sensory sources and limbic structures that influence tagging emotional and motivational significance to the stimulus. Aside from the visual field defects discussed in chapter 1, patients may experience image distortion or shifting, or persistence of an image when the eyes have already moved from

COGNITIVE AND LANGUAGE EVALUATION

Figure 2-6 Nondominant Hemisphere Higher Cortical Dysfunction

A. Constructional dyspraxia and spatial disorientation

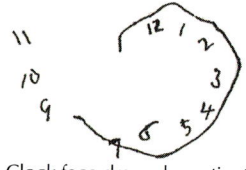
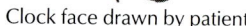
Clock face drawn by patient

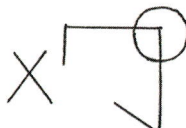
Patient asked to copy → Draws this

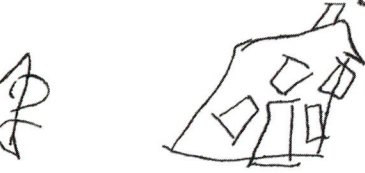
House drawn by patient

B. Neglect of left-sided stimuli

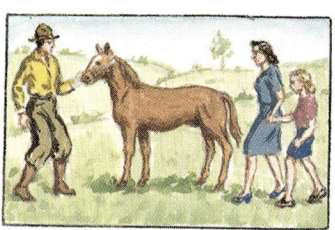

Patient shown picture → Sees this

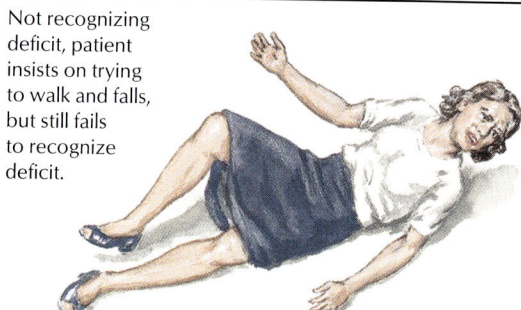

Patient shown printed page → Sees this

C. Anosognosia
(unawareness of deficit)

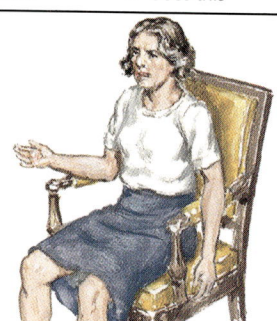

Patient with obvious left hemiplegia. Asked, "What is wrong with you?" Answers, "Nothing is wrong, I am perfectly all right."

Not recognizing deficit, patient insists on trying to walk and falls, but still fails to recognize deficit.

D. Motor impersistence

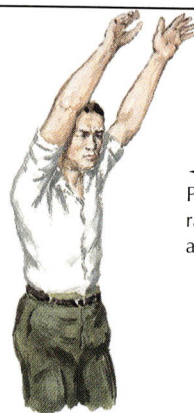
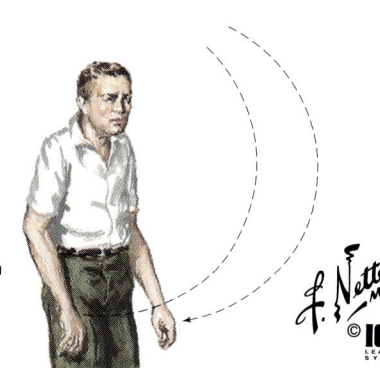

Patient asked to raise arms over head and to keep them up

Raises arms but then drops them quickly

E. Abnormal recognition of nonlanguage cues
(facial expression, voice tone, mood)

Patient shown picture. Asked, "Which is the happy face?"

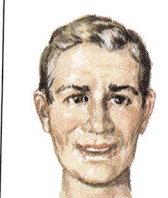 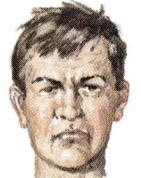 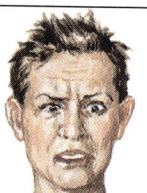 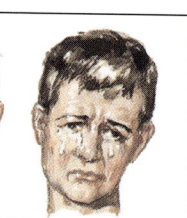

Patient answers, "I don't know, they are all the same."

NEUROLOGIC EXAMINATION

COGNITIVE AND LANGUAGE EVALUATION

Figure 2-7 Occipital Lobe Functional Anatomy

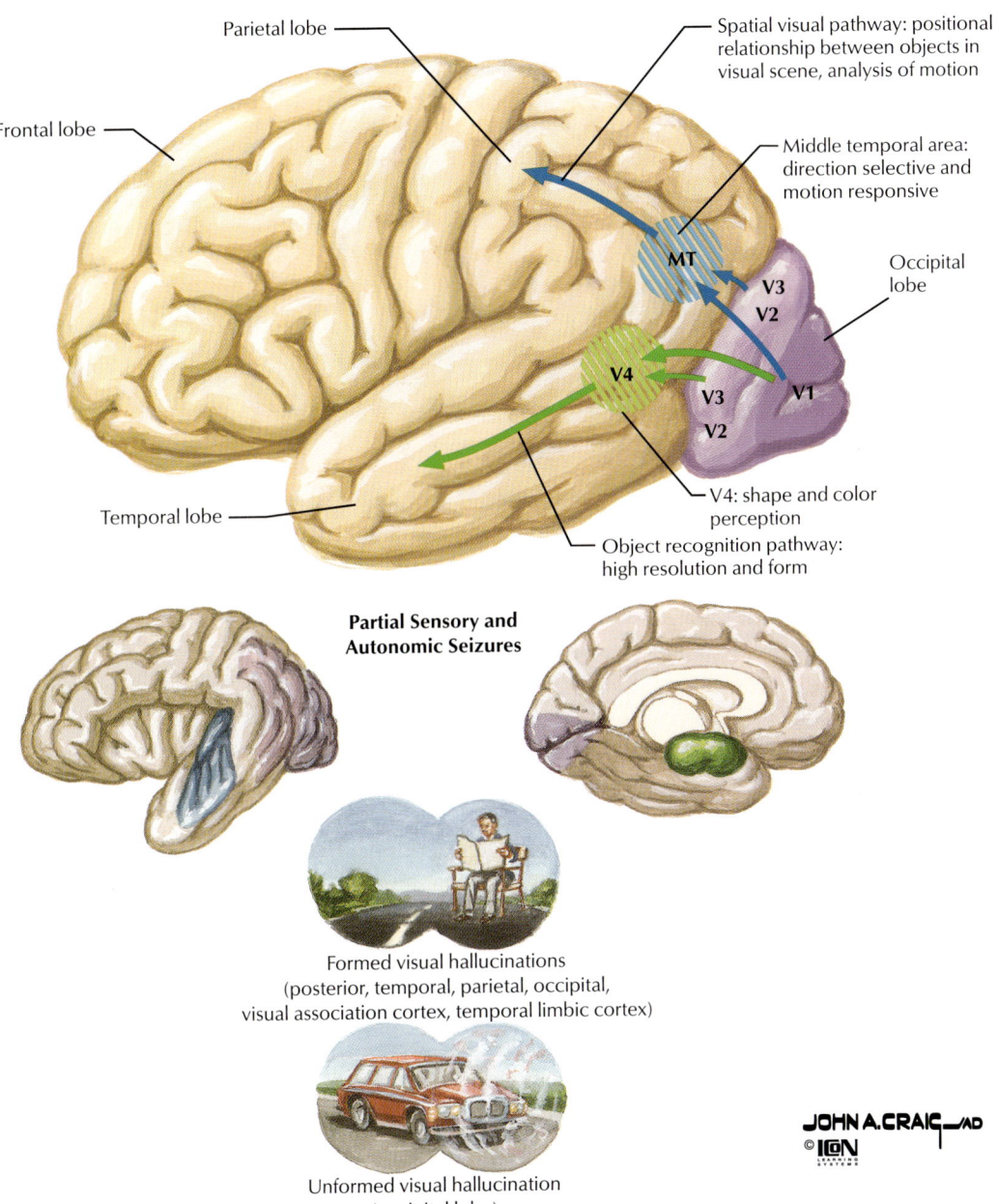

the object. Usually, these phenomena are observed in occipital and temporal lesions. More dramatic "realistic" images are described in patients with temporal lobe lesions and in some individuals without a specific cerebral structural abnormality. Bonnet syndrome applies to the latter group, usually elderly patients who often have severely compromised vision.

Visual agnosias are not related to visual perception but to the incorporation of visual data with other relevant information. Patients with the most basic form of visual agnosia cannot recognize objects shown to them but can easily recognize them by touch. Other rare agnosias include prosopagnosia, in which patients cannot recognize faces or understand the meaning of facial expression. In Balint syndrome, there is a profound inability to scan visual space or grasp an object in space. In these visual agnosia syndromes, visual information seems to be disconnected from brain areas that associate significance with that information. It is unclear whether this occurs in the somatosensory, language, or other higher-order visual areas. Most of the lesions that cause visual agnosias, such as diffuse anoxia after cardiac arrest or occipital lobe infarcts, are bilateral.

REFERENCES

Damasio AR, Damasio H, Van Hoesen GW. Prosopagnosia: anatomic basis and behavioral mechanisms. *Neurology.* 1982;32:331-341.

Damasio AR, Geschwind N. Anatomical localization in clinical neuropsychology. In: Vinken PJ, Bruyn GW, Klawans HL, eds. *Handbook of Clinical Neurology.* Vol 45. Amsterdam, The Netherlands: Elsevier; 1985:7-22.

Denny-Brown D. The frontal lobes and their functions. In: Feiling A, ed. *Modern Trends in Neurology.* New York, NY: Hoeberharper; 1951:13-89.

Landis T, Cummings JL, Benson F, Palmer EPL. Loss of topographic familiarity. An environmental agnosia. *Arch Neurol.* 1986;43:132-136.

Mesulam MM. *Principles of Behavioral Neurology.* Philadelphia, Pa: FA Davis; 1985.

Papez JW. A proposed mechanism of emotion. *Arch Neurol Psychiatry.* 1937;38:725-743.

Section II
NEURO-OPHTHALMOLOGY

Chapter 3
Retina and Optic Nerve 54

Chapter 4
**Optic Chiasm, Optic Tract, Lateral Geniculate
Nucleus, and Optic Radiations** .64

Chapter 5
Primary Visual Cortex 72

Chapter 6
Cranial Nerve III: Oculomotor .77

Chapter 7
Cranial Nerve IV: Trochlear 85

Chapter 8
Cranial Nerve VI: Abducens 89

Chapter 3
Retina and Optic Nerve

Ippolit C. A. Matjucha and Robert J. Updaw II

RETINA
Anatomy and Physiology

The retina, the neural tunic of the eye, contains 9 types of cells arranged in 10 distinct layers (Figure 3-1). Its function is 3-fold: to detect visible light, transduce the photic energy of light into neural signals, and perform an initial analysis of visual information before sending it to the brain for further processing. Many types of cells participate in accomplishing these tasks.

Vascular Supply

The outer retina receives blood via the choriocapillaris. The remaining retina, however has an additional vascular source; the central retinal artery sends branches into the eye through the optic disk (Figure 3-2). Although significant variations are encountered, in general, 4 branches of the central retinal artery emanate from the disk: superior nasal, superior temporal, inferior nasal, and inferior temporal.

Retinal Disease

The topographic layering of the retina allows a disease process (eg, inflammation) to destroy one group of photoreceptors and leave an immediately adjacent group unaffected. Visual field defects based on retinal disorders have sharp, steep borders that may be irregular or ragged edged.

The shape of visual field deficits due to **vascular compromise** is largely predictable, being relatively consistent with the location of the retinal occlusion. Because branch retinal arteriolar occlusions affect the nerve fiber layer, defects extend beyond the local occlusion in an outwardly expanding arcuate or sectoral pattern because all nerve fibers arcing through the ischemic area are affected. For example, with branch occlusions of the retinal artery supplying the superior retina, the inferior field of vision within that eye is lost.

Retinitis Pigmentosa

Frequently, a genetic disorder, retinitis pigmentosa, is characterized by rod and cone dystrophies and is often from a gene mutation for rhodopsin or peripherin, a glycoprotein on the photoreceptor outer segments. Retinitis pigmentosa is characterized by progressive night blindness (nyctalopia). Pigmentosa is named for the characteristic black clumps of pigment found within the peripheral retina known as *bone spicules*. As retinitis pigmentosa advances, only a central island of vision may remain, which may eventually be extinguished.

The pathognomonic retinal pattern of visual field loss in retinitis pigmentosa is characterized by the classic ring scotoma, with a midperipheral loss sparing the center and far periphery. Ring scotomata are encountered in other retinal diseases, particularly the toxic retinopathies of chloroquine, hydroxychloroquine, or phenothiazines.

Macular Degeneration

Few retinal diseases have more epidemiologic impact than age-related macular degeneration, an ischemic disorder. Macular degeneration produces painless loss of central vision in the elderly. Two types exist: a nonexudative or "dry" type, and an exudative or "wet" variety when choroidal neovascularization intrudes into the macular retina.

Characteristic of the nonexudative variant are retinal drusen (from the German term for geode crystals). Ophthalmoscopically, drusen are small, discrete, extracellular deposits recognized as yellow lesions clustered around the macula. These lesions gradually become larger, more numerous, and confluent, with adjacent retinal atrophy. Visual acuity and disturbed color vision loss ensues from the inability to support the metabolic activity of the photoreceptors.

RETINA AND OPTIC NERVE

Figure 3-1 — The Retina and the Photoreceptors

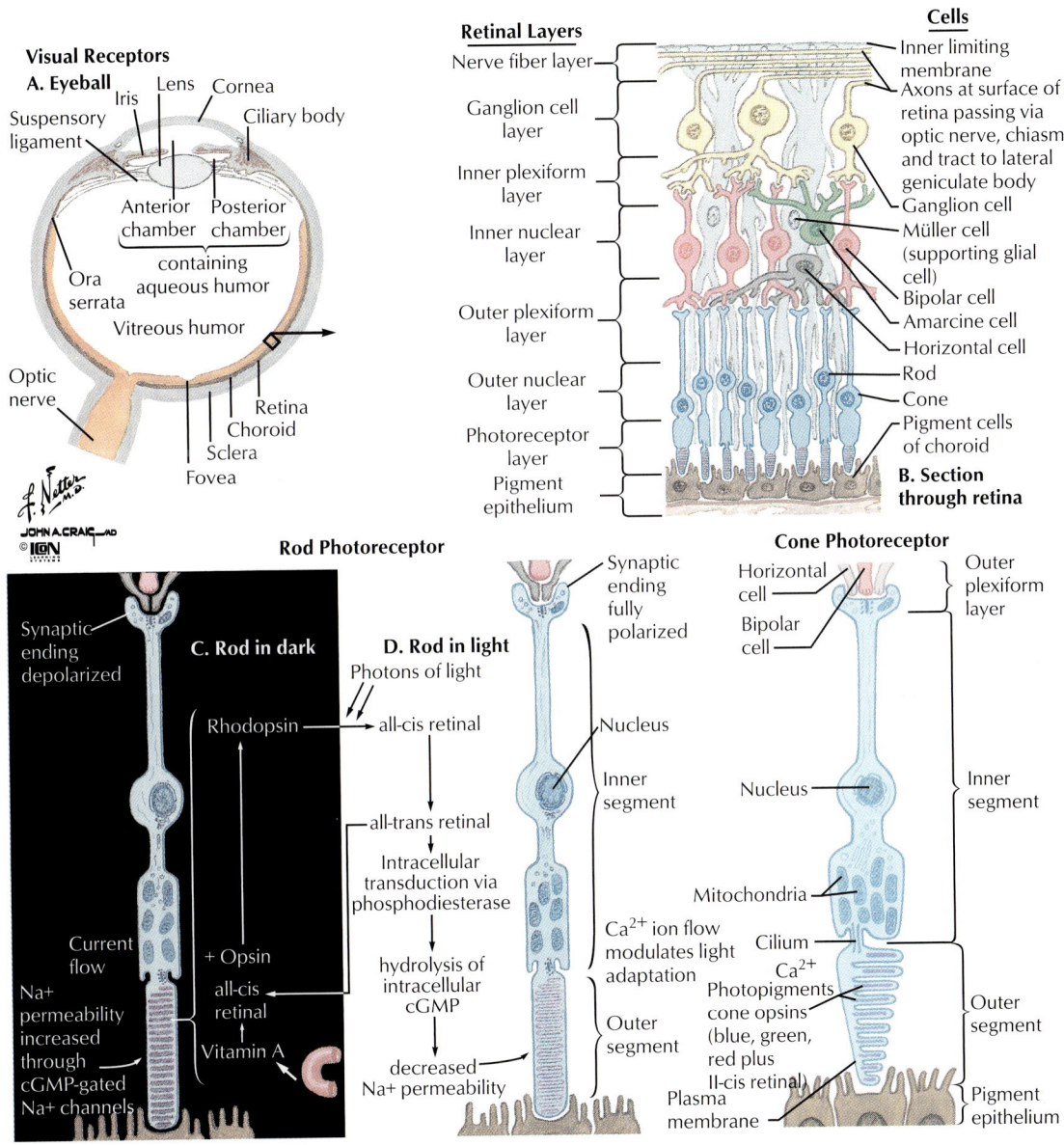

RETINA AND OPTIC NERVE

Figure 3-2   Retinal Architecture and Perimetry

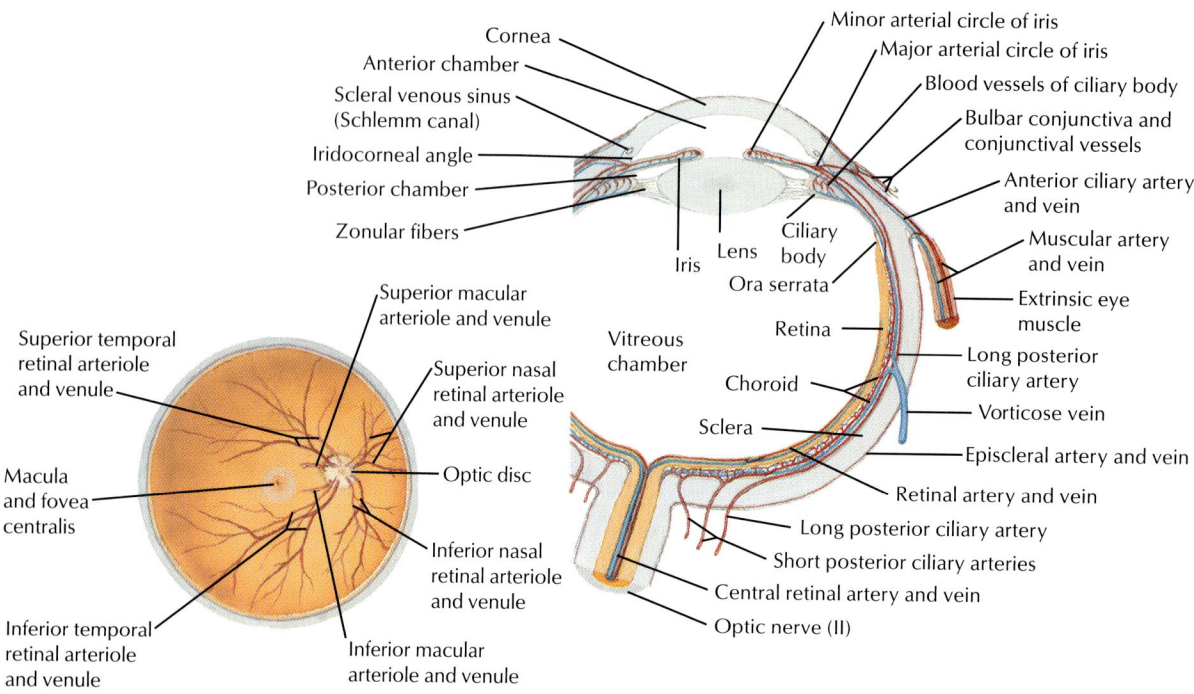

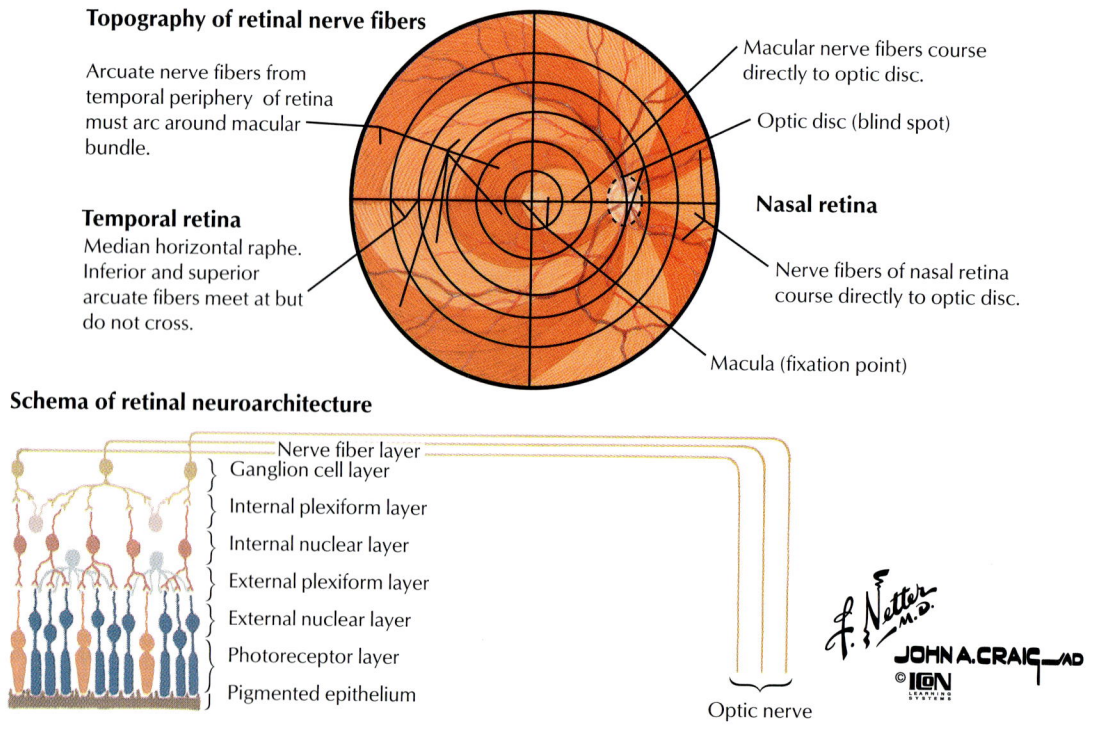

OPTIC NERVE

Anatomy of the Optic Disk and Nerve

The optic nerve nominally begins when the axons of the ganglion cells turn 90°, changing orientation from horizontal along the inner retinal surface to vertical through the retina and out of the eye via the scleral canal (Figure 3-3). The ganglion cells receive input from bipolar and amacrine cells. The gathering of axons at the canal forms the optic disk of the fundus, also called the *optic nerve head*.

Numerous axons carrying information from the foveal retina form a thick area in the nerve fiber layer as they gather at the temporal quadrant of the disk. This area, the papillomacular bundle, is located between the disk and the fovea. The papillomacular fibers enter the temporal optic disk; diseases that produce **temporal pallor** of the disk, particularly multiple sclerosis (MS), therefore produce a central scotoma on visual field testing (chapter 1).

The inferior and superior arcuate bundles, 2 additional groupings of retinal nerve fibers, relay information from the non–foveal macula and enter the disk at its inferior and superior poles. The remaining nerve fibers constitute the nasal nerve fiber bundle, entering the disk in a radial fashion. The more superior and inferior fibers of the nasal bundle contain axons from the temporal retinal periphery; the more central fibers contain axons from the nasal periphery.

The optic nerve begins at the optic disk and courses to the optic chiasm. It has several portions: intraocular, intraorbital, and intracranial. The first part of the intracranial segment runs through the bony optic canal. When the optic nerve leaves the interior of the eye, the axons pass through a reticulated opening in the sclera called the *lamina cribrosa* and then undergo a major anatomical change.

Its previously nonmyelinated fibers now become myelinated with CNS myelin, explaining why the optic nerve is affected by MS. The optic nerve is therefore misnamed; it is not a peripheral nerve but a white matter tract of the brain. It is also bathed in CSF and invested with arachnoid tissue, pia mater, and dura mater that fuses with orbital connective tissue, forming the optic nerve sheath. After leaving the optic canal, the optic nerves course below the frontal lobes before meeting at the optic chiasm, just above the pituitary gland.

Disorders

The many diseases affecting the optic nerve produce characteristic patterns of visual field loss, depending on where the optic nerve is affected. Generally, defects occur with disease of the disk or the anterior optic nerve, the orbital optic nerve, and the prechiasmal or "junctional" optic nerve. Glaucoma, optic neuritis, anterior ischemic optic neuropathy, optic nerve drusen, papilledema, and congenital dysplasia occur within the anterior optic nerve. Diseases of the orbital optic nerve include posterior ischemic optic neuropathy, optic neuritis, compressive optic neuropathy, toxic optic neuropathy, and genetic or metabolic optic neuropathies. Junctional optic nerve disease is usually due to compression.

Anterior Optic Nerve Pathoanatomical Correlations

Visual field defects from anterior optic nerve disease (eg, glaucoma) typically consist of paracentral, Bjerrum, Seidel, arcuate, nasal step, and altitudinal scotomata. The scotomata represent levels of depletion of the inferior or superior arcuate bundles. If the damage is minimal or small, an elongated blind spot (Seidel scotoma) or partial arcuate loss (Bjerrum scotoma) may result. With more significant disease, a complete arcuate scotoma or more extensive altitudinal loss involving the entire superior or inferior field nasal to the blind spot can be seen. Because of the horizontal raphe, such cases often show a sudden "step" change, called a *nasal step*, in the visual field on crossing the nasal horizontal meridian; it is a dependable sign of anterior optic nerve disease.

The **papillomacular bundle** consists of macular fibers entering the temporal aspect of the optic disk. As these neurons travel into the orbit, they comprise a central position in the orbital optic nerve. Because no central optic nerve artery exists, blood reaches these axons from vessels on the exterior of the nerve. A partial watershed of blood flow is produced, in which the most metabolically active axons on the optic nerve (the papillomacular bundle) are the farthest from

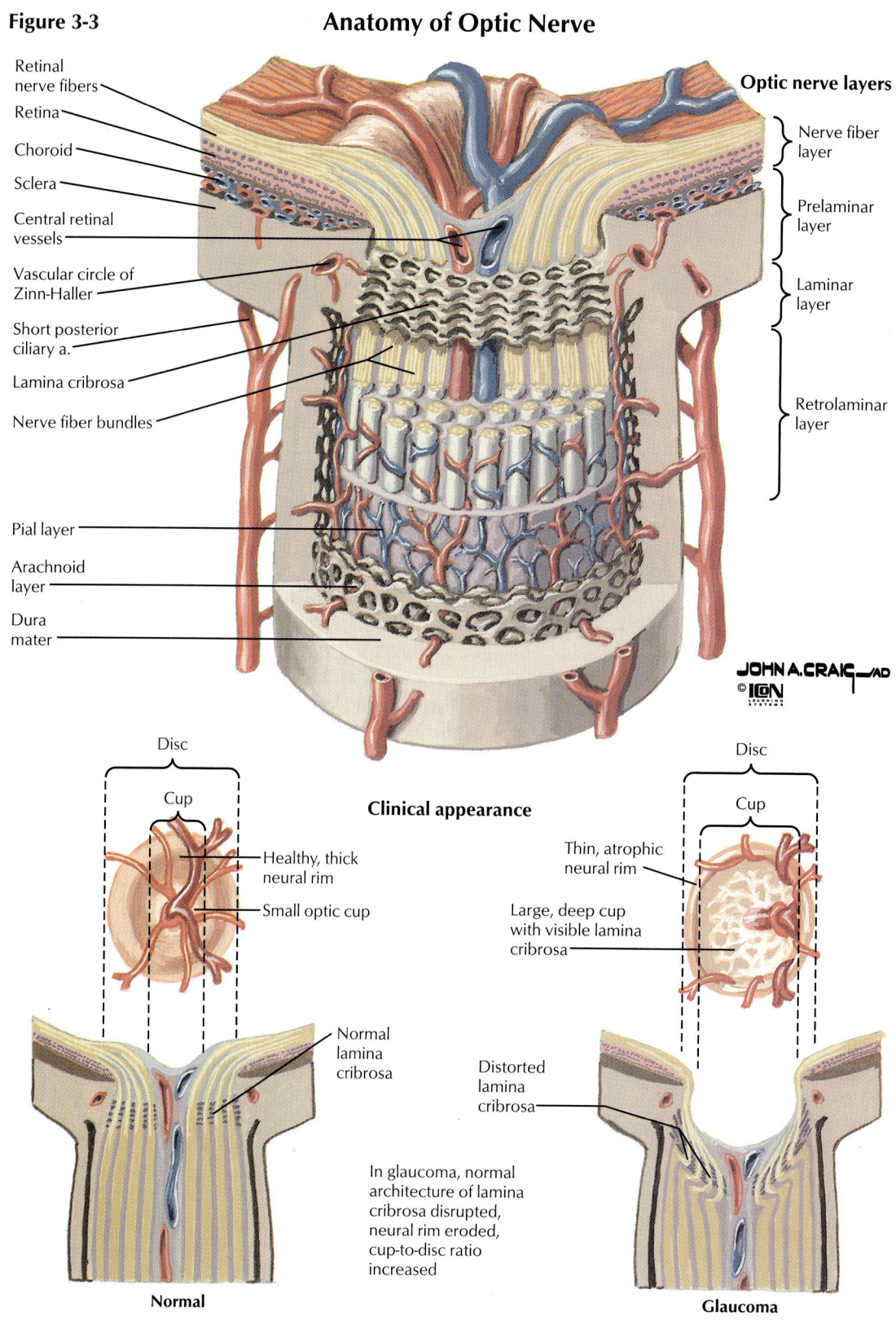
Figure 3-3. Anatomy of Optic Nerve

the blood supply. These neurons are therefore regarded as particularly fragile and prone to injury.

Hence, central and centrocecal (extending to the blind spot) scotomata are seen in metabolic, toxic, and compressive optic nerve diseases. Although the entire optic nerve is exposed to the effects of compression, toxic exposure, or metabolic disease, often only these core fibers are injured, producing the characteristic central scotoma.

Glaucoma

Glaucoma is a family of slowly progressive optic neuropathies usually related to high intraocular pressures and progressive cavitating ("cupping") atrophy of the optic disk. Visual loss starts in the midperiphery as circular or arcuate scotomata, which, over years in severe cases, first abolish most of the peripheral vision, and then abolish the central vision. No restorative therapy exists.

Treatment concentrates on slowing or stopping progression by decreasing intraocular pressure through medications, laser surgery, or ocular surgery. Most cases are asymptomatic until visual loss is severe; therefore, detection of patients at risk by routine screening of intraocular pressure and optic nerve contour is vital, especially for patients with a family history of glaucoma or another significant risk factor (eg, history of severe ocular trauma) (Figure 3-4).

Optic Neuritis

Often the presenting sign and one of the most common MS features, optic neuritis typically produces a brief prodrome of periocular pain, mounting over days and worsened by eye movements. Ensuing visual loss is often sudden and severe, with perceived worsening over days; however, the degree of visual loss varies. Examination demonstrates central vision, visual field, and color vision loss in the affected eye and a relative afferent pupillary defect; however, initially the optic nerve usually looks normal, until partial pallor begins some weeks later. Recovery of vision, typically to near normal, occurs mainly over a 2- or 3-month period.

Although MS produces visual loss by affecting the white matter within the visual pathways, the syndrome of **monocular visual loss with pain** usually means the lesion is within the orbital portion of the optic nerve. Therefore, central scotomata are the classic finding, although peripheral loss and scotomata more typical of anterior or junctional optic nerve lesions are routinely seen. Similarly, ensuing pallor of the optic disk is typically **temporal pallor**, involving fibers of the papillomacular bundle that occupies the central orbital nerve.

Intravenous methylprednisolone (1 g/d for 3 days, followed by oral prednisone) is recommended for accelerating visual recovery and providing some protective effect against new MS events, perhaps up to 2 years. However, it does not improve the eventual degree of recovery of the optic neuritis; possible inherent risks with this medication must be considered. Alternative treatment with oral prednisone alone is contraindicated because it may predispose to occurrence of MS relapse earlier than if the condition is left untreated.

Anterior Ischemic Optic Neuropathy

Anterior ischemic optic neuropathy is a stroke affecting the optic nerve at the disk. Patients usually experience sudden, severe, painless, monocular visual loss, often on awakening (Figure 3-5). Examination classically reveals an altitudinal (superior or inferior) visual field loss, with a unilaterally swollen, hemorrhagic disk.

Usually, the combination of constricted optic nerve anatomy (a small crowded disk) and nocturnal systemic hypotension are the responsible mechanisms. There is no recognized therapy for the involved eye. To prevent contralateral involvement, daily antiplatelet therapy (eg, 81 mg aspirin) is recommended.

Giant Cell Arteritis

One of the major neurologic emergencies, giant cell arteritis, places patients at risk for rapid—sometimes within a few days or hours—total visual loss in one or both eyes. Few cases of anterior ischemic optic neuropathy result from this serious disorder, which primarily affects individuals older than 65 years and rarely occurs in younger persons (Figure 3-5B). Some individuals have a premonitory warning of incipient visual loss with transient blurred vision that leads them

RETINA AND OPTIC NERVE

Figure 3-4 ## Optic Disc and Visual Field Changes in Glaucoma

Early

Right eye nasal side

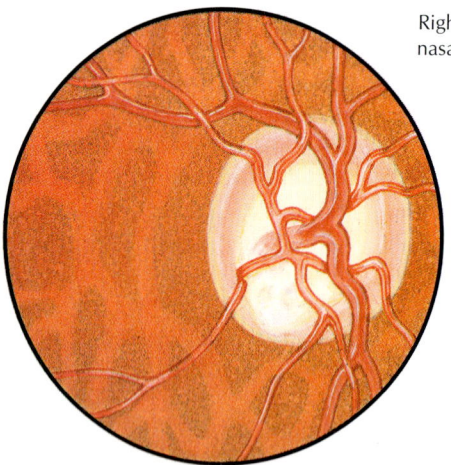
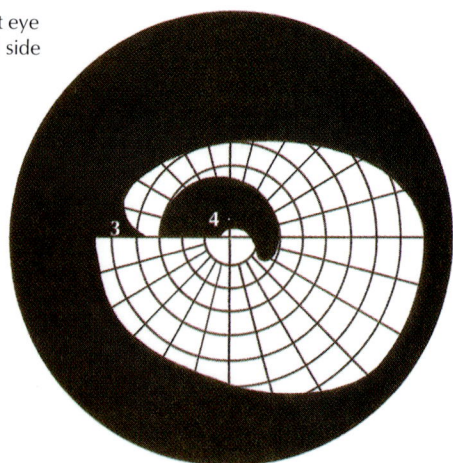

Funduscopy: notching of contour of physiologic cup in optic disc with slight focal pallor in area of notching; occurs almost invariably in superotemporal or inferotemporal (as shown) quadrants

Perimetry: slight enlargment of physiologic blind spot (1); development of a secondary, superonasal field defect (2) which corresponds to nerve fiber damage in area of inferotemporal notching

Minimally advanced

Right eye nasal side

Funduscopy: increased notching of rim of cup; thinning of rim of cup (enlargement of cup); deepening of cup; lamina cribrosa visible in deepest areas

Perimetry: localized constriction of superonasal visual field (3) because of progessive damage to inferotemporal fibers; superior arc-shaped scotoma (Bjerrum scotoma) develops (4)

JOHN A. CRAIG—AD
©ICON

RETINA AND OPTIC NERVE

Figure 3-5A
Multiple Sclerosis: Ocular Manifestations

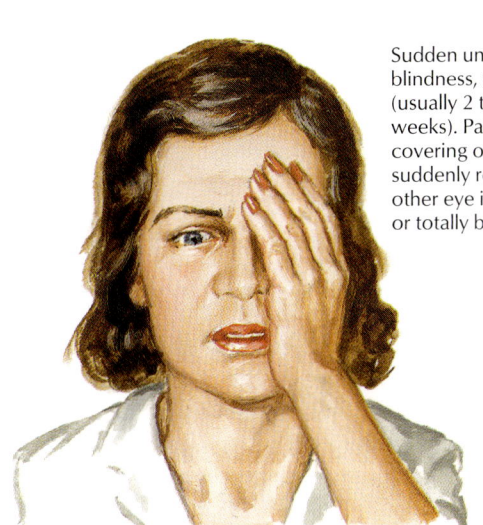

Sudden unilateral blindness, self-limited (usually 2 to 3 weeks). Patient covering one eye, suddenly realizes other eye is partially or totally blind.

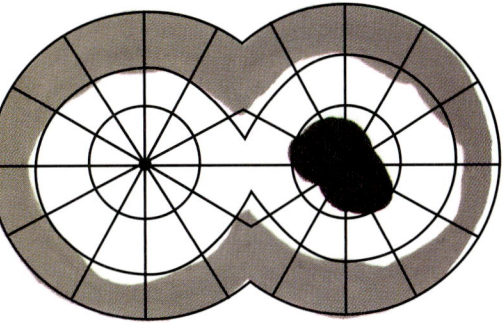

Visual fields reveal central scotoma due to acute retrobulbar neuritis.

Figure 3-5B
Giant Cell Arteritis: Ocular Manifestations

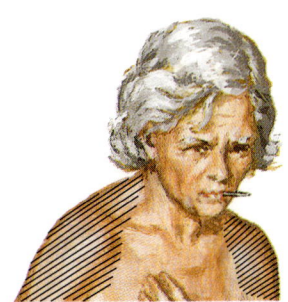

Senior citizen with sudden monocular visual blurring or blindness, associated with malaise, scalp tenderness, and myalgia. The erythrocyte sedimentation is very elevated, usually 60 to 120 min/h.

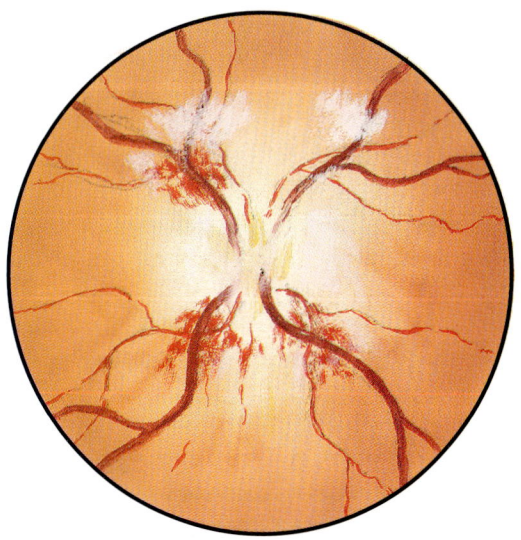

Anterior ischemic optic neuropathy

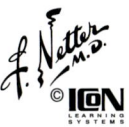

Neuro-ophthalmology

to seek care. Typically, patients may have noted general malaise, weight loss, and headaches with scalp tenderness, and they often have a preceding diagnosis of polymyalgia rheumatica. Sometimes, patients also report jaw claudication characterized by masticatory muscle pain with chewing. Rarely, these patients present with or later have a stroke, usually within the extracerebral portions of the vertebral artery. The primary examination finding is a prominent, thickened, and tender superficial temporal artery.

Every such patient requires immediate evaluation. ESR is an excellent screening test because most patients have significant increases, 60 to 110 mm/h, normal less than 20 mm/h. Ideally, an immediate temporal artery biopsy is indicated. However, because it is not often possible on an emergency basis, high-dose (80 mg/d) prednisone must be initiated pending the results of the biopsy. If the pathologic findings demonstrate giant cell granulomas and interruption of the elastic membrane, treatment must be maintained for at least 3 to 6 months. Usually, gradual dose reduction on an alternate-day basis lessens the well-known adverse effects of corticosteroids; disease activity is monitored by the ESR.

Papilledema

Papilledema (Figure 1-5A), optic nerve elevation and swelling, is usually due to high intracranial pressure. Often, patients have no symptoms of visual compromise, although with chronic intracranial pressure increases, some report visual obscurations with transient blurring, particularly with postural changes. Many primary pathophysiologic mechanisms are associated with papilledema, including CNS tumor (with edema or obstructive hydrocephalus), meningitis, certain medications (eg, tetracycline or vitamin A), or intracranial venous obstruction.

Papilledema is occasionally seen, without explanation, in obese women of childbearing age and is called **idiopathic intracranial hypertension** or **pseudotumor cerebri** (chapter 71). Treatment is directed against known causes. In the idiopathic group, treatment is initially deferred if the condition is mild with no progressive visual loss or debilitating headache.

When visual loss occurs, it starts with **blind spot enlargement** (Figure 1-5B), a nonspecific and often reversible change. In chronic or severe cases, visual field loss resembling that of glaucoma can ensue, sometimes rapidly. Treatment consists of acetazolamide (typically 1 g/d in divided doses) to reduce production of CSF; occasionally, other diuretics are used. When medical treatment fails, two surgical options exist: optic nerve sheath fenestration or lumboperitoneal CSF shunt.

TREATMENT

New classes of medication have been developed for the treatment of glaucoma, and new treatments attempting to slow macular degeneration range from novel lasers to simple dietary supplements. However, the goals of restorative or regenerative treatment for extensive retinal or optic nerve disease remain elusive.

FUTURE DIRECTIONS

Diagnostic advances in retinal and optic nerve disease have focused on new imaging and electrophysiologic modalities for these structures and on identification of genetic markers and other specific risk factors. Computer-driven laser scanning devices permit the determination of nerve-fiber layer thickness in the retina, allow tomographic optical "sectioning" of the retina, and may even analyze the neural content of the retina using the optical birefringence of the arrayed nerve fibers. These advanced techniques allow better detection and localization of structural abnormalities.

Gross whole-field (Ganzfeld) electroretinography is complemented by focal and multifocal techniques that test smaller areas of retina, so that focal but critical losses (ie, in the fovea) are not "masked out" by predominantly normal signals from most of the retina. Earlier and more certain diagnosis of more limited forms of retinal disease is therefore possible.

The slow task of finding dependable genetic markers for optic nerve and retinal diseases has experienced some small, remarkable successes (eg, Leber hereditary optic atrophy), suggesting hope in more common diseases. The study of patients with common eye diseases to seek out new risk factors (eg, thin corneas predisposing to glaucoma) continues to help determine which patients need the most aggressive treatment.

REFERENCES

Bron AJ, Tripathi RC, Tripathi BJ. *Wolff's Anatomy of the Eye and Orbit*. 8th ed. Boston, Mass: Chapman & Hall (Kluwer Academic); 1997.

Harrington DO, Drake MV. *The Visual Fields: Text and Atlas of Clinical Perimetry*. 6th ed. St. Louis, Mo: CV Mosby; 1991.

Hedges TR, Friedman D, Horton J, Newman SA, Striph G, Kay MC. Neuro-ophthalmology. In: Weingeist TA, Liesegang TJ, Slamovits TL, eds. *Basic and Clinical Science Course, 1997-1998*. San Francisco, Calif: American Academy of Ophthalmology; 1997:51-55.

Tripathi RC, Chalam KV, Chew EY, et al. Fundamentals and principles of ophthalmology. In: Weingeist TA, Liesegang TJ, Slamovits TL, eds. *Basic and Clinical Science Course, 1997-1998*. San Francisco, Calif: American Academy of Ophthalmology; 1997:76-92.

Chapter 4
Optic Chiasm, Optic Tract, Lateral Geniculate Nucleus, and Optic Radiations

Ippolit C. A. Matjucha and Robert J. Updaw II

OPTIC CHIASM

Clinical Vignette

A 51-year-old woman presented with worsening vision over many months. She reported no other significant medical history.

On checking visual acuity, the examiner discovered that the patient could see only the left half of the eye chart with her right eye and only the right half with her left eye. A gross confrontation visual field check confirmed a dense bitemporal hemianopia. The examiner also noted that the woman had facial hypertrichosis and enlargement of her brow, nose, lips, and jaw and that the patient's rings and shoes no longer fit properly. Acromegaly, as occurs from abnormally high circulating levels of human growth hormone produced by a pituitary tumor, was diagnosed. MRI confirmed the lesion compressing the optic chiasm.

Bitemporal hemianopsia is characteristic of an optic chiasm lesion, usually caused by pituitary tumors, although occasionally a craniopharyngioma is the primary lesion. The optic chiasm (from the Greek letter x) represents the "Great Divide" of the afferent visual system. Visual field defects are typically categorized into 3 anatomical areas. **Prechiasmatic** defects affect the visual field of the ipsilateral eye only and typically result from retinal or optic nerve pathology. **Chiasmatic** disorders classically lead to bitemporal hemianopia (also, *hemianopsia*), with loss of the right lateral field in the right eye and left lateral field in the left eye. **Postchiasmatic** defects produce homonymous hemianopias, with defects appearing more congruous (equal for both eyes) the farther posteriorly the lesion is located.

Anatomy

The optic chiasm is an X-shaped intersection of the optic nerve axons located above the pituitary body within the sella turcica of the sphenoid bone, which is covered by the diaphragm sellae (Figure 4-1). The chiasmatic cistern is located between the chiasm and the diaphragm sella. Superior to the chiasm is the third ventricle. The internal carotid arteries flank the optic chiasm laterally and then bifurcate into the anterior and middle cerebral arteries. The anterior cerebral arteries and the anterior communicating artery are anterior to the optic chiasm. Within the chiasm, axons from the temporal retina (nasal field) comprise its lateral aspect, remaining ipsilateral, whereas the nasal retinal fibers decussate, carrying the temporal field information to the contralateral side. Inferior nasal fibers decussate within the chiasm more anteriorly than superior ones. As the inferior nasal retinal fibers approach the posterior aspect o the chiasm, the fibers shift to occupy the lateral aspect of the contralateral optic tract.

Vascular Supply

The arterial blood supply of the optic chiasm is derived from the circle of Willis, particularly the carotid artery trunks and its branches, the superior hypophyseal arteries, derived from the supraclinoid trunk of the carotids. A "prechiasmal plexus," the hypophyseal portal system, and branches of the anterior cerebral arteries also contribute to the chiasmal blood supply.

OPTIC PATHWAYS

Figure 4-1

Anatomy and Relations of Optic Chiasm

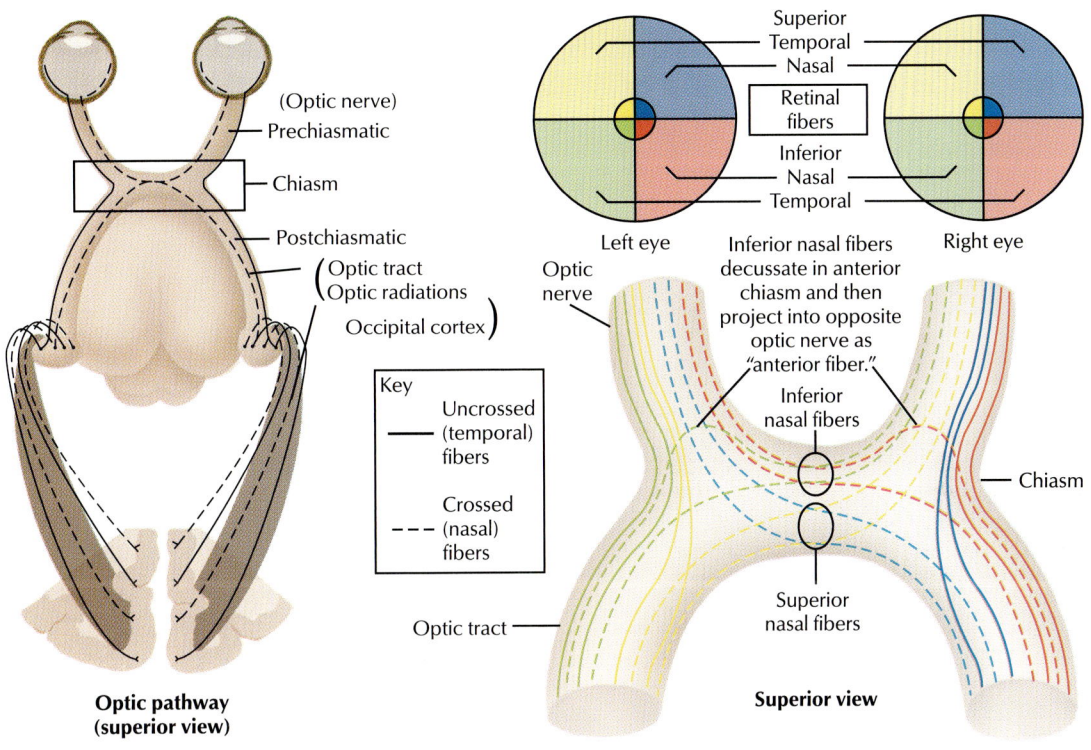

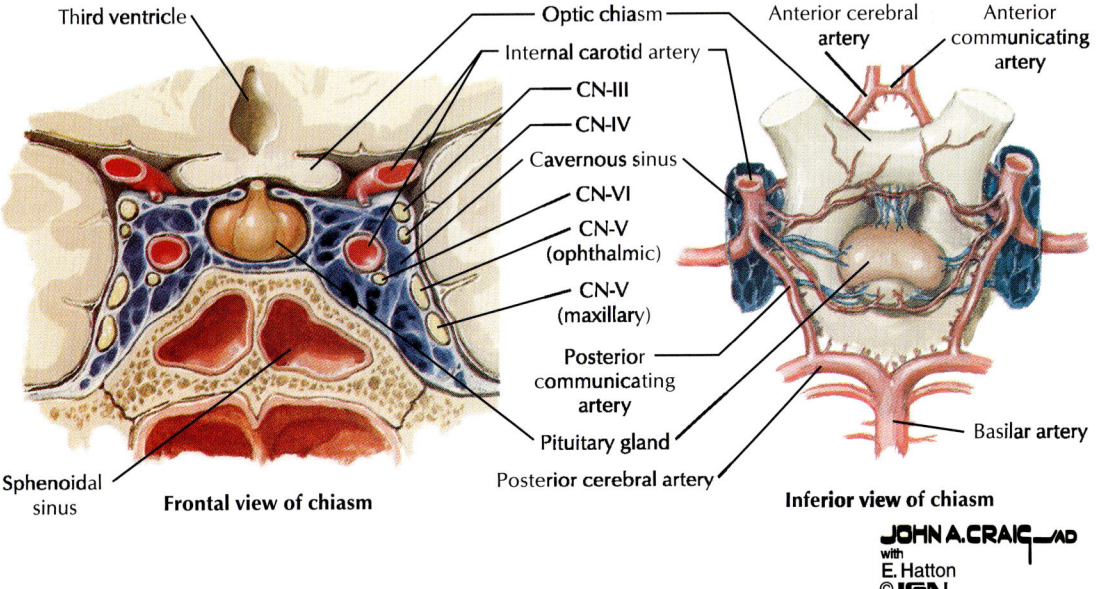

Neuro-ophthalmology

OPTIC PATHWAYS

Figure 4-2   Disorders Affecting Optic Chiasm

A. Lesions of anterior chiasm

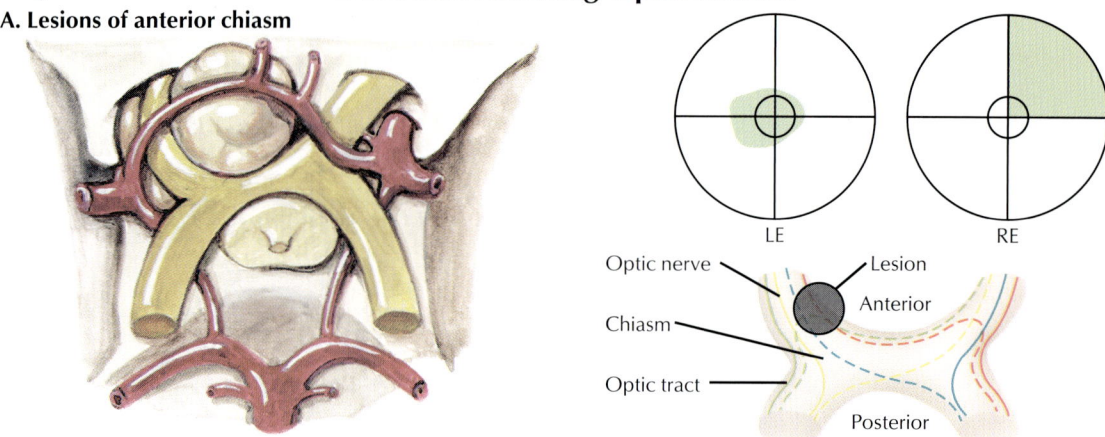

Anterior chiasm tumor compressing optic nerve at its entrance to chiasm results in junctional scotoma consisting of a central visual field loss in eye ipsilateral to lesion and a superior temporal defect in the opposite eye.

B. Lesions of central chiasm

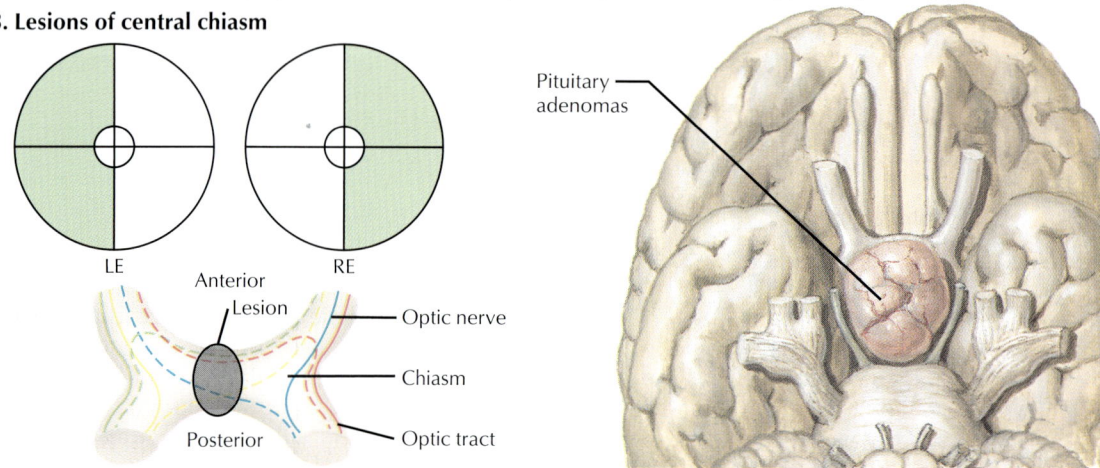

Pituitary adenomas are most common lesion to affect chiasm. Central lesions which compress mid chiasm affect crossing nasal retinal fibers, resulting in the typical bitemporal hemianopsia on visual field examination.

C. Lesions of posterior chiasm

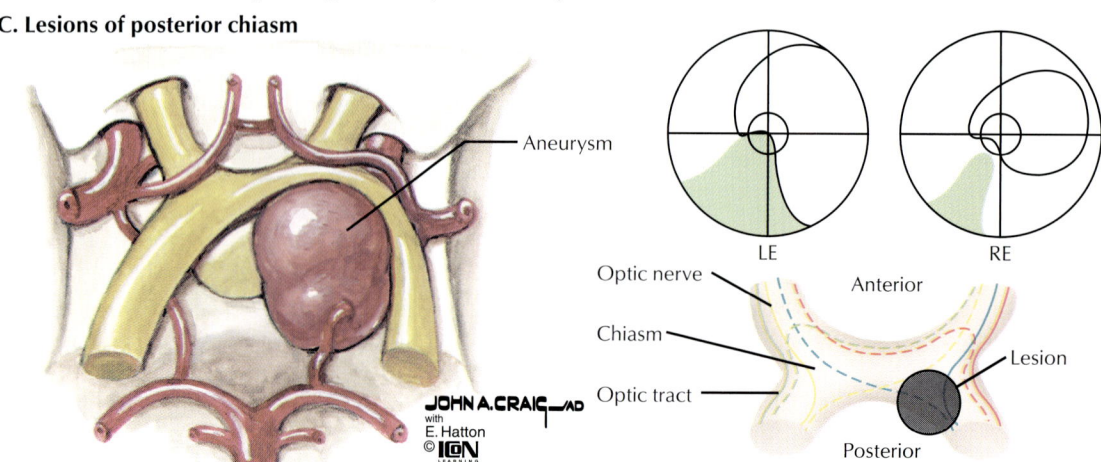

Posterior communicating artery aneurysm affecting posterior chiasm combines features of both a chiasmatic and an optic tract lesion, resulting in a posterior junctional scotoma—an incongruous (less dense in ipsilateral eye) hemianopic field loss contralateral to lesion.

Neuro-ophthalmology

Venous drainage comprises 2 primary areas: the superior aspect into the anterior cerebral veins and the inferior aspect draining into the infundibular plexus and thus to the paired basal veins of Rosenthal.

Disorders

Pituitary adenomas are generally benign neoplasms and the most common of the numerous diseases affecting the optic chiasm (Figure 4-2). Aneurysm, often of the anterior or posterior communicating artery, and trauma, especially from severe deceleration injury to the frontal skull, are other important etiologies.

Lesions of the anterior chiasm compress the optic nerve at its entrance to the chiasm, resulting in a **junctional scotoma**, a central visual field loss in the eye ipsilateral to the lesion and a superotemporal defect in the other, a combination of the visual field characteristics of an optic nerve lesion with chiasmal disease. The field loss in the contralateral eye is from involvement of the anterior chiasm; early crossing fibers from the inferonasal retina of the contralateral eye are affected. Because the inferior nasal fibers decussate in the anterior aspect of the chiasm, the scotoma of the contralateral eye is typically superotemporal. Central chiasmal lesions most commonly produce a bitemporal hemianopsia that ensues when the optic chiasm is compressed or damaged midsaggitally at its decussation. Such lesions preferentially affect the crossing nasal retinal fibers responsible for temporal vision, as in the vignette in this chapter.

Progressive visual field loss from an expanding sellar tumor characteristically begins in the upper temporal field, likely from preferential compression of the inferior chiasm by the underlying pituitary tumor exerting pressure on the chiasm through the diaphragm sellae. Typically, this deficit begins with visual acuity depression within the superotemporal quadrant, particularly affecting perception of colors and small objects; the remaining field remains normal. As the tumor enlarges, the upper temporal quadrant becomes an absolute peripheral depression, but central fixation is still spared. With further progression, the lower nasal field is affected. Finally, the superotemporal field is affected, and, if progression continues, the whole field disappears.

Posterior optic chiasm lesions lead to a **posterior junctional scotoma**, which displays the features of chiasmal and optic tract lesions. The classic finding is **incongruous** (less dense in the ipsilateral eye) **hemianopic visual field loss** contralateral to the lesion—from involvement of the nascent optic tract and an inferotemporal visual field loss in the ipsilateral eye—from pressure on the posterior chiasm affecting the late-crossing superotemporal retinal fibers. Such defects occur in disorders located near the anterior aspect of the third ventricle that approach the chiasm from its posteriomedial aspect. The incongruous nature of the hemianopic defect is caused by the incomplete intermixing of the decussating fibers on entering the optic tract with their corresponding uncrossed fibers from the contralateral eye.

OPTIC TRACT AND LATERAL GENICULATE NUCLEUS
Optic Tract

Axons contained within the optic tract are those emanating from the retinal ganglion cells, which have yet to synapse. Nevertheless, after they leave the chiasm for the optic tract, they nominally become part of the "posterior visual pathway" (Figure 4-3). Axons that leave the optic chiasm and go to the lateral geniculate nucleus (LGN) within the thalamus form the optic tract, which resembles a round band, approaching the LGN via the anterior limb of the internal capsule. It courses between the tuber cinerum and the anterior perforated substance, continuing posteriorly as a band of flattened fibers around the cerebral peduncles to synapse within the LGN.

A relatively small number of nonvisual retinal origin fibers within the optic tract accompany the optic nerve and chiasm and supply the afferent stimulus to the pupillomotor center within the pretectal nucleus. These axons for the pupillary fibers bypass the LGN laterally en route to the midbrain.

Lateral Geniculate Nucleus

The LGN is a thalamic relay nucleus that serves as the synapse point of the retinal ganglion cells. It comprises 6 gray matter layers separated by 5 white matter layers. The layers are folded over, forming a bend or small knee. Each

OPTIC PATHWAYS

Figure 4-3

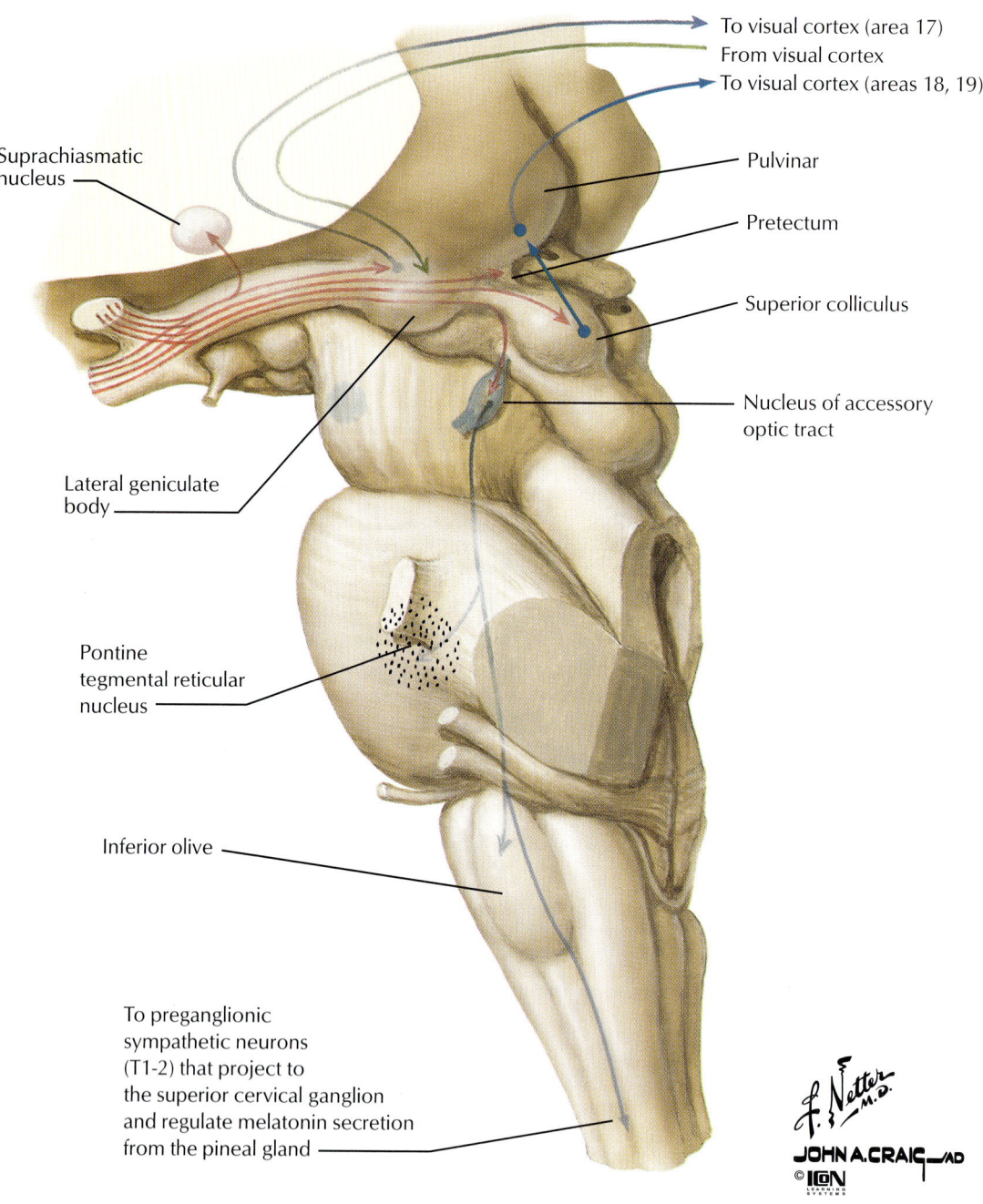

layer has a retinotopic organization, creating a map of the contralateral hemifield. The ratio of geniculate cells to retinal axons is approximately 1:1. Retinal input to the LGN comprises only one fifth of its afferent fibers. The remainder comes from the mesencephalic reticular formation, posterior parietal cortex, occipital cortex, and other thalamic nuclei. The LGN may use these nonretinal elements to "screen" the visual input, gating certain inputs to the visual cortex while blocking other signals, depending on the state of these other inputs.

OPTIC PATHWAYS

The same vessels that supply the posterior chiasm nourish the anterior one third of the optic tract: the internal carotid, middle cerebral, and posterior communicating arteries. The blood supply of the posterior two thirds of the optic tract is derived from the anterior choroidal artery, a branch of the internal carotid that runs posteriorly near the optic tract. The lateral geniculate body receives blood from the posterior cerebral artery and the posterior communicating arteries.

Disorders

Like all components of the posterior visual pathways, optic tract lesions are characterized by homonymous hemianopia. However, these lesions have a unique propensity to lead to combined homonymous hemianopia with pupillary changes and optic disk pallor. Total lesions of the optic tract, by affecting the pupillary afferents within the tract, produce a mild relative afferent papillary defect in the contralateral eye because slightly more crossed fibers exist within the tract from that eye than uncrossed fibers from the ipsilateral eye. When wallerian degeneration ensues, pallor characteristic of optic tract lesions develops in the optic disks. The ipsilateral eye, losing axons from the retina temporal to the fovea, has chiefly superior and inferior polar atrophy, whereas the contralateral eye, losing the interior of the papillomacular bundle and the axons from the retinal nasal to the optic nerve, has pallor in the temporal and nasal poles (**"bow tie" atrophy**).

As with the chiasm, neoplasms, aneurysms, and trauma are the typical lesion mechanisms. In the optic tract and LGN, strokes are relatively uncommon. Depending on the severity of the lesion, the field loss is a complete homonymous hemianopia or an incomplete incongruous one. In either instance, the visual field defect affects both eyes in the field of vision contralateral to the affected site. Incomplete lesions often produce wedge-shaped defects, with the point of the wedge encroaching on the center, a "dagger into fixation."

OPTIC RADIATIONS
Anatomy

The optic radiations are myelinated axons emanating from cell bodies in the LGN, coursing to the primary visual cortex. After they leave the lateral geniculate body, they continue through the posterior limb of the internal capsule. Most fibers take a fairly direct path to the calcarine cortex, following the curve of the internal capsule through the parietal lobe to the occipital lobe. However, the most inferior axons (Meyer loop) that carry visual information from the opposite superior field detour laterally around the lateral ventricles and through the posterior temporal lobe (Figure 4-4). Therefore, stroke or injury confined to this portion of the temporal lobe affects only this portion of the optic radiations. Meyer loop fibers rejoin the rest of the optic radiations after their detour.

Vascular Supply

Five primary arteries supply blood to the optic radiation: the anterior and posterior choroidal arteries, the middle and posterior cerebral arteries, and the calcarine artery (Figure 4-5). The anterior choroidal artery supplies the anterior portion of the optic radiations, the optic tract, and the lateral geniculate body. The anterior optic radiations are also fed by a meshwork of branches from the posterior choroidal arteries. The middle portion of the optic radiations, however, is fed via the deep optic branch of the middle cerebral artery, which lies lateral to the ventricle. The posterior portion of the optic radiation is fed by the posterior cerebral artery and one of its branches, the calcarine artery.

Disorders

Tumors, stroke, and demyelination are chief injury mechanisms to the optic radiations. Lesions confined to the temporal lobe can only affect the Meyer loop of the optic radiations. The resulting visual field defect is typically a superior wedge, with one side located at the vertical meridian, and the second edge being less sharp. This defect, resembling a "slice" removed from the superior visual field, has been termed a *"pie in the sky" defect*. When encountered, it provides strong evidence of a temporal lobe origin. Often, other neurologic deficits compatible with temporal lobe dysfunction confirm the visual field findings. Generally, these lesions are mildly incongruous.

Conversely, if a parietal lesion affects the optic radiations anteriorly, an inverse lesion sparing

OPTIC PATHWAYS

Figure 4-4

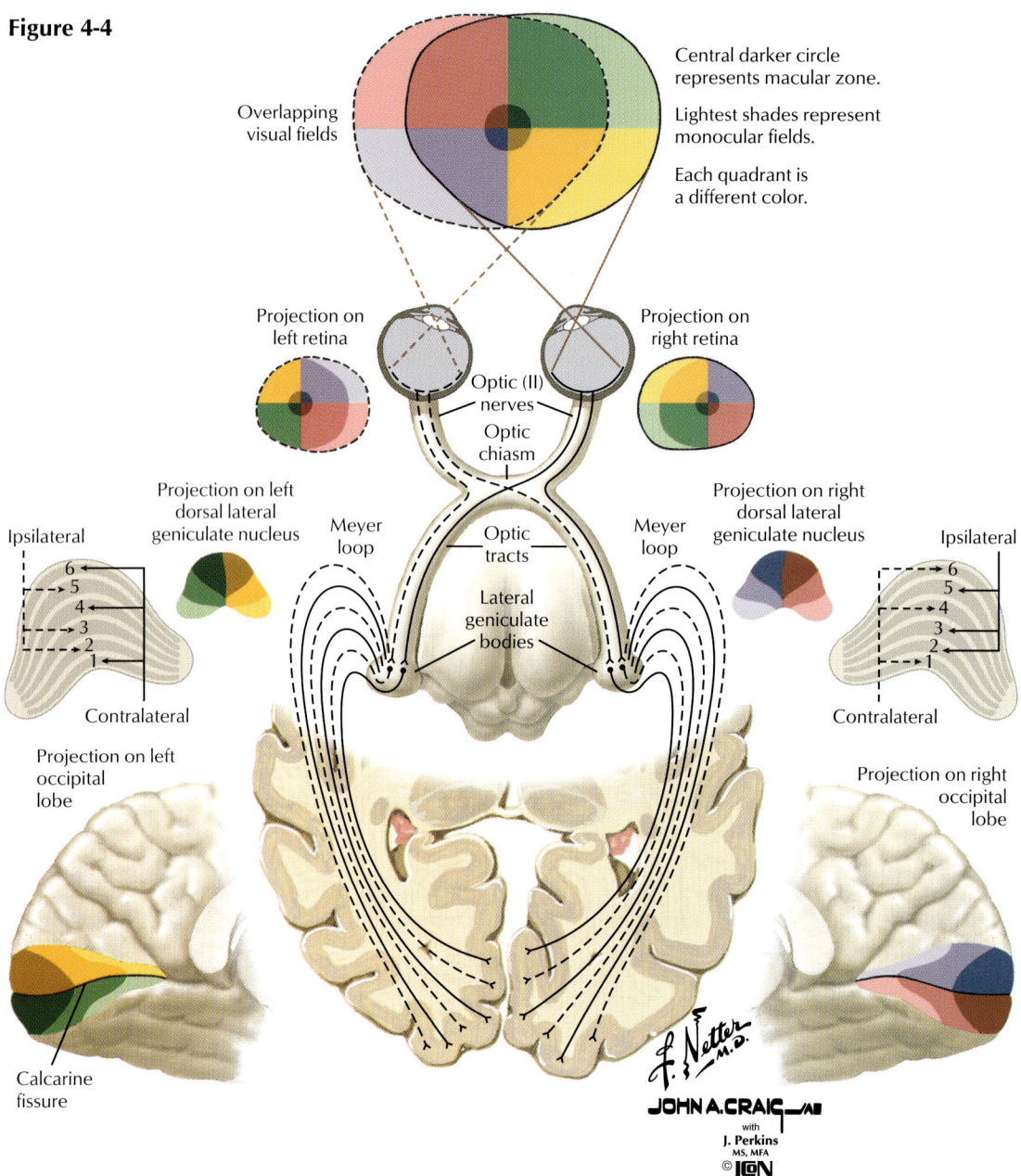

the temporal lobe "wedge" occurs; however, such lesions are rarely encountered. Occasionally, a larger or more posterior parietal lesion can affect all of the optic radiations when the Meyer loop has rejoined the other fibers, producing a complete homonymous hemianopia.

Complete hemianopias are "non-localizing"; by examining the visual field, there is no evidence whether they are secondary to a lesion at the level of the optic tract, lateral geniculate body, parietal lobe, or occipital lobe. However, the rare optic tract lesions also produce a mild contralateral relative afferent pupil defect and contralateral bow tie atrophy of the optic disk. Thus, when present, these additional findings help to localize the responsible lesion. Similarly, because areas within the parietal lobe contribute to pursuit eye movements, patients with a complete homonymous hemianopia from a parietal lesion may show altered or absent pursuit move-

OPTIC PATHWAYS

Figure 4-5   **Arteries of Brain: Inferior Views**

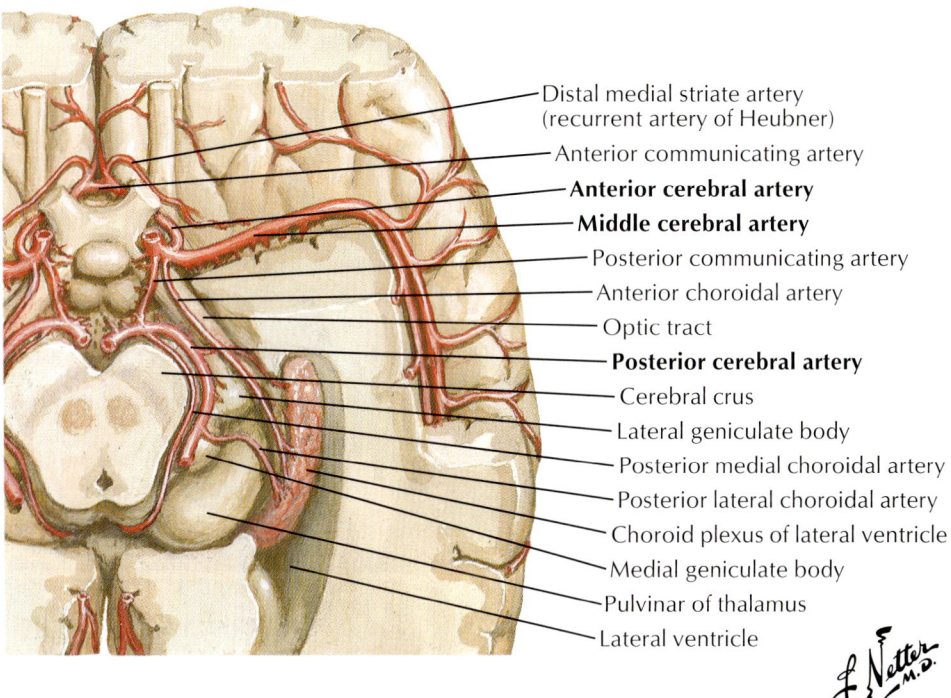

ments in the direction toward the lesion. Such defects are best demonstrated clinically with a standard optokinetic nystagmus drum.

FUTURE DIRECTIONS

Advances in diagnosis have focused on improved imaging techniques. For example, diffusion MRI scanning allows for better detection of early, focal brain edema after stroke. Functional MRI scanning, allowing the MRI scan to detect pH or neurochemical abnormalities focally, may become a practical addition to current diagnostic tools.

REFERENCES

Hedges TR, Friedman D, Horton J, Newman SA, Striph G, Kay MC. Neuro-ophthalmology. In: Weingeist TA, Liesegang TJ, Slamovits TL, eds. *Basic and Clinical Science Course, 1997-1998,* San Francisco, Calif: American Academy of Ophthalmology; 1997:55-70.

Miller NR, Newman NJ, eds. *Walsh and Hoyt's Clinical Neuro-ophthalmology.* 5th ed. Baltimore, Md: William & Wilkins; 1998.

Chapter 5
Primary Visual Cortex

Ippolit C. A. Matjucha and Robert J. Updaw II

Clinical Vignette

A 64-year-old gynecologist, while operating, suddenly had difficulty seeing to the right. He had to turn his head to see the full operative field. The next day, he saw his ophthalmologist, who found evidence of a dense right homonymous hemianopsia.

A subsequent neurologic consultation was otherwise unremarkable. MRI demonstrated a hypodensity in the left occipital lobe. ECG and transesophageal echocardiography results were normal. A 48-hour Holter monitor documented 7 periods of intermittent atrial fibrillation. Anticoagulation was initiated. The patient was advised to have his wife do all the driving.

This vignette typifies an embolus to the left posterior cerebral artery causing a left occipital lobe infarct. Although occasionally such patients improve, often individuals have no substantial resolution of function. Prevention of further strokes is needed, by treating the atrial fibrillation or, if unsuccessful, using anticoagulants to prevent further atrial thrombi from forming. Complete driving restriction is essential because of the total inability to perceive objects in the densely lost field.

ANATOMY

Axons of the optic radiations synapse with the primary visual cortex. A unique white stripe or stria (stripe of Gennari for the discovering anatomist), representing a myelin-rich cortical layer, is easily seen in gross sections through the cortex with its layered, highly structured organization of **V1**, also known as the ***primary visual cortex***, the ***striate cortex***, or ***Brodmann area 17***. Primarily located on the mesial surface of the occipital lobe within and surrounding the calcarine fissure, the most posterior aspect of V1 typically wraps around the posterior (occipital) pole for a short distance (Figure 5-1).

Microscopically, the visual cortex is arranged in 6 laminae, running from the surface to a depth of slightly greater than 2 mm. The most superficial, layer I, primarily contains glial cells. Layers II and III contain pyramidal cells and small interneurons. The thickest stria is layer IV, comprising almost half the depth of the visual cortex. Highly branched stellate cells exist superficially within layer IVa. The Gennari stripe comprises layer IVb, containing myelinated axons from afferent visual (geniculate) cells and cortical association fibers. Pyramidal and granule cells and giant pyramidal (Meynert) cells occur more deeply at IVc. Layer V is a densely cellular region with variously sized pyramidal cells. Layer VIa is a less cellular superficial portion, and layer VIb contains a varied neuronal population.

Vascular Supply

The blood supply of the striate cortex primarily derives from the **calcarine artery**, a branch of the **posterior cerebral artery**, and sometimes the **middle cerebral artery**, or anastamoses from it (Figure 5-2). Usually, the calcarine artery supplies most of the visual area. However, in 75% of cases, other arteries contribute: the posterior temporal or parietooccipital arteries, occasionally aided by the middle cerebral artery.

Topographic Organization

Specific anatomical correlations are the primary clinical features pertinent to the striate cortex: visual information from the left visual field in each eye is projected to the right visual cortex (and conversely); the superior visual field is projected into the inferior half of V1 (and con-

PRIMARY VISUAL CORTEX

Figure 5-1A **Functional Organization of the Cerebral Cortex**

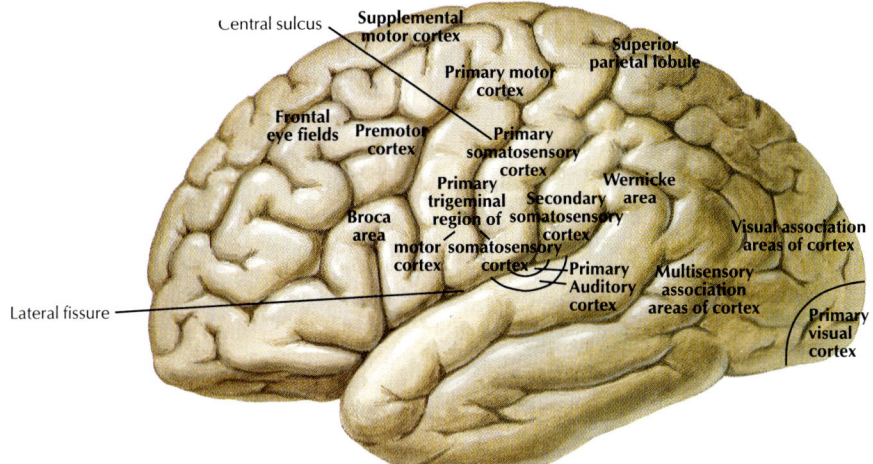

Figure 5-1B **Visual Cortex**

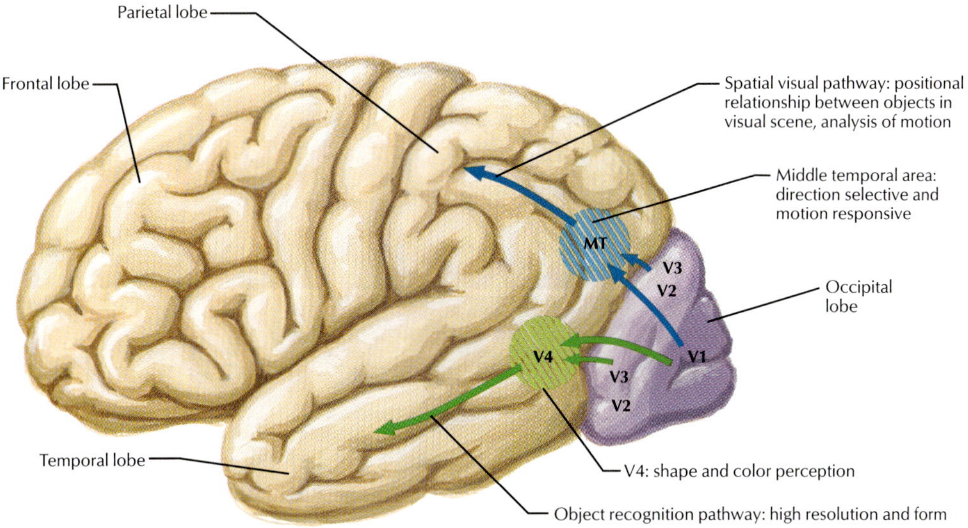

Figure 5-1C **Medial Aspect of the Cerebral Cortex**

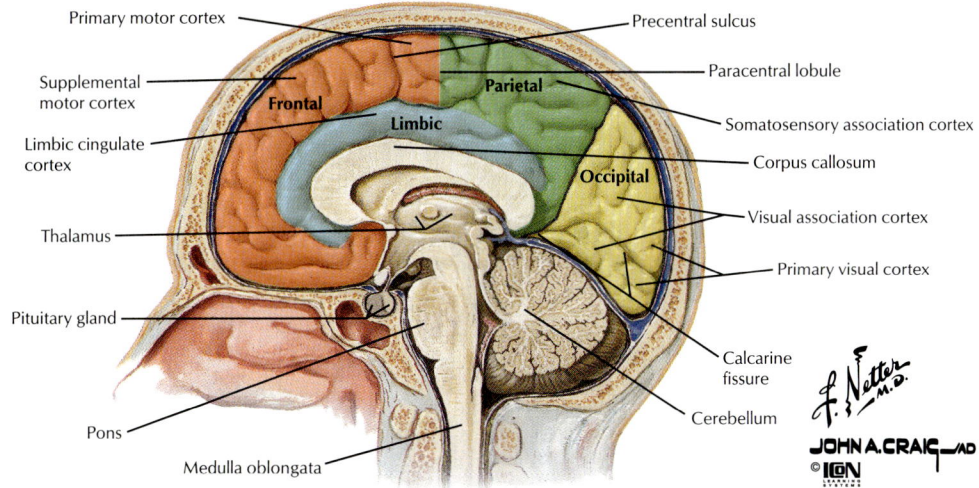

73

PRIMARY VISUAL CORTEX

Figure 5-2   **Arterial Supply of Cerebral Cortex**

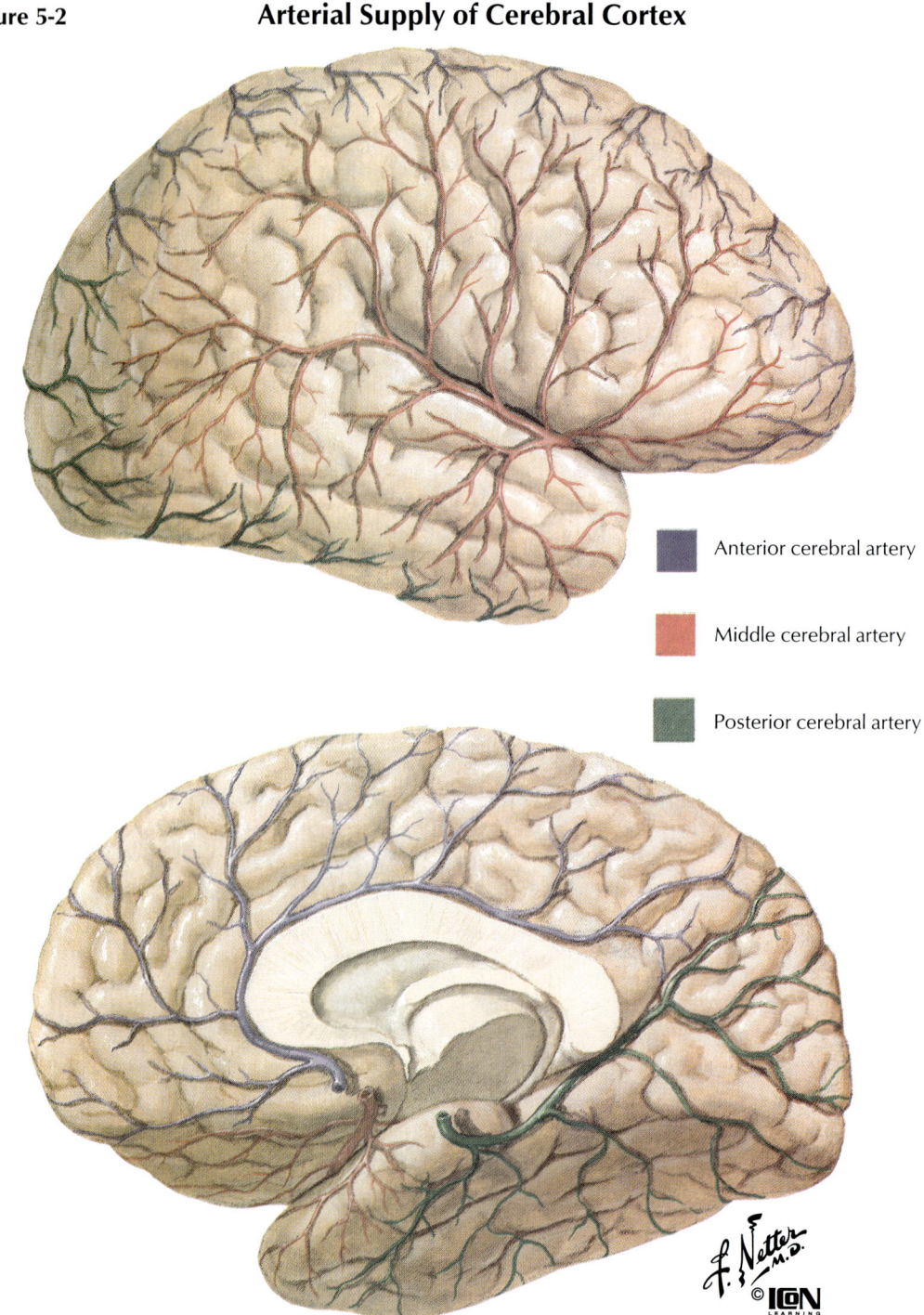

versely); and the most central visual field is projected most posteriorly, whereas the peripheral field is located anteriorly within V1.

"Cortical magnification" in V1 results in much more cortex dedicated to the central area than to the periphery. Up to 50% of the cortex may correspond to the central 10° of vision; in fact, the most central 1° of vision uses as much cortex posteriorly as the most peripheral 50°. Cortical magnification is considered a reflection of the evolutionary importance of precise central vision to survival.

Ocular dominance columns run at right angles to the cortical surface. Within a column, visual input is derived from one eye only; in the immediate neighboring cortical surface, perhaps only 0.5 mm from that column, another column deriving input from the other eye is encountered.

Monocular occlusion during the early postnatal period demonstrates that the columns of the occluded eye grow smaller, whereas the columns of the open eye enlarge. Subsequent uncovering of the occluded eye does not restore the equality of the columns, which is considered central to understanding critical periods in visual development. The failure of that development is designated *amblyopia*.

A hierarchy exists to the processing of visual information at a cellular level. The striate cortex has different cell types that respond to increasingly specific stimuli, including **simple cells,** which have the same light/dark, center/surround response profile as retina and lateral geniculate nucleus cells. Additionally, **complex and hypercomplex cells** respond best to a light stimulus that is not a spot but a line at a particular angle or a specific length to achieve an optimal cell response.

This hierarchical structure suggests that additional cell types, probably located in extrastriate association cortices, respond to more specific and complex stimuli until, eventually, the putative "grandmother cell"—the unique cell that fires when a picture of one's grandmother is seen—is encountered. Although instructive and fanciful, this concept is incorrect; single-neuron deaths in the brain occur daily, but the inability to recognize a single person when other individuals are recognized normally is not a described disease state. There may be "higher" association cortices, with groups of cells producing specific **patterns of neuronal activation** that represent the anatomical correlate for perceptual recognition.

DISEASES OF THE STRIATE CORTEX

Striate cortex lesions, like other neurologic lesions, can be classified into ischemic, neoplastic, and demyelinating disease; infection, especially from septic emboli, is rare. Clinical characteristics of visual field defects from V1 lesions provide a diagnostic set leading to an anatomical localization even before imaging procedures. The hemianopic visual field loss from V1 lesions, if incomplete, shows close congruence of deficit between the eyes. The small size and close proximity of the left and right ocular dominance columns make it impossible to selectively damage the visual field of only one eye.

The extreme temporal visual field of each eye represents an exception to this principle. Because the nasal visual field extends only approximately 65°, the remaining lateral field on each side is supplied solely by the ipsilateral eye. This "temporal crescent" of the visual field corresponds to the most anterior aspect of V1, abutting the occipitoparietal fissure, where ocular dominance columns are absent, because all input comes from the contralateral eye's nasal retina. Therefore, in a lesion of the anterior striate cortex, if only the most temporal 25° is affected, a "monocular homonymous defect" may result.

Because of the specialized nature of V1, lesions there affect vision and no other neurologic function. In addition to the extreme congruity of the visual field defects of the 2 eyes, striate cortex lesions have no signs of anterior visual pathway involvement, ie, no optic pallor and no relative afferent papillary defect. Typically, central acuity is not affected. This deficit isolation differs from parietal lesions that typically affect both visual field (homonymous contralateral loss) and eye movements (loss of contralateral lateral saccade, manifesting as uncorrected ipsilateral drift on testing with an opticokinetic nystagmus drum turning toward the affected side).

Rarely, bilateral occipital cortical lesions occur simultaneously. Generalized systemic hypotension, such as from a cardiac arrest or basilar or bilateral posterior cerebral artery occlusion, causes bilateral ischemic damage. Similarly, direct or contrecoup traumatic damage occurs when both occipital poles are injured. Initially, bilateral occipital pole lesions may be confused with bilateral optic nerve lesions because an apparent "central scotoma" is found in each eye. However, careful visual field mapping along the vertical axis demonstrates a discontinuity, a vertical step. The vertical step is expected because these cortical injuries should not be absolutely symmetric, so the extent of visual field loss should vary in size between the left and right hemifields. The size difference is seen most easily at the vertical meridian, resulting in a keyhole defect. Like temporal crescent defects, keyhole defects are characteristic of occipital lobe lesions.

Macular sparing in visual field defects is expected with incomplete striate cortex destruction and preservation of the posterolateral extension around the occipital pole, where the total loss of the cortex is certain (eg, surgical removal), and as a testing artifact from inconstant fixation of the tested eye on the target center. The anatomy of V1, with the most central visual field represented on the posterior pole rather than on the mesial occipital surface and often supplied by the middle rather than the posterior cerebral artery, may make it likely that even lesions affecting most of V1 may miss the most anterior, central vision area. Such sparing is due to relative anatomical and vascular isolation of that cortical area from areas representing more peripheral vision.

EXTRASTRIATE ASSOCIATION VISUAL AREAS

Brodmann areas 18 and 19, immediately adjacent to area 17, in the area surrounding the calcarine fissure, were termed the *parastriate* or *association visual cortex* on the assumption that they functioned to "associate" the visual data from V1 with brain areas regarding spatial orientation, recognition, and language. Human correlates of the described macaque areas remain uncertain.

In brief, areas V2 and V3 are adjacent to V1, sharing its retinotopic organization. V2 cells are driven by orientation of stimulus, whereas V3 contains cells that favor specific direction of stimulus motion. V2, V4, and VP (ventral parietal area) are influenced by stimulus color and thus may influence color vision. V5 or the middle temporal area seems to select for certain stimulus speeds. V6, perhaps correlated with the human parietooccipital visual cortex, varies from V1 in not having retinotopic organization or central magnification and may be a visual/somatosensory interface. The macaque medial superior temporal area seems to help decipher complex visual motion.

FUTURE DIRECTIONS

Research continues to describe new areas of visual association cortex that subserve specific aspects of vision, increasing the possibility of recognizing deficits experienced by patients with lesions in these areas and guiding investigations of poorly understood visual problems, such as visual hallucinations and palinopsia (persistence of visual sensation after the stimulus has ended or moved).

Advancing imaging techniques may help to improve sensitivity and precision in diagnosis. Specific protection of neurons after ischemic or traumatic injury remains at the far horizon of research, as do regenerative therapies for neural tissue.

REFERENCES

Horton JC, Hoyt WF. The representation of the visual field in human striate cortex: a revision of the classic Holmes map. *Arch Ophthalmol.* 1991;109:816-824.

Hubel DH. *Eye, Brain and Vision.* New York, NY: WH Freeman; 1995. Scientific American Library; No. 22.

Nicholls JG, Martin AR, Wallace BG, Fuchs PA. *From Neuron to Brain.* 4th ed. Sunderland, Mass: Sinauer Associates; 2001.

Chapter 6
Cranial Nerve III: Oculomotor

Ippolit C. A. Matjucha

Clinical Vignette

A 37-year-old woman presented with a 2-day history of disturbed vision on upward gaze, vertical binocular diplopia, and headache. One month previously, she had experienced the same symptoms for 5 days. Sinusitis was diagnosed, and an antibiotic was prescribed.

Examination demonstrated impaired upward gaze in the right eye and poor downward gaze and adduction. She had ptosis on the right, and the pupil was slightly larger and reacted poorly compared with the left.

MRI yielded normal results, but catheter angiography demonstrated a posterior communicating artery (P-com) aneurysm. At craniotomy that same night, the neurosurgeon clipping the 5 × 10-mm aneurysm reported fresh and old clot around the aneurysm that was compressing the right oculomotor nerve. The patient had an uneventful recovery, with gradual resolution of the neuro-ophthalmologic findings.

The oculomotor nerves course from the ventral midbrain to the orbits. CN-III provides the general somatic motor efferent innervation controlling upper lid elevation and most of the extraocular movements upward, medially, and downward. In addition, CN-III carries the general visceral motor (parasympathetic) efferent innervation responsible for pupillary constriction and accommodation (near focus) of the crystalline lens.

Any individual who has an oculomotor (CN-III) paresis must be evaluated for a P-com aneurysm (Figure 6-1A). Often, such patients present with a concomitant severe headache, described as the worst one they have ever had. When patients have diabetes and the pupil is unaffected, the lesion may be related to a microvasculopathy of CN-III (Figure 6-1B). However, this diagnosis of exclusion cannot be made until imaging studies rule out an aneurysm.

CLINICAL PRESENTATION

The following description from the early 20th century captures the classic presentation of a CN-III palsy:

> Oculo-motor paralysis ... presents a characteristic picture. The upper lid hangs loosely down (ptosis) and has to be drawn up with the finger to give a view of the eyeball, which is deflected strongly outward and somewhat down, because the two muscles not paralyzed—the [lateral] rectus and the superior oblique—draw it in this direction.

The pupil is dilated and immobile (paralysis of the sphincter pupillae), and the eye is focused for the far point and cannot accommodate for near by (paralysis of the ciliary muscle).*

ANATOMICAL CORRELATIONS
Oculomotor Nucleus

The CN-III nucleus is a lepidopteroid collection of 9 subnuclei located in the center of the rostral midbrain at the level of the superior colliculi (Figure 6-2). The most ventral of these subnuclei is the central caudate nucleus, a midline structure that innervates both levator palpebrae muscles. Because of the bilateral innervation, when CN-III is injured at the nucleus, the patient's eyelids exhibit bilateral blepharoptosis or are normal, depending on whether the injury extends to the central caudate nucleus.

Similarly, axons from the right and left medial columns, the subnuclei serving, respectively, the left and right superior rectus muscles, immediately decussate across the midline so each innervates the contralateral superior rectus—hence the clinical presentation of a nuclear CN-III palsy wherein the contralateral eye displays defective upward gaze, with the remaining ocular motor deficits seen ipsilaterally.

The other 6 subnuclei likewise form 3 left-and-right pairs but innervate ipsilateral extraocular

---
*Duane, page 310.

CRANIAL NERVE III: OCULOMOTOR

Figure 6-1A   **Ophthalmologic Manifestations of Cerebral Anerurysms**

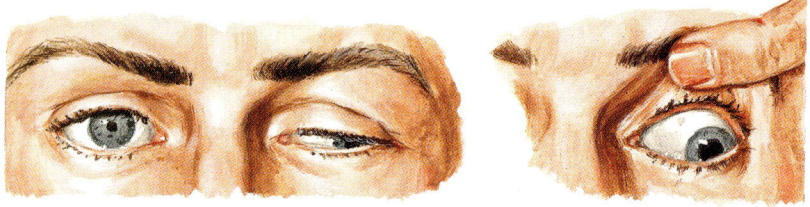

Oculomotor palsy: Ptosis, eye turns laterally and inferiorly, pupil dilated; common finding with cerebral aneurysms, especially carotid-posterior communicating aneurysms

Neuromuscular disorders
Abducens palsy: Affected eye turns medially. May be first manifestation of intracavernous carotid aneurysm. Pain above eye or on side of face may be secondary to trigeminal (V) nerve involvement.

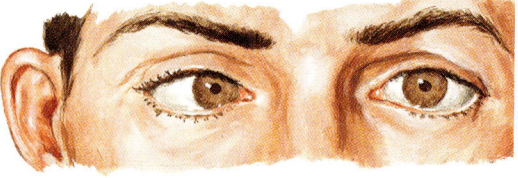

Retinal changes

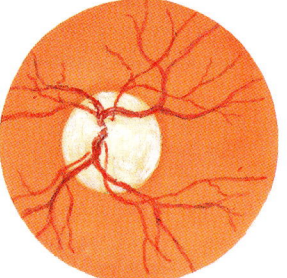

Optic atrophy may develop as a result of pressure on the optic (II) nerve from a supraclinoid carotid, ophthalmic, or anterior cerebral aneurysm.

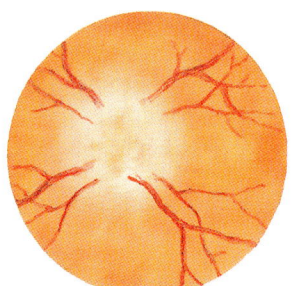

Papilledema may be caused by increased intracranial pressure secondary to rupture of a cerebral aneurysm.

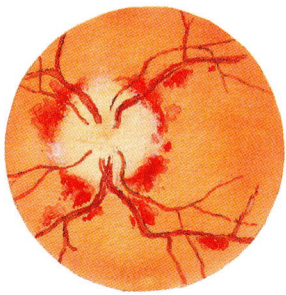

Hemorrhage into optic (II) nerve sheath after rupture of aneurysm may result in subhyaloid hemorrhage with blood around disc.

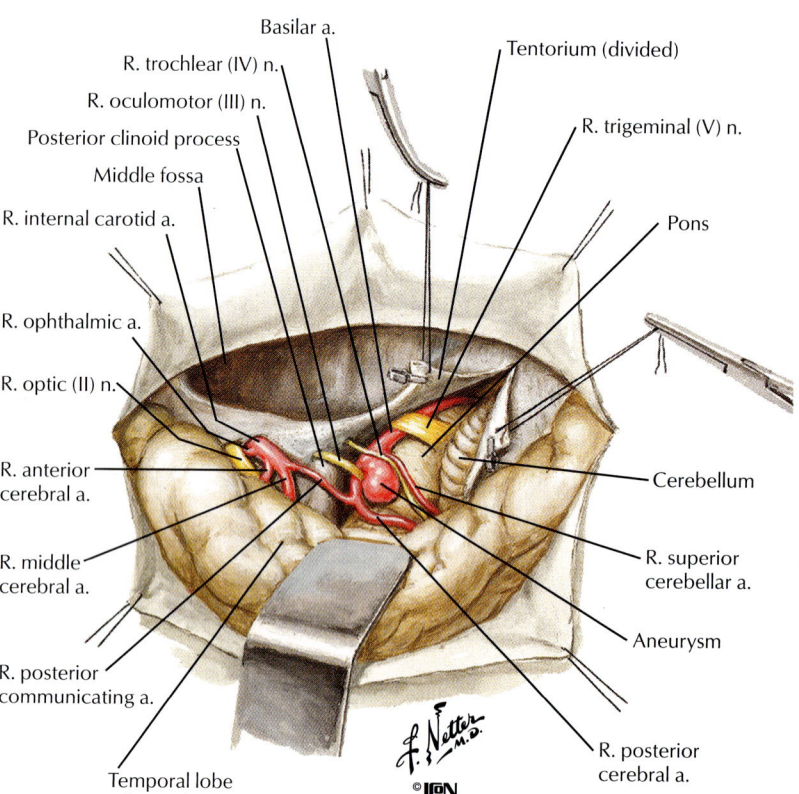

Neuro-ophthalmology

CRANIAL NERVE III: OCULOMOTOR

Figure 6-1B **Ocular Complications of Diabetes**

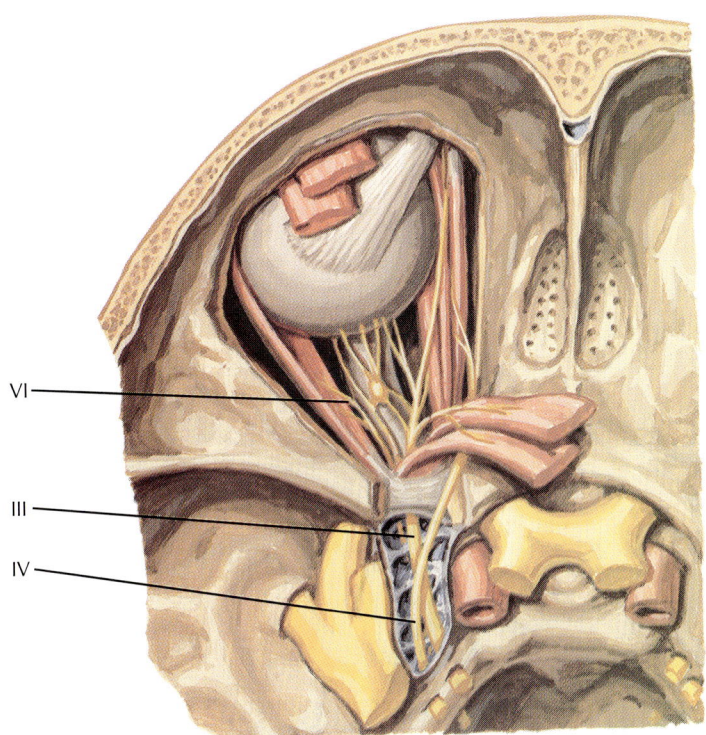

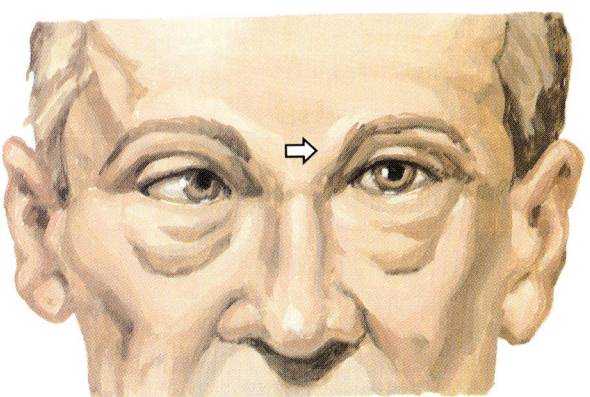

Attempted left gaze in left
sixth cranial nerve palsy

CRANIAL NERVE III: OCULOMOTOR

Figure 6-2

Oculomotor (III), Trochlear (IV), and Abducent (VI) Nerves: Schema

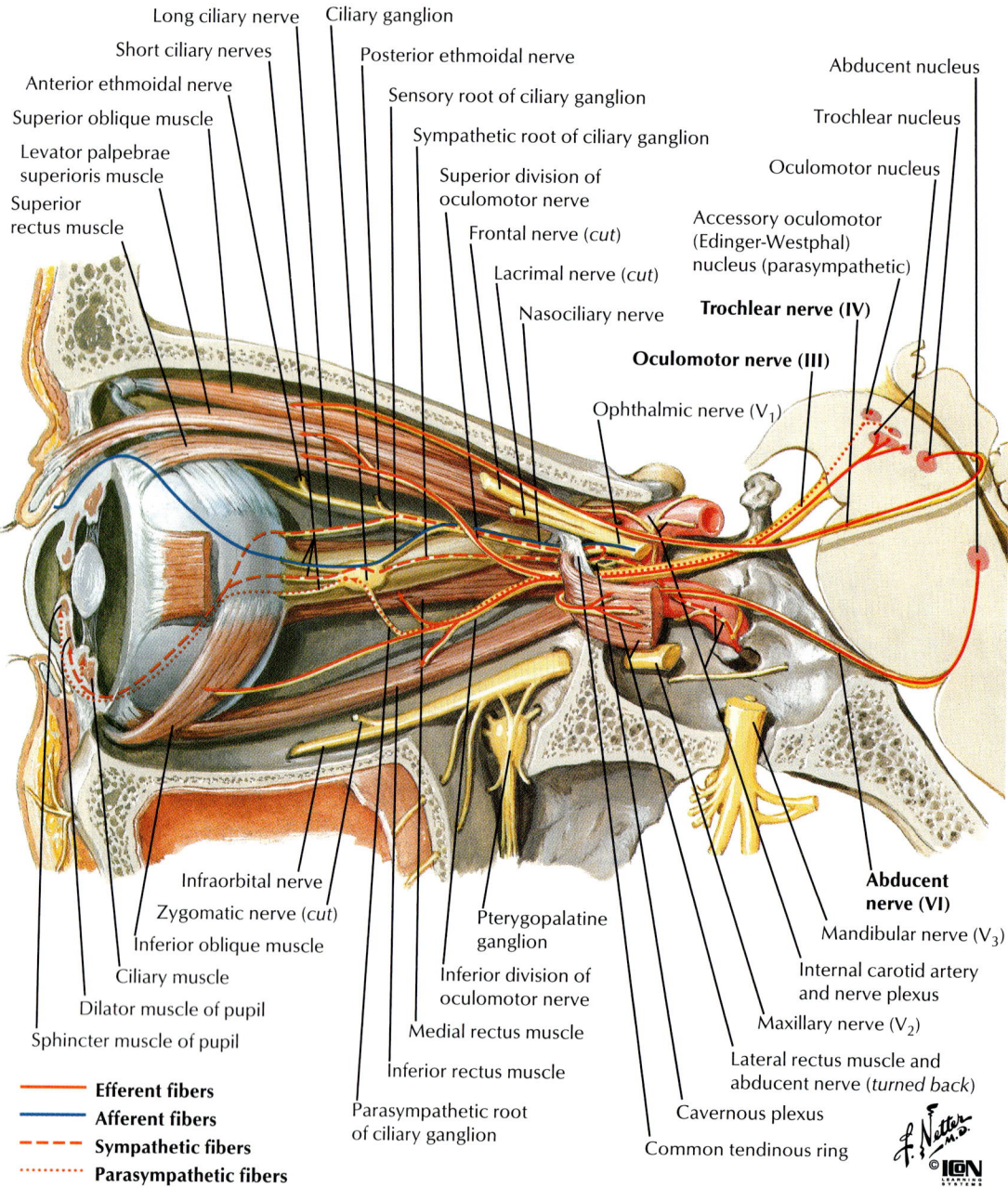

muscles. The ventral nucleus, intermediate column, and dorsal nuclei, respectively, control the medial rectus (eye adduction), inferior oblique (intortion and some elevation), and inferior rectus (depression).

The CN-III nucleus receives numerous afferents, including inputs from the paramedian pontine reticular formation for horizontal eye movement, the rostral interstitial nucleus of the medial longitudinal fasciculus for vertical and torsional movements, and the vestibular nuclei. Other afferents come from the superior colliculi, the occipital cortex, and the cerebellum.

Sometimes considered a subnucleus of CN-III, the **Edinger-Westphal nucleus** abuts the others rostrodorsally, residing at the ventral edge of periaqueductal gray matter. The Edinger-Westphal nucleus supplies the cholinergic efferents producing pupillary constriction and ciliary muscle contraction (lens accommodation). Afferents from the pretectal nuclei mediate the pupillary light reflex, whereas inputs influencing pupil constriction and lens accommodation in response to near visual stimulus originate from striate and prestriate cortex and the superior colliculus. When the pupillary fibers join the oculomotor nerve, they move exteriorly and dorsally within the nerve, a clinical continuation of the spatial relation of the Edinger-Westphal nucleus to CN-III.

Oculomotor Fasciculus

Axons from the CN-III nucleus gather into a fascicle and sweep ventrally in an arc curving toward the medial surface of the cerebral peduncle, passing through the red nucleus. The cerebral peduncle at this level carries the corticospinal tract axons that innervate the contralateral somatic musculature; the red nucleus provides secondary motor inputs contralaterally. Bordering the red nucleus is the superior cerebellar peduncle (brachium conjunctivum), caudally comprising cerebellocortical axons aiding motor control ipsilaterally, and the medial lemniscus laterally that relays contralateral somatic afferents.

CN-III fasciculus lesions at the red nucleus present as oculomotor palsy with crossed hemitremor, **Benedikt syndrome**. If the lesion extends to the medial lemniscus, there is also contralateral hypesthesia. Similar lesions with caudal extension also affect the brachium conjunctivum, producing ipsilateral cerebellar ataxia, called **Claude syndrome**. When damage extends ventrally into the basis pedunculi, corticospinal tract dysfunction causes **Weber syndrome**: hemiplegia contralateral to the CN-III palsy.

Subarachnoid Oculomotor Nerve

The nascent oculomotor nerve emerges from the medial surface of the cerebral peduncle to enter the interpeduncular cistern. It crosses the cistern for approximately 5 mm, passing under the posterior cerebral artery. It follows beneath the P-com for 10 mm, and then pierces the dura underneath the P-com en route to the cavernous sinus. This short segment of CN-III forms the pathophysiologic territory for an important pupillary finding in clinical neurology. Typically, in obtunded or comatose patients, when cerebral edema leads to uncal herniation, the ipsilateral anterior temporal lobe is pushed medially and downward through the tentorial window. The uncus of the temporal lobe compresses the ipsilateral posterior cerebral artery downward onto CN-III, with a resultant ipsilateral sluggish pupillary light reaction. With external compression of CN-III, pupillary motor fibers typically are affected earlier than extraocular motor fibers, an observation usually attributed to the exterior position of the pupil fibers on the surface of CN-III. As compression worsens, a fully dilated pupil develops. Shortly thereafter, other signs of oculomotor nerve dysfunction usually occur. Therefore, periodic checking of pupil function in comatose patients remains an indispensable clinical tool.

Cavernous Sinus and Superior Orbital Fissure

The cavernous sinus is part of the intracranial venous system. It receives blood from the ophthalmic vein and sphenoparietal sinus, transmitting this flow to the superior and inferior petrosal sinuses. The left and right cavernous sinuses are connected via the intracavernous plexus; they also communicate with the basilar sinus and the pterygoid and foramen ovale plexuses. The cavernous sinus resides lateral to the pituitary gland, resting atop the roof and lateral wall of the sphenoid sinus. Besides venous blood, the space con-

CRANIAL NERVE III: OCULOMOTOR

tains the intracavernous portions of CN-III, -IV, and -VI; the ophthalmic branch of CN-V and its maxillary nerve posteriorly; the internal carotid artery; and the sympathetic nerve fibers investing the adventitia of the internal carotid artery. CN-III, -IV, -VI and the ophthalmic nerve all leave the cavernous sinus to enter the orbit via the superior orbital fissure.

Given the confluence of these structures into this relatively small sinus, neurologic disorders in this area are prone to produce multiple CN palsies, often with pain in the ophthalmic distribution. If the pathologic process is extensive, signs of venous obstruction in the orbit also develop.

Orbit

CN-III typically divides into superior and inferior branches within the anterior cavernous sinus, thus entering the orbit as two distinct structures. The superior branch supplies the superior rectus and levator palpebrae muscles. The inferior branch provides somatic innervation to the medial and inferior recti and the inferior oblique and supplies the parasympathetic pupil inputs to the ciliary ganglion, located superiolaterally to the midorbital optic nerve. The parasympathetic axons from the Edinger-Westphal nucleus synapse here, with the postsynaptic neurons providing visceral motor control to the iris sphincter and the ciliary muscles via the short ciliary nerves.

At the orbital apex, the optic nerve and ophthalmic artery enter the orbit via the optic foramen just nasally to the superior orbital fissure.

DIFFERENTIAL DIAGNOSIS

Posterior communicating artery aneurysms are the most common cause of acute headaches with signs of CN-III palsy with pupillary involvement. The typical location of these aneurysms is the origin of P-com at the internal carotid artery (Figure 6-3). Up to 30% of acquired CN-III palsies develop from such aneurysms, and 90% of aneurysms present with CN-III palsy.

However, not all patients with acquired CN-III palsies have aneurysms. Pupillary findings provide a paramount distinguishing feature. In approximately 80% of CN-III palsy cases, the pupil is spared, and the cause is diabetes or other "microvascular" vasculopathies—not an aneurysm. Typically, these palsies have a favorable prognosis and uncomplicated recovery within 2 to 4 months.

Whether a spared pupil reliably excludes an aneurysm deserves discussion. Certainly, with instances of an incomplete extraocular CN-III palsy, the absence of pupil involvement must not be considered evidence of a benign etiology. This is particularly true in nonelderly patients with few microvascular risk factors. The relative ease of access to MRI and MRA has removed this concern. Still, two caveats exist about noninvasive neuroimaging: an aneurysmal complete extraocular CN-III palsy without pupillary involvement is exceedingly rare, but a negative noninvasive study does not guarantee absence of aneurysm.

Open or closed head injuries also may lead to oculomotor nerve palsies. The suspected locus of injury is the dural entrance, wherein the nerve is fixed in relation to the petrous bone, allowing a violent shift of the intracranial contents to produce traction injury to CN-III. Typically, these are associated with severe frontal deceleration impact (eg, unrestrained occupant in a motor vehicle accident) with loss of consciousness. In cases of CN-III palsies with pupillary involvement, concomitant with trivial injuries, an underlying pathology must be sought with appropriate imaging.

The prognosis for recovery in traumatic CN-III palsy is guarded; if recovery occurs, it is usually marked by **aberrant regeneration**. In such imperfect healing, axonal regrowth is misdirected such that nerve branches no longer innervate their expected muscle groups. The best-known example is the pseudo-Graefe sign, in which the branch of CN-III that normally innervates the inferior rectus now synkinetically innervates the levator palpebrae, causing the upper lid to lift on downward gaze (clinically simulating the lid lag, or Graefe sign, of Graves orbitopathy). Internal motor efferents can likewise be involved, resulting in a change of pupil size as gaze is shifted.

Duane syndrome is an example of a congenital aberrant innervation. In affected individuals, attempted lateral eye movement results in simultaneous stimulation of the medial and lateral recti, causing variable eye movement, measur-

CRANIAL NERVE III: OCULOMOTOR

Figure 6-3

Posterior Communicating Artery Aneurysm Compressing Cranial Nerve III

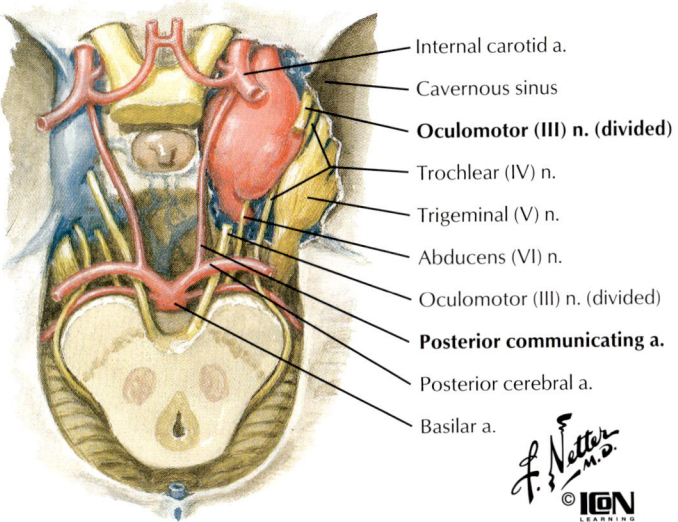

able globe retraction into the orbit, and consequent pseudoptosis. A prenatal abducens nerve dysgenesis or injury may result in subsequent misdirection in these cases. The congenital nature of this condition is most easily deduced by the absence of symptomatic diplopia in lateral gaze despite the presence of noncomitant strabismus.

Cavernous sinus thrombosis, often as a septic complication of central facial cellulitis, is a dreaded clinical entity. A septic phlebitis of the facial vein or pterygoid plexus is the usual intermediary between cellulitis and infectious thrombosis.

Acute pain occasionally develops associated with an **aneurysm**, especially at the origin of the meningohypophyseal trunk. Such aneurysms classically present with primary CN-III synkinesis, ie, aberrant regeneration without **antecedent palsy**. Because this type of aneurysm exists within a venous space, a ruptured aneurysm may produce a high-flow **carotid cavernous fistula**, a lesion having less devastating sequellae than ruptured subarachnoid aneurysms. However, one case of a subarachnoid aneurysm presenting with primary CN-III synkinesis has been reported.

Tolosa-Hunt syndrome is a painful ophthalmoplegia without venous obstruction that typically varies in degree over days. Sympathetic pupil dysfunction is often encountered when the carotid artery wall is involved and is noticeable because the associated CN-III palsy often spares the pupil. The usual etiology is an idiopathic cavernous sinus inflammation, although infection and tumor must be considered. Most instances relate to the spectrum of inflammatory pseudotumor. Neuroimaging confirms the diagnosis. Treatment with high-dose corticosteroids is indicated.

Cavernous sinus syndrome is usually a chronic noninflammatory process characterized by a cranial polyneuropathy. Typically, it affects CN-III, -IV, and -VI and the ophthalmic branch of CN-V. Slowly growing tumors within the cavernous sinus are in the differential. The clinical history often includes chronically increasing diplopia, sometimes with pain or numbness in the CN-V ophthalmic distribution. Therefore, any patient presenting with diplopia, initially thought to be related to a cranial mononeuropathy, must have careful examination of the adjacent CN to exclude involvement of other CNs. Similarly, patients presenting with new upper facial pain must always be checked for impaired eye movements and corneal hypesthesia to exclude early cavernous sinus syndrome. **Superior orbital fissure syndrome** is indistinguishable from cavernous sinus syndrome.

NEURO-OPHTHALMOLOGY

CRANIAL NERVE III: OCULOMOTOR

Lesions producing diminished vision with internal (ie, pupillary involvement) ophthalmoplegia, external ophthalmoplegia, and pain with corneal hypesthesia characterize **orbital apex syndrome**. In simplified terms, this syndrome clinically is characterized by findings of Tolosa-Hunt with a concomitant compressive optic neuropathy. Inflammation and tumor are the usual etiologies.

Because CN-III divides into superior and inferior rami just before its entrance into the orbit, ipsilateral dysfunction of the superior rectus and levator palpebrae muscles seems to indicate an orbital or anterior cavernous sinus pathologic site. However, more proximal intracranial disease is often responsible.

Inferior division palsies sometimes occur from a presumed orbital lesion. However, these palsies usually spare the pupil, the results of imaging studies are normal, and spontaneous recovery is observed—in all ways mimicking the microvascular CN-III palsies discussed in this chapter.

Adie tonic pupil is another example of aberrant regeneration affecting a facet of CN-III function with a probable intraorbital location within the ciliary ganglion. Typically, no specific etiology exists. In the acute setting, Adie pupil presents as unilateral parasympathetic ocular denervation, with consequent mydriasis and loss of accommodation but without ptosis or extraocular immobility. Patients report of photophobia in bright light and blurred near vision.

The postsynaptic axons reinnervate the iris sphincter and ciliary muscles. Their regeneration is apparently directed at random, such that previous ciliary fibers find their way to the iris or ciliary body. When regrowth is complete, over a few months, the resulting pupil is typically mid-dilated, constricts poorly to light, reacts slowly but more fully to accommodative stimulus, and redilates slowly, ie, tonically. Signs of incomplete iris reinnervation also occur, including irregular pupillary shape from persisting segmental denervation and a hypersensitivity to acetylcholine analogs from muscarinic receptor up-regulation.

REFERENCES

Arle JE, Abrahams JM, Zager EL, Taylor C, Galetta SL. Pupil-sparing third nerve palsy with preoperative improvement from a posterior communicating artery aneurysm. *Surg Neurol.* 2002;57:423-426.

Duane A. Motor anomalies of the eye. In: Fuchs HF. *Textbook of Ophthalmology.* 8th ed. Duane A, trans. Philadelphia, Pa: JB Lippincott; 1924:267-364.

McFadzean RM, Teasdale EM. Computerized tomography angiography in isolated third nerve palsies. *J Neurosurg.* 1998;88:679-684.

Miller NR, Newman NJ, eds. *Walsh and Hoyt's Clinical Neuro-ophthalmology.* 5th ed. Baltimore, Md: William & Wilkins; 1998.

Chapter 7
Cranial Nerve IV: Trochlear

Ippolit C. A. Matjucha

Clinical Vignette

A workman, bent over head-down, sustained a scalp laceration over the left occiput when a coworker dropped a tool from above. Diplopia and headache subsequently developed.

Examination revealed poor depression of the right eye in leftward gaze. Prismatic spectacle lenses were prescribed to alleviate the diplopia. After a few months, the patient reported that his vision had returned to normal.

This vignette describes a seemingly mild closed head injury with isolated injury to the trochlear nerve (CN-IV), often the most benign of the cranial neuropathies, particularly those related to extraocular muscle function. The CN-IV nuclei are located in the lower midbrain, off midline at the ventral edge of the periaqueductal gray, at the level of the inferior colliculi (Figure 7-1). The nuclei are crossed; the left trochlear nucleus innervates the right superior oblique and vice versa (Figure 1-2). The nucleus is ventrally bordered by the medial longitudinal fasciculus. The proximity of these structures predisposes to a syndrome of trochlear palsy with an internuclear ophthalmoplegia from lesions in the lower midbrain tegmentum.

Axons emanating from the trochlear nucleus arc laterally and dorsally into the tectum of the midbrain, where they cross the midline. These decussated fibers emerge beneath the inferior colliculus at the medial border of the brachium conjuctivum as CN-IV. The primary (central) neurons of the pupillary sympathetic chain pass through the midbrain in the central tegmental tract en route to the ciliospinal center of Budge-Waller.

CN-IV completely decussates and exits the brainstem from its dorsal aspect, a unique site among CNs. It enters the orbit via the superior orbital fissure and innervates the superior oblique muscle, which depresses the eye in adduction and intorts the eye.

CLINICAL PRESENTATION

Patients with trochlear palsy have impaired ability to depress the eye on the involved side, a hypertropia. Worse when the eye is in downward or medial gaze or when the head is inclined toward the side of palsy, it emphasizes the weakness of the depressor function of the superior oblique.

With a superior oblique palsy, head tilt toward the palsied side emphasizes the rotary component of the diplopia, magnifying the hypertropia because superior rectus action is unopposed. This pattern of incomitant strabismus is summarized as "hypertropia worse with gaze away and with tilt toward the affected side."

Patients with CN-IV palsy often adopt a secondary torticollis, offering a diagnostic clue. "The tilting of the head lowers the image on the side toward which the head is tilted ... so that the twin images are brought to the same level, and moreover it corrects the obliquity of the false image by inclining with it."* Because this posture minimizes the visual consequences of a CN-IV palsy, congenital CN-IV palsies are often undiagnosed for decades. Patients may have a diagnosis in adulthood after asthenopia or intermittent diplopia develops or when they seek treatment for torticollis. The characteristic head tilt in childhood photographs often confirms the congenital nature of the palsy.

---

*Duke-Elder, pages 4047-4048.

CRANIAL NERVE IV: TROCHLEAR

Figure 7-1A

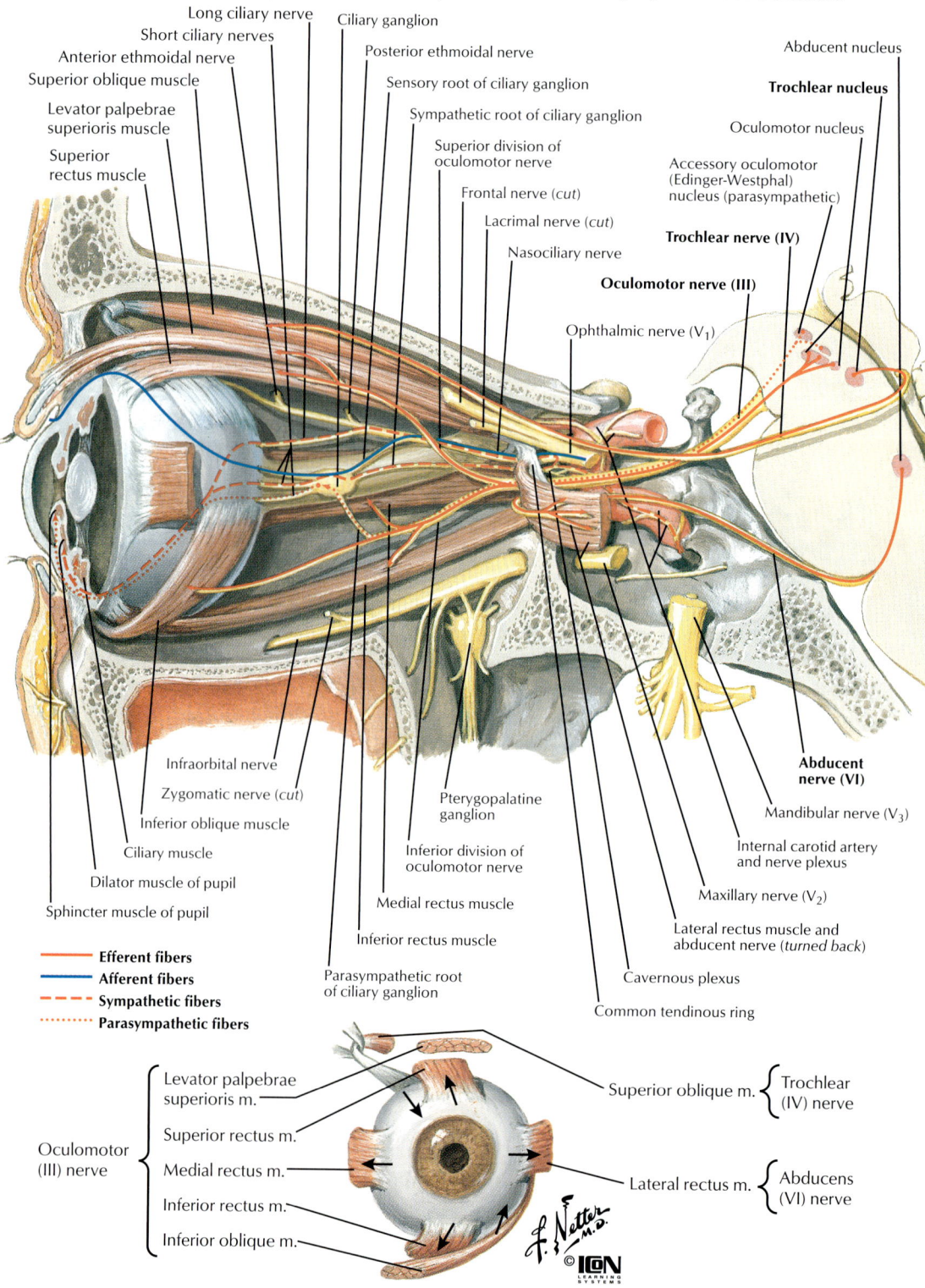

Oculomotor (III), Trochlear (IV), and Abducent (VI) Nerves: Schema

Neuro-ophthalmology

CRANIAL NERVE IV: TROCHLEAR

Figure 7-1B

Nerves of Orbit

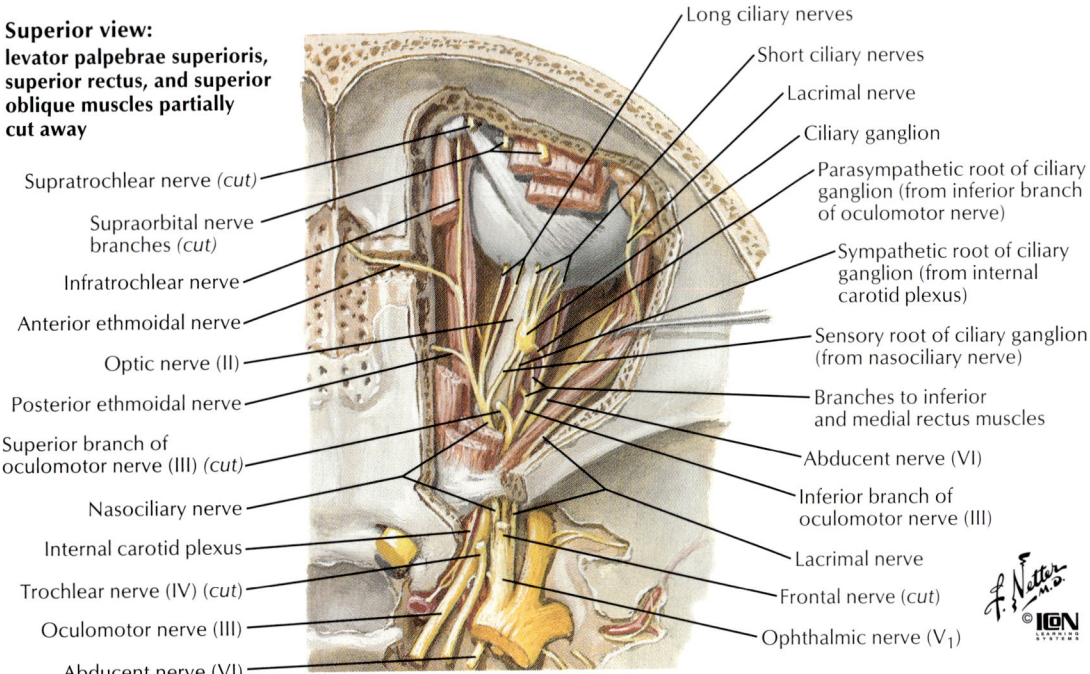

Superior view

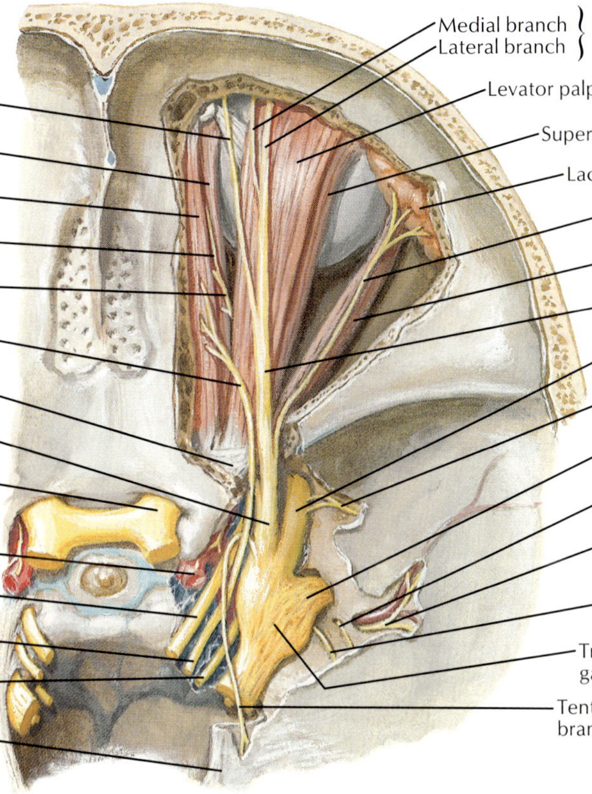

Supratrochlear nerve, Medial rectus muscle, Superior oblique muscle, Infratrochlear nerve, Nasociliary nerve, Trochlear nerve (IV), Common tendinous ring, Ophthalmic nerve (V₁), Optic nerve (II), Internal carotid artery and nerve plexus, Oculomotor nerve (III), Trochlear nerve (IV), Abducent nerve (VI), Tentorium cerebelli

Medial branch / Lateral branch — Supraorbital nerve, Levator palpebrae superioris muscle, Superior rectus muscle, Lacrimal gland, Lacrimal nerve, Lateral rectus muscle, Frontal nerve, Maxillary nerve (V₂), Meningeal branch of maxillary nerve, Mandibular nerve (V₃), Lesser petrosal nerve, Meningeal branch of mandibular nerve, Greater petrosal nerve, Trigeminal (semilunar) ganglion, Tentorial nerve (meningeal) branch of ophthalmic nerve

Superior view: levator palpebrae superioris, superior rectus, and superior oblique muscles partially cut away

Supratrochlear nerve (cut), Supraorbital nerve branches (cut), Infratrochlear nerve, Anterior ethmoidal nerve, Optic nerve (II), Posterior ethmoidal nerve, Superior branch of oculomotor nerve (III) (cut), Nasociliary nerve, Internal carotid plexus, Trochlear nerve (IV) (cut), Oculomotor nerve (III), Abducent nerve (VI)

Long ciliary nerves, Short ciliary nerves, Lacrimal nerve, Ciliary ganglion, Parasympathetic root of ciliary ganglion (from inferior branch of oculomotor nerve), Sympathetic root of ciliary ganglion (from internal carotid plexus), Sensory root of ciliary ganglion (from nasociliary nerve), Branches to inferior and medial rectus muscles, Abducent nerve (VI), Inferior branch of oculomotor nerve (III), Lacrimal nerve, Frontal nerve (cut), Ophthalmic nerve (V₁)

Neuro-ophthalmology

CRANIAL NERVE IV: TROCHLEAR

DIFFERENTIAL DIAGNOSIS

Midbrain Lesions

Traumatic unilateral and bilateral CN-IV palsies are frequently encountered. A high frontal impact creates contrecoup forces causing a traction injury at the origin of the nerves or a contusion injury of the tectum against the cerebellar tentorium. MRI demonstration of tectal subarachnoid hematoma in a traumatic trochlear palsy supports this theory. Similar force directions can be generated by deceleration in falls when the victim incurs occipital impact, or with coccygeal impact transmitted up a straight spinal column. The amount of force needed to produce traumatic CN-IV palsy seems variable.

Although an acquired trochlear palsy after minor head trauma prompts suspicion of an undiagnosed mass lesion, producing a "pathologic" palsy in an already damaged nerve, clinical experience includes patients with acquired CN-IV palsies who had relatively minor trauma but no preexisting pathology. CN-IV palsy has occurred in benign intracranial hypertension and after lumbar puncture—presumably due to tractional mechanisms—both with CN-VI coinvolvement, and in spontaneous intracranial hypotension with CN-III coinvolvement.

A lesion interrupting both the predecussation trochlear fasciculus and the ipsilateral sympathetics within the tectum produces an ipsilateral Horner syndrome with crossed CN-IV palsy. The confluence of the 2 trochlear fasciculi at their decussation provides a locus wherein a single lesion may produce bilateral trochlear palsies with the seeming paradox of no head tilt. These patients demonstrate a left hypertropia on right gaze and left head tilt, and right hypertropia on left gaze and right head tilt. They may adopt a chin-down head tilt. Various pathologies at the inferior dorsal midbrain cause bilateral CN-IV palsies.

Trochlear Nerve Lesions

After emerging below the corpora quadrigemina, CN-IV sweeps around the brainstem toward its ventral aspect, situated lateral and inferior to CN-III. After a distance of 75 mm, CN-IV enters the dura below the CN-III entrance, coming to the cavernous sinus via its lateral wall. At the superior orbital fissure, CN-IV courses superolaterally to the oculomotor nerve, entering the orbit.

Perhaps because of their relatively fixed location within the lateral wall of the cavernous sinus, the trochlear and trigeminal nerves can be injured concomitantly. Patients with a posteriorly draining carotid-cavernous fistula sometimes present with painful superior oblique dysfunction, presumably due to local cavernous distention.

DIAGNOSTIC APPROACH AND TREATMENT

A diagnosis is made when the characteristic pattern of worsening hypertropia in downward gaze, contralateral gaze, and ipsilateral head tilt is discovered. In patients with other CN coinvolvement, neuroimaging is required.

Patients with isolated CN-IV palsies may be observed for spontaneous improvement over 3 to 4 months, especially if the history indicates a likely etiology (trauma or known diabetes). Nonresolution over time usually prompts imaging unless congenital CN-IV palsy is strongly suggested by history and examination findings (eg, vertical fusional amplitude greater than 4 diopters).

Therapy may include the use of prismatic glasses to shift "second images" to line up with primary images, eliminating diplopia. However, the utility of prismatic glasses in CN-IV palsy is limited because only 1 prismatic strength can be ground into the spectacles, but different strengths are needed for different gazes. Many patients prefer strabismic surgical treatment of nonresolving palsies; it offers greater range of gaze without diplopia.

REFERENCES

Duke-Elder WS. *Neurology of Vision: Motor and Optical Anomalies.* St Louis, Mo: CV Mosby; 1949. Duke-Elder WS. *Text-book of Ophthalmology;* vol 4.

Jacobson DM, Warner JJ, Choucair AK, Ptacek LJ. Trochlear nerve palsy following minor head trauma: a sign of structural disorder. *J Clin Neuroophthalmol.* 1988;8:263-268.

Miller NR, Newman NJ, eds. *Walsh and Hoyt's Clinical Neuroophthalmology.* 5th ed. Baltimore, Md: Williams & Wilkins; 1998.

Chapter 8
Cranial Nerve VI: Abducens

Ippolit C. A. Matjucha

Clinical Vignette

A 78-year-old Asian-born woman was admitted to the hospital for worsening mentation and gait problems. Neuroimaging and initial eye examination results were negative. The patient became only partially responsive to verbal commands. A treating physician then noted that one eye no longer abducted normally; hours later, the patient could not abduct either eye, and fundus examination showed bilateral papilledema.

Lumbar puncture revealed markedly high intracranial pressure and chemical and cellular abnormalities of the CSF consistent with tubercular meningitis.

The sixth cranial nerve (CN-VI), similar to CN-IV, innervates a single extraocular muscle, the lateral rectus, which is the primary abductor for the eyes. Patients with CN-VI paresis have an inward deviation of the affected eye, a noncomitant esotropia. Temporal eye movement beyond midline is lost or reduced.

Patients with abducens palsies, especially partial and mild palsies, sometimes adopt a head turn toward the affected side to minimize diplopia by keeping the eye adducted. In more severe palsies, this strategy often fails or is uncomfortable given the large turn required, so patients present with one eye shut, patched, or covered.

The vignette at the beginning of this chapter of bilateral abducens nerve palsies is typical of leptomeningeal pathology, likely due to increased intracranial pressure. However, treatable chronic granulomatous inflammatory processes sometimes deserve consideration also.

ABDUCENS NUCLEUS

The CN-VI nucleus, located just beneath the facial colliculi in the inferior pons is enveloped by the turning CN-VII fascicular fibers of the facial genu and contains two physiologically—but not topographically—distinct groups of neurons (Figure 8-1). One group innervates the ipsilateral lateral rectus; the other sends axons across the midline to the contralateral medial longitudinal fasciculus (MLF). These latter axons ascend in the MLF to the ventral nucleus of the contralateral CN-III nuclear complex. These internuclear neurons control the near-simultaneous stimulation of the contralateral medial rectus during ipsilateral abducens nerve stimulation to produce lateral horizontal gaze.

ABDUCENS FASCICULUS

From its position laterally abutting the paramedian pontine reticular formation, the CN-VI nucleus first sends its motor afferents medially toward the MLF and then ventrally, passing through the paramedian pontine reticular formation and the undecussated corticospinal tract to reach the ventral surface of the brainstem at the inferior lip of the pons.

On exiting the ventral pons, the abducens nerve ascends between the pons and the clivus within the subarachanoid pontine cistern. After it enters the dura, CN-VI continues up the clivus to the posterior clinoid. It travels over the petrous ridge to lie beneath the inferior petrosal sinus and then enters the cavernous sinus via the Dorello canal, just medial to the Meckel cave, which houses the gasserian ganglion.

After CN-VI is within the cavernous sinus, it passes forward, adjacent to the internal lateral aspect of the carotid artery. Here, it likely, albeit briefly, carries the majority of the sympathetic axons to innervate the pupil. More anteriorly, the abducens passes these neurons onto the ophthalmic nerve to follow its nasociliary branch to the ciliary ganglion; the sympathetic fibers pass through the ganglion without synapse, entering

CRANIAL NERVE VI: ABDUCENS

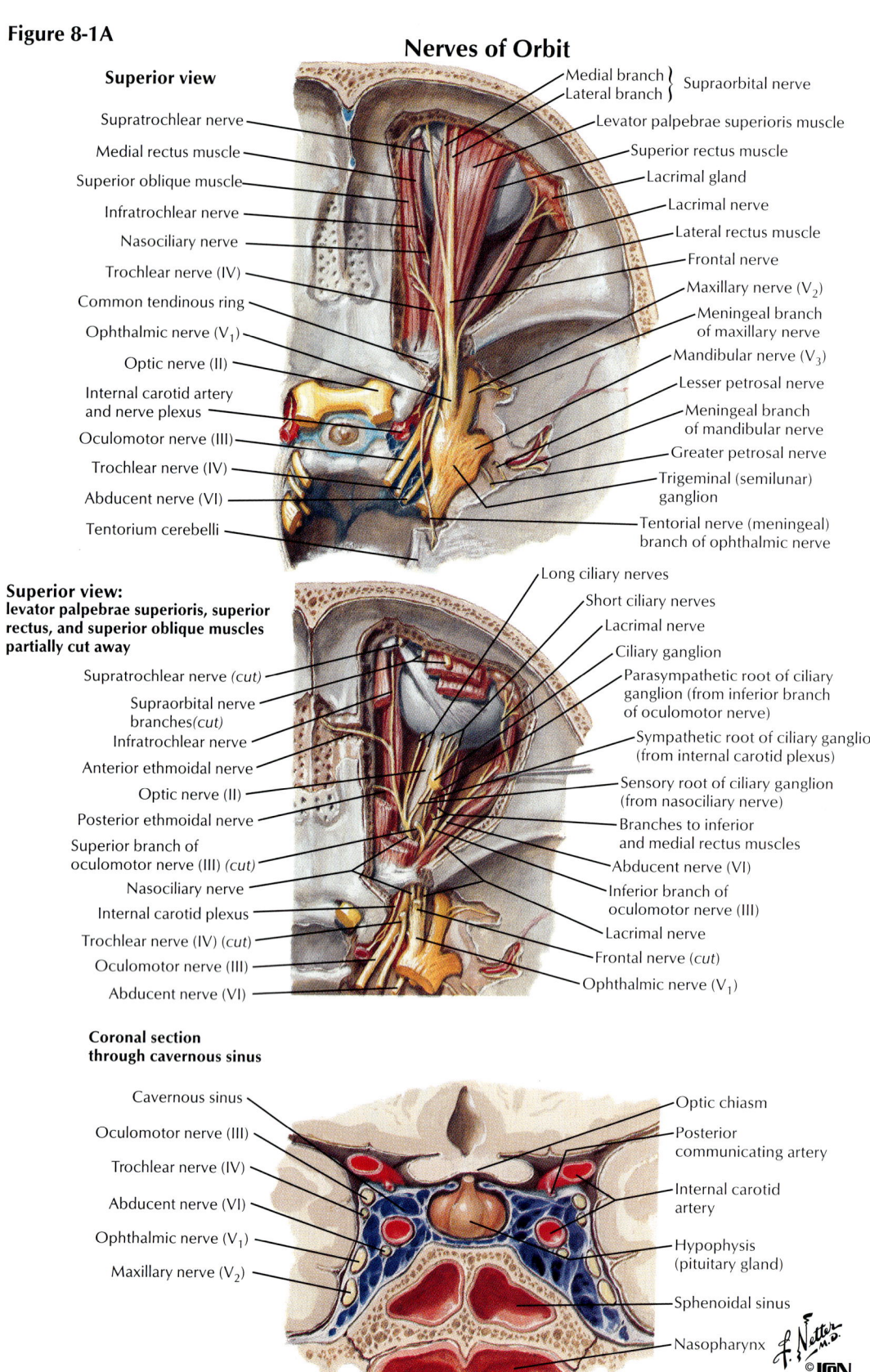

CRANIAL NERVE VI: ABDUCENS

Figure 8-1B   Central Control of Eye Movements

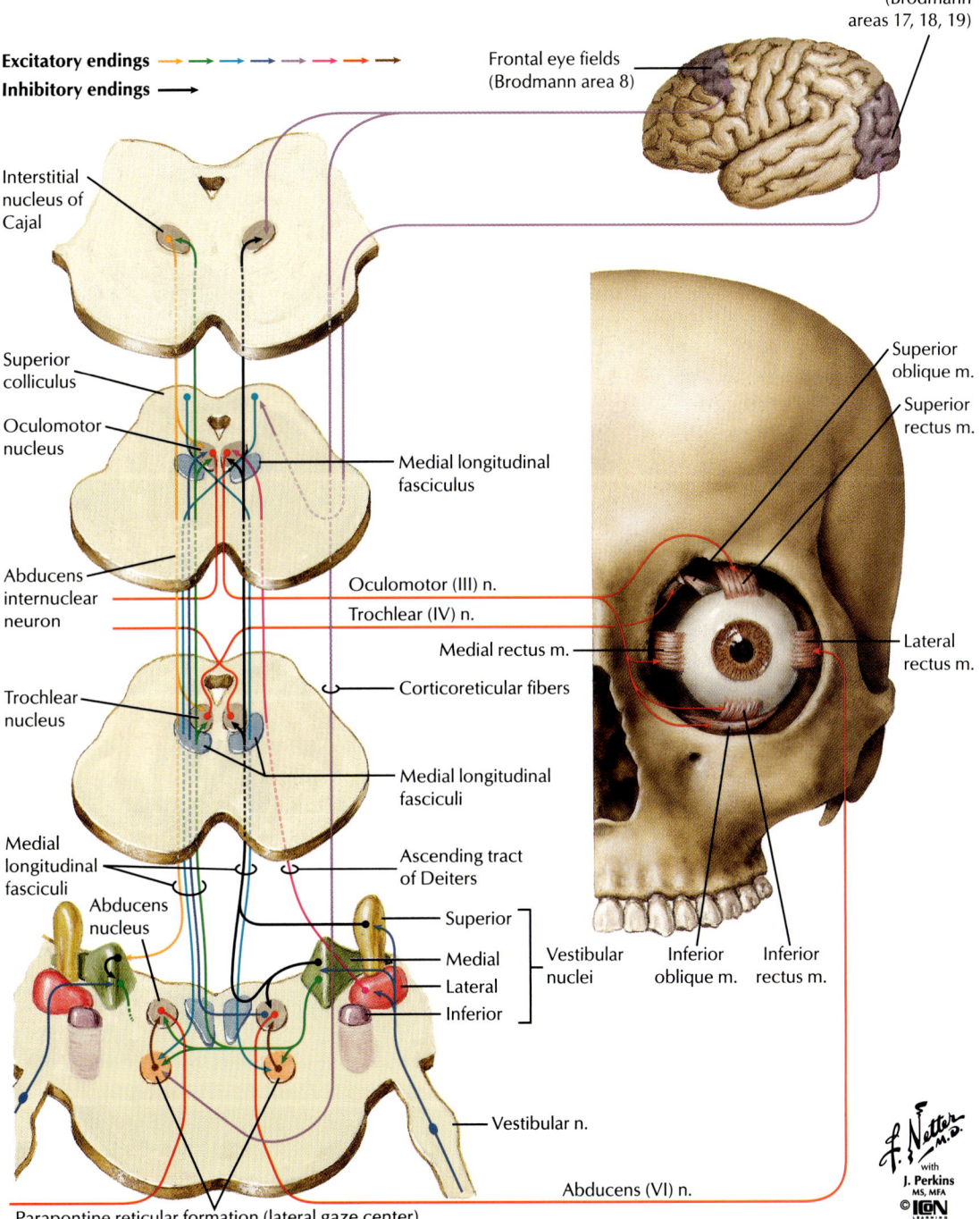

NEURO-OPHTHALMOLOGY

CRANIAL NERVE VI: ABDUCENS

the eye via the short ciliary nerves. Additional sympathetic fibers bypass the ciliary ganglion, entering the eye as the long ciliary nerves.

CLINICAL PRESENTATION

Primary nuclear CN-VI lesions typically have concomitant ipsilateral facial nerve involvement.

Interestingly, clinical lesions of the CN-VI nucleus do not result in isolated ipsilateral lateral rectus dysfunction. Instead, because there are 2 functionally separate types of neurons within the abducens nucleus, an ipsilateral gaze palsy develops, with inability to move both eyes to the affected side. This gaze palsy occurs because lesions involving the CN-VI nucleus affect neurons headed for the lateral rectus and the contralateral third nerve nucleus via the MLF.

Larger lesions affecting the CN-VI nucleus and the ipsilateral MLF interrupt the crossed internuclear neurons from the opposite CN-VI nucleus, with consequent inability to adduct the ipsilateral eye in horizontal gaze. This combined lesion produces the Fisher "one-and-a-half" syndrome: ipsilateral gaze palsy and internuclear ophthalmoplegia. As with other internuclear ophthalmoplegia variants, it can be distinguished from syndromes produced by true adduction palsy because patients maintain the ability to adduct both eyes for near stimulus (convergence). Convergence is spared in internuclear ophthalmoplegia because neither the upper midbrain pathways producing convergence nor CN-III is affected.

DIFFERENTIAL DIAGNOSIS
Arterial Vascular Syndromes

Paramedian basilar artery branch occlusion causes infarction of the medial and ventral structures of the inferior pons, producing ipsilateral gaze palsy (paramedian pontine reticular formation involvement), hemifacial paralysis (CN-VII), limb ataxia and nystagmus (involvement of middle cerebellar peduncle and possibly vestibular nuclei efferents), crossed paralysis (corticospinal tract), and crossed tactile hypesthesia (medial lemniscus). More focal lesions may produce **Raymond syndrome** (abduction palsy and crossed hemiplegia) from abducens fascicular injury at the corticospinal tract, whereas similar lesions with some lateral extension also involve the facial fasciculus, adding ipsilateral facial palsy to the presentation (**Millard-Gubler syndrome**).

Anterior inferior cerebellar artery occlusion typically produces more lateral damage characteristically to the vestibular nuclei, the auditory nerve, CN-VII, the paramedian pontine reticular formation, the spinothalamic tract, and the middle cerebellar peduncle and possibly extending dorsally to the cerebellar hemisphere and rostrally to the CN-V nucleus. The combined deficits produce a lateral inferior pontine syndrome of nystagmus (with beats or fast phase directed ipsilaterally), vertigo, gaze palsy, facial paralysis and hypesthesia, deafness, and ataxia, all with crossed analgesia.

Foville syndrome develops within this same territory. It is characterized by gaze or abducens palsy (CN-VI nucleus or fasciculus) with ipsilateral dysgeusia (nucleus of the tractus solitarius), facial analgesia (spinal tract of CN-V), Horner syndrome (central tegmental tract), and deafness (auditory nerve).

CN-VI, the carotid artery, and sympathetic pupil fibers are situated closely within the cavernous sinus, accounting for another syndrome. The expanding artery of **intracavernous carotid dissection** or **aneurysm** compresses the abducens nerve and the sympathetic fibers within the cavernous sinus, producing painful abducens palsy with ipsilateral Horner syndrome. Other pathologic processes within this region sometimes produce a similar clinical picture.

Other CN-VI Lesions

Processes that affect the anterior midline brain stem also deserve consideration in the differential diagnosis, including various posterior fossa tumors or inflammatory processes that affect the abducens nerve during its ascent of the clivus. Tumors such as chordoma that favor the midline skull base and grow slowly occasionally present as isolated or bilateral CN-VI palsy. Other tumors requiring consideration include meningiomas, chondrosarcomas, eosinophilic granulomas, nasopharyngeal carcinoma, and metastases. Although all these tumors may produce isolated CN-VI palsies, most often, they produce additional neurologic deficits.

Gradenigo syndrome is characterized by a painful abducens palsy resulting from mastoiditis and petrositis complicating chronic otitis media. The infectious process erodes the bone, affecting the abducens nerve and the gasserian ganglion; CN-VII is sometimes also involved as it passes through the mastoid bone en route to the stylomastoid foramen. A combined trigeminal-abducens-facial nerve syndrome can be produced by other entities, particularly tumors, that affect this region.

Unilateral or bilateral CN-VI palsy is also commonly recognized as a **false localizing sign** in patients with **increased intracranial pressure**, whether idiopathic or from tumor. A tumor distant from CN-VI can produce abducens palsies if intracranial pressure is increased sufficiently. The sharp turn of CN-VI across the petrous ridge may make it vulnerable. As the brain begins to cause downward brainstem herniation, CN-VI is stretched and loses function, perhaps from compressive ischemia. Similarly, downward shift of the pons in relation to the petrous ridge is thought to account for CN-VI palsies sometimes seen in intracranial hypotension, whether of spontaneous or post–lumbar puncture origin.

REFERENCES

Lyle DJ. *Neuro-ophthalmology*. Springfield, Ill.: Charles C Thomas; 1945.

Rizzo JF, Lessell S, eds. Neuro-ophthalmology. In: Albert DM, Jakobiec FA. *Principles and Practice of Ophthalmology*. Vol 4. Section XI. Philadelphia, Pa: WB Saunders; 1994:2387-2712.

Victor M, Ropper AH. *Adam's and Victor's Principles of Neurology*. 7th ed. New York, NY: McGraw-Hill; 2001.

Section III
CRANIAL NERVES

Chapter 9
Cranial Nerve I: Olfactory 96

Chapter 10
Cranial Nerve V: Trigeminal 101

Chapter 11
Cranial Nerve VII: Facial 112

Chapter 12
Cranial Nerve VIII: Vestibular 126

Chapter 13
Cranial Nerve VIII: Auditory 134

Chapter 14
**Cranial Nerve IX: Glossopharyngeal, and
Cranial Nerve X, Vagus: Swallowing** 143

Chapter 15
Cranial Nerve X, Vagus: Voice Disorders 153

Chapter 16
Cranial Nerve XI: Spinal Accessory 157

Chapter 17
Cranial Nerve XII: Hypoglossal 163

Chapter 9
Cranial Nerve I: Olfactory

Michal Vytopil and H. Royden Jones, Jr

Clinical Vignette

A 68-year-old widower reported to his girlfriend that he had been having difficulty smelling food for a few months. He was uncertain about the nature of the onset of this difficulty. His family had noted personality changes, especially disinhibition, although he denied it. He had no headaches, changes in vision, or seizures. He was no longer speaking with 2 of his 3 children.

Neurologic examination results demonstrated anosmia. His behavior was inappropriate, with almost complete fixation on sexual desires, stating that he wanted someone to help him so he could participate in such during most of his waking hours. However, his Mini-Mental Status Examination results were normal, he had no papilledema or optic atrophy, and his gait was normal, as was the remainder of the results of a complete neurologic examination.

Brain MRI demonstrated a large olfactory groove meningioma (Figure 9-1). The patient went to a neurosurgeon, who elected to observe the tumor; it did not change in size over a 2-year period.

The patient never regained his sense of smell, his behavior became increasingly inappropriate, and he declined neuropsychologic evaluation to determine whether he had cognitive impairment. His family began calling into question seemingly inappropriate financial decisions.

Although the benign neoplasm in this vignette had likely been present for years, it was not discovered until the patient became aware of his inability to smell. Family strife resulted from behavioral changes that were possibly related to the subfrontal tumor. Nevertheless, this previously astute individual functioned independently and adamantly declined further investigation except semi-annual neurologic visits to monitor tumor size.

The olfactory nerve (CN-I) provides the sense of smell. It is an important warning system because it enables identification of spoiled foods or noxious chemicals. Moreover, it significantly contributes to quality of life because it is largely responsible for many desirable sensations, such as food and beverage flavors. Unfortunately, many neurologists think of olfactory function testing (chapter 1) as somewhat redundant, and consequently, it is seldom performed adequately. Neglecting to perform smell evaluation may compromise rare patients. Occasional serious but treatable conditions, most notably olfactory groove meningiomas, may present with CN-I compromise as their first symptom.

When identifying odors, humans rely on volatile substances entering their nasal cavity to excite receptors. *Olfactory receptor cells* are bipolar sensory neurons whose dendrites form a delicate sensory carpet on the superior aspect of the nasal cavity (Figure 9-2). The thin, unmyelinated axons of the bipolar sensory cells collectively form CN-I and travel through the cribriform plate into the olfactory bulb at the base of the fronto-orbital lobe. Within the bulb, CN-I fibers synapse with the dendrites of the large mitral cells, whose axons constitute the olfactory tract passing along the base of the frontal lobe and projecting directly into the primary olfactory cortex in the temporal lobe without connecting to a thalamic nucleus (Figure 9-3). Although this may seem like an aberration to sensory connections, the direct relay to the limbic structures of the brain may have served an evolutionary function in lower animals and, later, primates. In humans, the primary olfactory cortex includes the uncus, hippocampal gyrus, amygdaloid complex, and entorhinal cortex.

CRANIAL NERVE I: OLFACTORY

Figure 9-1   **Subfrontal Meningioma**

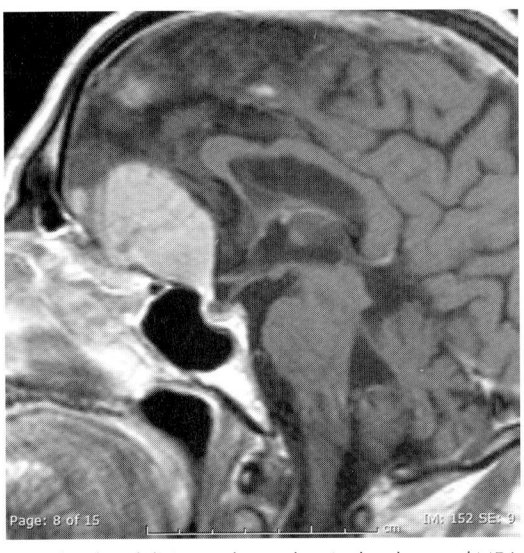
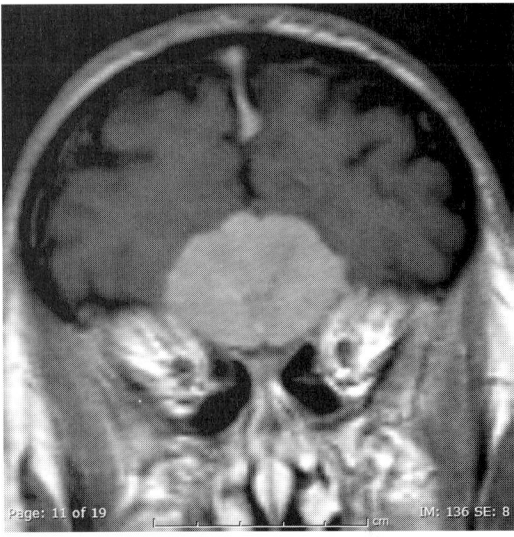

T1-weighted, gadolinium-enhanced sagittal and coronal MR images show a large enhancing mass on the skull base displacing and compressing the olfactory apparatus.

DIFFERENTIAL DIAGNOSIS

The sense of smell can be disrupted at any site along the olfactory pathway. Therefore, an olfactory impairment is not necessarily equivalent to a CN-I lesion. Several relatively common conditions that spare CN-I create various olfactory disturbances, including upper respiratory infections, nasal sinus disease, and, less frequently, damage to olfactory bulb, tract, or cortex.

Disturbances of smell are congenital or acquired, with the latter being more common. Although most olfactory dysfunctions occur bilaterally, unilateral anosmia is an important sign that should prompt MRI to exclude an olfactory groove tumor.

Congenital Disorder

In **Kallmann syndrome**, anosmia results from congenital hypoplasia of olfactory lobes and occurs in conjunction with hypogonadotropic hypogonadism. Most cases are sporadic, but familial cases have been reported suggesting various inheritances: X linked, autosomal dominant, or autosomal recessive. Some of the responsible genes have been identified. There is a strong predilection for males, even in sporadic and autosomal forms. In addition to the isolated primary olfactory form, Kallmann syndrome may be associated with other congenital deficits, such as cleft palate, lip/dental agenesis, and neural hearing loss.

Acquired Disorders

Together, **upper respiratory infection** and **nasal** and **paranasal sinus disease** account for more than 40% of olfactory disturbances and are the most frequent causes. These intranasal processes mechanically prevent volatile chemical stimuli from reaching the olfactory sensory epithelium and activating the receptors. Because they do not lead to direct damage to the CN-I pathways, they are called *transport* or *conductive olfactory disorders*. The high frequency of conductive disorders underscores the necessity for thorough otorhinolaryngologic evaluations in patients with an olfactory dysfunction.

Head trauma is responsible for approximately 20% of all cases of smell disturbances via direct damage to CN-I or the frontobasal cerebral cortex associated with olfaction. The incidence of

CRANIAL NERVE I: OLFACTORY

Figure 9-2

Olfactory Receptors

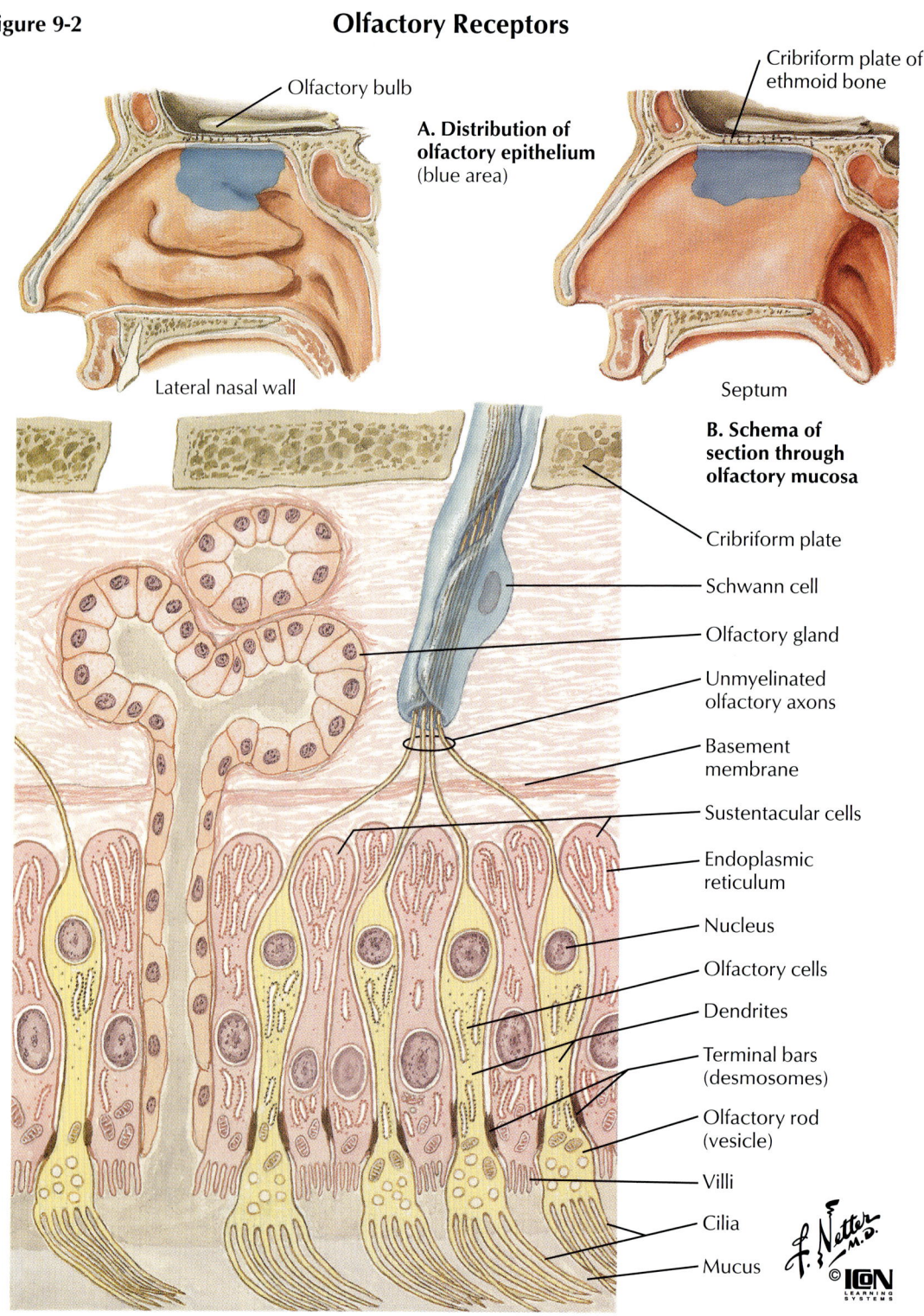

CRANIAL NERVE I: OLFACTORY

Figure 9-3   Olfactory Pathways

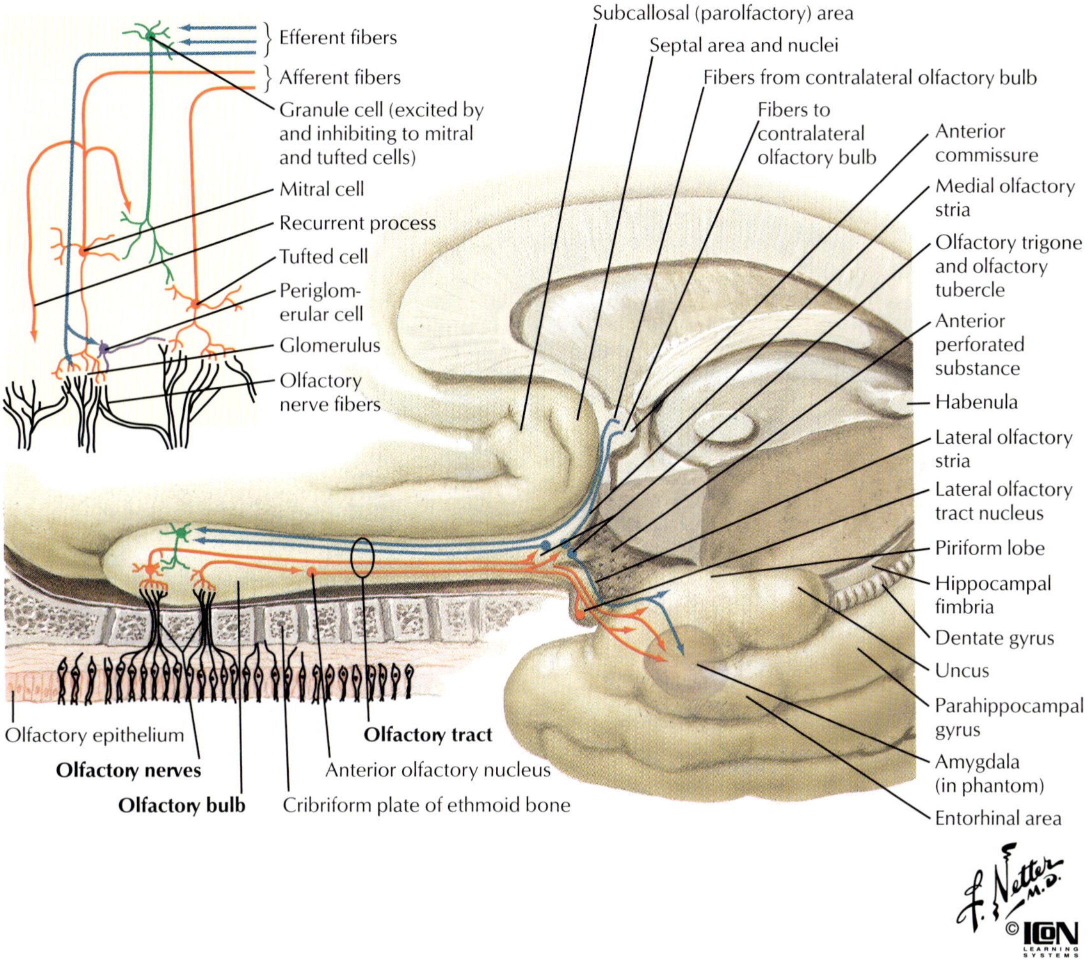

anosmia after head trauma is approximately 7% to 30%, depending on injury severity. Olfactory dysfunction after head trauma can present as unilateral or bilateral anosmia or hyposmia. It is hypothesized that most olfactory dysfunctions in blunt head trauma result from shearing of CN-I as it passes through the cribriform plate. Hence, occipital and side blows are more dangerous to olfaction than are frontal ones. More substantial damage, such as contusion of the olfactory bulb or cortical and subcortical olfactory areas, may occur in severe head traumas with anterior fossa fracture.

The average life span of olfactory receptor neurons is 30 days; they are continuously replaced by fresh cells growing into the olfactory sensory nerve. Recovery eventually occurs in some but not all individuals.

Olfactory groove meningiomas are rare but may result in significant morbidity unless diagnosed and treated early. Usually slow growing, they represent 8% to 18% of all intracranial meningiomas. Although unilateral or bilateral olfactory dysfunction is thought to be their first symptom, few patients present with disturbances in their sense of smell, probably because of a slow and orderly growth with resultant gradual decline in olfactory function. Moreover, because most meningiomas are unilateral and cause olfactory loss confined to the ipsilateral side, patients retain olfactory function on the contralateral side and are usually unaware of any loss.

CRANIAL NERVES

Consequently, most cases are not diagnosed until the tumor is large enough to cause other symptoms resulting from pressure on the frontal lobes and optic tracts, such as headache, visual disturbances, personality changes, and memory impairment. Therefore, early diagnosis of olfactory meningiomas remains challenging, and most tumors, as in the vignette, become relatively large (eg, >4 cm in diameter) at diagnosis.

An olfactory groove tumor, most often a meningioma, may rarely result in the **Foster-Kennedy syndrome**, characterized by unilateral optic atrophy and contralateral papilledema. Optic atrophy results from direct pressure of the neoplasm on the optic nerve, whereas increased intracranial pressure produces contralateral papilledema.

Other Entities

Normal **aging** is associated with a progressive decline in the ability to appreciate and discriminate odors.

Hallucinations of smell, although not disorders of CN-I, are important in differential diagnosis of an olfactory dysfunction. They can present in psychiatric conditions (depression, psychosis), as part of alcohol withdrawal syndrome, or in complex partial epilepsy (chapter 25). In the latter, hallucinations are called **uncinate crises**, are almost invariably of foul character, and often accompany symptoms typical for focal temporal lobe epilepsy, including staring and various automatisms.

Some **neurodegenerative disorders** are associated with an impaired sense of smell: Parkinson disease, Alzheimer disease, Huntington disease, and, inexplicably, motor neuron disease.

Olfactory discrimination can also be adversely affected by many **medications** and **drugs**, including opiates (codeine, morphine), antiepileptic drugs (carbamazepine, phenytoin), and immunosuppressive agents, that, similar to radiation, disrupt the physiologic turnover of receptor cells.

Abuse of cocaine via intranasal snorting may lead to septal perforation and direct trauma to CN-I.

REFERENCES

De Kruijk JR, Leffers P, Menheere PP, et al. Olfactory function after mild traumatic brain injury. *Brain Inj.* 2003;17:73-78.

Dode C, Levilliers J, Dupont JM, et al. Loss-of-function mutations in FGFR1 cause autosomal dominant Kallmann syndrome. *Nat Genet.* 2003;33:463-465.

Doty R. Olfaction. *Annu Rev Psychol.* 2001;52:423-452.

Doty RL, Yousem DM, Pham LT, et al. Olfactory dysfunction in patients with head trauma. *Arch Neurol.* 1997;54:1131-1140.

Finelli PF, Mair R. Disturbances of taste and smell. In: Bradley WG, Daroff RB, Fenichel GM, Marsden CD, eds. *Neurology in Clinical Practice: Principles of Diagnosis and Management.* 2nd ed. Boston, Mass: Butterworth-Heinemann; 1996:243-250.

Green P, Rohling ML, Iverson GL, et al. Relationships between olfactory discrimination and head injury severity. *Brain Inj.* 2003;17:479-496.

Rubin G, Ben David U, Gornish M, et al. Meningiomas of the anterior cranial fossa floor: review of 67 cases. *Acta Neurochir (Wien).* 1994;129:26-30.

Sweeney PJ, Hanson MR. The cranial neuropathies. In: Bradley WG, Daroff RB, Fenichel GM, Marsden CD, eds. *Neurology in Clinical Practice: Principles of Diagnosis and Management.* 2nd ed. Boston, Mass: Butterworth-Heinemann; 1996:1721-1732.

Turetsky BI, Moberg PJ, Yousem DM, et al. Reduced olfactory bulb volume in patients with schizophrenia. *Am J Psychiatry.* 2000;157:828-830.

Welge-Luessen A, Temmel A, Quint C, et al. Olfactory function in patients with olfactory groove meningioma. *J Neurol Neurosurg Psychiatry.* 2001;70:218-221.

Chapter 10
Cranial Nerve V: Trigeminal

Michal Vytopil and Edward Tarlov

ANATOMY

The trigeminal cranial nerve (CN-V) has 3 major divisions: ophthalmic, maxillary, and mandibular (Figures 10-1 and 10-2). CN-V is the major sensory nerve of the face, mouth, and nasal cavity. It also supplies motor and proprioceptive fibers to the muscles involved in chewing. It has a complex course originating within the pons from 2 nuclei, a large sensory and smaller motor give rise to sensory and motor roots that emerge from the midlateral pons. Both roots continue toward the trigeminal ganglion on the bottom of the middle cranial fossa, where the general sensory fibers have their cell bodies. Distal to the ganglion, the 3 sensory divisions exit the cranium through the superior orbital fissure, foramen rotundum, and foramen ovale. The motor component passes through the trigeminal ganglion and accompanies the mandibular division.

CN-V Nuclei

The **motor nucleus** is located in the mid pons, medial to the large sensory nucleus. The **sensory nucleus** is the largest, begins rostrally within the midbrain, and extends caudally through the pons and medulla into the second segment of the cervical spinal cord (Figure 10-3). It is subdivided into 3 portions. The mesencephalic portion contains cell bodies of sensory fibers carrying proprioceptive information from the masticatory muscles. The pontine trigeminal portion, also called the *principal sensory nucleus*, is thought to receive only tactile stimuli and, therefore, to subserve exclusively light touch. The spinal tract nucleus is considered primarily to relay pain and temperature.

Principal Sensory Component

The sensory component of CN-V conveys general sensation from the facial skin and scalp to the top of the head, tragus of the ear, and anterior wall of the external auditory meatus. Also, it provides general sensation from the mouth, including the tongue and teeth, nasal and paranasal sinuses, and meninges of the anterior and middle cranial fossae.

Trigeminal Ganglion

The cell bodies of almost all sensory CN-V fibers, with the exception of proprioceptive fibers, are located within the trigeminal ganglion. The ganglion sits in a depression, a **Meckel cave**, on the floor of the middle cranial fossa. Central processes of neuronal cell bodies constitute the large sensory root that enters the pons and projects into the pontine trigeminal and spinal tract nuclei. Peripheral processes divide into the 3 sensory divisions that exit the skull.

Sensory Divisions

The **ophthalmic division** collects touch, pain, temperature, and proprioceptive information from the upper third of the face, adjacent sinuses, and scalp regions. These nerve branches course posteriorly in the orbit toward the superior orbital fissure, where they enter the skull.

The **maxillary division** carries sensory information from the skin overlying the maxilla, side of the forehead, medial cheek, and side of the nose, upper lip, palate, upper teeth, nasopharynx, and meninges of the anterior and middle cranial fossae.

The **mandibular division** primarily provides sensory innervation for the skin overlying the lower jaw (with the exception of the angle of the jaw innervated by the second and third cervical nerves), cheeks, chin and lower lip, mucous membrane of the mouth, gums, inferior teeth, anterior two thirds of the tongue, side of the head, anterior wall of the external auditory meatus, external wall of the tympanic membrane, and temporomandibular joint.

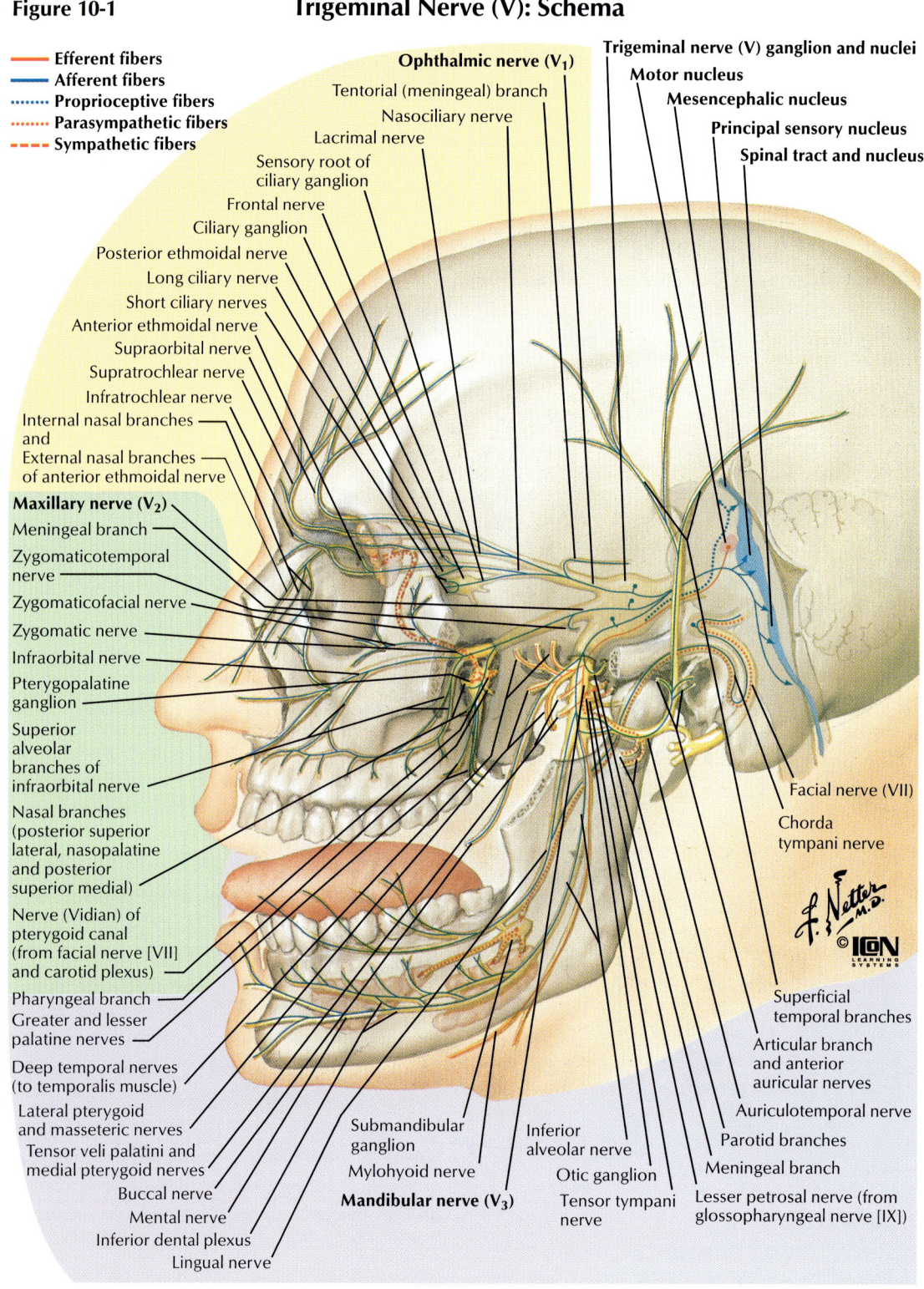

CRANIAL NERVE V: TRIGEMINAL

Figure 10-1

Trigeminal Nerve (V): Schema

CRANIAL NERVE V: TRIGEMINAL

Figure 10-2A   Ophthalmic (V$_1$) and Maxillary (V$_2$) Nerves Sensory

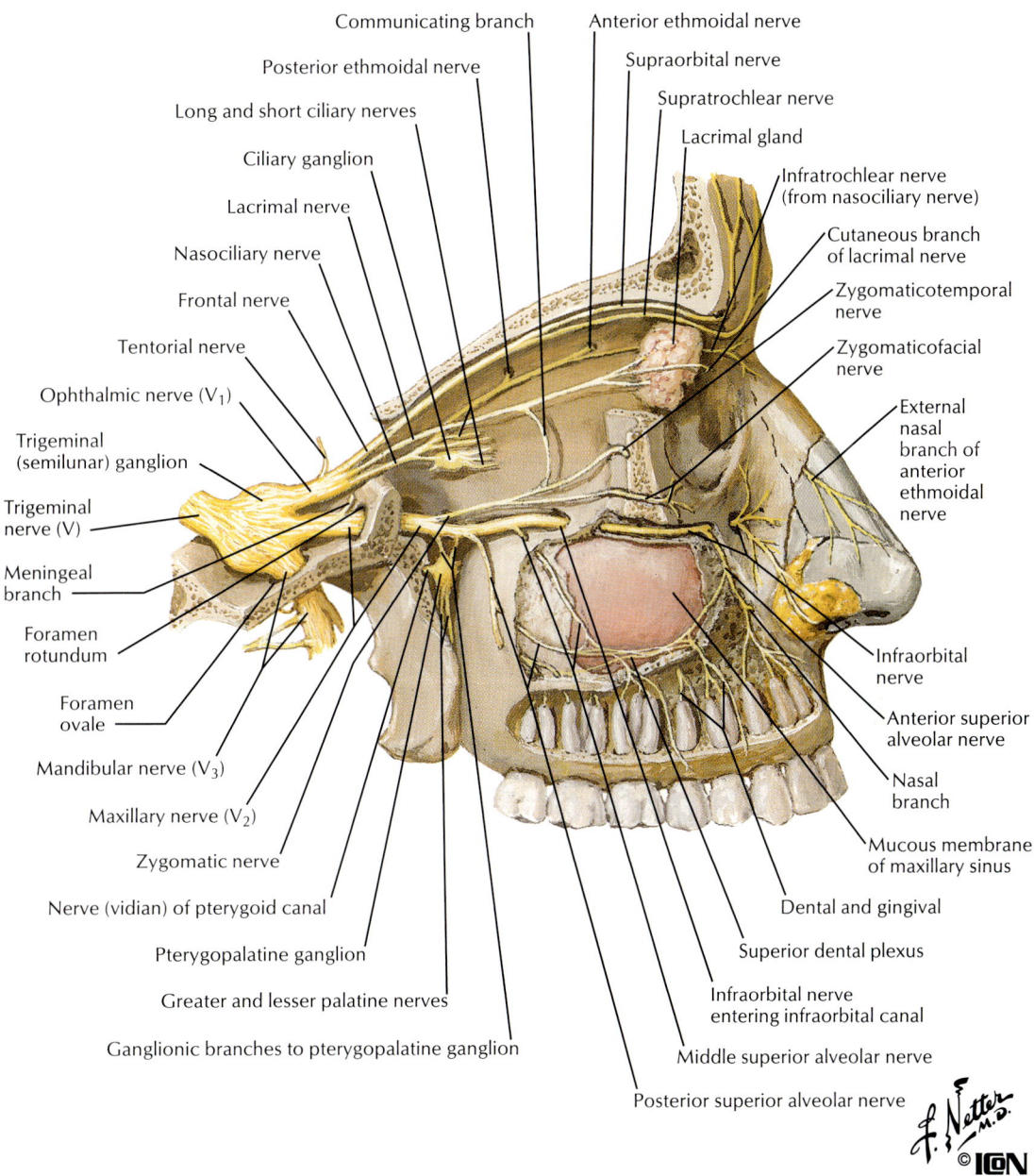

CRANIAL NERVES

103

CRANIAL NERVE V: TRIGEMINAL

Figure 10-2B   Mandibular Nerve (V₃) Sensory and Motor

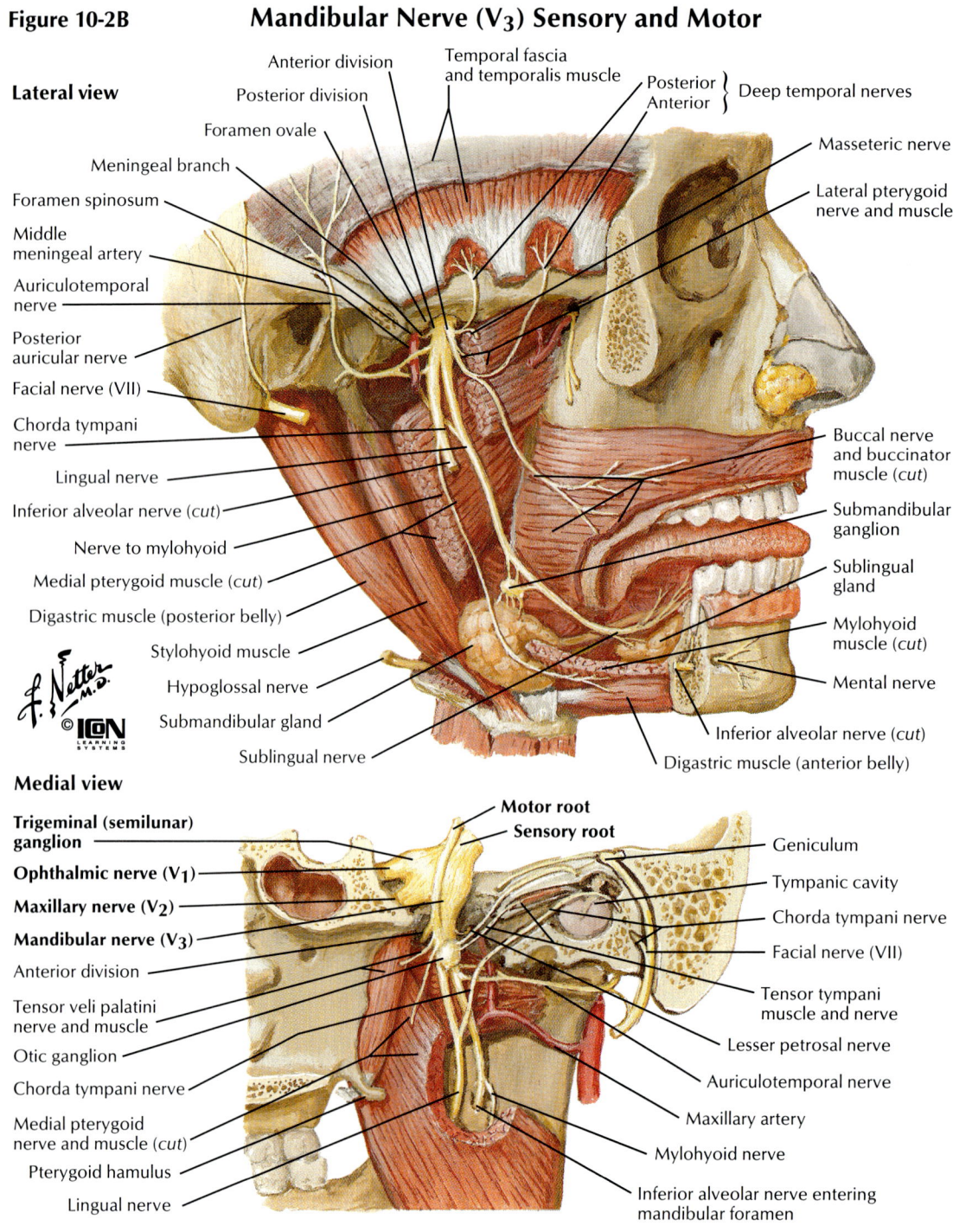

104

CRANIAL NERVE V: TRIGEMINAL

Figure 10-3 **Cranial Nerve Nuclei in Brainstem: Schema**

Posterior phantom view

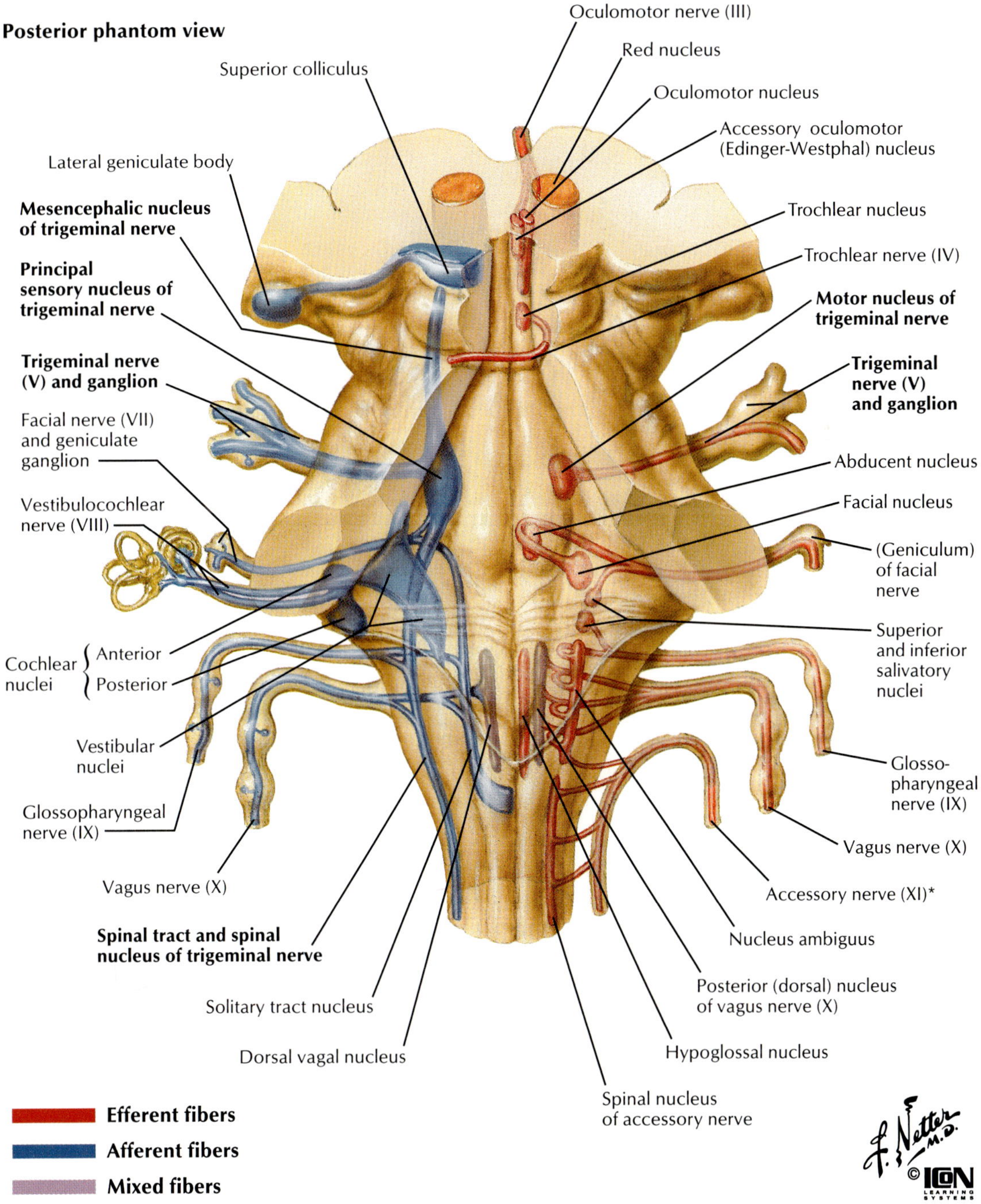

*Recent evidence suggests that the accessory nerve lacks a cranial root and has no connection to the vagus nerve. Verification of this finding awaits further investigation.

CRANIAL NERVES

105

CRANIAL NERVE V: TRIGEMINAL

Motor Component

The motor nucleus, originating within the mid pons, receives its major input from primary proprioceptive neurons in the mesencephalic subnucleus, creating a monosynaptic reflex arch similar to spinal reflexes, assessable by eliciting the jaw jerk. Motor nucleus axons exit the pons as the motor root medial to the sensory root, passing through the trigeminal ganglion and exiting the skull via the foramen ovale. Extracranially, this root combines with the sensory mandibular division forming the mandibular nerve, which provides branches innervating the muscles of mastication: the masseter, temporalis, medial and lateral pterygoid, mylohyoid, and anterior digastric muscles.

TRIGEMINAL NEURALGIA

Clinical Vignette

A 48-year-old woman experienced lightninglike attacks of electrical shock–like, intense pain in the left cheek. They usually occurred without warning but were often precipitated by talking, chewing, washing her face, or applying lipstick to the left upper lip. She was free of pain between attacks. Neurologic examination results were within normal limits.

Treatment with carbamazepine (200 mg 3 times daily) helped initially, but relapse necessitated dosage increases to 800 mg and 1000 mg/d. Although the patient's pain was controlled at the higher dosage, she became lethargic and forgetful and could not function.

The neurosurgical consultant advised microvascular decompression. Teflon was placed between the artery and the nerve to maintain decompression. Postoperatively, the patient experienced significant relief.

Disabling, brief paroxysms of pain within the CN-V distribution are some of the worst pains an individual may experience. Also called **tic douleureux**, trigeminal neuralgia is not diagnosable by any test, so diagnosis must come from its characteristic history. Patients are almost always adults and often senior citizens. Typically, they experience spontaneous, paroxysmal, unilateral, often provocable, disabling pain, usually in the lower face and primarily within the second or third trigeminal divisions, rarely involving the first division. Knowledge of the anatomy and facial distribution of CN-V and an awareness of the character of trigeminal neuralgia are essential for accurate diagnosis (Figure 10-4).

Typically, the pain is intermittent and rarely occurs at night. It may be provoked by simple daily activities, including talking, chewing, shaving, or drinking hot or cold liquids, or any facial touch or sensory stimulation.

In many patients, perhaps the majority, myelin loss within the posterior root of the CN-V leads to this pain. In younger individuals, a primary CNS demyelinating disorder, particularly multiple sclerosis, is occasionally operative. Another common cause is an artery that has lengthened during adult life and become tortuous. An ectatic loop of such an artery, usually a branch of the superior cerebellar artery, compresses the trigeminal posterior root, causing the pain. Trigeminal neuralgia can result from other conditions causing pressure on CN-V, including acoustic neuromas, meningiomas, AVM, or aneurysms compressing the posterior root of the CN-V.

MRI is generally appropriate, particularly in younger persons who may have unexpected multiple sclerosis. It also helps exclude the rare mass lesions previously mentioned.

Treatment

Several treatments are available for trigeminal neuralgia, regardless of the cause. Most patients respond initially to carbamazepine (600 mg daily), which stabilizes cell membranes and increases the threshold of neural stimulation. Phenytoin, gabapentin, and lioresal are also used. When these fail, surgery is considered.

If the diagnosis is accurate, surgical decompression is often successful. Effective surgical procedures include microvascular decompression of the trigeminal sensory root, percutaneous radiofrequency rhizotomy, and percutaneous trigeminal ganglion balloon compression. The latter two imply partial and irreversible destruction of the trigeminal ganglion.

Nonparoxysmal steady pain, post-traumatic pain, pain after dental procedures, and pain that is not strictly within the trigeminal zone, including pain at the vertex, side of the neck, or retroauricular sources, are not trigeminal neuralgia. These other types of pain do not respond effectively to trigeminal neuralgia treatments.

CRANIAL NERVE V: TRIGEMINAL

Figure 10-4

Trigeminal Neuralgia

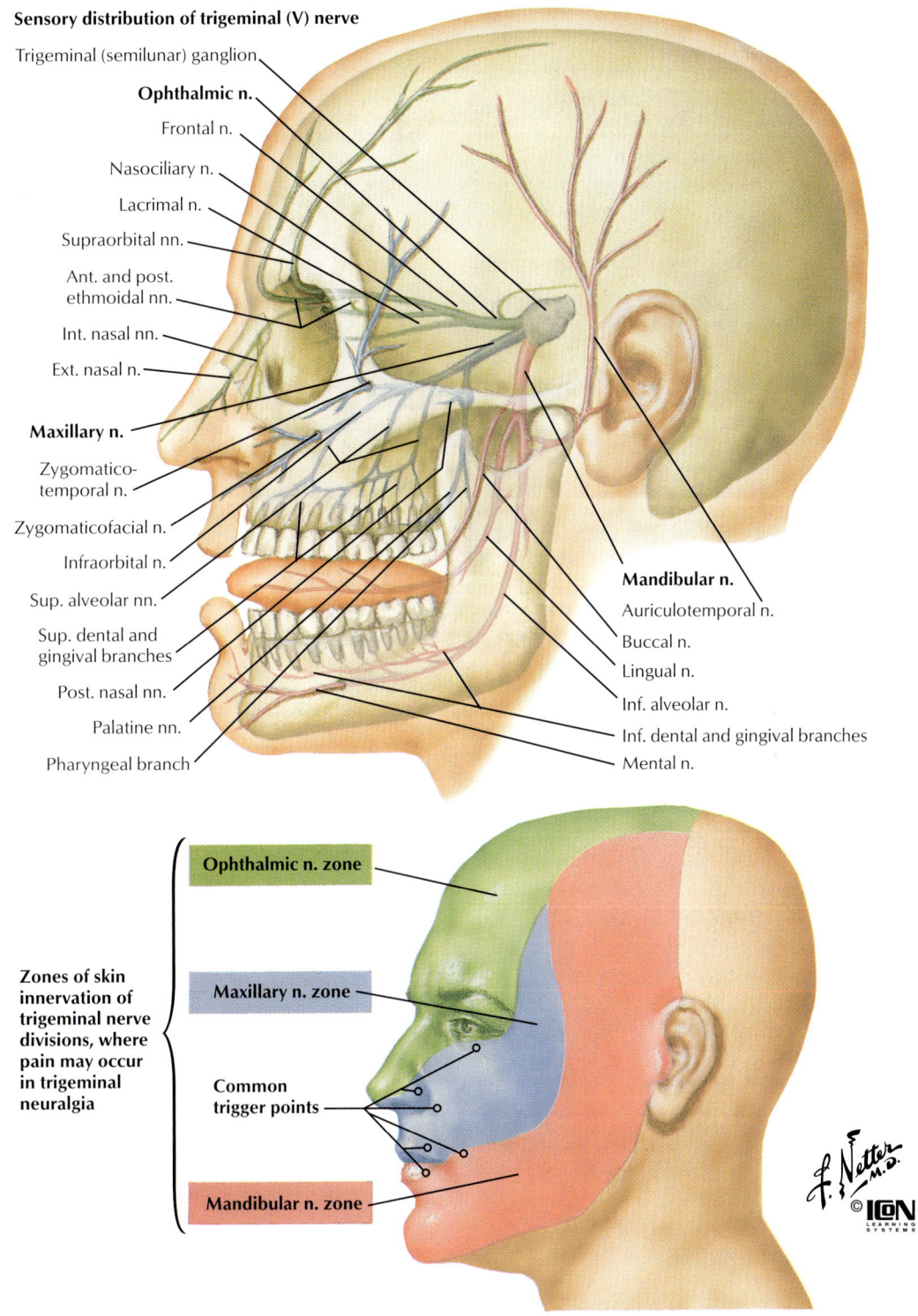

CRANIAL NERVE V: TRIGEMINAL

OTHER CN-V LESIONS
Clinical Presentation and Diagnostic Approach

Facial numbness is the most common symptom of CN-V neuropathy and may be produced by a lesion at any site along the sensory pathway: the nuclei within the brainstem, sensory root, trigeminal ganglion, or primary divisions of CN-V. The division or nerve in question is identified by testing sensation in the distribution of individual branches.

Unilateral loss of the corneal reflex is a clinically useful sign of CN-V neuropathy, although its localizing value is low. Masticatory weakness, difficult to test when the change is subtle, occurs when the motor nucleus, root, or mandibular division is damaged.

Facial pain, numbness, or both are the hallmarks of most CN-V lesions, including herpes zoster. The possibility of a neoplasm infiltrating the nerve must be considered with severe and persistent facial pain. Impairment of general sensation from the tongue and palate carried by CN-V may also cause taste disturbances, even though the special sensory fibers providing taste sensation are supplied by the facial and glossopharyngeal nerves. Both general and special sensation to the tongue and palate are necessary for fully functional taste.

Differential Diagnosis

The primary differential diagnosis includes herpes zoster, dental trauma, and other cranial injuries, the most frequent etiologies in developed countries, followed by neuropathies due to neoplasms and idiopathic causes. Worldwide, Hansen disease is a common cause of CN-V neuropathy (Table 10-1).

Clinical Entities

CN-V divisions and branches are exposed to injuries especially from invasive dental treatments, fractures of facial bones or the cranium, and other invasive procedures in the face and neck. Trauma is among the most common etiologies of CN-V lesions and typically results in anesthesia in the area supplied by the affected branch.

Herpes zoster ophthalmicus occurs when a latent varicella-zoster virus infection in the

Table 10-1
Differential Diagnosis of CN-V Lesion Origin

Brainstem:	stroke, brain stem gliomas, multiple sclerosis, or syringobulbia
Intracranial:	trigeminal neurinoma, acoustic neurinoma, meningioma, granuloma, metastasis, herpes zoster, carotid or basilar aneurysms, trigeminal sensory neuropathy
Skull base lesions:	metastasis, nasopharyngeal carcinoma, lymphoma, basilar meningitis
Trigeminal divisions and nerve branches:	trauma, metastasis, spreading skin tumor, salivary tumor, vasculitis, leprosy
Drug intoxication:	trichloroethylene, hydroxystilbamidine

trigeminal ganglion becomes reactivated, affecting the ophthalmic division. Most patients present with a characteristic periorbital vesicular rash and severe neuralgic pain within the ophthalmic division (Figure 10-5). Similar to other herpes zoster syndromes, the pain may precede eruption of cutaneous lesions. Permanent visual impairment is the most serious outcome of ophthalmic zoster infection. Antiviral agents such as acyclovir are the main therapy. Rarely, an ipsilateral middle cerebral artery infarction may subsequently develop in these patients.

In **trigeminal sensory neuropathy**, the trigeminal ganglion cell bodies are the primary pathologic target. Although the pathogenesis of this ganglionopathy is not understood, an association between trigeminal sensory neuropathy and connective tissue disorders is recognized. Presumably, circulating autoantibodies attack the ganglion cells whose blood-brain barrier is more permeable to large molecules than is the blood-brain barrier elsewhere in the peripheral nervous system. Systemic sclerosis and mixed connective tissue disorder typically have numbness that begins around the mouth and spreads slowly over months, involving all CN-V divisions, unilaterally or bilaterally. Sometimes the ophthalmic division is spared. In Sjögren syndrome, trigeminal involvement is common and usually seen as part of a more widespread sensory ganglionopathy.

CRANIAL NERVE V: TRIGEMINAL

Figure 10-5   Varicella Zoster with Probable Keratitis

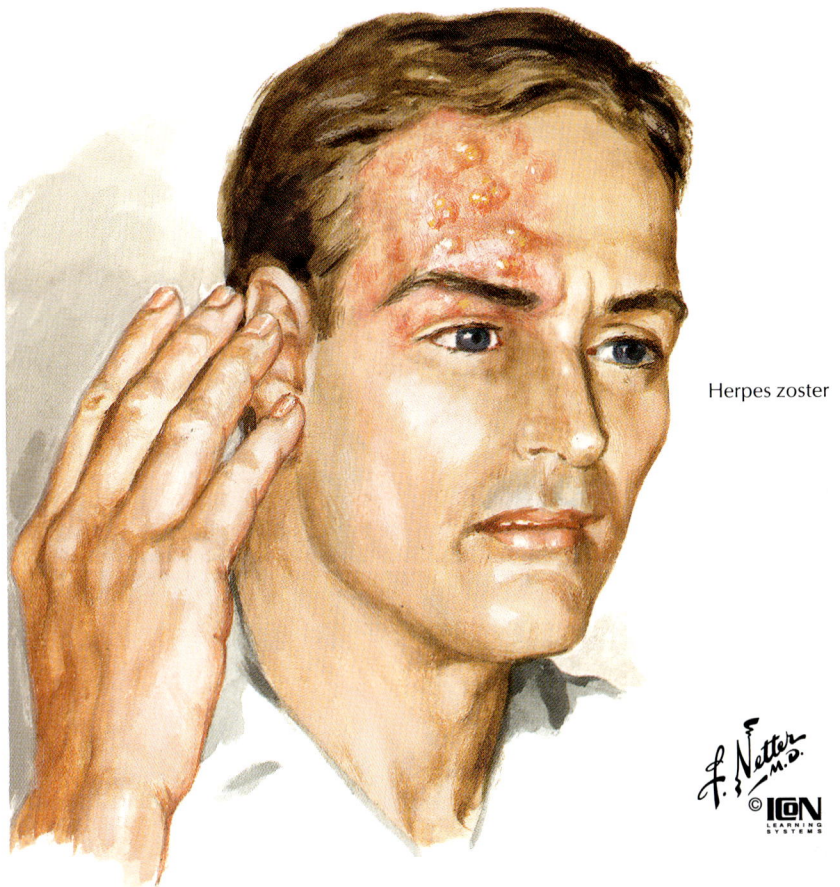

Herpes zoster

Trigeminal neurinomas are rare (0.2% of intracranial tumors and 2% to 3% of intracranial neurinomas), usually benign, well-demarcated, and slowly growing neoplasms. Most frequently, they arise near the trigeminal ganglion, usually extending into the middle and posterior cranial fossae. Rarely, they arise exclusively from one of the sensory divisions and spread extracranially. Rare instances of malignant schwannomas originating within the trigeminal ganglion are described. Most neurinomas reach a diameter of up to 2.5 cm before diagnosis because of their slow and asymptomatic growth. At presentation, patients typically report numbness and paresthesias within the CN-V distribution. Trigeminal neuralgia or burning intermittent pain is less common. Rarely, sensory problems are accompanied by other neurologic symptoms resulting from damage to adjacent structures. Thus, tumors growing downward into the posterior fossa may lead to cerebellar ataxia and lesions of CN-VII and CN-VIII, manifesting with facial palsy, tinnitus, or hearing loss. In contrast, neurinomas exerting pressure upward on the cavernous sinus lateral wall produce CN-II, -III, -IV, and -VI lesions.

Cerebellopontine angle tumors, typically acoustic neurinomas, initially involve CN-VIII (Figure 10-6). Enlarging tumors may compress the trigeminal sensory root and lead to facial numbness or pain with subsequent ipsilateral loss of corneal reflex.

Other neoplasms include meningiomas, epidermoids, lymphomas, hemangioblastomas, gangliocytomas, chondromas, and sarcomas. Tumors involving the face, such as squamous cell carcinoma, microcystic adenexal carci-

CRANIAL NERVE V: TRIGEMINAL

Figure 10-6   Acoustic Neurinoma Compressing Trigeminal Nerve*

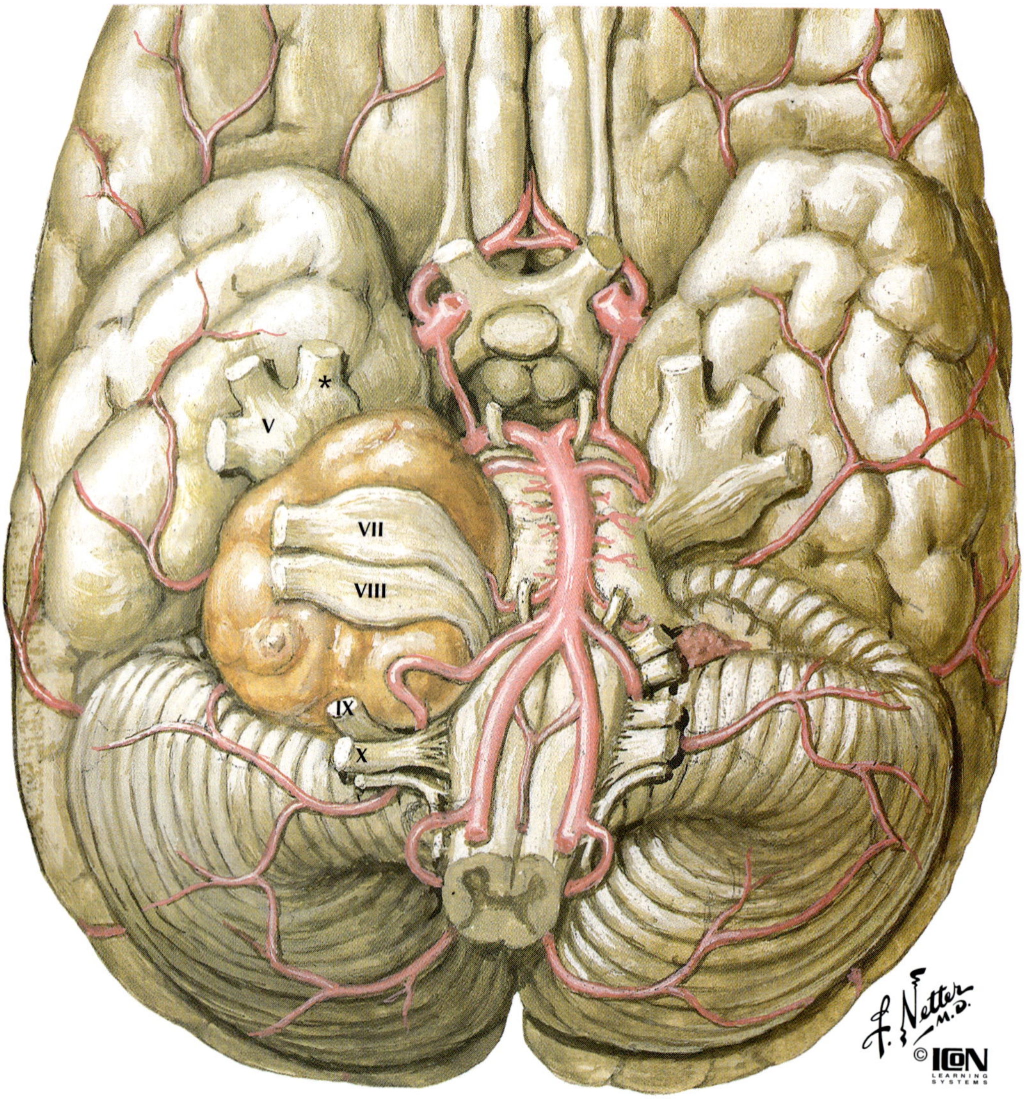

Large acoustic neurinoma filling cerebellopontine angle, distorting brainstem and cranial nerves V, VII, VIII, IX, X

noma, and keratoacanthoma, have a proclivity for invading cutaneous nerves because of their innate neurotropism. Similarly, certain skull base tumors, such as nasopharyngeal carcinoma, salivary gland adenocarcinoma, and metastatic disease, sometimes also invade various trigeminal divisions. The numb chin syndrome consists of unilateral numbness of the chin and adjacent lower lip. Although seemingly harmless, it is usually an ominous sign of primary or metastatic cancer involving the mandible, skull base, or leptomeninges. Lymphoproliferative malignancies and metastatic breast cancer are the most common etiologies.

REFERENCES

Elias WJ, Burchiel KJ. Trigeminal neuralgia and other neuropathic pain syndromes of the head and face. *Curr Pain Headache Rep.* 2002;6:115-124.

Hughes RAC. Diseases of the fifth cranial nerve. In: Dyck PJ, Thomas PK, Griffin JW, Low PA, Poduslo JF, eds. *Peripheral Neuropathy.* 3rd ed. Philadelphia, Pa: WB Saunders Co; 1993;801-817.

Loeser JD. Tic douloureux. *Pain Res Manag.* 2001;6:156-165.

Maillefert JF, Gazet-Maillefert MP, Tavernier C, et al. Numb chin syndrome. *Joint Bone Spine.* 2000;67:86-93.

Nager GT. Neurinomas of the trigeminal nerve. *Am J Otolaryngol.* 1984;5:301-333.

Rosenbaum R. Neuromuscular complications of connective tissue diseases. *Muscle Nerve.* 2001;24:154-169.

Rowe JG, Radatz MW, Walton L, et al. Gamma knife stereotactic radiosurgery for unilateral acoustic neuromas. *J Neurol Neurosurg Psychiatry.* 2003;74:1536-1542.

Severson EA, Baratz KH, Hodge DO, et al. Herpes zoster ophthalmicus in Olmsted County, Minnesota: have systemic antivirals made a difference? *Arch Ophthalmol.* 2003;121:386-390.

Starr CE, Pavan-Langston D. Varicella-zoster virus: mechanisms of pathogenicity and corneal disease. *Ophthalmol Clin North Am.* 2002;15:7-15.

Sweeney PJ, Hanson MR. The cranial neuropathies. In: Bradley WG, Daroff RB, Fenichel GM, Marsden CD, eds. *Neurology in Clinical Practice: Principles of Diagnosis and Management.* 2nd ed. Boston, Mass: Butterworth-Heinemann; 1996;1721-1732.

Chapter 11
Cranial Nerve VII: Facial

Michal Vytopil, Peter J. Catalano, and H. Royden Jones, Jr

Lesions of the facial nerve (CN-VII) are one of the most frequent cranial mononeuropathies. As one of the most complex cranial nerves, CN-VII has a long course, multiple functions, and 4 primary components. **Motor fibers** constitute the largest component and serve the primary function of CN-VII: innervating the muscles of facial expression. Unilateral, complete facial weakness is the hallmark of almost all facial neuropathies. CN-VII also contains **autonomic fibers** that initiate lacrimal, salivary, and mucous secretions; **special sensory** fibers that collect taste sensations from the anterior two thirds of the tongue; and **general sensory** fibers that innervate the external auditory canal and a small skin area behind the ear.

When a patient presents with facial weakness, differentiation should be made between **peripheral facial** nerve lesions and **CNS facial** processes. With the latter, when the patient is relaxed, subtle suggestions of a facial nerve lesion may be appreciated by noting the affected nasolabial fold flattening. Brain lesions are often associated with other findings that can help with localization. For example, a small lesion near the Broca area may result in motor aphasia and facial weakness. Larger lesions affecting a significant portion of a hemisphere, as with large hemispheric strokes, cause a constellation of symptoms, including face, arm, and leg weakness; gaze deviation; and neglect or aphasia. Posterior limb lesions of the internal capsule result in face, arm, and leg weakness.

ANATOMY
Intrapontine Portion

CN-VII consists of 2 primary roots (Figure 11-1). The larger division carries somatic motor fibers and has its origin within the facial nucleus in the caudal pons, where it lies adjacent to the spinal tract of the trigeminal nerve (CN-V). It then passes dorsally and rostrally, curves around the abducens nerve (CN-VI) nucleus (internal genu), and exits the brainstem at the bulbopontine angle between CN-VI and CN-VIII.

Its smaller component, the intermediate nerve of Wrisberg (the **nervus intermedius**), contains a combination of autonomic, special sensory (taste), and general sensory fibers. Its preganglionic parasympathetic fibers arise from the superior salivatory nucleus, relay through the pterygopalatine and submandibular ganglions, and eventually provide the efferent function for lacrimation and salivation. The other intermediate nerve fibers carrying taste and general somatic sensation have their primary cell bodies in the geniculate ganglion and terminate within the nucleus solitarius and the spinal tract of CN-V, respectively.

Peripheral CN-VII

Both roots of CN-VII leave the brainstem to enter the temporal bone via the internal auditory meatus, where they accompany the auditory nerve (CN-VIII) passing through the internal auditory canal (Figure 11-1). CN-VII continues to the periphery through the facial canal; this segment has 5 parts, based on their relation to surrounding anatomical structures. The **labyrinthine** segment passes above the labyrinth and leads anterolaterally to the **geniculate ganglion**, containing the cell bodies of CN-VII afferents. At this site, the canal abruptly turns posteriorly and forms the external genu of CN-VII. The **greater petrosal nerve** originates here; it carries **preganglionic parasympathetic** fibers to the pterygopalatine ganglion, where they synapse and subsequently direct **postganglionic fibers** to the lacrimal gland.

The **tympanic segment** of CN-VII travels posteriorly and laterally along the medial wall of the middle ear. At the posterior wall of the middle ear, the facial canal changes its course and travels inferiorly toward the exit at the stylomastoid foramen. This vertical portion is named the **mastoid segment**; it has 2 important branches: proximally, the **stapedius nerve** arises to innervate the stapedius muscle; more distally, the **chorda tympani** branches and exits the facial canal and, after traversing the middle ear, joins the lingual nerve belonging to the third division of CN-V. The **chorda tympani** contains **preganglionic parasympathetic** fibers that synapse within the submandibular ganglion to innervate the submandibular and sublingual glands. The **chorda tympani** also carries taste fibers. Their cell bodies originate within the geniculate ganglion, mediating taste sensation from the anterior two thirds of the tongue.

Soon after leaving the skull at the **stylomastoid foramen**, the distal CN-VII gives rise to several small motor branches innervating the posterior auricular, occipital, digastric, and stylohyoid muscles (Figure 11-2). The main motor trunk of CN-VII then passes through the parotid gland to terminate as the **temporal**, **zygomatic**, **buccal**, **mandibular**, and **cervical branches**. The first two innervate the muscles involved in moving the forehead, closing the eyes, and wrinkling the nose. Muscles of the lower face and neck are primarily innervated by the latter 2 branches. CN-VII subserves all muscles of facial expression except the levator palpebrae superioris, and therefore, CN-VII impairment, with a resultant asymmetric facies, is a major social and cosmetic impediment.

CLINICAL CORRELATIONS AND ENTITIES

CN-VII can be damaged at any level along its complex course. Almost all CN-VII pathologies, regardless of the lesion site, produce a facial musculature paralysis. The degree of facial paralysis with various dysfunctions of other CN-VII components causes symptoms that help to identify the lesion site.

An **upper motor neuron** dysfunction causes facial palsy by depriving the facial nucleus of its cortical input. Because there is bilateral innervation of the frontalis and orbicularis oculi, these muscles are spared with an upper motor neuron lesion such as a **cerebral infarct**. The mechanism of this phenomenon is not fully appreciated, but presumably, bilateral central innervation of the motor neurons for the upper face, in contrast to the classic contralateral input to the lower facial muscles, is responsible for this valuable clinical tool. In the uncommon circumstance where there is bilateral corticobulbar tract involvement, as in various suprabulbar palsies, facial movement is retained in response to emotional stimuli but absent as a voluntary effort.

Intramedullary pontine lesions affect the facial motor nucleus and often the contiguous fibers of CN-VI that traverse over the facial nucleus. These often lead to concomitant ipsilateral paralysis of facial expression with diminished lateral gaze as in a brainstem glioma.

Cerebellopontine (CP) angle tumors, if they are large acoustic neuromas, have conjoint CN-VIII and CN-VII fiber involvement manifested by diminished hearing, sometimes initially presenting with tinnitus and later presenting with peripheral facial paresis (Figure 11-3). Occasionally, when these lesions are large, concomitant involvement of the ipsilateral CN-V fibers causes unilateral facial numbness, sometimes only initially signaled by the loss of the corneal reflex.

In addition to an ipsilateral facial palsy, relatively proximal intracanicular CN-VII palsies have an associated motor fiber dysfunction of the stapedius muscles characteristically associated with **hyperacusis**, an increased sensitivity to sound that is particularly noticeable while using a telephone. When CN-VII is injured along its course from the facial nucleus to the geniculate ganglion, lacrimation, salivation, taste sensation for the anterior two thirds of the tongue, and somatic sensation for the external auditory canal are also impaired.

When the lesion is more distally situated, between the geniculate ganglion and the stapedius nerve, all of the above findings occur, but lacrimation is spared. If damage occurs between the stapedius nerve and the chorda tympani, salivation and taste are impaired, but changes in lacrimation and hyperacusis are not present. CN-VII lesions distal to the chorda tympani only produce ipsilateral facial weakness.

Clinical Vignette

An 18-year-old, previously healthy woman experienced modest pain in her right ear; 1 day later, voices

CRANIAL NERVE VII: FACIAL

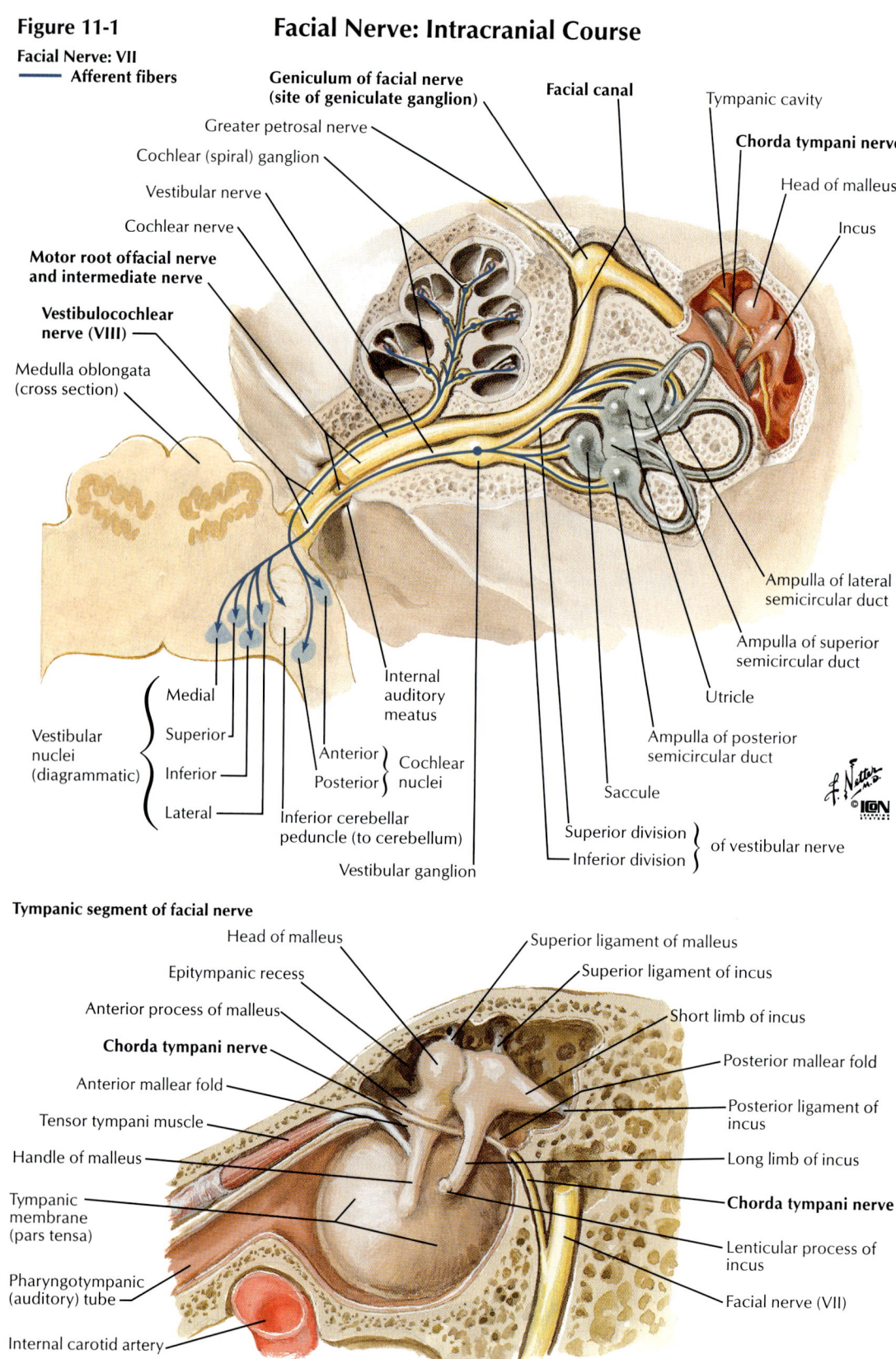

Figure 11-1
Facial Nerve: VII
— Afferent fibers

Facial Nerve: Intracranial Course

CRANIAL NERVE VII: FACIAL

Figure 11-2 Facial Nerve (VII): Schema

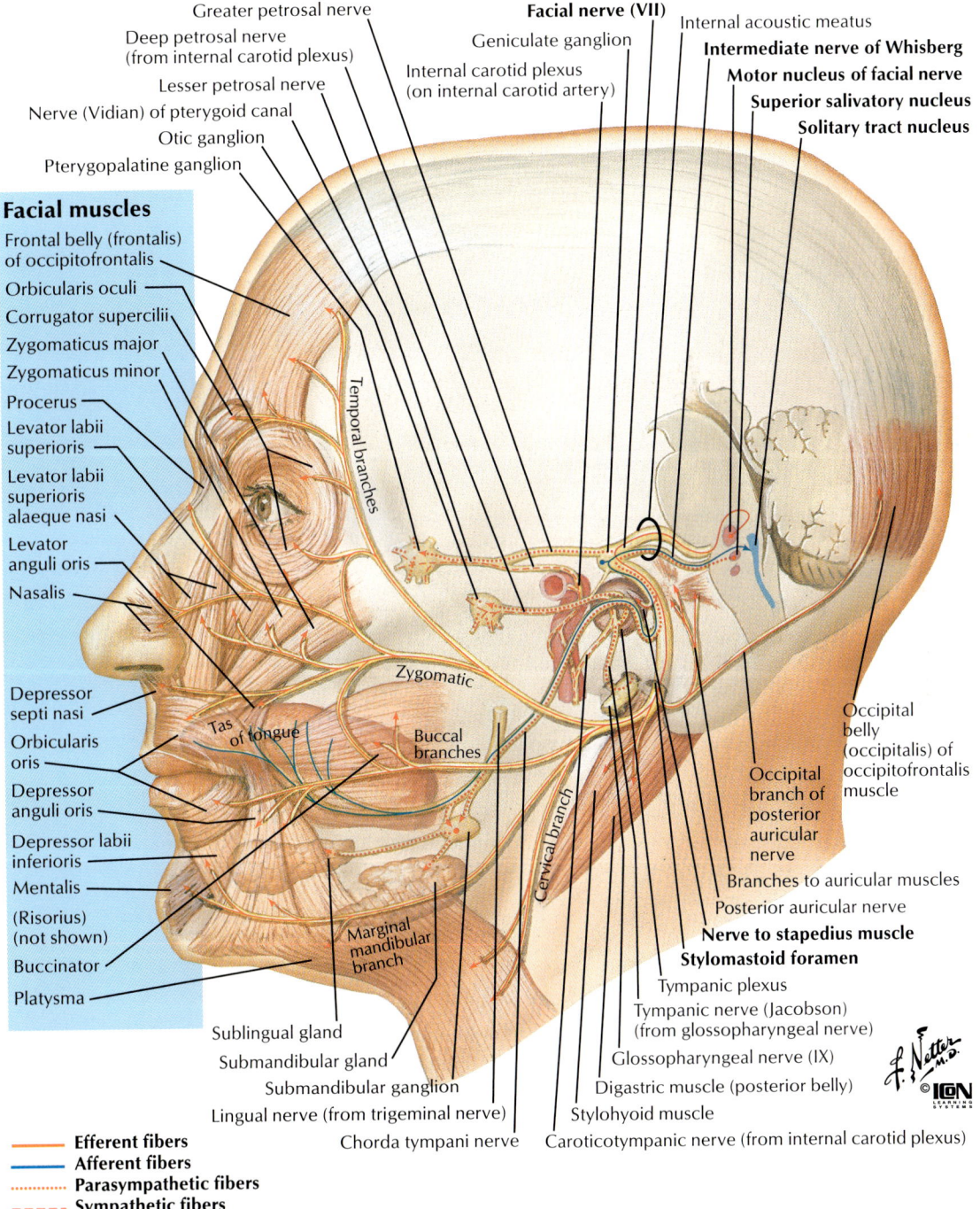

115

CRANIAL NERVE VII: FACIAL

Figure 11-3

Cerebellopontine Angle Tumor

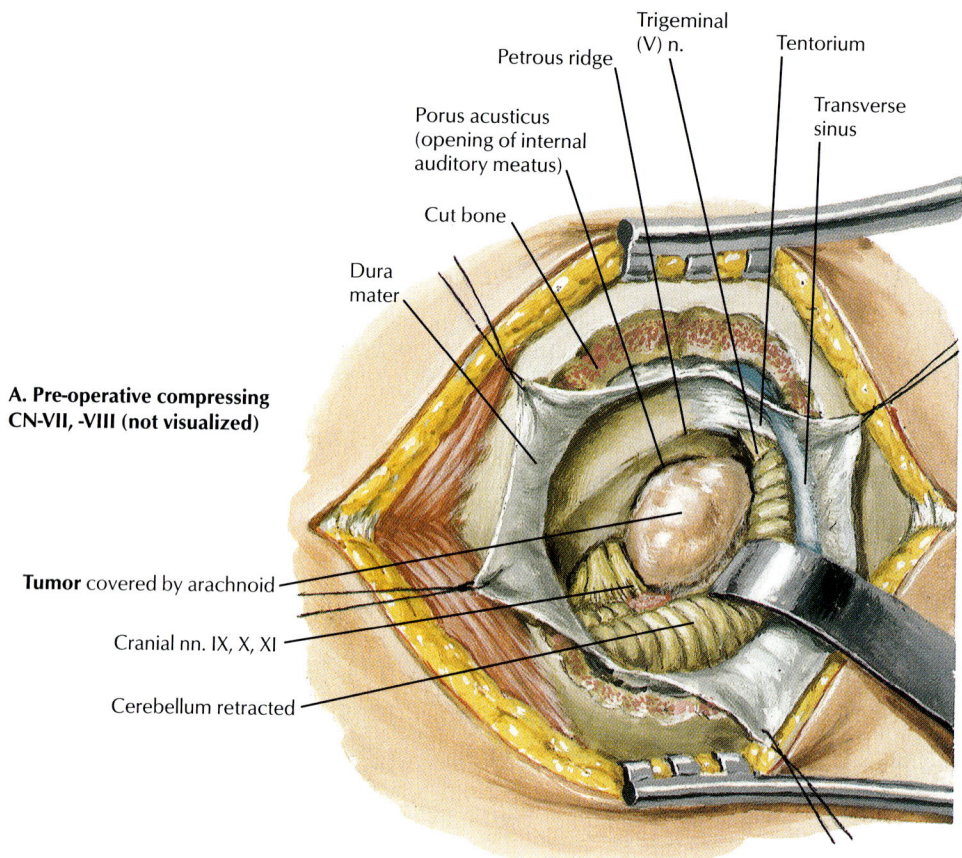

A. Pre-operative compressing CN-VII, -VIII (not visualized)

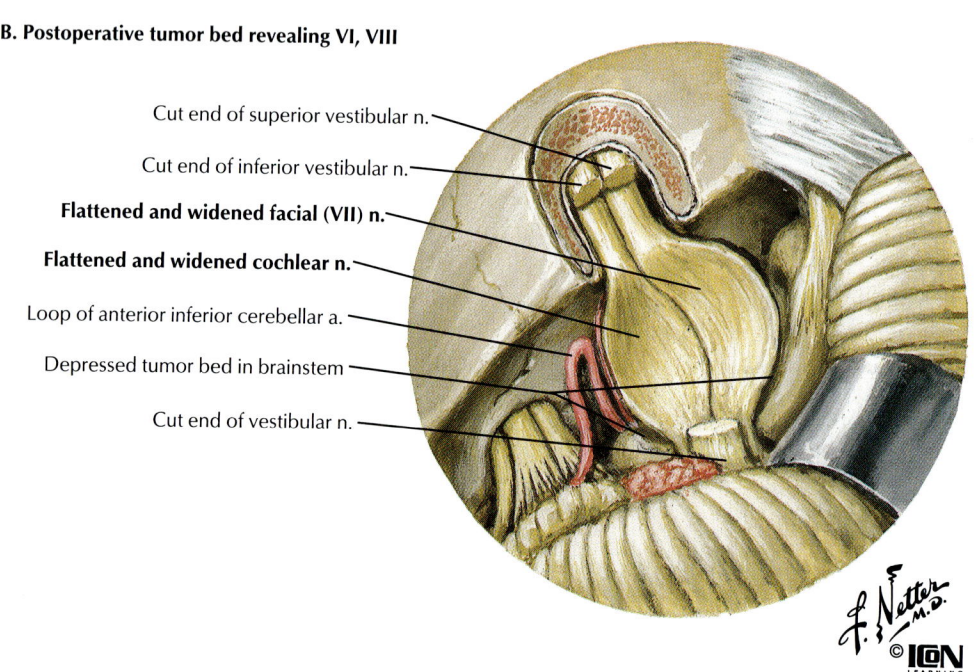

B. Postoperative tumor bed revealing VI, VIII

seemed to be louder than normal while she was talking on the phone. The next day, she noted that her right eye did not close, and she could not smile on that side. Tearing was diminished in her right eye, and she could not taste things on the right side of her tongue.

On examination, the patient was unable to wrinkle her forehead, smile on the right, or close her right eyelids, although the eye rolled upward when she attempted to do so. She had diminished tearing and loss of taste sensation on the anterior two thirds of the right side of her tongue. All other examination results were normal.

A steroid dose pack was given at the initial evaluation. The patient experienced gradual return of total CN-VII function over the next 2 months.

Idiopathic Facial Palsy

This vignette describes a benign, idiopathic facial palsy (Bell palsy) (Figure 11-4). The lesion had a proximal location, denoted by the loss of total motor function on one side of the patient's face involving the frontalis and orbicularis oculi muscles, the lower facial muscles, and the loss of stapedius muscle and lacrimal gland function. Her benign outcome is typical of 85% to 90% of individuals with acute and relatively total Bell palsy within a few days after symptom onset.

Bell palsy is one of the most common and distinctive entities in clinical neurology. Typically, patients present with acute unilateral weakness of all mimetic muscles, and the lesions evolve, often over several hours to just a few days. Although Bell palsy is usually benign, its dramatic appearance creates significant distress in many patients who are concerned that it may represent a stroke or that permanent facial disfigurement will result.

The pathogenesis of Bell palsy is generally thought to be associated with edema, entrapment, and resulting ischemia of CN-VII as it passes through its bony canal. The specific pathophysiology is unknown; a reactivation of herpes simplex and varicella-zoster virus latent infection within the geniculate ganglion is hypothesized. The combination of possible edema and infection provide the basis for treatment.

Clinical Presentation

Patients become aware of the weakness when a family member or friend notes the facial asymmetry, when they notice an inability to close an eye, or when they experience difficulty holding saliva, food, and fluids in the affected side of the mouth. Less commonly, decreased taste, or **hyperacusis**, is the first symptom. A preceding dull aching pain behind the ear is a common initial problem.

Facial asymmetry is unequivocally present; the affected frontalis is smooth and cannot be normally corrugated, whereas the angle of the mouth appears depressed even in repose. Eversion of the lower lid, responsible for excessive tearing (**epiphora**) in some patients, and an inability to completely close the eyelids (**lagophthalmos**) result from orbicularis oculi weakness. The **Bell phenomenon** refers to the eyeball turning up without eyelid closure despite attempted eye closure (Figure 11-4). Whether the palsy is accompanied by taste disturbances may help to distinguish lesions proximal and distal to the chorda tympani branch. For example, a pure motor lesion may suggest a lesion at the distal part of the facial canal or within the parotid gland, whereas when all 4 primary functions are affected, an unusual proximal lesion, or even a pontine lesion when concomitant ocular abduction is weak, is a possibility.

Differential Diagnosis

It is important to initially exclude other causes of unilateral facial paralysis and determine whether the lesion has an upper or a lower motor neuron source. Patients with upper motor neuron paralysis primarily present with an asymmetric smile, unilateral drooling, or both, whereas in peripheral facial palsy, all musculature innervated by CN-VII is affected.

Inflammatory conditions present with acute facial palsy. Facial palsy in **Lyme disease, sarcoidosis,** and **Guillain-Barré syndrome** is often but not always bilateral. Other features distinguishing these conditions are usually present. In some instances of **Ramsay-Hunt syndrome**, unilateral facial paralysis, secondary to herpes zoster, may precede the typical herpetic vesicles in the external auditory canal and is clinically indistinguishable from classic idiopathic Bell palsy. The diagnosis requires detection of a 4-fold increase in the antibody titer against the virus. The typically acute onset of Bell palsy is another critical differential feature in favor of an idiopathic or infectious mechanism versus the evolutionary nature of neoplastic processes.

CRANIAL NERVE VII: FACIAL

Figure 11-4
Course and distribution of facial (VII) nerve

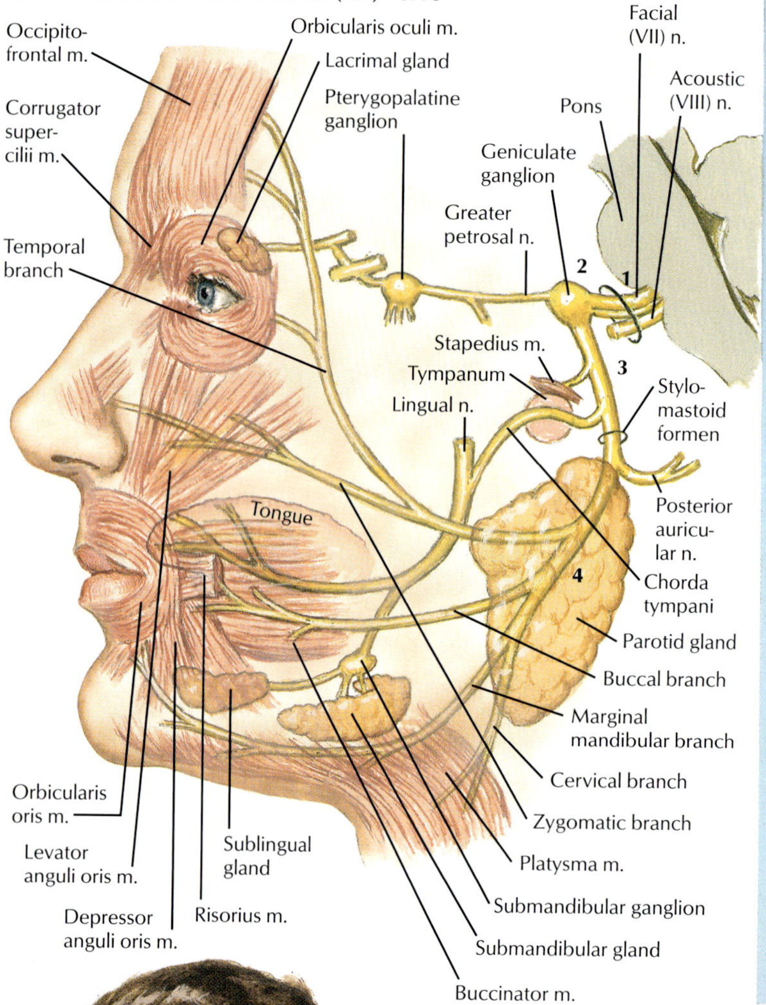

Bell Palsy

Sites of lesions and their manifestations

1. **Intracranial and/or internal auditory meatus.** All symptoms of 2, 3, and 4, plus deafness due to involvement of eighth cranial nerve.

2. **Geniculate ganglion.** All symptoms of 3 and 4, plus pain behind ear. Herpes of tympanum and of external auditory meatus may occur.

3. **Facial canal.** All symptoms of 4, plus loss of taste in anterior tongue and decreased salivation on affected side due to chorda tympani involvement. Hyperacusia due to effect on nerve branch to stapedius muscle.

4. **Below stylomastoid foramen (parotid gland tumor, trauma).** Facial paralysis (mouth draws to opposite side; on affected side, patient unable to close eye or wrinkle forehead; food collects between teeth and cheek due to paralysis of buccinator muscle).

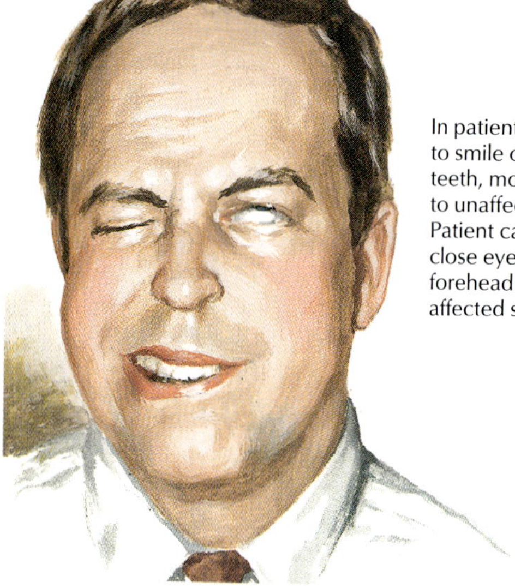

In patient's attempts to smile or bare teeth, mouth draws to unaffected side. Patient cannot wink, close eye, or wrinkle forehead on affected side.

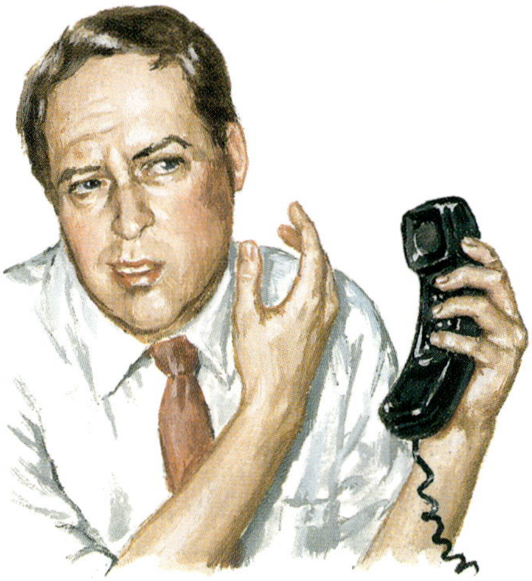

Hyperacusia: patient holds phone away from ear because of painful sensitivity to sound

CRANIAL NERVES

Slowly progressive evolution of a unilateral CN-VII weakness suggests a neoplasm. Neoplasms may be located proximally and focally, near the brainstem, and later may be associated with other cranial neuropathies, as with focal CP angle tumors. Or these may occur diffusely in the leptomeninges, such as with metastatic carcinoma or lymphoma and affect multiple cranial nerves, including the facial. An evolving, progressive *distal* CN-VII lesion suggests a parotid tumor.

Treatment and Prognosis

Treatment is controversial because of the good prognosis in most Bell palsy cases. **Corticosteroid use** seems to reduce the duration of paralysis and risk of permanent impairment. The typical regimen, if started within 7 days after the onset of palsy, is 1 mg/kg oral prednisone, up to 60 mg/d for 6 days and then tapering over the next 4 days. Limited evidence suggests that the combination of **acyclovir** and **prednisone** has greater complete recovery rates than prednisone alone. The common dosage of acyclovir is 2000 mg/d for 10 days. There is insufficient evidence to support primary surgical CN-VII decompression in Bell palsy.

Great care is required to protect the exposed cornea that is subject to trauma from incomplete eye closure. Additionally, a dry and unprotected cornea is susceptible to development of trophic defects. Therefore, eye patching, particularly at night, and artificial tears are warranted.

The recovery rate from Bell palsy follows 2 patterns: most patients begin to regain facial strength within 3 weeks after onset, but in some, the recovery is delayed until 3 to 6 months after onset. The overall prognosis is good; most patients (80-85%) recover completely, but the rest may have synkinesis, residual weakness, tearing, or contracture. Synkinesis is the most frequent permanent sequela, resulting from misdirection of regenerating axons that grow into muscles that they initially did not innervate. It clinically manifests as synchronized movement of different muscles that normally do not contract together. Typically, there is subtle eye closure with smiling, or a lip or chin twitch with blinking. This is rarely disabling.

The rate, completeness, and quality of recovery from Bell palsy are determined by the severity of the underlying CN-VII injury. The degree of injury ranges from mild (pure demyelinating conduction block) to severe (axon loss and resulting wallerian degeneration). With a demyelinating conduction block, the most common type (up to 90% of Bell palsy cases), there is no associated axon loss, and therefore, recovery is prompt, complete, and without synkinesis. The remaining patients have axonal damage with wallerian degeneration, resulting in slow and incomplete recovery that requires regenerating axons to reinnervate paralyzed muscles.

EMG provides valuable prognostic information, especially if it is not performed until approximately 3 weeks after onset. By then, it is possible to distinguish between nerve fibers that have undergone wallerian degeneration and those that are only temporarily blocked. A significantly reduced amplitude of CN-VII **compound muscle action potential** and abundant fibrillation potentials in facial muscles indicate the former, whereas a demyelinating conduction block is typically partially resolved by that time, evidenced by absent or scarce fibrillation potentials.

Infectious Facial Palsies

Varicella-Zoster Virus

Ramsay-Hunt syndrome, from reactivation of the varicella-zoster virus within the geniculate ganglion, is the second most common cause of atraumatic facial palsy. Clinically, it is characterized by the triad of acute facial palsy, neuralgic pain, and eruption of herpetic vesicles within the external auditory canal, ipsilateral palate, and anterior two thirds of the tongue. The areas of pain and rash are appropriate to the general sensory innervation of the afferent CN-VII branches. The geniculate ganglion cell bodies host the latent varicella-zoster virus infection.

The prognosis for Ramsay-Hunt syndrome is worse than that of idiopathic Bell palsy, with frequent complete paralysis, incomplete recovery, and residual synkinesis. Therefore, aggressive treatment with acyclovir (750 mg/d IV or 4000 mg/d oral), in combination with prednisone, is indicated. The best long-term results are obtained when treatment is started within 3 days after onset.

CRANIAL NERVE VII: FACIAL

Lyme Disease

Clinical Vignette

A 32-year-old woman presented with recent left facial drooping and an associated 1-week history of headaches and photosensitivity.

Her temperature was 38°C (100.6°F). There was a 10-cm circular rash on the medial aspect of her right thigh. Her neck was slightly rigid; no intraauricular vesicles were noted. Neurologic examination results demonstrated an isolated left peripheral CN-VII weakness.

Brain CT results were unremarkable. Lumbar puncture revealed a WBC count of 23/mm³, primarily lymphocytes, with a normal protein level and a slightly decreased glucose level. CSF and serum Lyme antibody test results were positive.

This vignette is typical of Bell palsy secondary to Lyme disease (neuroborreliosis). Although relatively uncommon, it should always be considered, particularly in endemic areas.

Facial paralysis is the most common focal manifestation of neuroborreliosis; 40% of these patients have cranial neuropathies, and approximately 80% have CN-VII involvement. Multiple cranial nerves are affected in one fifth of those with a cranial neuropathy; two thirds of this 20% with multiple cranial neuropathies primarily have bilateral facial palsy. Additional clues (ie, erythema migrans, possible exposure to disease transmitting ticks) suggesting neuroborreliosis in patients with acute facial palsy warrant further studies.

Essential studies include titers of anti–*Borrelia burgdorferi* antibodies in blood and CSF and standard CSF analyses. Although the latter may demonstrate a pleocytosis with lymphocytic predominance, the results of this analysis are sometimes normal. Facial paralysis may also occur before seroconversion, eg, early in the disease before antibody testing results become positive. When clinical suspicion of Lyme disease is high, follow-up serologic tests are indicated.

Although it is generally presumed that these CN-VII lesions are from basilar meningitis, some patients with Lyme disease have a pure motor facial paresis without dysgeusia, hyperacusis, or associated CSF pleocytosis. This suggests that the facial neuropathy in some patients results from a more distal CN-VII lesion.

Optimal treatment remains controversial; a regimen of oral or IV antibiotics is recommended. If meningitis is clearly present, treatment should be more aggressive. Facial palsy prognosis in Lyme disease is excellent; most patients recover completely.

Other Infections

Peripheral facial paralysis may occur with **infectious mononucleosis**, caused by Epstein-Barr virus, and **poliomyelitis**, caused by an enterovirus.

Several infectious conditions involving the temporal bone can also cause peripheral facial paralysis, such as acute and chronic **otitis media** and **osteomyelitis** of diverse etiologies, including tuberculosis and syphilis. Similarly, acute **bacterial** or **tuberculous meningitis** may affect multiple cranial nerves including CN-VII. **Leprosy** is a common cause of facial palsy in endemic areas.

Granulomatous Disorders

Sarcoidosis is a disease of unknown etiology characterized by histopathologic findings of nonnecrotizing granulomas within multiple organs. Unilateral or bilateral CN-VII palsy with hyperacusis and dysgeusia, thought to result from granulomatous meningitis, is the most frequent neurologic manifestation. The prognosis is favorable; most patients recover completely after steroid treatment.

Wegener granulomatosis is a systemic disease characterized by necrotizing, granulomatous lesions of the upper and lower respiratory tract, glomerulonephritis, and systemic necrotizing vasculitis. Of the primary systemic vasculitides, only Wegener granulomatosis is associated with a significant frequency of cranial neuropathies. CN-VII involvement, usually occurring in conjunction with other cranial neuropathies, may reflect direct granulomatous invasion of the temporal bone or granulomatous basilar meningitis. Because the 2-year fatality rate of untreated Wegener granulomatosis is greater than 90%, aggressive immunotherapy is warranted on diagnosis.

Traumatic Facial Palsy

Facial paralysis may occur in traumatic fractures of petrous temporal bone. Also, facial palsy may result from surgery of the middle ear, surgery of the parotid gland, or mastoidectomy.

Neoplasms

Several primary and metastatic malignancies may cause a facial palsy. **Carcinomatous meningitis** usually affects multiple cranial nerves; the most common sources are the lung, the breast, and gastrointestinal cancers and lymphomas. Typically, these tumors have an aggressive clinical course; those that present with an isolated CN-VII lesion soon demonstrate signs of multiple cranial or spinal nerve root involvement or both.

Certain benign tumors may exert chronic extrinsic pressure on CN-VII. **Schwannomas** from the vestibular portion of CN-VIII, typically occurring within the acoustic meatus at the CP angle, or less commonly **meningiomas** at similar sites, do not affect CN-VII initially. When they eventually do so, they tend to predominantly and subtly affect sensory fibers; motor fibers are more resilient to chronic deformation. Therefore, the only sign of CN-VII involvement may be relatively minor numbness behind the ear, on the floor of the ear canal, in the posterior inferior quadrant of the eardrum (Hitselberger sign), or a combination of these sites. The change in hearing leads to the diagnosis. Signs of a motor CN-VII lesion do not occur until these lesions become large.

Malignant distal infiltration of CN-VII is seen with parotid tumors (Figure 11-5).

Clinical Vignette

A 62-year-old man initially experienced subtle weakness of his left lower face while shaving. Within 2 months, he became aware of a more profound weakness of his entire left face, particularly his ability to close the left eye. He did not report any other symptoms. A neurologist reassured him that he had "benign" Bell palsy. When his symptoms seemed to worsen, he sought a second opinion.

Examination results demonstrated weakness in all left CN-VII divisions without synkinesis. The remainder of the head, neck, and otoscopic examination results were unremarkable. Audiologic test results were normal, including the left acoustic/stapedius reflex. A corneal reflex was sluggish on the left but present bilaterally. Palpation of the cheek demonstrated some fullness in the left parotid gland.

Biopsy results demonstrated a malignant parotid gland adenocarcinoma with extension beyond the capsule at surgery.

The absence of clinical hyperacusis and preservation of taste function in the patient in this vignette pointed to a pure motor lesion distal to the chorda tympani branch. Unfortunately, the progressive nature of the temporal profile of the illness was not appreciated at the first presentation. Whether the parotid tumor would have been identified before extending beyond its capsule is unknown but emphasizes the importance of determining the temporal profile of each patient's presentation, because early diagnosis can be lifesaving. This man died within a few years.

Uncommon Mass Lesions

Cholesteatomas are another rare mass lesion at the CP angle that deserve consideration in patients with slowly evolving facial paralysis. Other uncommon entities include pontine gliomas, arachnoid cysts, lipomas, and hemangiomas.

Neuromuscular Disorders With Facial Palsy

The motor portion of the CN-VII nucleus with nuclei of CN-V, -IX, -X, -XI, and -XII may be involved in various motor neuron diseases, such as **amyotrophic lateral sclerosis** and **bulbospinal muscular atrophy (Kennedy disease)**.

CN-VII is affected in 33% to 50% of **Guillain-Barré** syndrome cases, often bilaterally. Although usually first evident when limb weakness is severe, CN-VII lesions may develop at any disease stage, including as the presenting sign.

Miller-Fisher syndrome, a variant of Guillain-Barré syndrome, is characterized by ophthalmoplegia, ataxia, and areflexia. However, involvement of cranial nerves other than CN-III, IV, and VI occurs in more than 50% of cases. Facial weakness has been reported in approximately 25% of published Miller-Fisher syndrome cases, underscoring the important clinical overlap between classic ascending Guillain-Barré syndrome and Miller-Fisher syndrome.

Some primarily muscular diseases may cause bilateral facial weakness, typically accompanied by wasting. In adult-onset **myotonic dystrophy**, muscles innervated by CN-III and CN-V,

CRANIAL NERVE VII: FACIAL

Figure 11-5

Facial Nerve Branches and Parotid Gland

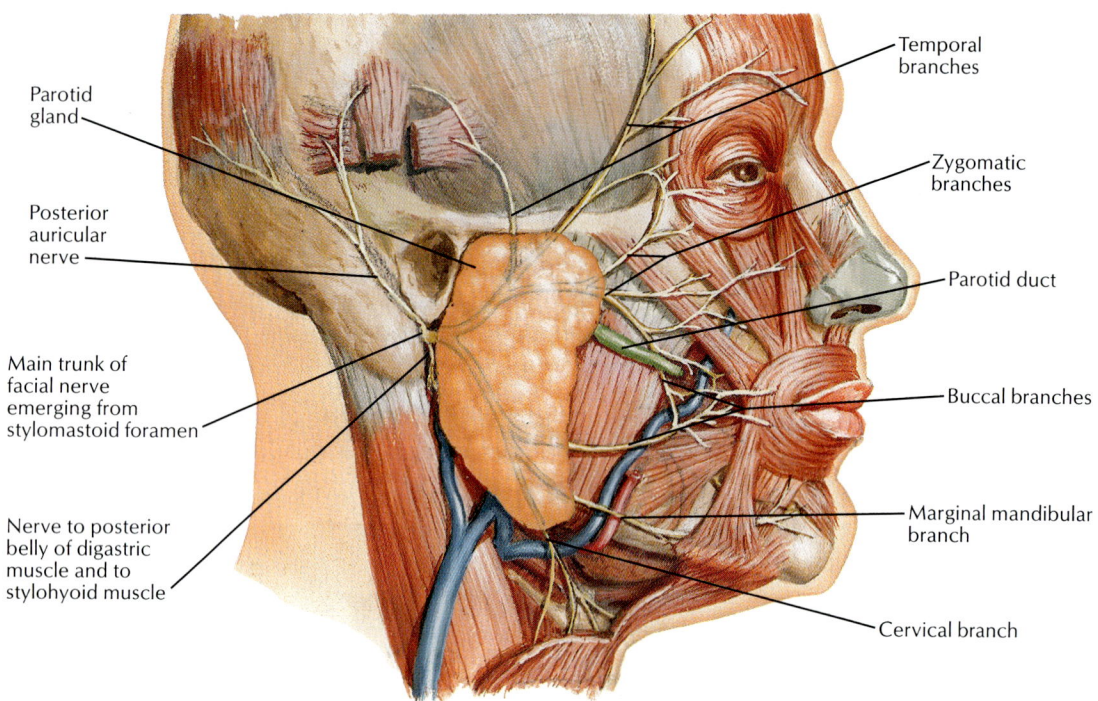

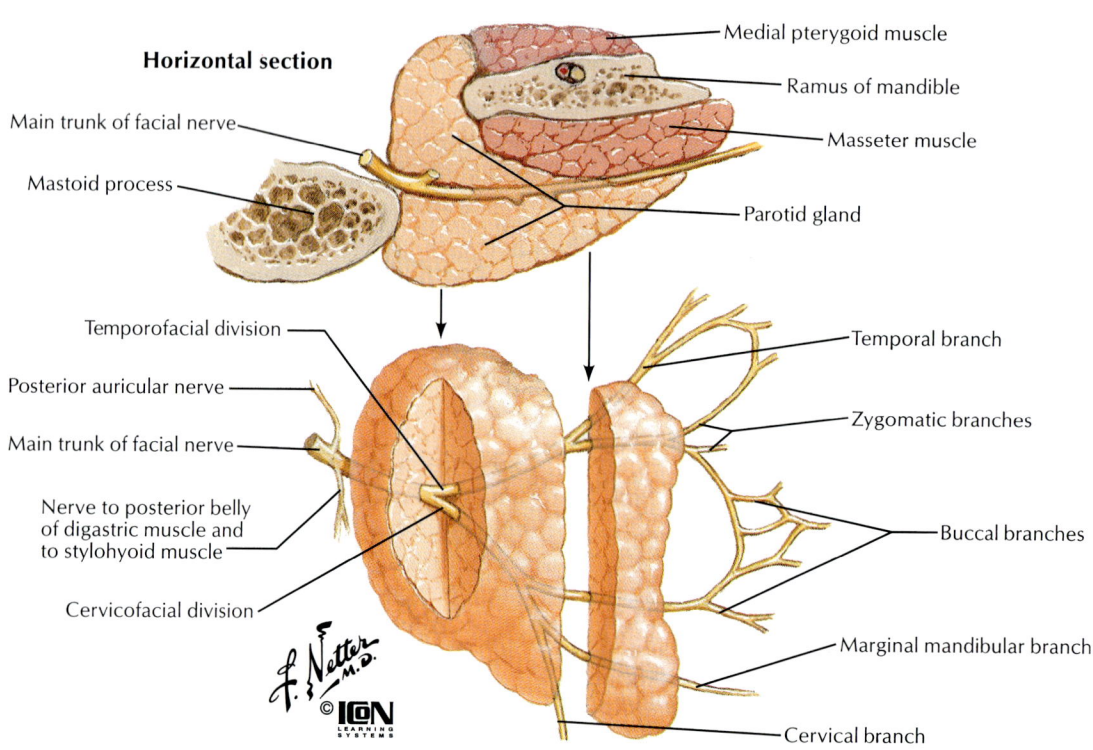

CRANIAL NERVE VII: FACIAL

Figure 11-6 **Seventh Nerve Hemangioma**

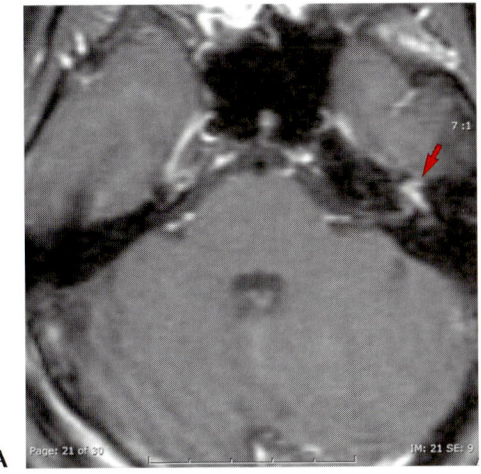
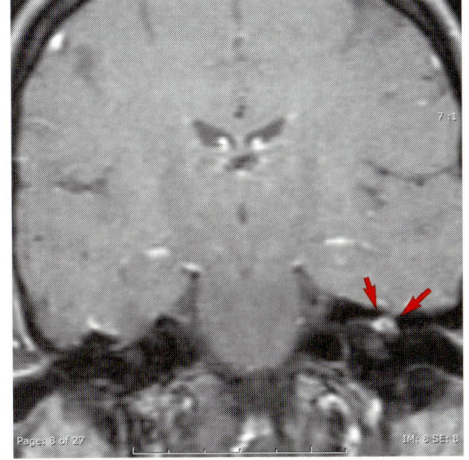
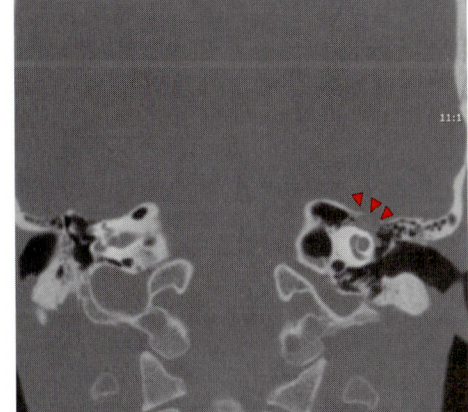
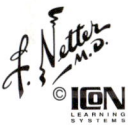

(**A** and **B**) Axial and coronal post–gadolinium-enhanced, T1-weighted, fat-saturated images demonstrate enlargement and enhancement of the geniculate ganglion (thin arrows). (**C**) Coronal thin section CT of petrous bone shows smooth enlargement of the geniculate region (arrowheads).

such as the levator palpebrae superioris and the temporalis, are also involved. Therefore, ptosis and jaw weakness often also occur. **Congenital myotonic dystrophy** may present with bilateral facial diplegia and is sometimes associated with severe neonatal hypotonia. Facial weakness occurs in 95% of patients with **facioscapulohumeral dystrophy** who are younger than 30 years. It affects predominantly the orbicularis oris and is often asymmetric. Although facial weakness is rarely the presenting problem, most patients with facioscapulohumeral dystrophy reveal long histories of difficulties whistling or blowing balloons. Therefore, facial involvement is likely to be an early, slowly progressing sign.

Recurrent CN-VII Palsy

Recurrence occurs in approximately 10% of Bell palsy cases, a circumstance necessitating extensive diagnostic evaluation to exclude underlying causes, especially neoplasms and basilar meningeal involvement.

Melkersson-Rosenthal syndrome, an autosomal dominant hereditary disorder, is characterized by a triad of facial palsy, facial edema, and a furrowed tongue (lingua plicata) but often exhibits an incomplete penetrance. Each component may occur independently or in combination. Patient history is characterized by recurrent attacks of facial paralysis, often beginning during childhood. Attacks can also include facial swelling, particularly affecting the upper lip. The tendency to recur is the only feature of facial paralysis that distinguishes it from most Bell palsy cases.

Hereditary liability to pressure palsies is an allelic disorder with the Charcot-Marie-Tooth IA neuropathy, caused by deletion of the region containing the peripheral-myelin-protein 22 gene. It manifests with recurrent acute painless palsies from nerve lesions at sites of compression or increased exposure. Although the typical presentation is of peroneal or ulnar neuropathy, recurrent facial paralysis occasionally occurs.

CN-VII Hyperactivity

Several positive symptoms occur from excessive reactivity of CN-VII; **synkinesis**, **facial myokymia**, and **hemifacial spasm** are the most frequent.

Synkinesis is frequently observed subsequent to aberrant reinnervation in patients with antecedent severe Bell palsy; an inappropriate facial movement results, ie, concomitant blinking while smiling. **Ephaptic transmission**, or "artificial synapse", may arise at a lesion site where depolarization of the injured fibers acts as a stimulus to the intact portion of the nerve.

Facial myokymia is characterized by subtle, continuous, undulating movement of facial muscles. The movements are usually unilateral, subtle, often confined to 1 to 2 facial muscles, and sometimes accompanied by facial contracture or weakness. Observed mainly in **multiple sclerosis**, it much less commonly reflects an intrinsic brainstem tumor, particularly **pontine gliomas**. In the former, it is usually self-limited and abates after several weeks. Some cases of facial myokymia are thought to be from an antibody-mediated specific subtype of voltage-gated potassium channels. The specific antibody identified in some patients with facial myokymia also occurs with Isaac syndrome.

Hemifacial spasm consists of intermittent paroxysms of rapid, irregular, clonic twitching facial movements. The attack typically starts around the eyes and spreads to other ipsilateral facial muscles, especially in the perioral region. It is strictly confined to muscles innervated by CN-VII; preceding CN-VII lesions are rare. Paroxysms are often induced by voluntary or reflex facial movements, stress, and fatigue and may persist during sleep. The most common pathogenetic mechanism of hemifacial spasm seems to be vascular compression of CN-VII by an aberrant arterial loop near the brainstem. Therefore, detailed imaging studies including MRA are essential for diagnosis of hemifacial spasm. Less frequent pathophysiologic mechanisms include tumors and localized infectious processes. Botox injections are an effective symptomatic treatment. Surgical decompression is an alternative sometimes leading to remission.

DIAGNOSTIC MODALITIES

Diagnostic modalities include imaging studies that may define the presence of contiguous or rarely intrinsic CN-VII lesions and testing modalities used to study the various functions of CN-VII.

Imaging Studies

The 2 primary imaging options are MRI and CT. MRI is best at imaging the CP angle and the parotid gland. CT is the choice to image the temporal bone and its facial (fallopian) canal. MRI must include primary and gadolinium enhancement images. The concentration of contrast agent within lesions is of diagnostic importance. A **proximal lesion at the CP angle** is easily identified with brain MRI. There may be unexpected relatively diffuse leptomeningeal enhancement when a facial neuropathy is the inciting lesion leading to a diagnosis of metastatic carcinoma or lymphoma.

Primary facial neuromas also strongly enhance with contrast. It is crucial that the ordering physician indicate a diagnosis of facial palsy, requesting an evaluation of CN-VII along its entire course, not just the intracranial portion.

Extracranial lesions must also be considered in the imaging evaluation of facial weakness/palsy. If the neoplasm appears to be distal to the stylomastoid foramen, as with a highly malignant **adenocarcinoma of parotid**

gland, MRI of the face may identify this tumor. Bone erosion or destruction versus remodeling is another important distinction that can be evaluated only on a bone window CT. Slow-growing benign lesions remodel bone, whereas bone erosion is more indicative of an aggressive or malignant process.

Intrinsic CN-VII Topognostic Testing Studies

Intrinsic CN-VII topognostic testing studies are based on the presence or absence of specific anatomical branch-point functions. With modern imaging studies, these are used less often but are occasionally valuable.

Motor fibers of CN-VII innervate the many striated facial muscles, including the stapedius. Its motor innervation is the most proximal branch of this group. An abnormality in the efferent limb of the **acoustic reflex** arc localizes the lesion proximal to this branch. The absence of a unilateral acoustic reflex suggests an afferent or efferent problem. If auditory function is normal on audiometric testing, the afferent arc is normal.

The **Schirmer test** of lacrimal flow depends on an intact geniculate ganglion, the site of the most proximal anatomical branch point along the course of CN-VII, giving rise to the greater superficial petrosal nerve. The greater superficial petrosal nerve carries autonomic fibers to the lacrimal gland. Decreased lacrimation based on Schirmer testing suggests a problem with the lacrimal gland, the greater superficial petrosal nerve, or CN-VII proximal to the ganglion. An associated facial palsy eliminates the former 2 possibilities.

REFERENCES

Ang KL, Jones NS. Melkersson-Rosenthal syndrome. *J Laryngol Otol.* 2002;116:386-388.

Grogan PM, Gronseth GS. Practice parameter: steroids, acyclovir, and surgery for Bell's palsy (an evidence-based review): report of the Quality Standards Subcommittee of the American Academy of Neurology. *Neurology.* 2001;56:830-836.

Grose C, Bonthius D, Afifi AK. Chickenpox and the geniculate ganglion: facial nerve palsy, Ramsay Hunt syndrome and acyclovir treatment. *Pediatr Infect Dis J.* 2002;21:615-617.

Hanson MR, Sweeney PJ. Disturbances of lower cranial nerves. In: Bradley WG, Daroff RB, Fenichel GM, Marsden CD, eds. *Neurology in Clinical Practice: Principles of Diagnosis and Management.* 2nd ed. Boston, Mass: Butterworth-Heinemann; 1996;251-263.

Keane JR. Bilateral seventh nerve palsy: analysis of 43 cases and review of the literature. *Neurology.* 1994;44:1198-1202.

Knox GW. Treatment controversies in Bell palsy. *Arch Otolaryngol Head Neck Surg.* 1998;124:821-823.

Renault F, Quijano-Roy S. Congenital and acquired facial palsies. In: Jones HR, De Vivo DC, Darras BT, eds. *Neuromuscular Disorders of Infancy, Childhood, and Adolescence: A Clinician's Approach.* Philadelphia, Pa: Butterworth-Heinemann; 2003;277-300.

Sweeney CJ, Gilden DH. Ramsay Hunt syndrome. *J Neurol Neurosurg Psychiatry.* 2001;71:149–154.

Sweeney PJ, Hanson MR. The cranial neuropathies. In: Bradley WG, Daroff RB, Fenichel GM, Marsden CD, eds. *Neurology in Clinical Practice: Principles of Diagnosis and Management.* 2nd ed. Boston, Mass: Butterworth-Heinemann; 1996;1721-1732.

Ter Bruggen JP, van der Meche FG, de Jager AE, et al. Ophthalmoplegic and lower cranial nerve variants merge into each other and into classical Guillain-Barre syndrome. *Muscle Nerve.* 1998;21:239-242.

Verzijl HT, van der Zwaag B, Cruysberg JR, et al. Mobius syndrome redefined: a syndrome of rhombencephalic maldevelopment. *Neurology.* 2003;61:327-333.

Chapter 12
Cranial Nerve VIII: Vestibular

Kinan K. Hreib, Judith White, and Marie C. Lucey

Clinical Vignette

A 65-year-old woman came to the emergency department with a chief complaint of "dizziness." At 3:00 AM, she had awoken to an odd feeling in her head, which was accompanied by nausea. As she turned to her right to ask her husband for help, she experienced a severe spinning sensation with increased nausea followed by vomiting. The symptoms lasted for a few minutes. However, in the car and subsequently in the emergency department, any head and neck movement precipitated recurrent symptoms. Her medical history included diabetes mellitus, hypertension, and a remote TIA manifested by right-sided weakness.

Her blood pressure was 180/90 mm Hg. She appeared pale and uncomfortable and refused to open her eyes or move her head during the examination. The findings of her neurologic examination were normal, with the exception that she was hesitant to get off the examining cart to allow gait testing. Brain MRI results were normal, excluding an acute cerebellar infarction. A subsequent otolith particle-repositioning (Epley) maneuver successfully alleviated her symptoms.

This vignette describes a classic case of an individual with acute benign paroxysmal positional vertigo (BPPV). In most patients, this annoying disorder can be successfully treated by a simple maneuver. However, the possibility of a stroke or other cerebellar lesion must be considered before making this diagnosis.

Dizziness is a common nonspecific symptom. In patients older than 75 years, it is the most common medical complaint that brings individuals to a physician; dizziness is the third most common symptom among all age groups. In the United States, there are 8 million visits annually for dizziness; chronic dizziness affects 16% of the self-reported population.

When patients report dizziness, one of the primary challenges is to define its precise character. Feeling faint or lightheaded and experiencing loss of equilibrium, vertigo, unsteady gait, and fainting can all be grouped under a patient's ill-defined description of "dizziness," although these symptoms often suggest different etiologies. Clarification of the precise historical details—onset, duration, positional and other exacerbating factors, and associated symptomatology—is essential to determine the likely cause.

Vertigo is the illusory perception of motion. Patients describe it as a sensation similar to that experienced on a merry-go-round. An inquiry as to whether things actually move in front of the patient's eyes helps the patient define this symptom. Determining whether vertigo is precisely present is helpful because any acute unilateral peripheral or central vestibular pathologic feature causes vertigo. Typical associated clinical findings include sudden precipitous onset, nausea and vomiting, nystagmus, and postural dysequilibrium.

Gaze-dependent nystagmus occurs in processes that affect the ipsilateral cerebellum. **Vertical nystagmus** seen **with upward gaze** is often the result of disease in the cerebellum or tegmentum. **Downward gaze vertical nystagmus** is most often found in processes at the foramen magnum level, especially Chiari malformations. *Optokinetic* nystagmus refers to a reflexive slow movement of the eye (**pursuit**) and a cortically driven corrective fast movement (**saccade**). Patients with parietal lobe lesions lose the fast, saccadic elements of the optokinetic response when the strip is moved in the direction of the abnormal hemisphere.

ANATOMY

The vestibulocochlear nerve, CN-VIII, is actually composed of 2 nerves: the vestibular and cochlear nerves. The vestibular nerve is responsible for efferent and afferent fibers that control balance and equilibrium. The cochlear nerve,

CRANIAL NERVE VIII: VESTIBULAR

Figure 12-1
Vestibular Receptors

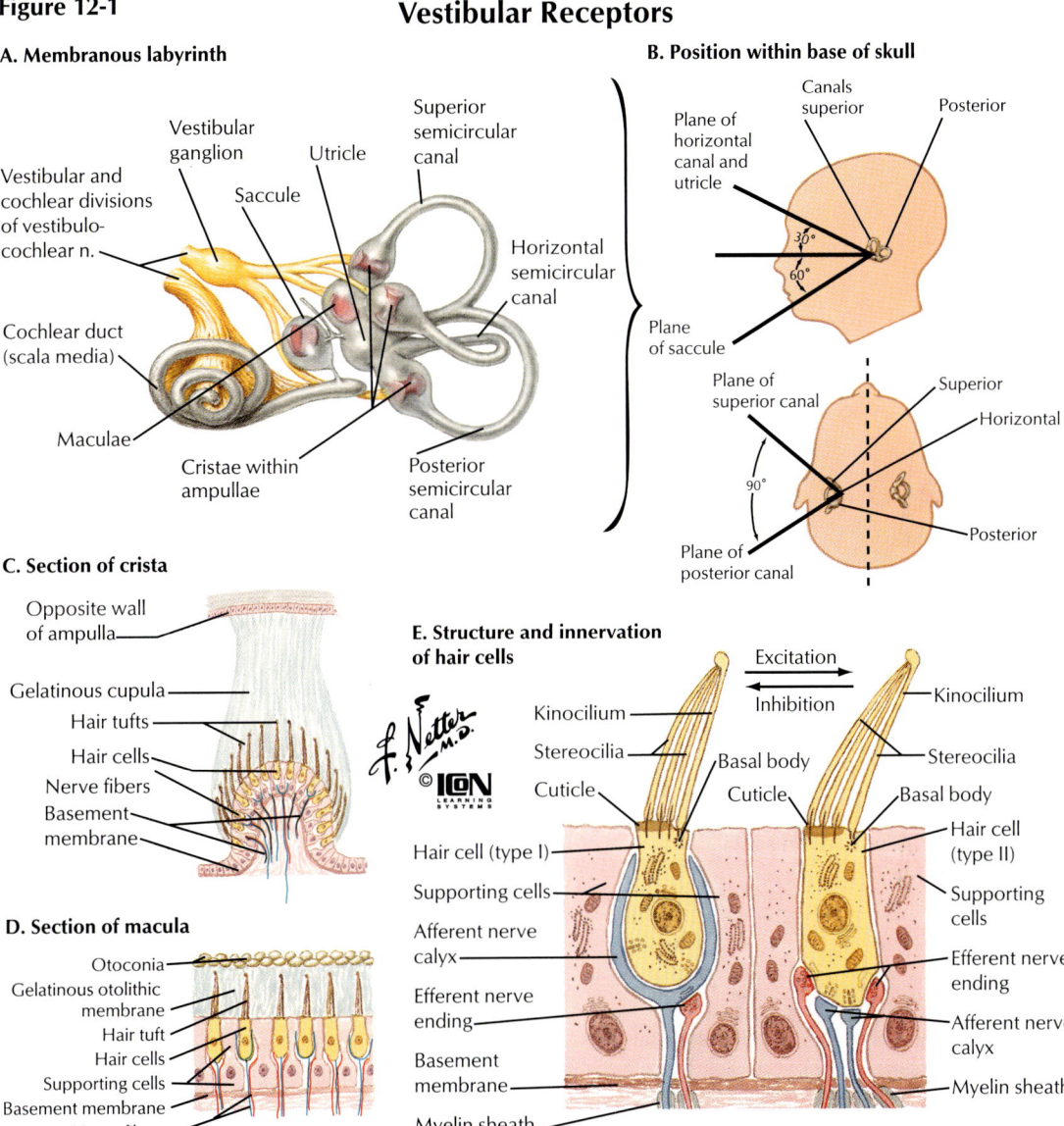

CRANIAL NERVE VIII: VESTIBULAR

also called the *auditory nerve*, carries the efferent and afferent fibers for hearing. The vestibular system provides specific sensory input and influences motor function in reference to postural control (Figures 11-1 and 12-1); the latter depends on interrelated mechanisms, including perception of position and motion in relation to gravity and orientation of the head and body in relation to vertical during quiet stance. Other vestibular functions include the selection of appropriate sensory cues for postural orientation in various sensory environments; this aids in controlling the center of gravity when the body is static or moving and stabilizes the head during bodily movements. Because the vestibular system primarily provides sensory information about the head on the body, the CNS must rely on other sensory modalities to determine overall body position and movement.

The visual system provides multiple information modes about head position and movement with respect to the environment, the direction of vertical, and low frequency information regarding slow or static tilts. Joint position and muscle stretch also contribute to the somatosensory system, which provides information about the relative alignment of body segments with each other and the support surface. Postural control involves the combination of the complex organization of this sensory information, a "central set" based on previous experience and biomechanical constraints. Normally, to maintain proper body alignment over the support base, the individual generates a motor output via the vestibulospinal and corticospinal systems.

During the patient's initial evaluation, it is important to differentiate a CNS lesion from a peripheral localization by determining whether any associated neurologic deficits exist (Figure 12-3).

CNS DISORDERS

Brainstem dysfunction typically includes prominent dysmetria, diplopia, dysphagia, dysarthria, perioral numbness, or weakness. Of patients with risk factors for stroke who present to emergency medical settings with isolated vertigo, nystagmus, and postural instability, 25% have an inferior cerebellum infarction within the territory of the posterior inferior cerebellar artery. The acute postural instability with a posterior inferior cerebellar artery infarction is usually so severe that independent ambulation is not possible. Similarly, patients with multiple sclerosis with lesions in the brainstem may present with acute vertigo and gait dysfunction.

In contrast, patients with peripheral vestibular disorders have preserved ambulation, although they may have feelings of dysequilibrium and be frightened to move as noted in the vignette. If carefully brought into the upright posture, most of these individuals can ambulate well.

Therefore, for patients presenting with vertigo who concomitantly cannot ambulate independently, and particularly those with vascular risk factors, brain imaging is mandated to rule out cerebellar infarction or multiple sclerosis. Other than difficulty walking, there may be no cerebellar or central findings with a posterior inferior cerebellar artery infarction. This diagnosis is particularly important because acute postinfarction swelling or hemorrhage within the cerebellar hemisphere can cause brainstem compression and death (chapters 20 and 62).

PERIPHERAL NERVOUS SYSTEM DISORDERS

Acute peripheral vestibular dysfunction causes vertigo by interrupting the normal tonic discharge of 1 labyrinth. The matched tonic input of both vestibular end organs is processed centrally to mediate head stability. Unilateral reduction in vestibular input is interpreted as turning. In the intact vestibular system, upright head rotation causes a reduction in horizontal semicircular canal firing rate on one side, paired with an increased firing rate on the other side. With acute unilateral vestibular loss, the reduced firing rate simulates the normal response to turning, generating fast phase nystagmus away from the affected ear. The nystagmus is usually more pronounced in gaze toward the affected side and reduced in gaze away from the affected side (law of Alexander). Veering or tilting toward the side of lesion may be present, from effects on the vestibular-spinal, vestibular-ocular, and vestibular-cerebellar pathways.

CRANIAL NERVE VIII: VESTIBULAR

Figure 12-2

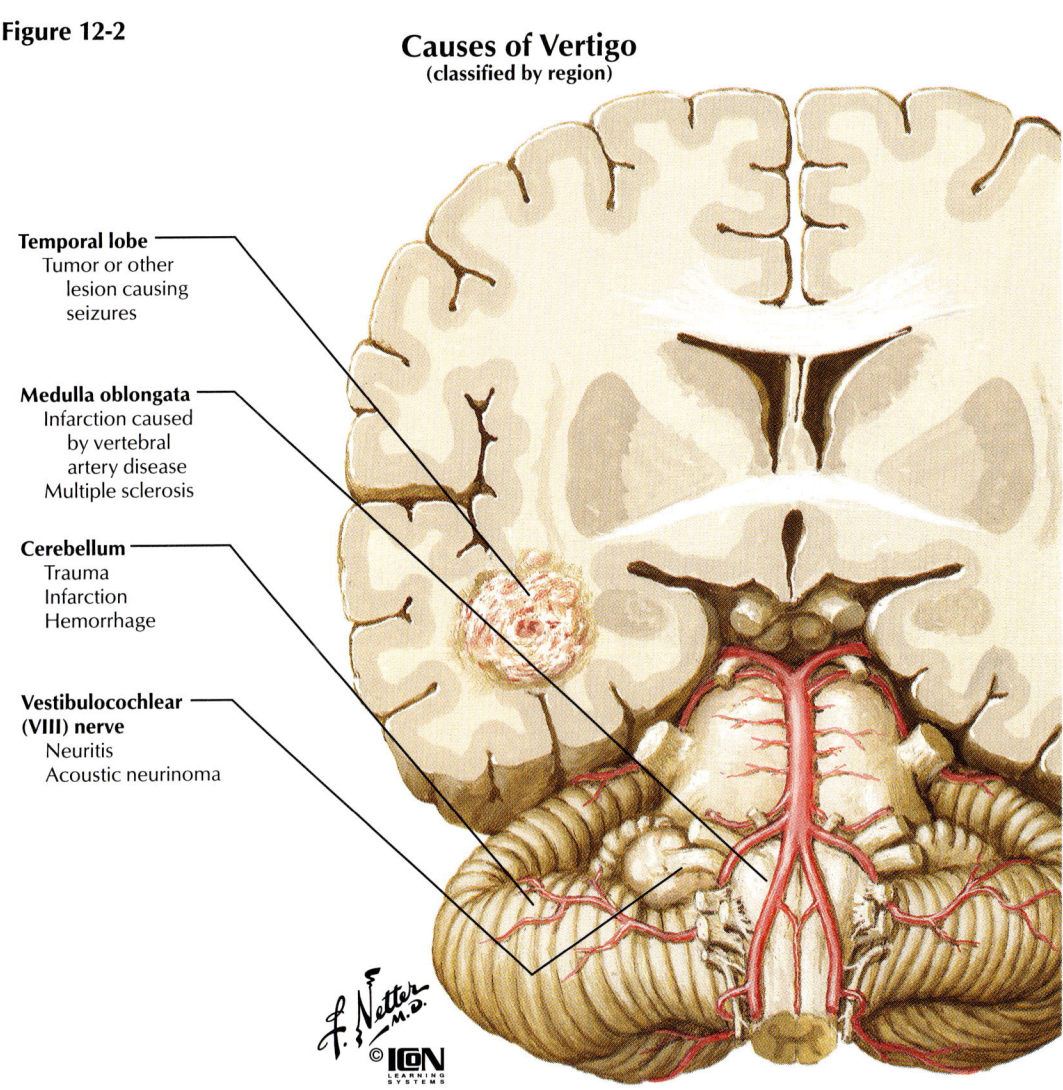

Causes of Vertigo
(classified by region)

Temporal lobe
  Tumor or other lesion causing seizures

Medulla oblongata
  Infarction caused by vertebral artery disease
  Multiple sclerosis

Cerebellum
  Trauma
  Infarction
  Hemorrhage

Vestibulocochlear (VIII) nerve
  Neuritis
  Acoustic neurinoma

ETIOLOGIC CLASSIFICATION OF PERIPHERAL VESTIBULOPATHIES

Etiologic classification of peripheral vestibulopathies is initially based on symptoms and the presence of hearing loss. When symptoms persist for days to weeks, and concomitant cochlear symptoms such as hearing loss and tinnitus are present, a diagnosis of **labyrinthitis** is made once other causes are excluded. Although labyrinthitis is presumably of viral origin, certain structural pathologic conditions including erosive cholesteatoma, temporal bone trauma or fistula, and central pathophysiologic mechanisms need to be excluded.

Ménière disease, secondary to an imbalance of the inner ear's endolymph, is characterized by recurrent episodes of vertigo lasting for hours, associated with hearing loss and tinnitus. Rarely, infectious processes, including syphilis, Lyme disease, and HIV, mimic Ménière disease. Similarly, certain central processes such as acoustic neuroma must be excluded. Studies suggest that bilateral Ménière disease may have an autoimmune basis.

CRANIAL NERVE VIII: VESTIBULAR

Vestibular neuritis is characterized by prolonged vertigo without hearing loss. This is a cranial mononeuropathy, limited to the vestibular division of CN-VIII. Diagnosis is often difficult in patients with recurrent true vertiginous episodes lasting hours, without associated cochlear symptomatology.

Initially, it is important to exclude vertebrobasilar TIAs, particularly in those with vascular risk factors, including young persons with recent neck injury predisposing the individual to a vertebral artery dissection. However, it is rare for vertigo to be the sole manifestation of a TIA, emphasizing the importance of a careful history. The patient may overlook seemingly less important symptoms that could lead to a diagnosis and may focus on the vertigo. Occasionally, early Ménière disease is diagnosed in some patients when hearing loss eventually develops.

TYPES OF VERTIGO

Benign paroxysmal positional vertigo is usually intense, short-lived, and reliably reproduced by positional maneuvers. Typically, patients with BPPV report rotational vertigo lasting for seconds when lying down, arising quickly, bending, looking up, or reaching or when extending the neck or lying back at the hairdresser or dentist. BPPV results from otoconial/statoconium (otolith) debris entering the semicircular canals and rendering them gravitationally sensitive. Normally, the canals respond to angular acceleration (turning) by the fluid in the canal transducing inertial momentum by pressing against the crista and stimulating the vestibular neurons. Solid debris acts as a plunger or weight, disrupting the normal function.

Immediate treatment with particle repositioning maneuvers is effective in 80% to 90% of cases (Figure 12-3). Although most cases of BPPV involve the posterior canal, rarely horizontal or anterior canal involvement will cause variation in the observed nystagmus pattern. Risk factors for BPPV include recent head trauma (which can be relatively minor), otologic surgery or disease, habitual unusual positioning such as is a daily occurrence for plumbers, mechanics, and yoga enthusiasts, or advanced age. Prevalence studies suggest that 10% of community-dwelling elderly may have BPPV.

Chronic vestibulopathies are less likely to cause vertigo, because their duration allows for CNS compensation. Acoustic neuromas and other slow-growing neoplasms affecting CN-VIII may cause unilateral tinnitus, hearing loss, and abnormal hypoactive caloric responses on electronystagmogram. However, these tumors rarely present with vertigo.

Bilateral vestibular problems do not typically cause vertigo. Because vestibular input is bilaterally reduced, there is no sensation of turning. However, disruption of bilateral vestibular input affects the vestibular-ocular reflex, which stabilizes visual perception during head motion. Vestibulotoxic agents, such as aminoglycosides, alcohol, and heavy metals, can also lead to transient or permanent vestibular damage. Bilateral vestibular hypo-function can occur in otherwise healthy adults (idiopathic) or can result from a genetic predisposition.

Oscillopsia, or failure to stabilize vision during head movement, can cause bobbing visual perception while walking, with decline in dynamic visual acuity. Because some patients call this "dizziness," the history differentiates such from true vertigo. Oscillopsia is typically seen in patients with the Arnold-Chiari syndrome, a developmental condition often associated with syringomyelia and syringobulbia. This symptom complex may also occur in patients with other lesions involving the brainstem, particularly at the foramen magnum. It may be rarely observed in patients with multiple sclerosis or those receiving ototoxic drugs. If it involves only 1 eye, the possibility of ocular muscle myokymia is a benign consideration.

DIAGNOSTIC APPROACH

When one sensory vestibular mechanism is absent, the remaining sensory inputs are used to elicit postural reactions. Other neurologic disorders including stroke, Parkinson disease, cerebellar pathologic conditions, or peripheral neuropathy may affect the potential of the CNS for compensation. Careful musculoskeletal evaluation can define the presence of impairments in muscle strength, particularly the large truncal and proximal lower extremity musculature, and in postural alignment, such as scoliosis, kyphosis, or lower extremity contractures.

CRANIAL NERVE VIII: VESTIBULAR

Figure 12-3

Canalith Repositioning
(Epley Maneuver)

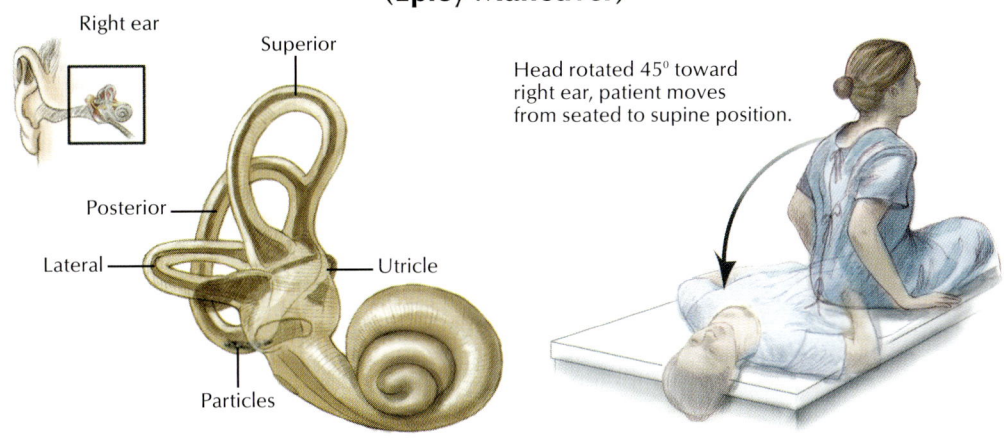

Head rotated 45° toward right ear, patient moves from seated to supine position.

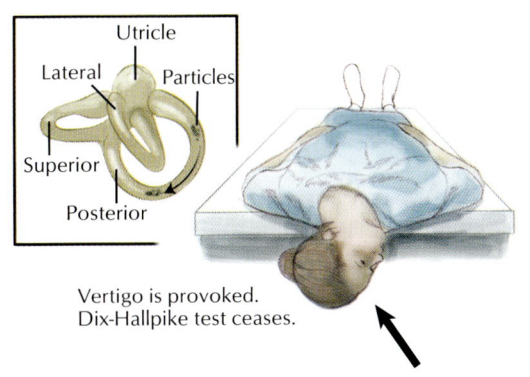

Vertigo is provoked. Dix-Hallpike test ceases.

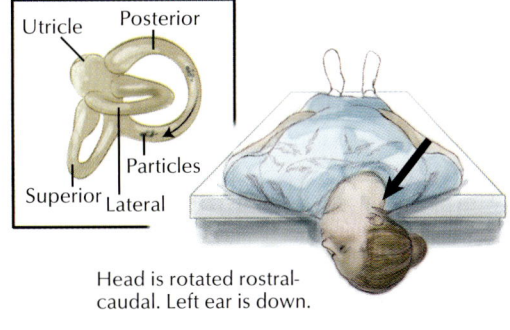

Head is rotated rostral-caudal. Left ear is down.

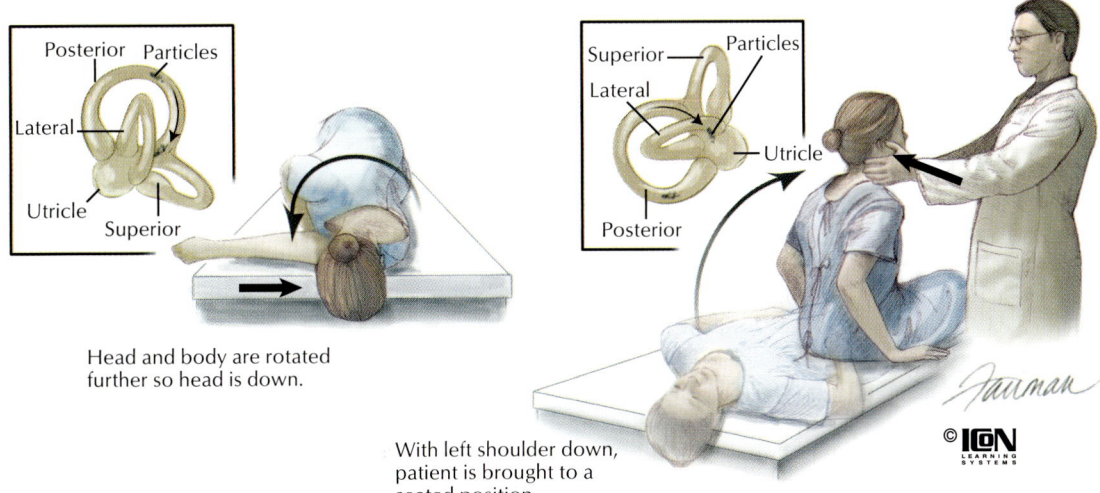

Head and body are rotated further so head is down.

With left shoulder down, patient is brought to a seated position.

CRANIAL NERVES

CRANIAL NERVE VIII: VESTIBULAR

Dynamic posturography is a complex testing modality providing useful information to define the extent to which a patient is able to use visual, somatosensory, and vestibular input for postural control. However, to date, the value of this test is still open to question, although it is sometimes a useful tool for designing rehabilitation strategies.

The clinical test of sensory interaction and balance uses a combination of 3 visual and 2 support surface conditions to clinically measure a patient's sensory interaction for postural stability. The **Romberg test**, sharpened Romberg with eyes open and eyes closed, and unilateral standing with eyes open and eyes closed are not specific for postural deficits secondary to vestibular pathologic conditions. However, patients with vestibular damage may demonstrate increased sway or falling during these tests.

Dynamic tests, such as floor walking with the eyes closed, measure tandem walking for up to 10 steps. Persons with acute or chronic vestibular disorders may fail this test based on established age-related norms.

Several performance tests are used to establish a baseline function analysis and measure outcome in individuals with impairments of static and dynamic postural control. These include the Timed Up and Go Test, the Dynamic Gait Index, and the Berg Balance Scale.

The **Timed Up and Go** test measures the time required to rise from a standard chair, walk 10 feet, return to that chair, and sit. The norm for neurologically intact, older adults is 10 to 12 seconds. The results may be a predictor for falls in community-dwelling elders. There is a maximum of 14 seconds for elders at minimal risk for falls and less than 30 seconds for elders who are dependent on assistance for ambulation in the community. There is no threshold established for patients with vestibular disorders.

The **Dynamic Gait Index** measures a patient's ability to modify gait in response to 8 different task demands during ambulation. Each task is given a score of 0 to −3, with a maximum of 24 points. A mean score of 21 ± 3 is defined for older adults with no neurologic impairments or history of imbalance. In contrast, a score of 11 ± 4 is found in older adults with a history of falls but no neurologic disorders.

The Berg Balance Scale, another useful evaluation modality, uses 14 test-specific items rated 0 to 4 that measure postural control during functionally related tasks. These require anticipatory abilities and are performed only while sitting and standing. Test score is a good predictor of elderly fall status. Scores less than 45 were associated with an increase risk for falls; scores less than 36 were associated with a 100% risk of falls.

TREATMENT
Rehabilitation

Many vestibular rehabilitation programs provide a range of treatment modalities aimed to facilitate acute recovery and ongoing compensation programs for patients with degrees of residual vestibular deficit. Some are useful for acute or chronic vestibular lesions and are equally applicable to vertigo, dizziness, and dysequilibrium.

Pharmacologic Therapy

Recent studies suggest that methylprednisolone significantly improves the recovery of peripheral vestibular neuritis, whereas valacyclovir does not. Treatment was begun with 100 mg daily with reduction by 20 mg every third day, eventually down to 10 mg daily. Vestibular suppressant medications such as meclizine, scopolamine, and benzodiazepines are useful for relief of acute symptoms of vertigo, dizziness, and dysequilibrium. However, long-term use interferes with central vestibular compensation mechanisms.

Nonpharmacologic Therapy

Vestibular compensation results from active neuronal changes in the cerebellum and the brainstem in response to sensory conflicts created by vestibular pathology. Despite spontaneous "recovery," patients still experience disequilibrium, motion-provoked vertigo, or both because the system, inhibited by the cerebellum, is unable to respond appropriately to labyrinthine input produced by normal head movement.

Because movement provokes symptoms of dysequilibrium and vertigo, patients with vestibular disorders may restrict their activity level and trunk and head movements to avoid these symptoms. This provides for greater short-term compensatory stability but interferes with long-term recovery if patients are not challenged to increase movement to facilitate vestibular compensation. Educating patients about vestibular function encourages and reassures them to safely increase their activity level even though early recovery movement provokes symptoms.

Initially, an assistive device such as a cane or walker may be recommended. Sensory input through the upper extremity from a cane or light touch through fingertips can reduce postural sway in patients without vestibular function.

Motor organization exercises also improve standing, ambulation, and functional activities such as moving at various speeds, changing directions, and maneuvering around obstacles. These exercises also help to promote normal timing and coordination to maintain stability.

Weekly therapy visits for 4 to 12 weeks help to monitor the effectiveness of assigned home exercise programs. Treatment success also depends on the nature of the primary underlying neurologic dysfunction. Peripheral vestibular disorders such as BPPV and stable vestibular hypofunction are most amenable to treatment. In contrast, individuals with primary CNS disorders have poorer outcomes. However, many of these patients still demonstrate reduced symptomatology with treatment.

Other factors influencing treatment effectiveness include the degree of initial disability and a more recent time of onset. Comorbidities, such as underlying musculoskeletal dysfunction and other neurologic impairments, and patient compliance also affect outcomes. Elderly patients often require longer treatment times to reach maximum benefit. Similarly, they generally require more therapist contact in addition to a home exercise program. Patients with chronic vestibular disorders may also find help through the Vestibular Disorders Association, http://www.vestibular.org.

REFERENCES

Fregley AR, Graybiel A, Smith MJ. Walk on floor eyes closed (WOFEC): a new addition to an ataxia test battery. *Aerospace Med.* 72;43:395-399.

Furman J, Cass S. Benign paroxysmal positional vertigo. *N Engl J Med.* 1999;341:1590-1596.

Furman J, Whitney S. Central causes of dizziness. *Phys Ther.* 2000;80:179-187.

Herdman S. Advances in the treatment of vestibular disorders. *Phys Ther.* 1997;77:602-618.

Horak F. Clinical measures of postural control in adults. *Phys Ther.* 1987;67:1881-1885.

Horak FB, Jones-Rycewiccz C, Black FO, Shumway-Cook A. Effects of vestibular rehabilitation on dizziness and imbalance. *Otolaryngol Head Neck Surg.* 1992;106:175-180.

Hotson J, Baloh R. Acute vestibular syndrome. *N Engl J Med.* 1998;339:680-685.

Norrving B, Magnusson M, Holtas S. Isolated acute vertigo in the elderly: vestibular or vascular disease? *Acta Neurol Scand.* 1995;91:43-48.

Mathias S, Nayak U, Issacs B. Balance in elderly patients: the "Get Up & Go" test. *Arch Phys Med Rehabil.* 1986;67:387-389.

Podsialdo D, Richardson S. The timed "Up & Go": a test of basic functional mobility for frail elderly persons. *J Am Geriatr Soc.* 1991;39:142-148.

Shumway-Cook A, Brauer S, Woollacott M. Predicting the probability for falls in community-dwelling older adults using the timed up and go test. *Phys Ther.* 2000;80:896-903.

Strupp M, Zingler VC, Arbusow V, et al. Methylprednisolone, valacyclovir, or the combination for vestibular neuritis. *N Engl J Med.* 2004;351:354-361.

Chapter 13
Cranial Nerve VIII: Auditory

Ellen Choi and Peter J. Catalano

Clinical Vignette

A 68-year-old man presented with sudden onset of unilateral right-sided hearing loss. He stated that this was preceded by several months of constant ringing in his right ear. He had a history of hypertension and type II diabetes mellitus that was well controlled by oral hypoglycemic agents. He had no recent head trauma or previous surgeries. His only medications included atenolol and glyburide. There was no family history of hearing loss. He did not have a history of excess noise exposure or recent travel. No other otolaryngologic symptoms were reported.

On examination, his tympanic membranes (TMs) were bilaterally normal. The Weber test lateralized the tuning fork to the side opposite his hearing loss. Rinne test results were normal. The rest of the head and neck examination findings were unremarkable.

CBC results were normal, and results of a fluorescent treponemal antibody absorption blood test were negative. Autoimmune screening tests were not ordered.

The patient received a baseline audiogram demonstrating a right ear sensorineural hearing deficit predominantly in the higher frequencies. Brain MRI failed to demonstrate any mass lesion. Because of its asymmetric distribution, a brainstem auditory evoked response (BAER) study was performed and revealed a prolonged interaural wave I-III latency, compatible with a retrocochlear process.

In this vignette, because of the patient's history of diabetes and the absence of a tumor or other more specific lesion, his sudden hearing loss may be attributed to a microvascular infarct of the auditory nerve. However, similar to other cardiovascular processes, there is no difference in the incidence of hearing loss between patients with and without diabetes; therefore, the etiology in this case is unknown.

ANATOMY

The vestibulocochlear nerve, CN-VIII, is actually composed of 2 nerves: the vestibular and cochlear nerves. The vestibular nerve is responsible for efferent and afferent fibers that control balance and equilibrium (chapter 12). The cochlear nerve, also called the auditory nerve, carries the efferent and afferent fibers for hearing. To understand dysfunction of the auditory nerve, a brief description of the human hearing mechanism is required.

Sound waves travel through the external auditory canal and vibrate the TM, which produces motion of the middle ear ossicles (incus, malleus, and stapes) (Figure 13-1). The vibrations are transmitted through the oval window at the footplate of the stapes, causing a fluid wave to travel through the endolymphatic fluid of the cochlea of the inner ear. The fluid waves vibrate the organ of Corti's basilar membrane, thus stimulating inner and outer hair cells. Hair cells, receptors of the sensorineural system, transmit action potentials to the bipolar neurons, the bodies of which are in the spiral ganglion.

Afferent fibers projecting toward the CNS comprise the auditory nerve (Figure 13-2). They travel to the dorsal and ventral cochlear nuclei located in the caudolateral part of the pons. Most of the secondary neurons project contralaterally over the midline to the superior olivary nucleus and then travel up the lateral lemniscus into the inferior colliculus of the midbrain. Decussating fibers from the cochlear nucleus to the superior olivary nucleus are located in the trapezoid bodies and also in the base of the pons. Fibers from the inferior colliculus continue to travel rostrally to the medial geniculate body of the thalamus and then terminate at the auditory cortex, located in the transverse temporal gyri of Heschl.

CRANIAL NERVE VIII: AUDITORY

Figure 13-1

Frontal section

Pathway of Sound Reception

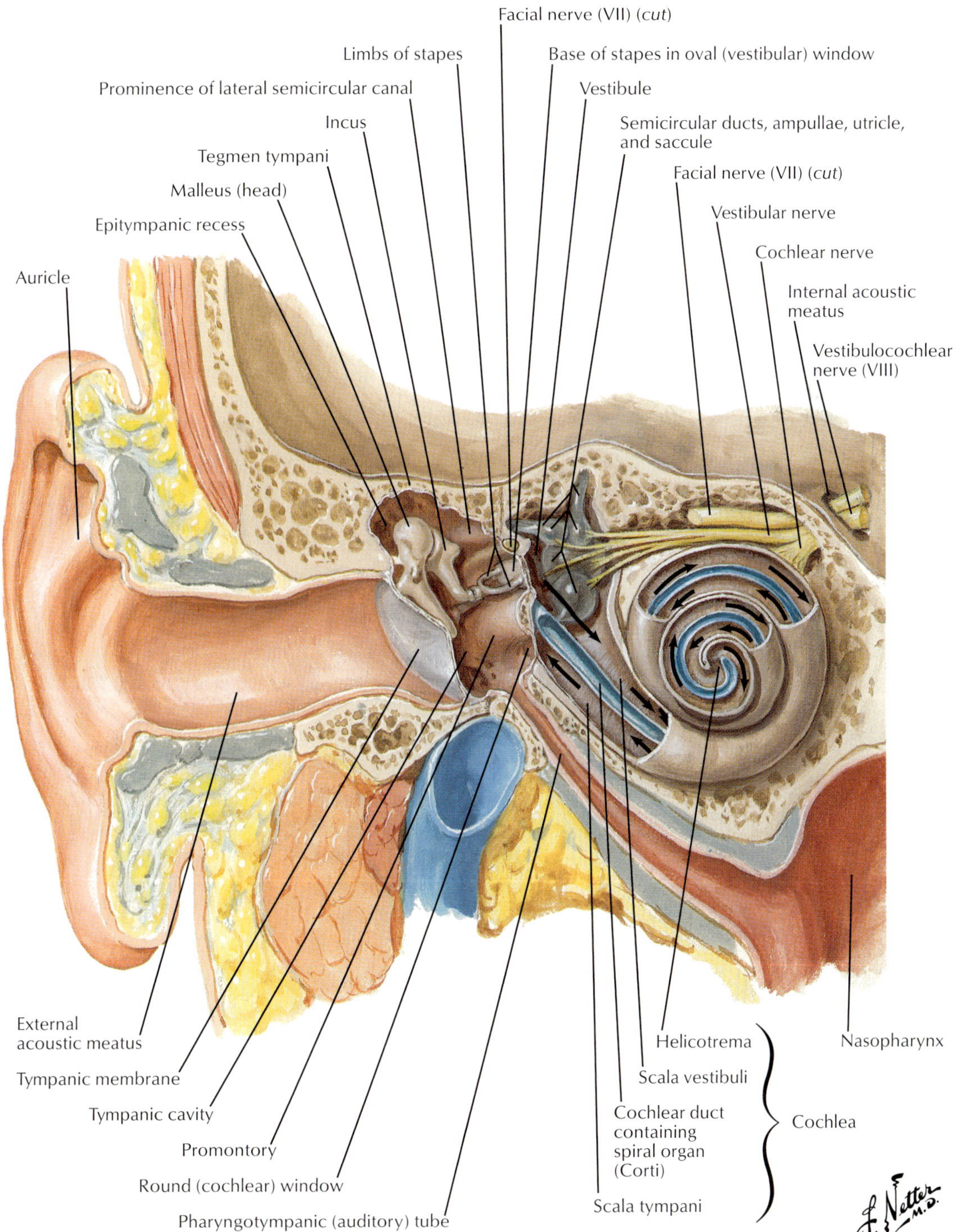

Note: Arrows indicate course of sound waves.

CRANIAL NERVES

135

CRANIAL NERVE VIII: AUDITORY

Figure 13-2

Afferent Auditory Pathways

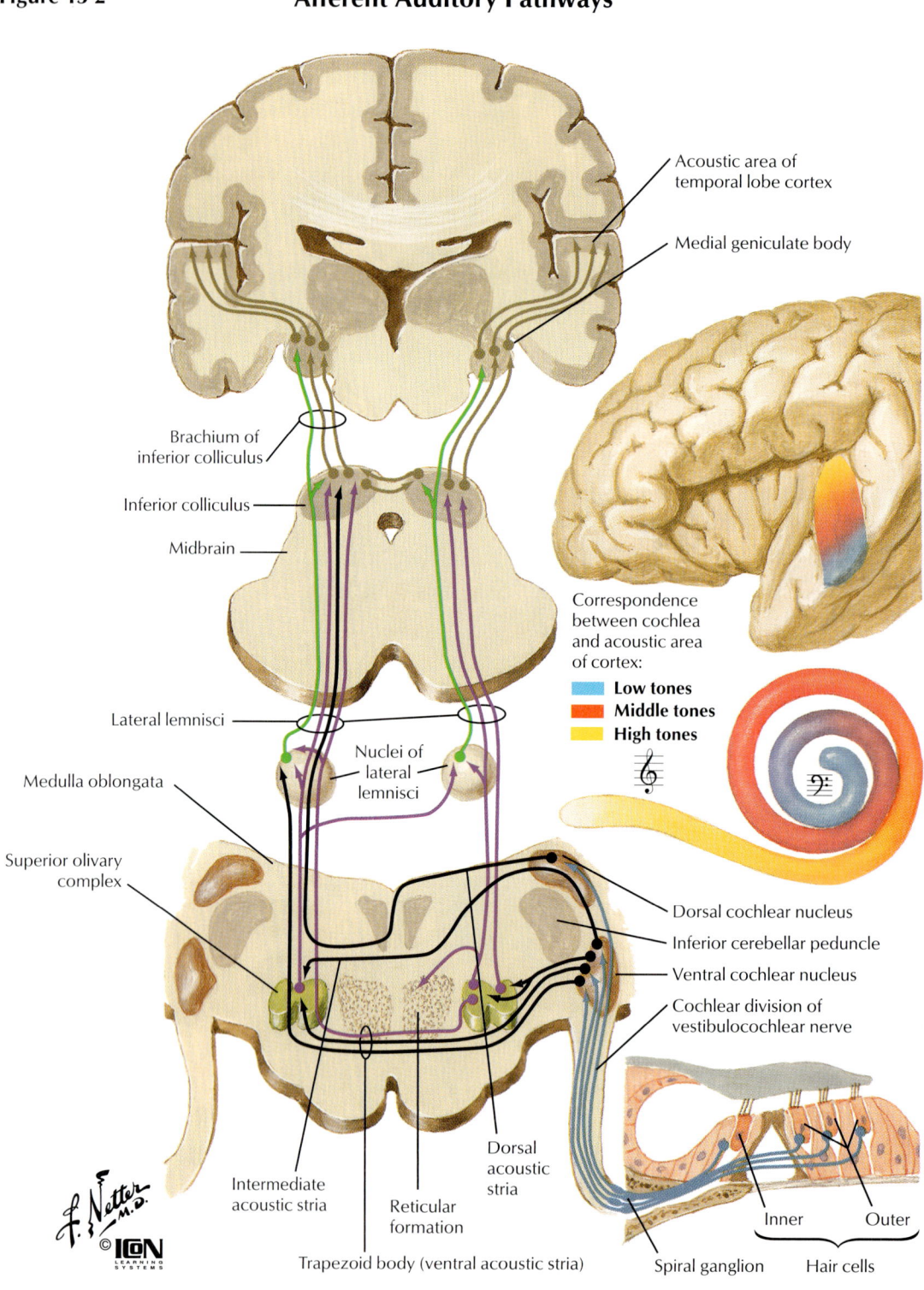

136

CRANIAL NERVES

CRANIAL NERVE VIII: AUDITORY

CLINICAL PRESENTATION
History

Auditory nerve dysfunction usually results in tinnitus, sensorineural hearing loss (SNHL), or both. SNHL is hearing deficit from dysfunction of the cochlea (sensory), the auditory nerve (neural), or any part of the central auditory pathway. Hearing loss can result from pathologic conditions anywhere along the anatomic pathway for hearing. It may involve the auditory nerve (eg, acoustic tumors), or the auditory nerve may be uninvolved (serous otitis media). A targeted history and physical examination narrow the diagnosis. The temporal profile of symptom onset (ie, sudden, progressive, fluctuating, or stable) is critical.

Tinnitus often presents concomitant with SNHL but can be the only presenting symptom. Tinnitus is classified into 2 subgroups. Subjective tinnitus, the most common, is heard solely by the patient. It can range from soft fluctuating ringing noise to loud constant roaring that can be debilitating. The cause is usually unknown; however, subjective tinnitus is associated with exposure to loud noise, ototoxic drugs (such as aspirin, cisplatinum, and aminoglycosides), acoustic tumors, Ménière disease, and cochlear otosclerosis. Objective tinnitus is heard by the patient and the examiner and is usually not a sign of auditory nerve dysfunction. Middle ear effusion, as in serous otitis media, can magnify vascular pulsations from the nearby internal carotid artery and produce vascular tinnitus. Pulsatile tinnitus is usually secondary to vascular causes, such as arteriovenous malformations or glomus tumors. Clicking tinnitus is secondary to temporomandibular joint disease, palatal myoclonus, or spontaneous contraction of the middle ear muscles.

Laterality of hearing loss is essential in the assessment. Bilateral hearing loss occurs in processes such as ototoxicity, noise exposure, and presbycusis (hearing loss related to aging). Unilateral hearing loss raises the concern of neoplastic, vascular, neurologic, or infectious etiologies. Fluctuation of hearing is seen in Ménière disease, whereas progressive or sudden hearing loss occurs with acoustic neuromas and viral neuritis, respectively.

Whether the hearing loss involves a process in the external or middle ear versus the inner ear must be determined. Only a few processes, such as otosclerosis and otitic meningitis, involve both areas. Typically, tinnitus and vertigo are inner ear symptoms and indicate involvement of the cochlea, vestibular labyrinth, or auditory nerve or a combination of these structures.

Hearing loss associated with otalgia, otorrhea, headache, and aural fullness is most likely inflammatory and can be confirmed on physical examination. Concomitant tinnitus, vertigo, or both suggest the ominous extension of the inflammatory process to the inner ear or beyond. In this setting, a formal audiogram is indicated to determine whether the perceived hearing loss is secondary to a middle ear effusion or an additional sensorineural component. The latter is an otolaryngologic emergency.

With both ototoxicity and Ménière disease, concomitant vestibular symptoms, tinnitus, aural fullness, or a combination of these symptoms may accompany hearing loss. In conditions such as presbycusis and noise-induced hearing loss, vestibular symptoms are less likely to be part of the presentation.

Neurologic or ophthalmologic complaints, or both, sometimes accompany primary otologic symptoms. These occur with diseases such as multiple sclerosis (MS) or expanding neoplastic lesions that may lead to combined facial nerve, trigeminal nerve, or ophthalmologic symptoms.

Systemic diseases can contribute to hearing loss and tinnitus. Ototoxic drugs (aminoglycosides, salicylates, or loop diuretics) are important causes of SNHL, tinnitus, and vestibular symptoms. Trauma to the temporal bone area, resulting in labyrinth or auditory nerve injury, can create auditory nerve dysfunction. Diving and flying may cause barotrauma, leading to rupture of the cochlear membranes with subsequent hearing loss. Occupational and recreational noise exposure damages the cochlea's outer hair cells, creating high-frequency hearing loss. It is also important to establish whether a family history of hearing loss exists because this can be an important mechanism.

Physical Examination

Cerumen impaction or foreign bodies are easily identified on inspection of the external audi-

CRANIAL NERVE VIII: AUDITORY

tory canal. Pneumatic otoscopy is used to assess quality (color, lucency, and mobility) of the TM and defines conductive hearing loss as a reason for hearing deficit. Decreased TM mobility can be attributed to ossicular fixation, such as otosclerosis, or middle ear effusion, as in otitis media. Middle ear or expanding jugular foramen tumors can present as a mass behind the TM and can cause conductive hearing loss.

Tuning fork tests assess whether the hearing loss is conductive or sensorineural (Figure 13-3) (chapter 1). During the head and neck examination, a complete cranial nerve examination must also be performed to assess other potential cranial nerve abnormalities. Facial nerve weakness may be attributed to viral infections, such as herpes zoster oticus, or expanding neoplasms in the internal auditory canal or cerebello-pontine angle, such as meningiomas or facial neuromas. Auscultation of the areas around the orbit and ear may detect pulsatile tinnitus.

Etiologies of SNHL

Ototoxic drugs, excess noise exposure, and autoimmune diseases affect the cochlea, the primary sensory organ of hearing, by damaging the hair cells within it. The quality of the hearing loss is usually described as decreased sensitivity to pure tones with preserved speech discrimination.

Hearing loss caused by retrocochlear lesions of the nerve fibers of CN-VIII or its central auditory projections begins as decreased speech discrimination with relatively normal pure tone sensitivity. Decreased speech discrimination is not exclusive to retrocochlear lesions; it is also observed with extensive hair cell damage.

DIAGNOSTIC APPROACH

Standard laboratory blood tests are not routinely obtained for hearing loss, unless a particular cause is suspected. Usually, the fluorescent treponemal antibody absorption blood test or the microhemagglutination test for *Treponema pallidum* or both should be ordered, because syphilis is often asymptomatic and is a treatable cause of SNHL. Routine tests for other systemic diseases are not useful unless prompted by the history and physical examination.

A basic audiogram with pure tones and speech discrimination evaluation determines the type and amount of hearing loss. (Serous effusion does not exclude a sensorineural component to the hearing loss.) Unilateral decrease or asymmetry in speech discrimination, high-frequency hearing loss, or acoustic reflex abnormalities suggest a retrocochlear lesion, warranting further testing.

Gadolinium-enhanced MRI is specifically indicated when history, symptoms, and audiometric tests strongly suggest retrocochlear disease. MRI is the diagnostic "gold standard" for tumors causing hearing loss. For patients presenting with asymmetric hearing loss, especially if sudden, MRI is warranted to exclude acoustic neuromas or other cerebellopontine tumors. MRI with gadolinium can detect 2- to 3-mm tumors within the temporal bone. It can also detect vascular disease and the lesions of MS.

Brainstem auditory evoked response is a useful objective and quantitative test when a retrocochlear deficit is suspected. It can suggest the site-of-lesion from the cochlea to the inferior colliculus in the pons. BAER studies were initially considered highly sensitive for retrocochlear causes; however, as with most tests, false-negative and false-positive results are possible. The BAER uses electrodes attached to the patient's head and clicking sounds emitted through earphones. The sounds elicit action potentials through the peripheral and central auditory pathways, and the EEG activity is measured and averaged by a computer. Right and left ear waveform morphologic appearance and latencies are compared. Interaural differences suggest pathologic conditions. Five wave peaks characterize the BAER, corresponding to specific anatomic points within the auditory pathway: I, CN-VIII action potential; II, cochlear nucleus; III, olivary complex; IV, lateral lemniscus; and V, inferior colliculus. A change in peak morphologic appearance and latency helps localize the pathologic condition.

DIFFERENTIAL DIAGNOSIS

Usually idiopathic, sudden SNHL is generally defined as loss that develops in 12 hours or less. However, a broad differential includes Ménière disease, neoplasms, vascular disorders, viral infections, MS, and rarely, hematologic disorders.

CRANIAL NERVE VIII: AUDITORY

Figure 13-3

Hearing Test: Weber and Rinne

Weber Test

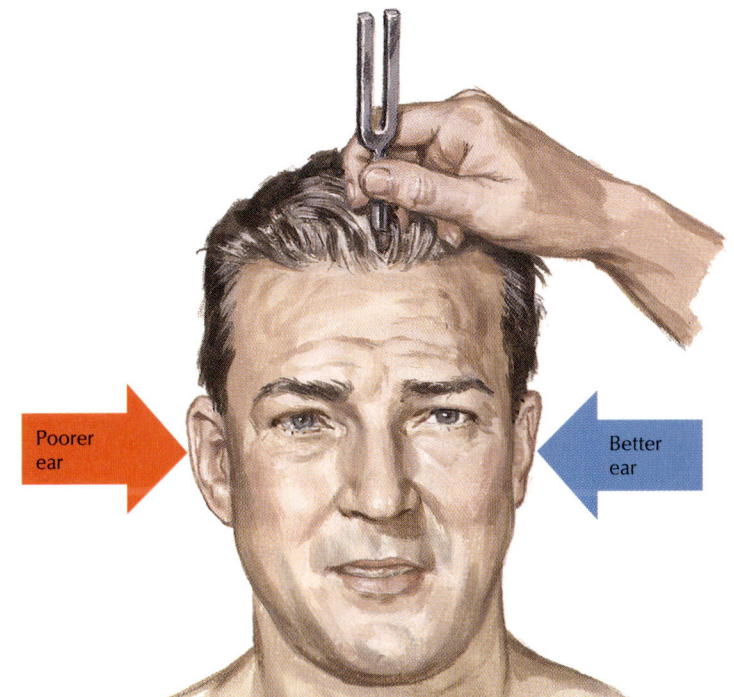

Tone referred to poorer ear indicates conductive impairment.

Tone referred to better ear indicated perceptive impairment.

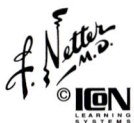

Rinne Test

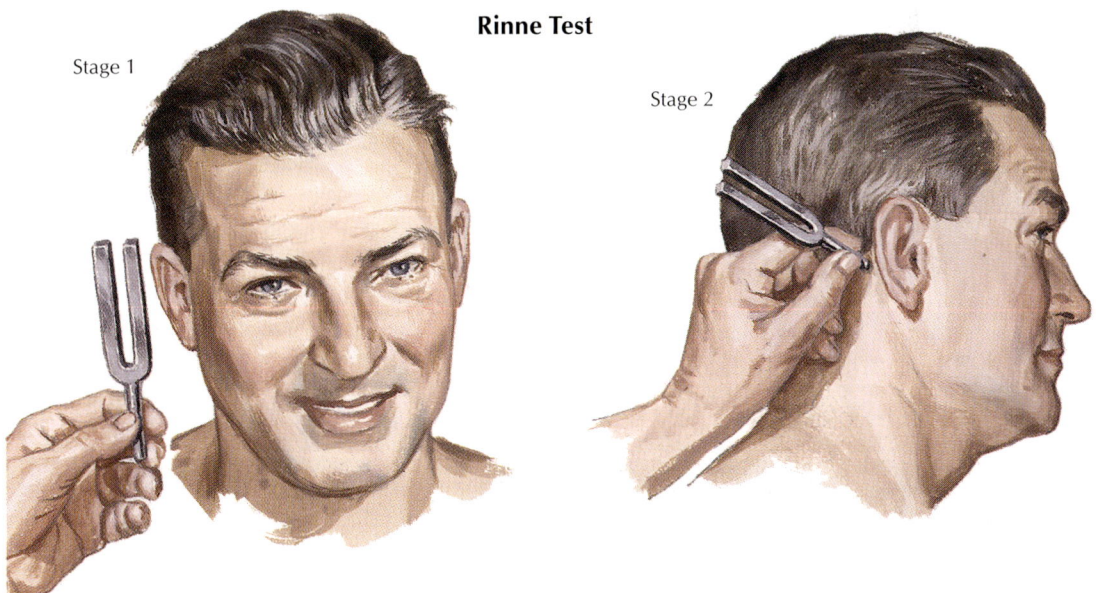

Tone heard longer by air conduction = Rinne positive: indicates perceptive loss
Tone heard longer by bone conduction = Rinne negative: indicates conductive loss

CRANIAL NERVES

CRANIAL NERVE VIII: AUDITORY

Figure 13-4
Vestibular Schwannoma

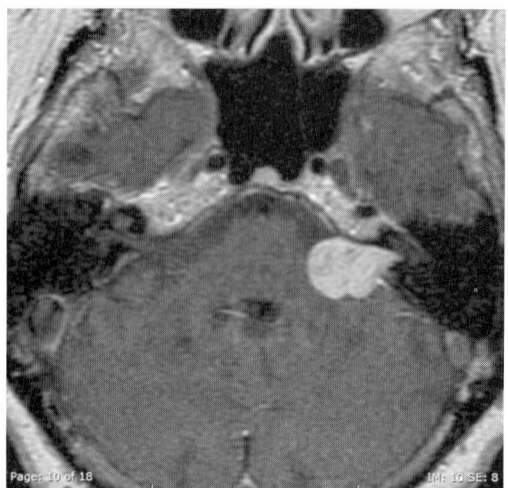

Axial T1-weighted, post-gadolinium-enhanced fat-saturated image shows an enhancing mass widening the medial left internal auditory canal and extending into the CP angle with distortion of the pons. The right side is normal (arrowhead).

© ICON LEARNING SYSTEMS

Ménière Disease

Ménière disease is an idiopathic process characterized by episodic vertigo, fluctuating SNHL, tinnitus, aural fullness, or a combination of these symptoms. Vestibular symptoms are usually the main complaint. Patients with Ménière disease likely constitute less than 5% of all patients with SNHL. However, a condition called cochlear Ménière produces only SNHL and is considered a "diagnosis of exclusion" because there are no specific tests for it.

Neoplasms

In any case of sudden, unilateral hearing loss, neoplastic lesions, although rare, belong in the differential until excluded by diagnostic and radiologic testing. Acoustic neuromas are benign tumors arising from the Schwann cells of CN-VIII and account for 6% of all intracranial tumors. These occur on the vestibular portion of CN-VIII, involving its adjacent cochlear division by compression against the bony walls of the internal auditory canal. Less commonly, neuromas can also arise directly from the cochlear nerve.

Hearing loss is the most commonly reported symptom, occurring in approximately 95% of patients during the disease. Progressive hearing loss generally results from stretching or compression of the cochlear nerve as the tumor grows. In contrast, when the hearing loss is precipitous, it is thought to be secondary to occlusion of the internal auditory artery supplying the cochlea. Tinnitus with acoustic neuromas is typically high pitched, continuous, and unilateral. Paradoxically, vestibular symptoms are not seen frequently with vestibular nerve Schwannomas because as these lesions grow, the contralateral vestibular system adjusts to the imbalance, preventing any prolonged vestibular symptoms. Larger tumors occasionally lead to facial or trigeminal nerve symptoms, such as facial paralysis or paresthesias, respectively.

Before MRI, BAERs were the diagnostic test of choice for acoustic neuromas, with a sensitivity of 93% to 98%; but, the sensitivity is significantly lower with tumors less than 1 cm (58%). With MRI, smaller tumors are detected in patients who have had normal BAERs.

Vascular Etiologies

Vertebrobasilar stroke is another cause of sudden, unilateral SNHL. This mechanism has potential devastating effects. Distinguishing whether hearing loss results from microvascular disease or a brainstem infarct is vital. The anterior inferior cerebellar artery supplies blood to the inferolateral portion of the pons, CN-VII, the spinal trigeminal tract, and the inferior cerebellum. A stroke from occlusion of this artery causes an infarct of the ipsilateral pons, creating a myriad of symptoms: ipsilateral hearing loss, vestibular symptoms, gait ataxia, facial paralysis, and contralateral loss of pain and temperature sensation in the extremities and the ipsilateral face.

CT is the initial imaging study of choice to exclude a hemorrhagic infarct, particularly within the cerebellum and brainstem. MRI provides better definition when available.

Unilateral hearing loss also occurs secondary to occlusion of the cochlear blood supply, including the internal auditory artery, a terminal branch of the anterior inferior cerebellar artery, or the basilar artery. Occlusion usually occurs secondary to compression by an acoustic neuroma in the internal auditory canal, but a thrombotic or embolic event can also occlude the artery.

Microvascular disease may also cause sudden, unilateral hearing loss and, depending on the patient's history, can be attributed to different systemic diseases. Atherosclerosis and hypertension may cause microvascular disease, causing hearing loss. Patients with diabetes have an increased incidence of SNHL. The link between diabetes and hearing loss makes intuitive sense, because neuropathic and microvascular disease processes exist in persons with diabetes.

Multiple Sclerosis

Patients with MS present with a variety of neurologic symptoms, depending on the location of the lesions. SNHL appears as a retrocochlear manifestation in approximately 4% to 10% of patients with MS. However, it is rare for SNHL to be the initial presentation. Usually, the hearing loss is sudden and resolves in weeks with treatment. If MS is suspected, CSF evaluation may be helpful; increased IgG index and oligoclonal bands in gel electrophoresis suggest MS. Audiometric testing can show normal or decreased speech discrimination in proportion with pure tone threshold. MRI is the radiologic study of choice because periventricular white matter lesions on the inferior colliculus or cochlear nucleus are visible on T2-weighted images.

Infections

Various viral and bacterial infections can cause sudden hearing loss. Herpes zoster oticus usually affects the facial nerve, creating herpetic skin eruption around the auricle and in the external auditory canal, and a facial palsy. Measles and mumps previously led to hearing loss, although vaccination for these childhood viruses has eliminated them in economically privileged countries.

Nonspecific viral processes, often following a flulike illness, are considered a common cause of sudden deafness, especially when no vestibular symptoms coexist. The mechanism of action of the presumed viral illness is unknown; therefore, this etiology is considered a "diagnosis of exclusion."

Otosyphilis is defined as a positive syphilis serologic result in the setting of unexplained SNHL. The hearing loss, usually a late manifestation of the disease, begins at higher frequencies and can progress to bilateral cochlear and vestibular dysfunction. The exact causal mechanism is unknown; however, proposed theories include microvascular disease, direct spirochetal infiltration of the perilymph, and temporal bone osteitis. Diagnostic tests for syphilis, a treatable cause of SNHL, include the fluorescent treponemal antibody absorption blood test.

Hematologic Disorders

Leukemia, sickle cell anemia, polycythemia, and macroglobulinemia can also cause sudden SNHL, usually from sludging, hemorrhage into the inner ear, or microthrombi. CBC can exclude hematologic etiology.

Presbycusis

The most common cause of slowly progressive, bilateral, symmetric, high-frequency hearing loss that develops with increasing age, presbycusis originates from a pathologic condition that decreases the number of hair cells within the organ of Corti. It has an almost universal incidence in the elderly. Multiple factors determine its progression rate. Three of the most common are genetic predisposition, nerve toxins, particularly medications, and history of long exposure to loud noises.

TREATMENT

When the primary causal mechanism for hearing loss is identified, such as an acoustic neuroma or syphilis, therapy is straightforward and potentially remediable depending on when the lesion is diagnosed in the illness course. In vascular lesions with infarction of the auditory nerve, there is no treatment. However, for common disorders such as presbycusis, a variety of high-technology, hearing-enhancing modalities can be designed to meet the patient's needs, with the aid of an otologist.

REFERENCES

Cummings CW, Haughey B. *Otolaryngology: Head and Neck Surgery*. 3rd ed. St Louis, Mo: Mosby-Year Book Inc; 1999.

Duck SW, Prazma J, Bennett PS, Pillsbury HC. Interaction between hypertension and diabetes mellitus in the pathogenesis of sensorineural hearing loss. *Laryngoscope*. 1997;107:1596-1605.

CRANIAL NERVE VIII: AUDITORY

Fletcher SD, Cheung SW. Syphilis and otolaryngology. *Otolaryngol Clin N Am.* 2003;36:595-605.

Ho SY, Kveton JF. Acoustic neuroma: assessment and management. *Otolaryngol Clin N Am.* 2002;35:393-404.

Rudick RA. Multiple sclerosis and demyelinating conditions of the central nervous system. In: Goldman L, Ausiello D, eds. *Cecil Textbook of Medicine.* 22nd ed. Philadelphia, Pa: WB Saunders Co; 2004:2320-2327.

Schmidt RJ, Sataloff RT, Newman J, Spiegel JR, Myers DL. The sensitivity of auditory brainstem response testing for the diagnosis of acoustic neuromas. *Arch Otolaryngol Head Neck Surg.* 2001;127:19-22.

Sismanis A. Pulsatile tinnitus. *Otolaryngol Clin N Am.* 2003;36:389-402.

Swartz MH. *Textbook of Physical Diagnosis: History and Examination.* 4th ed. Philadelphia, Pa: WB Saunders Co; 2002.

Chapter 14

Cranial Nerve IX, Glossopharyngeal, and Cranial Nerve X, Vagus: Swallowing

Eva M. Michalakis, Allison Gudis Jackson, and Peter J. Catalano

Clinical Vignette

A 70-year-old man with a history of hypertension and paroxysmal atrial fibrillation presented to the emergency department with acute onset of slurred speech, left-sided paresis, left neglect, and a left inferior quadrant anopsia. MRI revealed a right middle cerebral artery stroke. An initial oral peripheral and cranial nerve examination revealed bilateral depressed gag reflex and diminished soft palate elevation, left central facial weakness, reduced labial retraction, and tongue deviation to the right side with protrusion, ie, weakness of the left tongue movement. The patient was to receive nothing per mouth (NPO) and was referred to a speech pathologist.

Clinical swallowing evaluation demonstrated hoarse and moderately dysarthric speech that retained fair intelligibility. Graduated sized boluses of thin liquids, nectar thick liquids, and purees were administered. The patient had significant difficulty with oral containment, bolus formation, and posterior transport though the oral cavity, with left side greater than right. Posterior placement on the right side facilitated oral swallowing. He also had a reduced orolabial seal that benefited from a straw. Attempts to administer a soft solid bolus were unsuccessful. Because of the severity of oral deficits, he was not given solids; he had delayed triggering of oropharyngeal swallow.

There were mild vocal changes after liquids, characterized by a wet vocal quality, indicative of laryngeal penetration and possible silent aspiration. The patient was able to clear with cues to use a throat clear/re-swallow strategy. Use of a chin tuck swallowing posture with nectar thick liquids eliminated clinical signs of aspiration.

He was placed on a modified pureed diet with nectar thick liquids, and medications were crushed in applesauce. Aspiration precautions included remaining upright 90° during and 45 minutes after all oral intake, with single, small boluses. Swallowing strategies included a chin tuck swallowing posture and right posterior placement of food in the oral cavity to decrease anterior leakage and assist in oral transport. The patient was referred for a flexible endoscopic evaluation of swallowing with sensory testing, an objective assessment of swallowing function, to further assess dysphagia, exclude silent aspiration, determine appropriate diet modifications, and identify additional intervention strategies. The testing demonstrated bilateral vocal cord movement, right > left. Sensory testing revealed severe left laryngopharyngeal sensory deficit. Accordingly, and because of the silent aspiration, the patient remained at risk for aspiration pneumonia.

Swallowing functions are important to survival; malfunctioning prevents adequate nutrition intake and may predispose to significant aspiration with a risk for potentially fatal pneumonia. Dysphagia can be the presenting sign of several nervous system disorders that negatively affect swallowing.

Dysphagia may occur with CNS disorders including acute cerebral infarction, brainstem strokes, Parkinson disease, and bulbar disorders such as multiple sclerosis, motor neuron disease, syringobulbia, or primary pontomedullary or meningeal tumors. Similarly, peripheral disorders including peripheral nerve lesions (particularly Guillain-Barré syndrome), neuromuscular junction dysfunction (especially myasthenia gravis), and myopathies such as oculopharyngeal or myotonic dystrophy and dermatomyositis can also compromise swallowing function.

PHYSIOLOGY

Swallowing is a complex process involving motor control with sensory feedback from many anatomic structures within the oral cavity, pharynx, larynx, and esophagus (Figure 14-1). The trigeminal (CN-V), facial (CN-VII), glossopharyngeal (CN-IX), vagus (CN-X), and hypoglossal (CN-XII) cranial nerves are involved. "Normal

CRANIAL NERVES IX, X: GLOSSOPHARYNGEAL, VAGUS

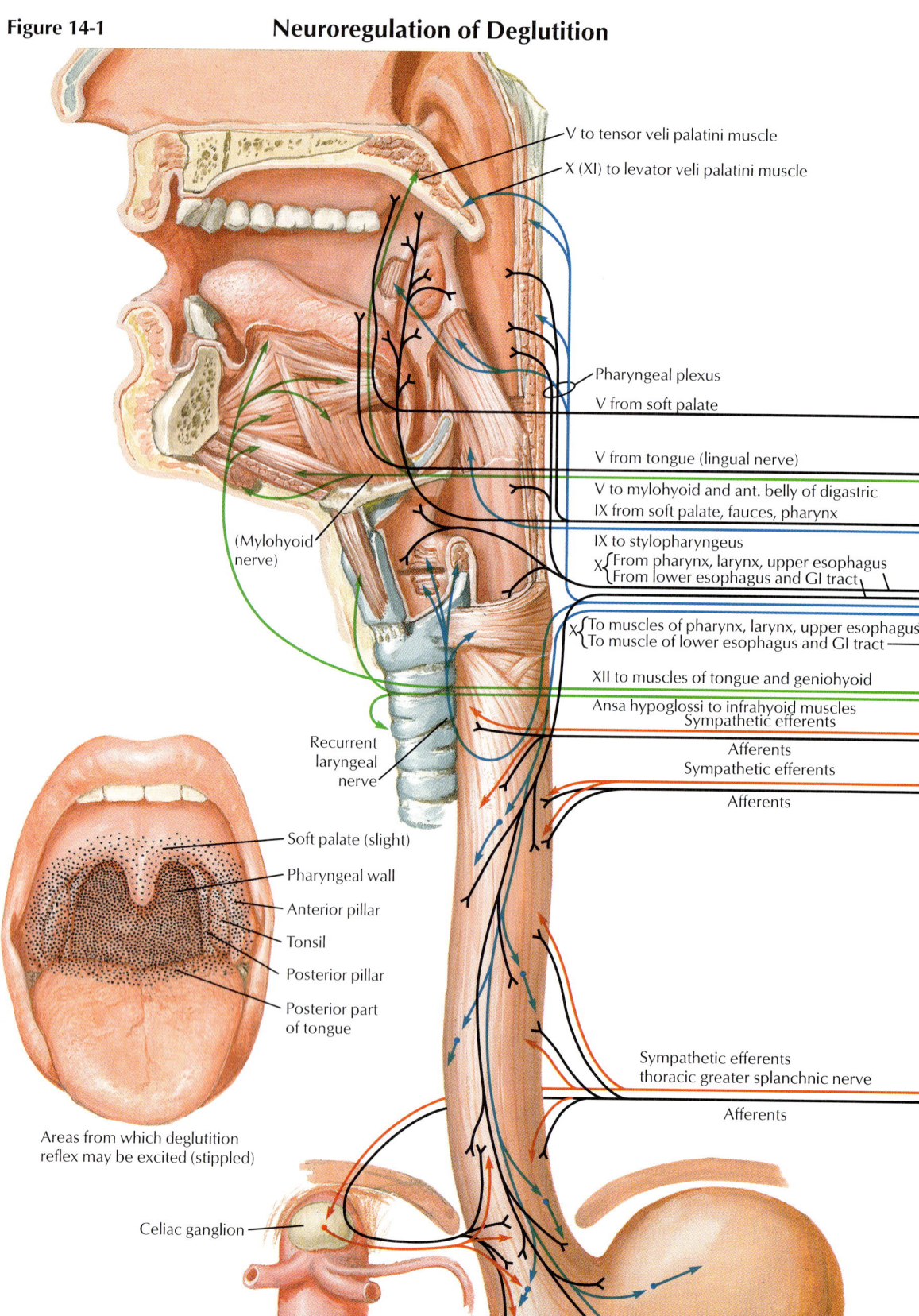

Figure 14-1. Neuroregulation of Deglutition

CRANIAL NERVES IX, X: GLOSSOPHARYNGEAL, VAGUS

Figure 14-1   **Neuroregulation of Deglutition (continued)**

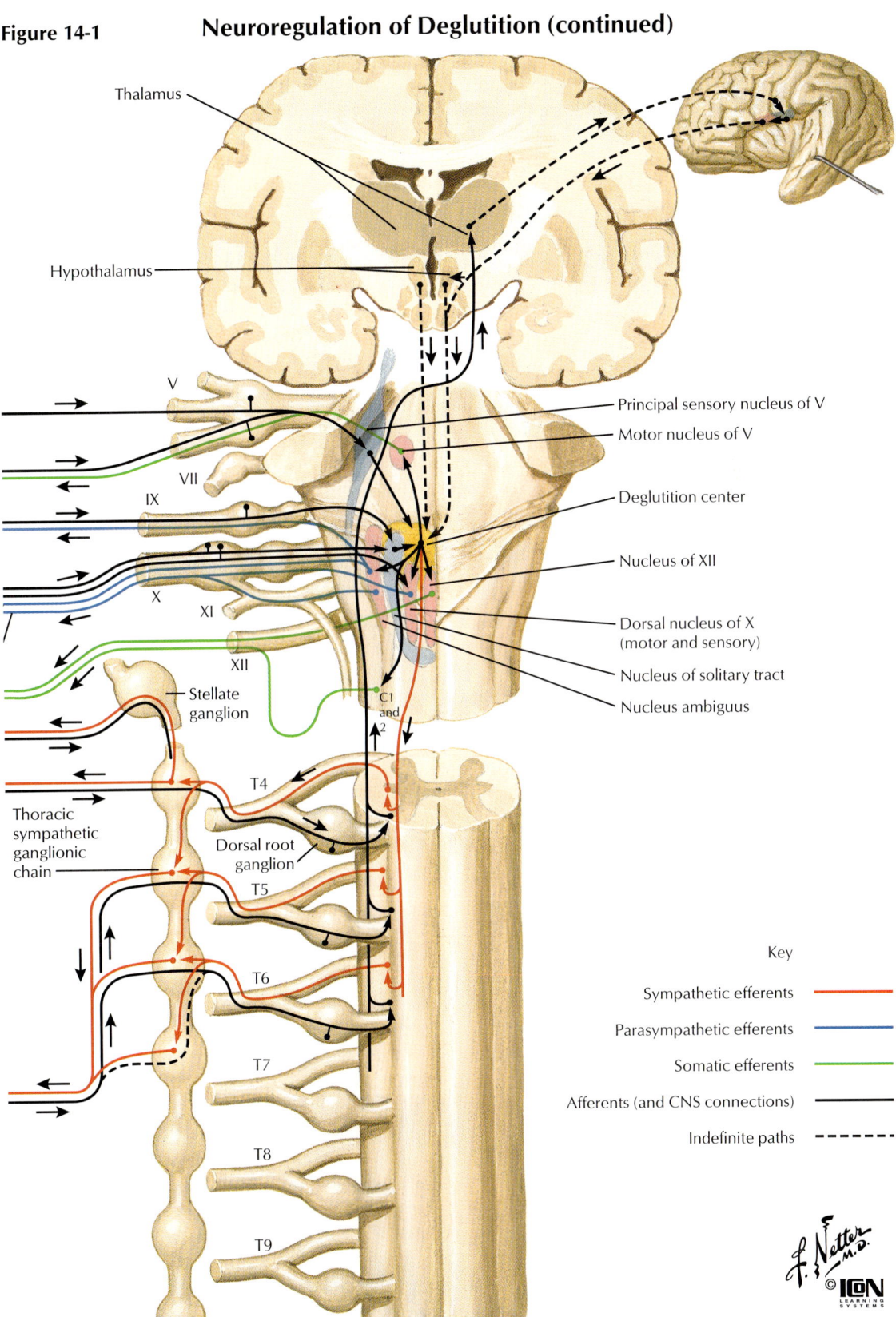

CRANIAL NERVES IX, X: GLOSSOPHARYNGEAL, VAGUS

swallow" comprises 2 major components, bolus transport and airway protection. The swallowing process is typically classifed into 4 phases.

The oral preparatory phase is voluntary motor function during which food or liquid is taken into the mouth, masticated (CN-V), and mixed with saliva to form a cohesive bolus (Figure 14-2). This phase requires coordination of lip closure and labial seal (CN-VII), tension in the labial and buccal musculature closing the anterior and lateral sulci (CN-VII), rotary mandible motion for chewing (CN-V_3), lateral rolling tongue motion (CN-XII) to position food, and bulging of the soft palate forward to seal the oral cavity posteriorly while widening the nasal airway to prepare food for the swallow (CN-IX). Tongue mobility is the most important neuromuscular function involved in this first phase. The mid and lower divisions of CN-V provide sensory feedback for positioning the bolus. Saliva derived from the parotid, sublingual, and submandibular glands, innervated by secretomotor fibers of CN-IX and -VII, contain digestive enzymes that act as an emollient to soften the bolus.

The oral phase of swallowing is initiated when the tongue (CN-XII) sequentially squeezes the bolus posteriorly against the hard palate, beginning propulsion into the oropharynx. Lips and buccal muscles contract (CN-V and CN-VII) with elevation of the velum (CN-V and CN-X) providing the valving process that generates pressure to seal the nasopharynx, preventing reflux and nasal regurgitation. CN-V is responsible for the afferent (sensory) feedback for the entire oral cavity and tongue. The soft palate (CN-IX) critical to containing the bolus within the oral cavity during the oral preparatory phase, moves posteriorly, allowing the bolus to pass through the faucial arches and simultaneously preventing the bolus from entering the nasopharynx. The swallowing reflex is triggered as the bolus passes the anterior tonsillar pillars, which initiates the pharyngeal phase.

Taste for the anterior two thirds of the tongue is carried by CN-VII, whereas the afferent CN-IX controls taste for the posterior one third of the tongue and the posterior pharyngeal wall. CN-X supplies primary innervation to the palatal muscles, pharyngeal constrictors, laryngeal musculature, and cricopharyngeus. Afferent fibers also provide critical sensory feedback from the larynx and esophageal inlet.

The pharyngeal phase begins with the bolus passing into the throat, triggering the swallowing reflex and causing several pharyngeal physiologic actions to occur simultaneously, allowing food to pass into the esophagus. Once pharyngeal swallowing is elicited, essential functions of airway protection occur. Intrinsic laryngeal muscles innervated by CN-X close the larynx at the aryepiglottic, false vocal, and true vocal folds, creating a seal to separate the airway from the digestive tract. The laryngeal vestibule is then protected from foreign material aspiration. The tongue (CN XII) is the major force pushing the bolus through the pharynx. Synergistic actions with CN-X produce pharyngeal peristalsis as it innervates the pharyngeal constrictors and carries afferents from the lower pharynx.

CN-IX mediates the sensory portion of the pharyngeal gag but innervates just 1 muscle, the stylopharyngeus. The absence of the gag reflex is not the sole indicator of a patient's swallowing abilities. A study of the risk of aspiration in 14 patients with dysphagia with absent gag reflex demonstrated that 86% tolerated a modified diet. Additionally, the gag reflex was absent in 13% of 69 nondysphagic control group individuals.

Poor airway protection and delayed triggering of pharyngeal swallow may cause aspiration. When swallowing is inefficient and aspiration occurs, a reflexive cough needs to occur as respiratory defense against foreign matter. The cough reflex is induced by irritation of afferent CN-IX and CN-X sensory fibers in the larynx, trachea, and larger bronchi (Figure 14-3). If a reflexive cough is not elicited in response to foreign material within the airway, **silent aspiration** results; it is radiographically documented in 50% of aspiration cases.

CN-IX is the primary afferent of the swallowing response, whereas CN-X is the secondary afferent; both nerves terminate in the **swallowing center** located in the medulla within the nucleus solitarius. Sensory events initiating swallowing occur with stimulation to jaw, posterior tongue, faucial pillars, and upper pharynx and are mediated through CN-V, CN-IX, and CN-X. These afferent fibers converge on the nucleus solitarius in the medulla and communicate with the nucleus ambiguous via interneurons stimulating the motor response.

The esophageal phase occurs with the passage of the bolus through the cricopharyngeal sphincter, moving over the closed airway and passing the pharyngoesophageal segment into the esophagus via the cricopharyngeal sphincter at the proximal esophagus (Figure 14-2). This area contains the cricopharyngeus muscle that normally keeps the esophagus closed. CN-X mediates the action of the cricopharyngeus, which relaxes to allow food to pass from the hypopharynx into the esophagus.

Elevation and anterior movement of the larynx is the significant mechanical force contributing to the opening of the cricopharyngeal sphincter, which in conjunction with the relaxation of the cricopharyngeus muscle opens the pharyngoesophageal segment, permitting the passage of food into the esophagus. The sphincter must otherwise remain closed to prevent the entrance of air into the stomach and reflux from the esophagus into the hypopharynx. CN-X, specifically the efferent fibers from the dorsal nucleus, innervate the involuntary muscles of the esophagus, stomach, small intestine, and portions of the large intestine.

CLINICAL PRESENTATION

Dysphagia, or difficulty swallowing, can result from many causes, including neurologic disorders; viral, bacterial, or fungal infections of the upper airway; surgeries or disease processes that do not directly involve the oral, pharyngeal, or laryngeal structures; and psychogenic mechanisms. Aging and medications may exacerbate dysphagia. Some antidepressant medications cause xerostomia (reduced salivary flow), affecting bolus formation. Medications causing drowsiness or lethargy may significantly affect swallowing. Common signs of dysphagia include pocketing of food in the oral cavity, drooling, wet vocal quality during meals, episodes of coughing with throat clearing, and shortness of breath during meals.

Aspiration, the primary concern when dealing with patients with dysphagia, is technically defined as entrance of a foreign substance below the level of the vocal cords, into the trachea. Aspiration is a dangerous precursor of aspiration pneumonia. Concomitant risk factors include chronic obstructive pulmonary disorders, congestive heart failure, feeding tubes, dependence for oral care and feeding, medications, decreased laryngopharyngeal sensation, and a reduced level of alertness. Any patient with aspiration risk needs to be placed on aspiration precautions and referred for swallowing evaluation before initiation of oral intake.

DIAGNOSTIC APPROACH

Formal assessment of swallowing function through various examinations evaluates the severity of dysfunction and identifies therapeutic strategies and intervention. Clinical swallowing evaluation includes the assessment of patient history combined with observations regarding mental and respiratory status. Oral, peripheral, and cranial nerve examinations are conducted. Various food consistencies are administered with close evaluation of the oral preparatory, oral, and pharyngeal phases of swallowing. Based on this evaluation, swallowing strategies may be implemented or the need for objective studies may be identified.

Flexible endoscopic evaluation of swallowing with sensory testing allows direct evaluation of motor and sensory aspects of the pharyngeal swallow. It requires transnasal passage of a fiberoptic laryngoscope into the hypopharynx to view the larynx and surrounding structures. Laryngeal airway protection and the integrity of the oropharyngeal swallow are assessed.

A comprehensive swallowing evaluation is then performed. The patient is given various food consistencies tinted with food coloring to enhance visualization. Similar to the modified barium swallow (MBS), compensatory strategies and postures are attempted when indicated to facilitate improved swallowing function and decrease the risk of aspiration pneumonia. Velopharyngeal closure, anatomy of the base of the tongue and hypopharynx, abduction and adduction of the vocal folds, pharyngeal musculature, and the patient's ability to manage secretions are assessed. Laryngopharyngeal reflux can also be visualized.

Modified barium swallow, also called videofluoroscopy or videopharyngogram, is a functional evaluation requiring active patient participation. Before scheduling MBS, laryngopharyngeal sen-

CRANIAL NERVES IX, X: GLOSSOPHARYNGEAL, VAGUS

Figure 14-2

Deglutition

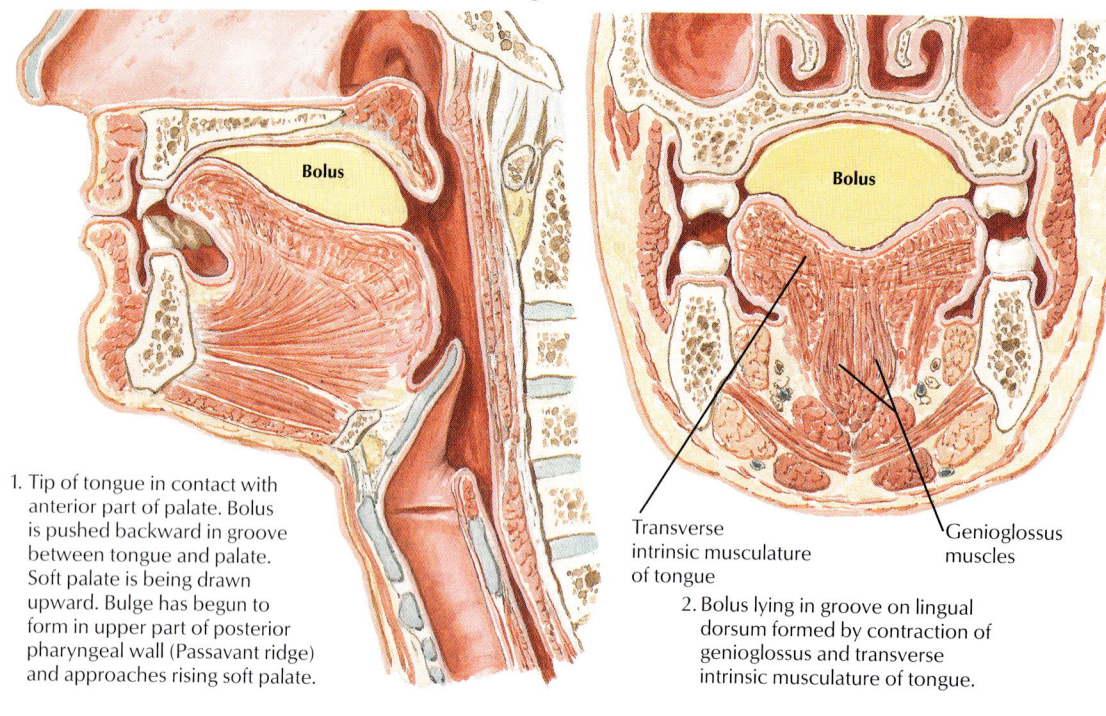

1. Tip of tongue in contact with anterior part of palate. Bolus is pushed backward in groove between tongue and palate. Soft palate is being drawn upward. Bulge has begun to form in upper part of posterior pharyngeal wall (Passavant ridge) and approaches rising soft palate.

2. Bolus lying in groove on lingual dorsum formed by contraction of genioglossus and transverse intrinsic musculature of tongue.

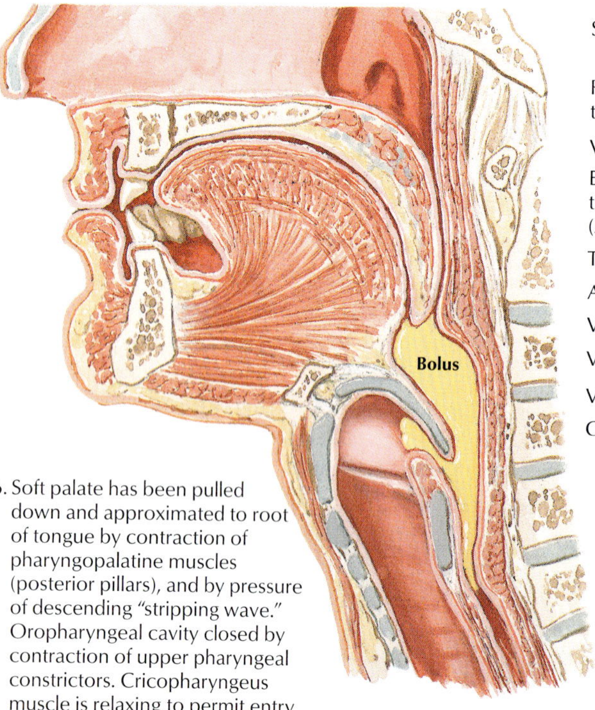

6. Soft palate has been pulled down and approximated to root of tongue by contraction of pharyngopalatine muscles (posterior pillars), and by pressure of descending "stripping wave." Oropharyngeal cavity closed by contraction of upper pharyngeal constrictors. Cricopharyngeus muscle is relaxing to permit entry of bolus into esophagus. Trickle of food enters also laryngeal aditus but is prevented from going farther by closure of ventricular folds.

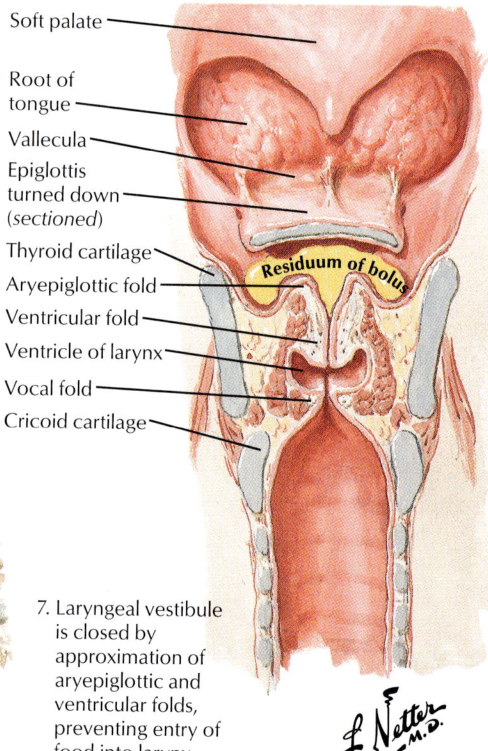

7. Laryngeal vestibule is closed by approximation of aryepiglottic and ventricular folds, preventing entry of food into larynx (coronal section: AP view).

CRANIAL NERVES IX, X: GLOSSOPHARYNGEAL, VAGUS

Figure 14-2 **Deglutition (continued)**

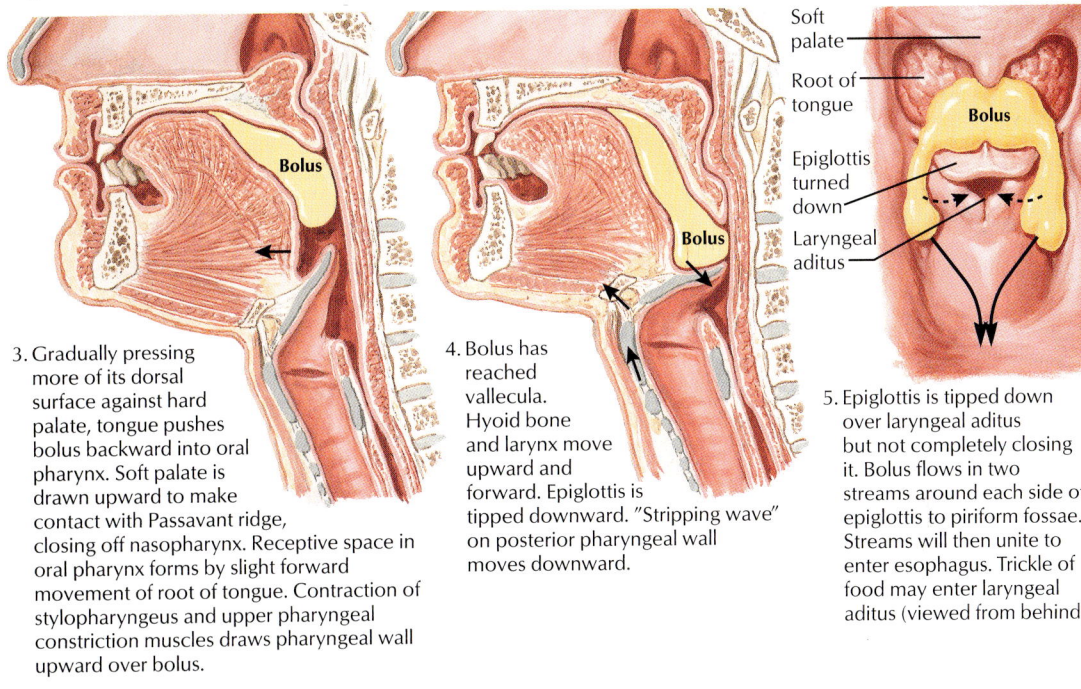

3. Gradually pressing more of its dorsal surface against hard palate, tongue pushes bolus backward into oral pharynx. Soft palate is drawn upward to make contact with Passavant ridge, closing off nasopharynx. Receptive space in oral pharynx forms by slight forward movement of root of tongue. Contraction of stylopharyngeus and upper pharyngeal constriction muscles draws pharyngeal wall upward over bolus.

4. Bolus has reached vallecula. Hyoid bone and larynx move upward and forward. Epiglottis is tipped downward. "Stripping wave" on posterior pharyngeal wall moves downward.

5. Epiglottis is tipped down over laryngeal aditus but not completely closing it. Bolus flows in two streams around each side of epiglottis to piriform fossae. Streams will then unite to enter esophagus. Trickle of food may enter laryngeal aditus (viewed from behind).

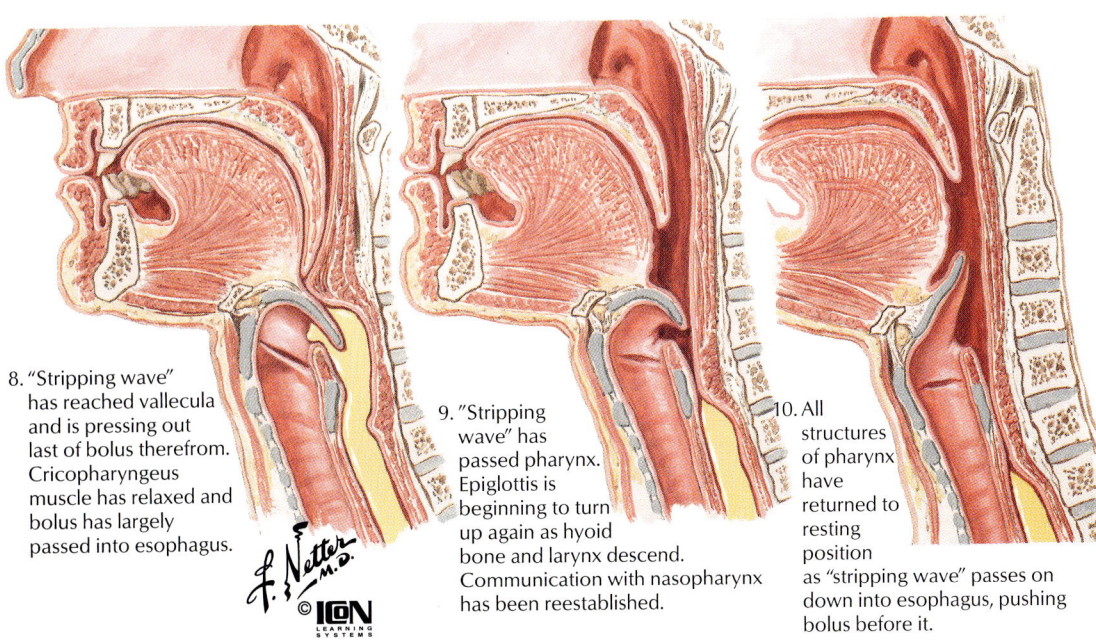

8. "Stripping wave" has reached vallecula and is pressing out last of bolus therefrom. Cricopharyngeus muscle has relaxed and bolus has largely passed into esophagus.

9. "Stripping wave" has passed pharynx. Epiglottis is beginning to turn up again as hyoid bone and larynx descend. Communication with nasopharynx has been reestablished.

10. All structures of pharynx have returned to resting position as "stripping wave" passes on down into esophagus, pushing bolus before it.

CRANIAL NERVES

CRANIAL NERVES IX, X: GLOSSOPHARYNGEAL, VAGUS

Figure 14-3A   Glossopharyngeal Nerve (IX): Schema

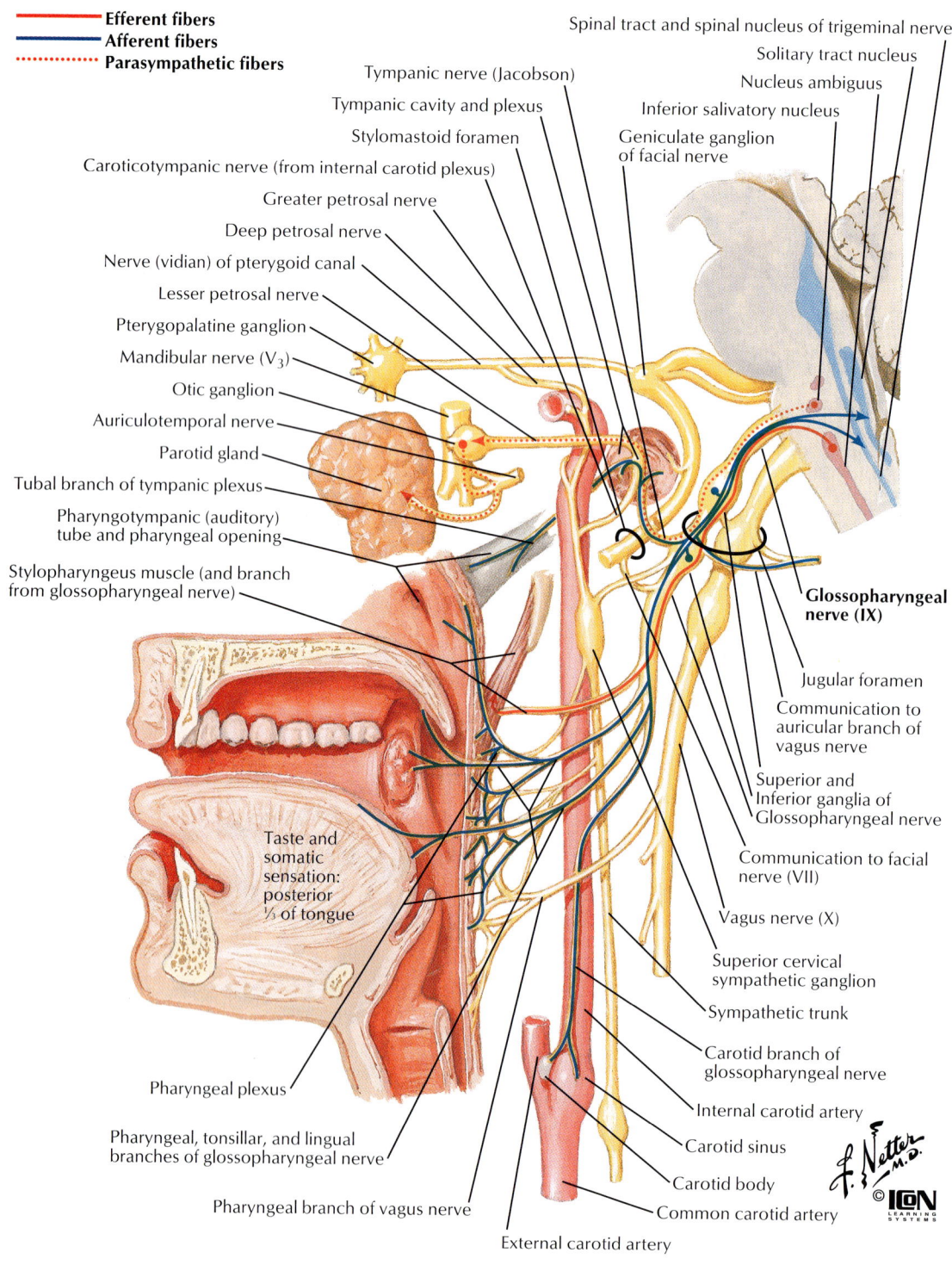

CRANIAL NERVES IX, X: GLOSSOPHARYNGEAL, VAGUS

Figure 14-3B   **Vagus Nerve (X): Schema**

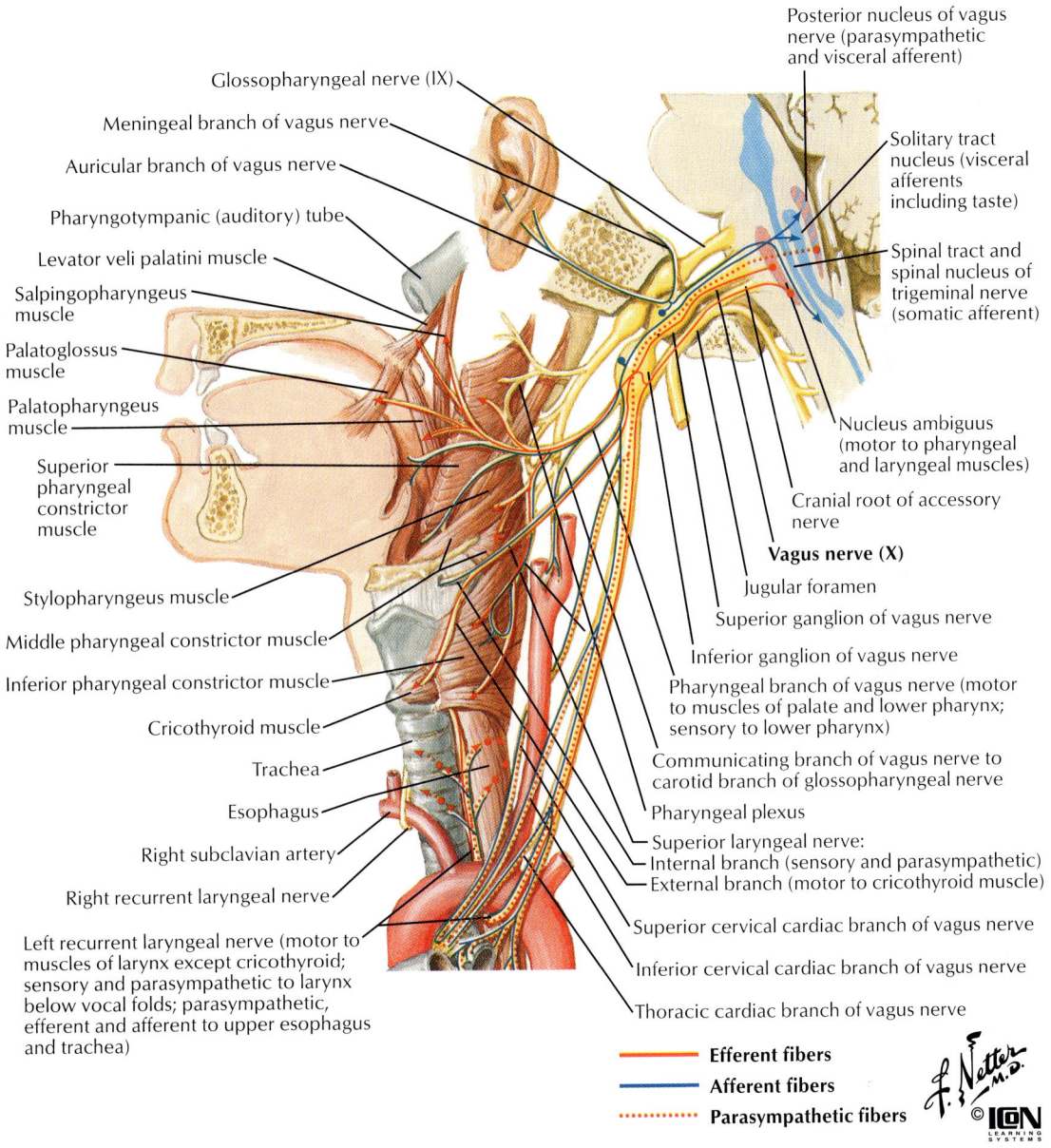

sation should be evaluated via flexible endoscopic evaluation of swallowing with sensory testing to assess the risk of barium aspiration. MBS, performed in conjunction with radiologic examination, differs from the standard barium swallow. Patients ingest graduated sized boluses of various consistencies mixed with barium in the upright position. The primary purpose of MBS is to determine appropriate therapeutic intervention strategies to facilitate safe and efficient swallowing function. Aspiration and silent aspiration can also be detected. Images are taken in lateral and anterior-posterior projections to focus on oropharyngeal swallowing anatomy and physiology, with screening for esophageal motility and esophageal or pharyngeal reflux. The patient need not be NPO for MBS.

TREATMENT

Patient candidacy for oral intake requires consideration of 3 major components: safety of swallow, efficiency and ability to maintain nutritional support through swallowing, and quality of life. For some patients, particularly those who are neurologically compromised, safety of swallow is grossly impaired, heightening the risk of aspiration pneumonia. Additionally, many of these patients are bedridden and have cognitive impairment or decreased levels of alertness. In this setting, even small amounts of aspiration cannot be tolerated. Other patients may present with a good swallow, but may fatigue with chewing and consecutive swallowing (as is seen with myasthenia gravis), which impedes swallowing safety and the potential to tolerate a full oral diet. Eating becomes hard work, making consumption of enough calories difficult.

Efficiency and ability to maintain nutritional support through swallowing is the second treatment consideration. Damage to descending corticobulbar fibers can occur from stroke, head injury, or multiple sclerosis. Stroke can result in mild-severe dysphagia depending on the site and size of the lesion and the accompanying deficits. Unilateral hemispheric stroke is a common, temporary cause of dysphagia. However, delayed oral transit times, delayed or absent triggering of the pharyngeal swallow, and poor pharyngeal bolus propulsion with decreased sensory awareness in the oral and pharyngeal cavities are common sequelae of stroke-induced dysphagia. They also increase the risk of aspiration.

Apraxia of the swallow mechanism with uncoordinated muscle movements, characterized by reduced bolus formation and inability to manipulate the bolus and trigger timely sequenced swallow, may also occur. If the nucleus ambiguus is damaged in a brainstem stroke, ipsilateral paralysis of the larynx, pharynx, and palate may lead to a severe pharyngeal phase dysphagia. If the nucleus ambiguus is spared, but there is unilateral tongue, face, or jaw weakness with concomitant loss of sensation in the affected side of the oral cavity, a more severe dysphagia may result.

Optimal management of neurogenic dysphagia requires a multidisciplinary approach. Clinicians must be aware of the natural history of the underlying disorder, with consideration for eventual improvement (ie, cerebrovascular accident versus further degeneration of the swallowing process as is typical for amyotrophic lateral sclerosis). Concomitant respiratory disorders and psychosocial aspects of eating must also be considered.

Placement of a percutaneous esophagogastrostomy can be lifesaving in neurologic disorders associated with severe dysphagia that have significant potential for recovery, such as brainstem strokes. Even in patients with fatal illness such as amyotrophic lateral sclerosis, a percutaneous esophagogastrostomy can provide sustained comfort and maintain nutrition while significantly lessening the risk of fatal aspiration pneumonia.

REFERENCES

Hughes TAT, Wiles CM. Clinical measurement of swallowing in health and in neurogenic dysphagia. *Q J Med.* 1996;89:109-116.

Langmore SE, Skarupski KA, Park PS, Fries BE. Predictors of aspiration pneumonia in nursing home residents. *Dysphagia.* 2002;17:298-307.

Larson C. Neurophysiology of speech and swallowing. *Semin Speech Lang.* 1985;6:275-289.

Logemann JA. *Evaluation and Treatment of Swallowing Disorders.* 2nd ed. Austin, Tex: Pro-Ed; 1998.

McConnell FMS, Cerenko D, Mendelson MS. Manofluorgraphic analysis of swallowing. *Otolaryngol Clin N Am.* 1988;21:625-635.

Zemlin WR. *Speech and Hearing Science: Anatomy and Physiology.* 4th ed. Boston, Mass: Allyn and Bacon; 1998.

Chapter 15
Cranial Nerve X, Vagus: Voice Disorders

Timothy D. Anderson

Clinical Vignette

A 62-year-old man with an unremarkable history except for 50 pack-years of cigarette smoking presented with a hoarse, breathy voice. He had lost his voice suddenly 3 months earlier but had gradually regained some vocal function. He noted that speaking tired him quickly and that he frequently ran out of breath in mid-sentence.

Physical examination revealed a healthy male in no apparent distress with a breathy, hoarse voice. The remainder of the examination showed normal findings. Otolaryngology consultation revealed left vocal fold paralysis with partial compensation. CT with contrast of the brain, neck, and upper chest showed a large mass in the left upper lung. A biopsy specimen revealed a primary lung adenocarcinoma.

Although the larynx is usually considered the source of speech, speech production requires precise coordination of multiple organ systems. Contraction of the abdominal musculature, diaphragm, and chest wall provides a power source for the voice. The larynx acts as a pressure regulator and vibratory source. The pharynx, tongue, nose, and mouth shape these vibrations into recognizable speech and singing. However, the larynx is the most easily injured of these systems, and most vocal problems originate within it.

ANATOMY OF THE LARYNX

The skeleton of the larynx consists of thyroid and cricoid cartilages. The arytenoid cartilages articulate with the posterior portion of the cricoid. Vocal ligaments stretch from the arytenoids to the thyroid cartilage. Muscles inserting on the arytenoids move the vocal folds and arytenoids together for speech and swallowing, and apart for respiration. Although the arytenoids' motion is multidimensional, knowledge of the intrinsic laryngeal muscles and their functions is important for diagnosis (Table 15-1). Note that the cricothyroid muscle is the only intrinsic laryngeal muscle innervated by the superior laryngeal nerve (SLN), and the posterior cricoarytenoid is the only vocal fold abductor.

The motor supply of the laryngeal muscles begins in the nucleus ambiguous (Figure 15-1). These fibers travel within the vagus nerve (CN-X) as it exits the cranium via the jugular foramen, traveling through the neck within the carotid sheath (Figure 15-2). High in the neck, the SLN

Table 15-1
Laryngeal Muscle Innervation, Action, and Vocal Function*

Muscle	Innervation	Action	Vocal Function
Lateral cricoarytenoid	RLN	Adduction	Speech
Posterior cricoarytenoid	RLN	Abduction	Respiration
Thyroarytenoid	RLN	Adduction and shortening	Fine voice control
Cricothyroid	SLN	Lengthening	Increase pitch

*RLN indicates recurrent laryngeal nerve; SLN, superior laryngeal nerve.

CRANIAL NERVE X, VAGUS: VOICE DISORDERS

Figure 15-1

Vagus Nerve (X): Schema

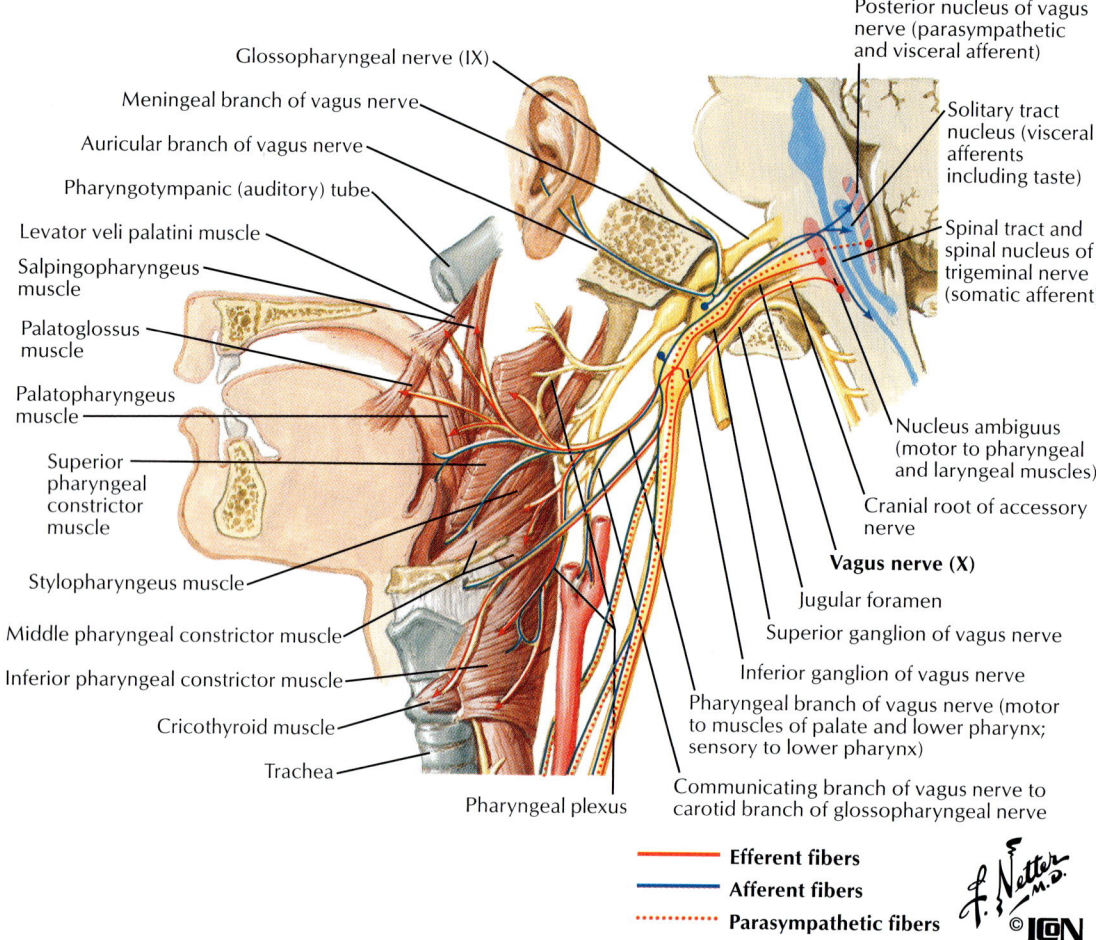

splits from CN-X and travels medially. It splits again into internal and external branches. The internal branch pierces the thyrohyoid membrane and provides sensory innervation to the pharynx and larynx. The external branch travels lower in the neck past the superior pole of the thyroid gland to innervate the cricothyroid muscle.

The recurrent laryngeal nerve (RLN) takes a more tortuous path. It separates from CN-X, loops around the aortic arch on the left and the brachiocephalic artery on the right, and travels back toward the larynx in the tracheoesophageal groove bilaterally. It passes under the thyroid gland and inserts into the larynx under the thyroid cartilage, innervating all other intrinsic laryngeal muscles. Both these nerves are vulnerable to injury and have distinct symptoms when injured.

DISORDERS OF VOICE
Recurrent Laryngeal Nerve

Recurrent laryngeal nerve damage usually causes vocal fold immobility on the side of injury. Depending on the position of the vocal fold, symptom severity varies greatly. The most common symptoms are a breathy, hoarse voice and ineffective cough. If the paralyzed vocal fold is in the midline, the only symptom may be vocal fatigue and slight breathiness. Most patients eventually compensate somewhat. The normal vocal fold may cross the midline slightly, or the patient may use muscles around the larynx to squeeze the vocal folds shut. If accessory muscles are used to speak, muscle fatigue and neck pain may develop after prolonged talking.

CRANIAL NERVE X, VAGUS: VOICE DISORDERS

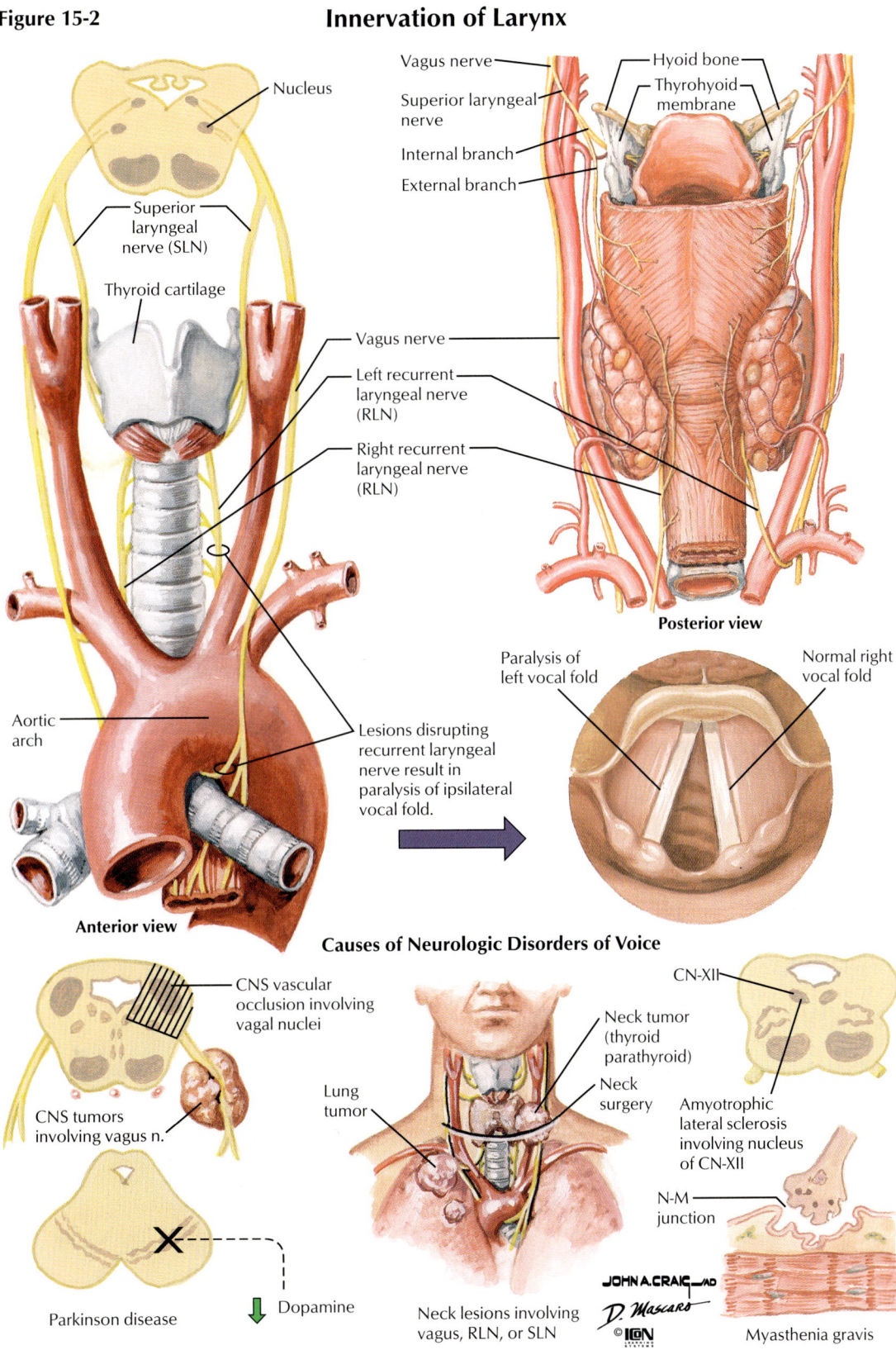

Figure 15-2. Innervation of Larynx

CRANIAL NERVE X, VAGUS: VOICE DISORDERS

Common causes of vocal fold paralysis include thyroid, lung, or neck tumors; cerebrovascular accidents; CN-X tumors; and surgery near CN-X or the RLN. Less common causes include thyroiditis (causing inflammation of the RLN), infectious diseases such as Lyme and syphilis, or diabetic or other neuropathies.

Diagnostic evaluation of vocal fold paralysis includes imaging of the brain, neck, and upper chest, serologic testing, and thyroid function tests; electromyography of the laryngeal muscles may confirm the diagnosis. Even with extensive investigation, the cause of vocal fold paralysis sometimes cannot be determined. Treatment is usually directed at moving the paralyzed vocal fold to the midline. Reinnervation procedures have been described but are not widely used because of inconsistent results.

Superior Laryngeal Nerve

The classic symptom of SLN dysfunction is the inability to raise the vocal pitch. Patients also frequently have weak voices that tire easily. If the injury includes the external SLN branch, patients may also have poor laryngeal sensation leading to aspiration. High CN-X lesions and cerebrovascular accidents cause combined SLN and RLN injuries. These patients are at high risk for aspiration because they can neither close the larynx nor sense when they are about to aspirate. Common causes of SLN dysfunction include thyroiditis and thyroid surgery. Infections such as Lyme and syphilis can also cause SLN dysfunction. However, most cases of SLN paresis are idiopathic.

Other Neurologic Disorders of the Larynx

Spasmodic dysphonia is a task-specific dystonia affecting the larynx. Patients have irregular voice breaks when trying to speak, but many can sing normally. Its cause is unknown. Treatment involves identifying the involved muscles and paralyzing them with injections of botulinum toxin.

Patients with **laryngeal tremor** have regular voice breaks and a tremulous voice. Laryngeal examination reveals regular contractions of the laryngeal muscles at rest and during phonation. Singing is not spared. It can be difficult to distinguish spasmodic dysphonia from tremor.

Although most common in Parkinson disease, vocal fold bowing can occur in several other neurologic disorders. The voice is weak and breathy, and accessory muscle compensation is common, causing neck pain and vocal fatigue. Medical treatment of the underlying disease is the first therapy. Speech therapy is also frequently successful. Surgery is sometimes necessary to straighten and strengthen the bowed vocal folds. **Neuromuscular disorders**, most commonly myasthenia gravis, can affect the laryngeal muscles. A rare form of myasthenia gravis isolated to the laryngeal muscles has been described. The most common symptom is vocal fatigue. Patients generally respond to medical therapy.

Other Neurologic Voice Disorders

Neurologic damage to other portions of the vocal production system can create voice complaints. Tongue dysarthria, from cerebrovascular accident, amyotrophic lateral sclerosis, or hypoglossal nerve damage, is one of the most common. Paralysis of the palatal muscles can give a hypernasal voice. Although tongue and pharyngeal neurologic disorders can cause voice problems, swallowing problems associated with these disorders are often more problematic and require urgent diagnosis and management (chapter 14).

REFERENCES

Anderson TD, Mirza N. Immediate percutaneous medialization for acute vocal fold immobility. *Laryngoscope.* 2001;111:1318-1321.

Berke GS, Gerratt B, Kreiman J, Jackson K. Treatment of Parkinson hypophonia with percutaneous collagen augmentation. *Laryngoscope.* 1999;109:1295-1299.

Boutsen F, Cannito MP, Taylor M, Bender B. Botox treatment in adductor spasmodic dysphonia: a meta-analysis. *J Speech Lang Hear Res.* 2002;45:469-481.

Chhetri DK, Gerratt BR, Kreiman J, Berke GS. Combined arytenoid adduction and laryngeal reinnervation in the treatment of vocal fold paralysis. *Laryngoscope.* 1999;109:1928-1936.

Dursun G, Sataloff RT, Spiegel JR, Mandel S, Heuer RJ, Rosen DC. Superior laryngeal nerve paresis and paralysis. *J Voice.* 1996;10:206-211.

Mao VH, Abaza M, Spiegel JR, Mandel S, Hawkshaw M, Heuer RJ, Sataloff RT. Laryngeal myasthenia gravis: report of 40 cases. *J Voice.* 2001;15:122-130.

Ramadan HH, Wax MK, Avery S. Outcome and changing cause of unilateral vocal cord paralysis. *Otolaryngol Head Neck Surg.* 1998;118:199-202.

Chapter 16
Cranial Nerve XI: Spinal Accessory

Michal Vytopil and H. Royden Jones, Jr

Clinical Vignette

A 23-year-old medical student noted swollen lymph nodes in the left posterior triangle of his neck. He was otherwise asymptomatic. The student health service told him there was nothing wrong except that he was overly concerned. Within a short time, he became quite fatigued. He sought an opinion from a respected internist. The presence of abnormal left posterior cervical and axillary nodes was confirmed; the remaining findings of his clinical examination were normal. Results of a mononucleosis spot test were normal and results of liver function studies were abnormal; therefore, excision of 1 cervical node was performed.

During the procedure, the surgeon queried the student about the risks of this minor operation. The student correctly replied that it is important to exercise caution so as not to cut the spinal accessory nerve (CN-XI) because paralysis of the trapezius muscle would result. When he returned to his rotation on the chief of surgery's service, the student was informed by the intern that the chief, on hearing about his missing student, commented that there was a 50% 5-year mortality rate among people undergoing this procedure.

The professor of pathology could not arrive at a diagnosis and sent the node to the Armed Forces Institute of Pathology and to the Mayo Clinic for more definitive opinions. They did not believe it represented a lymphoma; 6 weeks later, the test for infectious mononucleosis was positive. The editor of this text notes that it is now 44 years since he had this biopsy.

This vignette exemplifies that careful consideration of every patient complaint is warranted, even of those in the medical profession. The patient was labeled with "medical studentitis," and a peer created emotional turmoil for him until a benign mechanism was established. Occasionally, patients undergoing similar procedures experience iatrogenic laceration of CN-XI, sometimes leading to significant shoulder pain and atrophy of the unilateral trapezius muscle with some scapular winging. The more proximally innervated sternocleidomastoid muscle (SCM) is spared. Cervical lymph node biopsies may be the most common cause of CN-XI palsy.

Of the CNs, CN-XI is probably the least crucial despite its interesting, primarily motor, function for the neck and shoulder. It also has an intriguing functional array because one of the 2 major muscles it innervates, the SCM, originates on the occiput; when one side contracts it turns the head, seemingly paradoxically, in the opposite direction, ie, turning to the left requires a right SCM contraction and vice versa.

The uncommon patients who have conversion hysteria or malingering with a purported hemiparesis will not "be able" to turn the head to the "affected" side, even though each SCM is responsible for the contralateral function (the right SCM for a left hemiparesis, and vice versa). This anatomic paradox becomes a useful evaluative tool, especially when considering patients whose weakness is doubted. However, patients whose nonanatomical weakness is corroborated should not be abandoned. They may be calling for support or emotional help, as was one patient who later proved to be a victim of incest.

ANATOMY

CN-XI is primarily a motor nerve innervating the SCM and trapezius muscles in the neck and back (Figure 16-1). In contrast to other CNs, its lower motor neuron cell bodies are located primarily within the spinal cord. The accessory nucleus is a cell column within the lateral anterior gray column of the upper 5 or 6 cervical spinal cord segments. Proximally it lies nearly in line with the nucleus ambiguus and caudally within the dorsolateral ventral horn. Originating from the accessory nucleus, the rootlets emerge from the cord and unite to form the trunk of CN-XI. It

CRANIAL NERVE XI: SPINAL ACCESSORY

Figure 16-1

Accessory Nerve (XI): Schema

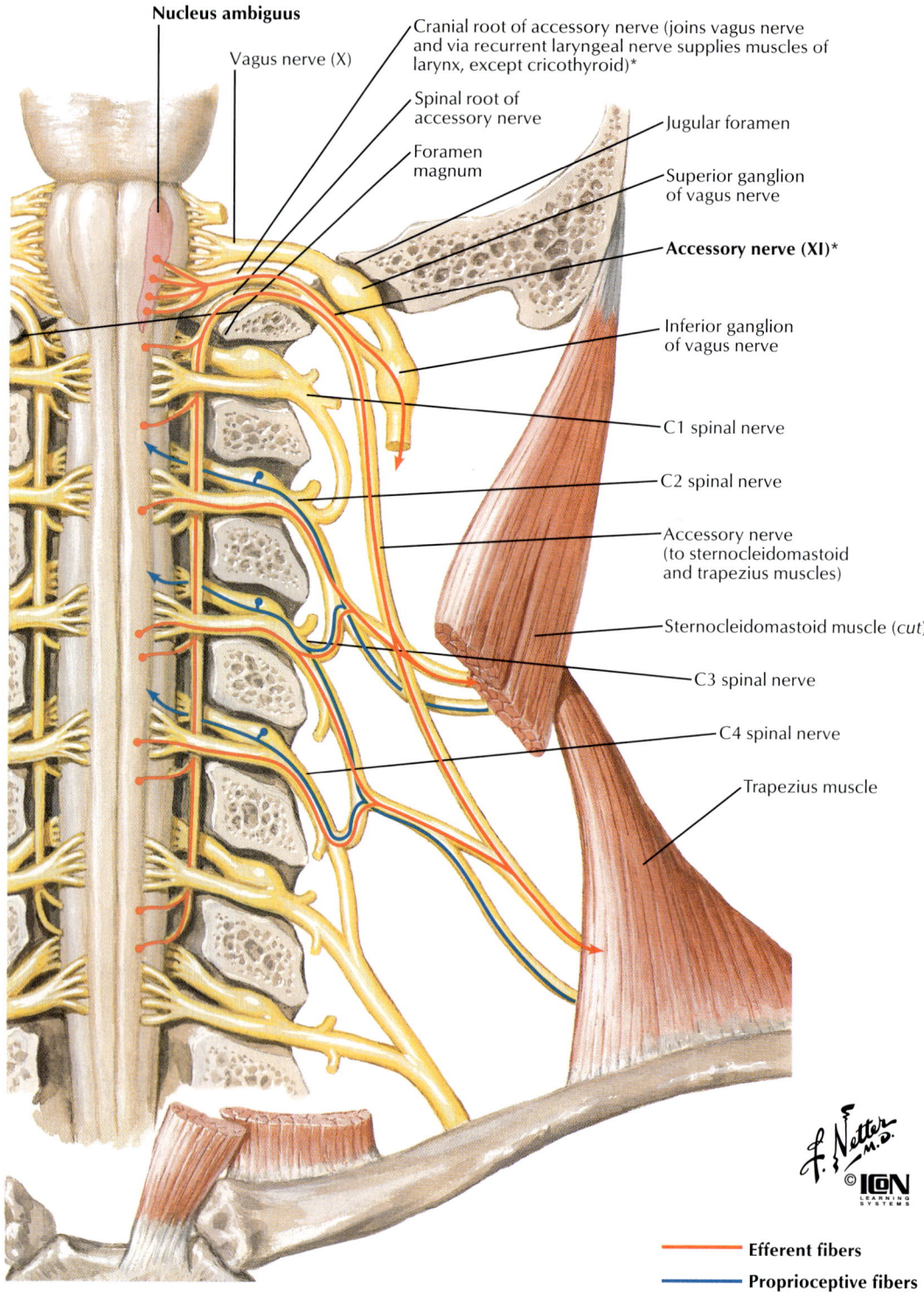

*Recent evidence suggests that the accessory nerve lacks a cranial root and has no connection to the vagus nerve. Verification of this finding awaits further investigation.

CRANIAL NERVE XI: SPINAL ACCESSORY

extends rostrally through the foramen magnum into the posterior cranial fossa. Intracranially, it accompanies caudal fibers of the vagus nerve (CN-X) and leaves the skull through the jugular foramen.

CN-XI then descends in close proximity to the internal carotid artery and internal jugular vein (Figure 16-2). During its extracranial course, CN-XI is joined by some fibers derived from the third and fourth upper cervical ventral rami. Some of these cervical fibers may innervate the caudal trapezius, whereas the proximal trapezius and the entire SCM muscle may be primarily innervated by CN-XI. Having emerged from the midpoint of the posterior border of the SCM, CN-XI crosses the posterior triangle of the neck superficial to the levator scapulae. Importantly, this is where CN-XI is closely related to the superficial cervical lymph nodes. Further caudally, approximately 5 cm above the clavicle, it passes into the anterior border of the trapezius muscle, which it also innervates.

There is a minor afferent component to CN-XI. These fibers seem to have a primary proprioceptive function for the 2 muscles that CN-XI innervates.

CN-XI is described as having a cranial root in addition to the spinal roots described above. The cranial root consists of a few fibers originating in the caudal portion of the nucleus ambiguus, which run with the 11th CN intracranially, then through the jugular foramen.

CLINICAL PRESENTATION AND DIAGNOSTIC APPROACH

Lesions located intracranially or proximally to the innervation of the SCM cause weakness of the SCM and the trapezius. Damage to the nerve in the posterior triangle of the neck spares the SCM and results in weakness of the trapezius only. If the SCM is weak, the patient experiences weakness when turning the head to the opposite side.

Involvement of the trapezius manifests as drooping of the shoulder and mild scapular winging away from the chest wall with slight lateral displacement. Weakness in shoulder elevation and arm abduction above horizontal is typical. Winging is apparent, with arms hanging along the trunk, and becomes accentuated when patients abduct the arms. In contrast, scapular winging from long thoracic nerve palsy with weakness of serratus anterior is most prominent on forward elevation of the arms (Figure 16-3).

Typically, the patient often also experiences a painful paresis secondary to direct nerve injury during various procedures or disorders or, if delayed, by entrapment of the nerve within scar tissue or structural lesions such as tumors.

EMG is important for confirming that the observed lesion is confined to the distribution of CN-XI. Additionally, a gadolinium-enhanced MRI is appropriate if any question exists of a lesion more widespread than a simple CN-XI neuropathy.

DIFFERENTIAL DIAGNOSIS

The close association of CN-XI with superficial cervical lymph nodes renders it vulnerable to iatrogenic damage during various **surgical procedures** within the posterior triangle, including lymph node biopsy and radical neck surgical dissection. Damage also rarely occurs after **carotid endarterectomy** or **jugular vein cannulation** because of the nerve's proximity to large neck vessels. Various disorders at the anatomical level of the anterior horn cell are within the differential, including **motor neuron disease**, **syringomyelia**, and **poliomyelitis**.

Intraspinal and intracranial portions of CN-XI may be affected by intrinsic spinal cord lesions, posterior fossa meningiomas, or metastases. Benign tumors such as an enplaque meningioma at the base of the brain or metastatic tumors at the jugular foramen or foramen magnum may impinge on CN-XI; however, they usually concomitantly affect CN-X and sometimes even the hypoglossal nerve that exits through the adjacent hypoglossal foramen. Rarely, radiation injury affects CN-XI with treatment of adjacent tumors.

Because most individuals with CN-XI palsies present with shoulder or neck pain or both, lesions at the level of the cervical nerve roots or brachial plexus require consideration. Patients with neuralgic amyotrophy may have concomitant involvement of CN-XI and the phrenic nerve. These plexopathies and radiculopathies have an acute onset.

CRANIAL NERVE XI: SPINAL ACCESSORY

Figure 16-2

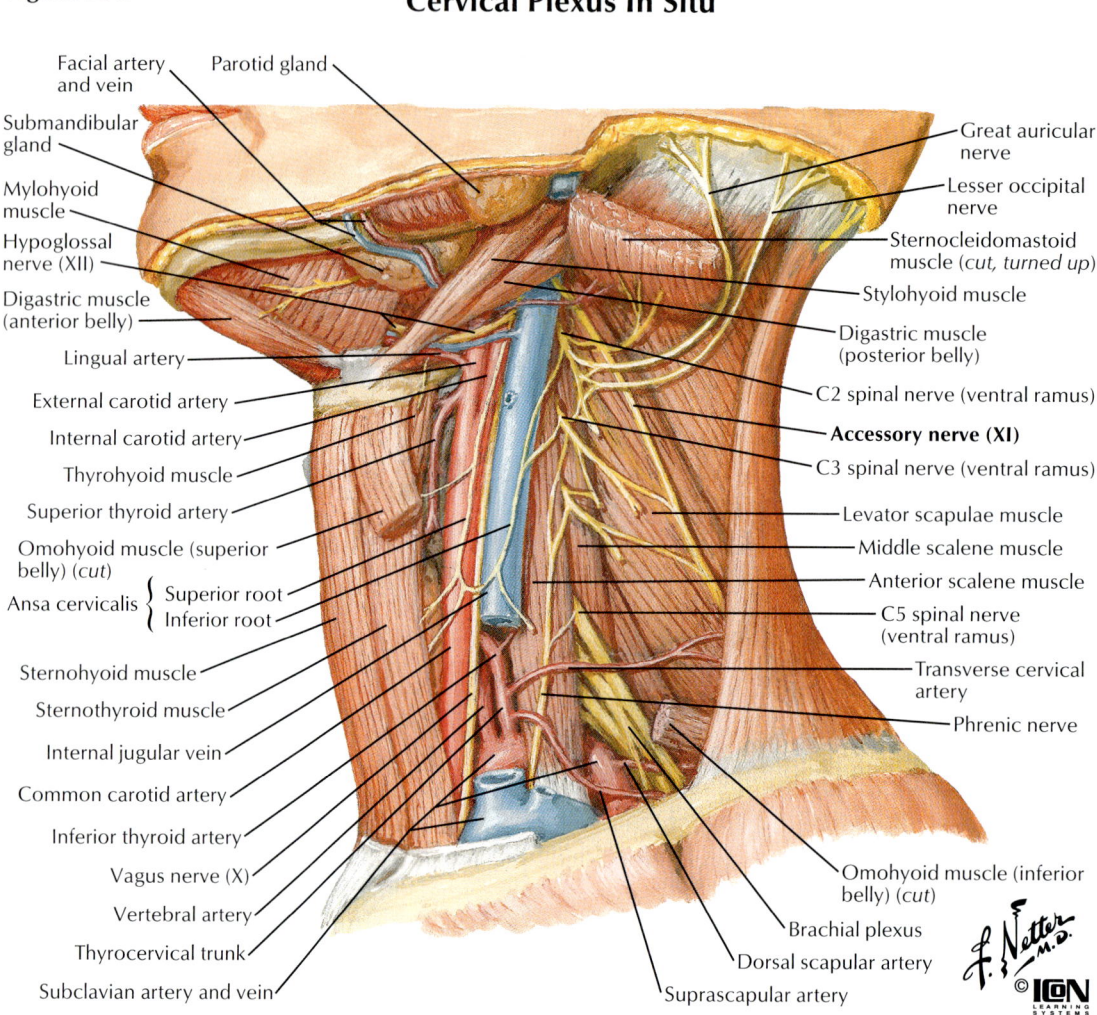

Cervical Plexus In Situ

PROGNOSIS

For patients with benign traumatic lesions, the likelihood of reinnervation is good unless the 2 CN-XI segments are widely separated. Sometimes surgical exploration is helpful. The time frame for reinnervation is similar to that for any peripheral nerve: 1 mm per day or 3 cm per month.

CRANIAL NERVE XI: SPINAL ACCESSORY

Figure 16-3 **Clinical Findings in Cranial Nerve XI Damage**

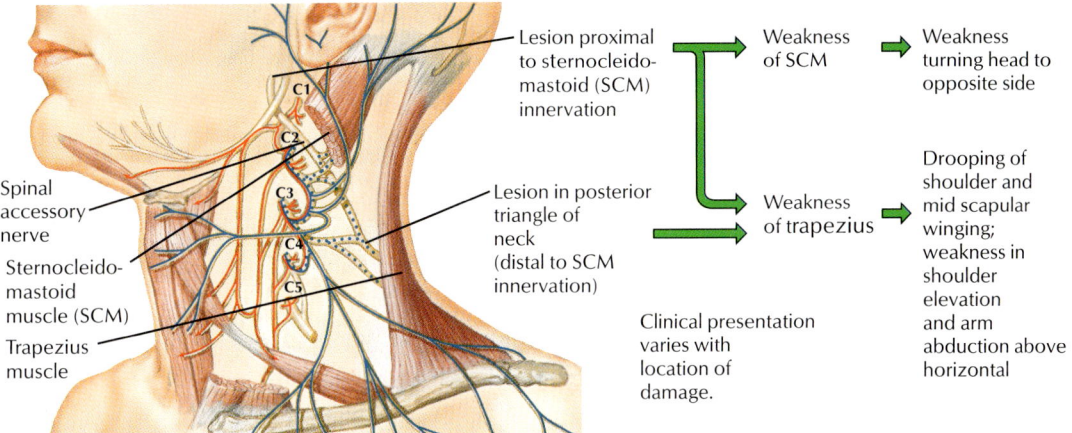

Comparison of clinical findings in CN-XI and long thoracic nerve damage

CN-XI damage

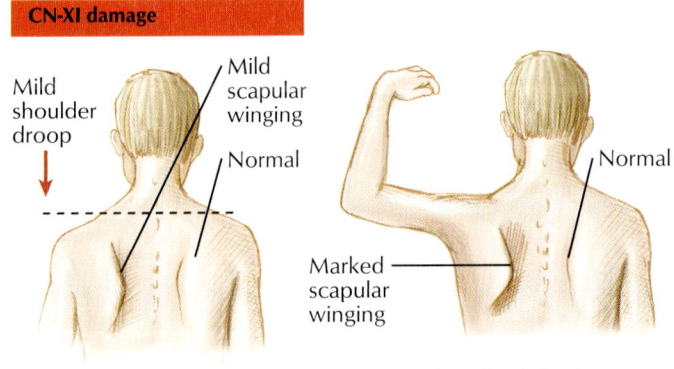

Spinal accessory (CN-XI) nerve lesions cause weakness of trapezius muscle on involved side and present with mild shoulder droop. Weakness of shoulder elevation and scapular winging most pronounced on arm abduction

Long thoracic nerve damage

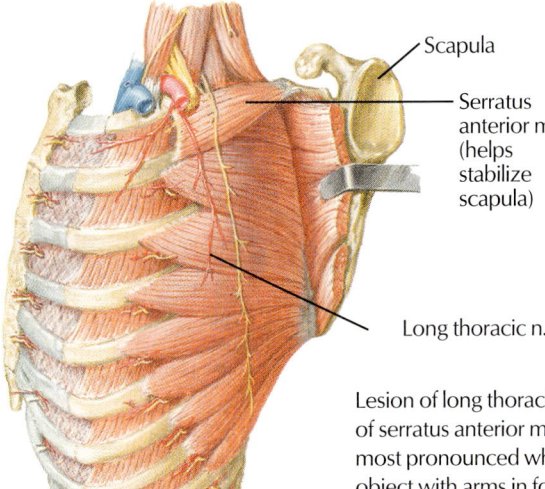

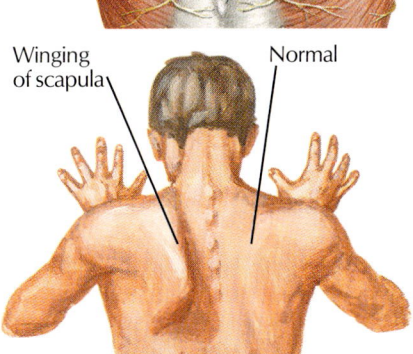

Lesion of long thoracic nerve causes weakness of serratus anterior muscles with winging of scapula most pronounced when pushing against stationary object with arms in forward elevation.

CRANIAL NERVES

CRANIAL NERVE XI: SPINAL ACCESSORY

REFERENCES

Berger PS, Bataini JP. Radiation-induced cranial nerve palsy. *Cancer.* 1977;40:152-155.

Brown H. Anatomy of the spinal accessory nerve plexus: relevance to head and neck cancer and atherosclerosis. *Exp Biol Med (Maywood)* 2002;227:570-578.

Finsterer J, Erdorf M, Mamoli B, et al. Needle electromyography of bulbar muscles in patients with amyotrophic lateral sclerosis: evidence of subclinical involvement. *Neurology.* 1998;51:1417-1422.

Friedenberg SM, Zimprich T, Harper CM. The natural history of long thoracic and spinal accessory neuropathies. *Muscle Nerve.* 2002;25:535-539.

Hanson MR, Sweeney PJ. Disturbances of lower cranial nerves. In: Bradley WG, Daroff RB, Fenichel GM, Marsden CD, eds. *Neurology in Clinical Practice: Principles of Diagnosis and Management.* 2nd ed. Boston, Mass: Butterworth-Heinemann; 1996:251-263.

Kim DH, Cho YJ, Tiel RL, et al. Surgical outcomes of 111 spinal accessory nerve injuries. *Neurosurgery.* 2003;53:1106-1112.

Sarma S, Sekhar LN, Schessel DA. Nonvestibular schwannomas of the brain: a 7-year experience. *Neurosurgery.* 2002;50:437-448.

Sweeney PJ, Hanson MR. The cranial neuropathies. In: Bradley WG, Daroff RB, Fenichel GM, Marsden CD, eds. *Neurology in Clinical Practice: Principles of Diagnosis and Management.* 2nd ed. Boston, Mass: Butterworth-Heinemann; 1996:1721-1732.

Thomas PK, Mathias CJ. Diseases of the ninth, tenth, eleventh, and twelfth cranial nerves (1993). In: Dyck PJ, Thomas PK, Griffin JW, Low PA, Poduslo JF, eds. *Peripheral Neuropathy.* 3rd ed. Philadelphia, Pa: WB Saunders Co; 1993:869-885.

Wilson-Pauwels L, Akesson EJ, Stewart PA. Accessory nerve. In: Wilson-Pauwels L, Akesson EJ, Stewart PA, eds. *Cranial Nerves: Anatomy and Clinical Comments.* Philadelphia, Pa: BC Decker; 1988:139-145.

Woodward G, Venkatesh R. Spinal accessory neuropathy and internal jugular thrombosis after carotid endarterectomy. *J Neurol Neurosurg Psychiatry.* 2000;68:111-112.

Chapter 17
Cranial Nerve XII: Hypoglossal

Michal Vytopil and H. Royden Jones, Jr

Despite being the most distal of the 12 paired CNs, the hypoglossal nerve (CN-XII) controls what is teleologically an important human function: the final common pathway for language implementation. Phylogenetically, CN-XII has major significance because of its role in food intake. As with any CN, CN-XII is susceptible to numerous pathologic processes.

ANATOMY

CN-XII carries motor fibers that supply all intrinsic and most extrinsic tongue muscles, ie, the hyoglossus, styloglossus, genioglossus, and geniohyoid (Figure 17-1). Its fibers originate from the hypoglossal nucleus beneath the floor of the fourth ventricle. In its intramedullary course, CN-XII axons pass ventrally to the lateral side of the medial lemniscus emerging from the medulla in the ventrolateral sulcus between the olive and the pyramid. The rootlets unite to form CN-XII, which exits the skull through the hypoglossal foramen within the posterior cranial fossa.

After exiting the skull, CN-XII runs medial to CN-IX, -X, and -XI. It continues between the internal carotid artery and internal jugular vein, and deep into the posterior belly of the digastric muscle. It then loops anteriorly, coursing on the lateral surface of the hyoglossus muscle, and later, it divides to supply the intrinsic and extrinsic muscles of the ipsilateral tongue.

The anterior primary ramus of the spinal nerve C1 sends fibers to accompany CN-XII for a short distance; these fibers later connect with the fibers of C2 and C3 anterior primary rami, forming a loop called *ansa cervicalis*. This innervates the scalenus group, rectus capitis, longus capitis, longus colli, and the levator scapulae muscles of the neck.

Clinical Vignette

A 67-year-old man presented with a 2-week history of slurring of speech and difficulty swallowing liquids. Two months earlier, he had experienced a few transient episodes of aphasia lasting 15 to 20 minutes consistent with a diagnosis of transient ischemic attacks of the left carotid system. Severe bilateral carotid stenosis was diagnosed. Sequential carotid endarterectomies were performed 6 days apart at another hospital. Immediately after the second surgery, the patient noted speech and swallowing difficulties.

Neurologic examination demonstrated dysarthric speech, particularly for lingual sounds. The patient had bilateral tongue weakness with inability to protrude or elevate the tongue but no atrophy or fasciculation. EMG 5 weeks after surgery demonstrated considerable diminution in the number of motor units with fibrillation potentials confined to the tongue and infrahyoid muscles. The patient's speech and swallowing gradually improved over the subsequent 6 months.

The close proximity of CN-XII to the carotid artery makes it vulnerable to concomitant lesions. Typically, acute carotid artery dissection is accompanied by signs of Horner syndrome, an associated cranial XII neuropathy, or both, and sometimes by dysgeusia. However, swallowing and speech functions are not greatly affected until bilateral lesions develop, as in the vignette in this chapter. Both CN-XII nerves were damaged sequentially by the carotid endarterectomies.

CLINICAL PRESENTATION

Straight protrusion of the tongue is accomplished by balanced action of both genioglossus muscles. Therefore, bilateral CN-XII lesions impair tongue protrusion causing dysarthria and swallowing difficulties. Unilateral CN-XII lesions do not interfere with swallowing or speech but cause the tongue to deviate toward the side of the lesion when the patient attempts to protrude the tongue (Figure 17-2). A lower motor neuron lesion of CN-XII typically results in atrophy, fasciculation, and increased furrowing of the ipsilat-

CRANIAL NERVE XII: HYPOGLOSSAL

Figure 17-1A Hypoglossal Nerve (XII): Schema

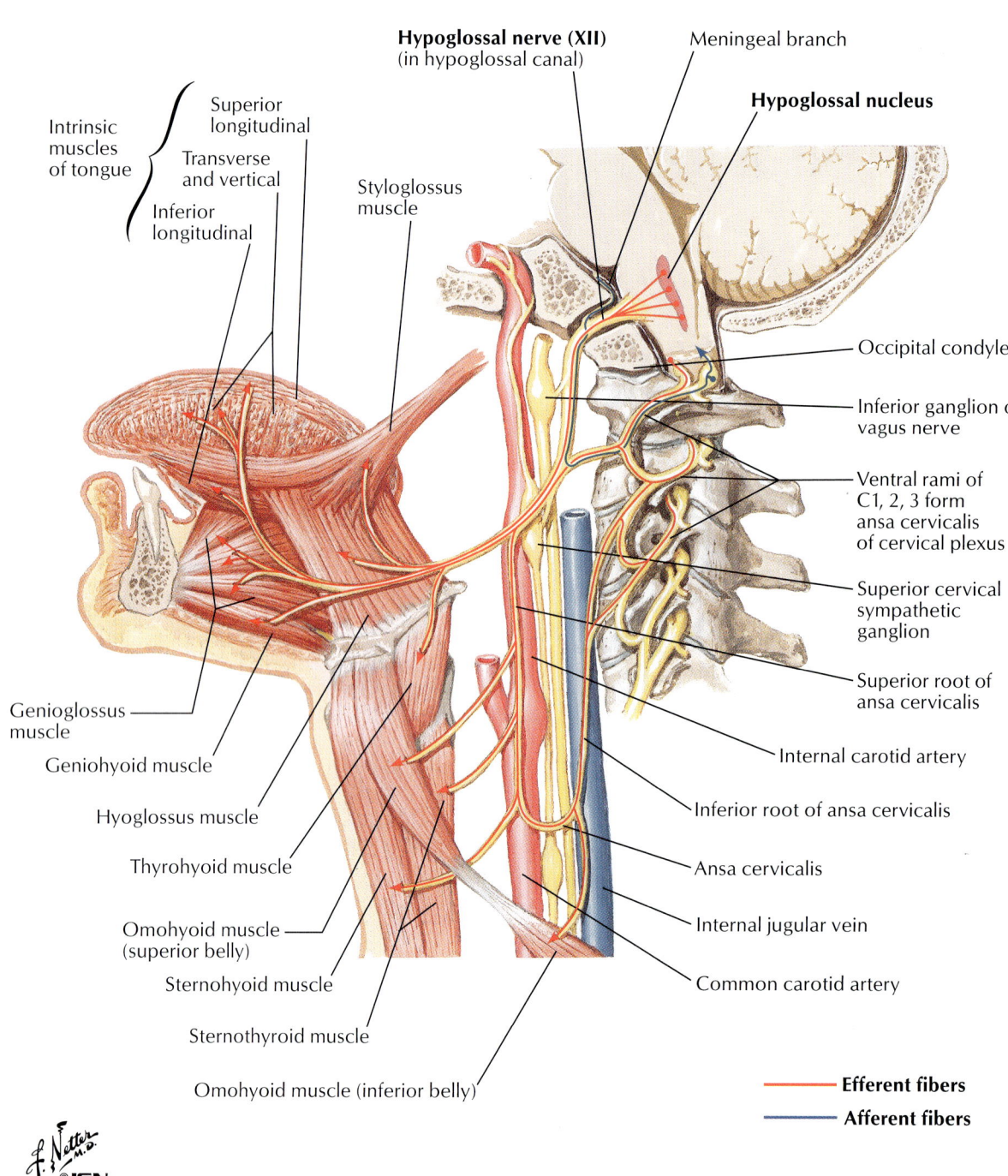

164

CRANIAL NERVE XII: HYPOGLOSSAL

Figure 17-1B   ## Hypoglossal Nerve Intermedullary Course

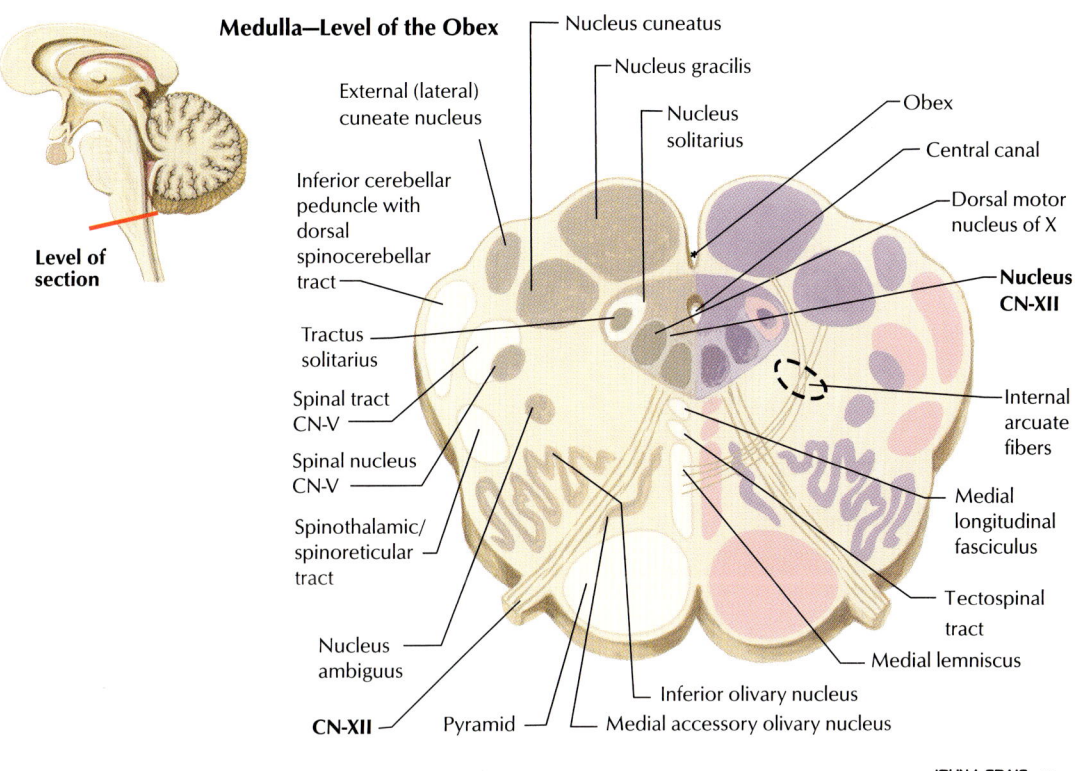

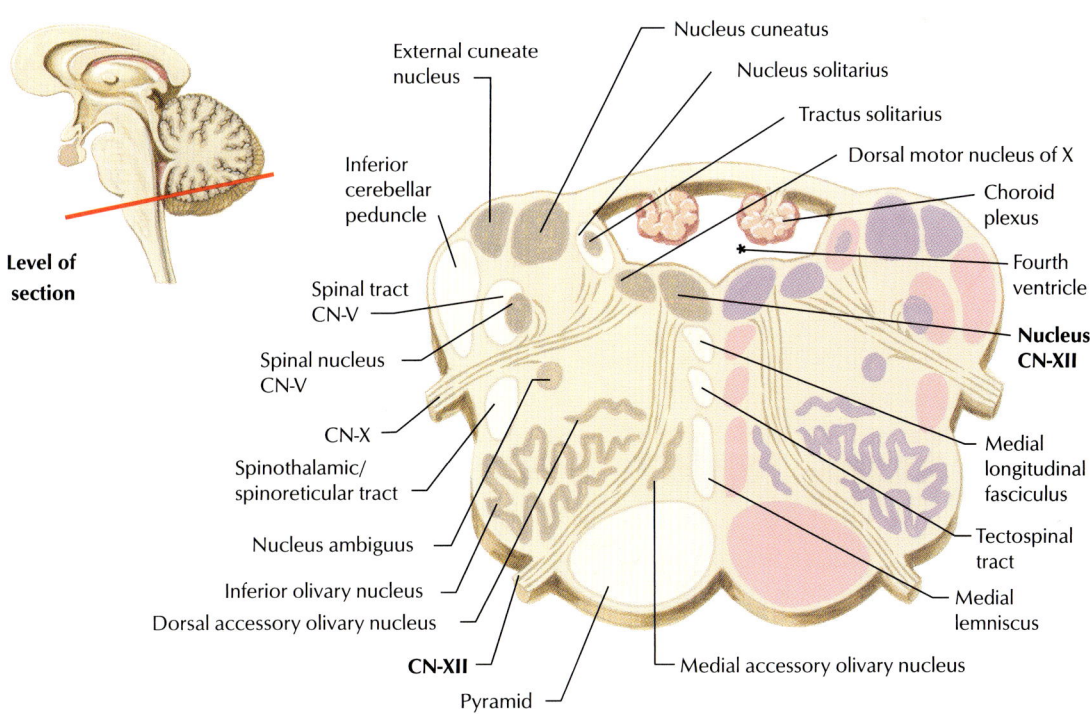

CRANIAL NERVES

CRANIAL NERVE XII: HYPOGLOSSAL

Figure 17-2

Hypoglossal Nerve (CN-XII)

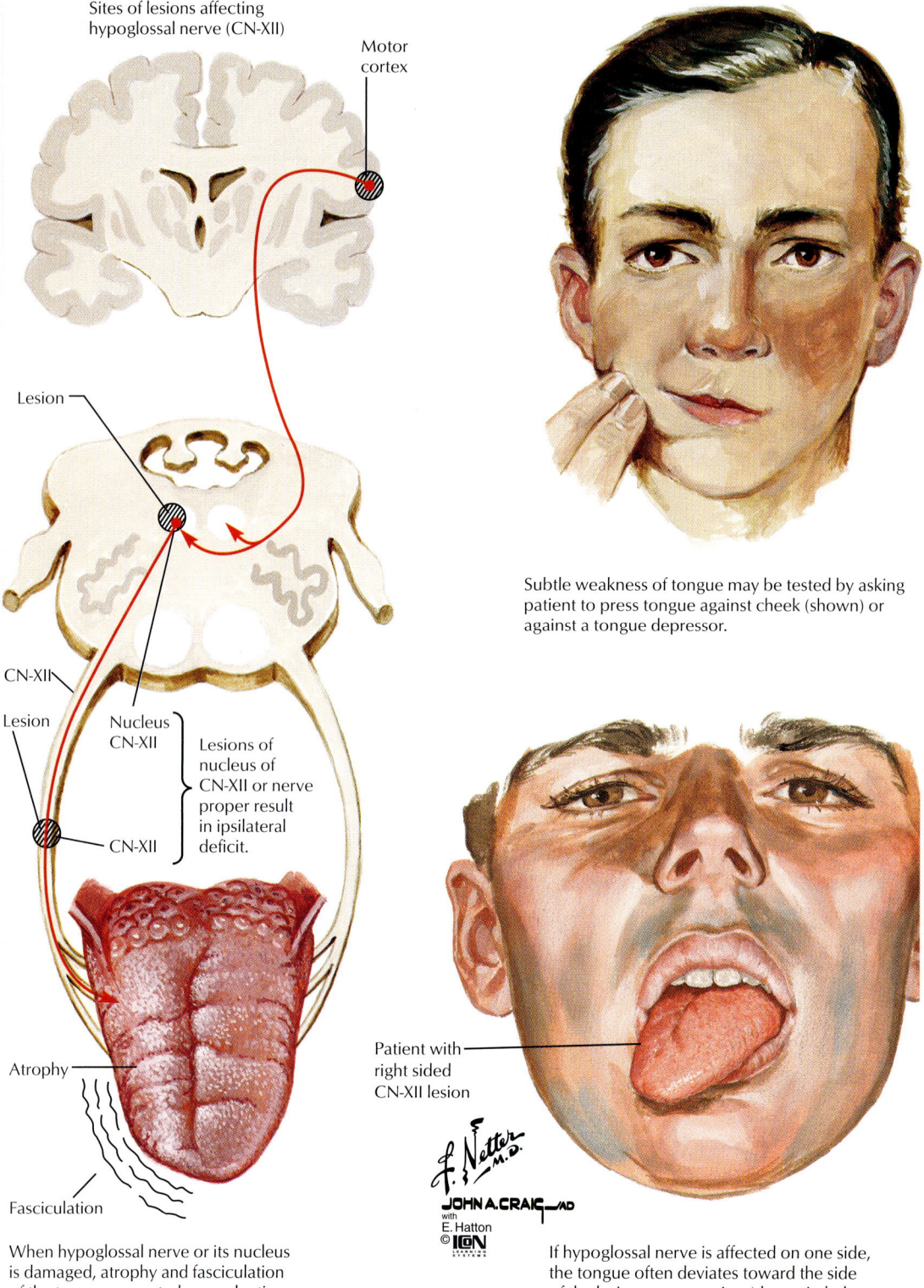

Sites of lesions affecting hypoglossal nerve (CN-XII)

Motor cortex

Lesion

CN-XII

Lesion

Nucleus CN-XII

CN-XII

Lesions of nucleus of CN-XII or nerve proper result in ipsilateral deficit.

Atrophy

Fasciculation

When hypoglossal nerve or its nucleus is damaged, atrophy and fasciculation of the tongue are noted on evaluation.

Subtle weakness of tongue may be tested by asking patient to press tongue against cheek (shown) or against a tongue depressor.

Patient with right sided CN-XII lesion

If hypoglossal nerve is affected on one side, the tongue often deviates toward the side of the lesion on protrusion (due to imbalance of genioglossus contraction).

CRANIAL NERVES

eral side of the tongue. In contrast, a unilateral upper motor neuron lesion may result in deviation of the tongue contralateral to the lesion without evidence of atrophy or fasciculation.

DIFFERENTIAL DIAGNOSIS

Anterior horn cell disorders may affect the hypoglossal nucleus, as in **motor neuron disease** or **poliomyelitis**. Other intramedullary processes such as **syringobulbia** or **intramedullary tumors** may also lead to a tongue paresis. Syringobulbia is frequently associated with the **Arnold-Chiari malformation**. Lower motor neuron tongue weakness of sudden onset may be a manifestation of a rare form of **brainstem infarction** but is usually accompanied by other features, most notably contralateral hemiparesis and involvement of other lower CNs.

Although tongue weakness secondary to intrinsic medullary lesions is usually bilateral and is accompanied by other features, isolated unilateral hypoglossal paralysis should always suggest a **neoplasm**. A primary tumor of CN-XII, such as **neurinoma**, may be the cause. **Intracranial metastases**, particularly bronchial or breast carcinomas, lymphomas, or benign lesions such as **meningiomas**, **chordomas**, or **cholesteatomas** occasionally affect CN-XII. **Glomus jugulare tumor**, a relatively rare lesion, occasionally presents in this clinical context. Sometimes, no mechanism is identified.

Neck trauma with or without **spontaneous dissection of the internal carotid** is a rare cause of CN-XII neuropathy. Similar to some other CNs, CN-XII may be affected by **radiation therapy**.

Glossodynia is a controversial syndrome characterized by burning pain in the tongue. The condition occurs in middle-aged patients and occurs more frequently in women. Although vitamin B deficiency, including B_{12}, has been suggested as a cause, most cases are thought to be psychogenic.

DIAGNOSTIC APPROACH

MRI of the brain base and neck are the diagnostic tests of choice. If these tests do not define evidence of a specific mass lesion, leptomeningeal enhancement should be checked. The latter is typically seen with metastatic tumors, sarcoidosis, or other rare leptomeningeal infiltrating lesions such as tuberculosis.

CSF analysis is indicated if an infiltrative process is clinically suspected or suggested from MRI. CSF analysis must include routine studies and cytologic analysis for malignant cells.

EMG is indicated when the above studies are unremarkable. Unfortunately, an asymmetrically atrophied tongue is most commonly the presenting sign of motor neuron disease.

REFERENCES

Berger PS, Bataini JP. Radiation-induced cranial nerve palsy. *Cancer*. 1977;40:152-155.

Combarros O, Alvarez de Arcaya A, Berciano J. Isolated unilateral hypoglossal nerve palsy: nine cases. *J Neurol*. 1998;245:98-100.

DePaul R, Abbs JH, Caligiuri M, et al. Hypoglossal, trigeminal, and facial motoneuron involvement in amyotrophic lateral sclerosis. *Neurology*. 1988;38:281-283.

Gutrecht JA, Jones HR. Bilateral hypoglossal nerve injury after bilateral carotid endarterectomy. *Stroke*. 1988;19:261-262.

Hanson MR, Sweeney PJ. Disturbances of lower cranial nerves. In: Bradley WG, Daroff RB, Fenichel GM, Marsden CD, eds. *Neurology in Clinical Practice: Principles of Diagnosis and Management*. 2nd ed. Boston, Mass: Butterworth-Heinemann; 1996:251-263.

King AD, Leung SF, Teo P, et al. Hypoglossal nerve palsy in nasopharyngeal carcinoma. *Head Neck*. 1999;21:614-619.

Sarma S, Sekhar LN, Schessel DA. Nonvestibular schwannomas of the brain: a 7-year experience. *Neurosurgery*. 2002;50:437-448.

Spector GJ, Druck NS, Gado M. Neurologic manifestations of glomus tumors in the head and neck. *Arch Neurol*. 1976;33:270-274.

Sweeney PJ, Hanson MR. The cranial neuropathies. In: Bradley WG, Daroff RB, Fenichel GM, Marsden CD, eds. *Neurology in Clinical Practice: Principles of Diagnosis and Management*. 2nd ed. Boston, Mass: Butterworth-Heinemann; 1996:1721-1732.

Thomas PK, Mathias CJ. Diseases of the ninth, tenth, eleventh, and twelfth cranial nerves (1993). In: Dyck PJ, Thomas PK, Griffin JW, Low PA, Poduslo JF, eds. *Peripheral Neuropathy*. 3rd ed. Philadelphia, Pa: WB Saunders Co; 1993:869-885.

Wesselmann U, Reich SG. The dynias. *Semin Neurol*. 1996;16:63-74.

Wilson-Pauwels L, Akesson EJ, Stewart PA. Accessory nerve. In: Wilson-Pauwels L, Akesson EJ, Stewart PA, eds. *Cranial Nerves: Anatomy and Clinical Comments*. Philadelphia, Pa: BC Decker; 1988:147-151.

Section IV
HEADACHE

Chapter 18
Primary and Secondary Headache 170

Chapter 18
Primary and Secondary Headache

Jose A. Gutrecht and Edward Tarlov

Clinical Vignette

A 40-year-old woman presented to her internist because of increasing severity of long-standing headaches. These headaches occurred without warning and were characterized by unilateral, throbbing pain aggravated by minor physical activities such as bending over or climbing stairs. She had nausea, photophobia, and was unable to work for 1 to 2 days until the headache subsided. Chocolate often precipitated a headache, and the patient's family history was positive for migraines. Her neurologic and general medical examination was normal. CT scan of the brain was normal.

Headache is one of the most common symptoms in medicine, often a primary presenting complaint. It can be the presentation in many primary neurologic illnesses and in some serious systemic disorders. The preceding vignette is typical of one of the most common headache syndromes (migraine) that bring patients to medical attention. More serious causes requiring specific treatment must not be overlooked, such as brain tumors, ruptured aneurysms, low cerebrospinal pressure syndromes, subdural hematoma, meningitis, and temporal arteritis. The primary pain-sensitive structures in the head include the leptomeninges, arteries, and nasal sinuses (Figure 18-1).

Assessment of a patient presenting with a significant headache starts with the detailed history. Essential characteristics should be defined: any premonitory symptoms, manner of onset (eg, precipitous or gradual), provoking factors, pain characteristics, the associated clinical circumstances and symptoms, duration, and degree of disability. Family and social history, current medications, drug allergies, and review of systems are also paramount. A detailed neurologic and general medical examination is essential to the evaluation, particularly with individuals having a recent or precipitous onset or experiencing changes in headache characteristics. Ancillary laboratory and neuroradiologic testing are often indicated.

Headache syndromes must first be classified as primary, without significant underlying neurologic pathology, or secondary to some cerebral or extracerebral pathology. The differentiation between primary and secondary is critical; it dictates the diagnostic approach and guides treatment and prognosis.

PRIMARY HEADACHE DISORDERS
Migraine

Migraine is the most common type of headache that leads patients to seek medical care. Its prevalence is almost 10% (30 million persons) in the US population, with a female to male ratio of 3:1. First-degree relatives of patients with migraine seem to be at higher risk. Frequently, migraine begins during puberty. It is more prevalent in individuals aged 25 to 55 years and is one of the leading causes of chronic suffering and disability in this population.

Patients with migraine often have prodromal symptoms of emotional or mood disturbances such as irritability, elation or depression, general symptoms of fatigue, thirst, anorexia, fluid retention, food cravings, or other neurologic phenomena, including drowsiness or even enhanced alertness (Figure 18-2). Many individuals with migraine have premonitory focal disturbances that mimic a TIA or stroke. Of migraine patients, approximately 15% have an aura preceding the pain phase. This presentation was formerly referred to as *classic migraine*; however, the new classification system identifies it as **migraine with aura**. The aura comprises focal neurologic symptoms, most commonly visual (>95% of all auras).

PRIMARY AND SECONDARY HEADACHE

Figure 18-1 Pain—Sensitive Structures and Pain Referral

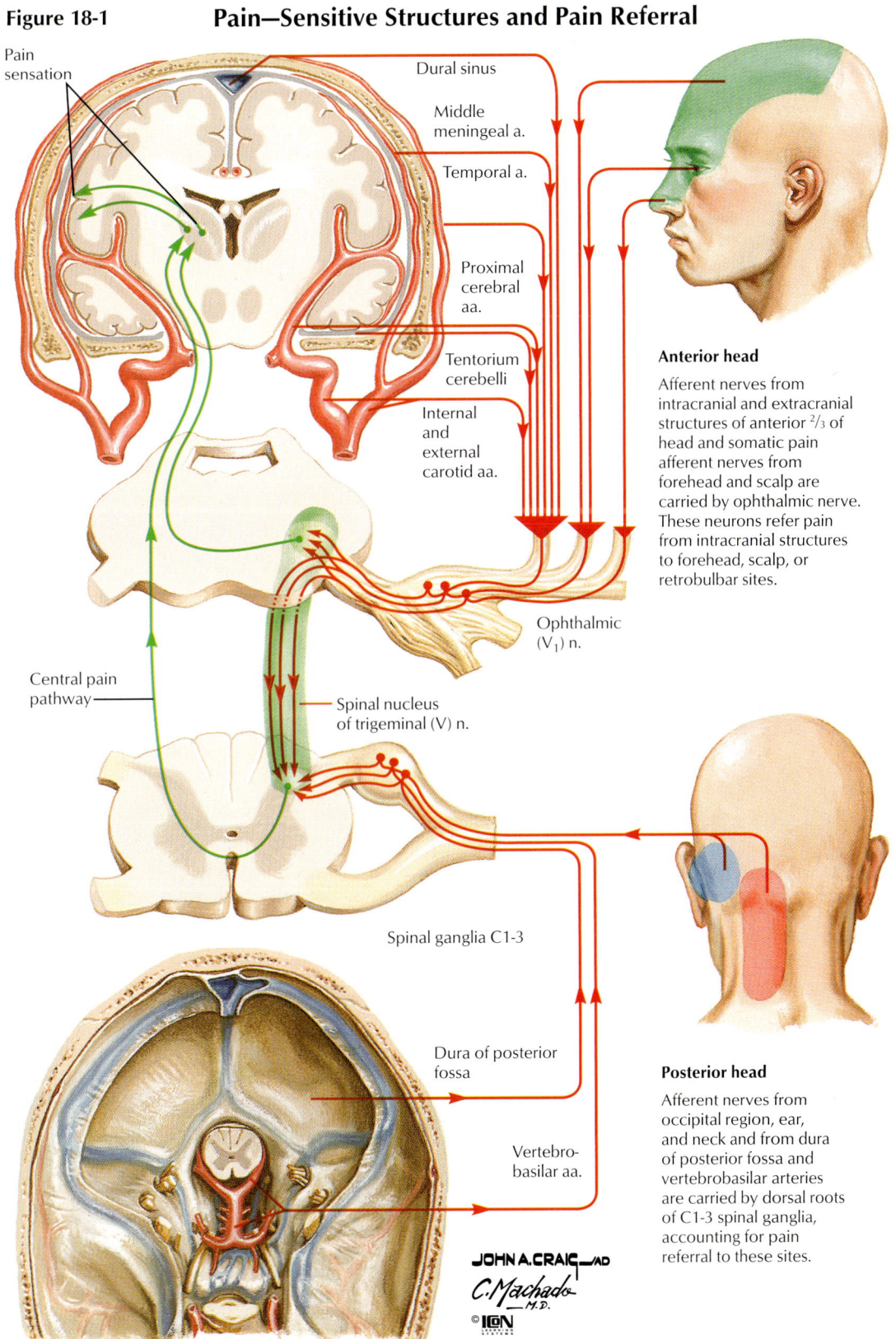

Anterior head

Afferent nerves from intracranial and extracranial structures of anterior 2/3 of head and somatic pain afferent nerves from forehead and scalp are carried by ophthalmic nerve. These neurons refer pain from intracranial structures to forehead, scalp, or retrobulbar sites.

Posterior head

Afferent nerves from occipital region, ear, and neck and from dura of posterior fossa and vertebrobasilar arteries are carried by dorsal roots of C1-3 spinal ganglia, accounting for pain referral to these sites.

HEADACHE

PRIMARY AND SECONDARY HEADACHE

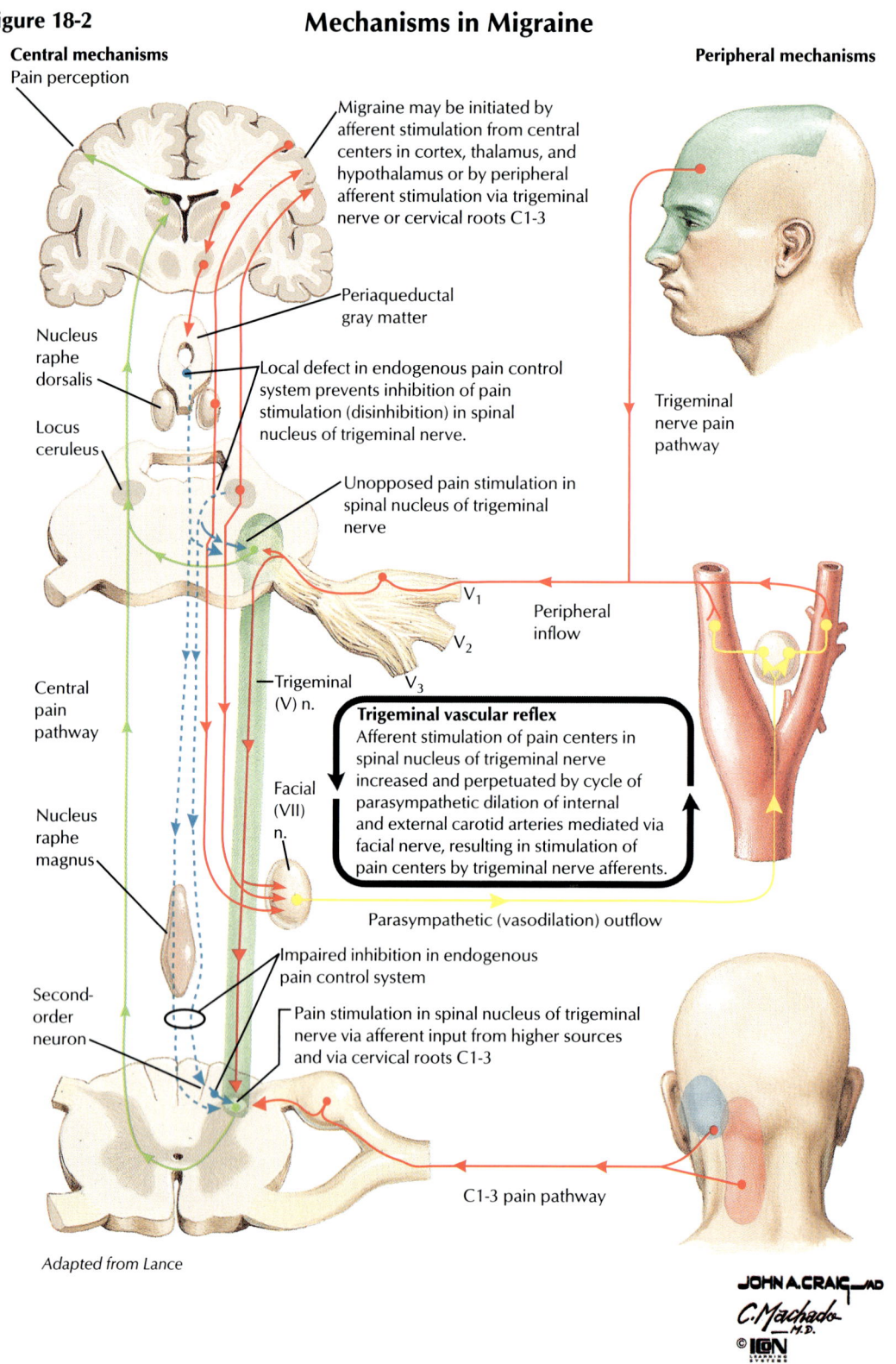

Figure 18-2. Mechanisms in Migraine

PRIMARY AND SECONDARY HEADACHE

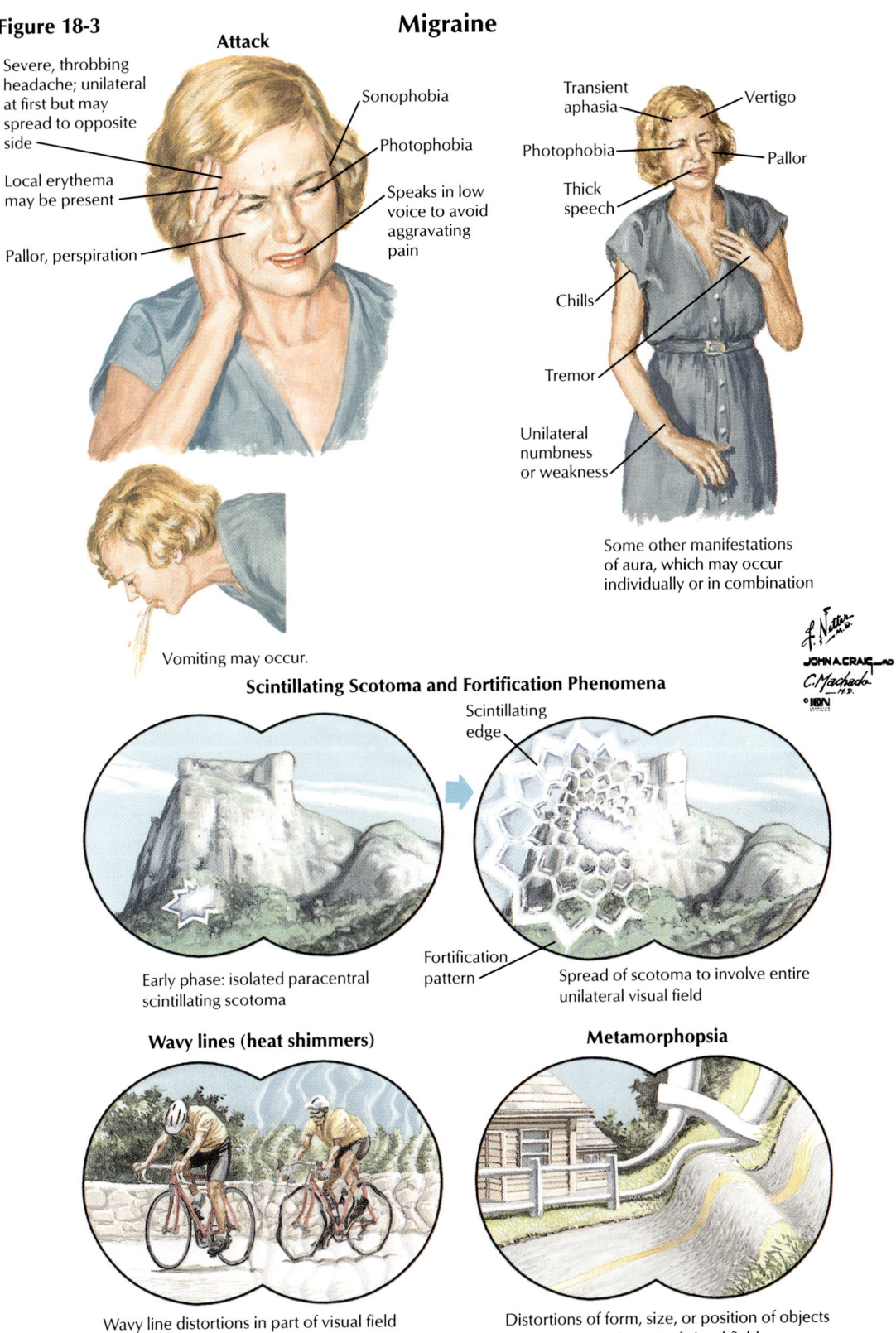

Figure 18-3

Migraine

Attack

- Severe, throbbing headache; unilateral at first but may spread to opposite side
- Local erythema may be present
- Pallor, perspiration
- Sonophobia
- Photophobia
- Speaks in low voice to avoid aggravating pain

Vomiting may occur.

- Transient aphasia
- Photophobia
- Thick speech
- Chills
- Tremor
- Unilateral numbness or weakness
- Vertigo
- Pallor

Some other manifestations of aura, which may occur individually or in combination

Scintillating Scotoma and Fortification Phenomena

- Early phase: isolated paracentral scintillating scotoma
- Scintillating edge
- Fortification pattern
- Spread of scotoma to involve entire unilateral visual field

Wavy lines (heat shimmers)

Wavy line distortions in part of visual field similar to shimmers above hot pavement

Metamorphopsia

Distortions of form, size, or position of objects or environment in part of visual field

HEADACHE

173

These visual phenomena occur in a homonymous or hemifield distribution. Typically, scotomata, either scintillating simple flashes often called *stars* (phosphenes) or geometric patterns known as a *fortification spectra* characterize these symptoms.

Other types of migrainous auras include sensory, motor, or rarely, involvement of higher cortical functions, including language. Most auras develop slowly over several to 20 minutes, involve anatomically different areas, and last less than 1 hour. For example, the patient may initially experience numbness in the fingers that gradually spreads up the arm to the face and sometimes even down the leg. Occasionally, in some individuals, the auras may not be followed by the headache phase. Less commonly, the aura phase consists of a more complex symptomatology. For example, in **basilar artery migraine**, symptoms may include dysarthria, vertigo, ataxia, diplopia, and hearing deficits. In **confusional migraine**, cognitive deficits are more prominent. Ocular nerve palsies are the hallmark of **ophthalmoplegic migraine**. **Hemiplegic migraine** has a variably prominent unilateral weakness.

Careful neurologic evaluation is mandatory before migraine can be safely diagnosed in individuals with a focal aura; this diagnosis, in these circumstances, is one of exclusion. The pathophysiology of the aura may be related to neuronal events of "spreading depression" and concomitant decrease in cerebral blood flood. Although auras are thought to typify migraine and to help differentiate migraines from other headaches, most migraine patients never experience an aura.

The pain phase and its associated symptoms support the clinical classification of headaches as migraine. According to the 1988 guidelines of the Headache Classification Committee of the International Headache Society, the headache must last 4 to 72 hours (either untreated or unsuccessfully treated) and must be associated with nausea and/or vomiting, or photophobia, and/or phonophobia. The headache must be characterized by 2 of the following 4 symptom characteristics: unilateral location, throbbing pulsatile quality, moderate or worse degree of severity, or intensified by routine physical activity. These criteria must be met for at least 5 separate episodes. Concomitantly, it is crucial for the physician to ensure that specific organic pathophysiologic mechanisms are excluded before confirming a diagnosis of migraine. Therefore, careful evaluation of the patient presenting with the first few headaches is essential. Similarly, any change in the character of the individual headaches warrants a fresh investigation of the underlying mechanism.

Migraine pathophysiology is related to a combination of meningeal blood vessel dilatation, secondary activation of trigeminal pathways, and subsequent release of vasoactive neuropeptides (Figure 18-3). These promote neurogenic inflammation and pain perception at thalamic and cortical brain levels.

Special Considerations

Two thirds of **women** with migraines primarily experience them just before or during menses. These headaches are often associated with other premenstrual dysphoric symptoms. Estrogen withdrawal most likely influences this major migraine subgroup.

Migraine may worsen early in **pregnancy** but tends to improve during the later trimesters, particularly in women with migraine primarily related to their menstrual cycle. Migraine prevalence decreases with age. Women with migraines that occur earlier in life generally experience a significant decrease in episode frequency after menopause.

Great care must be used in the evaluation and treatment of "*migraine*" headache in the **elderly**. The incidence of headaches as a manifestation of other illnesses significantly increases with age. Headaches may occur as an adverse effect of medications, and the use of antimigraine medication may be more hazardous.

Treatment

There are 2 primary steps in the care of migraine patients: treatment of an acute headache and prevention of subsequent events. The initial goal is prompt pain relief without recurrence, with minimal, if any, untoward adverse effects, while restoring baseline function. For mild to moderately severe nondisabling pain, oral NSAIDs, acetylsalicylic acid (aspirin), or acetaminophen is recommended for short-term treatment. Caffeine may enhance the effect of these various medications. Antiemetics are often useful in conjunction with analgesics.

However, in patients with more severe disabling migraines, oral, injectable, intranasal, or quick-dissolve oral serotonin 1B/1D receptor agonist ("triptan") preparations are the medications of choice. Standard doses are 6.25 to 12.5 mg almotriptan, 25 to 100 mg sumatriptan, 10 mg rizatriptan (5 mg if the patient is taking a β blocker), and 2.5 to 5 mg zolmitriptan. These doses may be repeated after 2 hours if necessary. These preparations are also recommended for patients with milder headaches whose migraines are disabling because they are refractory to the simpler analgesics. When the above-mentioned therapeutic options are ineffective in patients with the most severe migraines, opiate category medications such as intranasal butorphanol or IM meperidine are often used in EDs. However, the possibility of untoward sedation and more importantly, subsequent overuse and dependence, must be considered. Nonnarcotic treatments, such as ketorolac and antiemetics, are still preferred.

Prophylactic treatment, the other aspect of the migraine therapeutic algorithm, is indicated for patients with frequent headache (>3 disabling headaches/month lasting more than 1-3 days). Other indications for preventive therapies include poor response or adverse effects from immediate treatment medications, need for medications with potential for abuse and dependency, or patient preference when one migraine can significantly interfere with daily activities or responsibilities. Various antidepressants, β blockers, calcium channel blockers, sodium valproate, and methysergide are the most effective medications. Experimentation often dictates the most effective medication for the individual patient.

Cluster Headache

Clinical Vignette

A 36-year-old man reported, "For the last 10 days, I have had an absolutely terrible pain behind my left eye that wakes me up every night in the early morning hours, almost like clockwork." He stated, "The pain is intense, I have tearing from the eye, and my nose feels congested. I am told my eye looks red." Occasionally, the pain occurred in the daytime. "I become very restless during the episode, which generally lasts no more than 1 hour. A few years ago, I had similar headaches for about 4 or 5 weeks."

As evident from the initial interview, a cluster headache is one of the most severe headaches a patient can experience, with the exception of an acute ruptured berry aneurysm. Fortunately, cluster headaches occur much less commonly than migraine, to which they are unrelated. These recurrent headaches usually first occur in the third decade, affecting men more often than women (male to female ratio is 2-7:1). Unlike in migraine, a family history of cluster headache is uncommon. Distinctive clinical features include abrupt recurrence once or twice daily, often awakening the patient from sleep. These headaches are always severe with a unilateral distribution around one eye and orbit, lasting up to 1 hour. Most patients with cluster headaches experience concomitant autonomic dysfunction, including partial Horner syndrome, lacrimation, and nasal congestion ipsilateral to the headache (Figure 18-4). Patients are often restless during the episode. Alcohol ingestion is a frequent precipitant.

The periodicity of cluster headaches, likely from dysfunction at the medial hypothalamic areas of the brain, is one of the most important diagnostic characteristics. The patient reports a clinical course of daily headache recurrence for 6 to 12 weeks, with periods of cluster recurring every several months to few years. The underlying pathophysiology seems to be activation of the trigeminal vascular and parasympathetic systems.

Like migraine, the 2 parts to the treatment algorithm are short-term and preventive therapy. Effective short-term headache therapies include sublingual triptan, 25 to 50 mg oral indomethacin 3 times daily, or oxygen inhalation at 4 to 6 L/min for 15 minutes. Preventive therapy must also be used. Verapamil is the drug of choice for prophylaxis of cluster headaches. Other beneficial drugs include sodium valproate, lithium, short-term corticosteroids, and methysergide, although now in short supply. In 10% of the patients with cluster headaches, a chronic form develops; combined-drug programs may be advised for these patients. Very rarely, in well-selected patients, surgical ablation

PRIMARY AND SECONDARY HEADACHE

Figure 18-4 Cluster Headache and Chronic Paroxysmal Hemicrania

Cluster headache

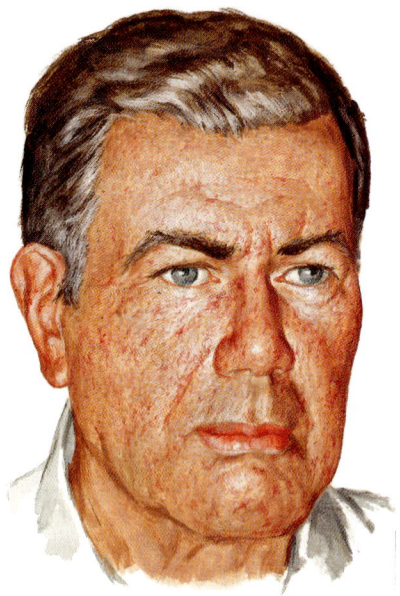
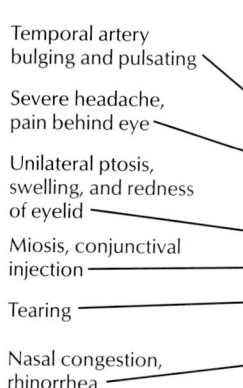

- Temporal artery bulging and pulsating
- Severe headache, pain behind eye
- Unilateral ptosis, swelling, and redness of eyelid
- Miosis, conjunctival injection
- Tearing
- Nasal congestion, rhinorrhea
- Flushing of side of face, sweating

Large, strong, muscular man typical patient. Face may have peau d'orange skin, telangiectasis.

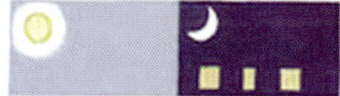

Attacks typically nocturnal; average frequency 1-3 in 24 hours, lasting 15 minutes-3 hours

Chronic paroxysmal hemicrania (CHP)

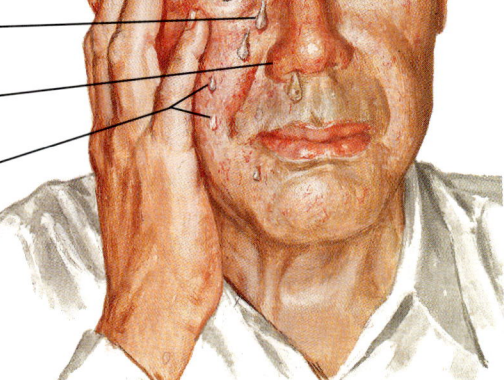

Attacks typically nocturnal; average frequency 10-30 in 24 hours, lasting 5-20 minutes

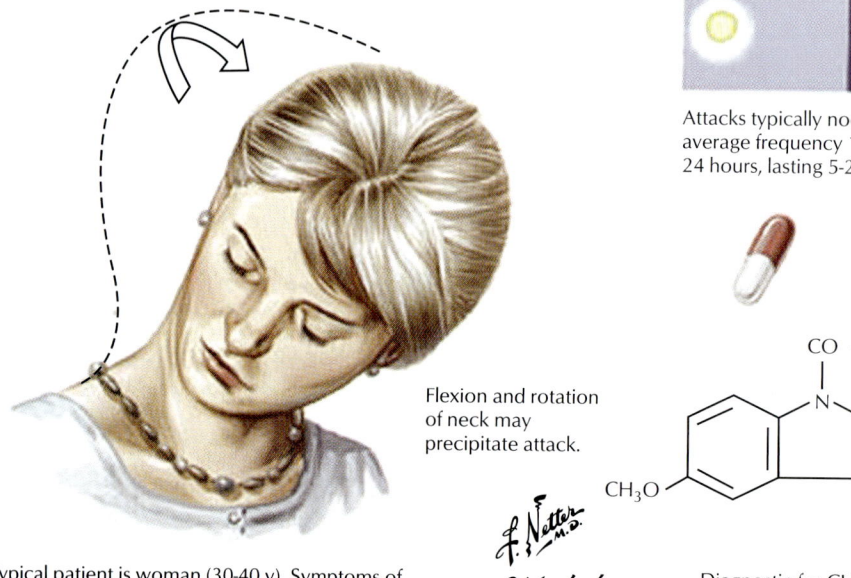

Flexion and rotation of neck may precipitate attack.

Typical patient is woman (30-40 y). Symptoms of unilateral headache (lacrimation, rhinorrhea, and miosis), which are common in cluster, are absent in CHP.

Diagnostic for CHP, prompt and absolute response to indomethacin

HEADACHE

176

or radiofrequency rhizotomy of the trigeminal nerve offer other options.

Tension Headache

Tension headache is the most common headache type. In 1988, the Headache Classification Committee of the International Headache Society determined that a diagnosis of tension headache requires the presence of at least 2 of the following pain characteristics: a nonpulsating quality, mild or moderate nondisabling intensity, bilateral location, and no aggravation by routine physical activity. In addition, these patients do not experience nausea or vomiting and have no photophobia or phonophobia. Tension headaches last fewer than 7 days.

Careful evaluation is indicated in every patient suspected of having tension headache. Exclusion of structural, infectious, or metabolic disorders is essential. Although sometimes features of migraine are present, they are a minor part of the clinical picture. Specific triggering factors are also less common than with migraine. Chronic tension headaches are diagnosed when they recur more than 15 times per month. The precise pathophysiology is unknown. It is probably a heterogeneous disorder with various etiologic factors, including pericranial muscular tension (Figure 18-5), oromandibular dysfunction, psychosocial stress, anxiety, depression, and analgesic drug overuse. Tension headache treatment usually requires only over-the-counter analgesics, including NSAIDs, and nonpharmacologic intervention, including relaxation techniques, massage, or heat application. Prophylactic medication is indicated for frequent recurrence.

Chronic Daily Headaches

Some individuals experience frequent tension ("rebound") headaches. If they recur more than 15 days per month, the diagnosis of chronic tension-type headache or chronic daily headaches applies. Patients with migraines recurring more than 15 days per month are said to have either *chronic migraine* or *transformed migraine*. Many patients in these 2 clinical groups repeatedly and inappropriately use acute headache medications for longer than 3 months, complicating treatment. Medications known to have potential for abuse are analgesics, ergotamine, barbiturates, and opiates.

Patient education is of utmost importance. The patient must understand the pathophysiologic mechanisms and agree to cooperate if treatment is to succeed. Step 1 is withdrawal of the offending medication. Patient support mechanisms to control anxiety and a management plan for headache recurrence are needed. Hospitalization with a series of IV dihydroergotamine treatments may be necessary for short-term pain control. Comorbid etiologic factors—depression, psychosocial stresses, and poor sleep—require attention. Follow-up prophylactic treatments for both groups may be nonpharmacologic, including emotional support, counseling, physical therapy, relaxation exercises, heat, or massage. Antidepressants often provide the key pharmacologic treatment.

Paroxysmal Hemicranias

These are unusual primary headaches, unilateral and short lived (<1 hour), which occur in a chronic or episodic manner. Typically, the pain has a severe throbbing or boring quality and often recurs during the same day. These headaches are associated with ipsilateral cranial autonomic dysfunction but occur more often in women than men. Furthermore, these headaches have a greater daily recurrence and less of a cluster pattern than cluster headaches. They usually respond well to 25 to 50 mg indomethacin 3 times daily.

Hypnic Headaches

Headaches of this type tend to occur in the elderly population and affect women more than men, particularly at night, waking patients during REM stages of sleep. Such headaches are generalized, throbbing, and without autonomic features. They may last up to 1 hour and may recur through the night.

Cold Stimulus Headaches

These are the classic "ice cream headaches." Typically, these benign headaches occur during the rapid ingestion of cold food or drink, are located in the forehead, and subside in a few minutes without medication.

PRIMARY AND SECONDARY HEADACHE

Figure 18-5

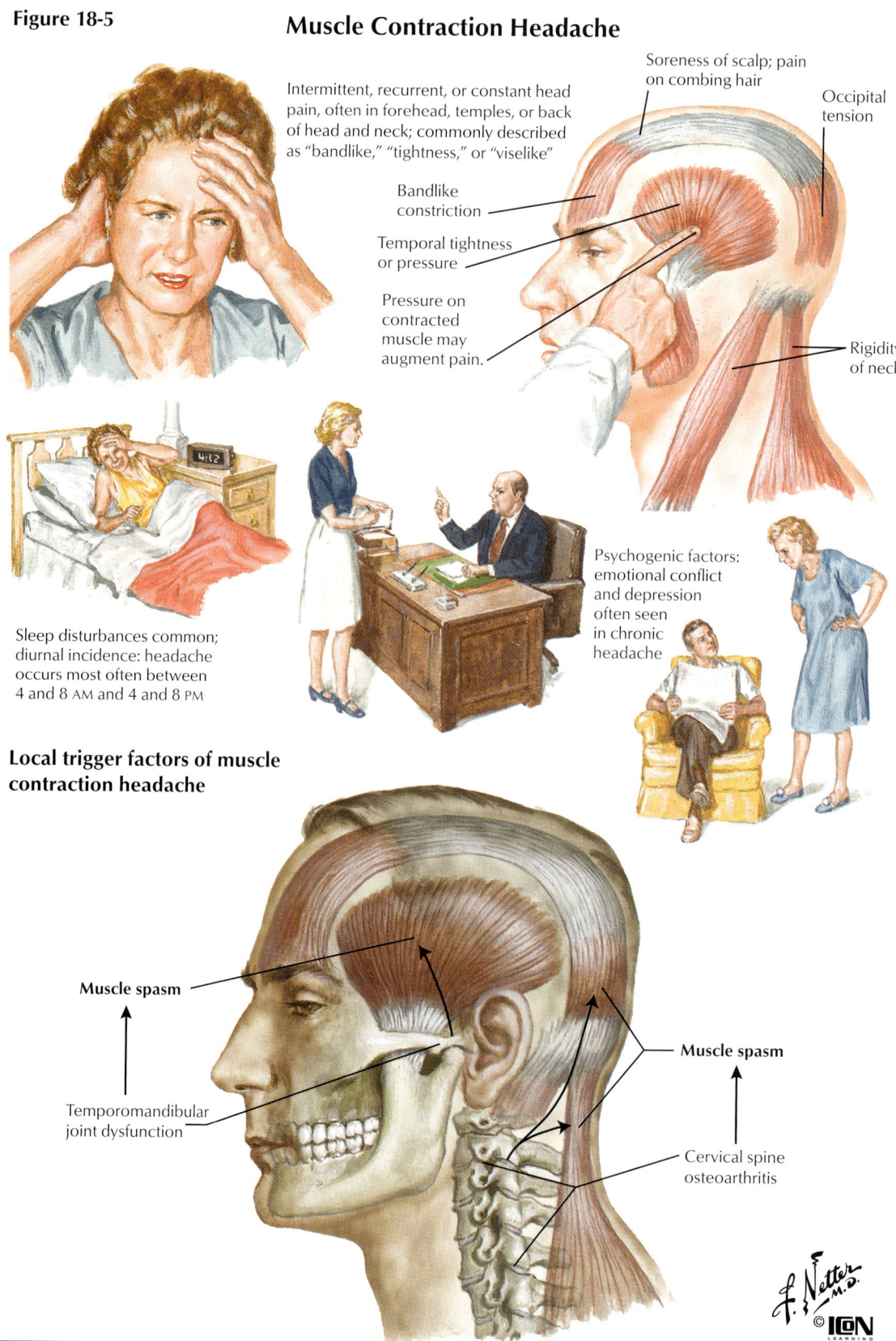

Benign Exertional Headaches

Physical exercise is always the precipitating factor in benign exertional headaches. They may develop during acute straining (eg, weight lifting) or after sustained exercise such as running. These headaches are usually generalized and throbbing and often respond to 25 to 50 mg indomethacin 3 times daily taken either after the exercise or prophylactically once a typical pattern is established. β Blockers may also be used. However, the possibility of serious disorders such as arterial dissection, aneurysmal rupture, and even an intracranial mass must be excluded. CT, MRI, and MRA may be appropriate.

Benign Cough Headaches

These brief, generalized headaches typically occur in an older population and may represent another variety of exertional headaches. They respond to 25 to 50 mg indomethacin 3 times daily.

Coital Headaches

Typically, these headaches develop as dull, generalized pain during sexual activity or as an acute severe pain during orgasm. As with other paroxysmal headaches, such as cough or exertional types, a search for underlying systemic or intracranial pathology, particularly a ruptured aneurysm, is needed before diagnosing a benign process. Administering 25 to 50 mg indomethacin 3 times daily is useful for many individuals if ingested before the activity.

SECONDARY HEADACHE DISORDERS

Although most headaches occur in the absence of underlying intracranial or systemic pathology, some result from more serious illness. The neurologist is often the initial physician contacted by such patients. Because of the painful nature of the headaches, the clinical presentation may be the patient's only expressed concern. A careful history is mandatory to achieve an accurate diagnosis and eventual patient management. The temporal profile and age at headache onset, sex, family history, precipitating factors (triggers), pain character, and associated symptoms require analysis. The history is followed by neurologic examination and testing essential to patient management. Often, immediate laboratory, neuroradiologic testing, or both are crucial.

Whether this approach applies to every patient with headaches is debatable. However, with the widespread availability and relatively inexpensive nature of brain CT, it is judicious to image patients who have experienced recent onset of a significant headache, including those with normal clinical examinations. Significant neurologic disorders, such as subarachnoid hemorrhage in all age groups, a third ventricular cyst in younger individuals, or subdural hematomas in the elderly, provide examples wherein brain CT may diagnose serious neurologic conditions when the most careful neurologic examinations are normal.

Giant Cell (Temporal) Arteritis

Clinical Vignette

A 70-year-old man reported a recent onset of mild, generalized headaches. The patient's history further revealed some malaise, slight fever, and weight loss. He had significant blurred vision, affecting his ability to read with his left eye. Fortunately, his eyesight returned fully within 20 minutes. This led him to seek medical attention. Questionable tenderness over the temporal arteries was noted on neurologic examination, the results of which were otherwise normal. A temporal artery biopsy demonstrated the classic findings of giant cell arteritis. The symptoms resolved with treatment with corticosteroids in gradually diminishing doses during the next 8 months.

Headache is the most common and prominent presenting symptom of giant cell arteritis, also called *temporal arteritis*, a serious disorder in the elderly with potentially major complications, particularly permanent blindness. The patient in the above vignette is a classic example whose early identification and treatment prevent blindness from developing. The pain is usually nonspecific, throbbing or continuous, and sometimes so mild that its potential significance is easily overlooked. These patients may have subtle and intermittent visual blurring early in the illness (Figure 18-6). Systemic complaints including general malaise, myalgias, and arthralgias are common, frequently providing important diagnostic clues. Although often present, temporal artery tenderness may be relatively minor.

PRIMARY AND SECONDARY HEADACHE

Figure 18-6

Giant-Cell (Temporal) Arteritis, Polymyalgia Rheumatica

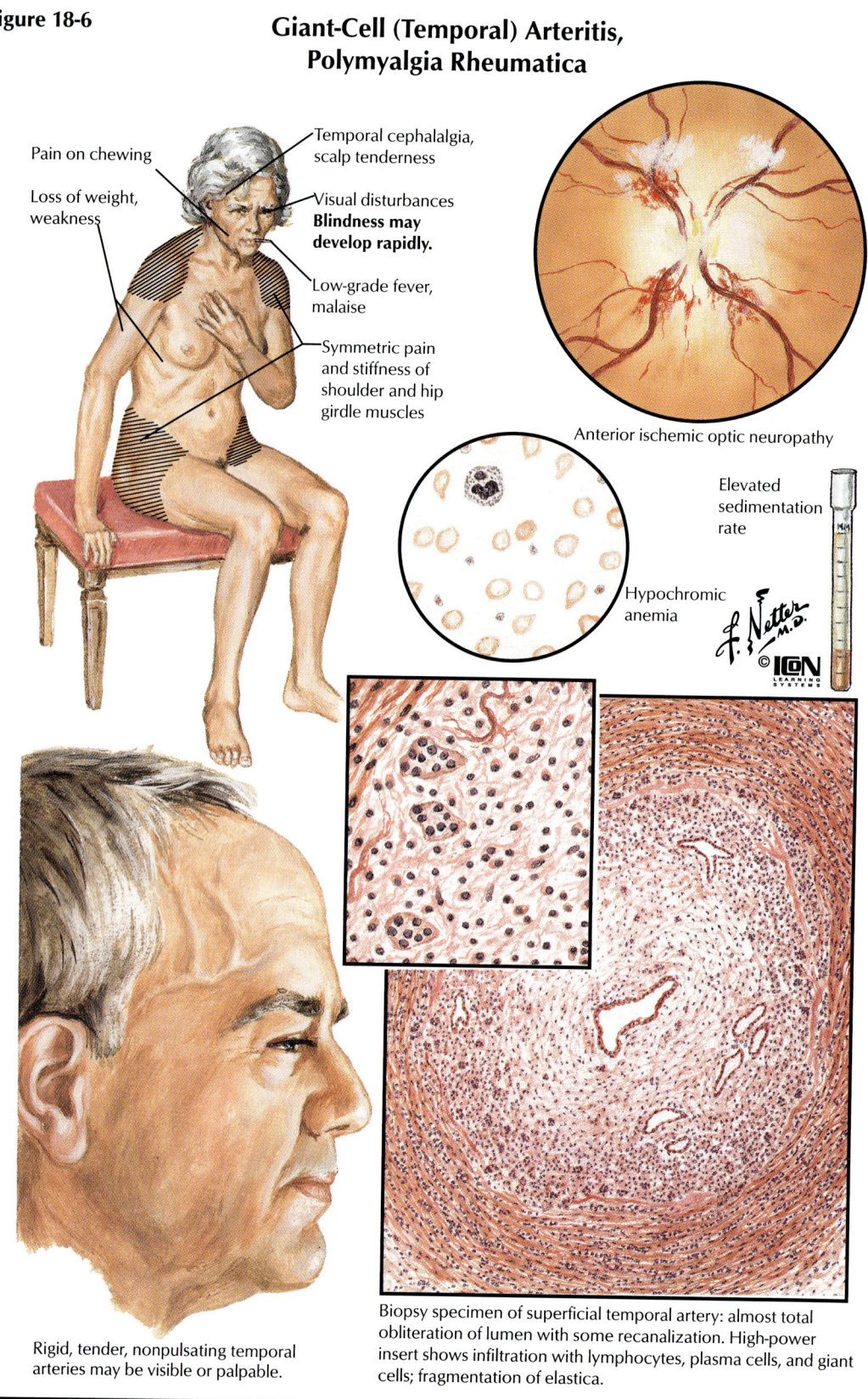

Biopsy specimen of superficial temporal artery: almost total obliteration of lumen with some recanalization. High-power insert shows infiltration with lymphocytes, plasma cells, and giant cells; fragmentation of elastica.

Early diagnosis is paramount because the arteritis may precipitously cause unilateral or bilateral permanent visual loss. Furthermore, the arteritis may be widespread with involvement beyond the temporal arteries to the extracerebral vertebral artery with an uncommon potential for posterior circulation stroke.

ESR and C-reactive protein evaluation provides the laboratory means supporting this potential diagnosis. Typically, the ESR is significantly increased to 60 to 110 mm/h, although there are rare exceptions. Biopsy of a long temporal artery segment is indicated in every patient suspected of having temporal arteritis. Because temporal arteritis is a chronic disorder, it requires relatively long-term corticosteroid treatment. Prompt diagnosis and treatment initiation are required to prevent serious complications. Treatment must not be delayed by the biopsy. Corticosteroid treatment does not alter the pathologic findings if the biopsy is performed within a few days of therapy initiation. The usual treatment of giant cell arteritis is oral corticosteroids. The initial dose is 40 to 60 mg/d prednisone, continued for 1 to 2 years at smaller doses.

Brain Hemorrhage, Infections, and Tumors

Subdural, intracerebral hematoma; subarachnoid hemorrhage; meningitis; and brain tumors are important causes of secondary headaches. Each of these entities needs consideration in patients who experience the recent onset of a new, different type, or changing pattern of headaches. Each of these important disorders is discussed elsewhere in this text; however, a few comments are warranted here.

Every individual who has a precipitous onset of **"the worst headache of my life"** warrants a careful evaluation in the ED, or the neurologist's or primary care physician's office. A careful general evaluation is essential, including whether the patient is febrile. A neurologic examination should evaluate mental status, language function, muscle stretch reflexes, and plantar stimulation for Babinski signs and should search for signs of meningismus, pupillary changes, or extraocular muscle palsies. A careful funduscopic examination should evaluate for increased intracranial pressure, papilledema, or subhyaloid hemorrhages. Regardless of the findings, emergency imaging is also needed: CT, possibly with MRI or MRA if there is concern about hemorrhage. If these are normal and no evidence of a mass lesion exists, a CSF analysis is indicated to check for a subarachnoid hemorrhage or signs of an infectious process (chapters 24, 63, and 64).

Idiopathic Intracranial Hypertension (Pseudotumor Cerebri)

Considered a nonspecific headache syndrome, pseudotumor cerebri is usually associated with diplopia, papilledema, and an associated otherwise benign increased intracranial CSF pressure. Typical patients are young, morbidly obese, otherwise healthy women. Neuroimaging studies are mandatory to exclude the other possible causes of increased intracranial pressure (chapter 71).

Low CSF Pressure Headache

Clinical Vignette

A vigorous, healthy, 61-year-old physician noted the onset of progressively severe headaches over a 3-week period. These were precipitated by going down stairs, straining, and sneezing and were particularly excruciating while landing on a lake in a float plane. This jarring produced such severe pressurelike headaches each time the plane bounced on the water surface that this gentleman chose to seek further diagnostic evaluation. Until then, he had ignored the initial headaches because he was in otherwise excellent health. His neurologic examination was normal despite his severe pain each time he bent forward.

The results of initial MRI studies were unremarkable; however, there was marked leptomeningeal enhancement after the administration of gadolinium. CSF demonstrated RBCs and WBCs with a slightly increased protein level. Cytology results were normal. The results of intracerebral and cervical MRA studies were normal.

The headache that occurs subsequent to a lumbar puncture for CSF analysis or spinal anesthesia is the classic example of a low CSF pressure headache. Occasionally, a similar headache occurs subsequent to a closed head injury such as walking into a low doorway or from a contact-sport injury. Typically, the patient does not immediately associate the onset of the pain with the previous trauma. Therefore, this history is not recalled until detailed inquiry by the suspicious physician based on headache characteristics.

Typically, these headaches develop soon after the spinal tap, although they may be less precipitous after an injury. Generally, they occur during the waking hours and worsen when the patient assumes the upright posture, clearing almost completely with recumbence. Often, the headache is associated with nausea, vomiting, and neck pain, which all clear on recumbence. Usually, the headache subsides with bed rest in a few days, but it can persist. A **blood patch** injected at the lumbar puncture site, sealing the leak, almost universally improves post–lumbar puncture headaches, providing credence to the theory that they are secondary to a CSF leak. Although leptomeningeal enhancement is classically seen with either a malignancy or infectious infiltration, the relatively smooth characteristics of the findings in the preceding vignette were typical for a benign dural leak. A diagnosis of presumed traumatic leptomeningeal tear with CSF leak and subsequent low-pressure syndrome was made. A therapeutic trial of an autologous blood dural patch was successful, with relief of all symptoms within 1 week.

The chronic type of low CSF pressure headache usually has a less obvious and ill-defined initiating event. Operative spinal procedures, a Valsalva test, or even coughing are known to precipitate this condition. Unfortunately, many of the provoking events seem minor to the patient and are forgotten.

MRI with gadolinium demonstrates diffuse pachymeningeal enhancement in most low CSF pressure headaches. This can be striking and may be confused with leptomeningeal inflammatory or neoplastic processes. Bed rest is the initial treatment. Caffeine may help. A search for a CSF leak and its specific treatment is sometimes necessary. Sometimes, a blood patch in the lumbar spine can provide relief in these individuals, despite no identifiable source. Occasionally, such headaches are resistant to therapy and become disabling.

Cranial Neuralgias

This group of patients experience brief but exceedingly severe paroxysms of head pain in the distribution of a specific cranial nerve, particularly the trigeminal.

Trigeminal Neuralgia

Clinical Vignette

A 48-year-old woman developed electrical shock-like attacks of intense pain in the left cheek. They usually came without warning but were often precipitated by talking, chewing, or washing her face or applying lipstick to the left upper lip. Between the attacks, she was free of pain. Neurologic examination was normal. Treatment with 600 mg/d carbamazepine was initiated. This initially helped; however, a relapse of pain required increasing dosages to 1000 mg/d. Although her pain was now controlled, she became lethargic and forgetful with these higher medication levels.

A neurosurgeon was consulted, and microvascular decompression was advised. At craniotomy, an ectatic loop of the superior cerebellar artery was found markedly compressing the trigeminal posterior root. The artery was gently displaced from the vicinity of the nerve and a cushion of Teflon placed between the artery and the nerve. Postoperatively, she experienced significant relief, stopped carbamazepine, and regained her former quality of life.

Five years later, her pain recurred. Although initially mild, it again became severe. After neurosurgical consultation, a percutaneous radiofrequency lesion was performed. This provided pain relief with an accompanying mild sensory loss in the left cheek and lips. Her lasting relief of pain was extremely welcome.

A careful history is the key to the diagnosis of this uncommon but eminently treatable facial neuralgia. Trigeminal neuralgia, also called *tic douloureux*, is a disabling, lancinating, or electrical-like facial pain that occurs in the trigeminal nerve distribution (Figure 18-7). It is one of the worst pains humans experience. This condition is not defined by any test, requires that the clinician recognize the entity, and is diagnosed by its primary historical attributes. The patient, almost always an adult and often a senior citizen, experiences paroxysmal and frequently provokable intermittent unilateral pain that rarely occurs during sleep. It primarily involves the second or third divisions of the trigeminal nerve and occasionally the first division. Characteristically, it is provoked by talking, chewing, shaving, drinking hot or cold liquids, or any form of sensory facial stimulation. The pain is invariably unilateral; when it affects both sides of the face, it does not do so concomitantly.

In perhaps the majority of individuals, an idiopathic loss of myelin insulation within the poste-

PRIMARY AND SECONDARY HEADACHE

Figure 18-7   **Cutaneous Nerves of Head and Neck**

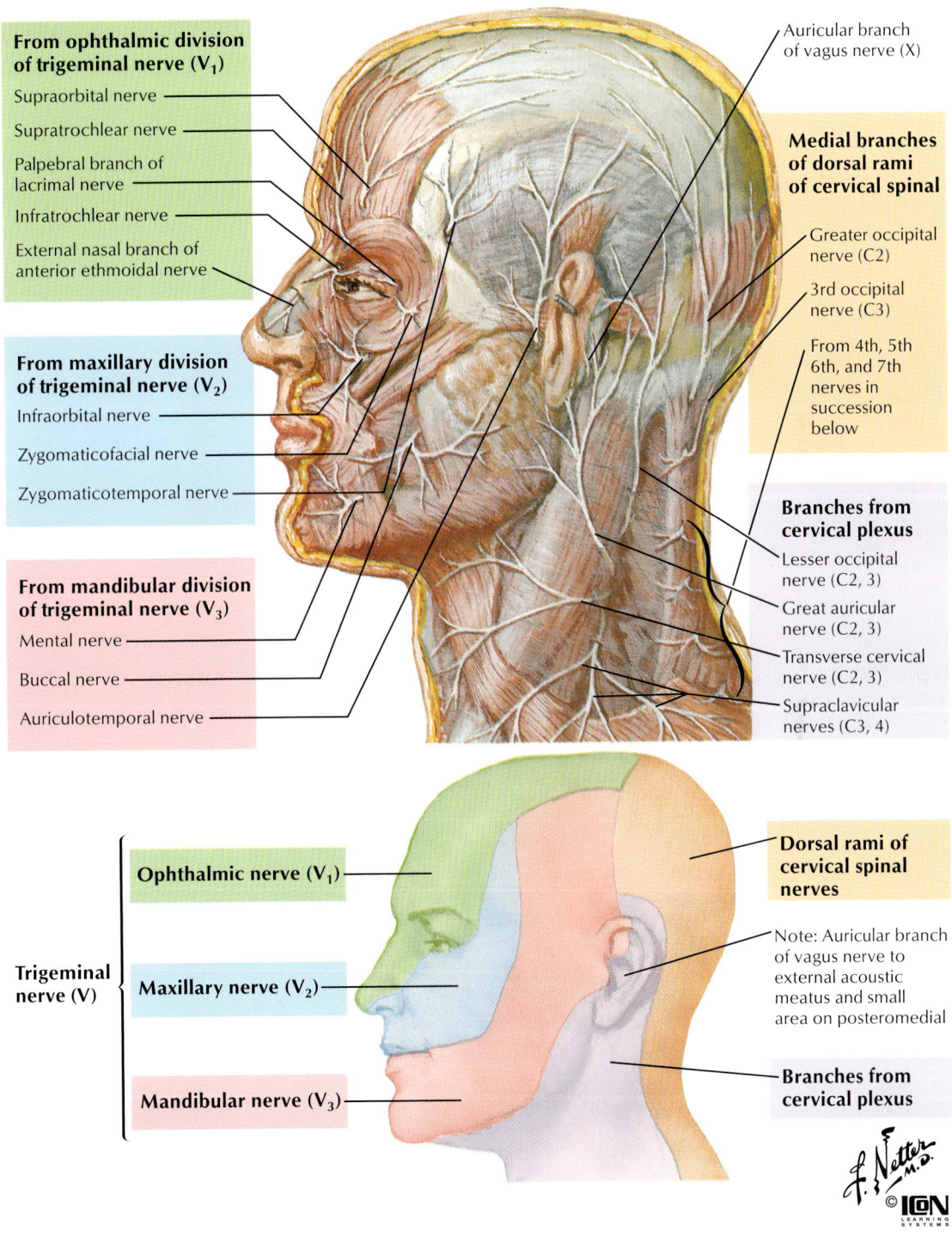

HEADACHE

183

PRIMARY AND SECONDARY HEADACHE

Figure 18-8

Suboccipital Triangle

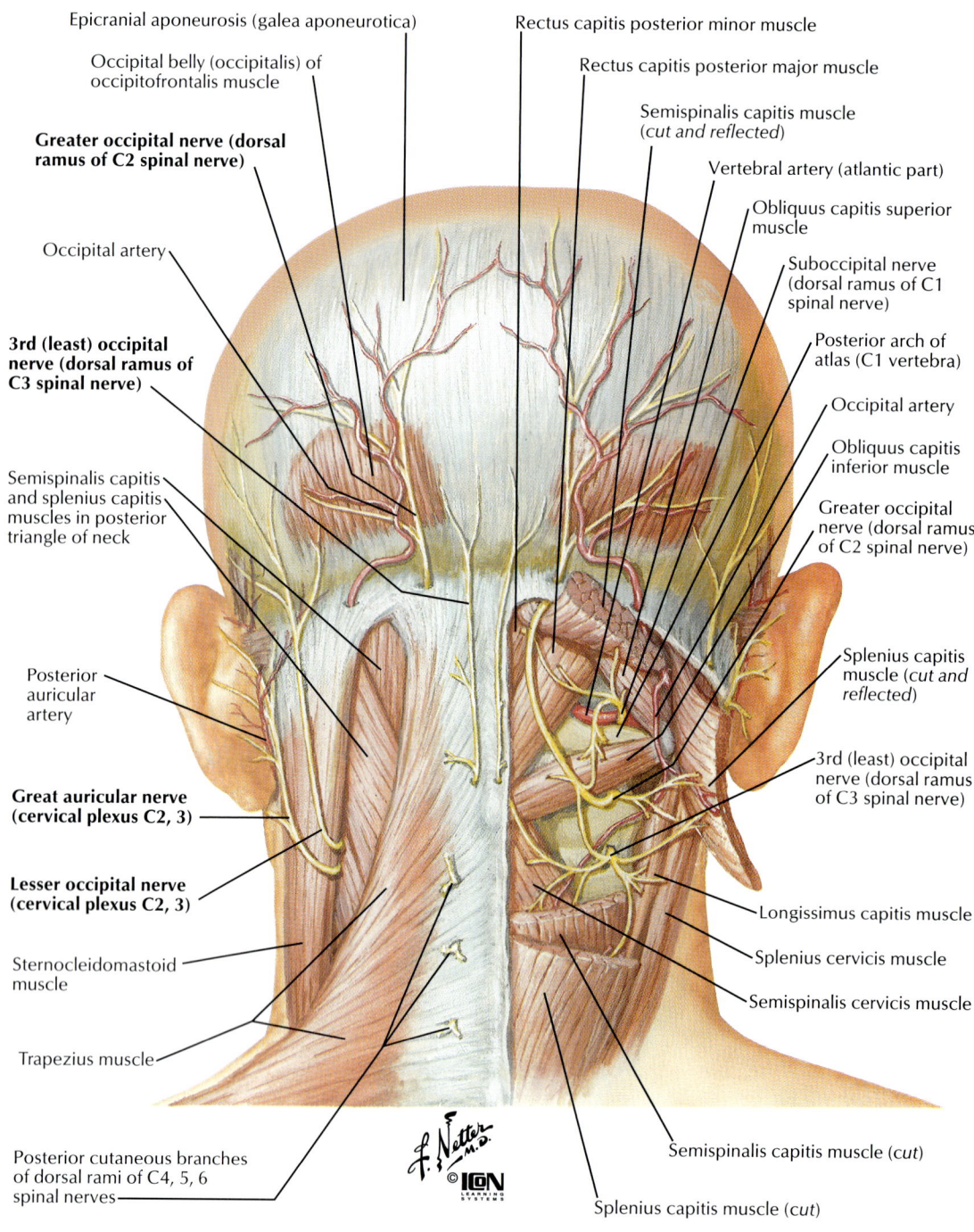

HEADACHE

184

rior root of the trigeminal nerve causes the pain. When it occurs in a young adult, the primary demyelination of multiple sclerosis is often the mechanism. Another cause is an artery that has lengthened during adult life and become tortuous. An ectatic loop of such an artery, usually a branch of the superior cerebellar artery, compresses the trigeminal posterior root causing the pain. Rarely, trigeminal neuralgia results from other conditions causing pressure on the trigeminal nerve, including acoustic neuroma, meningioma, arteriovenous malformation, or an aneurysm pressing on the trigeminal posterior root. These various etiologies suggest that external pressure on the root or a primary or secondary form of demyelination (eg, multiple sclerosis) may cause trigeminal neuralgia. Mass lesions of the gasserian (trigeminal) ganglion need to be excluded via MRI.

Several treatments are available. Most patients respond initially to the use of carbamazepine, which stabilizes cell membranes and raises the threshold of neural stimulation. Phenytoin, gabapentin, oxcarbazepine, and baclofen may be useful. In many individuals, adverse effects of these therapies—lethargy, loss of mental acuity, drowsiness, hematologic effects and others—are troublesome. Several surgical approaches are available for patients who cannot tolerate medical therapy: trigeminal radiofrequency lesioning by percutaneous electrode technique, microvascular decompression in the posterior cranial fossa (which can often relieve the tic pain with less sensory loss than that of the radiofrequency lesion), open trigeminal rhizotomy in the posterior cranial fossa, and a form of focused beam radiation by gamma knife therapy.

Trigeminal neuralgia can recur after any procedure and does so at a lifetime rate of 15% to 20%. Recurrences can be treated with further or subsequent radiofrequency ablation. An ipsilateral hearing loss is the occasional adverse effect of the decompressive surgery, relating to the delicate anatomic relationship between the auditory and trigeminal nerves. The operation carries a 1% risk of death or stroke.

Accurate diagnosis is essential to successful surgical relief. Steady pain, posttraumatic pain, pain after dental procedures, and pain that is not in the trigeminal zone, including pain over the top of the head, on the side of the neck, and behind the ear are not trigeminal neuralgia and will not be effectively treated by these procedures. Knowledge of the anatomy of the trigeminal nerve and its facial distribution and an appreciation of the paroxysmal, provokable, and unilateral character of trigeminal neuralgia is essential for accurate diagnosis and initiation of therapy.

Glossopharyngeal Neuralgia

Unlike trigeminal neuralgia, glossopharyngeal neuralgia is rare. The pain is paroxysmal, recurrent, severe, and generally located in the tonsillar area, deep within the throat in the sensory distribution of CN-IX. Swallowing is usually the primary triggering mechanism. Occasionally, patients experience bradycardia during the pain paroxysms, sometimes causing loss of consciousness. Medical treatment is similar to that for trigeminal neuralgia. Rhizotomy or decompression of CN-IX may be necessary in severe, medically intractable cases.

Occipital Neuralgia

Occipital neuralgia is the least common of the cranial neuralgias. Similar in pain characteristics to trigeminal neuralgia, it is differentiated by location to the unilateral posterior scalp innervated by the second cervical dermatome (C2) (Figure 18-8).

Infectious Mechanisms

Meningitis is an infectious disease process that must be considered in anyone having an acute-onset headache. Typically, these individuals have a concomitant fever and stiff neck (meningismus) as detailed in chapter 63.

Herpes zoster (shingles) is a viral process that is a "reactivation" of the virus within the gasserian ganglion. It is a relatively rare etiology for an acute-onset severe headache. Typically, these patients report a severe, sometimes excruciating, boring head pain or neuralgia. Usually, the rash precedes the onset of the headache, but, in other instances, intense head pain can antedate the skin lesions by a few days. The classic vesicles can sometimes vary from very few easily overlooked lesions to an extensive vesicular rash. After the dermatologic changes appear, treatment with acyclovir is needed. There is an increased incidence in patients who are immunosuppressed, those with AIDS or receiving immunosuppressive medications, and those with underlying neoplasms, particularly lymphoma.

Contiguous Structure Headaches

The last group of head pain etiologies is not secondary to inherent brain, vascular, and leptomeningeal structures as discussed in the sections on tumors, stroke, or neuralgias. Contiguous anatomical structures such as the nasal sinuses or teeth may be responsible.

Nasal Sinus Infection

Often, a patient with headache presents with a self-diagnosis of "sinus headaches." This entity must be considered in each patient presenting with headache. Most "sinus headaches" represent a variety of tension headache.

The typical patient with active nasal sinus infection experiences a deep boring discomfort in the maxillary or ethmoid facial region, or both. With acute infections, there is often percussion tenderness, a purulent nasal discharge, and, if the infection is severe, fever. In contrast, sphenoid sinus infection is more easily masked, presenting with only a deep-seated headache, and poses the greatest risk for a parameningeal focus to later provide a source for bacterial meningitis. Diagnosis depends on CT, MRI, or both. Appropriate antibiotic treatment is usually effective.

Dental Infection

An abscessed tooth, primarily in the upper jaw, is a relatively common cause of facial and head pain. Although the diagnosis is usually obvious to patients, on occasion they may not initially seek a dental opinion but come to a physician first. Sometimes, the evaluation by the dentist does not uncover the diseased tooth. Therefore, the neurologist must consider a primary dental source as an unusual cause for some instances of head and facial pain. A careful dental evaluation may be diagnostic when no other mechanism is identified by the neurologic physician.

REFERENCES

Cady R, Dodick DW. Diagnosis and treatment of migraine. *Mayo Clin Proc.* 2002;77:266-261.

Headache Classification Committee of the International Headache Society. Classification and diagnostic criteria for headache disorders, cranial neuralgia, and facial pain. *Cephalalgia.* 1988;8(suppl 7):1-96.

Olesen J, Tfelt-Hansen P, Welch KMA. *The Headaches.* 2nd ed. Philadelphia, Pa: Lippincott Williams & Wilkins; 2000.

Silberstein SD, Lipton RB, Dalessio DJ. *Wolff's Headache and Other Head Pain.* 7th ed. Oxford, England: Oxford University Press; 2001.

Section V
CEREBROVASCULAR DISORDERS

Chapter 19
Arterial Supply to the Brain and Meninges 188

Chapter 20
Ischemic Stroke 195

Chapter 21
Endarterectomy for Extracranial Carotid Artery Atherosclerosis 218

Chapter 22
Cerebral Venous Thrombosis 223

Chapter 23
Intracerebral Hemorrhage 234

Chapter 24
Cerebral Aneurysms and Subarachnoid Hemorrhage 248

Chapter 19
Arterial Supply to the Brain and Meninges

Aaron C. Heide and Claudia J. Chaves

THE CAROTID ARTERY SYSTEM

The brain and meninges are supplied by arteries derived from the common carotid artery (CCA) and vertebrobasilar system. The right CCA usually originates from the brachiocephalic trunk, while the left CCA originates directly from the aortic arch. Both vertebral arteries (VAs) originate from the subclavian arteries. The morphologic variants of the CCA and VAs usually are not clinically significant.

The CCA bifurcates at approximately the level of the sixth cervical vertebrae into the external and internal carotid arteries. The external carotid artery (ECA) supplies the neck, face, and scalp. The internal carotid artery (ICA) and its branches are mostly responsible for the arterial supply of the anterior two thirds of the brain (anterior circulation).

The vertebrobasilar and posterior cerebral arteries (PCAs) supply blood to the brainstem, cerebellum, occipital lobes, and posterior portions of the temporal and parietal lobes (posterior circulation) (Figure 19-1).

External Carotid Artery

At its origin, the ECA deviates anteriorly and medially in relation to the ICA in the neck, providing many branches to the neck (superior thyroid, ascending pharyngeal arteries) and face (lingual and facial arteries). As the artery ascends, occipital and posterior auricular branches supply the scalp in the occipital region and behind the ear, respectively. The occipital artery also has several meningeal branches that supply the meninges of the posterior fossa and dura. Within the substance of the parotid gland, the ECA divides into its 2 terminal branches: the superficial temporal and maxillary arteries.

The **superficial temporal artery** is the main supply to the scalp over the frontoparietal convexity and its underlying muscles. The more proximal branches also supply the masseter muscle. The superficial temporal artery is commonly involved in giant cell arteritis, an important consideration for headaches in the elderly because, if it goes untreated, it may lead to blindness (chapter 18).

The **maxillary artery** supplies the face and through its middle meningeal branch provides most of the blood supply to the dura mater covering the brain. The middle meningeal artery is often implicated in the formation of epidural hematomas in patients with skull fracture.

The ECA occasionally has an important role by supplying collateral flow in ICA occlusive disease. Variable anastomoses develop between its branches (facial, maxillary, and superficial temporal arteries) and the ophthalmic artery.

Internal Carotid Artery

There are 4 ICA segments: cervical, petrous, cavernous, and supraclinoid. The **cervical segment** ascends vertically in the neck, posterior and slightly medial to the ECA. Significant atherosclerotic disease is usually located at the ICA origin, with potential for artery-to-artery embolism, stenosis with eventual occlusion, or both. This segment does not have branches, unlike the ECA, allowing differentiation between those vessels on imaging scans.

The ICA enters the skull through the carotid canal within the petrous bone. This **petrous segment** ICA has 2 small branches, the caroticotympanic and pterygoid branches, which are usually clinically irrelevant.

The **cavernous segment**, usually called the *carotid siphon* because of its shape, is the portion of the ICA within the cavernous sinus. Of its many branches, the ophthalmic artery is the most significant. The **ophthalmic artery** arises

ARTERIAL SUPPLY TO THE BRAIN AND MENINGES

Figure 19-1   Arteries to Brain and Meninges

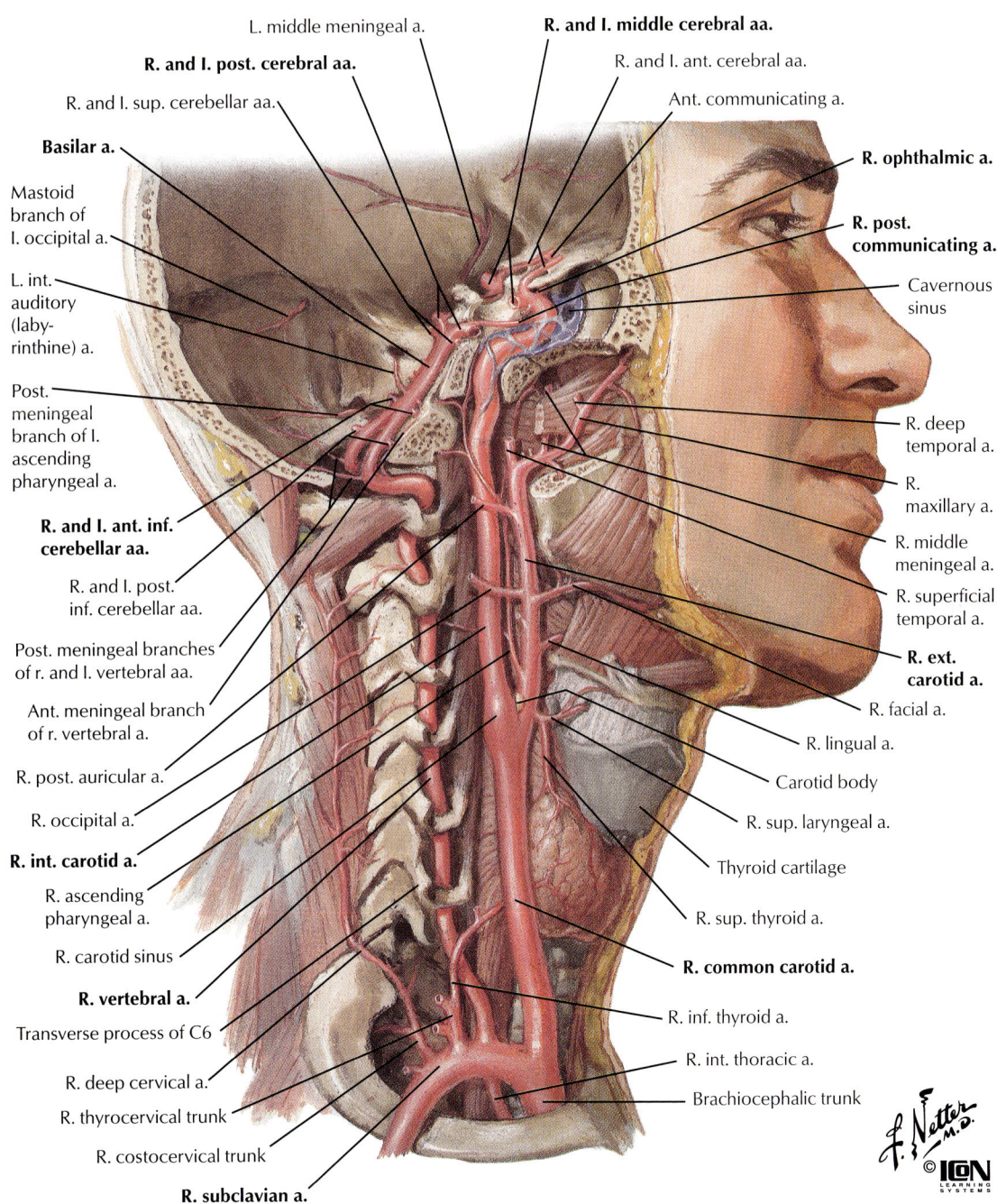

CEREBROVASCULAR DISORDERS

ARTERIAL SUPPLY TO THE BRAIN AND MENINGES

from the ICA just before it emerges from the cavernous sinus and passes through the optic canal into the orbit just below and lateral to the optic nerve. It supplies the globe and orbital contents through its 3 major branches: the ocular (**central retinal** and **ciliary arteries**), orbital, and extraorbital branches. The ophthalmic artery forms extensive anastomoses with branches of the ECA, which become an important source of collateral flow in ICA occlusive disease.

The supraclinoid segment is the last portion of the ICA. It begins when this segment penetrates the dura. The **posterior communicating artery** (P-com) and the **anterior choroidal artery** are the 2 important branches originating at this level. The ICA then bifurcates into the **anterior cerebral artery** (ACA) and **middle cerebral artery** (MCA).

The P-com is often hypoplastic. When present, it travels posteriorly to communicate with the posterior circulation at the level of the PCA. The P-com also provides the **thalamoperforate** branches that supply the anterior and medial thalamus, parts of the cerebral peduncles, and important collateral pathways in extensive vertebrobasilar disease or carotid artery occlusive lesions allowing collateral flow from the anterior to the posterior circulation or vice versa.

The **anterior choroidal artery** arises from the posterior surface of the ICA just above the P-com origin. This artery supplies an extensive cerebral area, including the visual system (optic tract, portions of the lateral geniculate body, optic radiations), genu and posterior limb of the internal capsule, basal ganglia (medial globus pallidus, tail of the caudate), the diencephalon (portions of the lateral thalamus and subthalamus), the midbrain (substantia nigra and portions of the cerebral peduncle), the medial temporal lobe (uncus, pyriform cortex, amygdala), and the choroidal plexus of the temporal horn and atrium.

The **ACA** travels medially and anteriorly toward the interhemispheric fissure. It supplies the anterior portions of the basal ganglia and internal capsule and most of the mesial portions of the frontal and parietal lobes.

The first segment of the ACA, the **A1 segment**, begins at the carotid bifurcation, terminating at the level of the **anterior communicating artery**, which connects both A1 segments and constitutes an important collateral pathway in carotid artery occlusive disease. It provides an opportunity for cross-flow from the opposite side toward the hypoperfused hemisphere. Occasionally, only a single A1 exists where one ICA supplies both ACAs, termed an *azygous* ACA. The **recurrent artery of Heubner** is the most important branch of the A1 segment, which supplies the anteroinferior portion of the head of the caudate nucleus, the putamen, and the anterior limb of the internal capsule.

The **ACA** continues as the A2 segment, where the **orbitofrontal branch** arises and travels around the genu of the corpus callosum to the orbital and medial surface of the frontal lobe, and the frontopolar branch supplies the rest of the medial surface of the frontal lobe. The ACA then gives off its 2 major branches, the pericallosal artery that runs just above the corpus callosum and the callosomarginal artery that outlines the cingulate gyrus. These 2 arteries supply the mesial portions of the frontal and parietal lobes.

One of the major fail-safe systems within the cerebral circulation is the circle of Willis, formed by the confluence of both ACAs, the anterior communicating artery, the cavernous carotid, the P-coms, and both PCAs. When a single vessel becomes significantly diseased even with total occlusion, ie, 1 cervical ICA, this vascular network sometimes provides a viable option for ongoing perfusion without development of a cerebral infarction. Each of these vessels, at their respective junctions and origins, are primary sites for the origin of a berry aneurysm, the major source for development of subarachnoid hemorrhage.

The **MCA** originates from the supraclinoid carotid stem and is a classic site for large-sized cerebral artery emboli to lodge, sometimes amenable to emergent intraarterial thrombolytic therapy. Subsequently, it travels laterally as the main-stem **M1 segment**, giving off **lenticulostriate** branches to the basal ganglia. As the MCA approaches the sylvian fissure, it usually divides into 2 large trunks, the superior and inferior divisions. Occasionally, the MCA trifurcates, and a middle trunk is also present. Different branches supply the **frontal** (orbitofrontal, ascending frontal, precentral, and central branches), **pari-**

etal (anterior and posterior parietal and angular branches), and **temporal** (anterior and posterior temporal) lobes. The orbitofrontal, ascending frontal, precentral, and central branches usually arise from the superior division of the MCA, while the angular, anterior, and posterior temporal branches arise from the inferior division. The anterior and posterior parietal branches can arise from either division (Figures 19-2).

VERTEBROBASILAR ARTERIES

The VAs originate from the subclavian arteries (Figure 19-2). They have 2 portions, extracranial and intracranial. After their origin, the **extracranial VAs** travel posteriorly and enter the transverse foramen of the cervical vertebrae, usually through C6 and extending superiorly to C1. This area is the most likely site of VA dissection. At the atlas, the VAs turn sharply posteriorly before traveling rostrally, piercing the posterior atlanto-occipital membrane and dura mater to enter the intracranial cavity through the foramen magnum; this segment is occasionally affected by temporal arteritis.

The **intracranial VAs** course anteriorly, first lateral to the medulla, then ventral to the hypoglossal nerve to the midline base of the brainstem. At the pontomedullary junction, the confluence of the 2 VAs forms the **basilar artery** (Figure 19-3).

The **lateral medullary** branches, **posterior-inferior cerebellar arteries**, and **anterior** and **posterior spinal arteries** are the most important VA branches. The medullary arteries supply the lateral portions of the medulla. The posterior-inferior cerebellar arteries primarily supply the posterior and inferior regions of the cerebellum but also a small portion of most of the dorsum of the medulla. It is the most common site for embolic occlusion within this group of vessels, resulting in classic Wallenberg syndrome.

The **anterior spinal artery** is often a single vessel running the full length of the spinal cord in the anteromedial sulcus. It also supplies the medial portions of the medulla; however, adequate collateral circulation in this anatomic substrate must exist, because primary clinically apparent medial medullary infarction is rare. In contrast, the anterior spinal artery within the cord is crucial to spinal cord function; its occlusion leads to the anterior spinal artery syndrome. The **posterior spinal arteries** arise from the posterior-inferior cerebellar arteries or intracranial VAs and run downward along the posterior and lateral aspect of the spinal cord, supplying these cord areas.

Often, asymmetry between VAs is seen, with deviation of the basilar artery toward the hypoplastic side. The **basilar artery** courses rostrally on the anterior surface of the pons, and along the clivus. It is particularly prone to atherosclerotic deposition throughout its length, which, at its extreme can cause formation of a fusiform aneurysm. When the basilar artery reaches the level of the cerebral peduncles, it terminates by dividing into the 2 PCAs. At this site, the basilar is most likely to be occluded by an embolus leading to the classic "top of the basilar" syndrome. Similarly, this is the most common site for berry aneurysms within the vertebrobasilar system.

The most important branches of the basilar artery are the **anterior inferior cerebellar arteries**, **superior cerebellar arteries** (SCAs), and the **paramedian arteries**. The anterior inferior cerebellar arteries usually arise from the midportion of the basilar artery and supply the brachium pontis, lateral pontine tegmentum, flocculus, and anteroinferior portions of the cerebellum. Often, the internal auditory artery arises from the anterior inferior cerebellar arteries and supplies the vestibular and cochlear structures. The SCAs arise from the distal portion of the basilar artery before it bifurcates into the PCAs. During their course around the midbrain, the SCAs provide branches that supply the superior lateral pontine tegmentum and the tectum of the midbrain. Then, the SCAs course toward the cerebellum, supplying the superior vermis and lateral portion of the cerebellar hemispheres. The SCA also irrigates most of the cerebellar nuclei and the majority of the cerebellar white matter.

The PCA supplies portions of the temporal, parietal, and occipital lobes; and the thalamus, midbrain, and other deep structures, including the choroid plexus and ependyma of the third and lateral ventricles.

CEREBRAL SINUSES AND VEINS

Surrounded by dura, cerebral sinuses and veins are the venous structures of the brain. They typically contain inpouchings of arachnoid cells,

ARTERIAL SUPPLY TO THE BRAIN AND MENINGES

Figure 19-2 **Arteries of Brain (Lateral and Medial Views)**

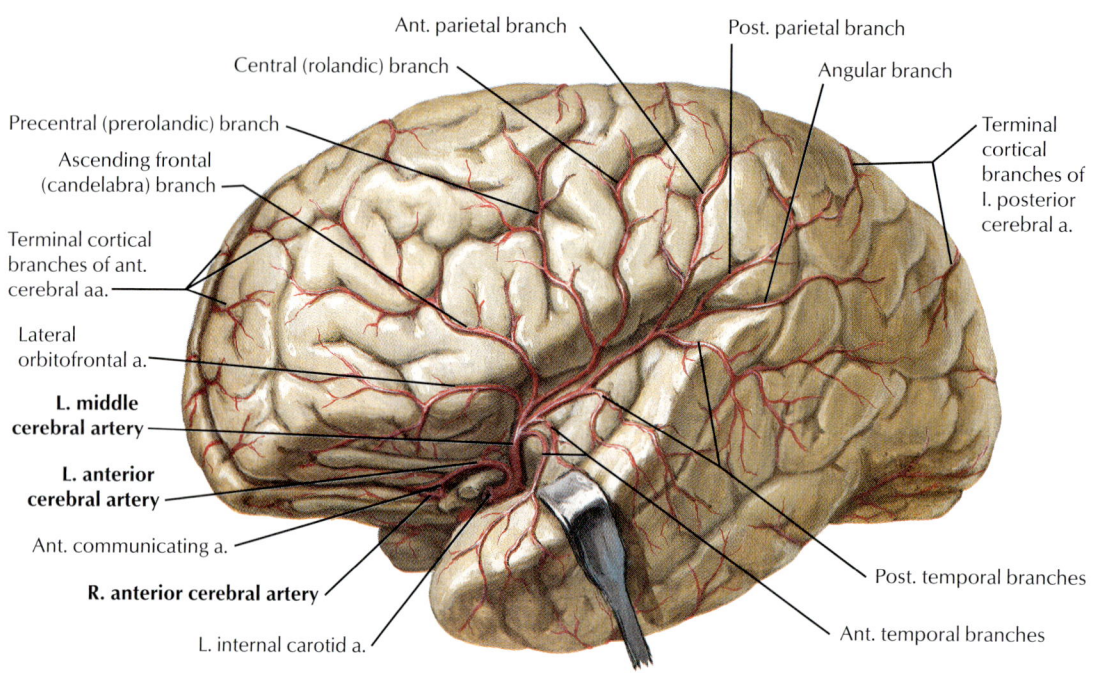

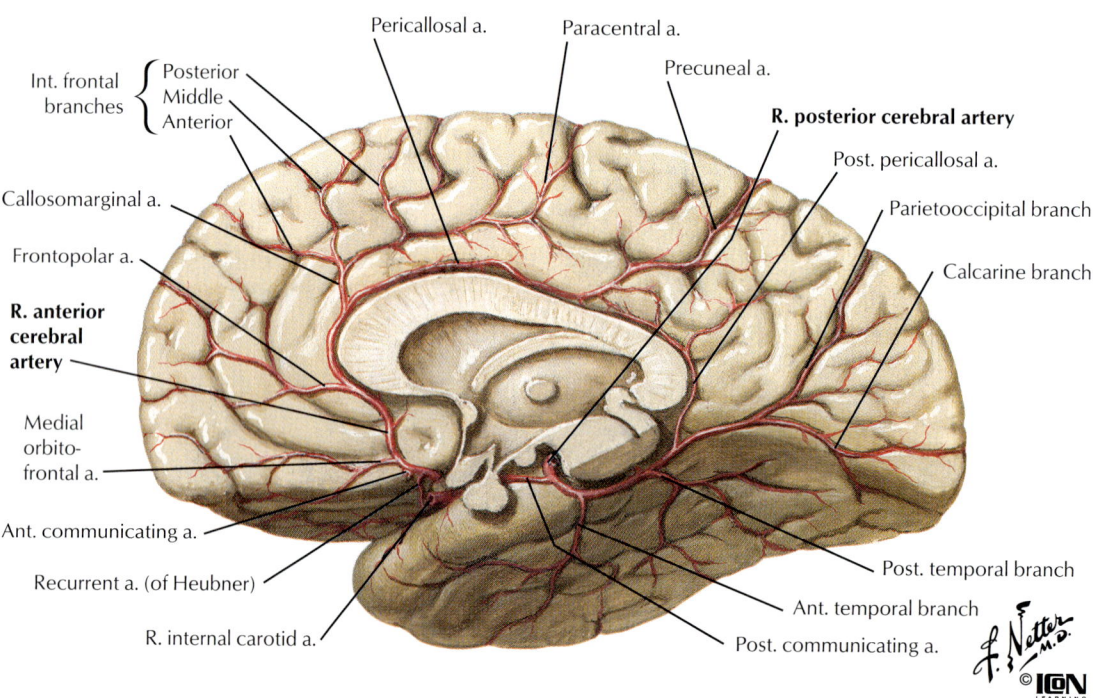

Cerebrovascular Disorders

ARTERIAL SUPPLY TO THE BRAIN AND MENINGES

Figure 19-3

Arteries of Brain: Inferior Views

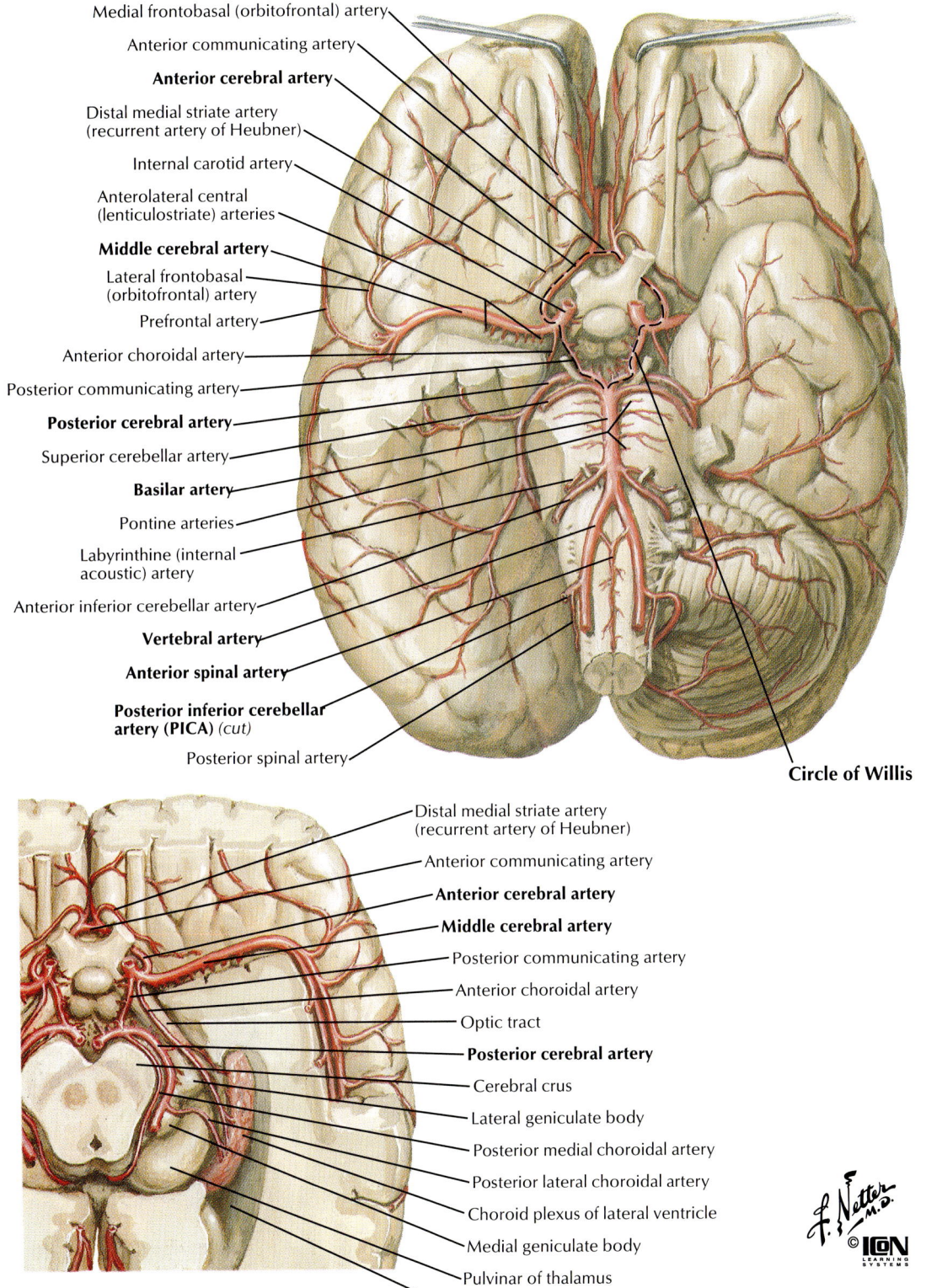

CEREBROVASCULAR DISORDERS

193

called *arachnoid granulations*, which allow CSF drainage. These granulations function as one-way valves and are pressure dependent. Malfunction of these valves can occur in subarachnoid hemorrhage or meningitis, leading to normal pressure hydrocephalus (chapter 58). The main venous sinuses include the **superior and inferior sagittal sinuses**, the **straight sinus**, the **transverse sinuses**, the **sigmoid sinuses**, the **occipital sinus**, the **cavernous sinuses**, the **superior and inferior petrosal sinuses**, and the **sphenoparietal sinuses**.

The superior sagittal sinus is located within the midline of the cerebral hemispheres surrounded by dura and tethered to the inner table of the skull via the pachymeninges. It runs posteriorly from the foramen cecum to the occipitocerebellar junction. The superior sagittal sinus drains the frontal and parietal lobes through the superior cerebral veins, the largest of which is the rolandic vein in the central sulcus. This sinus often drains into the right transverse sinus.

The inferior sagittal sinus parallels the corpus callosum, traveling in the inferior portion of the falx cerebri, draining the region of the medial hemispheres and cingulate gyrus. It drains into the straight sinus.

The straight sinus is formed by the intersection of the inferior sagittal sinus and the great vein of Galen. The vein of Galen drains many smaller venous channels including the choroidal, lateral ventricular, and thalamostriate veins and the basal vein of Rosenthal. These veins drain the choroid plexus, lateral ventricle, basal ganglia, thalamus, and medial temporal lobes. The straight sinus often drains into the left transverse sinus.

The transverse sinuses lie in the grooves of the occipital bone and run laterally and forward for a short distance before diving down to become the sigmoid sinuses. Each transverse sinus receives blood from the superior petrosal sinuses, mastoid and condyloid emissary veins, inferior cerebral and cerebellar veins, and diploic veins.

The sigmoid sinuses are the continuation of the transverse sinuses and end at the jugular foramina, becoming the internal jugular veins.

The cavernous sinus is an intricate venous channel interconnecting with its contralateral partner via intercavernous channels around the infundibulum. The cavernous sinus is important for the structures that it drains and for the structures that run through it. Laterally in the cavernous sinus wall are CN-III, -IV, and -V (V1 and V2 segments), and through its center runs the intracavernous portion of the ICA, sympathetic plexus, and CN-VI. The cavernous sinuses drain into paired superior and inferior petrosal sinuses that, in turn, drain into the transverse sinus and internal jugular vein, respectively.

The superior petrosal sinus connects the cavernous with the transverse sinus. It drains the tympanic cavity, cerebellum, and inferior portions of the cerebrum. The inferior petrosal sinus connects the cavernous sinus with the internal jugular vein and drains the inner ear, medulla, pons, and cerebellum.

The sphenopalatine sinuses lie below the lesser wings of the sphenoid bone and drain the dura mater into the cavernous sinuses.

REFERENCE

Netter FM. *The Netter Collection of Medical Illustrations.* Vol 1: *Nervous System.* Part 1: *Anatomy and Physiology.* Teterboro, NJ: Icon Learning Systems; 2001.

Chapter 20
Ischemic Stroke

Claudia J. Chaves and H. Royden Jones, Jr

Ischemic stroke is the third most frequent cause of mortality in the United States and a common cause of prolonged morbidity. Often considered a single entity, it represents a constellation of etiologies and mechanisms. New technology has improved understanding of stroke pathophysiology that may eventually translate into more specific treatment and better outcomes.

ETIOLOGY AND PATHOPHYSIOLOGY

The most common ischemic stroke etiologies are large artery occlusive disease, cardioembolism, and small vessel disease.

Large Artery Occlusive Disease

Atherosclerosis causes stenosis or occlusion of the extracranial and intracranial arteries and is directly responsible for a significant percentage of cerebral ischemic events. Atheroma formation involves the progressive deposition of fatty materials and fibrous tissue in the subintimal layer of the large and medium arteries, occurring most frequently at branching points (Figure 20-1). Intraplaque hemorrhage, subintimal necrosis with ulcer formation, and calcium deposition can cause enlargement of the atherosclerotic plaque with consequent worsening of the degree of arterial narrowing.

The disruption of the endothelial surface also triggers thrombus formation within the arterial lumen, due to the activation of nearby platelets by the subendothelial collagen. When the platelets become activated, they release thromboxane A_2, causing further platelet aggregation (Figure 20-2). The development of a fibrin network stabilizes the platelet aggregate, forming a "white thrombus." If the thrombus develops further, RBCs become enmeshed in the platelet-fibrin aggregate, forming a "red thrombus." Either the white or red thrombus can dislodge and embolize to distal arterial branches.

The most frequent sites for carotid system atherosclerosis are the origin of the internal carotid artery (ICA) and the carotid siphon at the base of the brain (Figure 20-3). The main stem of the middle cerebral artery (MCA) and ACA are less often affected than the ICA in the general population, although in Asian, Hispanic, and African-American populations, intracranial atherosclerosis is more common than carotid disease. In the vertebrobasilar system, the origins of the vertebral arteries in the neck and the distal portion of the intracranial vertebral arteries are the most commonly affected areas. The basilar artery and origins of the posterior cerebral arteries (PCAs) are other frequently affected sites.

The main risk factors for large artery disease are arterial hypertension, diabetes, hypercholesterolemia, and smoking. The role of high levels of homocysteine as a risk factor for large artery occlusive disease has been posited and is being investigated.

Large artery disease can cause ischemic strokes by 2 mechanisms: intra-arterial embolism and, less commonly, hemodynamic ischemia, causing hypoperfusion.

Cardiac Embolism

Several types of cardiac disease lead to cerebral embolism: cardiac arrhythmias, ischemic heart disease, valvular disease, dilated cardiomyopathies, atrial septal abnormalities, and intracardiac tumors (Figure 20-4A). Cardiac arrhythmias including chronic or paroxysmal atrial fibrillation (AF) and sick sinus syndrome (in particular bradytachycardia syndrome) are the most embologenic rhythms. Often, stroke is the first sign of AF. Because this arrhythmia is often intermittent, careful patient monitoring is needed to identify the presence of paroxysmal atrial fibrilla-

ISCHEMIC STROKE

Figure 20-1 — Atherosclerosis, Thrombosis, and Embolism

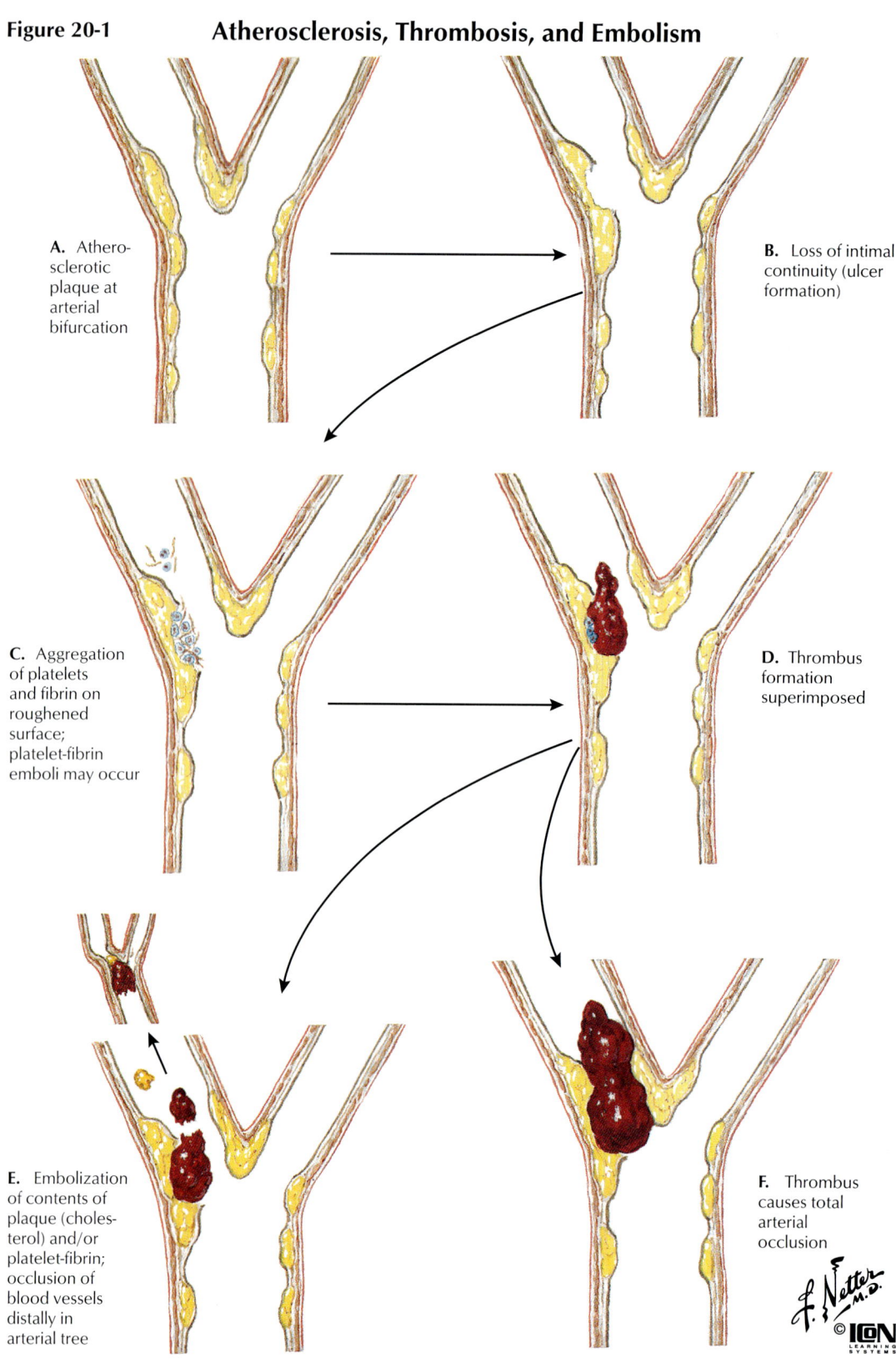

CEREBROVASCULAR DISORDERS

ISCHEMIC STROKE

Figure 20-2　　Role of Platelets in Arterial Thrombosis

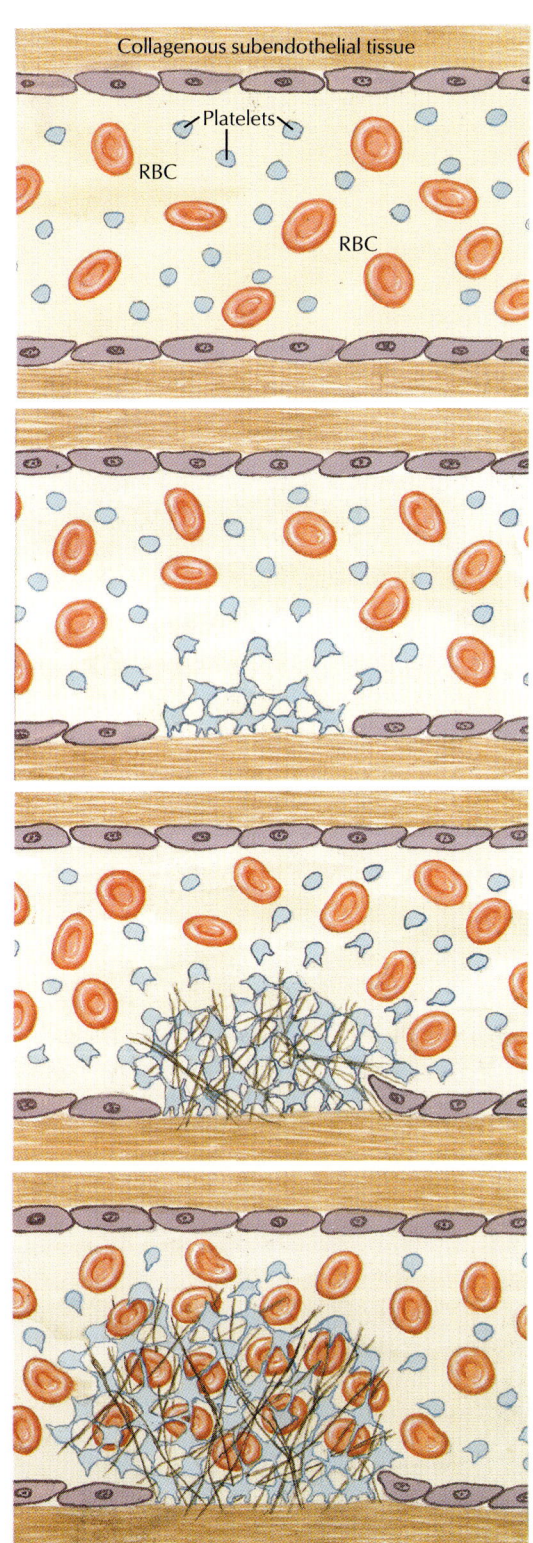

Platelets circulating in blood contain thromboxane A$_2$, a substance that promotes their aggregation, while vascular endothelium secretes prostacyclin, an aggregation inhibitor that balances this effect. These products are synthesized after conversion of arachidonic acid into intermediate endoperoxides by cyclooxygenase enzymes.

If endothelial continuity is interrupted by trauma, atherosclerosis, etc, subsurface collagen is exposed to blood and stimulates adhesion of platelets to vessel wall. Platelets then discharge thromboxane A$_2$, causing aggregation of adjacent platelets.

As more platelets aggregate, fibrin network develops and stabilizes mass into "white thrombus," which then retracts into vascular wall. In some cases, endothelium may later heal over with or without narrowing of lumen.

If thrombus develops further, red blood cells become enmeshed in platelet-fibrin aggregate to form "red thrombus," which may grow and block vessel lumen. Either platelet-fibrin aggregates or more fully formed clots may break off, with embolization into distal arterial branches.

CEREBROVASCULAR DISORDERS

197

ISCHEMIC STROKE

Figure 20-3
Extracranial Occlusive Disease of Vertebral and Subclavian Arteries

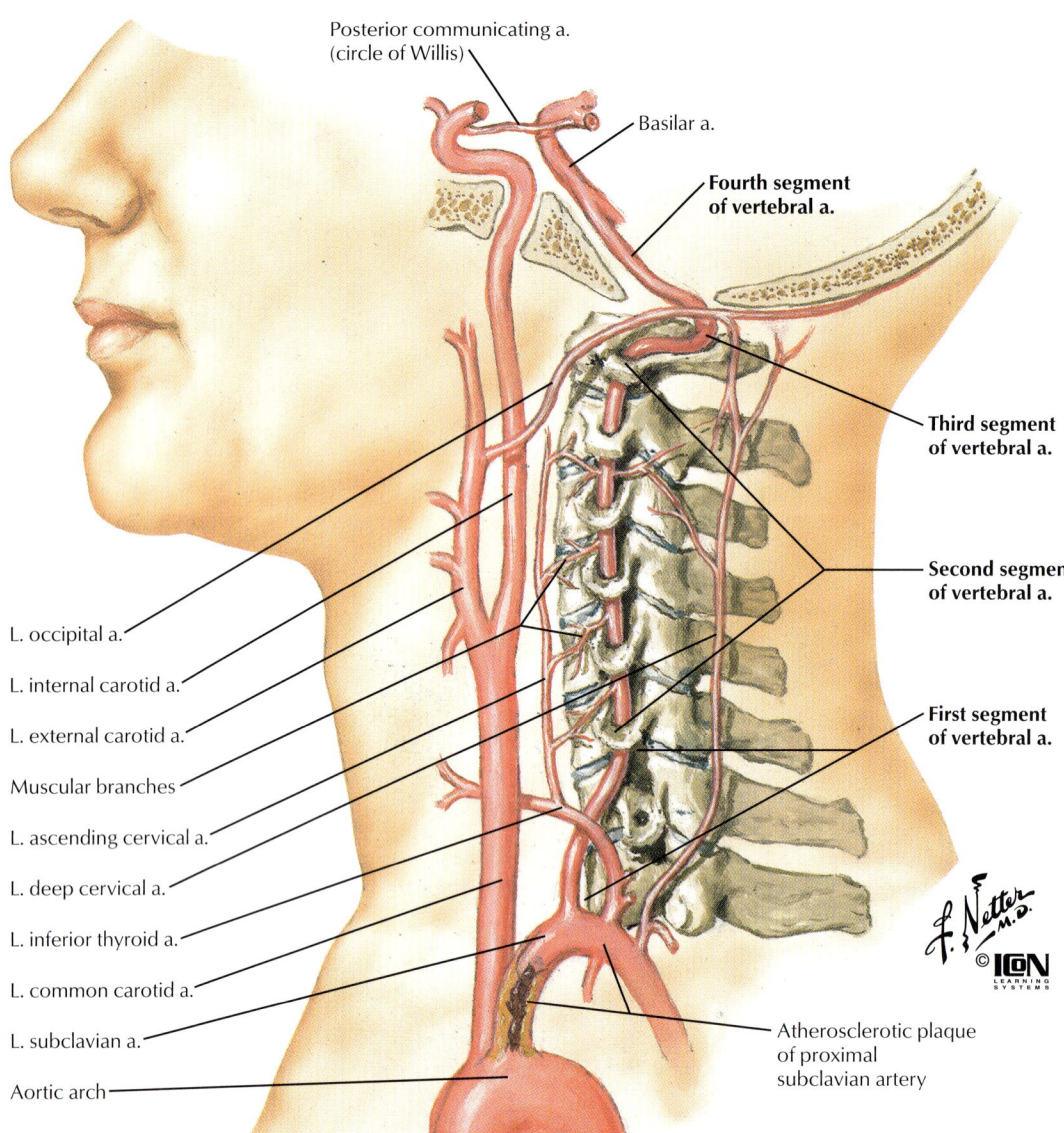

tion, which predisposes to a significant risk for another stroke.

Within the first 4 weeks of myocardial infarction (MI), particularly when ischemia involves the anterior heart wall, there is a higher risk of embolic stroke. More remote MIs can be a potential embologenic source, particularly in patients in whom akinetic segments or left ventricular aneurysm develops.

Rheumatic valvular disease, mechanical prosthetic heart valves, and infective endocarditis are well-known cardiac sources of embolism. Three other relatively common abnormalities, mitral valve prolapse, mitral annulus calcification, and bicuspid aortic valve have suspected embologenic potential. However, these diagnoses should be considered as potential causes of stroke only after other etiologies are excluded.

CEREBROVASCULAR DISORDERS

ISCHEMIC STROKE

Mural thrombi are common in patients with dilated cardiomyopathies. Brain embolism is estimated to occur in approximately 15% of these patients.

Patent foramen ovale (PFO) and atrial septal aneurysm are risk factors for stroke. A meta-analysis of case-control studies comparing younger patients (younger than 55 years) to ischemic stroke and nonstroke control patients showed an odds ratio for stroke of 3.1 for PFO and of 6.1 for atrial septal aneurysm. Potential mechanisms for stroke included paradoxical embolism, direct embolization from thrombi formed within the PFO or atrial septal aneurysm, and thrombus formation caused by atrial arrhythmias thought to be more prevalent in this population.

Atrial myxomas, although rare, are important causes of embolic strokes. These tumor emboli frequently affect the vasa vasorum leading to the development of multiple and peripheral cerebral aneurysms similar to mycotic aneurysms.

Small Vessel Disease (Lacunes)

Lipohyalinosis and fibrinoid necrosis affecting the small penetrating arteries are the anatomic substrate of small vessel disease. Occlusion of these arteries causes small (1-20 mm), discrete, and often irregular lesions called *lacunes* to develop. Lacunes occur most often in the basal ganglia, thalamus, pons, internal capsule, and cerebral white matter. Arterial hypertension and diabetes are the main risk factors.

Arterial Dissection

Dissection or tear within the extracranial ICA, particularly its pharyngeal and distal segments, or the extracranial vertebral artery, mainly in its first and third segments, are the 2 commonly affected vessels (Figure 20-3). Dissection occurring between the intima and media usually causes stenosis or occlusion of the affected artery, whereas dissection between the media and adventitia is associated with aneurysmal dilatation. Congenital abnormalities in the media or elastica of the arteries as seen in Marfan syndrome, fibromuscular dysplasia, and cystic medial necrosis can predispose patients to arterial dissection. Although often associated with acute trauma, arterial dissection may result from seemingly innocuous incidents, such as a fall while hiking or skiing, sports activities, particularly wrestling or diving into a wave, and paroxysms of coughing.

Less Common Stroke Etiologies (Figure 20-3A)

Although frequently considered in the differential diagnosis of ischemic stroke, arteritis is a rare stroke etiology. Usually, CNS vasculitis presents as an encephalopathy with multifocal signs.

Cocaine, amphetamine, and heroin are the most frequent drugs associated with ischemic strokes. Vasoconstriction and vasculitis are posited as the mechanisms.

Hematologic disorders such as polycythemia, sickle cell disease, and thrombocytosis (usually >1,000,000/dL) can cause ischemic strokes by increasing blood viscosity, coagulability, or both. Antithrombin III, protein S, protein C deficiencies, factor V Leiden, and prothrombin gene mutation are usually associated with venous and not arterial thrombosis.

CLINICAL PRESENTATION
Large Artery Occlusive Disease
Carotid Artery Disease

Clinical Vignette

A 58-year-old white man with history of hypercholesterolemia and 50-pack-year smoking presented with a 10-day history of 2 transient episodes affecting the right side of his body. While sitting, he felt that his right leg was numb and that it did not belong to him. This TIA lasted 10 minutes, after which he returned to normal. A week later, he had another episode of numbness and lack of control of the movements involving both his right arm and leg, which lasted for 1½ hours; soon thereafter, he played golf.

The patient came to the ED 3 days later. Brain MRI with diffusion-weighted imaging demonstrated 2 small strokes in the left frontal and parietal lobes. Head and neck MRA was remarkable for a 70% to 80% stenosis on the left ICA, confirmed by carotid ultrasound. Heparin was administered on admission. A right carotid artery endarterectomy was successful; the TIAs ceased.

Clinical Vignette

A 65-year-old white man with history of arterial hypertension, high cholesterol, and a 65-pack-year smoking history presented with a 1-month history of recur-

ISCHEMIC STROKE

rent 1- to 2-minute episodes of shaking of his left extremities that occurred only on standing. His BP was 110/80 mm Hg, and neurologic examination results showed a left pronator drift but were otherwise normal.

Head CT showed small strokes in the border zone territory between the right MCA and ACA and right MCA and PCA. Head and neck computed tomography angiography (CTA) demonstrated a right ICA occlusion. Computed tomography perfusion showed hypoperfusion in the right MCA territory, worse in the border zone areas. Collateral flow through the right ophthalmic, anterior communicating, and posterior communicating arteries was detected by transcranial Doppler and conventional angiogram. His antihypertensive medication dose was decreased, with a consequent increase in systolic BP to 140 to 150 mm Hg. No further episodes occurred.

Large artery ICA disease predisposes to TIAs, strokes, or both by 2 mechanisms: intra-arterial embolism (the first vignette) and hypoperfusion (the second vignette). Identification of the exact mechanism has important therapeutic implications.

TIAs are common in patients with carotid artery disease and usually precede stroke onset by a few days or months. TIAs caused by intra-arterial embolism from a carotid source may not be stereotypical. TIA symptoms vary, depending on which ICA branch is involved. For example, patients can have a transient expressive aphasia, sometimes with weakness of the right hand and mouth in one episode, or the latter in isolation, only to experience right leg weakness with another event. This depends on whether the MCA is the destination in the first example or the ACA territory is the destination of the emboli in the latter (Figure 20-4, part a). In contrast, hemodynamic TIAs are often stereotypical and posturally related and are usually seen in patients with tight ICA stenosis or occlusion. "Limb-shaking" TIA is a classic example of a hemodynamic TIA. In this condition, patients present with recurrent, irregular, and involuntary movements of the contralateral arm, leg, or both, usually triggered by postural changes and lasting a few minutes. These differ from a focal seizure, where the movements are more regular and rhythmic.

An important clue of ICA disease is an episode of transient monocular blindness (TMB) (Figure 20-4, part a). *TMB* refers to the occurrence of temporary unilateral visual loss that is often classically described by careful observers as a "shade descending over one eye," but most frequently as a "fog" or "blur" in one eye, lasting 1 to 5 minutes. It often occurs spontaneously but sometimes is triggered by position changes. Positive phenomena such as sparkles, lights, or colors are typical of migrainous events and help to differentiate benign visual changes, ie, migraine equivalents, from the more serious TMB, which may be a precursor of a cerebral infarct within the carotid artery vasculature, ie, the MCA or the ACA. Rarely, with critical ipsilateral internal carotid stenosis, patients report spontaneous loss of vision when they step outside on a bright day, such as with snow on a sunlit background. Temporal arteritis must be considered in the differential diagnosis of TMB.

Frequently, patients cannot precisely describe whether they lost vision in one eye because they have not known to cover the unaffected eye during the event. If they do cover the unaffected eye, individuals with a carotid artery source TMB are unable to see when the normal eye is covered, because the affected artery is totally non-operational during the ischemia. In contrast, patients partially lose vision in both eyes with a vertebral basilar system embolus to one of the PCAs because of homonymous hemianopsia, ie, if there is a right homonymous field deficit, the patient may inadvertently say they have lost right-sided vision, and it is not until they perform the cover test of the "unaffected" left eye that they realize the seemingly abnormal right eye has retained vision within the distribution of the unaffected left homonymous field (Figure 20-4, part b).

As in the first vignette, strokes from intra-arterial embolism from ICA disease are usually cortically based. Symptoms depend on whether branches of the MCA, ACA, or both are involved. PCA territory may rarely be affected by intra-arterial emboli from ipsilateral ICA stenosis or occlusion when patients have a persistent fetal PCA.

Hemodynamic strokes, like the one in the second vignette, usually involve the border zone territory between ACA and MCA (anterior border zone), MCA and PCA (posterior border zone), or between deep and superficial perforators (subcortical border zone) causing typical clinical symptoms (Table 20-1).

ISCHEMIC STROKE

Figure 20-4 Ocular Signs of Large Vessel Disease

Ocular Signs of Carotid Artery Ischemia (Transient Monocular Blindness [TMB])

Other Causes of Transient Monocular Blindness

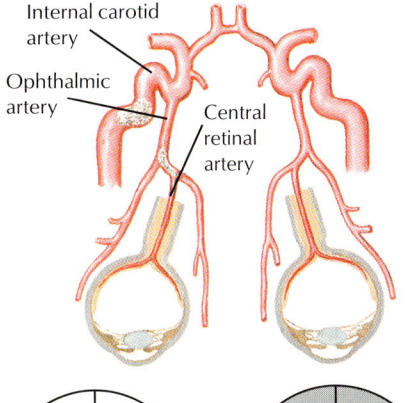
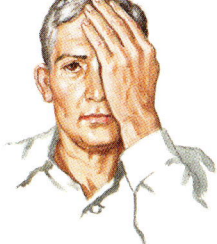
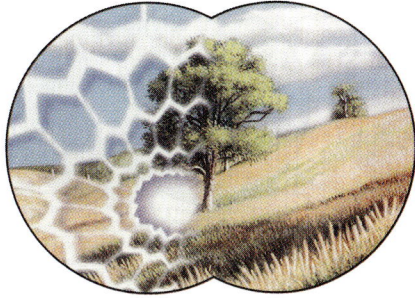

Covering one eye may reveal unsuspected monocular vision loss

Typical scintillating scotoma helps to diagnose TMB due to migraine.

Erythrocyte sedimentation rate should be obtained to rule out TMB due to temporal arteritis.

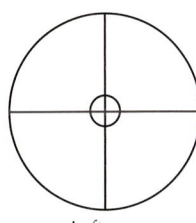
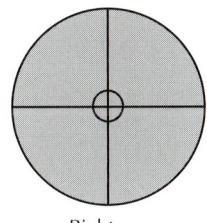

Left eye — Right eye

Episodes generally transient (3-5 min). Visual fields during episode show monocular decreased vision.

Ocular Signs Due to Posterior Cerebral Artery Ischemia
Temporal lobe

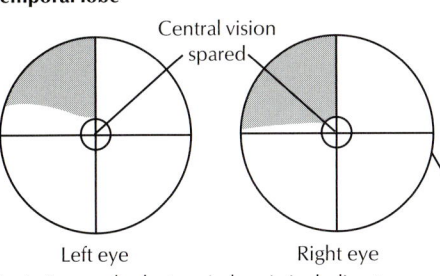

Central vision spared

Left eye — Right eye

Posterior cerebral artery ischemia including temporal lobe optic radiations often presents as a homonymous quadrantanopia.

Occipital lobe

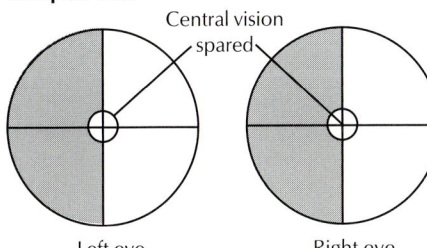

Central vision spared

Left eye — Right eye

Posterior cerebral artery ischemia involving occipital lobe may present as a homonymous hemianopia, which patient may interpret as "poor vision" in eye oppsite ischemic lobe.

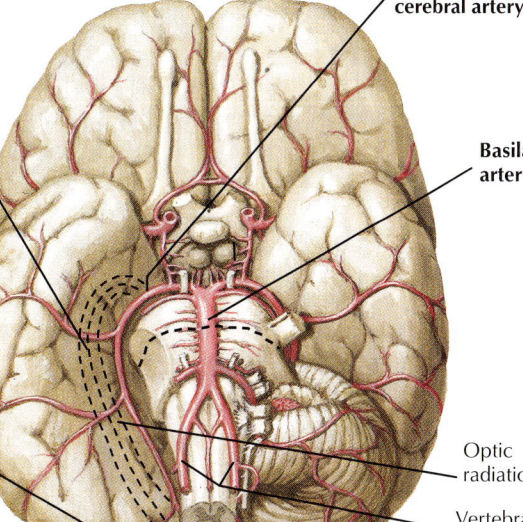

Fundus examination may reveal signs of retinal ischemia in ischemic optic neuritis.

Posterior cerebral artery

Basilar artery

Optic radiations

Vertebral arteries

CEREBROVASCULAR DISORDERS

201

ISCHEMIC STROKE

Table 20-1
Clinical Symptoms in Patients With Border Zone Strokes

Stroke Location	Clinical Symptoms
Anterior border zone	Contralateral weakness (proximal > distal), sparing face, transcortical motor aphasia (left-sided infarcts), mood disturbances (right-sided infarcts)
Posterior border zone	Homonymous hemianopsia, lower-quadrant anopsia, transcortical sensory aphasia (left-sided infarcts), hemineglect, and anosognosia (right-sided infarcts)
Subcortical border zone	Brachiofacial hemiparesis with or without sensory loss, subcortical aphasia (left-sided infarcts)

Intracranial MCA and ACA Disease

Clinical Vignette

A 73-year-old man with history of diabetes mellitus and arterial hypertension presented to the ED with history of mild right-sided weakness first noticed on awakening 2 days previously. This hemiparesis progressed to a right hemiplegia with dysarthria within 48 hours without change in the patient's level of consciousness.

Head CT demonstrated a stroke involving the left centrum semiovale. Head CTA showed a distal M1 segment stenosis. The patient was treated with heparin and warfarin.

This vignette describes a classic course of subcortical infarct from poor perfusion of the lenticulostriate vessels secondary to a fixed lesion in the ipsilateral MCA. The patient's symptoms evolved from relatively mild hemiparesis to complete paralysis within 2 days. Unlike large MCA infarctions, there was no impairment of the patient's level of consciousness despite the progressive nature of the neurologic deficit. Loss of consciousness would have occurred with an MCA lesion wherein cerebral edema developed secondary to infarction of a large amount of cerebral cortex.

Intrinsic occlusive disease of the MCA and ACA are more common in Asians, Hispanics, and African-Americans than in whites and are more common in women than in men. Arterial hypertension, diabetes, and smoking are the most common risk factors, with a lower incidence of high cholesterol and associated coronary and peripheral vascular disease. Although TIAs can occur, they are not as common as in patients with ICA disease and usually occur over a shorter period of time, often days. When strokes occur, initial symptoms are typically noticed on awakening and often fluctuate during the day, supporting a hemodynamic mechanism.

Neurologic findings vary by the location of the occlusion and presence of collateral circulation (Figure 20-5). A large MCA stroke is usually seen in patients with MCA main stem occlusion without good collateral flow, whereas deep or parasylvian strokes are the most common presentation when enough collateral flow is present over the convexities.

Contralateral motor weakness involving the foot more than the thigh and shoulder, with relative sparing of the hand and face is the typical presentation of distal ACA branch occlusion. Conversely, prominent cognitive and behavioral changes associated with contralateral hemiparesis predominate in patients with proximal ACA occlusions, due to the involvement of the artery of Heubner.

Vertebrobasilar Disease

Clinical Vignette

A 76-year-old white man with history significant for high cholesterol and a previous MI had an acute onset of vertigo associated with vomiting and gait difficulties 2 days before admission. On admission, he had acute onset of slurred speech and lack of right arm coordination.

Head CT demonstrated an old right posterior-inferior cerebellar artery (PICA) stroke and a subacute left PICA stroke. Head MRI with diffusion-weighted imag-

ISCHEMIC STROKE

Figure 20-5 Occlusion of Middle and Anterior Cerebral Arteries

Lesion		Artery occluded	Infarct, surface	Infarct, coronal section	Clinical manifestations
Middle cerebral artery	Entire territory	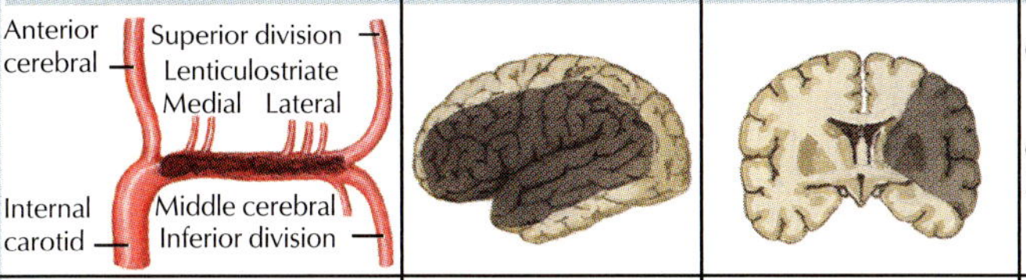 Anterior cerebral; Superior division; Lenticulostriate Medial Lateral; Internal carotid; Middle cerebral Inferior division			Contralateral gaze palsy, hemiplegia, hemisensory loss, spatial neglect, hemianopsia Global aphasia (if on left side) May lead to coma secondary to edema
	Deep				Contralateral hemiplegia, hemisensory loss Transcortical motor and/or sensory aphasia (if on left side)
	Parasylvian				Contralateral weakness and sensory loss of face and hand Conduction aphasia, apraxia, and Gerstmann syndrome (if on left side) Constructional dyspraxia (if on right side)
	Superior division				Contralateral hemiplegia, hemisensory loss, gaze palsy, spatial neglect Broca aphasia (if on left side)
	Inferior division				Contralateral hemianopsia or upper quadrant anopsia Wernicke aphasia (if on left side) Constructional dyspraxia (if on right side)
Anterior cerebral artery	Entire territory				Incontinence Contralateral hemiplegia Abulia Transcortical motor aphasia or motor and sensory aphasia Left limb dyspraxia
	Distal				Contralateral weakness of leg, hip, foot, and shoulder Sensory loss in foot Transcortical motor aphasia or motor and sensory aphasia Left limb dyspraxia

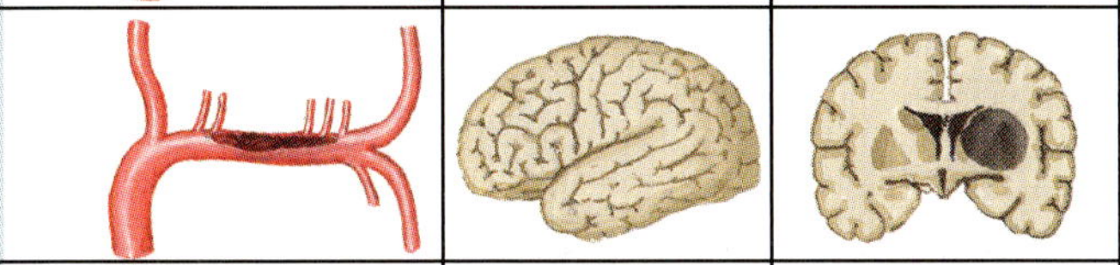

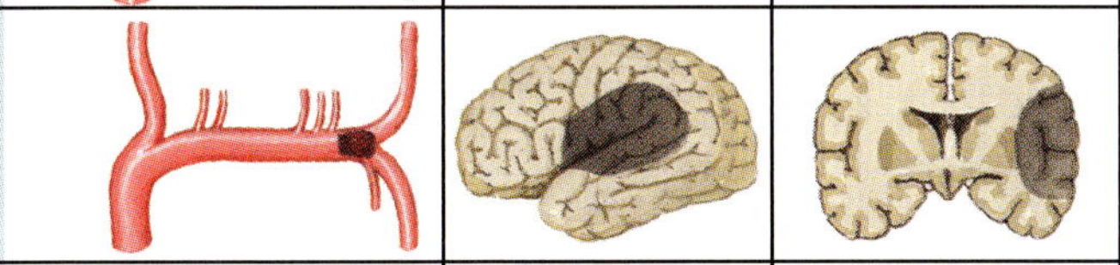

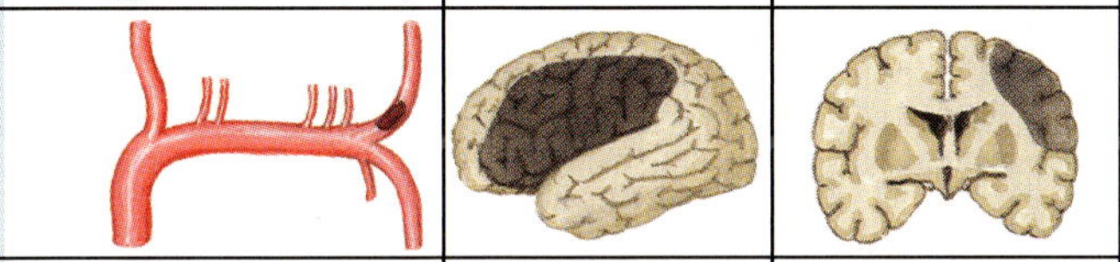

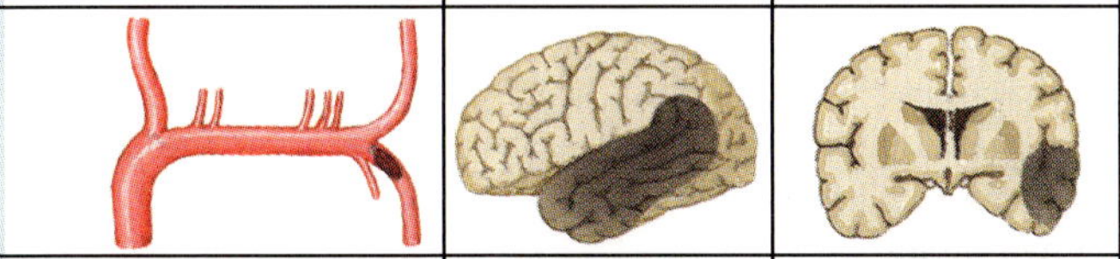

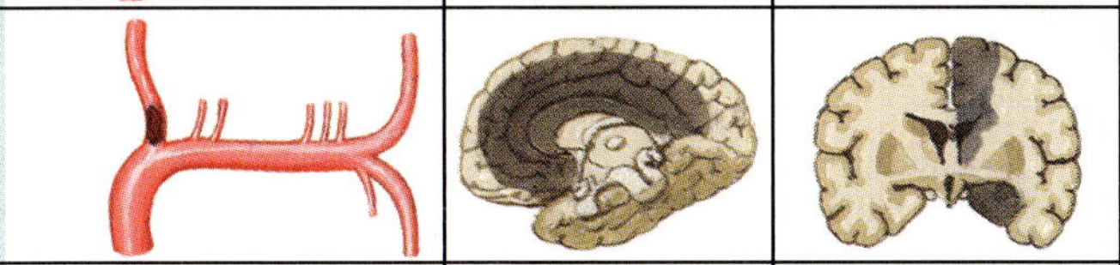

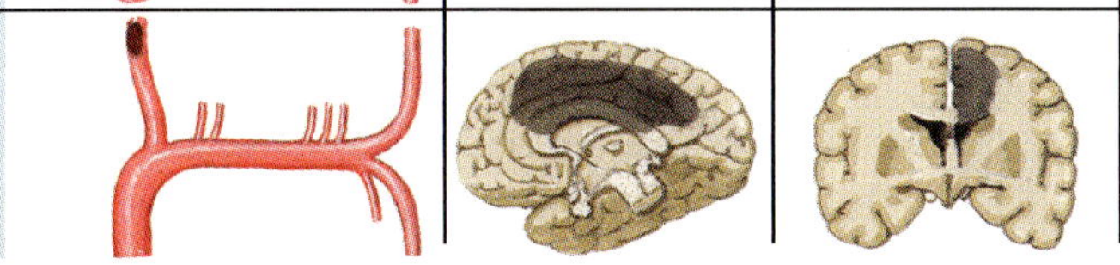

ing showed a new right superior cerebellar artery stroke. Head and neck CTA showed occlusion of the left vertebral artery (VA) origin, a hypoplastic right vertebral artery, and an embolus in the mid-distal portion of the basilar artery.

He was treated with heparin and subsequently warfarin. CTA 2 months later showed resolution of the basilar artery embolus. Clinically, the patient improved significantly.

As with carotid artery disorders, evaluation of patients with vertebrobasilar TIAs or strokes requires consideration of the pathophysiologic potential for anatomic substrate of each artery. The vertebral arteries originate from the subclavian arteries in the neck. Although stenosis or occlusion of the proximal subclavian arteries and the vertebral arteries at their origin can affect vertebral blood flow, it rarely causes symptoms because of the concomitant development of adequate collateral circulation within the neck through the thyrocervical and costocervical

CEREBROVASCULAR DISORDERS

ISCHEMIC STROKE

trunks and other subclavian artery branches eventually flowing into the distal vertebral artery. More often, patients with subclavian and concomitant vertebral stenosis at its origin from the subclavian have symptoms related only to upper extremity ischemia. They report pain, coolness, and weakness of the ipsilateral arm. Rarely does atherosclerotic disease at the vertebral origins, even when bilateral, cause chronic significant low flow to the vertebrobasilar system with resultant vertigo. Although hypothetically possible, it is conjectural whether true subclavian steal occurs that leads to definitive neurologic symptoms with ipsilateral arm exercise.

When stenosis or occlusion of the VA origin leads to TIAs, stroke, or both, intra-arterial embolism is the commonly recognized mechanism. The embolus usually lodges in the distal vertebral artery, causing a PICA stroke or "top of the basilar syndrome," respectively (Table 20-2).

Intracranial VA atherosclerotic disease most often occurs in the arterial portions that supply the lateral medulla and posterior inferior cerebellum. Therefore, occlusion of the distal portion of this artery usually presents as Wallenberg syndrome or cerebellar PICA syndrome. When intra-arterial embolism occurs, the distal portion of the basilar artery is usually affected with a PCA or "top of the basilar syndrome" (Figure 20-6A).

Atherosclerosis of the basilar artery often affects its proximal portion, although stenosis can also occur in its middle and distal portions. Most patients experience TIAs characterized by transient double vision, dizziness, and weakness affecting both legs or alternating between the right and left side that can be elicited by careful questioning. As in other occlusive large artery disease, some patients develop prominent headaches in the weeks before symptom onset. The headache is thought to be from collateral flow development; in patients with basilar disease, it is located in the occipital area. When stroke occurs, the most commonly affected area is the basis pons, causing bilateral, often asymmetric hemiparesis, pseudobulbar syndrome, abnormalities of eye movements (VI nerve palsy, unilateral or bilateral internuclear ophthalmoplegia, ipsilateral conjugate gaze palsy, "one and one-half syndrome"), nystagmus, and sometimes coma (Figure 20-6B).

Embolus to the distal basilar artery leads to the classic top of the basilar syndrome. Affected

Table 20-2
Clinical Manifestations of Ischemia in the Vertebrobasilar System According to the Artery Involved*

Involved Artery	Ischemic Manifestations
Lateral medullary artery (Wallenberg syndrome)	Ipsilateral limb ataxia and Horner syndrome, crossed sensory loss, vertigo, dysphagia, hoarseness
PICA	Vertigo, nausea, vomiting, gait ataxia
ACA	Gait and limb ataxia, dysfunction of ipsilateral CN-V, -VII, -VIII
SCA	Dysarthria and limb ataxia
Right PCA	Contralateral visual field cut and sensory loss, visual neglect, prosopagnosia (inability to recognize faces)
Left PCA	Contralateral visual field cut and sensory loss, alexia without agraphia, anomic or transcortical sensory aphasia, impaired memory and visual agnosia
Top of the basilar syndrome	Rostral brainstem—somnolence, vivid hallucinations, dreamlike behavior, and oculomotor dysfunction Temporal + occipital regions—hemianopsia, fragments of Balint syndrome, agitated behavior, and amnestic dysfunction

*PCA indicates posterior cerebral arteries; PICA, posterior-inferior cerebellar artery; SCA, superior cerebellar artery.

ISCHEMIC STROKE

Figure 20-6A Occlusion of "Top of Basilar" and Posterior Cerebral Arteries

- Internal carotid a.
- Middle cerebral a.
- Posterior communicating a.
- Thalamoperforating aa. to medial thalamus
- Thalamoperforating aa. to lateral thalamus
- Posterior cerebral a.
- Superior cerebellar a.
- Basilar a. and obstruction
- Anterior inferior cerebellar a.
- Vertebral a

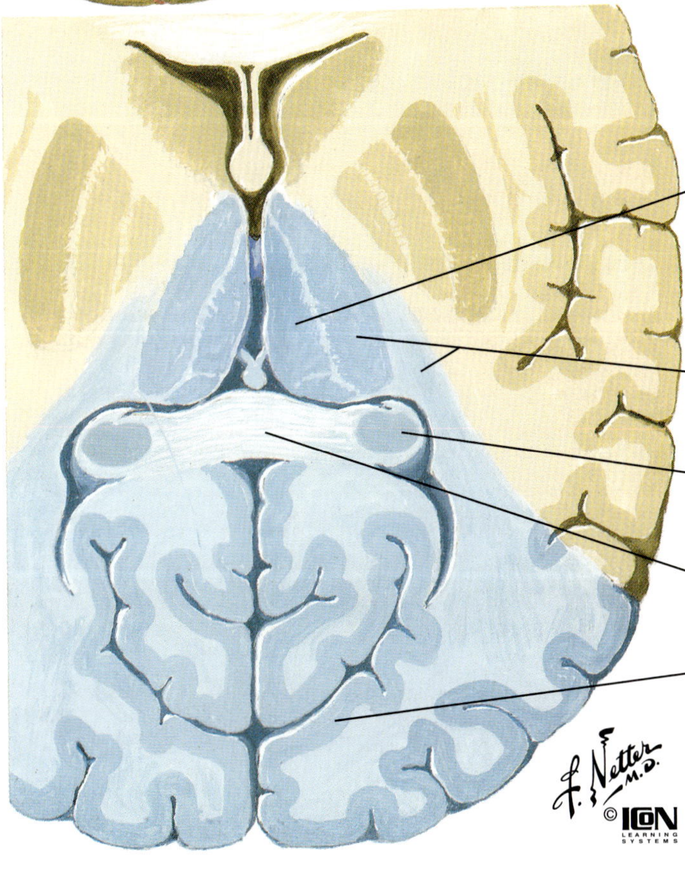

Areas supplied by posterior cerebral arteries (blue) and clinical manifestations of infarction

- **Medial thalamus and midbrain**
  - Hypersomnolence
  - Small, nonreactive pupils
  - Bilateral third cranial nerve palsy
  - Behavioral alterations
  - Hallucinosis
- **Lateral thalamus and posterior limb of internal capsule**
  - Hemisensory loss
- **Hippocampus and medial temporal lobes**
  - Memory loss
- **Splenium of corpus callosum**
  - Alexia without agraphia
- **Calcarine area**
  - Hemianopsia (or bilateral blindness if both posterior cerebral arteries occluded)

CEREBROVASCULAR DISORDERS

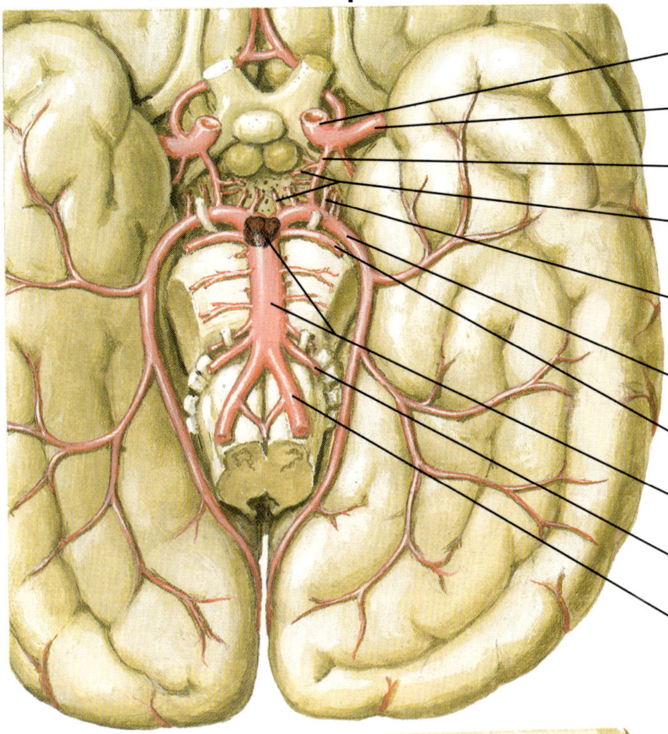

ISCHEMIC STROKE

Figure 20-6B

Ischemia in Vertebrobasilar Territory: Clinical Manifestations

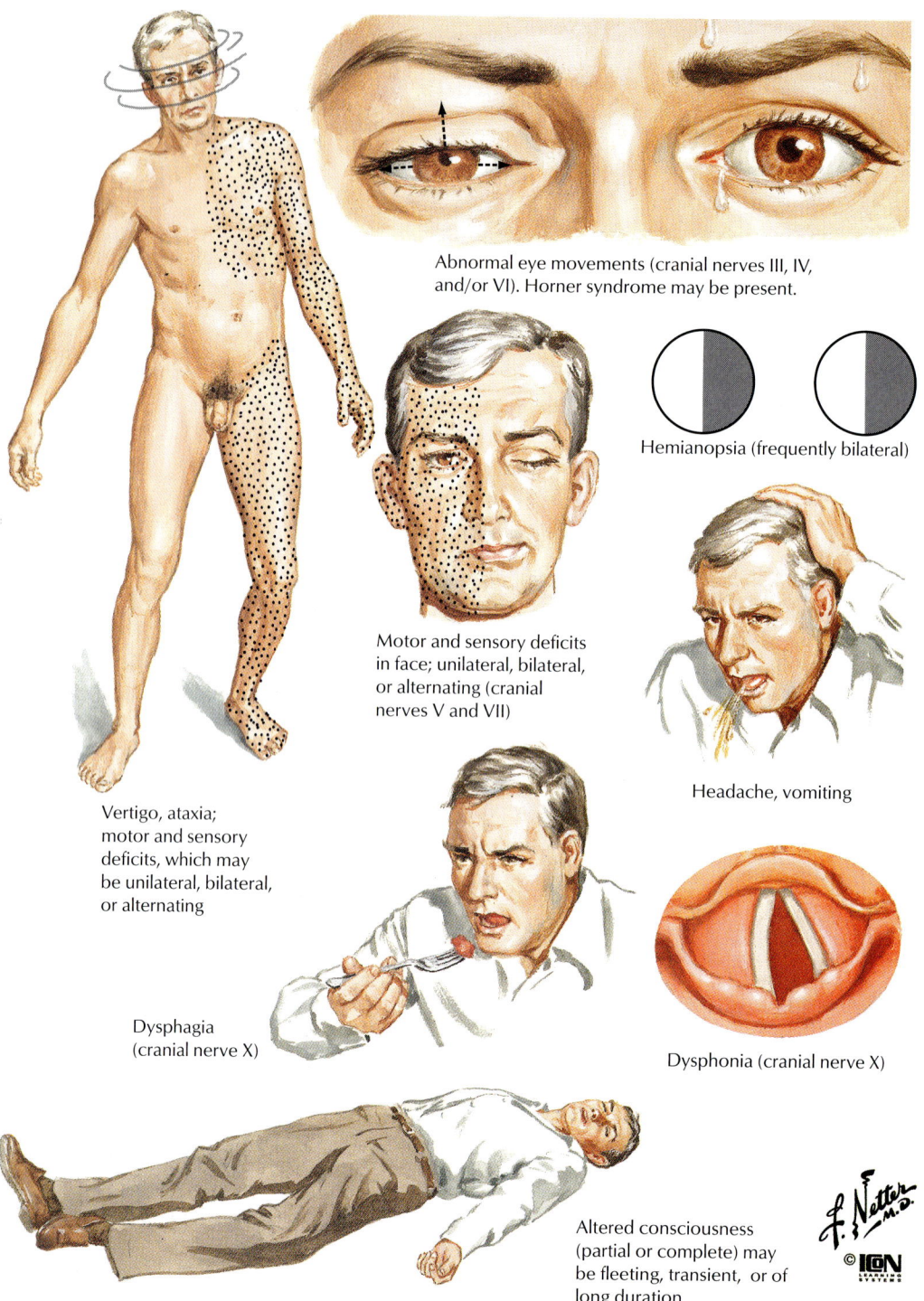

Abnormal eye movements (cranial nerves III, IV, and/or VI). Horner syndrome may be present.

Hemianopsia (frequently bilateral)

Motor and sensory deficits in face; unilateral, bilateral, or alternating (cranial nerves V and VII)

Headache, vomiting

Vertigo, ataxia; motor and sensory deficits, which may be unilateral, bilateral, or alternating

Dysphagia (cranial nerve X)

Dysphonia (cranial nerve X)

Altered consciousness (partial or complete) may be fleeting, transient, or of long duration.

CEREBROVASCULAR DISORDERS

areas are the rostral brainstem, dependent on branches from distal basilar artery; regions of the temporal lobe and thalamus, related to lesions of the bilateral PCAs; and the temporal and occipital lobes. Clinical presentation includes bilateral homonymous hemianopsias, confusion, and inability to form new memory. In contrast, when the embolus moves past the basilar tip and just one PCA is occluded, patients characteristically develop unilateral homonymous hemianopsia.

Most often, infarcts related to PCA disease are embolic, usually derived from a cardiac source or sometimes intra-arterial embolism. Intrinsic PCA stenosis occurs but is rare. Clinical symptoms usually consist of transient episodes of visual field cut, associated sometimes with contralateral hemisensory symptoms that precede the stroke onset by weeks or days, sometimes mimicking intrinsic MCA disease with a presumed fetal trigeminal artery. When headaches occur, they are often retro-orbital or above the eye. In addition to visual and sensory abnormalities, patients with left PCA stroke often have concurrent alexia (inability to read) without agraphia (preserved writing), anomic or transcortical sensory aphasia, impaired memory, and associative visual agnosia (recognition). Patients with right PCA stroke often have associated visual neglect and prosopagnosia (difficulty in recognizing familiar faces).

Cardioembolic Disease

Clinical Vignette

A 59-year-old physician suddenly had difficulty driving; his wife noted that their car almost hit objects on the right side. When questioned, he agreed that he was having difficulty seeing to the right. When this did not improve overnight, he was evaluated in the ED, revealing a dense right homonymous hemianopsia. Otherwise, neurologic and general physical examination results were normal.

Brain CT demonstrated a left occipital lobe hypodensity compatible with PCA infarction. MRI confirmed these findings, and MRA revealed a clot occluding the PCA origin. A 48-hour Holter monitor demonstrated intermittent AF.

Warfarin sodium was administered with careful monitoring. His right homonymous hemianopsia did not improve; therefore, he was told not to drive. Otherwise, he successfully compensated for this loss of vision.

Atrial fibrillation is one of the most common sources of cardiac embolism (Figure 20-7). It sometimes has a paroxysmal presence; however, whether persistent or intermittent, it has a major potential for further cerebral emboli. Therefore, when patients present with an acute stroke onset, particularly those suggestive of a cardioembolic mechanism, even when their initial cardiac evaluation results are unremarkable, it is prudent to obtain a Holter monitor. When AF is demonstrated, long-term anticoagulant or antiplatelet therapy is indicated. Patients who have homonymous hemianopsia must be counseled not to drive. Despite binocular vision, they can no longer perceive half of their visual fields.

Strokes secondary to cardiac sources typically present with acute onset of focal neurologic deficits, such as sudden loss of hand control or drooping of the mouth, often associated with forms of language dysfunction. Cerebral emboli are most clinically apparent during the day because patients can often provide a precise time of acute neurologic deficit onset. Often, these occur during patient activity, as in patients with intra-arterial or cardiac emboli. Emboli do occur while individuals are asleep, but the classic abrupt onset is only readily perceived when it immediately interferes with activity.

Anterior carotid and posterior vertebrobasilar circulations can be affected with emboli, the former 4 times more common because it receives 80% of cerebral blood flow. Furthermore, a history of TIAs, strokes, or both, affecting carotid and vertebrobasilar territories at different times, increases the possibility of cardiac embolism. The vessels more often affected by cardiac emboli are the MCA and its branches, the distal portion of the intracranial vertebral artery, distal basilar (top of the basilar syndrome), and PCA territory.

Typically, there is a history of significant cardiac arrhythmia, most commonly AF, coronary artery disease, or both. Emboli from a recent MI typically occur within a few weeks of the acute event. However, patients with prior anterior myocardial wall infarctions may develop a segmental defect with a hypokinetic myocardial wall or even an aneurysm. Such lesions can provide a

ISCHEMIC STROKE

Figure 20-7
Cardiac Sources of Cerebral Emboli

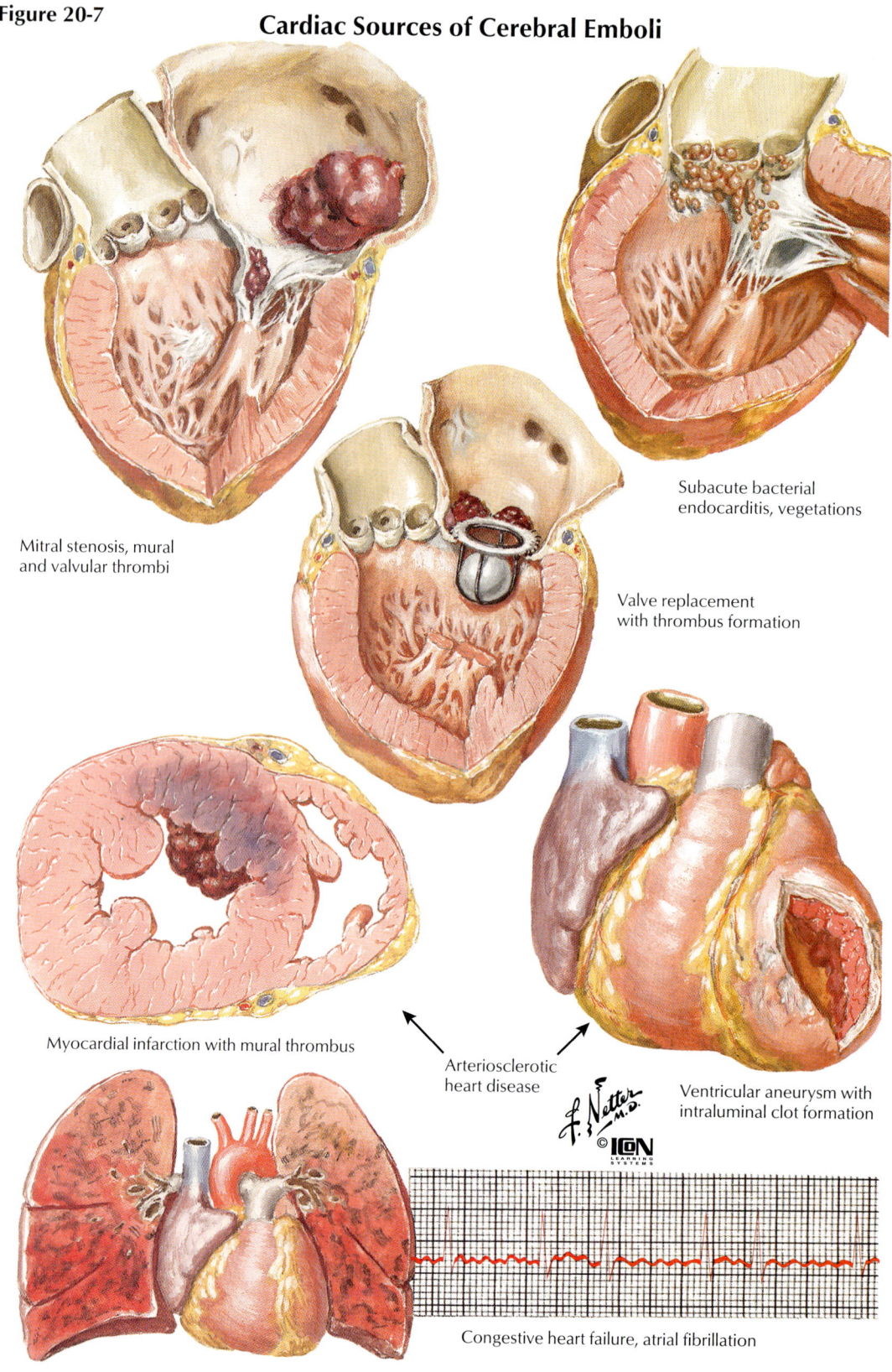

nidus for platelet thrombus formation with later potential for embolus formation.

Infective endocarditis presents with TIA or stroke in approximately 15% of patients; eventually 30% of individuals with infective endocarditis experience a major neurologic complication. Individuals with valvular heart disease are particularly at risk especially after various bodily invasive procedures, some as innocuous as dental cleaning. Patients who inject illicit drugs intravenously are also at major risk for infective endocarditis. Systemic symptoms, such as fever, weight loss, and malaise, and signs of microemboli to the nail beds and conjunctiva commonly occur with endocarditis, and rarely with primary atrial myxomas. It is important to seek evidence of systemic signs of these treatable entities in any stroke patient.

Clinical Vignette

A previously healthy 41-year-old woman had a right facial droop and difficulty speaking. One day previously, she had made a 10-hour car trip. Symptoms persisted. At the ED, neurologic examination confirmed these findings. Cardiac examination results were normal.

Brain MRI with diffusion-weighted imaging showed a small left insular stroke. Head and neck MRA results were normal. Transesophageal echocardiography (TEE) showed a PFO, and her hypercoagulable screen was remarkable for protein S deficiency. Symptoms gradually improved, clearing completely within 72 hours. She was treated with warfarin.

Despite a clinically normal cardiac examination at the emergency medicine evaluation of this woman's stroke, TEE confirmed a congenital lesion. The symptom complex acuity was consistent with a cardioembolic source, justifying a careful heart evaluation. In patients of her age group, PFO is the most likely associated condition with embolic stroke.

Patent foramen ovale and the less common atrial septal defect usually do not cause cardiac symptomatology, so the diagnosis, which requires TEE, is not appreciated until the embolic event occurs. The diagnostic consideration is particularly appropriate with patients who experience a stroke and have factors predisposing to deep venous thrombosis. Any venue that predisposes to increased right-sided pulmonary circulation pressure, decreasing the normal left-to-right intracardiac gradients, prompts venous clots to cross into the left atrium and thus paradoxically into the systemic circulation.

Patients at risk include those who are nonambulatory from prolonged bed rest, eg, because of a severe lumbosacral radiculopathy, or conversely, seemingly healthy persons in supposedly inconsequential settings, such as during prolonged inactivity on transoceanic flights. Valsalva maneuvers with straining that increase venous return and right heart pressures also change the intra-atrial pressure hemodynamics, eg, lifting heavy objects, straining at stool, and orgasm. Associated hematologic abnormalities, as defined in the "hypercoagulable screen" are occasionally demonstrated in the PFO cerebrovascular population. These lesions may predispose to occult venous thrombosis within the lower deep venous system of the extremities or the inferior vena cava in otherwise healthy individuals.

Prognosis depends on the site and extent of the initial brain damage. Often, larger-sized emboli, typical of patients with AF, may leave a significant deficit with an incomplete recovery. Identification of the precise pathophysiologic mechanism and treatment thereof is critical to prevent subsequent emboli so common in patients whose AF is not identified.

Lacunar Small Vessel Disease

Clinical Vignette

A 71-year-old woman with significant history of poorly controlled arterial hypertension developed a subacute-onset, initially evolving, left hemiparesis over 48 hours. She presented 2 weeks later when she had not fully recovered. There was no history of headache or sensory, visual, or language dysfunction. Neurologic examination demonstrated a pure motor hemiparesis, brisk right-sided muscle stretch reflexes, a right Babinski sign, and absolutely no sensory loss.

Brain MRI showed a lacune within the right pons. MRA of the head and neck were normal. The patient was treated with clopidogrel to inhibit platelet aggregation and gradually improved during a 2-week stay at the rehabilitation unit, but she still had a slight tendency to circumduct her leg while walking, even 6 months later.

Lacunar strokes affecting the internal capsule, thalamus, striatum, or brainstem (Figure 20-8) can

ISCHEMIC STROKE

Figure 20-8   Lacunar Infarction

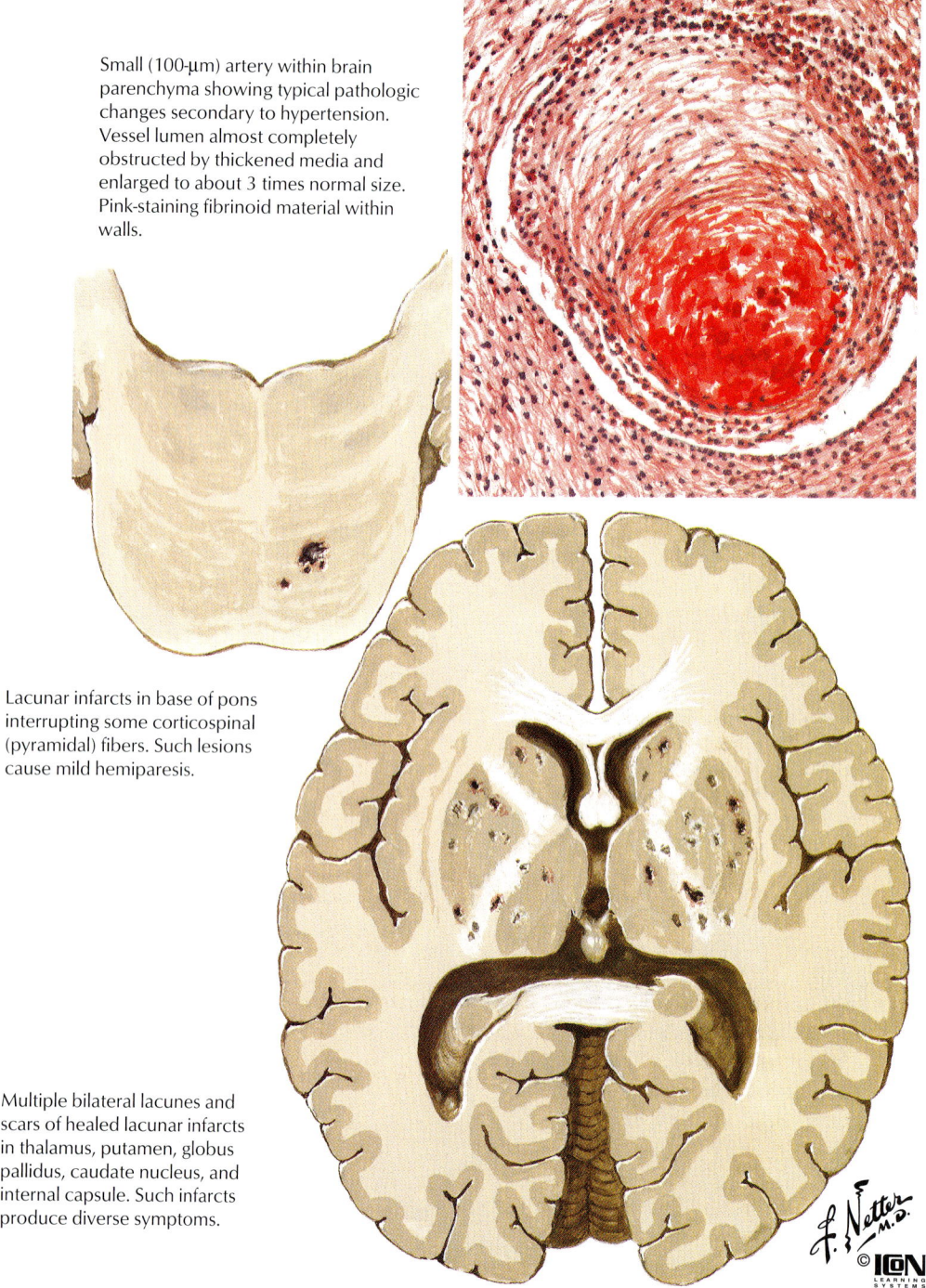

Small (100-μm) artery within brain parenchyma showing typical pathologic changes secondary to hypertension. Vessel lumen almost completely obstructed by thickened media and enlarged to about 3 times normal size. Pink-staining fibrinoid material within walls.

Lacunar infarcts in base of pons interrupting some corticospinal (pyramidal) fibers. Such lesions cause mild hemiparesis.

Multiple bilateral lacunes and scars of healed lacunar infarcts in thalamus, putamen, globus pallidus, caudate nucleus, and internal capsule. Such infarcts produce diverse symptoms.

CEREBROVASCULAR DISORDERS

often be clinically distinguished from embolic disease by the tendency toward a more insidious onset with deficit progression over 2 to 4 days. Additionally, lacunar deficits have a relatively typical distribution; they affect the entire side of the body with either motor or sensory loss, unlike the propensity for middle cerebral cortical branch occlusions to have a primary deficit involving the face and hand but not the leg.

Patients experiencing lacunar strokes can present with TIA or stroke just as with embolic cerebrovascular disorders. TIAs precede strokes in 15% to 20% of these instances. TIAs are stereotypical, but unlike those secondary to large artery disease, they tend to occur over 2 to 5 days and in clusters, sometimes with several over a 24-hour period and occasionally in crescendo fashion. Signs and symptoms vary according to the location of the ischemia (Table 20-3).

If affected individuals have hypertension, diabetes, or both, proper treatment of those conditions is essential to prevent further strokes. However, not all patients with lacunar disease have identifiable vascular risk factors, leaving empirical use of antiplatelet therapy as an option.

Arterial Dissection

Clinical Vignette

A 42-year-old man with no vascular risk factors presented with acute-onset left-sided weakness and numbness. Symptoms were preceded by a severe nonspecific right-sided neck and retro-orbital pain for 1 week after he had had a relatively inconsequential fall. Examination revealed evidence of a spastic left hemiparesis and hemineglect of the left arm more than the leg.

Head CT showed a complete right MCA stroke, and CTA showed tapering of the right ICA 2 cm above the bifurcation, suggestive of arterial dissection.

Extracranial carotid artery dissection occurs predominantly in patients aged 20 to 50 years. The characteristic clinical presentation is unilateral neck or face pain followed a few days later by acute onset of neurologic signs. In patients with carotid dissection, pain is usually referred to the eye, temple, or forehead. Ipsilateral Horner syndrome occurs in 40% to 50% of patients. Pulsatile tinnitus is common. Often, a history of minor trauma exists (violent coughing, cervical manipulation, whiplash injury, etc) in the days preceding symptom onset. As in the preceding vignette, benign traumatic events can cause a slight intima tear in the carotid or vertebral arteries, leading to platelet fibrin aggregation with potential for developing artery-to-artery emboli.

Similar to the carotid artery within the neck, the extracranial VA has a significant potential for sustaining traumatic dissection (Figure 20-3). Dissection usually occurs in the distal extracranial portion, also called the *third segment*, just before it penetrates the dura at the skull base. In those patients, pain is usually referred to the neck or back of the head and usually precedes the onset of neurologic signs by days, rarely weeks.

Table 20-3
Most Frequent Lacunar Syndromes and Their Locations

Clinical Syndrome	Location
Pure motor stroke: weakness equally involving face, arm, and leg	Internal capsule (posterior limb) or basis pontis
Pure sensory stroke: numbness or paresthesia equally involving face, arm, and leg and usually trunk	Lateral thalamus (posteroventral nucleus)
Sensorimotor stroke: combination of pure motor/pure sensory symptoms and findings	Thalamus internal capsule
Ataxic hemiparesis: weakness and incoordination in the arm and/or leg	Basis pontis or internal capsule
Dysarthria-clumsy hand: facial weakness, severe dysarthria and dysphagia, slight weakness, and clumsiness of the hand	Basis pontis

TIAs are more common in ICA than on VA dissections. In ICA dissection, TIAs usually involve the ipsilateral eye and cerebral hemisphere. When they occur in VA dissection, the most common symptoms are dizziness, diplopia, gait unsteadiness, and dysarthria. In extracranial ICA and VA dissections, strokes are usually caused by intra-arterial embolism, affecting more often the MCA and distal VA territories, PICA and lateral medullary strokes, respectively.

DIAGNOSTIC APPROACH

For every patient evaluated with history and examination suggestive of ischemic stroke or TIA, the location and mechanism of the lesion should be considered.

Anatomical Site

The precise anatomical location of an acute TIA or stroke can frequently be presumed by the history and neurologic examination findings. However, confirmation with an imaging study is needed and often provides more specific etiologic information. For example, occasionally intracerebral or subdural hematomas, or other structural lesions including benign and malignant tumors are found on brain CT and MRI in patients presenting with seemingly typical cerebrovascular events. Obtaining these studies soon after the event is particularly useful, because findings may modify the evaluation and potential therapy.

Brain CT examination is the initial study of choice for individuals presenting with an acute focal neurologic deficit. Most importantly, head CT can acutely show a hyperdense MCA sign in patients with emboli to the MCA stem, with immediate therapeutic implications if there is no evidence of sulcal effacement or loss of gray-white matter differentiation, typical of patients with large ischemic infarcts. However, usually head CT is normal within the first few hours of an ischemic stroke. In contrast, if a primary cerebral hemorrhage or a hemorrhagic infarct causes symptoms, it will be immediately detected as blood appears as a hyperdense area on head CT like a large focal embolus in the MCA stem.

Diffusion-weighted MRI is the most sensitive and specific test for acute ischemia, and abnormalities have been demonstrated as early as 1 hour after symptom onset (Figure 20-9). Other MRI sequences, such as FLAIR and T2-weighted imaging, can also show the area of stroke, often 6 to 12 hours after onset of symptoms.

Etiologic Mechanism

To define the specific pathophysiologic mechanism for a TIA or stroke, patency of the extracranial and intracranial arteries, the character of their endothelial surface, and the adequacy of cerebral perfusion are required. Complete assessment of cardiac function is also essential, including the electrical stability of the cardiac rhythm, myocardial contractility, valvular status, and whether a PFO is present.

Ultrasound, especially of the carotid arteries at their bifurcation in the neck, and transcranial Doppler of the intracranial vessels can functionally assess cerebral flow and determine the presence of a critical stenosis. MRA or CTA of the head and neck are appropriate to assess patency of the intracranial and extracranial arteries, particularly for critical stenosis within the cervical or intracerebral circulation. Cerebral perfusion is easily assessed with CT perfusion or MRI perfusion. The advantages and disadvantages of these studies require consideration (Table 20-4). Renal failure or pacemaker devices limit the imaging studies that can be performed in patients with TIAs and strokes (Table 20-5).

Subsequently, TEE is the choice because it provides more detailed information than the transthoracic approach, particularly about the intra-atrial septum and aortic arch.

Information gathered from imaging studies allows confirmation of 1 of 3 primary carotid or vertebrobasilar stroke mechanisms: large artery disease with intra-arterial embolism, small vessel disease, and large artery disease with hemodynamic ischemia. Echocardiography in these cases is optional and depends on the cardiac history and apparent risk factors. However, when other tests are unrevealing, TEE is essential to define the presence of occult potential cardiac or aortic arch embolic sources (Figure 20-10).

A hypercoagulable screen, including protein C, protein S, anticardiolipin antibodies, lupus anticoagulant, factor II DNA, factor V Leiden, and antithrombin III are typically evaluated in pa-

ISCHEMIC STROKE

Figure 20-9A   **Arterial Imaging With CT and MRI**

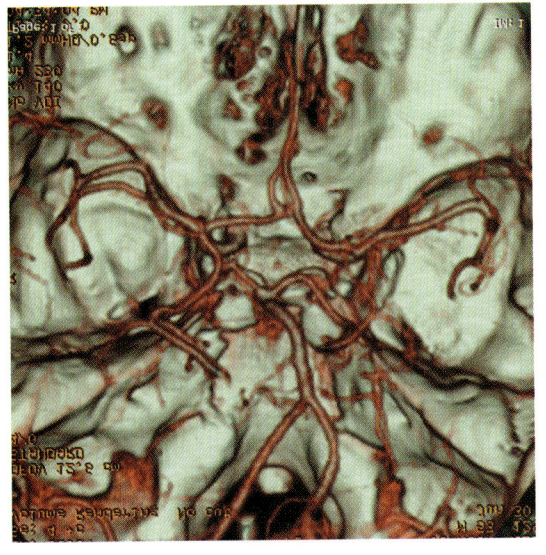

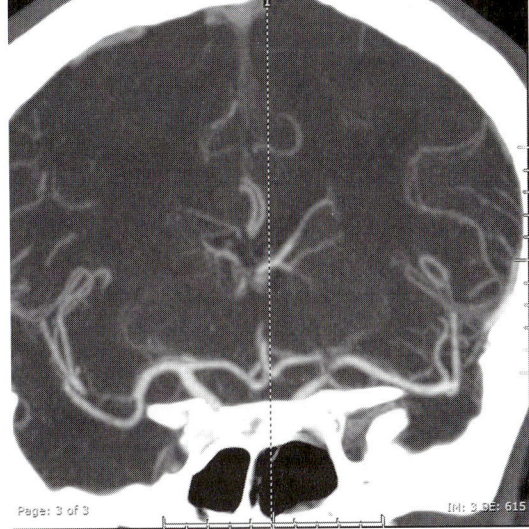

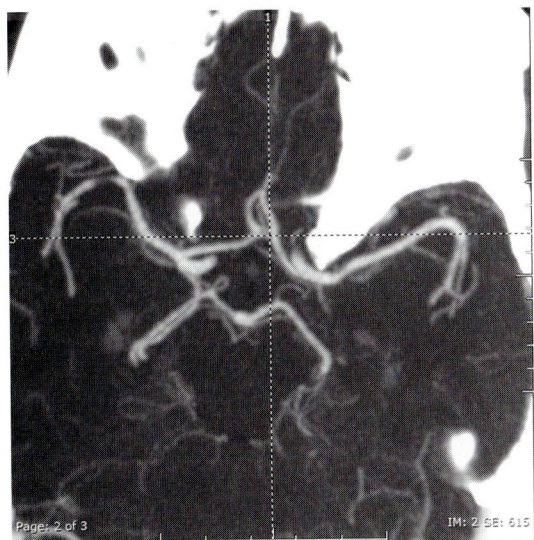

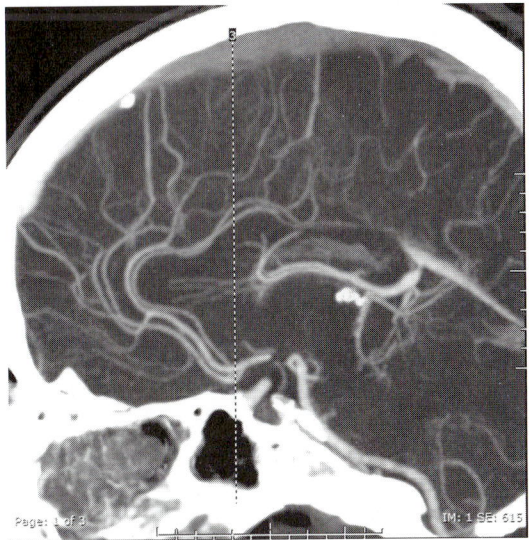

(**A**) 3-D reconstructed image of the Circle of Willis on computed tomography angiography (CTA). (**B-D**) Reconstructed CTA images of intercerebral vessels in 3 planes: coronal, axial, and sagittal.

tients younger than 50 years and in patients of any age without identifiable risk factors.

TREATMENT

The treatment of ischemic TIAs and strokes is best classified into prophylactic treatment of TIAs and strokes with anticoagulation or antiplatelet agents, acute treatment of ischemic strokes with thrombolysis, and surgical treatment.

Prophylactic Treatment of TIAs and Strokes
Anticoagulation

Standard heparin consists of a mixture of glycosaminoglycans with molecular weights from 3000 to 30,000 d. Low-molecular-weight he-

ISCHEMIC STROKE

Figure 20-9B — Arterial Imaging With CT and MRI (continued)

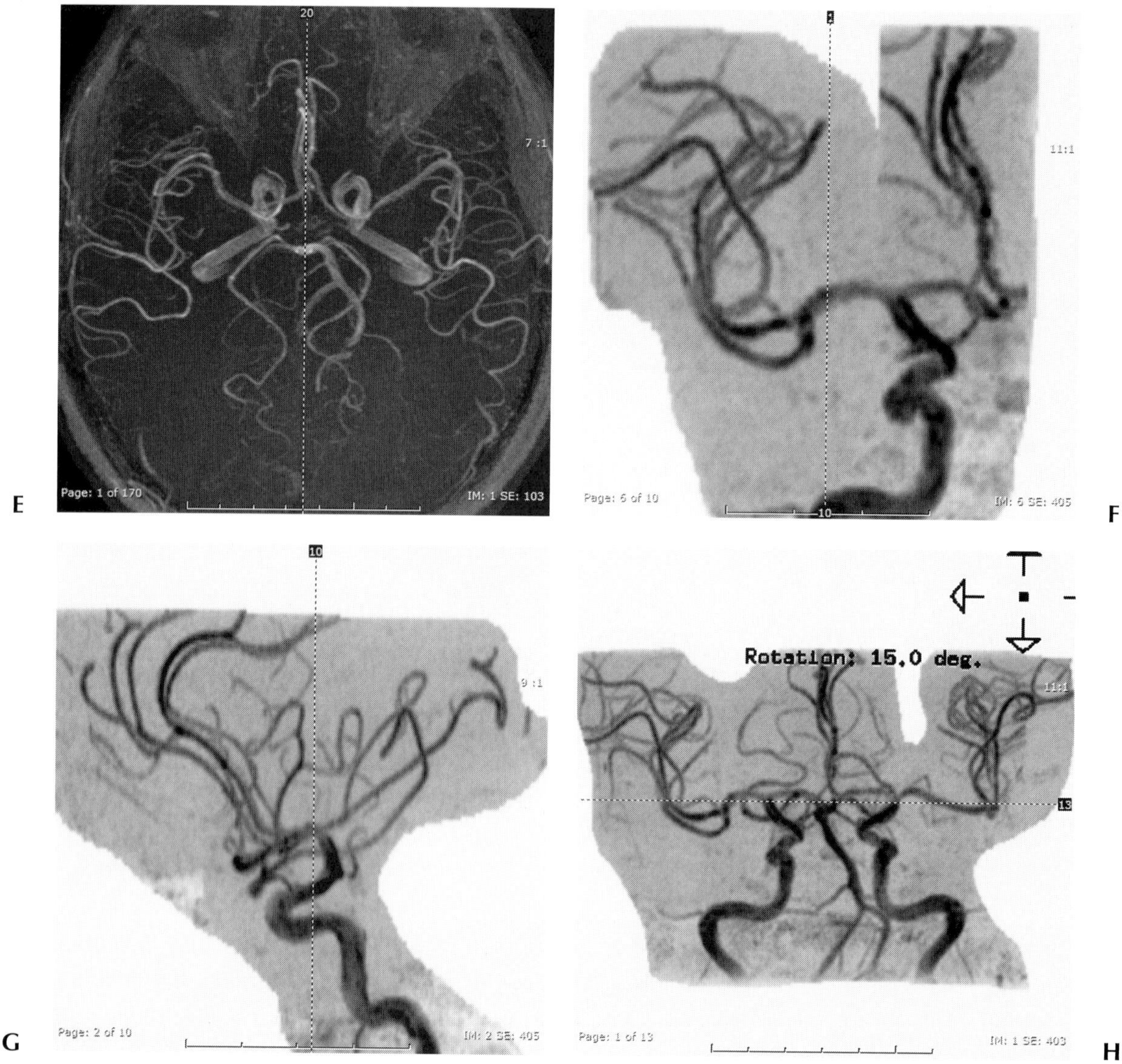

(**E-H**) Reconstructed magnetic resonance angiography (MRA) in several planes. **E** and **H** are composites of all proximal vessels, whereas **F** and **G** are images of the right internal carotid circulation.

parins (LMWHs) are fragments of standard heparin with a mean molecular weight of 5000 d. Heparinoids are natural or semisynthetic sulfated aminoglycosans structurally related to heparin, but similar in size to LMWHs. Each exerts anticoagulant activity by activating antithrombin III, which inhibits clotting factor Xa. Heparins larger than 5000 d also inhibit thrombin formation.

Despite its common use, few randomized trials have studied the effect of heparin on stroke mortality, morbidity, and early recurrence. Results are controversial; some showed beneficial effect of IV heparin in preventing stroke progression, but

ISCHEMIC STROKE

Table 20-4
Advantages and Disadvantages of Different Neurologic Imaging Techniques*

Imaging Method	Advantages	Disadvantages
MRI/MRA	DWI and PWI demonstrate the area of stroke and the area at risk (penumbra), respectively.	Prolonged test (30-60 min); patient must cooperate or sedation is required. Cannot be performed in patients with PCM. MRA can overestimate tight stenosis as an occluded vessel.
CTA/CTP	Images can be obtained rapidly (<5 min).	Patient must have normal renal function because CTA and CTP require high doses of contrast, 100 and 50 mL, respectively.
Ultrasonograhy of the neck	Easy to perform, can be done at the bedside	No detailed information about the vertebral arteries
TCD	Easy to perform, even at the bedside	Poor transtemporal windows limit the information about the intracranial vessels.

*CTA indicates computed tomography angiography; CTP, computed tomography perfusion; DWI, diffusion-weighted imaging; PCM, pacemaker; PWI, perfusion-weighted imaging; TCD, transcranial Doppler.

Table 20-5
Guidelines for Imaging in Ischemic Stroke/TIA Apropos to Patient Renal Function and Pacemaker Presence*

	Abnormal Renal Function	
Normal Renal Function	No PCM	+ PCM
CT of the head, CT perfusion, and CTA of head and neck *or*	MRI of head + DWI/PWI, MRA of the head and neck *or*	Head CT, US and TCD
MRI of the head + DWI/PWI, MRA of the head and neck *or*	CT or MRI of the head, US and TCD	
CT or MRI of the head, US and TCD		

*CTA indicates computed tomography angiography; DWI, diffusion-weighted imaging; PCM, pacemaker; PWI, perfusion-weighted imaging; TCD, transcranial Doppler; US, ultrasonography.

Figure 20-10 Uncommon Cardiac Mechanisms in Stroke

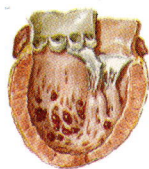
Myocardiopathy with thrombi

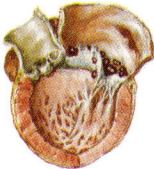
Mitral valve prolapse with clots

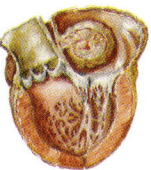
Atrial myxomatous tumor emboli

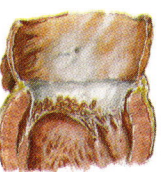
Marantic emboli

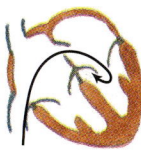
Probe-patent foramen ovale transmitting venous clots

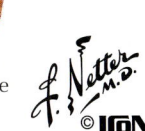

CEREBROVASCULAR DISORDERS

ISCHEMIC STROKE

not in reducing mortality. One study showed no benefit of heparin versus placebo for prevention of stroke progression, but patients with cardioembolic stroke were excluded.

Regarding prevention of recurrent events, a protective response of IV heparin was shown in a small randomized trial in patients with cardioembolic strokes. IV heparin prevented recurrent embolic events and hemorrhages. However, another trial, where subcutaneous heparin treatment was utilized, showed the reduced rate of recurrent stroke was balanced by increased numbers of hemorrhagic strokes. No conclusion can be drawn about the use of IV heparin.

More data are available about LMWH and heparinoids in patients with ischemic stroke. Subcutaneous nadroparin, a LMWH, had better outcomes at 6 months compared with placebo in a Chinese population. However, there was no difference in death or dependence at 3 months. A prospective study comparing dalteparin, a LMWH, with aspirin given within 30 hours of AF-associated stroke showed no differences between death and physical dependence at 3 months. A randomized double-blind study using IV danaparoid, a heparinoid, in patients with ischemic stroke showed no significant effect, although higher rates of favorable and very favorable outcomes were seen at day 7 in all treated patients. Hence, there is no evidence that LMWH and heparinoid reduced morbidity or mortality when used within the first 48 hours of onset in patients with ischemic stroke.

Warfarin has significant benefit compared with placebo for primary and secondary stroke prevention in patients with AF. As primary stroke prevention, patients with AF have an annual stroke rate of 4.5% when treated with placebo compared with only 1.4% in the group treated with warfarin. Benefit is more significant in patients with AF and a prior ischemic event, with an annual stroke rate of 4% in patients receiving warfarin compared with 12% in patients receiving placebo. The benefit of warfarin over placebo has also been documented in patients with prosthetic heart valves and anterior MI.

Warfarin for prevention of recurrent strokes in patients with noncardioembolic stroke is more controversial. One trial showed no benefit for warfarin compared with aspirin in patients with noncardioembolic strokes and excluded patients with severe carotid artery stenosis. Most patients in this trial had small vessel disease (56%) or stroke of unclear etiology (26.1%). Therefore, a definitive conclusion is lacking for patients with intracranial disease. A trial comparing warfarin versus aspirin in stroke prevention for patients with intracranial disease is ongoing.

Antiplatelet

Antiplatelet drugs include aspirin, ticlopidine, clopidogrel, and a combination of dipyridamole and low-dose aspirin. Aspirin is the oldest antiplatelet drug and probably the most often prescribed drug worldwide. It inhibits the cyclooxygenase enzyme preventing production of thromboxane A_2. A metaanalysis of 10 trials in which different aspirin doses were compared with placebo showed an overall benefit for aspirin with a relative risk reduction of 13% for vascular events. The most common US dose used is 325 mg/d, with a range of 81 to 650 mg/d.

Ticlopidine works by inhibiting platelet aggregation induced by adenosine diphosphate. One study showed a 30.2% relative risk reduction of stroke, nonfatal or vascular death for ticlopidine (250 mg twice daily) compared with placebo. Compared with high doses of aspirin, there was a 21% relative risk reduction of fatal and nonfatal stroke in 3 years with ticlopidine. However, more adverse effects, such as diarrhea, skin rash, and severe but reversible neutropenia were seen with ticlopidine.

The mechanism of action of clopidogrel is similar to that of ticlopidine. Compared with 325 mg aspirin, clopidogrel (75 mg once daily) showed a relative stroke risk reduction of 8%. In that study, clopidogrel was as safe as aspirin and safer than ticlopidine.

The combination of a low dose of aspirin (50 mg) and sustained-release dypiridamole (400 mg/d) is more effective than either drug alone. The relative reduction of stroke risk was 37% for aspirin and dypiridamole combined, 18.1% for aspirin, and 16.3% for dypiridamole. Dypiridamole inhibits platelet aggregation induced by the phosphodiesterase.

Acute Treatment of Ischemic Strokes

Acute treatment of patients with ischemic stroke includes general measures and, in selected patients, thrombolysis. Deep venous thrombosis prophylaxis, monitoring and control of BP and blood sugars, aggressive treatment of hyperthermia and any associated infection, strict fluid management and aspiration precautions are basic, but important measures in the first few days of acute stroke.

A randomized double-blind trial of IV recombinant tissue plasminogen activator (rt-PA) in patients with ischemic stroke treated within the first 3 hours of symptom onset showed a 12% absolute (32% relative) increase in the number of patients with minimal or no disability in the rt-PA group at 3 months. The benefit was present even when the different stroke subtypes were analyzed. Because of this report, patients arriving to the hospital within the first 3 hours of stroke onset are considered for IV rt-PA administration after it is confirmed that no contraindications exist (Table 20-6).

Intra-arterial rt-PA has been used in selected cases beyond the 3-hour window or in patients within the 3-hour time limit with recent major surgeries. Further studies are necessary to confirm its benefit and safety in these groups.

FUTURE DIRECTIONS

Modern technology has improved the understanding of stroke and TIA pathophysiology, which will translate into a more rational therapeutic approach. Improving stroke outcome with more potent antiplatelet drugs in the acute setting, such as the GPIIb/IIIa antagonists is an area of focus for the next few years.

Endovascular techniques, such as angioplasty and stents, will likely change the management approach for some patients with extracranial and intracranial disease. A trial comparing the efficacy of carotid endarterectomy (chapter 21) versus carotid angioplasty-stent for stroke prevention in patients with ICA stenosis is ongoing. Angioplasty and stents have also been used for intracranial artery stenosis in patients who failed medical treatment, but results are mixed. Future randomized studies are needed to determine its benefit.

Table 20-6
Contraindications for IV rt-PA*

Strong Contraindications for IV rt-PA

1. Symptoms minor or rapidly improving
2. Other stroke or serious head trauma within the past 3 months
3. Major surgery within the past 14 days
4. Known history of intracranial hemorrhage
5. Sustained systolic BP >185 mm Hg
6. Sustained diastolic pressure >110 mm Hg
7. Symptoms suggestive of subarachnoid hemorrhage
8. Gastrointestinal or urinary tract hemorrhage within 21 days
9. Arterial puncture at noncompressible site within 7 days
10. Received heparin within 48 h and had increased PTT
11. Platelet count <100,000 µL

Relative Contraindications

1. Seizure at onset of stroke
2. Serum glucose <50 mg/dL or >400 mg/dL
3. Hemorrhagic eye disorder
4. Myocardial infarction in the previous 6 weeks
5. Suspected septic embolism
6. Infective endocarditis
7. INR >1.7

*INR indicates international normalized ratio; PTT, partial thromboplastin time; rt-PA, recombinant tissue plasminogen activator.

REFERENCES

Caplan LR. *Posterior Circulation Disease: Clinical Findings, Diagnosis and Management.* Cambridge, Mass: Blackwell Science; 1996.

Caplan LR. *Stroke: A Clinical Approach.* Stoneham, Mass: Butterworth-Heinemann; 1993.

Chaves CJ, Caplan LR. Heparin and oral anticoagulants in the treatment of brain ischemia. *J Neurol Sci.* 2000;173:3-9.

Fisher CM. Lacunar strokes and infarcts: a review. *Neurology.* 1982;32:871-876.

Fisher M, Prichard JW, Warach S. New magnetic resonance techniques for acute ischemic stroke. *JAMA.* 1995;274:908-911.

Jones HR, Caplan LR, Come PC, Swinton N, Breslin DR. Cerebral emboli of paradoxical origin: report of five cases and review of the literature. *Ann Neurol.* 1983;13:314-319.

Jones HR, Siekert RG. Neurological manifestations of infective endocarditis: review of clinical and therapeutic challenges. *Brain.* 1989;112:1295-1315.

Mohr JP, Caplan LR, Melski D, et al. The Harvard Cooperative Stroke Registry. *Neurology.* 1978;28:754-762.

The National Institute of neurological Disorders and Stroke rt-PA Stroke Study Group. Tissue plaminogen activator for acute ischemic stroke. *N Engl J Med.* 1995;333:1581-1587.

Chapter 21
Endarterectomy for Extracranial Carotid Artery Atherosclerosis

Edward R. Jewell, Harold J. Welch, and Kevin B. Raftery

Clinical Vignette

A 62-year-old right-handed man with diabetes and hypertension was writing when he suddenly dropped his pen and was unable to pick it up. He tried to call a colleague but spoke in a nonsensical "ragtime" manner. An associate noted that the right side of his face was drooping. All symptoms resolved in approximately 5 minutes.

Evaluation in the ED demonstrated a pleasant but anxious obese man with a BP of 146/92 mm Hg, a normal sinus rhythm, a loud left internal carotid artery (ICA) bruit, and normal cardiac examination results. The results of a detailed neurologic examination were normal, with no neurologic deficits.

Brain imaging study results were normal; however, there was greater than 90% stenosis of the left ICA at its origin. Carotid endarterectomy (CEA) demonstrated a ruptured atherosclerotic plaque with much fibrin platelet debris. The patient's recovery was uneventful. He had no further TIAs and died 10 years later of cardiac failure after sustaining multiple myocardial infarctions.

The patient in this vignette is the ideal CEA candidate. He had no cerebral damage demonstrated by brain imaging, a critically tight carotid stenosis, and no associated cardiac risk factors. Despite later development of recurrent myocardial ischemia, he never experienced another TIA or stroke.

Carotid endarterectomy was introduced in 1954 as a logical procedure for the prevention of ischemic stroke distal to the carotid artery stenosis. However, the appropriateness of the operation became a matter of controversy in the 1980s because of lack of data showing its efficacy in preventing strokes. In the early 1990s, several trials compared surgical versus medical treatment for patients with symptomatic carotid artery disease. The North American Symptomatic Carotid Endarterectomy Trial (NASCET) showed that among symptomatic patients with 70% to 99% ICA stenosis, those who underwent CEA had a 17% absolute risk reduction and a 65% relative risk reduction of ipsilateral stroke at 2 years ($P<.001$). Those findings were also documented by the European Carotid Surgery Trial and the Veterans Affairs Cooperative Studies Symptomatic Stenosis Trial. Since then, CEA has been the treatment of choice in patients with symptomatic high-grade stenosis who have a reasonable surgical risk.

The benefit of CEA in symptomatic patients with less than 70% stenosis is not as significant; therefore, surgical treatment is not recommended with one primary exception. An obviously ulcerated plaque, serving as a nidus for formation of platelet thromboemboli, despite the lack of critical stenosis, creates special circumstances. NASCET showed that among symptomatic patients with stenosis of 50% to 69%, the 5-year rate of ipsilateral stroke was 15.7% among patients treated surgically and 22.2% among those treated medically ($P = .045$). Furthermore, patients with less than 50% stenosis had a rate of ipsilateral stroke that was not significantly different ($P = .16$) from patients treated surgically (14.9%) or medically (18.7%).

The Asymptomatic Carotid Atherosclerosis Study demonstrated that among asymptomatic patients with stenosis greater than 60% who had CEA, there was an absolute risk reduction in ipsilateral stroke of 5.9% over 5 years and a 53% relative risk reduction. The stroke risk reduction was more prominent in men and independent of the degree of stenosis or contralateral disease. Even though this trial showed a modest, statistically significant improvement with surgery compared with nonoperative clinical management, the benefit was small. Therefore, other aspects need consideration before the decision for surgery is made, including patient age and overall health, and the precise morbidity and mortality during CEA in the specific institution with each surgeon. Any perioperative morbidity or mortality greater than 5% negates any potential benefit from CEA.

SURGICAL MANAGEMENT

In 1954, the first well-publicized carotid operation reported successful treatment of a 66-year-old woman who had experienced 33 episodes of right hemiparesis secondary to left carotid stenosis. By the early 1970s, 20,000 CEAs per year were performed in the United States. Within another decade, that number rose to greater than 100,000. This remarkable increase in performance led to controversy about its indications and to studies of the risk factors inherent with this procedure. Studies of regional, hospital-specific, and most importantly, individual surgeon risk were compiled. It is possible to perform CEA, one of the more common operations by vascular surgeons, with a mortality rate of less than 1% and a concomitant stroke rate of 1%. A complication rate of less than 3% to 5% is thought to ensure overall patient benefit. Other complications include postoperative hemorrhage (1%), CN injuries (2-5%), and a small risk of postoperative cardiac complications. Most patients can go home the day after surgery.

Surgical Technique

A skillful surgeon is crucial to the success of CEA. Often, symptomatic patients have loose atherosclerotic debris within the **ulcerated** base of the carotid artery. If the surgery is performed in a rough manner, it can result in distal embolization to a derived cerebral vessel. Patients with asymptomatic disease may also have loosely adherent platelet fibrin clumps in the carotid artery. To avoid embolization of this debris to the brain, dissecting the "patient away from the artery" is recommended, rather than the artery away from the patient, to try not to disturb the artery unnecessarily during the dissection.

The patient's head is turned slightly to the contralateral side, providing more extensive exposure of the carotid artery, and is elevated to decrease venous bleeding (Figure 21-1). The surgical incision is made along the anterior border of the sternocleidomastoid muscle, and superiorly curved gently posteriorly to avoid injuring the ramus mandibularis. The dissection is carried through the platysma, and the jugular vein is dissected free, allowing visualization of the vagus nerve. The proximal common carotid is exposed. Extreme care is taken not to disturb the arteries because it is assumed that loose debris exists in all arteries.

The proximal external and internal carotid arteries are visualized well above the diseased area. The artery is a bluer shade above the atherosclerotic disease, which typically is localized to the bifurcation area. Once the exposure is ideal, the patient is given 5000 U IV heparin. Initially, the ICA is clamped distally to prevent embolization. Subsequently, the common carotid and then the external carotid are clamped. An arteriotomy is then made in the common carotid and extended up the ICA well above the diseased area. Next, a straight shunt is placed to bypass the diseased areas and maintain cerebral blood flow. During shunt placement, it is crucial to ensure there is no loose debris in the artery proximally or distally. Some surgeons use other effective methods for cerebral protection, including EEG monitoring, measurement of back pressures, or regional anesthesia (Figure 21-2).

The amount of disease determines the plane of endarterectomy, most commonly at the external elastic lamina. Importantly, the surgeon can carefully sculpt the distal end point with scissors, decreasing the need for tacking sutures distally. Almost invariably, the entire diseased segment with its atheromatous debris can be successfully removed. If the artery is large, a primary closure is reasonable. However, if this would lead to more narrowing than acceptable, synthetic or vein patching is a reasonable alternative. It is essential to ensure that there is no postoperative bleeding; it is poorly tolerated in the neck, especially because of the potential for tracheal dis-

ENDARTERECTOMY FOR EXTRACRANIAL CAROTID ARTERY ATHEROSCLEROSIS

Figure 21-1

Endarterectomy for Extracranial Carotid Artery Atherosclerosis

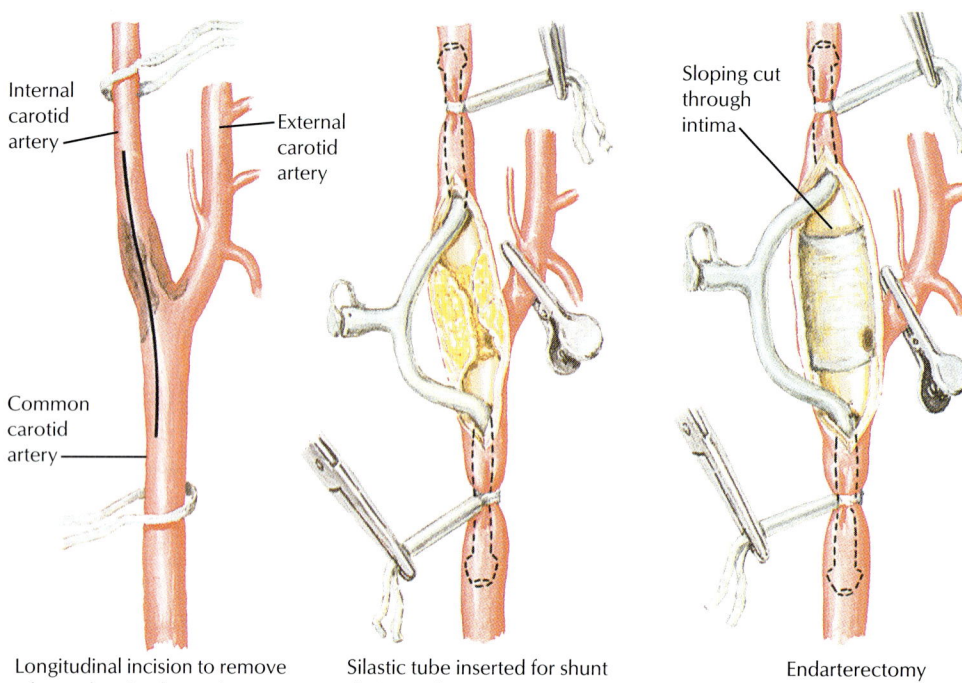

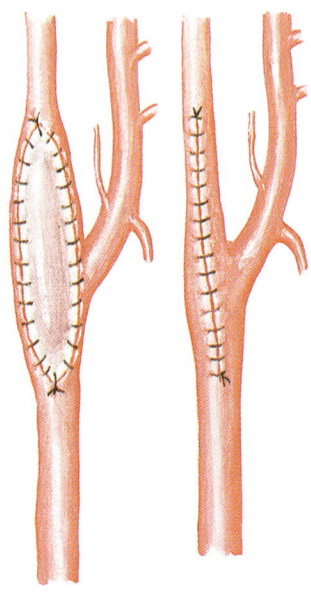

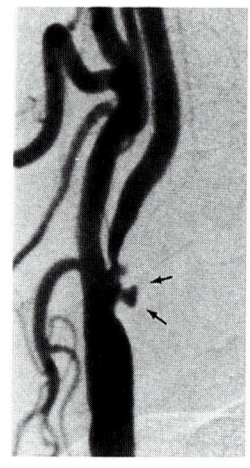

CEREBROVASCULAR DISORDERS

ENDARTERECTOMY FOR EXTRACRANIAL CAROTID ARTERY ATHEROSCLEROSIS

Figure 21-2   **Cerebrovascular Emboli Protection Device**

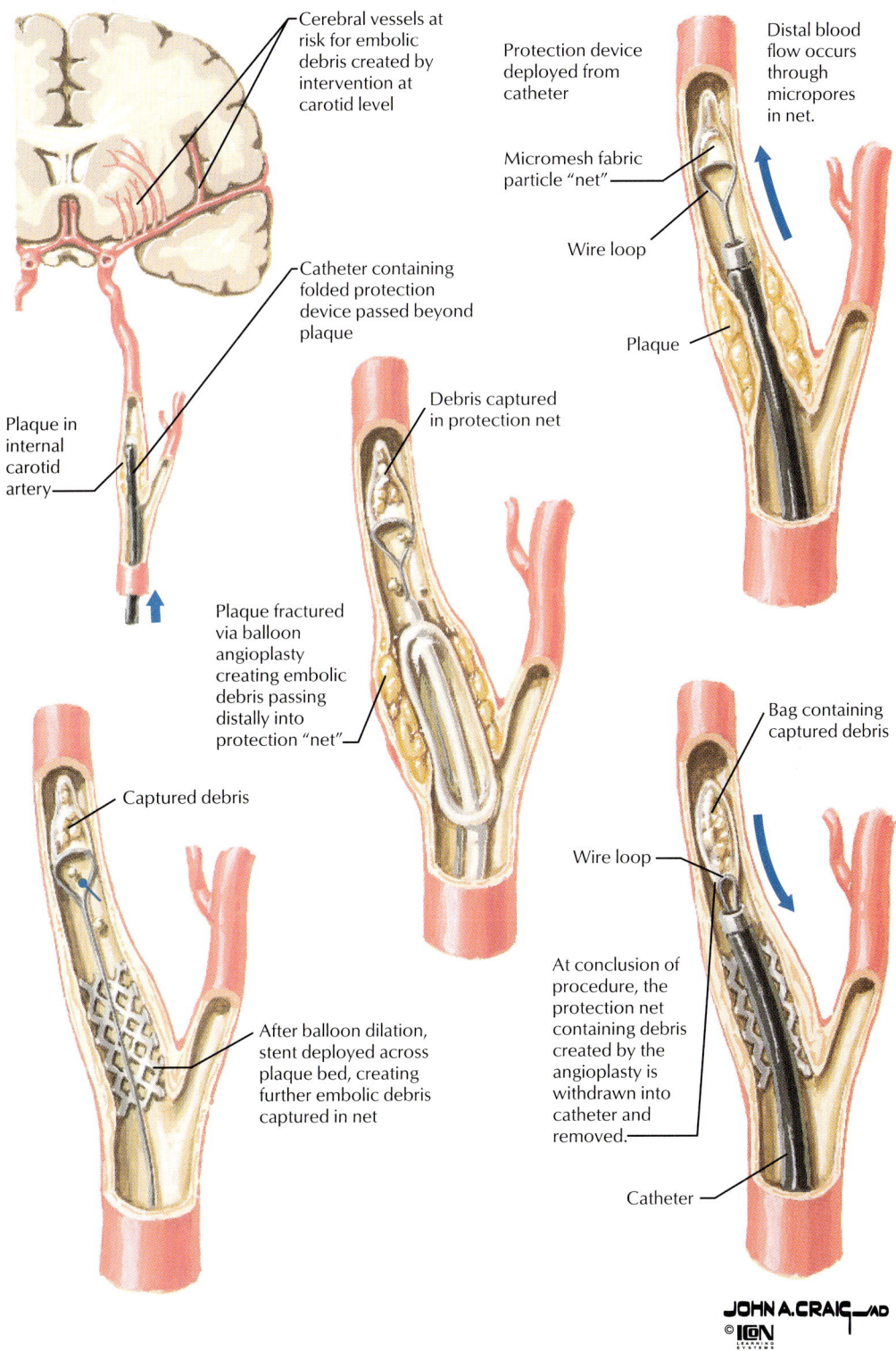

CEREBROVASCULAR DISORDERS

placement with subsequent acute respiratory distress that may be difficult to treat.

Carotid endarterectomy is an elegant procedure. When carefully performed, the inside of the artery looks amazingly perfect. These operations are durable; a recurrent plaque rarely requires reoperation.

Percutaneous angioplasty is an option for patients with symptomatic or asymptomatic carotid atherosclerosis. Results of series comparing traditional CEA with angioplasty are emerging. More data defining the appropriate indications for each are anticipated.

REFERENCES

Barnett HJ, Taylor DW, Eliasziw M, et al. Benefit of carotid endarterectomy in patients with symptomatic moderate or severe stenosis. North American Symptomatic Carotid Endarterectomy Trial Collaborators. *N Engl J Med.* 1998;339:1415-1425.

Eastcott HH, Pickering GM, Rob CG. Reconstruction of internal carotid artery in a patient with intermittent attacks of hemiplegia. *Lancet.* 1954;267:994-996.

Executive Committee for the Asymptomatic Carotid Atherosclerosis Study. Endarterectomy for asymptomatic carotid artery stenosis. *JAMA.* 1995;273:1421-1428.

North American Symptomatic Carotid Endarterectomy Trial Collaborators. Beneficial effect of carotid endarterectomy in symptomatic patients with high-grade stenosis. *N Engl J Med.* 1991;325:445-453.

Chapter 22
Cerebral Venous Thrombosis

Gregory Allam

Clinical Vignette

A 34-year-old man presented to the hospital after 1 week of increasing occipital headache, stiff neck, and chills. Brain CT and CSF analysis were normal; however, the patient was admitted to the hospital for worsening confusion and behavioral changes. Soon after admission, he had a generalized tonic-clonic seizure and underwent intubation.

A brain MRI demonstrated bilateral frontal hemorrhagic infarctions with edema and a sagittal sinus thrombosis. Because of obtundation and signs of increased intracranial pressure (ICP), mannitol and an IV heparin infusion were started. A continuous intrasinus infusion of urokinase was given over 2 days. The thrombosis resolved, and he recovered consciousness.

Eventually, the patient was discharged from the hospital on warfarin and anticonvulsants, with only minor left-sided sensory changes and mild left leg weakness. Unfortunately, he did not continue the prescribed anticoagulants and was readmitted 20 days later with pleuritic chest pain and shortness of breath. Bilateral deep vein thrombosis and a pulmonary embolism were diagnosed. An infrarenal inferior vena cava filter was inserted, and anticoagulation was resumed. The patient had a positive test result for anticardiolipin antibodies. This led to diagnosis of an anticardiolipin antibody syndrome, confirming the need for long-term systemic anticoagulation.

When venous drainage of the brain is compromised, the arterial flow creates back-pressure into the tissue capillaries causing capillary congestion, interstitial edema, decreased tissue perfusion, and ultimately ischemia. Eventually, capillaries rupture, causing hematomas to form. This process of cerebral venous congestion, infarction (not conforming to strict arterial territories) and hemorrhage, is the hallmark of cerebral sinus thrombosis.

The causes of cerebral venous thrombosis vary (Table 22-1), but many relate to transient or permanent hypercoagulable states with dehydration acting as a common precipitating event. A thorough investigation for such etiologies is crucial to directing long-term treatment and anticipating potential comorbidities.

Attention should be given to signs of meningitis, ie, fever, stiff neck, and rash. Examining the ears, sinuses, and face for infection or discharge may provide clues to possible septic venous thrombosis. Physical evidence or a history of head or neck trauma is important. Ocular pain, proptosis, and chemosis, often with combinations of cranial neuropathies, are significant signs that may indicate a basal skull or cavernous sinus thrombosis.

Table 22-1
Causes of Venous Sinus Thrombosis

Hypercoagulable states; anticardiolipin antibody syndrome, etc
Trauma
Parameningeal infection of the face, eye, ear, mastoids, or sinuses
Meningitis, subdural empyema, brain abscess
Pregnancy, oral contraceptive medications
Dehydration
Infiltrative malignancies
Ulcerative colitis
Systemic lupus erythematosus
Jugular trauma or canalization
HIV infection
Nephrotic syndrome
Behçet disease

ANATOMY

Although complex, cerebral venous system anatomy is best considered in 3 levels: the dural-based posterosuperior group, the dural an-

CEREBRAL VENOUS THROMBOSIS

Figure 22-1A

Venous Sinuses of Dura Mater: Normal Venous Sinuses

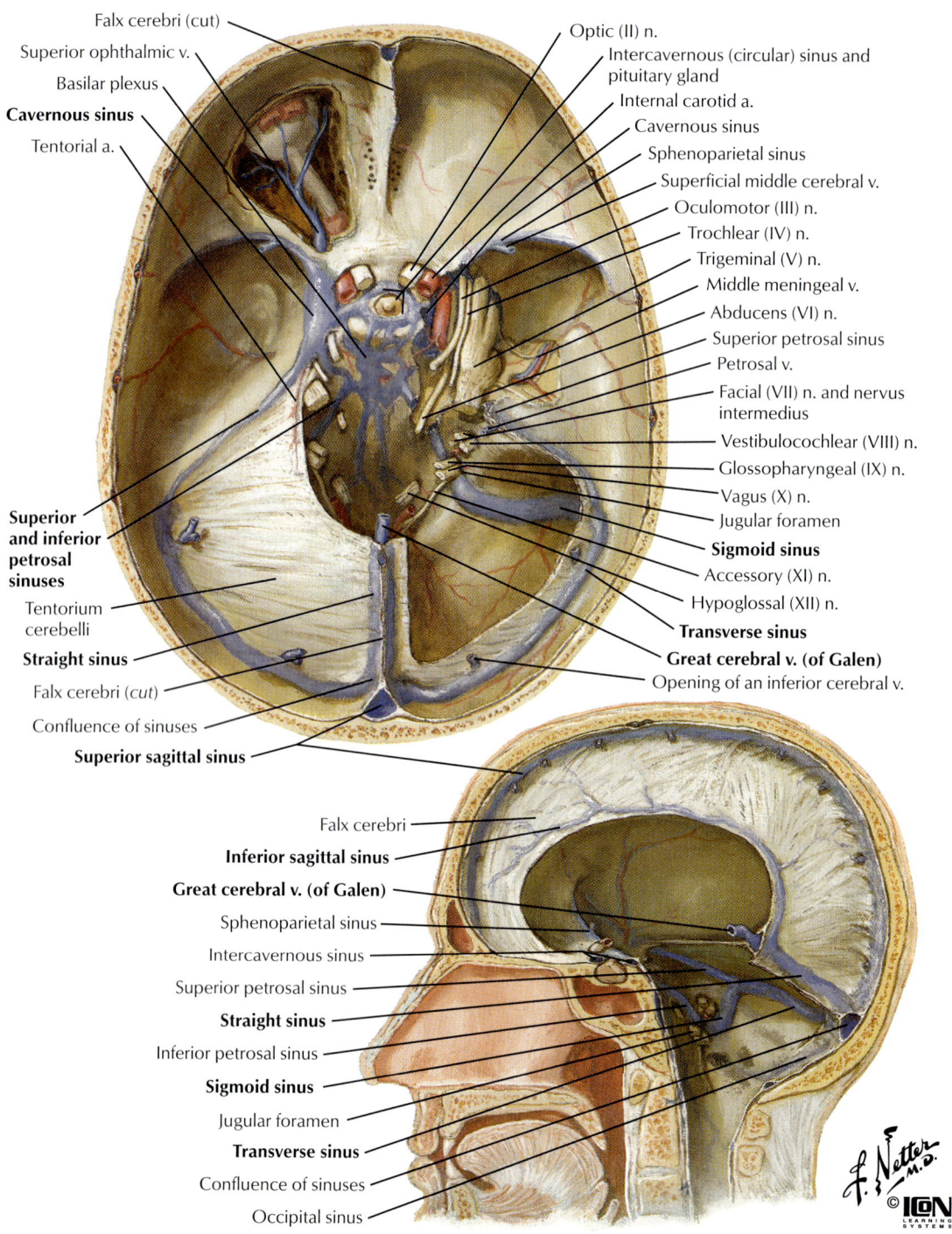

CEREBROVASCULAR DISORDERS

CEREBRAL VENOUS THROMBOSIS

Figure 22-1B   Deep and Subpendymal Veins of Brain

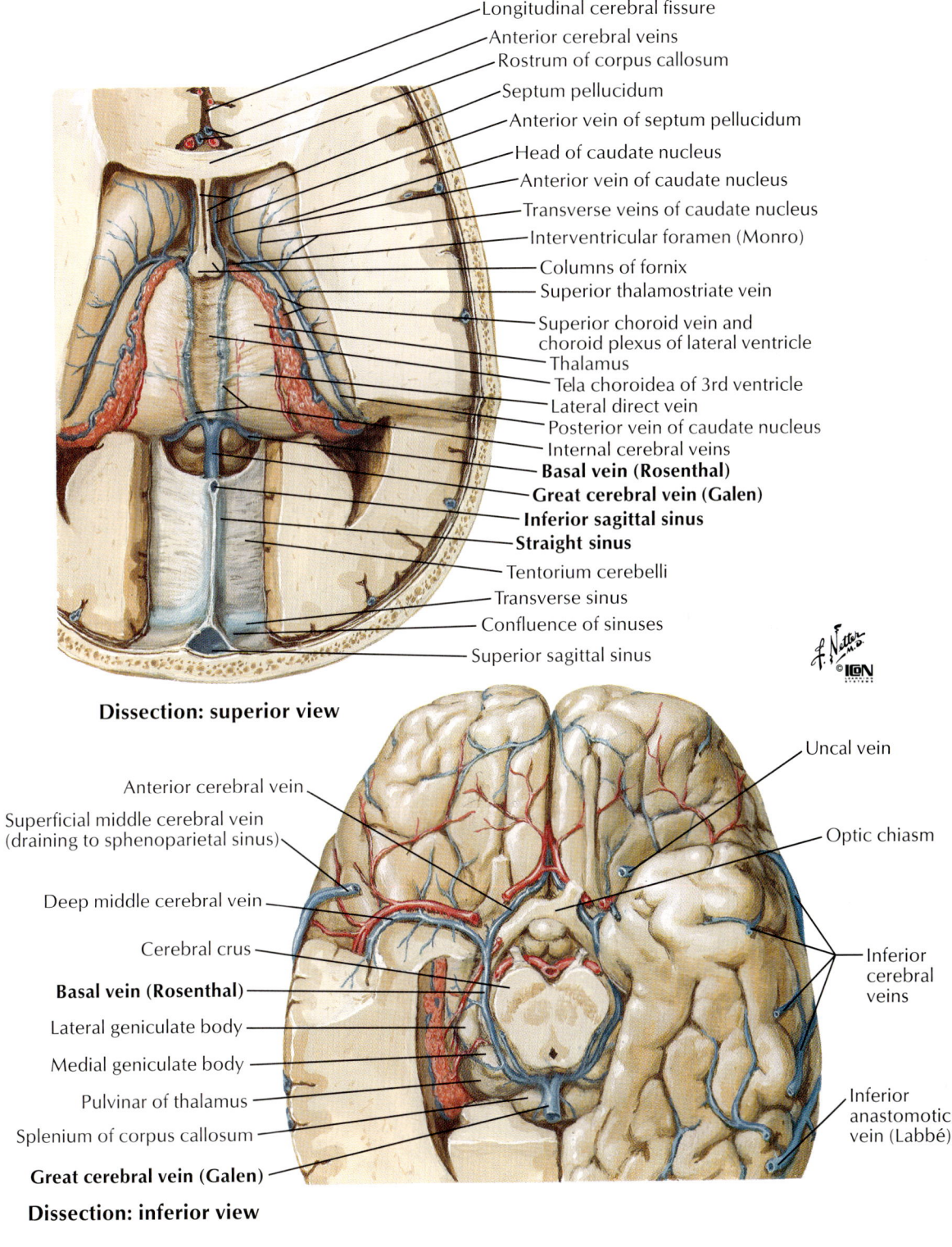

CEREBROVASCULAR DISORDERS

225

CEREBRAL VENOUS THROMBOSIS

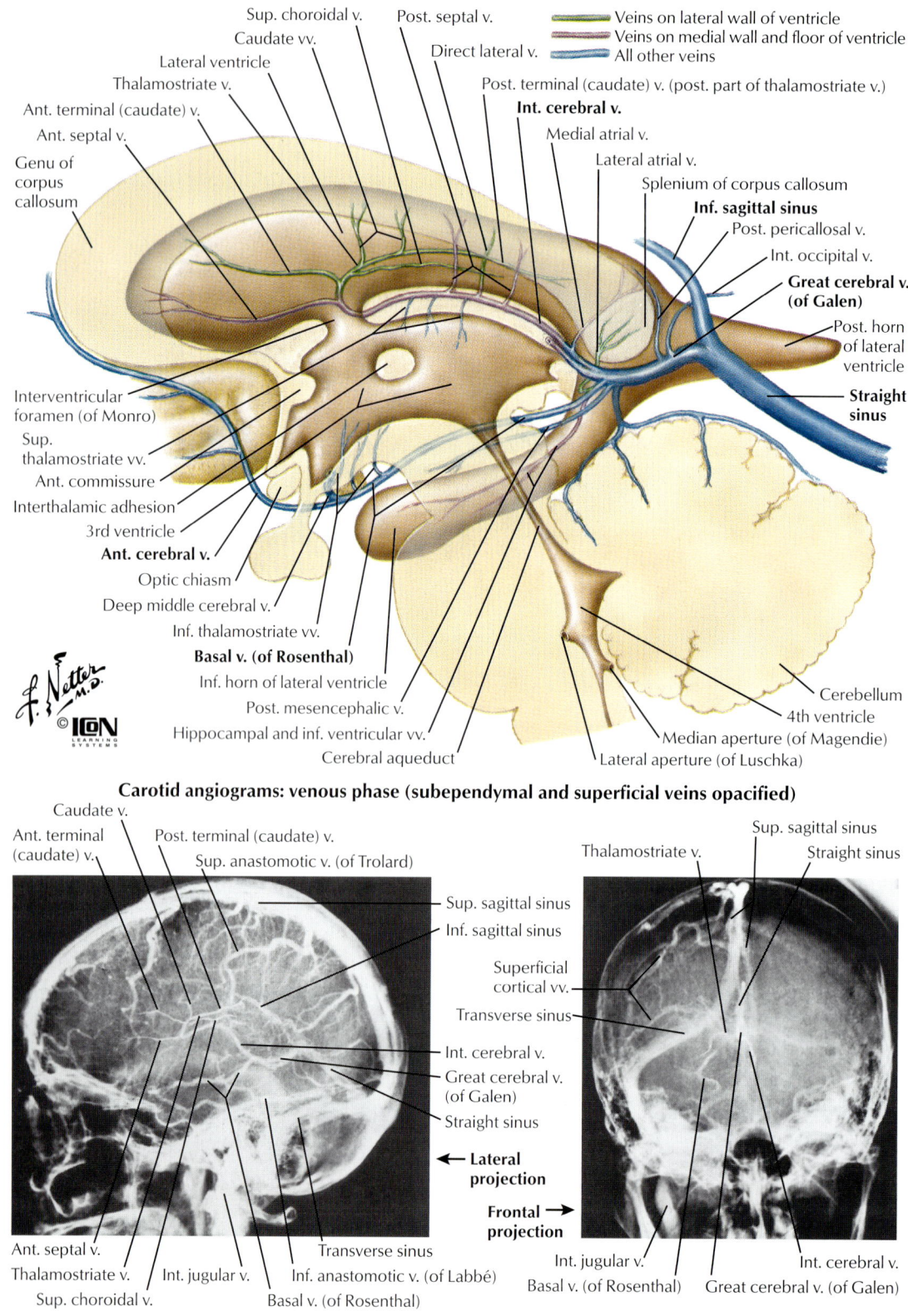

Figure 22-1C — Subependymal Veins

CEREBROVASCULAR DISORDERS

CEREBRAL VENOUS THROMBOSIS

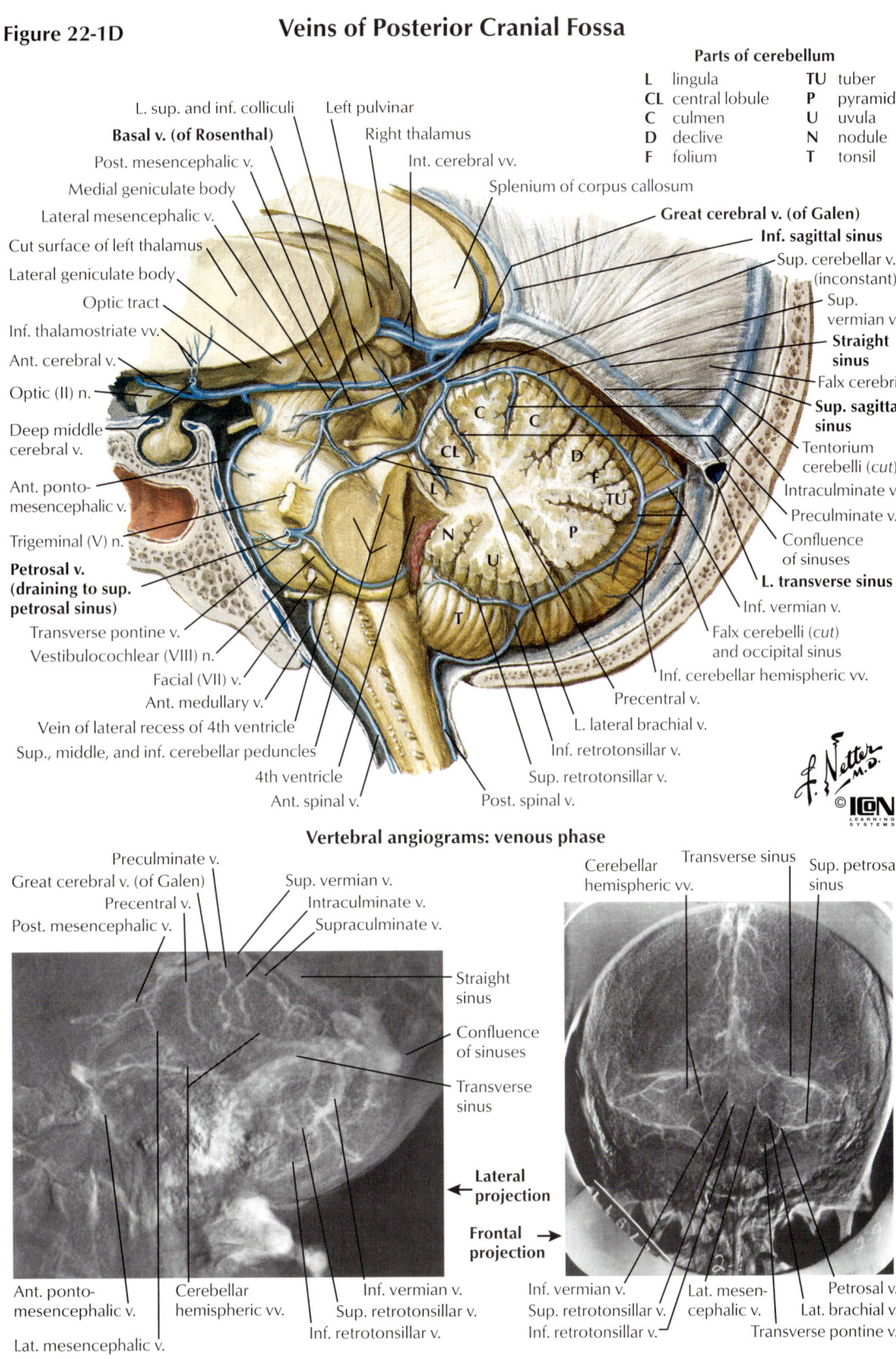

Figure 22-1D — Veins of Posterior Cranial Fossa

CEREBROVASCULAR DISORDERS

CEREBRAL VENOUS THROMBOSIS

teroinferior or basal group, and the deep veins of the brain.

The dura is formed of 2 layers, one abutting the inner calvarium and the other forming the outer meningeal covering. These layers separate in the midsagittal and transverse planes to form dural venous sinuses that drain into the jugular veins. A single **superior sagittal sinus** joins the often asymmetric but paired transverse sinus at the confluence of sinuses or **trocular herophili** (Figure 22-1). The transverse sinuses run laterally from the occipital bone to the middle cerebral fossa along the tentorium cerebelli. The right is often larger and is continuous with the superior sagittal sinus. The left usually curves out laterally as an extension of the single midline straight sinus. The straight sinus runs downward from near the splenium of the corpus callosum to the occipital protuberance. The **sigmoid sinus** curves down toward the skull base from the transverse sinus and joins the inferior petrosal sinus at the jugular foramen to form the jugular vein.

The **straight sinus** (Figures 22-1A through D) is formed by the splayed falx layered over the cerebellar tentorium. The inferior sagittal sinus runs in the fold of the lower arch of the falx cerebri and joins the cerebral vein of Galen in the proximity of the posterior horns of the lateral ventricles to form the straight sinus. The superior and inferior sagittal sinuses provide drainage for the cerebral hemispheres.

The **great cerebral vein of Galen** drains, through paired internal cerebral veins, the brainstem, cerebellum, posterior frontal and anterior parietal lobes, and thalamus; through the paired basal vein of Rosenthal, it drains the limbic system, hippocampus, and mesencephalon.

The **cavernous sinus** runs posteriorly at the brain base from the sphenoid bone in the area of the superior orbital fissure to the petrous temporal bone (Figure 22-2). Cavernous sinus tributaries include cerebral veins and the ophthalmic vein. The cavernous sinus drains along the medial upper layer of the tentorium and through the

Figure 22-2   **Cavernous Sinus and Its Cranial Nerves**

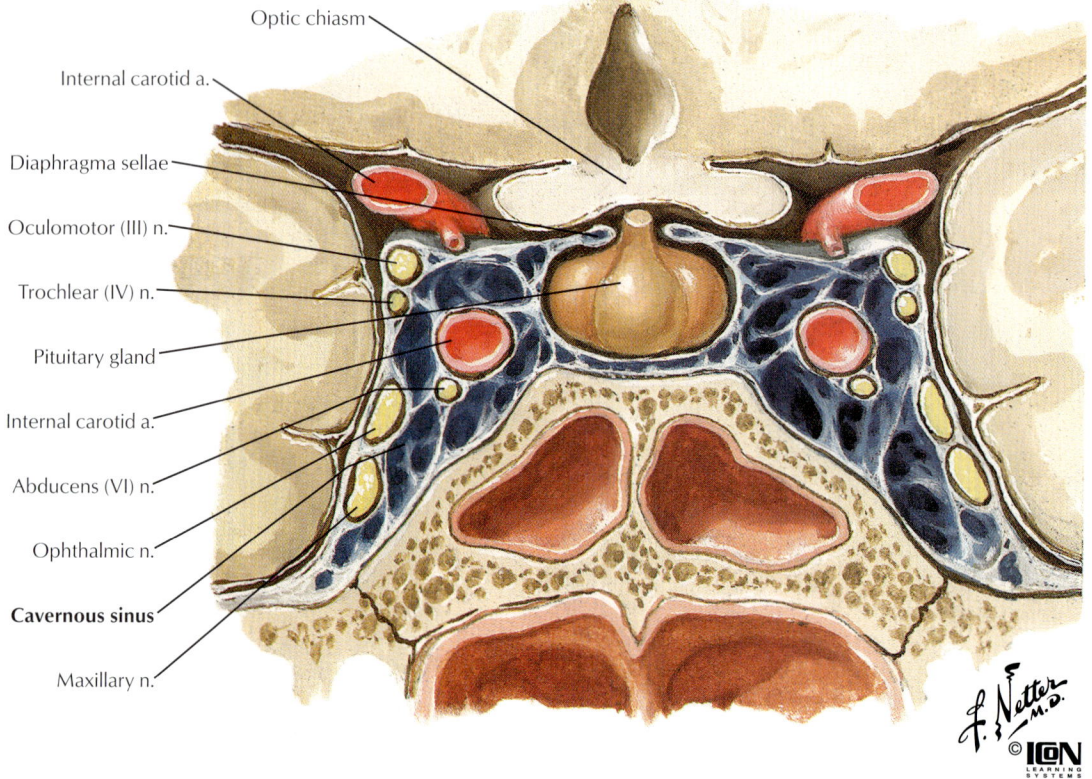

CEREBROVASCULAR DISORDERS

superior petrosal sinus, coursing posteriorly to the transverse sinus. The cavernous sinus houses the carotid artery; the oculomotor, trochlear, and abducens nerves; and the ophthalmic division of the trigeminal nerve. A mesh of venous sinuses around the pituitary and the anterior skull base connects the 2 cavernous sinuses across the midline. The **superior petrosal sinus** drains the anterior brainstem and the anterior superior and inferior cerebellar hemispheres. Below the tentorium, along the skull base, the **inferior petrosal sinus** links the cavernous sinus to the sigmoid sinus (Figure 22-1A).

CLINICAL PRESENTATION

The neurologic presentation is protean; general features depend on the location of venous thrombosis and the abruptness of occlusion. In most patients, the earliest sign is an evolving, constant, diffuse headache that worsens with recumbency. Blurred vision from papilledema is often present but, unless persisting for weeks, rarely leads to significant or permanent visual loss. Sudden brief spells of visual obscuration can occur with abrupt positional changes and are thought to represent transiently decreased perfusion of swollen optic nerves. Slowed cognition or encephalopathy without localized brain lesions or focal neurologic signs may occur with long-standing cerebral thrombosis of gradual evolution.

In patients who have a more abrupt onset of cortical vein or superficial venous sinus thrombosis, cortically based, often hemorrhagic lesions with focal neurologic signs and focal or generalized seizures develop. With involvement of the deep cerebral veins or more than two thirds of the superior sagittal sinus, obtundation, cortical, or decerebrate posturing and coma are the presenting signs. They reflect bihemispheric, bithalamic, basal ganglionic, or brainstem dysfunction. Combinations of painful cranial neuropathies with little involvement of consciousness occur with basal skull (jugular vein, cavernous, or petrosal sinus) sinus thrombosis.

In **superior sagittal sinus thrombosis** (SSST), increased venous pressure from decreased drainage initially causes generalized headaches with paroxysms of pain occurring with any Valsalva-like maneuver, ie, coughing, sneezing, straining, lifting, or bending. Blurred vision may occur secondary to optic nerve head edema or associated exudates involving the macula. Permanent visual compromise is unusual and only happens when papilledema persists for weeks. Light-headedness, transient blindness, and tinnitus can occur with sudden head elevation from lying or bending positions, similar to pseudotumor cerebri.

Intracerebral cortically based hemorrhages, common with SSST, are often associated with focal neurologic signs and seizures. Confusion, behavioral changes, somnolence, and coma may occur as thrombosis propagates within the sinus and ICP increases. These signs usually develop after the clot extends into the posterior third of the sinus. In most SSSTs, one of the lateral sinuses is concomitantly involved (Figure 22-4).

Occasionally, **isolated cortical vein thrombosis** is seen without sagittal sinus involvement. The clinical picture is similar to sagittal sinus thrombosis with headaches, focal neurologic dysfunction, and seizure. However, it lacks increased ICP or papilledema. Underlying causes are similar to sagittal sinus thrombosis, and treatment follows the same principles. Neuroimaging shows isolated, often hemorrhagic, ischemic lesions that do not follow defined arterial territory boundaries.

Deep **cerebral vein thrombosis** is present in 40% of superior sagittal sinus cases. When it is present with SSST, it is more likely to produce coma, pupillary abnormalities, ophthalmoplegia, and increased ICP than SSST alone.

Sole or predominant deep venous system involvement mostly occurs in children but is reported in adults with presentations ranging from isolated drowsiness or obtundation to coma with bilateral posturing and ocular abnormalities. Survivors experience bilateral weakness, rigidity, dystonia or athetosis, memory loss, personality changes, and various neuropsychologic disturbances.

The clinical presentation in a **base of the skull sinus thrombosis** is usually similar to that of painful cranial neuropathies. **Cavernous sinus thrombosis** is often septic from facial, orbital, or middle ear infections (Figure 22-3). It leads to eye pain, proptosis, and chemosis. Varying degrees of ophthalmoplegia are present secondary

CEREBRAL VENOUS THROMBOSIS

Figure 22-3

Intracranial Complications

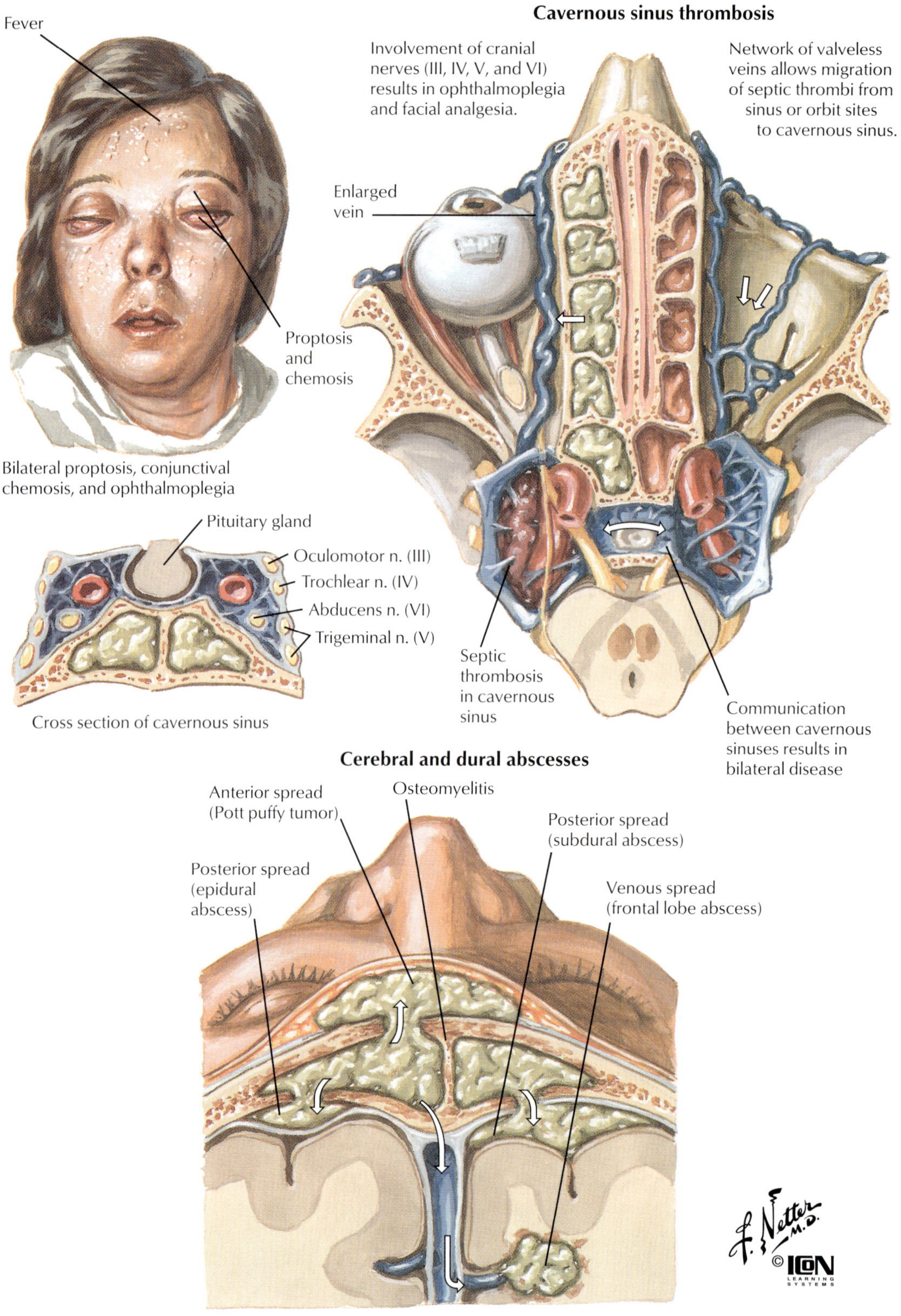

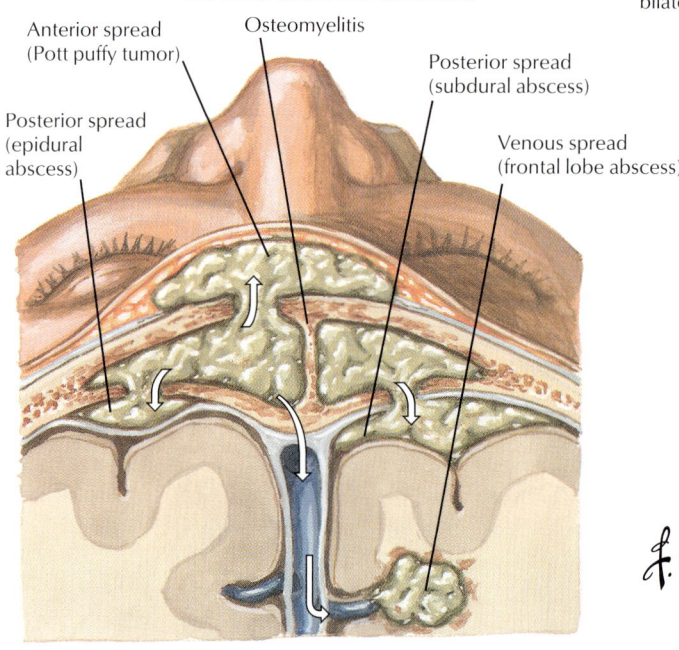

Cavernous sinus thrombosis

Fever

Involvement of cranial nerves (III, IV, V, and VI) results in ophthalmoplegia and facial analgesia.

Network of valveless veins allows migration of septic thrombi from sinus or orbit sites to cavernous sinus.

Enlarged vein

Proptosis and chemosis

Bilateral proptosis, conjunctival chemosis, and ophthalmoplegia

Pituitary gland
Oculomotor n. (III)
Trochlear n. (IV)
Abducens n. (VI)
Trigeminal n. (V)

Cross section of cavernous sinus

Septic thrombosis in cavernous sinus

Communication between cavernous sinuses results in bilateral disease

Cerebral and dural abscesses

Anterior spread (Pott puffy tumor)
Osteomyelitis
Posterior spread (subdural abscess)
Posterior spread (epidural abscess)
Venous spread (frontal lobe abscess)

CEREBROVASCULAR DISORDERS

CEREBRAL VENOUS THROMBOSIS

Figure 22-4   **Sagittal Sinus Thrombosis**

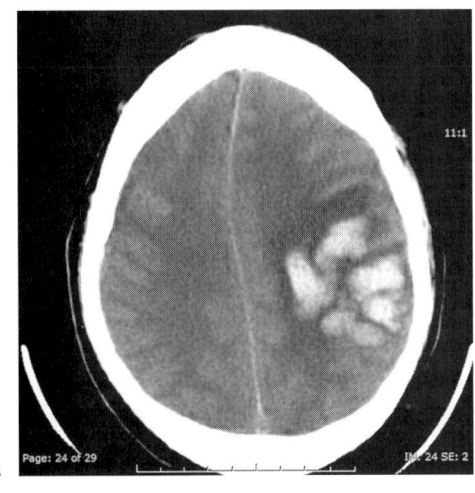
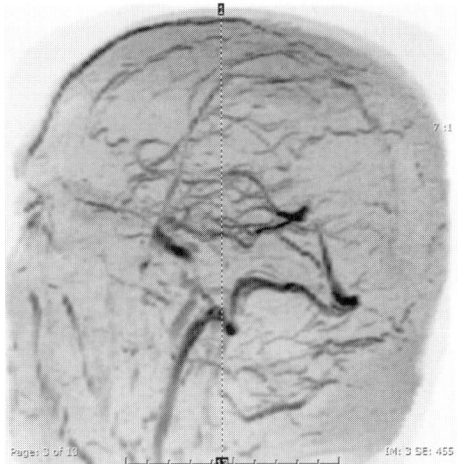
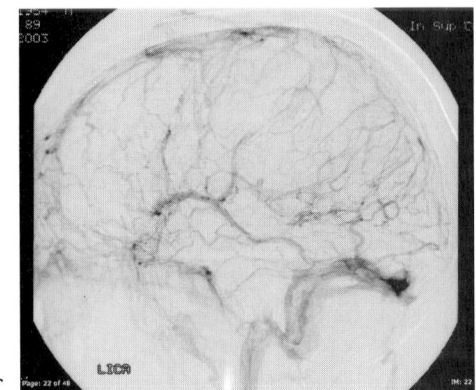
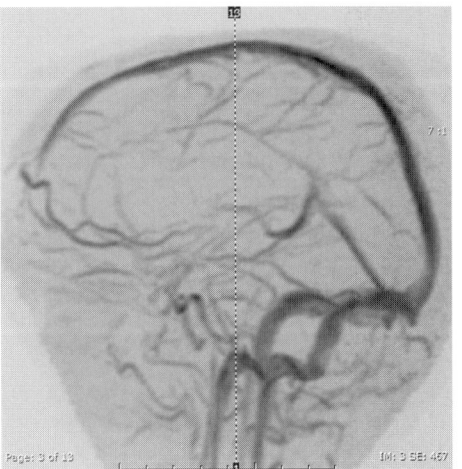

(**A**) CT 2 days after admission showing left posterior frontal parietal patchy hemorrhage within the ischemic region. (**B**) Magnetic resonance venography (MRV) demonstrates absence of flow in posterior sagittal sinus and some cortical veins (arrowheads). (**C**) Digital angiogram, venous phase confirms the MRV findings. (**D**) Normal MRV for comparison.

to involvement of CN-III, -IV, and -VI running through the lateral portion of the cavernous sinus. Because the ophthalmic division of the trigeminal nerve (V1) also courses through this sinus, forehead sensory changes are occasionally seen.

Inferior petrosal sinus thrombosis causes retro-orbital pain, trigeminal V1 sensory changes, and abducens nerve palsy (Gradenigo syndrome; CN-V, -VI). Localized thrombosis involving the internal jugular vein may be an extension of transverse or sigmoid sinus thrombosis or may result from catheterization or trauma. This often presents with CN-IX, -X, and -XI dysfunction (jugular foramen or Vernet syndrome).

DIAGNOSTIC APPROACH

Patients with cerebral venous thrombosis always should be examined for hypercoagulable states. Blood studies should include prothrombin time, partial thromboplastin time, platelet count, protein C and S quantification, lupus anticoagulant, anticardiolipin antibodies, homocysteine levels, and DNA testing for factor V or the Leiden factor and the prothrombin gene mutation.

Cerebral sinus thrombosis is often clinically diagnosed based on a detailed history and corroborating physical findings. Imaging studies confirm the diagnosis and guide treatment.

The pressure and protein content of CSF are increased. RBCs, xanthochromia, and pleocytosis are commonly seen, especially in cases of septic sinus thrombosis or cases associated with meningitis. Normal CSF analysis, although rare, does not exclude the disease.

Acutely, brain CT without contrast is obtained to assess for intracranial hemorrhage. It may reveal irregularly shaped hemorrhagic strokes in the paramedian cortex along the length of the sagittal sinus without conforming to arterial distributions. The "empty delta sign," where contrast partially fills the sinus, leaving an unenhanced island of clot within the occipital confluence, occurs in 50% of cases. Over the brain convexities, thrombosed cortical vessels sometime appear as hyperintense coiled or serpiginous signals. Diffuse edema and narrowed lateral ventricles may be apparent with or without hemorrhagic lesions.

MRI and magnetic resonance venography are standard imaging techniques (Figure 22-4). They have largely replaced angiography in confirming a cerebral sinus thrombosis diagnosis. Cerebral angiography with a prolonged venous phase is reserved for cases not clearly diagnosed by MRI or CT and for consideration of thrombolysis.

TREATMENT

The management of sagittal sinus thrombosis consists of hydration, anticoagulation, and treatment of underlying causes. Early volume repletion is of utmost importance because dehydration enhances clot propagation.

Heparin is given to make partial thromboplastin time double the control value. Anticoagulation is indicated despite hemorrhagic infarctions because the overall outcome is improved and intracranial hemorrhage is rarely worsened. Low-molecular-weight heparin has also been used with safety and efficacy. However, clinical follow-up and repeated brain CT to monitor the size and location of cerebral hemorrhages are advised. Warfarin is given for long-term anticoagulation and is started after 24 hours of heparin treatment or after the patient is stable. When indefinite anticoagulation is not needed, the duration of warfarin treatment remains unclear; accepted practice is 3 to 6 months.

When the precipitating cause is resolved, it is best to confirm that headache and papilledema are controlled and to use magnetic resonance venography to ensure at least partial recanalization of the sagittal sinus before discontinuing oral anticoagulants. Seizures occur in the acute phase in up to 30% of patients; they are usually focal but can be generalized. Recurrent seizures should be treated promptly because they may cause clinical deterioration and increased mortality. Up to 10% of patients may experience pulmonary embolism. This should be suspected with sudden respiratory deterioration and increased oxygen needs.

If deterioration continues despite IV anticoagulation, a more invasive approach with in situ clot thrombolysis is advocated. A femoral venous catheter thread through the jugular vein to the transverse or sagittal sinus is used. An initial attempt at partial thrombolysis is usually followed by a continuous 12-hour intrasinus infusion. Some patients have shown significant neurologic recovery despite increased bleeding complications. Monitoring hematomas remains necessary because expanding hemorrhagic infarcts may cause shift and herniation necessitating acute treatment of increased ICP with osmotic agents or hyperventilation. Surgical evacuation of intracranial hemorrhage is rarely required. To decrease potential bleeding complications, rheolytic mechanical thrombectomy catheters alone or in combination with low doses of thrombolytic agents have been pursued with some success. Numerous cases of thrombolytic treatment show significant clinical improvement even in patients with several hemorrhagic infarcts or days of obtundation or coma.

PROGNOSIS

With anticoagulation, 80% of patients have good recovery, with little or no residual disability. Poor outcomes correlate with deterioration after admission and patients' presenting with coma or obtundation and multiple cerebral hemorrhages, especially if present for days. Before the advent of anticoagulation, the mortality rate was 30% to 50%. A mortality rate of 6% to 10% remains in the acute phase; aggressive treatment with intrasinus thrombolysis may or may not change this.

Long-term complications include focal or generalized seizures, headaches, and papilledema with visual loss, with a 10% rate of occurrence for each. Seizures may necessitate continued anticonvulsant therapy despite resolution of all other symptoms and sinus recanalization. Headache usually resolves with increasing recanalization and better venous drainage and often does not necessitate long-term therapy.

Papilledema should be followed with serial visual fields by an ophthalmologist. If not controlled, progressive visual loss (accurate mid-peripheral field constriction and central visual loss with widening blind spot) is a danger, secondary to gradual optic nerve atrophy. Treatment of papilledema involves lumboperitoneal shunting, serial spinal taps, carbonic anhydrase inhibitors, or optic nerve fenestration into the orbit to relieve locally increased CSF pressure that otherwise would be transmitted to the optic nerve. Optic nerve fenestration is safe, is associated with few complications, and rarely reoccludes. It is done unilaterally, with positive effects on both eyes. The exact mechanism is unknown and is not thought to relate to general reduction of overall CSF pressure because many cases still demonstrate high lumbar puncture pressures after fenestration.

REFERENCES

Baker MD, Opatowsky MJ, Wilson JA, Glazier SS, Morris PP. Rheolytic catheter and thrombolysis of dural venous sinus thrombosis: a case series. *Neurosurgery*. 2001;48:487-494.

De Bruijn SF, De Haan RJ, Stam J. Clinical features and prognostic factors of cerebral venous sinus thrombosis in a prospective series of 59 patients. For The Cerebral Venous Sinus Thrombosis Study Group. *J Neurol Neurosurg Psychiatry*. 2001;70:105-108.

DeBruijn SF, Stam J. Randomized placebo-controlled trial of anticoagulation treatment with low molecular weight heparin for cerebral sinus thrombosis. *Stroke*. 1999;30:481-482.

Einhaupl KM, Villringer A, Meister W, et al. Heparin treatment in sinus venous thrombosis. *Lancet*. 1991;338:597-600.

Ferro JM, Lopes MB, Rosas MJ, Fontes J, Cerebral Venous Thrombosis Portuguese Collaborative Study Group. Long-term prognosis of cerebral vein and dural sinus thrombosis: results of the VENOPORT study. *Cerebrovasc Dis*. 2002;13:272-278.

Haley EC, Brasmear HR, Barth JT, Cail WS, Kassell NF. Deep cerebral venous thrombosis: clinical, neuroradiological and neuropsychological correlates. *Arch Neurol*. 1989;46:337-340.

Horton JC, Seiff SR, Pitts LH, Weinstein PR, Rosenblum ML, Hoyt WF: Decompression of the optic nerve sheath for vision-threatening papilledema caused by dural sinus occlusion. *Neurosurgery*. 1992;31:203-212.

Mehraein S, Schmidtke K, Villringer A, Valdueza JM, Masuhr F. Heparin treatment in cerebral sinus and venous thrombosis: patients at risk of fatal outcome. *Cerebrovasc Dis*. 2003;15:17-21.

Preter M, Tzourio C, Ameri A, et al. Long-term prognosis in cerebral venous thrombosis: follow-up of 77 patients. *Stroke*. 1996;27:243-246.

Wasay M, Bakshi R, Kojan S, Bobustuc G, Dubey N, Unwin DH. Nonrandomized comparison of local urokinase thrombolysis versus systemic heparin anticoagulation for superior sagittal sinus thrombosis. *Stroke*. 2001;32:2310-2317.

Chapter 23
Intracerebral Hemorrhage

Kinan K. Hreib and H. Royden Jones, Jr

Clinical Vignette

A 72-year-old woman with history of hypertension noticed tingling in her right arm. Within 30 minutes, her right leg buckled and she fell. Her husband helped her up. She was able to walk without support. She rested, but within an hour, she noted speech difficulties and more definite right-sided weakness.

She was brought to the ED and was noted to have mild right arm weakness and some word-finding difficulties. Her blood pressure was 140/80 mm Hg. She got up to go to the bathroom, walked approximately 10 ft, and collapsed on the floor. She was then globally aphasic, with left gaze deviation (ie, paralysis of gaze to the right) and right hemiplegia. Within 10 minutes, she became unresponsive.

She underwent intubation and was taken for brain CT, which demonstrated a large left putaminal hemorrhage. Soon thereafter, she had bilaterally dilated unresponsive pupils. The vestibular-ocular reflex was lost. Within another 10 minutes, she was determined brain dead.

The preceding vignette demonstrates the classic presentation of a primary intracerebral hemorrhage (ICH), one of the most common forms of cerebral hemorrhage, with a rapidly evolving focal neurologic deficit. Its progressively increasing size led to increased intracranial pressure with downward herniation of the uncus onto the brainstem and irreversible neurologic damage. The only means to avoid this untreatable condition is appropriate therapy of hypertension, its major risk factor.

There are 2 forms of intrinsic cerebral hemorrhage, primary ICH, which has a predilection to affect the striatum, thalamus, midbrain, pons, and cerebellum, and subarachnoid hemorrhage (chapter 24). Together, they comprise approximately 10% of all strokes, although improved control of hypertension has decreased the number of patients experiencing ICH.

Better recognition of "warning leaks" has somewhat improved early diagnosis and made successful treatment of some patients possible before a major hemorrhage, with its 50% mortality rate, occurs. Most cerebral aneurysms are related to both congenital and acquired factors. Typically, berry aneurysms arise at the bifurcations of major proximal vessels within the carotid and vertebrobasilar circulations, such as the anterior communicating, middle cerebral, posterior communicating, and top of the basilar arteries (Figure 23-1). In contrast, mycotic aneurysms that typically are acquired, mainly from septic emboli of infective endocarditis, are found more distally within the cerebral circulation.

PATHOPHYSIOLOGY

Intracranial hemorrhage is a rapidly evolving process that may progress over hours or days. The pressure effects of the initial hemorrhage lead to additional bleeding from surrounding vessels that were not involved within the first bleed. This cascade causes growth of the hematoma. The underlying pathology responsible for a primary ICH is attributable to either of 2 processes: miliary aneurysms or primary degeneration of the blood vessel smooth muscle medial wall layer. The presence of miliary aneurysms is directly related to hypertension (Figure 23-2). With degeneration of the smooth muscle wall, an ICH may occur without development of a miliary aneurysm. Other factors, yet undiscovered, may also contribute to ICH development or conversely protect some individuals from having a hemorrhage, despite the presence of hypertension. Most primary ICHs are attributed to degeneration of the cerebral blood vessel wall, creating the hematoma.

INTRACEREBRAL HEMORRHAGE

Figure 23-1

Typical Sites of Cerebral Aneurysms

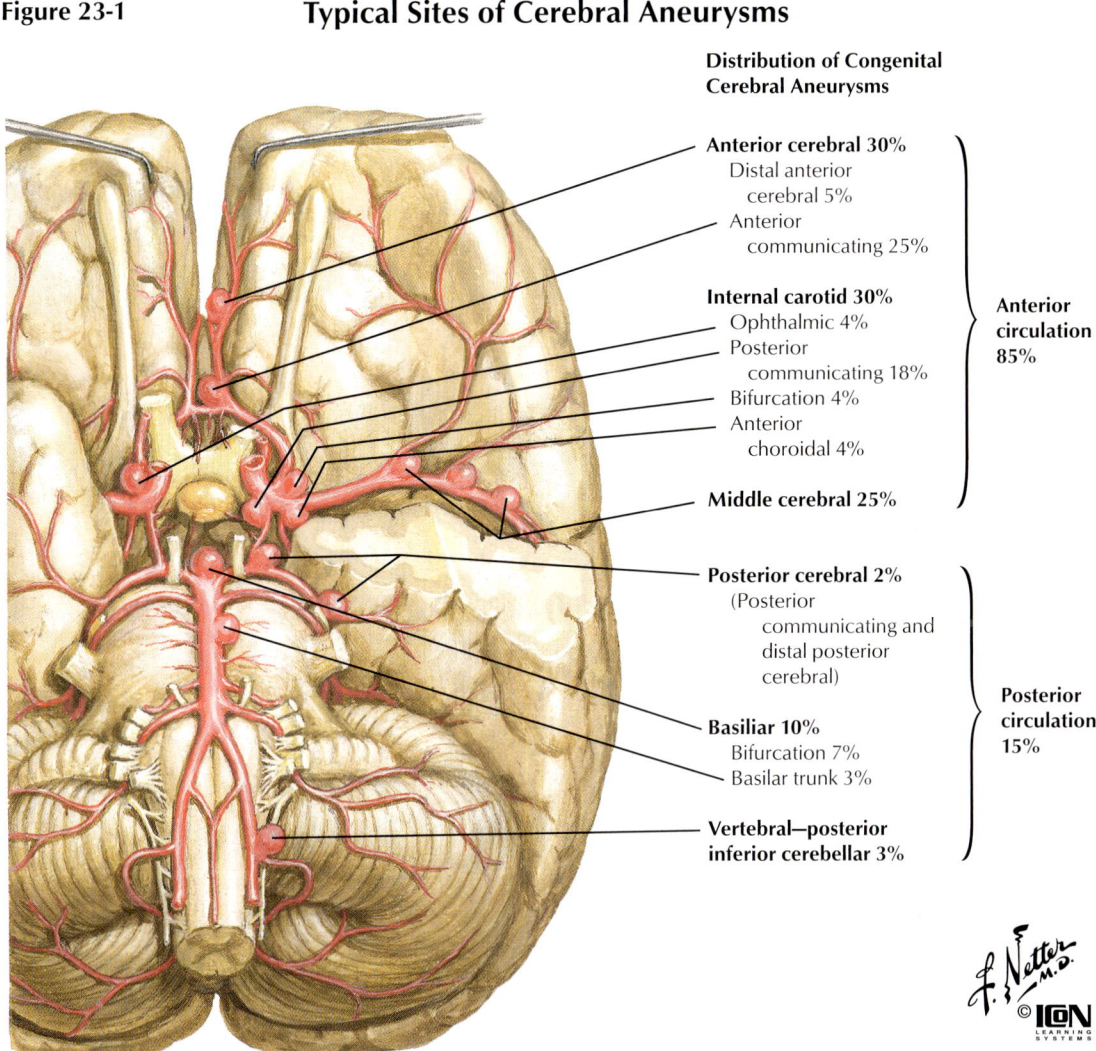

Distribution of Congenital Cerebral Aneurysms

- **Anterior cerebral 30%**
  - Distal anterior cerebral 5%
  - Anterior communicating 25%
- **Internal carotid 30%**
  - Ophthalmic 4%
  - Posterior communicating 18%
  - Bifurcation 4%
  - Anterior choroidal 4%
- **Middle cerebral 25%**

} Anterior circulation 85%

- **Posterior cerebral 2%** (Posterior communicating and distal posterior cerebral)
- **Basilar 10%**
  - Bifurcation 7%
  - Basilar trunk 3%
- **Vertebral–posterior inferior cerebellar 3%**

} Posterior circulation 15%

Intracranial hemorrhage contrasts with hemorrhagic brain infarct (HBI), where hemorrhage is secondary to an embolic cerebral infarct. When the embolus initially obstructs the specific artery, there is brain ischemia, and the distal portion of the same vessel wall becomes ischemic. Subsequently, when the embolus fragments and passes through the ischemic portion of the vessel, the endothelium of the vascular wall and the endothelium of the blood-brain barrier are compromised from ischemia. Therefore, the affected vessel no longer tolerates normal arterial perfusion pressures. Subsequent reperfusion into the damaged brain leads to leakage and sometimes gross hemorrhage through the damaged vessel into the recently infarcted brain. It is estimated that a petechial HBI, which allows leakage of erythrocytes into the brain, develops in 50% to 80% of patients with embolic infarcts. Although it is often implied that cardioembolic strokes are more likely to be associated with development an HBI, some investigators suggest that any large infarct, regardless of mechanism, may predispose to development of an HBI. The use of IV heparin may also

CEREBROVASCULAR DISORDERS

INTRACEREBRAL HEMORRHAGE

Figure 23-2   **Intracerebral Hemorrhage (Hypertensive): Pathogenesis**

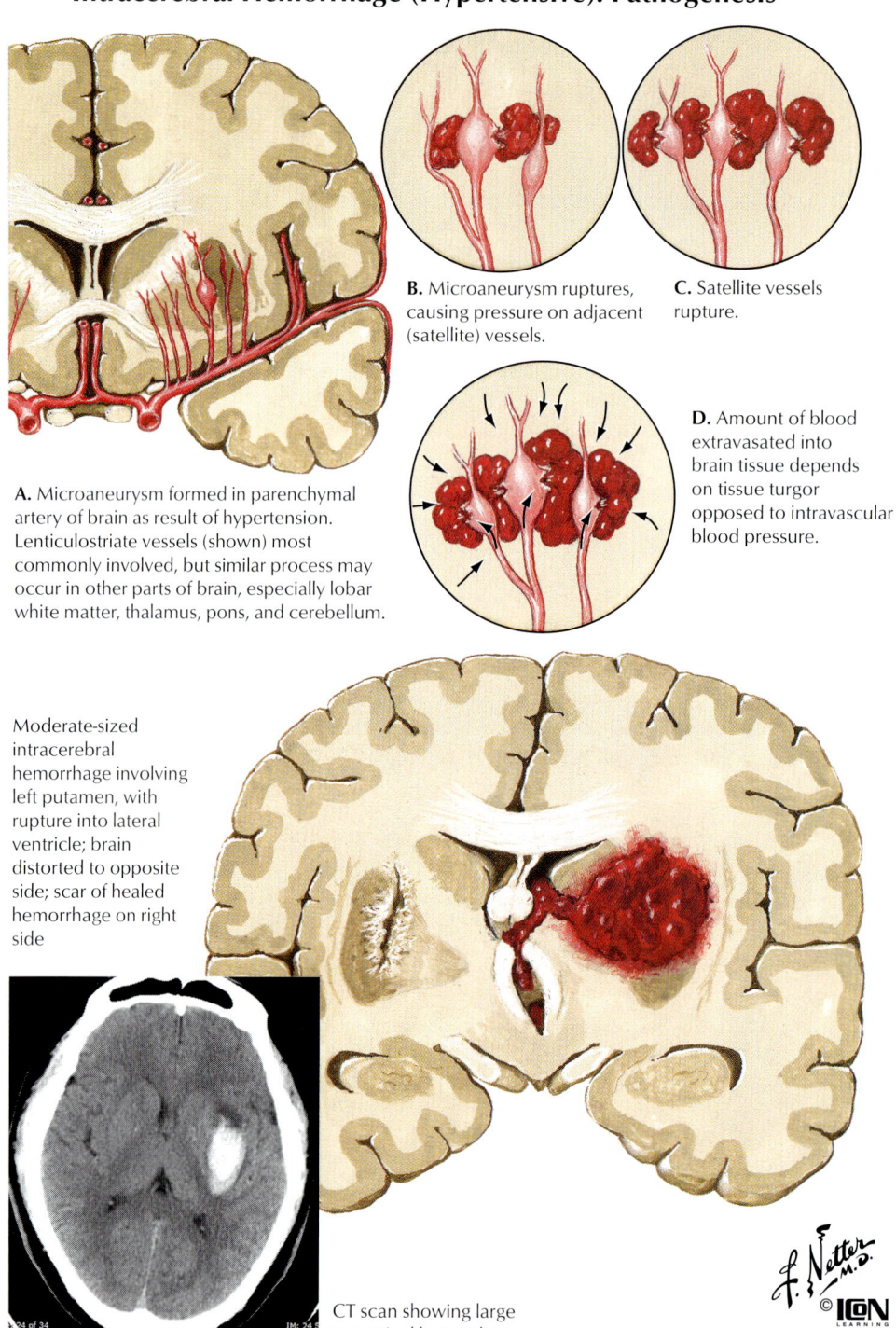

A. Microaneurysm formed in parenchymal artery of brain as result of hypertension. Lenticulostriate vessels (shown) most commonly involved, but similar process may occur in other parts of brain, especially lobar white matter, thalamus, pons, and cerebellum.

B. Microaneurysm ruptures, causing pressure on adjacent (satellite) vessels.

C. Satellite vessels rupture.

D. Amount of blood extravasated into brain tissue depends on tissue turgor opposed to intravascular blood pressure.

Moderate-sized intracerebral hemorrhage involving left putamen, with rupture into lateral ventricle; brain distorted to opposite side; scar of healed hemorrhage on right side

CT scan showing large putaminal hemorrhage

CEREBROVASCULAR DISORDERS

promote the development of HBI. However, the presence of petechial hemorrhage does not seem to worsen neurologic outcome. Few patients with embolic stroke have a true cerebral hemorrhage at the infarct site, although the precise incidence is unknown.

The highest risk for ICH is in persons older than 65 years. The incidence of ICH corresponds to 7% and 11% of all strokes, according to the Framingham Study and Lausanne, Switzerland Stroke Registry, respectively.

CLINICAL PRESENTATION

Intraparenchymal hemorrhages vary in presentation depending on the site of the bleed (Figure 23-3). In approximately 60% of patients, neurologic symptoms develop gradually or stepwise over a period of hours. To some extent, the location and size of the hematoma predict clinical outcome. Some small hemorrhages lead to significant long-term deficits due to disconnection syndromes.

Headache occurs at presentation in approximately 40% of patients with an ICH. It is uncommon for a headache to occur subsequently even within a few days after the ictus. The ICHs most commonly presenting with headache are located at the brain surface and within the cerebellum. Depression of consciousness level and vomiting occur in 50% of patients, particularly those with large cerebellar bleeds. Seizures occur at onset in up to 10% of individuals with ICH; most commonly, they occur with bleeds in the anterior circulation, especially with lobar hemorrhages. However, even patients with deep hemorrhages can have seizures. The subsequent risk for seizures in ICH patients is up to 29% for those with lobar hemorrhages but only 4% for those with deep hemorrhages. Other symptoms include fever without obvious infection. A description of some of the most common symptoms at different sites of ICH follows.

Supratentorial Hemorrhage

Putaminal Hemorrhages

The most common ICH, putaminal hemorrhages, are usually classified into anterior, middle, and posterior lesions. **Anterior putaminal** hemorrhage often causes motor weakness. If the ICH is on in the left, abulia and aphasia are common accompaniments. When the lesion occurs on the right, significant behavioral changes often occur, including disinhibition, poor insight and judgment, and occasionally violent behavior. Metabolic studies suggest that these symptoms result from disconnection from the frontal lobe. Often, deficits from anterior putaminal hemorrhages are reversible. Similarly, hemorrhages within the caudate can lead to cognitive and behavioral problems thought to relate to disconnection from the frontal cortex.

A hemorrhage within the **midputamen** results in severe deficits, often with poor recovery. Here, the ICH compresses and undercuts nearby cortical structures, causing global aphasia if involving the left hemisphere and severe neglect if involving the right.

With a **posterior putaminal** hemorrhage, a combination of sensory deficits, visual field difficulties, limb ataxia, and behavioral changes often results. Some putaminal hemorrhages present with abnormal, although often short-lived, movements. Some large putaminal hemorrhages, or smaller hemorrhages that are medially located, dissect toward the ventricle, with resultant intraventricular hemorrhage. For example, a striatal ICH within the head of the caudate may present with rapid deterioration due to increased intracranial pressure from blood leaking into the ventricular system. Primary intraventricular hemorrhage does not affect surrounding brain tissue. Most cases present as rapidly progressive neurologic syndromes with nausea, vomiting, stupor, and seizure. In less acute cases, the patient may present with headaches, confusion, and somnolence.

Thalamic Hemorrhages

Clinically, thalamic ICHs are classified into posterior-inferior, posterior-lateral, and dorsal-medial. Somnolence is one of the most common presentations of **medial-posterior and inferior thalamic bleeds**. Profound somnolence is usually the result of bilateral involvement with probable damage to the reticular activating system, but often, persistent hypokinetic behavior can result from disconnection from the frontal lobe.

With **inferior-lateral thalamic** hemorrhage, there is some weakness and clumsiness and, occasionally, tremors and choreoathetoid move-

INTRACEREBRAL HEMORRHAGE

Figure 23-3

Intracerebral Hemorrhage: Clinical Manifestations Related to Site

Pathology	CT scan	Pupils	Eye movements	Motor and sensory deficits	Other
Caudate nucleus (blood in ventricle)		Sometimes ipsilaterally constricted	Conjugate deviation to side of lesion; slight ptosis	Contralateral hemiparesis, often transient	Headache, confusion
Putamen (small hemorrhage)		Normal	Conjugate deviation to side of lesion	Contralateral hemiparesis and hemisensory loss	Aphasia (if lesion on left side)
Putamen (large hemorrhage)		In presence of herniation, pupil dialated on side of lesion	Conjugate deviation to side of lesion	Contralateral hemiparesis and hemisensory loss	Decreased consciousness
Thalamus		Constricted, poorly reactive to light bilaterally	Both lids retracted; eyes positioned downward and medially; cannot look upward	Slight contralateral hemiparesis, but greater hemisensory loss	Aphasia (if lesion on left side)
Occipital lobar white matter		Normal	Normal	Mild, transient hemiparesis	Contralateral hemianopsia
Pons		Constricted, reactive to light	No horizontal movements; vertical movements preserved	Quadriplegia	Coma
Cerebellum		Slight constriction on side of lesion	Slight deviation to opposite side; movements toward side of lesion impaired, or sixth cranial nerve palsy	Ipsilateral limb ataxia; no hemiparesis	Gait ataxia, vomiting

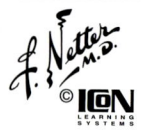

CEREBROVASCULAR DISORDERS

ments. Tremors are likely related to disruption of projections from the cerebellum and dentate nucleus. Disruption of the fibers of the ansa lenticularis are likely responsible for the choreoathetoid movements.

More **lateral thalamic** hemorrhages involving the ventral posteromedial and ventral posterolateral thalamic nuclei usually primarily cause unilateral sensory symptoms but occasionally motor involvement when the hemorrhage extends laterally to involve the internal capsule. Eye movement abnormalities, small pupils, ptosis, chorea, and dystonia also occur.

Hematomas involving the **dorsal-medial thalamic** area usually cause prominent memory problems and behavioral changes thought to relate to dissociated frontal cortex, cingulate gyrus, and amygdalar connections.

Speech and language deficits are the least consistent symptoms of thalamic hemorrhages. Paraphasia, naming difficulties, or a perceived inability to comprehend, with preservation of repetition, is typical of **thalamic aphasia**. In patients with right thalamic hemorrhage, deficits are often similar to those observed in patients with cortical involvement such as neglect, depending on the size of the hematoma. Vivid hallucinations, visual and less often auditory, can occur in the days after an ICH.

Lobar Hemorrhages

After the putamen, the most common site for a primary hemorrhage is one of the 4 major parts of the cerebral cortex. The parietal and occipital areas are most frequently involved. Evidence is inconclusive on whether a difference exists in the contribution of hypertension to lobar versus subcortical hemorrhages. Primary amyloid angiopathy is another frequent nonhypertensive mechanism for intracerebral lobar hemorrhage. Other less common causes include vascular malformations, primary and metastatic malignancies, sympathomimetic drugs, anticoagulants, irreversible antiplatelet and fibrinolytic agents, and sinus thrombosis.

Typically missed by angiography and diagnosed at pathologic inspection after the hematoma removal, occult vascular malformations are possibly the most underdiagnosed causes of lobar hemorrhages. The most common occult vascular lesions include small AVMs and cavernous angiomas.

Lobar hemorrhages often present with headaches and vomiting. Seizures at the onset of lobar hemorrhage are common, particularly with posterior parietal or frontal lobe hemorrhages. Functionally, patients with lobar hemorrhage may have better outcomes than those with deep hemorrhages. However, prognosis depends on hematoma size, level of consciousness, and presence of intraventricular blood. Mortality rates range from 12% to 30% compared with 25% to 42% in deep basal ganglionic and thalamic hemorrhages and up to 97% in pontine hemorrhages.

Frontal ICHs. Intracranial hemorrhages in the superior aspect of the frontal lobe are usually smaller and cause weakness to the contralateral leg. Inferior frontal hemorrhages are larger, causing a depressed level of consciousness, hemiplegia, hemisensory deficits, and horizontal gaze paresis. Language can also be affected. Apathy and abulia can occur and may be prominent.

Parietal Hematomas. Often, the most striking clinical presentation is a cortical neglect syndrome, with hemorrhage in the right hemisphere. However, because extension into subcortical areas often occurs, weakness and a true hemianopsia may be present. More medial hemorrhages can cause altered consciousness early in the ICH course.

Occipital Hematomas. Although headaches are prominent in many lobar hemorrhages, those occurring with occipital hemorrhage are particularly severe. The most obvious neurologic deficit is homonymous hemianopsia. Few patients present with other visual changes, including flashes of bright lights and palinopsia (afterimages). Other deficits indicative of more anterior hemorrhage include extinction, dysgraphia, and dyslexia. An occipital hematoma is the least likely ICH to be related to hypertension.

Temporal Hematomas. Neurologic deficits in temporal hematomas depend on whether the dominant side is involved and whether there is extension into the surrounding subcortical areas or adjacent frontal lobe. Fluent aphasia is the most prominent deficit from isolated left temporal lobe hemorrhage, often associated with paraphasia and poor comprehension. In contrast, right temporal hemorrhages are often associated with relatively minor problems, most commonly confusion.

Infratentorial Hemorrhages
Cerebellar Hemorrhage

Clinical Vignette

A 58-year-old woman with substantial history of arterial hypertension presented to the ED with a 1-hour duration of acute-onset headache, gait unsteadiness, and left arm incoordination.

On examination, the patient was alert and oriented but had left-sided dysmetria, gait ataxia, and left-sided CN-VI and CN-VII palsies. Her BP was 200/110 mm Hg. STAT head CT showed a 3-cm cerebellar hemorrhage with slight compression of the fourth ventricle. Antihypertensive treatment aiming for a MAP of 100 to 120 mm Hg was initiated.

Within 30 minutes after the CT, the patient's level of consciousness deteriorated, necessitating intubation. She was brought immediately to the operating room for evacuation of the hematoma and responded well. One month later, her examination results were remarkable; only mild clumsiness on her left arm and a slight wide-based gait persisted.

Patients with cerebellar hemorrhages can deteriorate rapidly, even "in front of one's eyes," as in the preceding vignette, but can respond exceptionally well with very expeditious surgical intervention. Most cerebellar hemorrhages are associated with hypertension. However, approximately 10% of primary cerebellar hemorrhages are caused by AVM, tumors, and blood dyscrasias, most often associated with the use of warfarin. Headache, spinning vertigo, nausea, vomiting, and, most commonly, unsteady gait characterize the typical presentation. Some headaches are occipital, but many involve the orbital and supraorbital areas. The most reliable symptoms of a hemispheric cerebellar hemorrhage include ipsilateral limb ataxia and ipsilateral peripheral CN-VI and CN-VII palsies with horizontal nystagmus.

The less common vermian hemorrhages often resemble a pontine hemorrhage. However, because they often progress rapidly to coma, it is difficult to know what specific early clinical signs are predictive. Cranial nerve palsies are related to involvement of adjacent pontine structures or nerve stretching secondary to increased cerebellar pressure. In hypertensive bleeds involving the vermis or the cerebellar hemispheres, the superior cerebellar artery is most often involved.

Unlike supratentorial bleeds, in which a small hemorrhage is often well tolerated, infratentorial ICH within the posterior fossa often leads to rapid neurologic deterioration and death. Patients with hemorrhages larger than 3 cm may deteriorate rapidly with development of an acute hydrocephalus. With a cerebellar bleed, there is also a risk of rebleeding, a rupture into the fourth ventricle, and hemorrhagic edema development, which, in combination, often lead to a devastating outcome. Patients with hemorrhage or ischemic infarct in the cerebellum must be treated in the ICU with close attention to any worsening of neurologic function, including incipient signs of increased intracranial pressure. Most commonly, deterioration occurs within 36 hours. However, a few reports describe deterioration more than 10 days after the initial hemorrhage, attesting to the need for ongoing close observations and sometimes more aggressive treatment.

The threshold should be low for evacuating a hematoma or necrotic tissue that has created an acute cerebellar mass. The major goal is decompression of the posterior fossa to prevent blockage of the fourth ventricle and compression of the adjacent brainstem. Fortunately, if impending brainstem compression is recognized early, there are often only minimal residual deficits, subsequent to surgery, even with extensive cerebellar evacuation and decompression. The potentially positive recovery reflects that intracerebellar hemorrhages typically spare the deep cerebellar nuclei from direct damage, as does the surgical procedure.

Pontine/Midbrain Hemorrhage

Pontine and midbrain hemorrhages are relatively uncommon but have the most devastating outcome compared with other sites of primary intracranial hemorrhages. Three distinct vascular territories in the pons dictate the clinical presentation. The **paramedian penetrators**, arising directly from the basilar trunk, are the primary arteries supplying the midline pons or midbrain within this anatomical site. ICH here causes bilateral damage and thus is often fatal.

Another group of small arteries, the **short penetrators**, courses laterally, supplying the lateral basis pontis, where a hemorrhage may predominantly cause unilateral bulbar symptoms, including profound dysphagia. The third important group supplying the pons, the **long circumferential arteries**, arises from the anterior inferior cerebellar artery and primarily supplies the lateral tegmentum. ICH within this segment sometimes leads to relatively minor symptoms, including facial numbness and ataxia secondary to involvement of the spinal trigeminal and vestibular nuclei. However, if some of the nearby intrinsic pontine nuclei, such as the cochlear and facial nuclei, are also affected, a more serious outcome results.

Clinical presentation of pontine hemorrhages often has a relatively gradual course evolving over hours. Neurologic deficits, including horizontal gaze paresis, small sluggish pupils, quadriparesis, and coma, are the expected clinical signs. Additionally, certain unique eye findings, including ocular bobbing and the one-and-a-half syndrome, provide excellent diagnostic clues to pontine ICH. Some patients also experience twitching of the limbs and face. Rippling of torso muscles and an irregular breathing pattern and pulse, with an increase in body temperature, have also been observed. Vivid, sometimes frightening hallucinations of moving human figures, called **peduncular hallucinosis**, occur relatively often in patients whose ICHs involve the tegmentum.

DIFFERENTIAL DIAGNOSIS

Many systemic disorders predispose to the occurrence of an ICH; hypertension is the most common associated illness (Tables 23-1 and 23-2 and Figures 23-4 and 25-5). Although hypertension is considered an important risk factor for ICH, studies are inconsistent in estimating the risk of hypertension as a primary ICH cause. Some suggest that up to 90% of patients had hypertension at the time of ICH, whereas others suggest only 25% of ICHs truly result from hypertension. Other important risk factors include smoking, alcohol consumption, black race, and

Table 23-1
Common Causes of Intracerebral Hemorrhage

1. Primary intracerebral hemorrhage
    Hypertension
    Idiopathic
2. Aneurysm
    AVM
    Cavernous angioma
3. Embolic infarct
4. Anticoagulant therapy

Table 23-2
Uncommon Causes of Intracerebral Hemorrhage*

1. Endocarditis
2. Venous sinus thrombosis
3. Malignancy: primary, metastatic
4. Blood diathesis
    DIC, ITP, TTP
    Leukemia
    Multiple myeloma
    Sickle cell disease
5. Other hematologic disorders, particularly coagulopathies
    Hemophilia
    von Willebrand factor deficiency
    Afibrinogenemia
6. Vasculitis
    Polyarteritis nodosa
    Systemic lupus erythematosus
    Wegener granulomatosis
    Takayasu arteritis
    Temporal arteritis
    Chemical vasculitis
    Primary CNS vasculitis
    Sympathomimetics (amphetamine, cocaine, phenylpropanolamine)
7. Systemic disorders
    Sarcoidosis
    Behçet syndrome
    CNS infectious, particularly herpes zoster
8. Trauma

*DIC indicates disseminated intravascular coagulation; ITP, idiopathic thrombocytopenia; TTP, thrombotic thrombocytopenia.

INTRACEREBRAL HEMORRHAGE

Figure 23-4   ## Common Causes of Intracerebral Hemorrhage
Thalamic Hemorrhage Secondary to AVM

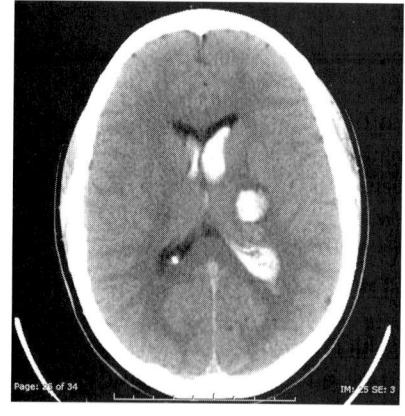
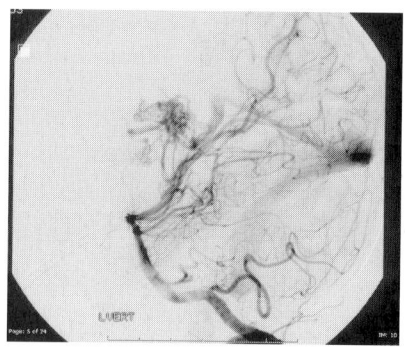

(**A**) CT with thalamic hemorrhage and blood in ventricles. (**B**) Lateral vertebral angiogram with thalamic AVM.

Cavernous Hemangioma

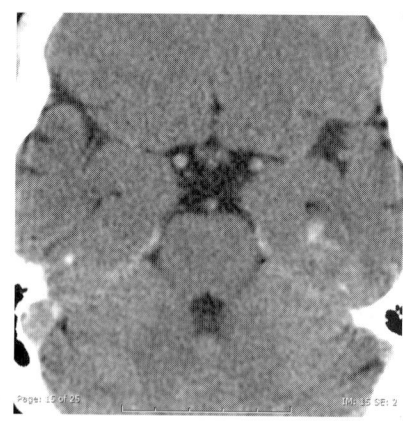
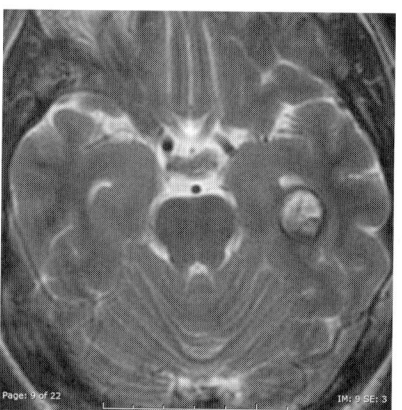

(**C**) CT with small acute hemorrhage. (**D**) T2-weighted MR with variable intensity pattern and black halo (paramagnetic effect of iron, Fe^{3+}).

Infarct With Late Petechial Hemorrhage

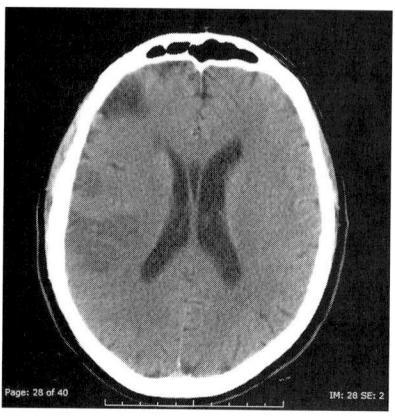
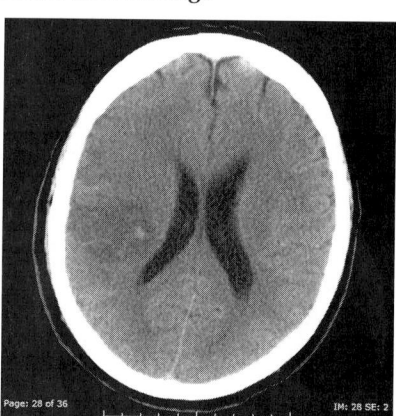

(**E**) CT of early infarct shows lucency caused by infarct. (**F**) CT 2 days after showing small hemorrhage within the infarct.

INTRACEREBRAL HEMORRHAGE

Figure 23-5   Uncommon Causes of Intracerebral Hemorrhage

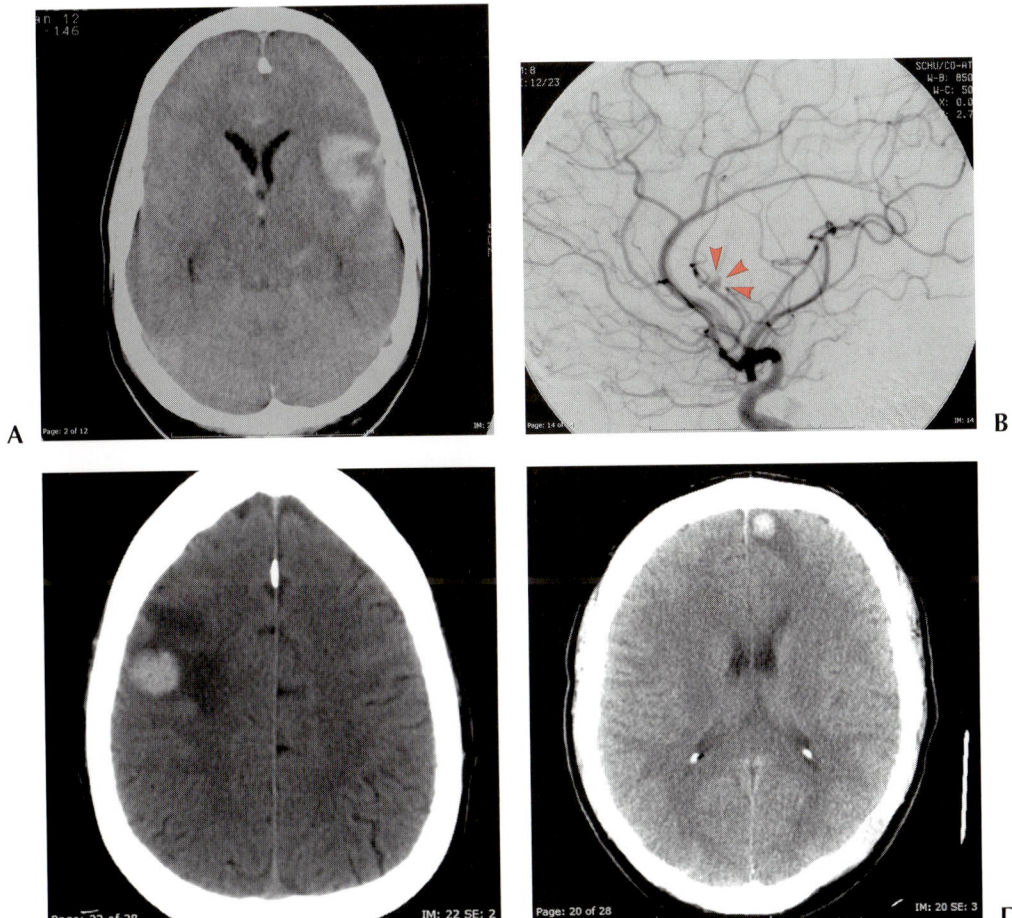

(**A**) CT with blood in left sylvian fissure. (**B**) Lateral left internal carotid angiogram with small distal MCA aneurysm (arrowheads). (**C**) CT showing dense right frontal subcortical mass with edema representing a hemorrhagic colon cancer metastases. (**D**) CT showing small left frontal hemorrhage in a patient with leukemia and bleeding diathesis.

low total serum cholesterol levels. Patients who sustained an ICH and concomitantly had low serum cholesterol levels also had high diastolic pressure. This association suggests that low cholesterol may weaken the arterial wall and, with increased blood pressure, cause its deterioration.

When hypertension is not an important risk factor for the ICH, imaging studies are essential to investigate the possibilities of underlying predisposing pathology, such as tumors (Table 23-3), AVMs, and cavernous angiomas. Imaging studies such as CT and MRI are often performed in the acute setting, and follow-up studies may help with the diagnosis. A single small hemorrhage from a metastatic lesion may be difficult to diagnose at presentation. Melanoma and hypernephromas are hemorrhagic tumors that may be confused with a primary ICH unless evidence of other lesions is identified. They may suggest metastatic disease or previous bleeds from amyloid angiography.

Atypical ICH location must prompt further investigations to exclude systemic disorders. Fol-

INTRACEREBRAL HEMORRHAGE

Table 23-3
Tumors Causing Intracerebral Hemorrhage*

Primary CNS	Metastatic
Mixed glioma	Melanoma
Epidermoid cyst	Kidney
Pituitary adenoma	Lung
Oligodendroglioma	Breast
Ependymoma	Osteogenic sarcoma
Choroid plexus papilloma	Ovary
Meningioma	Colon
Craniopharyngioma	
Glioblastoma	
Astrocytoma	

*In order of frequency.

low-up studies using contrast are often helpful. A detailed dermatologic examination may reveal irregularly pigmented lesions suggesting melanoma, and ultrasound may reveal a renal tumor. Generally, however, follow-up studies may be diagnostic only after blood has been reabsorbed and changing signal characteristics allow the underlying lesion to be more evident.

Antithrombotic- and Anticoagulant-Induced ICH

Whether the use of aspirin promotes ICH is unclear, but the Physician's Health Study report suggested increased risk. There were 13 hemorrhagic strokes in the treatment group and 6 in the placebo group, but this increase was not seen in many other clinical trials testing the benefits of aspirin for the prevention of stroke. Several trials using warfarin for stroke prevention in patients with atrial fibrillation have demonstrated intracerebral bleeding rates of 0.5 to 1.8 per year. The highest risk for bleeding was seen in patients older than 75 years. The combination of coumadin and aspirin suggested similar rates of systemic bleeding, approximately 2.4 per year, and no difference in rates of ICH. The use of intravenous heparin in the setting of acute stroke has not been systematically studied.

A few studies have suggested no risk of ICH or a risk of approximately 2%, especially when heparin is used in the setting of an acute stroke. The International Stroke Trial used subcutaneous heparin at 12,500 U twice daily versus 5000 U twice daily or a combination of subcutaneous heparin and aspirin. At 14 days, the risk of ICH was 1.8% for the high heparin dose and 0.7% for the low heparin dose. Rates were similar when heparin was combined with aspirin. Even heparinoid formulation in stroke treatment has shown a risk of ICH of 2.4% versus 0.8% for controls.

Amyloid Angiopathy

Amyloid angiopathy, an uncommon vasculopathy, is considered a significant risk factor for spontaneous ICH in the elderly. However, in North America, as a cause for ICH, it is documented in patients as young as 60 years. In the familial forms of amyloid angiopathy reported in Icelandic and Dutch families, the mean age for ICH occurrence is as young as 30 years. Unlike primary ICH, amyloid angiopathy leads to minor and large hemorrhages within the cortex and the corona radiata. It routinely spares the basal ganglia, the thalamus, and the brainstem. In contrast, in the familial forms of amyloid angiopathy, an ICH may also affect the brainstem, the cerebellum, and the more typical cortical and subcortical loci.

Many patients present with MRI evidence of previous asymptomatic small hemorrhages; typically, patients recover from these small hemorrhages (Figure 23-6). However, a succession of small intracranial hemorrhages within a short time period can cause death. In some patients, the presence of subcortical white matter disease may be a reflection of chronic ischemia from amyloid-laden arterioles. On MRI and CT scans, these changes may suggest a higher risk for future hemorrhages and therefore a more cautionary approach to anticoagulation or the potential use of thrombolytic agents.

Endocarditis

The true incidence of endocarditis is unknown. Rheumatic heart disease was formerly

INTRACEREBRAL HEMORRHAGE

Figure 23-6   Amyloid Angiopathy

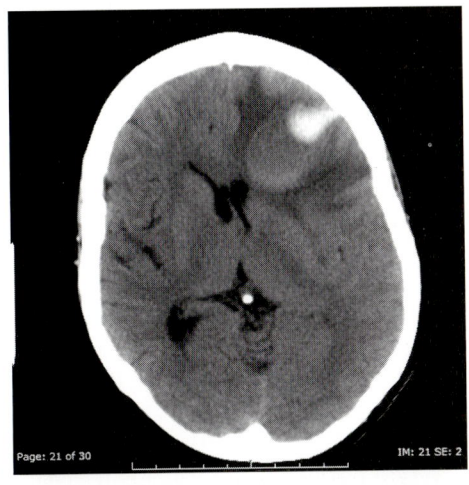
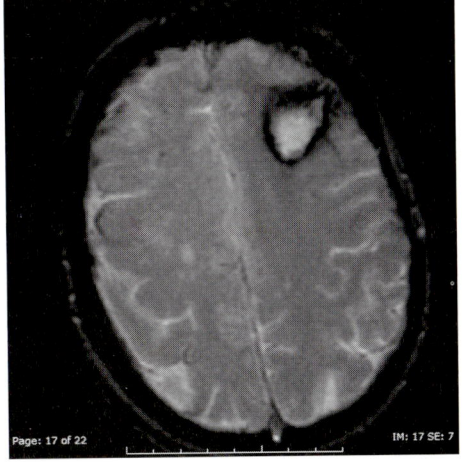

(**A**) CT with moderate-sized left frontal hematoma with edema. (**B**) GRE MRI shows high-intensity lesion with a hypointense rim representing blood products. (**C**) GRE MRI showing multiple small paramagnetic lesions consistent with multiple small previous hemorrhages (arrows).

the primary cause of bacterial endocarditis; the most common agent was *Streptococcus viridans*. More virulent forms of endocarditis emerged as the use of intravenous drugs increased. Furthermore, the use of implanted long-term catheters or other similar devices during routine hospital stays, particularly in patients who are immunocompromised, has increased the risk of infections. *Staphylococcus aureus* and fungal infections are surpassing streptococcal bacteria as causes for valvular infection.

Mitral and aortic valves are especially vulnerable. The mitral valve is more consistently associated with neurologic complications than is the aortic valve. In one study, more than 28% of those with bacterial endocarditis had neurologic complications. Mortality was 77% with staphylococcal infections and 36% with streptococcal infections. Cerebral infarctions occurred in 50% of patients, ICH occurred in 2.1%, and subarachnoid hemorrhage occurred in 0.8%.

Intracerebral hemorrhage in bacterial endocarditis is usually located superficially in the more distal vessels rather than at the primary vessel source near the base of the brain, as with berry aneurysms. However, the more peripheral locations are not protective, because ICHs there are no less devastating than the more typical deeper hemorrhages. The presumed hemorrhage mechanism is a ruptured mycotic

CEREBROVASCULAR DISORDERS

aneurysm. However, this type of lesion may be present in only 12% of patients with bacterial endocarditis. Bacterial mycotic aneurysms are often small and also located peripherally, unlike berry and fungal mycotic aneurysms found at bifurcations in the circle of Willis.

Pathologic studies demonstrate that the more common cause of ICH is a pyogenic arteritis resulting in blood vessel wall erosion rather than a classic mycotic aneurysm. Furthermore, many investigators observed that in patients receiving anticoagulation as treatment of a presumed ischemic stroke, there were more clinically significant hemorrhages. In one report, ICH occurred in 24% of patients receiving anticoagulation in the setting of ischemic infarcts caused by endocarditis.

Varied clinical profiles of TIA, stroke, and subarachnoid hemorrhage also typify the presentation of an atrial myxoma. Therefore, a cardiac embolic evaluation, including transesophageal echocardiography and ECG, seems to be a reasonable initial testing approach.

Vasculitis

Several rare disorders causing necrotizing vasculitis are uncommonly associated with brain hemorrhages, including polyarteritis nodosa and diffuse vasculitis, which most commonly lead to a mononeuritis multiplex, but rarely cerebral infarct with hemorrhage. Primary CNS angiitis is commonly associated with ICH. The disease course is usually subacute and presents with mental status changes, headaches, focal deficits, and seizures. Systemic lupus erythematosus is another disorder with a variable degree of CNS involvement. Autopsy series, however, suggest a high frequency of subarachnoid hemorrhage and, to a lesser extent, ICH and subdural hemorrhage. Wegener granulomatosis is another rare vasculitide with potential for ICH. Sarcoidosis and Behçet disease are other unusual systemic disorders rarely leading to cerebral hemorrhage.

Moyamoya

Moyamoya is a rare primary angiopathy associated with cerebral vascular occlusive disease. The carotid siphons and middle cerebral arteries are the vessels typically involved in the 2 forms of moyamoya. The familial form, most commonly seen in Japan, affects children aged around 10 years. These children often experience recurring bouts of hemiplegia or aphasia. Some symptoms may stutter or progress over a few weeks. The atherosclerotic form occurs in older patients, who may present with recurring TIAs or ICHs. Early in the disease, symptoms may be misinterpreted, and MRI findings are often unspecific. Careful observation for flow voids within the major vessels may demonstrate abnormalities that can prompt further investigation, including angiography. ICH most likely occurs in the older-patient form because of small friable vessels sprouting within the basal ganglia.

MANAGEMENT AND PROGNOSIS

Many patients with a primary ICH have a relatively progressive course during the initial illness phases. Although some patients initially experience a modest neurologic deficit, they may rapidly progress during the first 24 hours. CT demonstrates that ICH can recur or worsen up to 7 days after the ictus. As in the first vignette in this chapter, after the progression begins, it is often rapid and fatal, particularly if the hemorrhage extends to the ventricular system. An enlarging ICH leads to sudden volume increases with subsequent mass effect, further damaging surrounding brain structures and potentially leading to increased cerebral edema with possible tentorial herniation. Vasogenic edema, usually developing within the first 24 hours, leads to further mass effect. Blood in the ventricular system may also cause acute hydrocephalus. Concomitant infection, fever, hyperglycemia or hypoglycemia, excessive increase in blood pressure, and other medical conditions all worsen outcome.

The potentially increasing mass effect is the most devastating ICH consequence. The nidus of the bleed is often small compared with the amount of blood that has developed by the time the patient has CT. In the acute setting, management aims to decrease the mass effect. Although this is seemingly a logical approach, there is little agreement on methodology.

Deep-seated basal ganglia, thalamic, or brainstem hemorrhages are difficult to evacuate without disrupting surrounding normal structures. Many neurosurgeons also suggest that the emergent evacuation of superficial lobar ICH must be tempered. Injudicious brain decompression by hematoma evacuation may lead to unnecessary additional damage to islands of normal functioning brain. However, when a nondominant hemispheric or cerebellar ICH threatens impending tentorial herniation and before the patient's level of consciousness deteriorates, emergent surgery may be lifesaving, and the patient may have a reasonably good recovery.

In practice, treatment is often dictated by the last positive or negative outcome. Clinical trials are few and often inconclusive. Some demonstrate that best medical management and aggressive surgical treatment had similar outcomes. Patients who have smaller hematomas (smaller than 20 cm^3) seem to do generally well without surgical evacuation. However, larger hematomas (larger than 40 cm^3) do poorly, even when evacuated surgically. Hematomas between 20 and 40 cm^3 may do best after surgical evacuation. The evacuation method also matters: microsurgical ICH evacuations may have better outcomes.

Few neurosurgeons have investigated the benefits of evacuating deep hematomas using a continuous infusion and suction method. Thrombolytic agents such as tissue plasminogen activator have been infused into the hematoma. Although they produce more rapid hematoma resolution, the long-term clinical outcome seems unchanged.

Generally, the therapeutic approach must be individualized. In patients with intraventricular blood and early hydrocephalus, placement of a temporary external drain should be considered. Where the hematoma is exerting mass effect, the early use of mannitol may provide temporary relief. With superficial hematomas and declining neurologic function, surgical evacuation should always be considered.

The overall mortality of patients with ICH is approximately 50%. With the exception of the occasional patient with an ICH secondary to amyloid angiopathy, long-term follow up suggests no significant increase in risk for recurrent ICH. Nevertheless, just 1 instance of an ICH portends only a 50% chance to achieve independent activities of daily living. Initial presentation is predictive of outcome. Individuals who present with coma and signs of herniation have poor prognoses. Increasing levels of intracranial pressure with concurrent brainstem Duret hemorrhages often lead to reticular activating system damage. Under these circumstances, even the most rapid intervention to drain intraventricular blood proves unsatisfactory. Patients in whom hydrocephalus does not develop have better outcomes.

The size of the initial hematoma, as defined by CT, is also predictive of outcome. There is a mortality rate of approximately 50% to 75% in patients who have more than 40 cm of blood on CT at presentation. If the patient survives the bleed, the ultimate neurologic recovery depends on the hemorrhage location and residual deficits.

REFERENCES

Caplan LR. *Caplan's Stroke: A Clinical Approach*. 3rd ed. Woburn, Mass: Butterworth-Heinemann, 2000.

Dennis MS. Outcome after brain haemorrhage. *Cerebrovasc Dis*. 2003;16(suppl 1):9-13.

Fisher CM. Pathological observations in hypertensive cerebral hemorrhage. *J Neuropathol Exp Neurol*. 1971;30:536-550.

Garcia JH, Ho KL. Pathology of hypertensive arteriopathy. *Neurosurg Clin North Am*. 1992;3:497-507.

Garibi J, Bilbao G, Pomposo I, Hostalot C. Prognostic factors in a series of 185 consecutive spontaneous supratentorial intracerebral haematomas. *Br J Neurosurg*. 2002;16:355-361.

Kaneko M, Tanaka K, Shimada T, et al. Long term evaluation of ultra-early operation for hypertensive intracerebral hemorrhage in 100 cases. *J Neurosurg*. 1983;58:838-842.

Kase CS. Intracerebral hemorrhage: non-hypertensive causes. *Stroke*. 1986;17:590-595.

Mayer SA. Intracerebral hemorrhage: natural history and rationale of ultra early hemostatic therapy. *Intensive Care Med*. 2002;28(suppl 2):S235-S240.

Skidmore CT, Andrefsky J. Spontaneous intracerebral hemorrhage: epidemiology, pathophysiology, and medical management. *Neurosurg Clin North Am*. 2002;13:281-288.

Woo D, Broderick JP. Spontaneous intracerebral hemorrhage: epidemiology and clinical presentation. *Neurosurg Clin North Am*. 2002;13:265-279.

Chapter 24
Cerebral Aneurysms and Subarachnoid Hemorrhage

Carlos A. David

Clinical Vignette

A 36-year-old teacher suddenly experienced a terrible pain in her neck radiating into her forehead. The headache was so severe that she initially thought someone had stabbed her. She became nauseated, vomited, and went to the nurse's office. Although advised to go to the hospital, she chose to go home and rest over the weekend. Three days later, when the pain had not significantly improved, she agreed to seek medical care.

No new symptoms had developed since onset. In the ED, the patient reported that this was the worst pain she had ever experienced. Her initial neurologic examination results and brain CT were normal. The attending neurologist wished to perform a CSF examination, but the patient demurred. Angiography demonstrated a large posterior communicating aneurysm that was successfully clipped the next morning. The patient's postoperative course was uneventful.

Subarachnoid hemorrhage (SAH) refers to bleeding beneath the arachnoid coverings of the brain surface and within the contained cisterns. The most common age is between the fifth and seventh decades of life. There are multiple etiologies for SAH, primarily classified into aneurysmal causes and spontaneous nonaneurysmal mechanisms. Nonaneurysmal SAHs include AVMs, angiographically occult vascular malformations (cavernous malformation or angioma), idiopathic and iatrogenic coagulopathies, bacterial endocarditis and other central nervous system infections, inflammatory processes such as granulomatous angiitis, venous thrombosis, arterial dissections, occasional tumors, hypertension, and drug abuse. In addition, pathologic processes within the spinal canal can rarely lead to SAH, including spinal AVMs and spinal neoplasms such as myxopapillary ependymomas. Nevertheless, a ruptured intracranial aneurysm is the most preponderant cause of spontaneous SAH. One study of acute SAH in more than 6300 patients demonstrated that 51% of the patients harbored a ruptured intracranial aneurysm. Despite the normal neurologic examination results and head CT in the vignette, the patient's history was so compelling for a ruptured aneurysm or **warning leak** of same that her neurologist proceeded with the evaluation to find a large treatable berry aneurysm.

Subarachnoid hemorrhage is a catastrophic neurologic event having a precipitous onset, frequently without any premonitory warning. In North America, 28,000 patients per year experience a ruptured aneurysm. Slightly more than half die shortly after rupture. Among those who survive to reach a hospital, there is an additional 20% to 25% chance of further ruptures within the first 2 weeks. Overall mortality during the first month is approximately 50%; of those patients who survive, less than half have a favorable outcome.

Aneurysmal SAH, although catastrophic, can often be treated successfully. When an aneurysm is identified before rupture, treatment can be curative, preventing the devastating effects of a SAH. Recognition of SAH, accurate diagnosis, and timely treatment are essential.

Crucial points in taking the history of patients with a recent headache are the abruptness of pain onset and the severity of discomfort. Lack of abnormality on the neurologic examination does not exclude a symptomatic aneurysm, and therefore, the attending physician must carefully and fully evaluate such patients. Furthermore, as in the vignette in this chapter, a mild hemorrhage may not be observed with CT after just 24 hours. Therefore, negative CT at 24 to 72 hours does not exclude a diagnosis of ruptured aneurysm. This is the ideal opportunity to identify the aneurysm and save the patient's life, because a second bleed is also associated with the 50% mortality rate.

CLINICAL PRESENTATION

The classic symptom of SAH is the "worst headache of one's life." Headaches associated with aneurysm rupture are frequently sudden in onset and even described as a severe thunderclap, excruciating and unbearable. The headache peaks rapidly and is frequently associated with pain extending across the head and toward the neck. The headache is usually global, with a constant viselike ache and occasionally associated throbbing characteristics. Occasionally, there is a unilateral ache or a retro-orbital stabbing-like pain; when these occur in a fleeting manner, suspicion must be raised regarding a possible posterior communicating artery aneurysm.

Nausea and vomiting, neck pain, and altered consciousness are often associated with the headache. Approximately 30% of patients are found to be confused and lethargic after the ictus. During the moment of rupture, there is transient loss of consciousness in up to 35% to 40% of individuals. At the time of rupture, approximately one fourth of patients become comatose.

Seizurelike activity may be observed. The incidence of true seizure activity in patients with SAH is estimated as 20%. When seizures occur, they are most commonly associated with aneurysms that have ruptured and caused an intracerebral hematoma, most commonly associated with middle cerebral artery and anterior communicating artery aneurysms.

Unfortunately, many patients recall having a sentinel hemorrhage or warning leak with a fleeting, severe headache within the 2 to 3 weeks before the major hemorrhage. In retrospect, this headache is usually somewhat milder. Frequently, there is no associated meningismus, leading patients or physicians to ignore the symptoms until a catastrophic return announces the major rupture. When evaluating patients with SAH or sudden severe headache, special attention should be focused on the level of consciousness, signs of meningismus, focal neurological signs such as hemiparesis or cranial nerve palsy, and possible systemic effects (Figure 24-1). Meningismus frequently occurs, associated with nuchal rigidity. The Brudzinski maneuver is an excellent means of evaluation. The examiner flexes the patient's neck, precipitating hip flexion and knee extension and hamstring pain.

Examination of the optic fundi frequently discloses retinal or preretinal hemorrhage, subhyaloid hemorrhages, and occasional papilledema (Figure 24-2). Hemorrhage into the vitreous results in Terson syndrome, most commonly seen in anterior circulation aneurysms. A frequent cause of visual loss in these patients, it is often not noticed until 1 to 2 weeks later, when the patient has regained an appropriate level of consciousness and reports visual loss. The long-term prognosis for vision in this situation is fairly good; however, a vitrectomy is occasionally required.

When the aneurysm ruptures and dissects into adjacent brain tissue, various focal deficits may also be found on examination.

DIFFERENTIAL DIAGNOSIS

Patients presenting with a sudden apoplectic-type headache with associated meningismus or altered mental status must be considered to have a SAH until proven otherwise. However, SAH symptoms are sometimes confused with other disorders, including migraine headaches, hypertension, meningitis and other systemic infections, cervical spine disorders, vertigo, and syncope. The various vascular headache syndromes are most commonly confused.

Although **migraine** headaches are often characterized by severe pain at their maximum, careful history reveals that they typically have a gradual onset, followed by progression in degree of pain that, over hours, becomes so severe that nausea and vomiting develop. Many are preceded by a classic aura of seeing fortification spectra or scintillating lights minutes before the headache occurs.

Cluster headache is another benign but severe headache type with a well-defined clinical presentation. Typically, these headaches primarily affect men, awakening them from sleep with

CEREBRAL ANEURYSMS AND SUBARACHNOID HEMORRHAGE

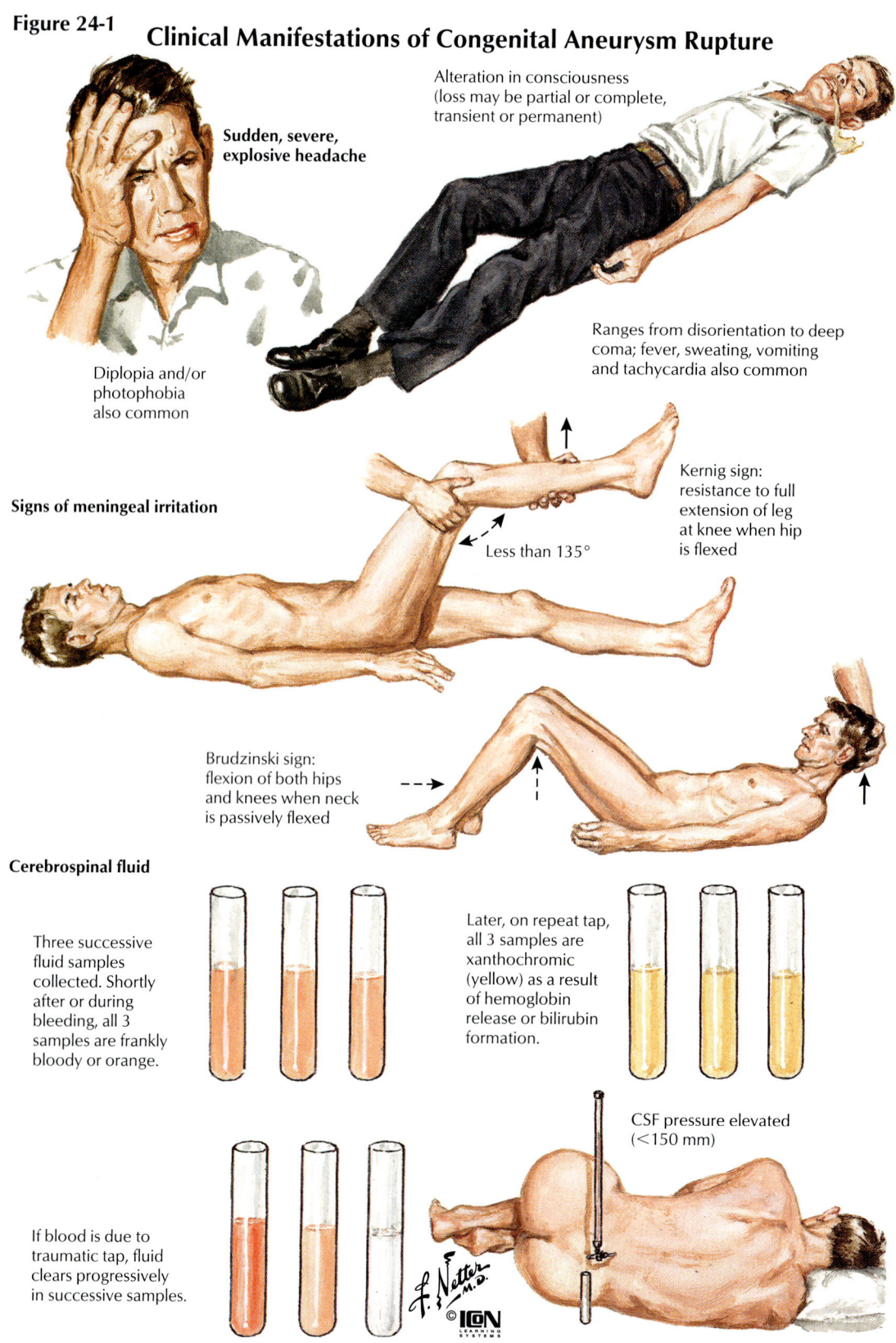

Figure 24-1: Clinical Manifestations of Congenital Aneurysm Rupture

CEREBRAL ANEURYSMS AND SUBARACHNOID HEMORRHAGE

Figure 24-2 Ophthalmologic Manifestations of Cerebral Aneurysms

A. Neuromuscular disorders

Abducens nerve palsy: affected eye turns medially. May be first manifestation of intracavernous carotid aneurysm. Pain above eye or on side of face may be secondary to trigeminal (V) nerve involvement.

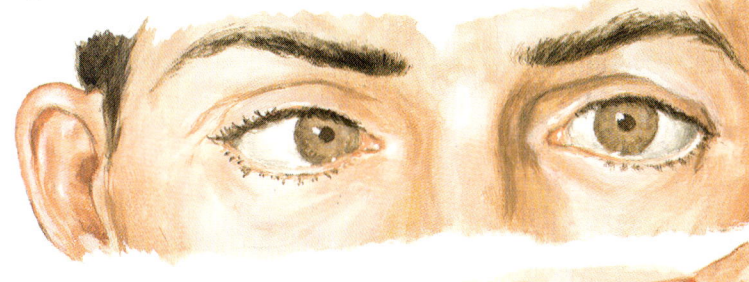

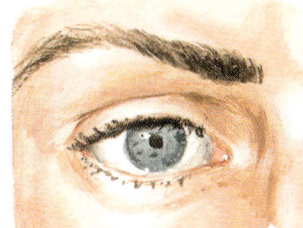 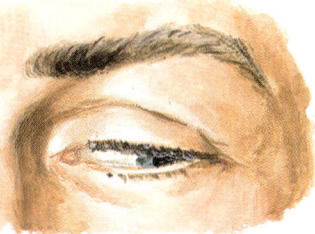 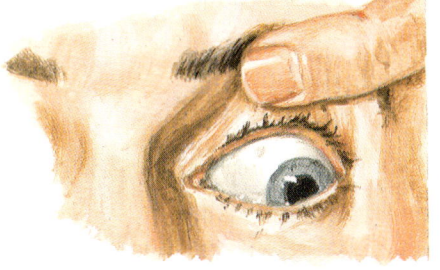

Oculomotor nerve palsy: ptosis, eye turns laterally and inferiorly, pupil dilated. Common finding with cerebral aneurysms, especially carotid-posterior communicating aneurysms.

B. Visual field disturbances

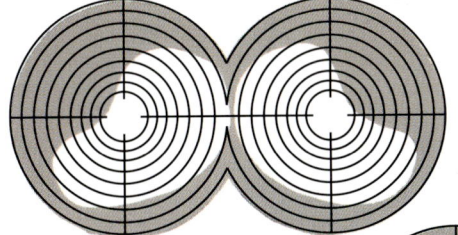 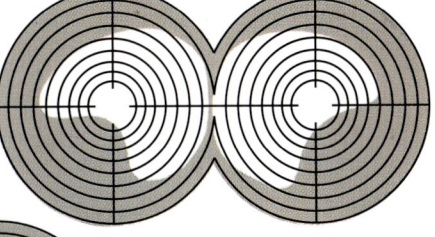

Superior bitemporal quadrantanopia caused by supraclinoid carotid aneurysm compressing optic chiasm from below

Inferior bitemporal quadrantanopia caused by compression of optic chiasm from above

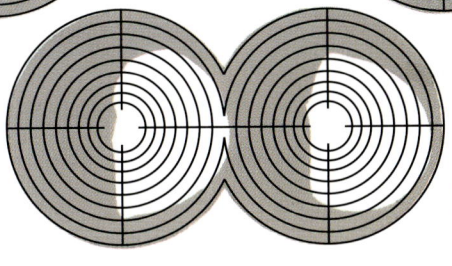

Right (or left) homonymous hemianopsia caused by compression of optic tract. Unilateral amaurosis may occur if optic (II) nerve is compressed.

C. Retinal changes

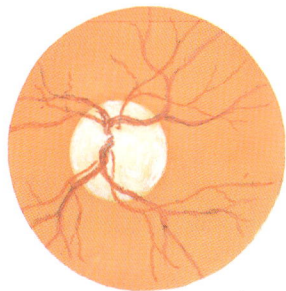 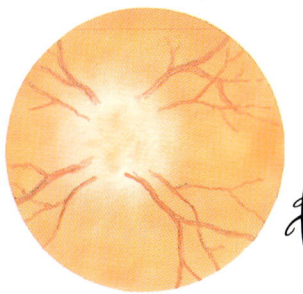 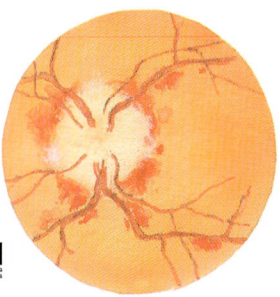

Optic atrophy may develop as result of pressure on optic (II) nerve from a supraclinoid carotid, ophthalmic, or anterior cerebral aneurysm.

Papilledema may be caused by increased intracranial pressure secondary to rupture of cerebral aneurysm.

Hemorrhage into optic (II) nerve sheath after rupture of aneurysm may result in subhyaloid hemorrhage, with blood around disc.

CEREBROVASCULAR DISORDERS

a terrible unilateral periorbital and frontal pain. These are almost always associated with conjunctival injection, watering of the eye, and nasal stuffiness. They have a limited time course, usually lasting less than 45 to 60 minutes, but then may recur at least nightly and sometimes a few times within 1 day. They occur in a temporal **cluster** for 6 to 8 weeks. When this pattern is established, the diagnosis is secure. However, when the patient first experiences this headache in early midlife, a careful evaluation is indicated to exclude SAH. A therapeutic response to inhalation of 100% oxygen is diagnostic.

Paroxysmal hemicrania is a related discomfort with an equal sexual distribution. Its response to indomethacin is a specific therapeutic diagnostic modality.

Orgasmic postcoital or **exercise-induced headaches** are another group of benign headaches that occur during sexual intercourse or with significant exercise. Those related to sexual activity generally occur precipitously at the peak of orgasm. These incapacitating severe headaches mimic the onset of an acute SAH. Such patients require the same full evaluation provided to other patients presenting with similar symptoms. **Orgasmic** or **postcoital** headache becomes a diagnosis of exclusion. Similar headaches also occur during strenuous physical exercise.

DIAGNOSTIC APPROACH

The clinical diagnosis of SAH is best confirmed with brain CT. Its sensitivity is highest in the first 24 hours after headache onset. A mild hemorrhage may wash away within 24 hours. However, approximately 50% of severe SAHs are still visible on CT 1 week after the ictus, and almost one third are still seen after 2 weeks. CT confirms the SAH and frequently highlights associated issues such as hydrocephalus, intraparenchymal hematoma, intraventricular hemorrhage, or subdural hemorrhage.

Whenever the clinical suspicion of SAH exists but CT is negative, a lumbar puncture must be performed. A nontraumatic tap is crucial. When the presence of blood in the CSF does not clear between the first and fourth tubes, this is particularly suggestive of SAH (Figure 24-1). However, a more sensitive indicator is CSF xanthochromia, which represents the lysis of erythrocytes within the CSF. This renders the CSF a yellowish color, is frequently present within 1 to 3 hours after a SAH and often persists for approximately 2 to 3 weeks.

When an SAH is confirmed by CT or lumbar puncture, the source of the hemorrhage must be confirmed. This is best achieved with a 4-vessel cerebral arteriogram. An aneurysmal source is found in 80% to 85% of these arteriograms. If arteriography is negative after SAH, a repeat study should be performed approximately 10 days later. Although reliance on CT angiography rather than catheter angiography has been increasing, cerebral arteriography remains the accepted standard for evaluating patients with SAH.

To ensure proper communication, predict outcomes, and guide management, a clinical grade for each SAH is needed. Several grading scales are available; the most widely used system is the Hunt-Hess scale (Table 24-1).

PATHOPHYSIOLOGY
Intracranial Aneurysms

Subtypes of intracranial aneurysms include saccular or berry, fusiform, dissecting, traumatic, and infectious (mycotic) aneurysms. Frequently associated with a SAH, saccular aneurysms are by far the most common type. They are usually spherical in shape but frequently have asymmetric outpouching and multilobulated characteristics, both providing potential rupture sites for the

Table 24-1
Hunt-Hess Grading Scale for Berry Aneurysms

Grade	Description
1	Asymptomatic, or mild headache and slight nuchal rigidity
2	Moderate to severe headache, nuchal rigidity, cranial nerve deficit
3	Mild focal deficit, lethargy, confusion
4	Stupor, hemiparesis, early decerebration
5	Deep coma, decerebrate rigidity, moribund appearance

CEREBRAL ANEURYSMS AND SUBARACHNOID HEMORRHAGE

aneurysm. The aneurysmal fundus or body is connected to the parent vessel via a small neck region, and as the aneurysm grows, this neck region may broaden and incorporate branch vessels.

Intracranial aneurysms characteristically occur at branch points of major cerebral arteries. Almost 85% of aneurysms are found in the anterior circulation, 15% within the posterior circulation (Figure 24-3). Overall, the most common sites are the anterior communicating artery followed by the posterior communicating artery and the middle cerebral artery bifurcation.

Within the posterior circulation, the most preponderant site is the basilar artery bifurcation.

Aneurysms are frequently classified according to their size, with small being smaller than 10 mm, large being 10 to 25 mm, and giant being larger than 25 mm. At presentation, most are small, with only 2% found to be giant (Figure 24-4). Although controversy remains regarding the association of size and the incidence of rupture, 7 mm seems to be the minimal size at the time of rupture. Overall, ruptured aneurysms are larger than unruptured aneurysms.

Figure 24-3   **Typical Sites of Cerebral Aneurysms**

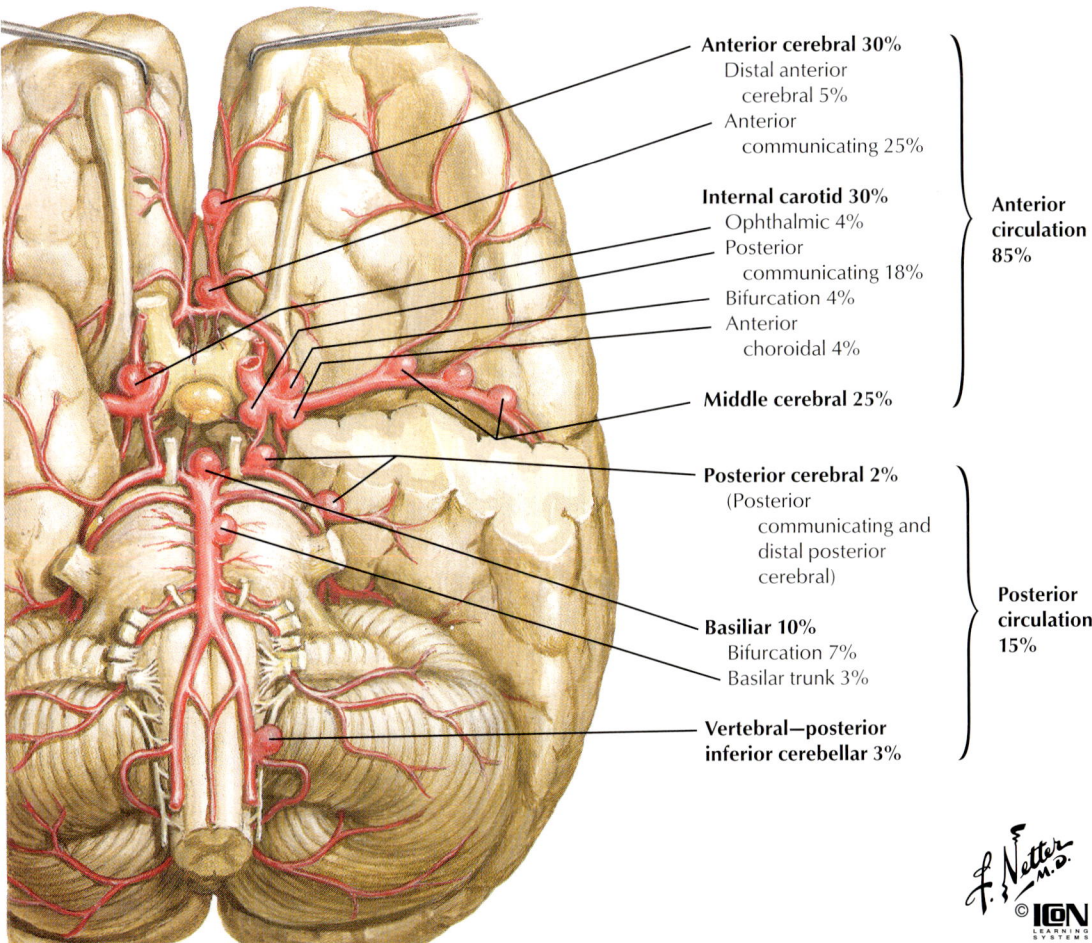

CEREBROVASCULAR DISORDERS

253

CEREBRAL ANEURYSMS AND SUBARACHNOID HEMORRHAGE

Figure 24-4

Giant Congenital Aneurysms

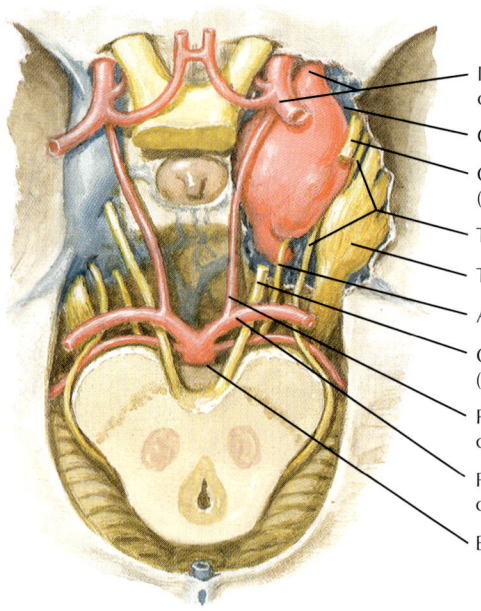

Labels: Internal carotid a.; Cavernous sinus; Oculomotor (III) n. (divided); Trochlear (IV) n.; Trigeminal (V) n.; Abducens (VI) n.; Oculomotor (III) n. (divided); Posterior communicating a.; Posterior cerebral a.; Basilar a.

A. Intracavernous (infraclinoid) internal carotid aneurysm compressing abducens (VI) nerve. Oculomotor (III), trochlear (IV), and trigeminal (V) nerves may also be affected. Trigeminal involvement may cause facial pain.

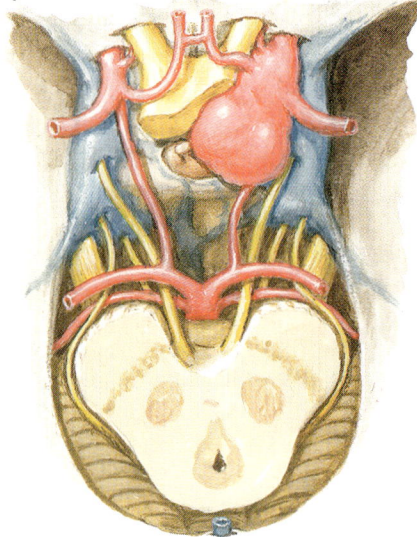

B. Aneurysm of supraclinoid segment of internal carotid artery elevating optic chiasm, distorting infundibulum and compressing oculomotor (III) nerve

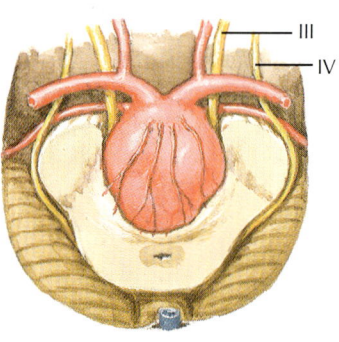

C. Aneurysm of basilar bifurcation projecting posteriorly, invading peduncles and compressing cerebral aqueduct. Corticospinal tracts may be affected, resulting in paralysis or paresis.

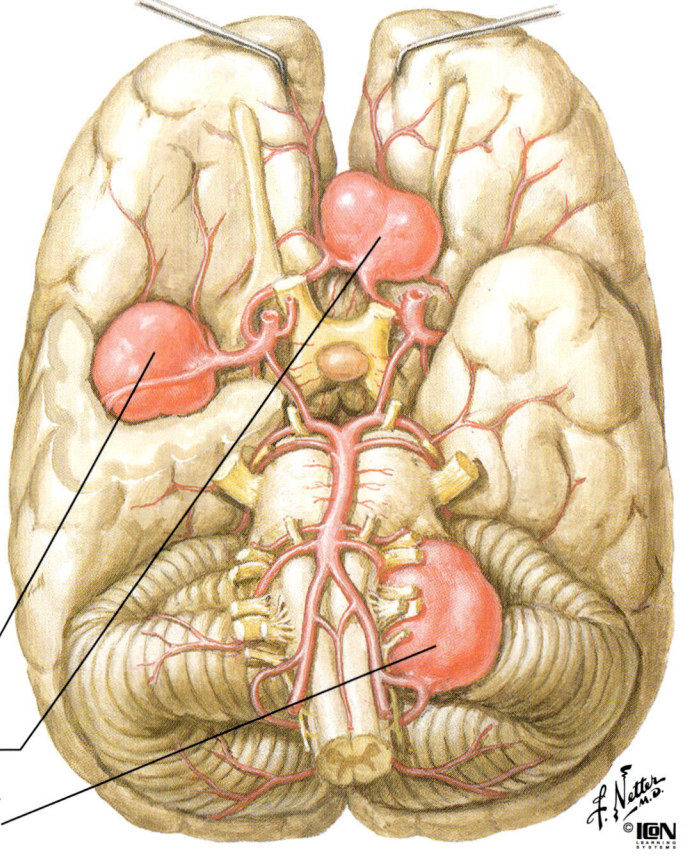

D. Aneurysm of middle cerebral artery

E. Aneurysm of anterior cerebral-anterior communicating arteries

F. Aneurysm of posterior inferior cerebellar artery

CEREBROVASCULAR DISORDERS

CEREBRAL ANEURYSMS AND SUBARACHNOID HEMORRHAGE

Aneurysms occur in approximately 5% of the adult population, somewhat more commonly in women. The causes of intracranial aneurysm formation and rupture are not well understood; however, it is thought that intracranial aneurysms form over a relatively short period and either rupture or undergo a stabilizing change resulting in an unruptured aneurysm. Pathologic examination of ruptured aneurysms obtained at autopsy demonstrates loss of the internal elastic lamina, disorganization of normal vascular architecture, and reduced collagen content. In contrast, unruptured aneurysms have nearly twice the collagen content of the normal arterial wall, resulting in increased thickness of the aneurysmal wall, which may be responsible for the observed relative stability and low rupture rate.

Perimesencephalic Subarachnoid Hemorrhage

Of patients presenting with spontaneous SAH, approximately 15% to 20% have negative arteriograms. Repeated arteriography may discern another 7% of patients that do harbor a cerebral aneurysm. However, a specific subset of individuals displays a separate disorder; they have a typical and specific CT distribution of SAH that occurs over the anterior aspect of the brainstem or perimesencephalic regions.

These forms of SAH, termed *benign perimesencephalic SAH*, occur typically in younger males who are nonhypertensive and who do not look as ill as typical patients with an aneurysmal SAH. Although the clinical presentation is similar to that of an aneurysmal SAH, symptom onset is more gradual, and patients generally do well. When these patients have a typical presentation and characteristic CT findings and a good quality angiogram that is negative, a follow-up arteriogram is not always needed. The entity of brainstem or perimesencephalic SAH seems to represent a clinically benign disorder of unknown cause.

Ruptured Aneurysms

The peak incidence of aneurysmal SAH is in the sixth decade of life. Only 20% of aneurysm ruptures occur in patients aged between 15 and 45 years. No predisposing activity has been identified, and aneurysmal SAH is equally distributed in sleep, routine daily activities, and strenuous activity.

Nearly 50% of patients who have a SAH, when properly questioned, relate a history of a **warning leak with headache** or symptoms around 2 to 3 weeks before the major hemorrhage. Nearly half of these individuals die before arriving at the hospital. Many of the initial survivors also succumb to a repeat hemorrhage after presenting to the hospital. The peak incidence of subsequent hemorrhage occurs in the first 24 hours, but the subsequent daily risk continues such that approximately 20% to 25% have rebled within the first 2 weeks of presentation. Mortality associated with the second hemorrhage is nearly 70%.

Risk Factors

Risk factors associated with aneurysmal rupture include cigarette smoking, oral contraceptive use, alcohol consumption, pregnancy, and childbirth. Possible diurnal blood pressure variations are associated with a circadian rhythm for aneurysm rupture. Most ruptures seem to occur early in the morning or evening, but few occur in the middle of the night. There also seems to be preponderance during the winter months or when there are drastic changes in barometric pressure. The most likely cause of rupture is hemodynamic stress associated with the biomechanical and structural weakness within the blood vessel and aneurysmal wall.

MANAGEMENT
Complications of the Ruptured Aneurysm

Specific therapeutic issues pertain to aneurysms, primarily securing them to prevent rebleeding, management of increased intracranial pressure (ICP) and hydrocephalus, and treatment of cerebral vasospasm. Associated medical sequelae lead to other management issues noted below.

Rebleeding

Rebleeding is the major cause of poor outcome after SAH. The second hemorrhage is associated with a 70% mortality rate. If untreated, the risk of subsequent aneurysm rupture is approximately 4% in the first 24 hours and 1.5%

CEREBRAL ANEURYSMS AND SUBARACHNOID HEMORRHAGE

per subsequent day, leading to an approximately 27% incidence of subsequent aneurysmal rupture within the first 2 weeks of hemorrhage. The rebleeding rate decreases to approximately 3% to 5% per year. The major goal in SAH treatment is to prevent rebleeding by methodologies designed to obliterate an aneurysm. Although the rebleeding risk can be somewhat decreased pharmacologically in the short term, the only definitive prevention is direct obliteration using surgical or endovascular techniques. Previous beliefs regarding the timing of aneurysm occlusion have been replaced by a general attitude that early and expeditious aneurysm occlusion must be performed when feasible.

Hydrocephalus

Up to 25% of patients with SAH develop an associated cerebral edema with ventriculomegaly secondary to an accompanying acute hydrocephalus, independent of grading after the aneurysm rupture, that worsens if left untreated. There is no consensus on the management of hydrocephalus and intraventricular hemorrhage. However, external ventricular drainage is recommended in conjunction with early aneurysm occlusion. Many patients can be weaned off the ventricular drainage later in their hospital course. Chronic hydrocephalus develops in only 25% of patients who survive an aneurysm rupture. Of patients with acute hydrocephalus who require ventricular drainage, approximately one half will ultimately require a ventricular-peritoneal shunt.

Cerebral Vasospasm

Cerebral vasospasm, a poorly understood problem, is the most feared and difficult issue associated with SAH. This represents a pathologic change within the cerebral vessels leading to vascular narrowing with decreased cerebral blood flow and subsequent stroke. Vasospasm is correlated with poor clinical grade and larger degrees of hemorrhage. It is thought that the products of blood decomposition within the CSF spaces results in an imbalance between vascular relaxing factor and constricting factors resulting in vessel spasm and narrowing. Typically, vasospasm develops about the fourth day after SAH and usually peaks between 7 and 10 days.

Management includes the use of calcium channel blockers such as nimodipine, decreasing ICP with ventricular drainage, and augmenting cerebral circulation. The latter is best achieved with **triple-H therapy**, consisting of hypervolemia, hemodilution, and hypertensive therapy. Hypervolemia is easily achieved using volume expanders, such as albumen and crystalloid fluids. Hemodilution frequently occurs passively with an optimum hematocrit goal between 30% and 33%. Hypertensive therapy, when needed, may be instituted using a-adrenergic agonists such as phenylephrine hydrochloride (Neo-Synephrine). The goal is to prevent the development of permanent neurologic deficits by reversing deficits as they occur. Transcranial Doppler ultrasonography is of value for detecting the presence and degree of vasospasm and for monitoring its response to therapy. Transcranial Doppler ultrasonography provides real-time information regarding blood flow velocities, which in turn correlates with the degree of vessel spasm. Occasionally, ischemic deficits continue to develop despite aggressive triple-H therapy. In this setting, endovascular maneuvers, such as intraarterial papaverine or intracranial angioplasty, can be used with excellent results.

Systemic Complications

Subarachnoid hemorrhage concomitantly results in a catastrophic assault on the entire physiologic system; frequently, these patients are the most clinically ill within the entire hospital. A multisystem therapeutic approach is necessary.

At the moment of SAH, experimental evidence suggests a **massive surge in ICP** rising to such an extent that it overcomes MAP, resulting in a momentary **global arrest in cerebral circulation**. As the increased ICP begins to wane, the circulation is reinstituted, at which point a small fibrin plug is created, sealing the aneurysm and preventing further bleeding.

The massive ICP increase affects the hypothalamus; when combined with the associated global ischemia, there is a **massive neuroendocrine response**. Consequently, there is a **catecholamine surge** leading to cardiac and pulmonary injury. **Cardiac abnormalities** may be identified on ECG in up to 50% of patients at admission, including bizarre T-wave abnormalities,

ST-segment depressions, prominent U waves, or prolongation of the QT interval. Cardiac arrhythmias and myocardial injury may develop.

Other patients may present with **acute respiratory distress syndrome** from massive pulmonary edema, termed *neurogenic pulmonary edema*. It may result in an associated hypoxia and may contribute to the overall system failure.

There is usually an associated acute **hypertension** on presentation and a clinical suspicion that the hypertension may be secondary to the Cushing response associated with increased ICP. Cerebral circulation must be maintained. Management of hypertension in this setting requires treatment of the increased ICP such as ventricular drainage of the CSF rather than the use of antihypertensive medications.

Frequently, abnormalities of **electrolytes** are also noted, particularly hyponatremia. Usually associated with a salt wasting state rather than a syndrome of inappropriate antidiuretic hormone, hyponatremia should be managed accordingly.

Unruptured Aneurysms

The diagnosis of an unruptured intracranial aneurysm is frequently approached with anxiety and recommendations for expeditious treatment when considering the high morbidity and mortality associated with SAH. However, increasing evidence suggests a basic pathologic difference between unruptured and ruptured aneurysms; the risk of SAH from smaller unruptured aneurysms may be small.

The natural history of unruptured aneurysms is not completely understood. Unruptured aneurysms may be classified into symptomatic unruptured aneurysms and asymptomatic unruptured aneurysms. Symptomatic unruptured aneurysms often require treatment because the presenting symptom frequently is the harbinger of an oncoming bleeding episode. Various symptoms can be described, most from compression of neural structures: cranial nerve deficits, especially of CN-III, headaches, and eye pain, as well as hemiparesis or motor deficits from giant aneurysms. Some aneurysms develop intraaneurysmal thrombosis that may lead to thromboembolic stroke or transient ischemic attacks.

The number of unruptured aneurysms receiving medical attention has increased significantly with the advent of imaging studies such as CT angiography and MRA. Traditionally, patients with unruptured aneurysms were thought to have a high risk of bleeding and were therefore considered for obliteration therapies. However, the International Study of Unruptured Intracranial Aneurysms raised concerns about treating all unruptured aneurysms. Despite criticisms regarding this report, conventional thinking and management of truly asymptomatic unruptured aneurysms is being reexamined.

Truly asymptomatic unruptured aneurysms are less prone to bleeding than symptomatic unruptured aneurysms. These lesions are frequently discovered during investigation of other neurologic complaints or screening of high-risk patients, such as those with a familial history of aneurysms, connective tissue disorders, or polycystic kidney disease. Their natural history has been the focus of much controversy, mainly stemming from the International Study of Unruptured Intracranial Aneurysms. An initially suggested hemorrhage risk of approximately 0.05% per year in patients with aneurysms smaller than 10 mm has been supplanted via further analysis, with a low risk associated with aneurysms smaller than 7 mm. It is recommended that aneurysms larger than 7 mm should be treated. Aneurysms smaller than 7 mm should be considered for treatment in patients with a familial history of SAH, patients who have had SAH associated with a separate aneurysm, and very young patients for whom the lifetime risk may become significant.

Saccular Aneurysms

The obliteration and elimination of saccular aneurysms from the circulation has undergone a revolutionary change. Less invasive endovascular routes have provided an attractive alternative, particularly in elderly and high-risk patients, to traditional treatment with surgical clipping of the aneurysm via craniotomy.

Despite the enthusiasm for endovascular approaches, studies suggest a 20% to 30% recurrence rate. Furthermore, this treatment frequently results in less than 100% obliteration of the aneurysm. The remaining unanswered question is whether the 1% to 2% remnants of aneurysms frequently associated with endovascular coil obliteration pose a risk of subsequent SAH.

In contrast, surgical clipping has withstood the test of time. When a neurosurgeon successfully secures an aneurysm by clipping it, the recurrence risk is less than 1%. However, the risks incurred with surgical clipping of an aneurysm are slightly higher than those incurred with endovascular obliteration, particularly with aneurysms of the posterior circulation.

Technical Aspects of Surgical Clipping

Craniotomy and aneurysm obliteration by clipping is the most effective treatment available. Aneurysms completely obliterated using this technique almost never recur. Overall, surgical treatment of unruptured aneurysms is associated with 3% mortality and 7% morbidity. The following discussion illustrates these lesions' anatomical complexities and unique features.

The development of the surgical microscope and microsurgical instrumentation and the evolution of skull base techniques have revolutionized treatment of cerebral aneurysms. Magnification and brilliant illumination of very narrow exposure windows has allowed the preservation of small perforating vessels that serve as strategic end arteries of eloquent brain regions that are not visible to the naked eye. The advent and evolution of skull base techniques in which bone is removed to obviate any brain retraction and manipulation has also facilitated the treatment of aneurysms, particularly the more complex and giant variety.

Craniotomy

Depending on the location, size, and shape of the aneurysm, many approaches can be used (Figures 24-5 and 24-6). Most anterior circulation aneurysms can be approached via a pterional craniotomy, a fundamental approach in aneurysm surgery. It encompasses the frontal and temporal regions and is centered on the pterion. During the craniotomy, a piece of skull is separated from the cranium, removing a segment of the frontal temporal bone based on the pterion. The sylvian wing is exposed. After the dura is opened, the frontal and temporal lobes are seen in the region of the sylvian fissure. The surgical microscope is brought into the field to accomplish the remaining surgery with magnified vision.

Intracranial Surgical Dissection

The neurosurgeon proceeds to the natural arachnoidal and cisternal compartments where the appropriate vessels and the parent vessel are exposed, and then dissection of the aneurysm, particularly its neck, is performed. When all branches and perforating vessels are dissected free, an appropriate aneurysm clip is placed across the aneurysm neck, sealing the aneurysm from the parent vessel circulation. When the aneurysm is exposed, inspection is performed to ensure that no perforating branch arteries are occluded or injured, and then the aneurysm is completely clipped. When the aneurysm is secured, it can be punctured to allow it to collapse and relieve mass effect if present. Adjuncts to the surgical treatment of aneurysms are beyond this scope of this text but include temporary clipping, cerebral bypasses, aneurysmorrhaphy, and, in some cases, full hypothermic cardiac arrest. With microsurgical technology and various temporary and permanent aneurysm clips available and the establishment of skull base and revascularization techniques, management of once inoperable lesions has become routine.

Endovascular Therapy

Advances in the design of microcatheters, embolization devices, and digital radiographic software have greatly extended the capability of intravascular navigation and transvascular catheter-directed therapies. The new discipline of interventional neuroradiology or endovascular surgery has emerged.

The development and clinical experience with the Guglielmi detachable coil technology is extensive, and follow-up is available beyond 10 years. In many patients, aneurysm endovascular coil occlusion is a valuable alternative to surgery. Procedural morbidity ranges between 6% and 19%. Overall, 82% of patients experience favorable outcomes.

However, endovascular procedures seem to be less successful when the degree of complete obliteration and recurrence is compared with

CEREBRAL ANEURYSMS AND SUBARACHNOID HEMORRHAGE

Figure 24-5

Frontotemporal Approach for Internal Carotid, Ophthalmic, Anterior Communicating, and Middle Cerebral Aneurysms

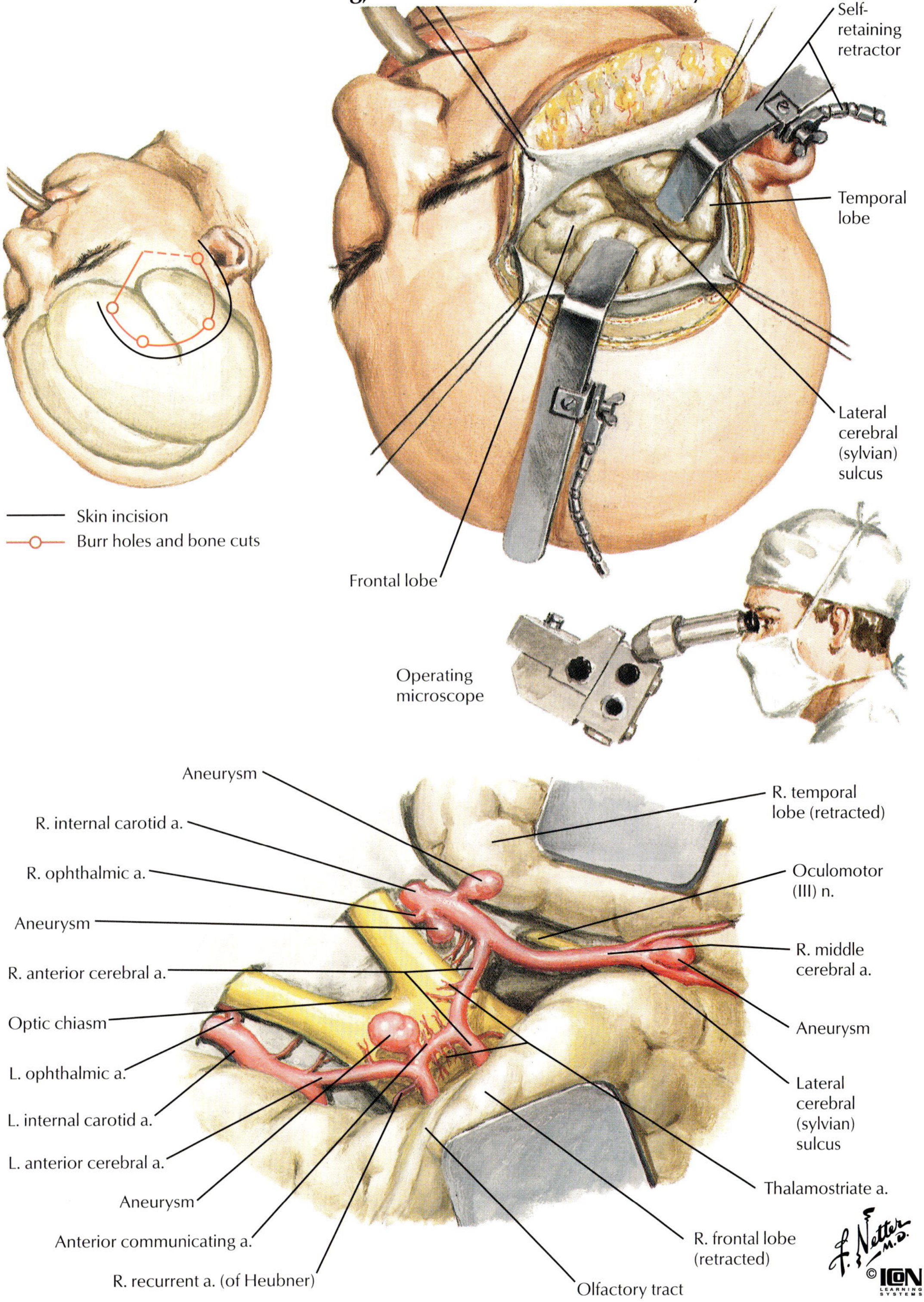

Labels (top illustrations):
- Self-retaining retractor
- Temporal lobe
- Lateral cerebral (sylvian) sulcus
- Frontal lobe
- Skin incision
- Burr holes and bone cuts
- Operating microscope

Labels (bottom illustration):
- Aneurysm
- R. internal carotid a.
- R. ophthalmic a.
- Aneurysm
- R. anterior cerebral a.
- Optic chiasm
- L. ophthalmic a.
- L. internal carotid a.
- L. anterior cerebral a.
- Aneurysm
- Anterior communicating a.
- R. recurrent a. (of Heubner)
- Olfactory tract
- R. frontal lobe (retracted)
- Thalamostriate a.
- Lateral cerebral (sylvian) sulcus
- Aneurysm
- R. middle cerebral a.
- Oculomotor (III) n.
- R. temporal lobe (retracted)

CEREBROVASCULAR DISORDERS

CEREBRAL ANEURYSMS AND SUBARACHNOID HEMORRHAGE

Figure 24-6   **Posterior Approach for Vertebral and Posterior Inferior Cerebellar Aneurysms**

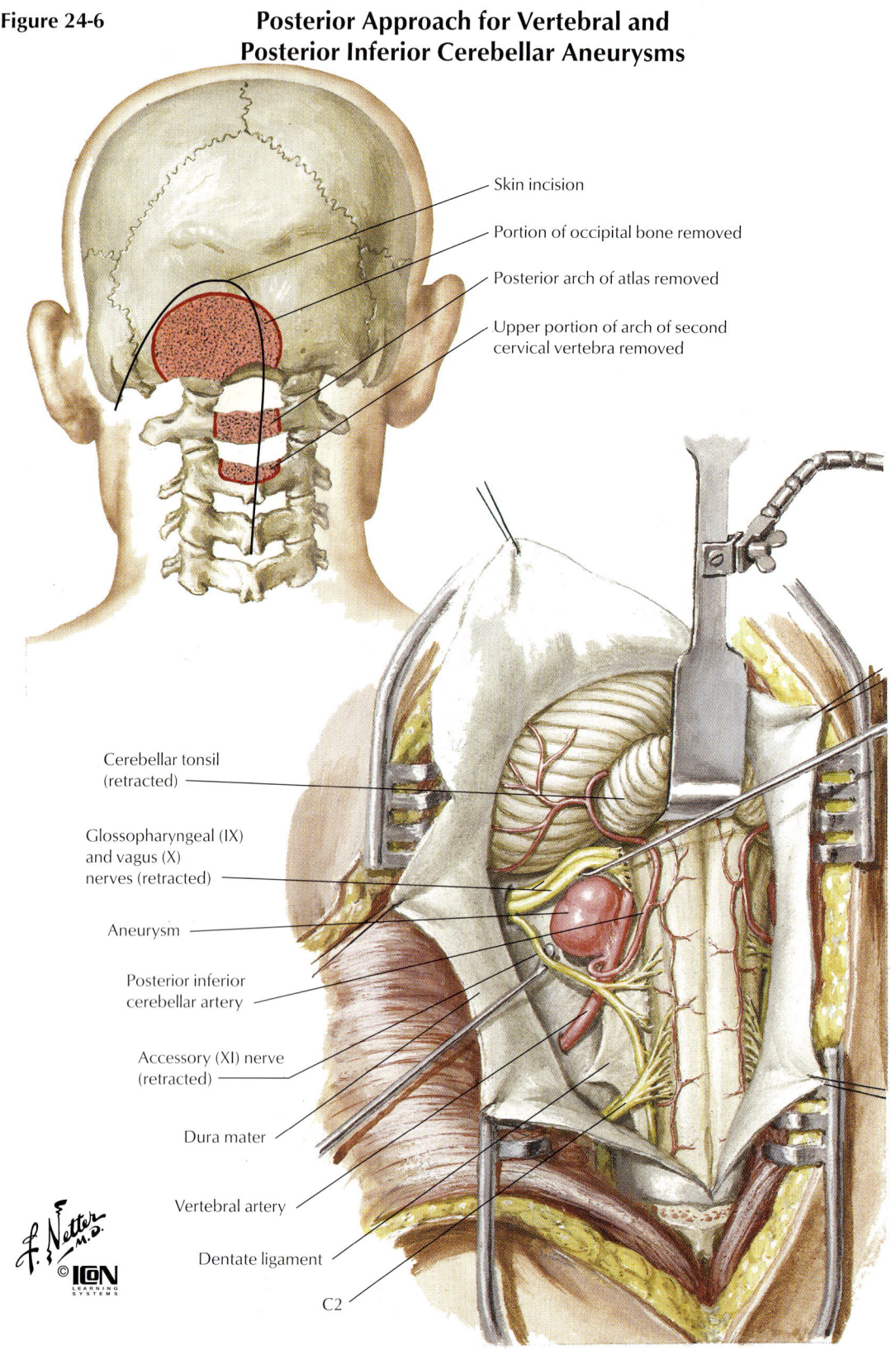

CEREBROVASCULAR DISORDERS

260

surgical procedures. Complete aneurysm occlusion is achieved in only 50% of cases. When near-complete occlusions are included, this level increases to 85% to 90%. A second limitation to endovascular procedures is aneurysm recurrence; approximately 16% to 32% of these aneurysms can recur, depending on the location, degree of compaction, and morphology of the aneurysm when primarily treated. Patients may require repeated treatment or even surgical treatment with removal of the coils.

The technique is based on microcatheter navigation within the vascular system. After a formal cerebral arteriogram is performed, the morphology, size, and shape of the aneurysm are studied, in particular the neck and dome size and ratios. A microcatheter is navigated through the vascular tree to the parent vessel and into the aneurysm itself. While in the aneurysm, various Guglielmi detachable coils are selected to fill the dome of the aneurysm. When deployed into the aneurysm, they are electrically detached. The nature of these coils provides for the filling of the aneurysm with the coil itself and promotion of thrombosis leading to aneurysm occlusion.

Collaboration between neurosurgeons and interventional neuroradiologists will increase the number of patients who can be safely treated with either technique or after one technique fails. The value of this collaborative effort cannot be overemphasized, particularly with the more complex aneurysms and those within the posterior circulation. The 2 techniques complement each other. In some instances, the primary treatment may be coiling of Guglielmi detachable coils. Others require surgical obliteration, and some aneurysms, because of their complex structures, giant size, or involvement of critical perforating branches, are not amenable to either treatment but require combined neurosurgical/neuroendovascular skills to achieve treatment success.

REFERENCES

Bederson JB, Ward I, Wiebers DO, et al. Recommendations for the management of patients with unruptured intracranial aneurysms: a statement for healthcare professionals from the stroke council of the American Heart Association. *Stroke.* 2000;31:2742-2750.

Eskridge J, Song J, and participants. Endovascular embolization of 150 basilar tip aneurysms with Guglielmi-detachable coils: results of the food and drug administration multi-center clinical trial. *J Neurosurg.* 1998;89:81-86.

International Study of Unruptured Intracranial Aneurysms Investigators. Unruptured intracranial aneurysms: risk of rupture and risk of surgical intervention. *N Engl J Med.* 1998;339:1725-1733.

International Subarachnoid Hemorrhage Aneurysm Collaborative Group. International subarachnoid aneurysm trial (ISAT) of neurosurgical clipping vs endovascular coiling in 2,143 patients with ruptured intracranial aneurysms: a randomized trial. *Lancet.* 2002;360:1267-1274.

Section VI
EPILEPSY AND SYNCOPE

Chapter 25
Epilepsy and Syncope 264

Chapter 26
Surgical Treatments for Epilepsy 281

Chapter 25
Epilepsy and Syncope

Joel M. Oster, Jose A. Gutrecht, and Paul T. Gross

EPILEPSY

Epilepsy is one of the most common and potentially serious neurologic disorders. Its prevalence is estimated as 1 in 200 persons. It affects all ages and is generally a chronic problem with high cost to the patient because of personal, social, and economic impact, often affecting the ability to hold jobs and drive. Epilepsy is generally defined as an illness with recurrent seizures. The clinical manifestations are initiated by an abnormal electrical discharge within the brain. The underlying pathophysiology is complex and not completely defined.

The diagnosis of epilepsy is primarily clinical, based on patient and witness history of the individual's events and on the neurologic examination. An abnormal EEG may substantiate a suspected diagnosis. Specific EEG epileptiform waveform abnormalities, particularly focal or generalized spikes or spike-and-wave discharges, are highly associated with seizures (Figure 25-1). Many other EEG changes are not specific for seizures and are of little help in differentiating epileptic from nonepileptic events. Epilepsy is a treatable disease, often with a specific correctable medical or surgical pathology. Accurate diagnosis must be the predominant goal in approaching a patient with seizures of recent onset. MRI and neuroimaging studies are critical to define any potentially treatable structural brain disease (Figure 25-2). Laboratory testing may assist in the evaluation and treatment.

Patients with chronic forms of epilepsy require ongoing medical treatment. Failure of medical therapy or quality-of-life issues may necessitate intensive patient evaluation for consideration for surgery. Surgical removal of carefully selected areas of the diseased brain may provide improvement and often a cure.

Partial Seizures
Simple Partial Seizures

Clinical Vignette

A 38-year-old previously healthy man consulted a neurologist because for the previous 6 months he had experienced episodes of clonic movements starting in the left thumb, spreading to the left arm and face. Each event lasted 1 to 2 minutes. The patient was alert and responsive throughout each episode and had a good recollection of them. On examination, he had mild clumsiness of his left hand and hyperactive muscle stretch reflexes in his left arm.

This history represents a typical simple partial seizure (SPS). During the episode, patients are conscious, aware of their surroundings, and able to respond appropriately. Partial seizures originate and develop within a discrete area of the cerebral cortex (Figure 25-3). They have a jacksonian march wherein the cortical epileptic discharges spread from the frontal motor area controlling the thumb to adjacent areas subserving the arm and face. The brain area involved determines the clinical signature of the event. Symptoms may be motor, as in the above vignette, when the origin is in the frontal lobe, somatosensory when discharges arise from the parietal lobe, or visual when they begin in the occipital lobe. However, the relation of focal cortical location to clinical expression is not absolute. Seizures may start in a cerebral cortical area that is clinically "silent," and the ictal symptoms may represent the result of the discharge spreading to a neighboring cortical area. SPSs may occasionally also have autonomic, psychic, or cognitive manifestations. By definition, these simple ictal events do not include any change in level of consciousness. It is this preserved responsiveness to the external environment that characterizes SPSs.

EPILEPSY AND SYNCOPE

Figure 25-1   Origin and Spread of Seizures

Normal firing pattern of cortical neurons

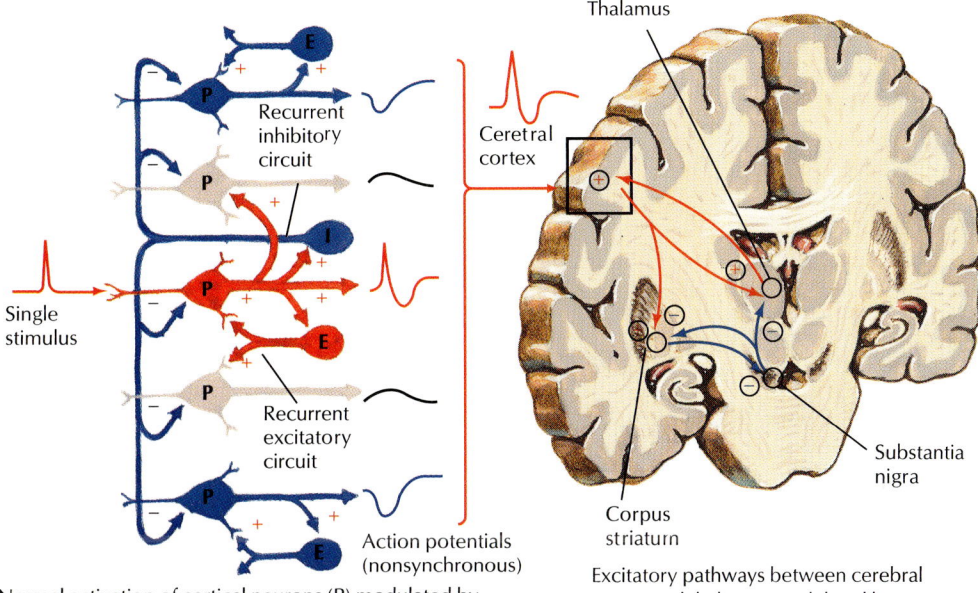

Normal activation of cortical neurons (P) modulated by excitatory (E) and inhibitory (I) feedback circuits

Excitatory pathways between cerebral cortex and thalamus modulated by tonic midbrain inhibitory stimuli

Epileptic firing pattern of cortical neurons

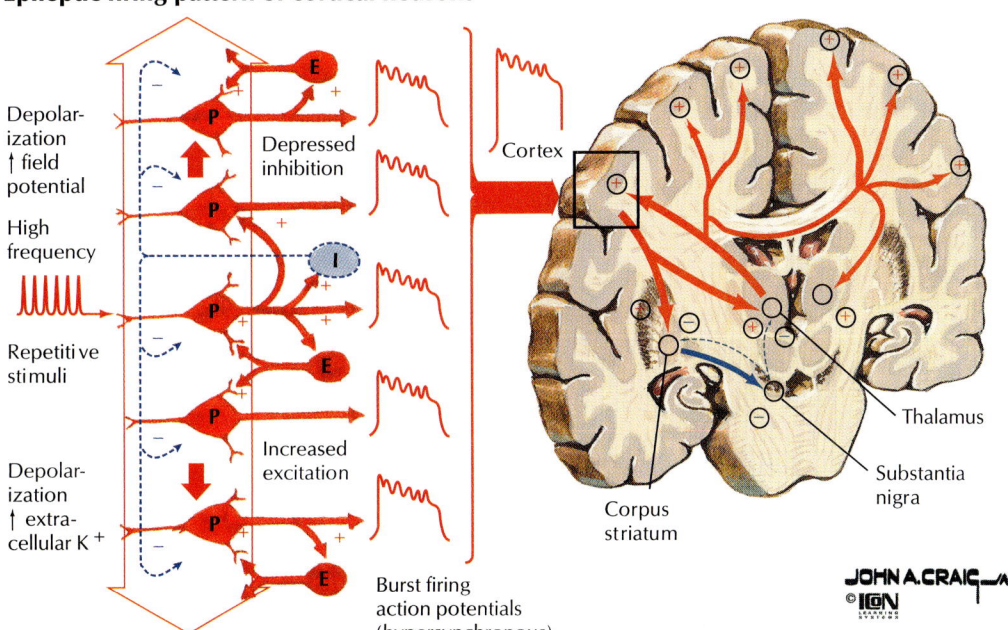

Repetitive cortical activation potentiates excitatory transmission and depresses inhibitory transmission, creating self-perpetuating excitatory circuit (burst) and facilitating excitation (recruitment) of neighboring neurons.

Cortical bursts to corpus striatum and thalamus block inhibitory projections and create self-perpetuating feedback circuit.

EPILEPSY AND SYNCOPE

Figure 25-2 — Neuroimaging Studies

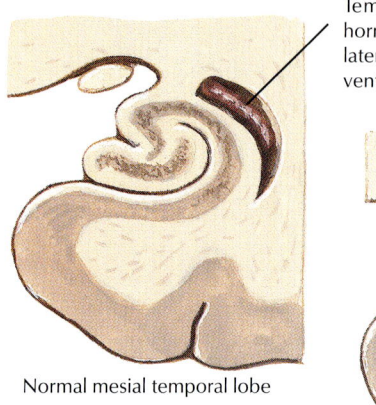

Normal mesial temporal lobe

Temporal horn of lateral ventricle

Cell loss and atrophy

Mesial temporal sclerosis (hippocampal atrophy)

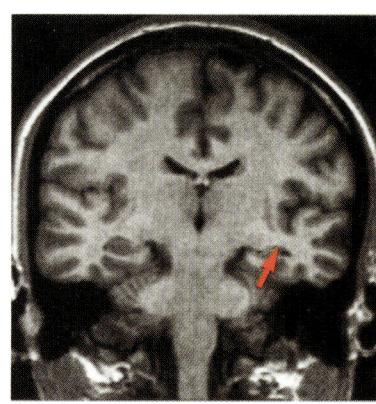

MRI: Mesial temporal sclerosis

PET scans

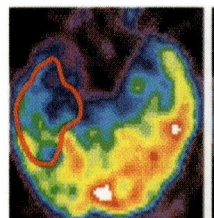 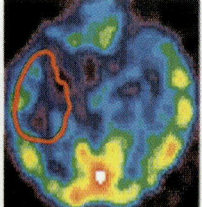 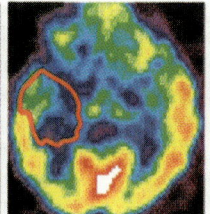 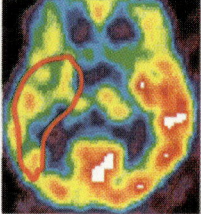 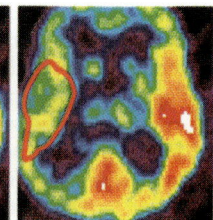

Interictal study shows areas of hypometabolism* in temporal lobe of patient with temporal lobe epilepsy. Blue and green represent low metabolism; red and white, high metabolism.

SPECT scans

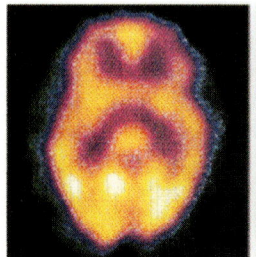 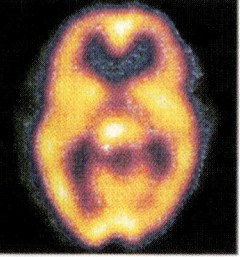 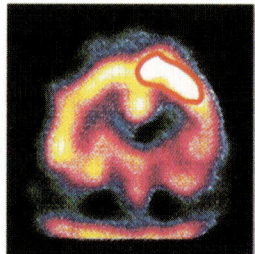 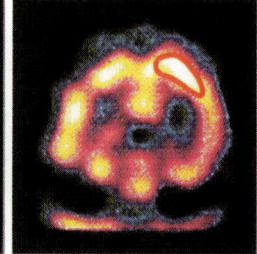

Interictal (baseline) study shows symmetrical blood flow.

Ictal study shows increased frontal blood flow* in patient with frontal lobe epilepsy.

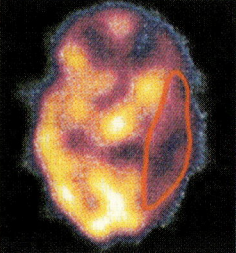 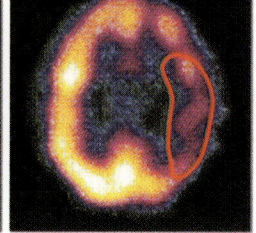

Postictal study shows decreased temporal blood flow* in patient with temporal lobe epilepsy.

* Areas of interest circled in red.

EPILEPSY AND SYNCOPE

Figure 25-3 Classification of Partial Seizures

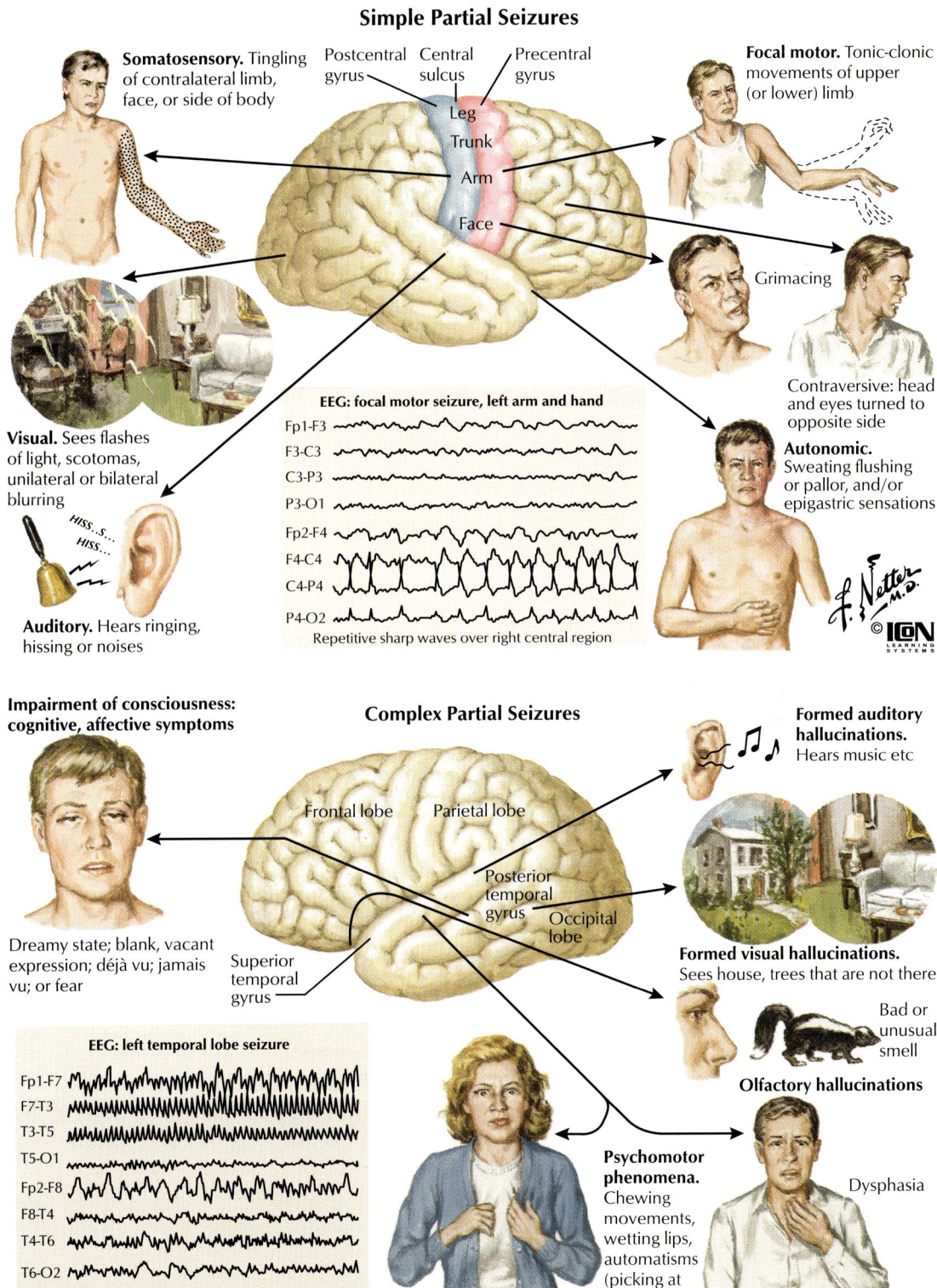

Sometimes, the clonic phase of a partial motor seizure may continue uninterrupted for some time, with no progression into other body segments for long periods. This type of seizure is known as *epilepsia partialis continua*, or *Kojewnikoff syndrome*, discussed below.

The clinical evaluation of patients with partial epilepsy must include an EEG, a neuroimaging test, and laboratory testing. The EEG is of paramount importance for the correct diagnosis and classification of the ictal events. Although the neurologist may diagnose a seizure disorder from the clinical description, the EEG may serve as an important confirmatory test when the episode is not well described. However, a routine EEG recording may be normal in patients with unequivocal seizure disorders.

The **EEG hallmark** of partial epilepsy is focal spikes or spike-and-wave discharges. The EEG should be recorded during both wakefulness and sleep. A definitive result is often obtained during sleep because it may activate epileptiform discharges and increase the probability of making the correct diagnosis and defining the focal origin (Figure 25-4). In patients with epilepsia partialis continua, the EEG contains spike-wave discharges in a variably continuous manner, often in the contralateral frontal lobe. A small number of individuals in the healthy population have an abnormal EEG containing focal spikes. Repeated recordings may be necessary if the nature of the episode is unclear and, in particular, if psychogenic nonepileptic seizures are suspected. At best, the EEG may capture an ongoing seizure and greatly clarify its origin. It may also help to localize the epileptogenic pathology, guiding surgery if medical treatment fails.

Neuroimaging studies, especially MRI, are vital to the evaluation of new-onset or changing-pattern seizures. Brain CT is a useful screening technique when MRI is not available. The onset of new partial seizures strongly suggests the development of a new pathologic process, including tumors (primary or metastatic) or abscess in the adult population, stroke from vasculitis or emboli in older age groups, and focal encephalitis such as Rasmussen encephalitis in children, herpes simplex in children or adults, or head trauma (Figure 25-5). However, sometimes a patient with a lesion, eg, mesial temporal sclerosis or an AVM, does not present with partial seizures until adulthood. Rarely, the cause of acute-onset partial seizures may be identified by laboratory studies (eg, nonketotic hyperglycemia).

Complex Partial Seizures

Clinical Vignette

A 27-year-old woman presented with a 7-year history of 6 episodes of a feeling of confusion followed by repetitive lip smacking, chewing motions, and semi-purposeful movements of her hands. During these events, she did not respond to questions appropriately. Each episode lasted 5 minutes. She was amnestic for most of the time during each seizure and confused for 1 to 2 hours after each seizure. Between episodes, she felt well. Her medical history included a few febrile convulsions at the age of 2 years. The neurologic examination results were normal.

This patient's history represents a typical example of complex partial seizures (CPSs). The clinical manifestations of the seizure include changes in alertness, level of consciousness, and partial amnesia (Figure 25-3). Automatic, involuntary, stereotyped, repetitive, facial, and lingual and oropharyngeal movements and gestures are often present. Patients often perform simple motor tasks and even may walk during the seizure. CPSs are usually of temporal lobe origin. They generally arise from mesial, temporal structures. Sometimes they originate in the inferior frontal lobe or other extralimbic temporal structures and spread via the uncinate fasciculus to the mesial temporal lobe.

Partial seizures of frontal lobe origin may have unusual clinical presentations frequently confused with a CPS of temporal origin, including a brief aura with fast generalization. Typically, these seizures manifest as versive head and eye movements with tonic posturing of arms. Rarely, a fall is the only clinical feature. Seizures originating in the frontal lobe may occur at night and often produce odd behaviors suggestive of psychogenic nonepileptic seizures.

Because complex seizures are of focal origin, patient evaluation is similar to that undertaken for an SPS. Typically, the interictal EEG (ie, obtained between seizures) reveals spike discharges in one or both anterior temporal lobes.

EPILEPSY AND SYNCOPE

Figure 25-4

Electroencephalography

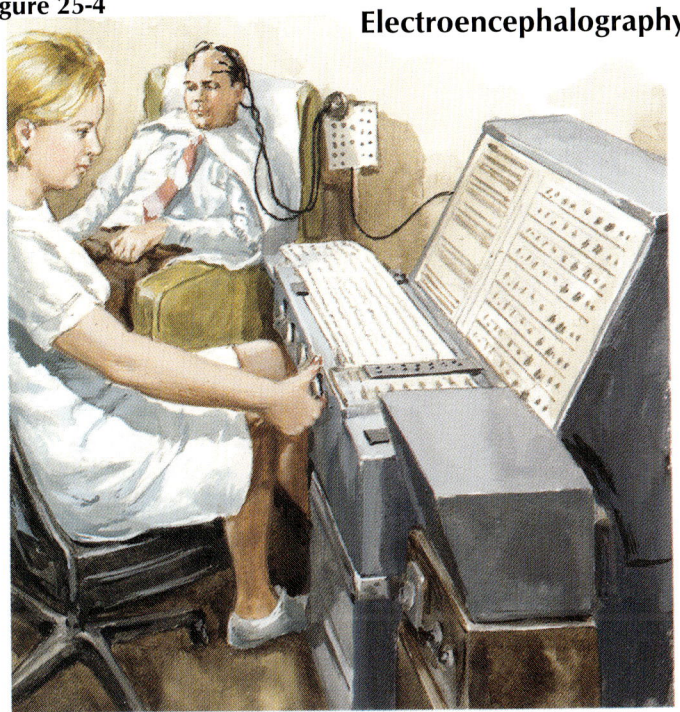

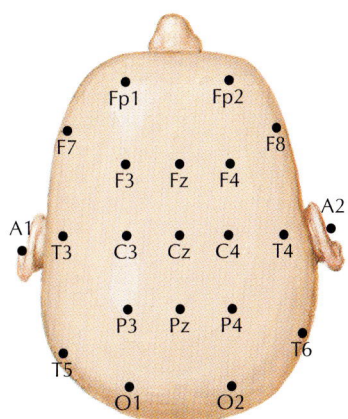

Electrode placement and lead identification

Odd numbers, left side
Even numbers, right side
z locations, midline

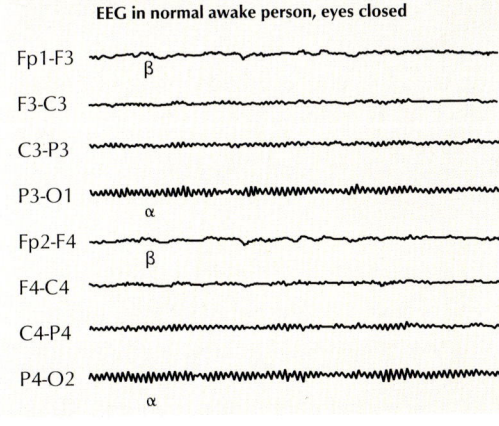

EEG in normal awake person, eyes closed

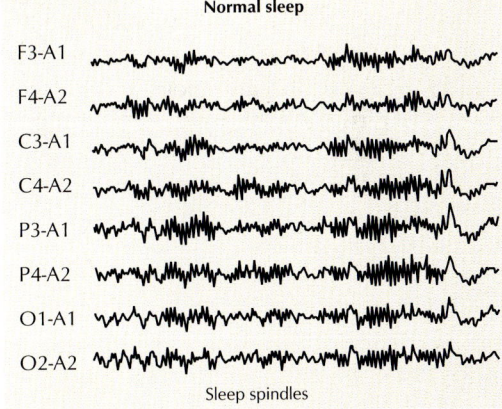

Normal sleep

Sleep spindles

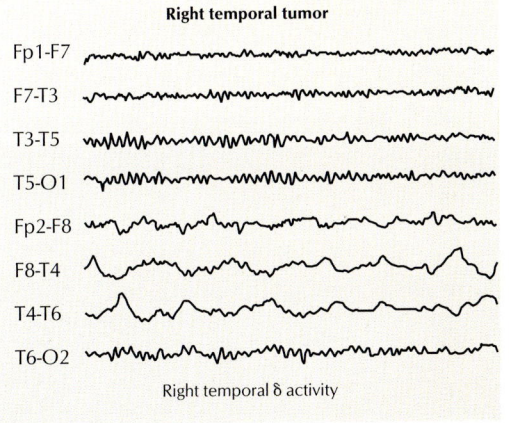

Right temporal tumor

Right temporal δ activity

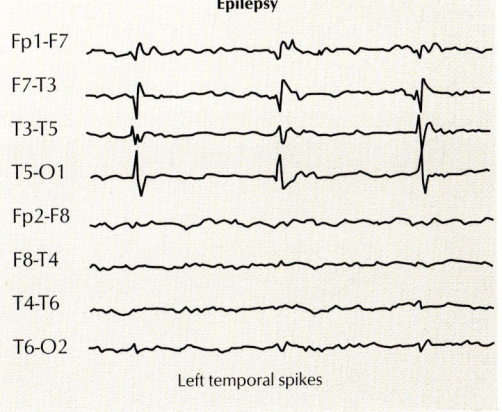

Epilepsy

Left temporal spikes

EPILEPSY AND SYNCOPE

Figure 25-5

Causes of Seizures
Primary

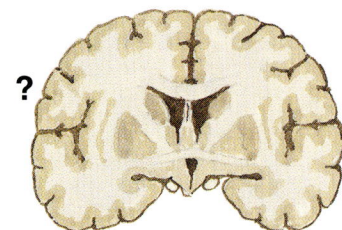

? ? Unknown (genetic or biochemical predisposition)

Intracranial

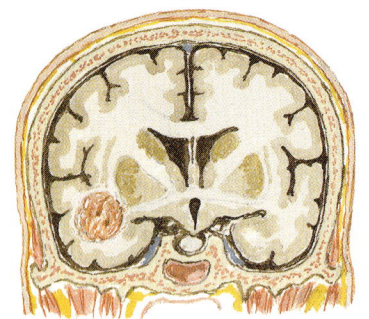

Tumor

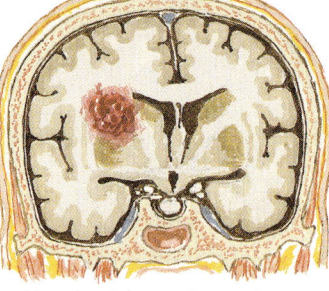

Vascular (infarct or hemorrhage)

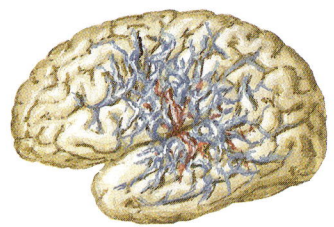

Arteriovenous malformation

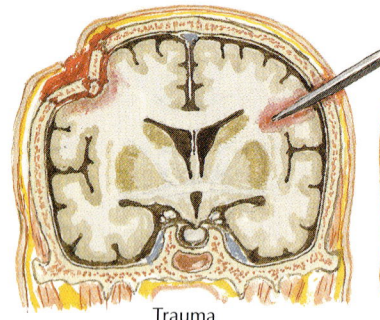

Trauma (depressed fracture, penetrating wound)

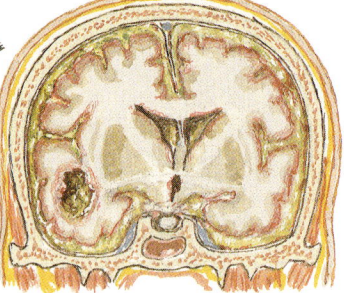

Infection (abscess, encephalitis)

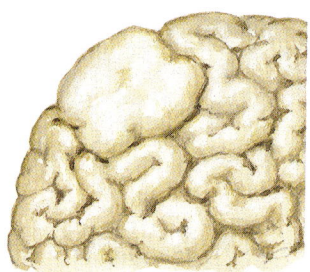

Congenital and hereditary diseases (tuberous sclerosis)

Extracranial

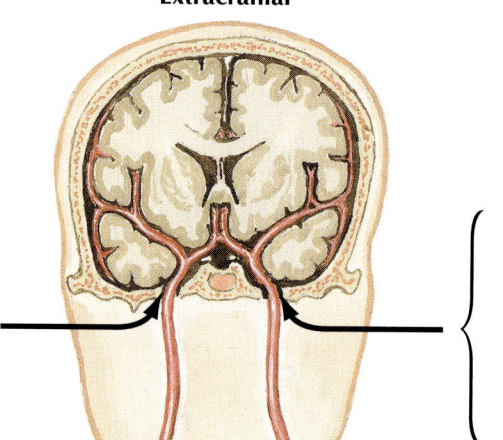

Metabolic
Electrolyte
Biochemical
Inborn errors of metabolism

Anoxia
Hypoglycemia
Drugs
Drug withdrawal
Alcohol withdrawal

The ictal EEG is usually abnormal, with recurrent focal spikes or rhythmic activity. Brain MRI should be obtained, with special attention given to the temporal lobes because these patients often have mesial temporal lobe sclerosis with cell loss and atrophy (Figure 25-5).

Partial Seizures with Secondary Generalization

Sometimes an SCS or a CPS develops into a generalized tonic-clonic convulsion. Because the initial partial symptoms may be brief or may not be recalled or witnessed, careful attention to the history is necessary to distinguish this from primary generalized tonic-clonic convulsions. Capturing a seizure with continuous EEG recordings may be the only way to differentiate them. The evaluation of patients with a focal lesion are described above.

Generalized Seizures
Tonic-Clonic (Grand Mal) Seizures

> **Clinical Vignette**
>
> *The wife of a 46-year-old man reported an event in which he suddenly cried out, extended his arms and legs, and then displayed rhythmic generalized jerking of all 4 extremities. He was unresponsive and unconscious, his face turned blue, and he later became limp. He bit his tongue and was incontinent of urine. Gradually, he woke up, reporting of muscle soreness. He was taken to his physician's office. Neurologic examination results were normal later that day. The patient had no recollection of the event.*

This type of seizure represents the classic picture that the public and medical community generically perceive as epilepsy. Typically, these tonic-clonic (grand mal) seizures are preceded by nonspecific, vaguely defined prodromes lasting up to hours. If these seizures have a specific aura, a focal origin with secondary generalization is most probable.

Grand mal seizures start with loss of consciousness, a cry, generalized tonic muscle contraction, and a fall (Figure 25-6). Autonomic signs are often present during the tonic phase, including tachycardia, hypertension, cyanosis, salivation, sweating, and incontinence. The tonic muscle contraction becomes interrupted relatively soon and is followed by the clonic phase of the seizure; the relaxation periods progressively lengthen, and the seizure eventually abates. Patients may remain stuporous for a moment and eventually awaken confused with postictal complaints of headaches, lethargy, disorientation, and myalgia that may persist for a few days.

A single generalized grand mal seizure does not warrant the diagnosis of epilepsy. In the vignette above, the patient later admitted that during the previous year, he was worried about his business and had been abusing alcohol and sedatives. He had recently discontinued these and had not had alcohol or sedatives for 48 hours. EEG and neuroimaging studies were normal. The seizure described above represents a reactive type of generalized grand mal seizure, ie, secondary to drug withdrawal. Similar seizures may occur from withdrawal from other drugs or various metabolic, infectious, and traumatic conditions.

Absence (Petit Mal) Seizures

> **Clinical Vignette**
>
> *A 10-year-old boy was brought to his pediatrician because of poor attention in class. The teacher noted that the child had brief (less than 15 seconds) episodes of impaired alertness and responsiveness. Some eye flutter and occasional facial twitching were noted during the episodes. The child seemed normal on termination of the episodes and was unaware of any problem. The family history was positive for seizures in a cousin. The neurologic examination results were normal. EEG demonstrated the classic 3-Hz spike-and-wave pattern.*

This is a typical history of a child with generalized absence (petit mal) seizures. Petit mal epilepsy is the classic example of benign primary generalized epilepsy (Figure 25-7). These seizures tend to remit in adulthood. The patient's brief lapse in consciousness is the main feature. Typically, these seizures start as a clinically generalized event without an aura (the presence of such would indicate a partial origin of the seizure) or any postictal symptoms. Although automatic movements may be observed, they are generally simple and brief. The neurologic examination results are usually normal.

EEG provides the best diagnostic confirmation. It typically demonstrates brief generalized bilaterally synchronous 3-Hz spike-and-wave discharges. Hyperventilation may precipitate these

EPILEPSY AND SYNCOPE

Figure 25-6

Generalized Tonic-Clonic Seizures

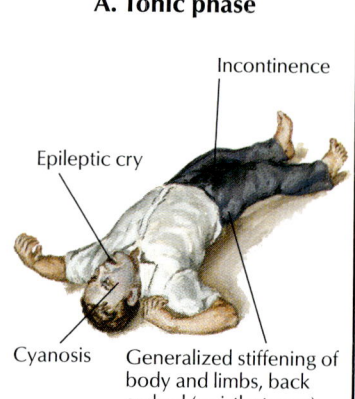
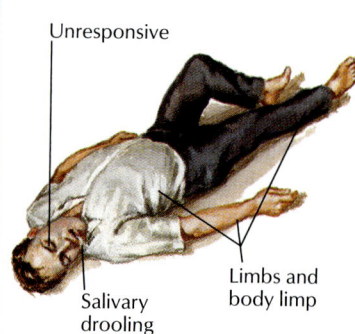
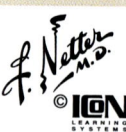

seizures and the classic epileptiform changes during EEG recording. There is neither focal interictal EEG epileptic activity nor focal initiation of the spike-and-wave pattern.

Atypical Absence Seizures

Atypical absence seizures differ from typical absence seizures because motor symptoms are more prominent and sometimes have a focal preponderance. Usually beginning during childhood, atypical absence seizures tend to occur over a longer lifetime period than classic petit mal seizures. Additionally, some patients have postictal confusion. Children with atypical absence seizures tend to have multifocal or generalized cerebral pathology, clinically associated with a lag in attaining normal developmental milestones.

The EEG demonstrates a slow (1.5- to 2.5-Hz) spike-and-wave pattern. This clinical constellation and its associated seizures and EEG pattern are characteristic of the **Lennox-Gastaut syndrome**, an example of an epileptic syndrome described below. Generally, these patients also have other types of seizures. Treatment of the seizures of this syndrome is difficult and usually requires multiple anticonvulsants.

Myoclonic Seizures

Clinical Vignette

A 17-year-old girl reported a history of unprovoked massive muscle jerks involving either arm for approximately 1 year. These tended to occur in the morning. This patient also had 2 recent unexplained falls. She did not report lapse of consciousness during the falls. Her neurologic examination results were normal.

EPILEPSY AND SYNCOPE

Figure 25-7 — Absence (Petit Mal) Seizures

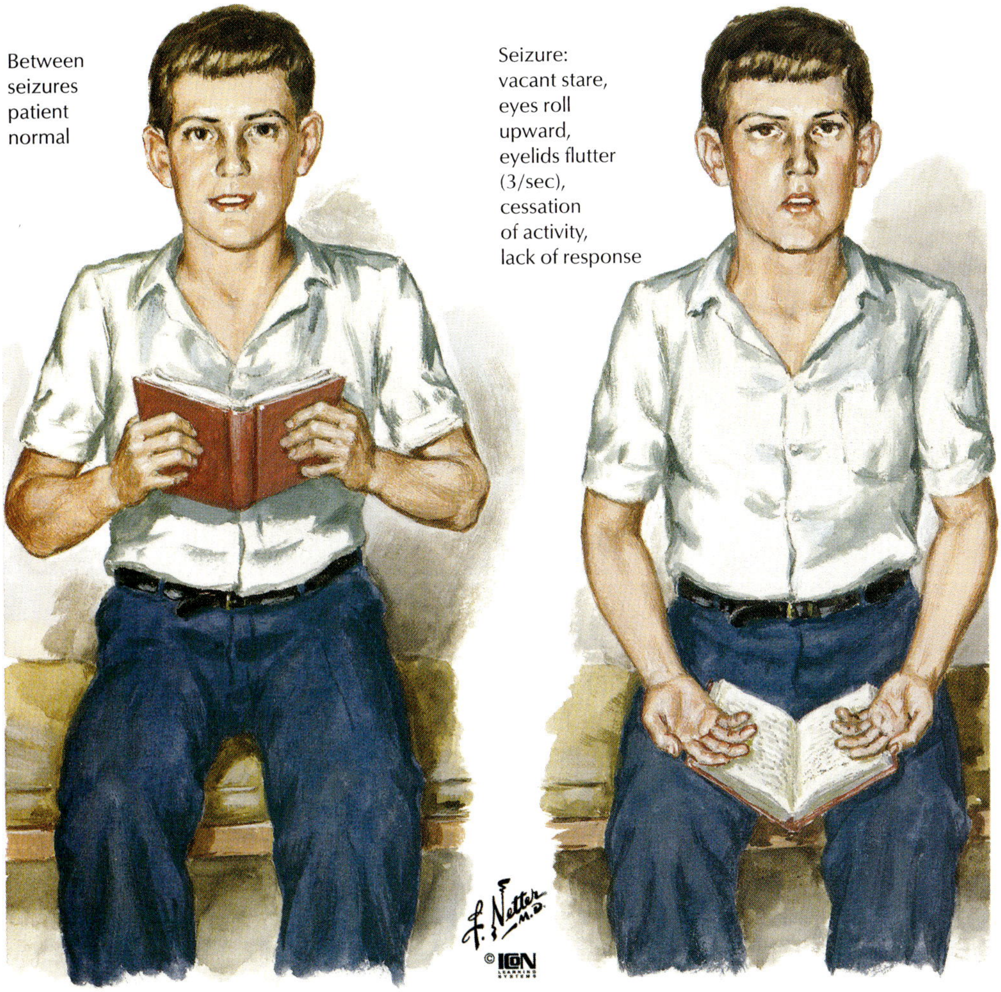

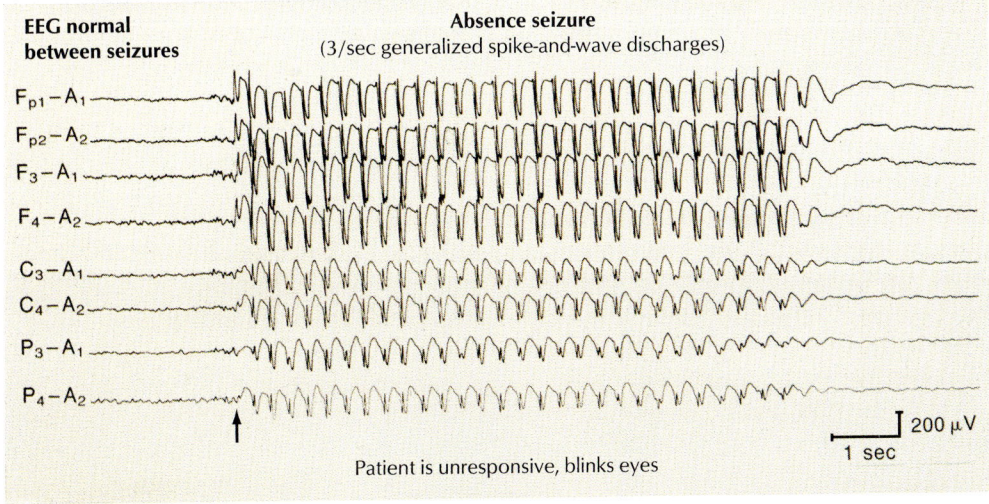

This history is typical of myoclonic seizures. The patient has a primary generalized epilepsy called *juvenile myoclonic epilepsy*. These myoclonic seizures usually begin during the teenage years. Many of these patients have occasional generalized seizures.

EEGs typically demonstrate bilaterally synchronous, irregular spike-wave or polyspike discharges at variable repetition rates at 4 to 6 Hz but no focal epileptic discharges. Paradoxically, the EEG discharges usually have no clinical myoclonic accompaniment. This condition usually responds well to antiepileptic medication and sometimes remits spontaneously in later years.

Myoclonic seizures also may occur in children with a variety of epileptic syndromes such as the Lennox-Gastaut syndrome, infantile spasms (West syndrome), and early myoclonic encephalopathy. Myoclonus also may be a part of CNS storage diseases. In the past, myoclonus occurred as a significant manifestation of a rare late form of measles, subacute sclerosing panencephalitis. This illness presented with poor school performance, mental changes, and myoclonus in teenagers, with periodic EEG complexes occurring regularly every several seconds.

In the adult population, myoclonus is one of the classic findings in the prion-caused dementing illness spongiform encephalopathy (Creutzfeldt-Jakob disease). This disease usually occurs in middle to late life. The EEG in Creutzfeldt-Jakob disease has a classic appearance with periodic sharp and slow wave complexes recurring usually at 1 to 2 Hz. The background EEG is abnormal.

Myoclonus is also a nonspecific term that describes brief nonepileptic muscle jerks. They may involve a body segment or be generalized, may be single or repetitive, and may be spontaneous or provoked by sensory stimulation (reflex) or limb action. One of the most frequently observed settings for myoclonus is the postanoxic syndrome in patients who experienced cardiac arrest. Prognosis is poor for individuals resuscitated after significant irreversible brain damage who display myoclonus.

Epileptic Syndromes

Stereotypic seizures at a particular age and associated with fairly distinct EEG abnormalities or a symptom complex constitute the epileptic syndromes. The seizures in these syndromes may be classified into reactive, the best known being benign febrile convulsions; primary or idiopathic, exemplified by childhood absence (petit mal) epilepsy; and secondary or symptomatic, eg, infantile spasms or West syndrome.

Benign Febrile Convulsions

Benign febrile convulsions occur in otherwise healthy children at the age of 6 months to 5 years. Up to 5% of healthy children in the US experience at least 1 febrile convulsion, usually early during a benign febrile illness. The seizures are brief, simple, and without localizing or lateralizing preponderance. Interictal EEGs are always normal. If not, other seizure mechanisms should be considered. The long-term prognosis is usually excellent if no seizures occur in nonfebrile circumstances.

Benign Childhood Epilepsy With Centrotemporal (Rolandic) Spikes

Benign childhood epilepsy with centrotemporal (rolandic) spikes is a primary (idiopathic) epileptic syndrome that develops during the first decade of life. Typically, these children have partial seizures characterized by unilateral perioral sensory or minor motor activity associated with dysarthria or speech arrest, salivation, and preserved consciousness. Nocturnal generalized convulsions may occur.

EEG shows distinctive high-amplitude spikes or sharp waves with an unusual surface positive-negative polarity over the centrotemporal (rolandic) cortex and midtemporal areas. These epileptiform transients may repeat for a few seconds, shifting in preponderance from side to side. Although the etiology is unknown, autosomal dominant inheritance is suggested. The prognosis is excellent for this benign type of epilepsy.

Infantile Spasms (West Syndrome)

West syndrome is an example of a secondary (symptomatic) generalized epileptic syndrome occurring during the first year of life. There is a concomitant arrest of psychomotor development. These seizures are characterized by brief jerks followed by a tonic phase and a subsequent period of generalized atonia lasting approximately 1 minute or associated with flexion-extension spasms.

The chaotic appearance of a typical EEG, called *hypsarrhythmia*, shows high-amplitude slow wave activity with mixed high-amplitude sharp or spike discharges. The EEG correlate of the spasm is a sudden appearance of high-amplitude slow waves followed by an electrodecremental period with low-voltage fast activity. The prognosis is poor. The primary treatment is corticotropin administration.

Status Epilepticus

Clinical Vignette

A 32-year-old man with a history of posttraumatic recurrent partial motor seizures, occasionally leading to generalized tonic-clonic seizures and drug noncompliance, was brought to the ED with recurrent seizures. His wife stated that the day before admission, he had experienced a few episodes of jerking of his hand. During the early morning hours, the patient's wife was awakened to find her husband having a generalized grand mal convulsion. Although to her he seemed to have been "coming out" of this event, he then proceeded to have another tonic-clonic seizure. Thereafter, he remained deeply stuporous. In the ED, his phenytoin level was 1.4 µg/mL. He was treated with IV phenytoin.

Generalized convulsive status epilepticus (GCSE) is defined as unremitting seizures without recovery of consciousness lasting 30 minutes or longer (Figure 25-8). One of the most common and life-threatening neurologic emergencies, GCSE mandates immediate treatment because of the potential for irreversible CNS damage, ie, neuronal loss secondary to anoxia and systemic metabolic and autonomic dysfunction. Medical complications such as cardiac arrhythmias, pulmonary edema, and renal failure sometimes occur during or after GCSE. The GCSE mortality rate approaches 30%. Unfortunately, the history in the final vignette in this chapter is common in patients with partial motor seizures with secondary generalization who do not comply with antiepileptic therapy and progress to status epilepticus.

Treatment of GCSE treatment requires maintenance of an adequate airway, breathing, and blood circulation and termination of the seizures. Etiologic mechanisms requiring prompt treatment include anticonvulsant or other medication withdrawal, illicit toxic drugs, hypoglycemia, hyponatremia, and hypocalcemia. GCSE may be the first manifestation of acute cerebral pathology.

The initial therapy, a benzodiazepine or phenytoin, often depends on whether the patient is actively seizing. Both first-line medications are frequently utilized within a short time. Intravenous lorazepam at 1 to 2 mg/min up to 8 mg or diazepam up to 20 mg is most often the initial therapy. An infusion of phenytoin (at 50 mg/min) or fosphenytoin (at an equivalence of 150 mg phenytoin/min) up to 20 mg/kg must also be started promptly because the benzodiazepines have a short-term effect. Phenytoin should not be given with a glucose solution because phenytoin will precipitate out. ECG monitoring is required because these drugs can affect cardiac conduction if given too rapidly. These patients often need assisted ventilation.

If seizures persist, additional phenytoin (5-10 mg/kg) may be given, or phenobarbital (at 50-100 mg/min, up to 20 mg/kg) may be added. If these are ineffective, barbiturate anesthesia with sodium pentobarbital at a loading dose of 5 to 15 mg/kg followed by 0.5 to 5 $mg \cdot kg^{-1} \cdot h^{-1}$ with EEG monitoring is suggested. Benzodiazepines such as midazolam or propofol infusions are sometimes used before barbiturate anesthesia is initiated.

Nonconvulsive status epilepticus or **absence status epilepticus** is another form of continued seizures without motor accompaniments. Typically, patients are poorly responsive with decreased alertness or obtundation. EEG reveals mostly continuous generalized spike-and-wave activity, the so-called spike-wave stupor. Intravenous benzodiazepine administration, the treatment of choice, is generally effective.

Complex partial seizures may recur frequently and occasionally evolve into **complex partial status epilepticus**, in which patients do not regain full consciousness between seizures. Prompt treatment as prescribed for GCSE is necessary. An SPS may evolve into epilepsia partialis continua, as described above. Long-term anticonvulsant therapy is usually needed in patients who have experienced status epilepticus.

EPILEPSY AND SYNCOPE

Figure 25-8 — Status Epilepticus

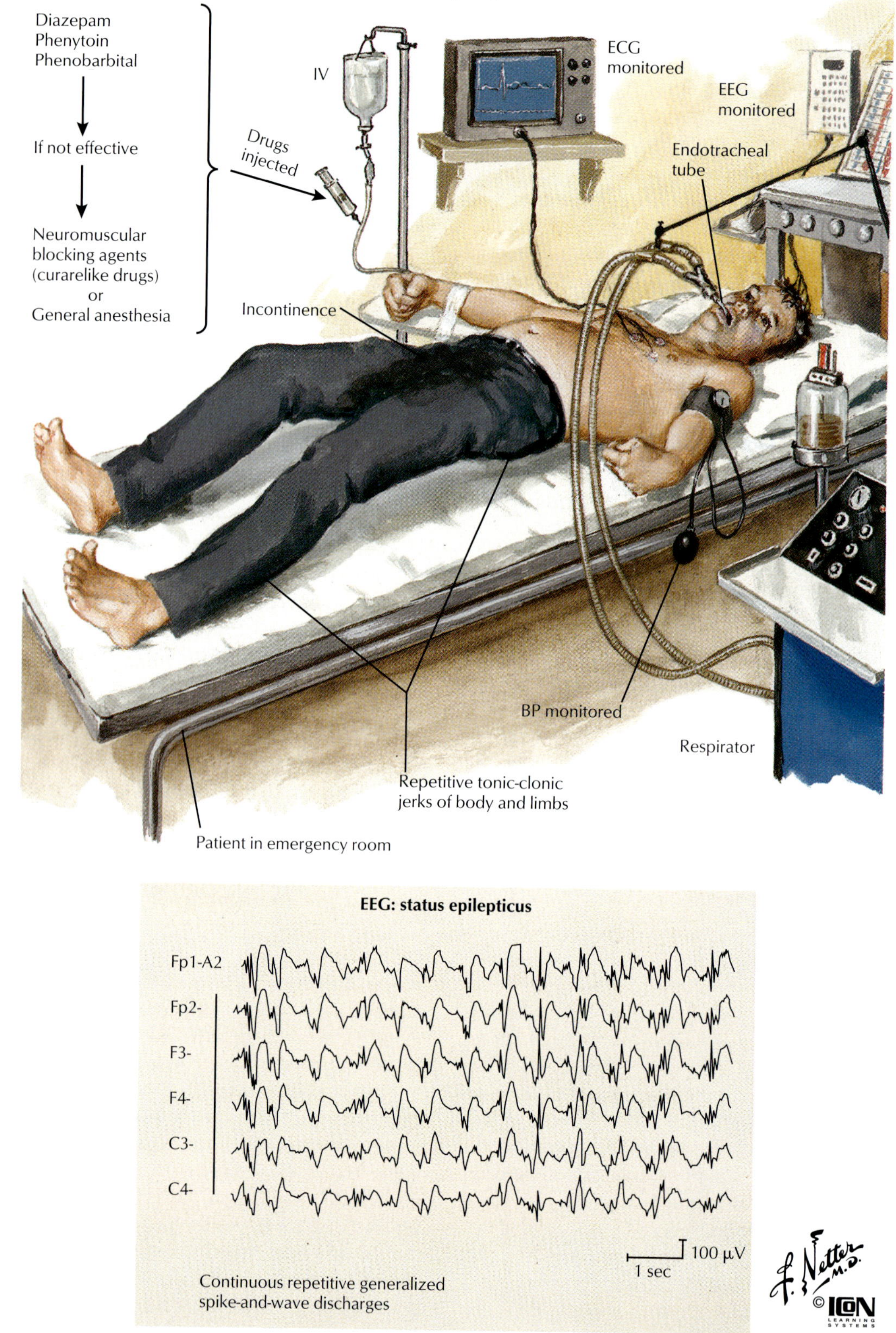

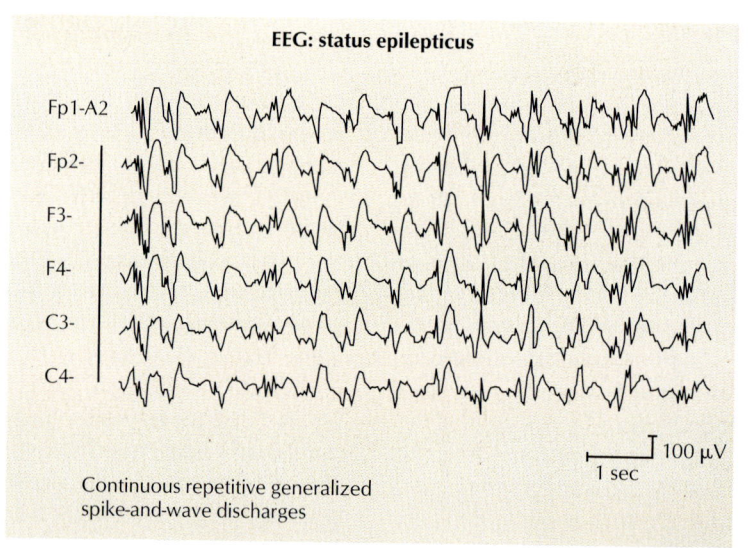

Continuous repetitive generalized spike-and-wave discharges

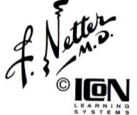

Antiepileptic Therapy

The goal of antiepileptic treatment is total seizure control. The most important step in seizure treatment is identification and treatment of the pathophysiologic mechanism. Examples include resection of a tumor, correction of a metabolic imbalance, and treatment of a CNS infection. Appropriate therapy may stop seizure recurrence.

Unfortunately, most seizures occur within chronic neurologic processes not amenable to specific therapy and therefore require long-term treatment. Ideally, seizure medication would have 100% efficacy, no adverse effects, little interaction with other drugs, easy compliance, and low cost. Unfortunately, no such anticonvulsant medication exists, so treatment must balance seizure control with quality of life.

Generally, seizure type suggests the choice of drug. Phenytoin and carbamazepine are the drugs of choice for partial seizures with or without generalization. A common dosage of **phenytoin** is 300 to 400 mg orally per day. Because phenytoin has a long half-life, it can be given once or twice daily in adults, thereby reducing the risk of missed midday dosages. Optimum seizure control occurs with blood levels of 10 to 20 µg/mL. With drug concentrations greater than the therapeutic range, adverse effects develop. Often mild, they mimic alcohol intoxication: dizziness, nystagmus, ataxia, slurred speech, and confusion. Prolonged use in youth may produce facial feature coarsening and gingival hyperplasia. Acute idiosyncratic reactions occur in approximately 10% of patients and vary from a mild morbilliform rash to a rare severe exfoliative dermatitis. As with other anticonvulsants, teratogenic effects may occur. Phenytoin interacts with numerous drugs of many classes. Phenytoin has zero-order kinetics, so small dosage changes may create large changes in serum concentrations.

Carbamazepine is another common and generally well-tolerated choice for partial seizures, with a usual dose of 600 to 1000 mg/d. The therapeutic blood serum level is 4 to 12 µg/mL. Early adverse reactions are dizziness, nausea, and drowsiness. Hypersensitive allergic reactions may occur, as with phenytoin, early in treatment. Serious drug complications may result from bone marrow suppression.

Oxcarbazepine is an antiepileptic drug that is converted to an active metabolite but does not require periodic blood counts. Hyponatremia sometimes occurs. Adverse reactions include psychomotor slowing and sedation. It may be better tolerated than carbamazepine, with less sedation. A typical starting dosage is 300 mg twice daily, increased gradually to 600 mg twice daily. Occasionally, higher dosages are used but should not exceed 2400 mg daily.

Phenobarbital and **primidone** had been used for years to treat a variety of epileptic seizures. Sedation is a prevalent adverse effect and has contributed to their decreased use. The usual dosage is 30 to 60 mg 3 times daily or 90 to 180 mg daily, usually at bedtime. Therapeutic levels usually range from 20 to 40 µg/mL.

Lamotrigine is a newer antiepileptic drug recommended as an adjunct medication for partial seizures in adults and for partial and generalized seizures in children. The usual adult maintenance dose is 300 to 500 mg/d in divided doses. It must be introduced at low doses with slow increases to achieve maintenance levels in several weeks. Rash is a potentially serious adverse effect, particularly in children, and may be more likely if lamotrigine is used with other antiepileptic drugs. Other adverse effects include nausea, dizziness, and ataxia. Interactions with other antiepileptic drugs must be carefully monitored.

Ethosuximide, usually well tolerated, is indicated for absence (petit mal) seizures. A common dose is 250 to 1000 mg/d according to age and response. The therapeutic blood level is 40 to 100 µg/mL.

Divalproex sodium is another drug commonly used for either generalized or partial seizures. It is also useful for myoclonic seizures; it is commonly given in a dosage of 500 to 2000 mg/d. The therapeutic blood level is 50 to 100 µg/mL. Adverse effects include dizziness, asthenia, tremor, weight gain, and hair loss. More serious effects include liver toxicity, pancreatitis, and teratogenic effects.

Several other drugs are recommended as adjunctive to the first-line medications mentioned above: gabapentin (Neurontin), topiramate, levetiracetam, tiagabine, and zonisamide. Because they have different mechanisms of action, they may complement the first-line drugs. They decrease seizure frequency and improve quality of life without adding untoward side effects or producing new ones in some patients.

All anticonvulsants have variable **teratogenic effects**. Significant caution is advised for their use in women of childbearing age. Use of these medications must include risk-benefit analysis, especially during the first trimester of pregnancy. Detailed discussions with patients about the potential teratogenic effects in this clinical setting are essential. Tests to detect neural tube and other anticonvulsant-induced congenital defects should be considered routine prenatal care.

Surgical treatment may be an option for individuals whose seizures are unresponsive to medical therapy. Patients who cannot take prescribed medications because of adverse effects or quality-of-life issues are also candidates for consideration of surgical treatment.

Patients with CPSs and underlying unilateral mesial temporal sclerosis, hamartoma, or other congenital pathologic processes frequently obtain excellent results after temporal lobectomy or lesion resection. Individuals with CPSs but no obvious underlying pathology may also be good surgical candidates. Patients must undergo detailed studies in specialized centers to clearly delineate the area producing the seizure. This requires long-term scalp EEG monitoring, sometimes with intracranial leads, PET, or SPECT. Wada testing to determine the dominant language hemisphere, neuropsychometric testing, and psychiatric evaluations are also indicated. Small cortical resections and palliative surgeries such as callosotomy and vagal nerve stimulation have been shown to be useful.

SYNCOPE

Syncope is defined as a brief and transient loss of consciousness from cerebral hypoperfusion. Lightheadedness, visual dimming, paleness, cold sweating, nausea, and a feeling of warmth are common premonitory symptoms (Figure 25-9). These are followed by loss of consciousness and postural muscle tone and, if the patient is standing, a fall. Significant trauma and fractures occur in approximately 5% of these patients. In contrast to patients who lose consciousness from a convulsion, individuals who have syncope generally have no confusion after the episode. Typically, they have good recollection of premonitory symptoms. Loss of consciousness lasts just a few seconds. Occasionally, a few clonic twitches or a brief generalized seizure occurs at the end of the episode.

An EEG recorded during syncope demonstrates early depression of α activity followed by slow wave activity in the Θ range and soon after in the δ range. Transient EEG voltage depression may follow. Elderly patients may be amnestic for the event. Almost 20% of people have had 1 syncopal episode in their lifetime.

Syncope may be classified as having cardiac or noncardiac origin. Cardiac syncope may be further subclassified into reflex, from orthostatic hypotension or cardiac disease. Noncardiac syncope is subclassified as neurologic, metabolic, psychiatric, or idiopathic. The most common type, cardiac reflex syncope, has three subtypes: vasovagal (called *neurocardiogenic* or *vasodepressor*), situational (eg, micturition, Valsalva, ocular compression, venipuncture, fear, exertion), and carotid hypersensitivity.

Vasovagal cardiac reflex syncope is the most commonly seen syncope in neurologic practice. Its pathophysiology is unresolved. The reflex is initiated by an intense sympathetic activation (eg, a painful stimulus or fear) with increase of blood pressure, tachycardia, decreased cardiac filling ("empty heart"), and powerful cardiac contractions that stimulate heart mechanoreceptors. Subsequently, cardiac inhibitor pathway activation causes a short-term increase of vagal activity and withdrawal of sympathetic activity, known as the *Bezold-Jarisch reflex*. The loss of consciousness, secondary to cerebral hypoperfusion, is primarily from a combination of profound bradycardia or arterial pressure collapse.

Vasovagal syncope often occurs while assuming the upright posture. In these instances, diminished blood return from the lower limbs and viscera and a subsequent pooling of blood in the lower body result in decreased cardiac filling and initiation of the cascade of events.

The clinical examination of a patient with presumed syncope aims first to exclude serious illnesses, sometimes associated with acute loss of

EPILEPSY AND SYNCOPE

Figure 25-9   Syncope: Four-Step Management Approach

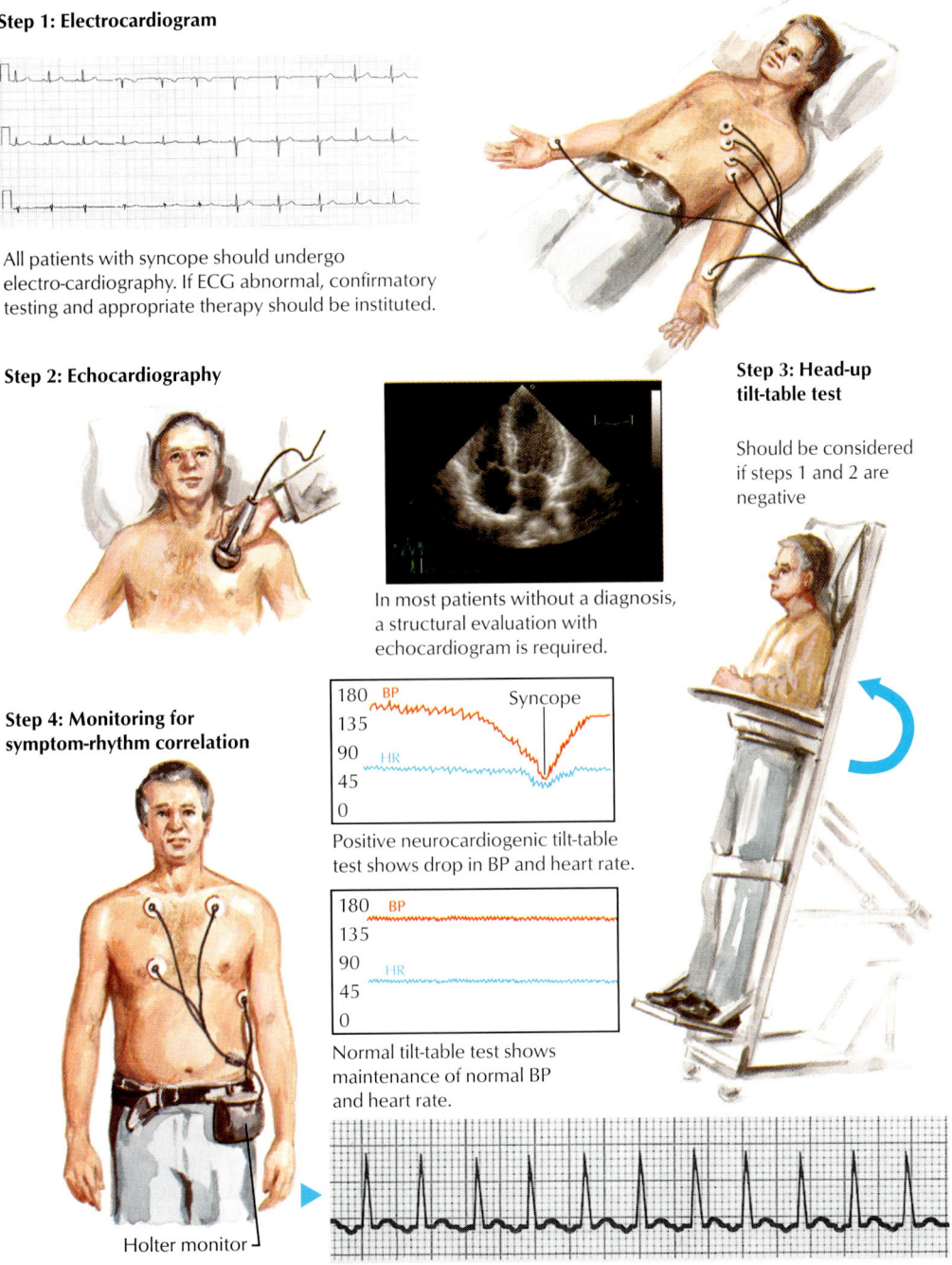

Step 1: Electrocardiogram

All patients with syncope should undergo electro-cardiography. If ECG abnormal, confirmatory testing and appropriate therapy should be instituted.

Step 2: Echocardiography

In most patients without a diagnosis, a structural evaluation with echocardiogram is required.

Step 3: Head-up tilt-table test

Should be considered if steps 1 and 2 are negative

Positive neurocardiogenic tilt-table test shows drop in BP and heart rate.

Normal tilt-table test shows maintenance of normal BP and heart rate.

Step 4: Monitoring for symptom-rhythm correlation

Holter monitor

Ambulatory monitoring recommended for patients with negative evaluation; duration of monitoring dependent on frequency of episodes; for daily symptoms, 48-hour monitor adequate

consciousness, including structural heart disease, such as valvular aortic stenosis, cardiac rhythm disturbances, coronary artery disease, and cardiomyopathies with compromised cardiac output. Patients with syncope from heart disease have a higher mortality rate than individuals with other causes of syncope. Evaluation must include a detailed history and physical examination with particular attention to the heart, an ECG, Holter monitor, other forms of cardiac event monitoring, echocardiography, treadmill exercise test, and electrophysiologic testing.

Orthostatic hypotension is a common cause of syncope. A tilt table test is essential to the evaluation of these patients and to the investigation of syncope of unclear origin. The causes of orthostatic hypotension vary and merit further evaluation. Medications of many classes are common causes of hypotension leading to syncope. Dehydration and hypovolemia are other, easily excluded, common pathophysiologic mechanisms.

Hyperventilation with associated hypocapnia is a rare cause of syncope. Metabolic causes of syncope include hypoglycemia and hypoxia. Psychogenic syncope sometimes can be difficult to document. It is best excluded by a careful history, witnessing the event, or both.

Primary neurologic causes of syncope are uncommon and usually have other associated symptoms. Peripheral neuropathies are the most common neurologic causes of syncope associated with orthostatic hypotension, particularly in patients with neuropathies secondary to diabetes and rarely primary amyloidosis. Central nervous diseases such as multiple system atrophy with parkinsonian, cerebellar, or mixed features, previously called *Shy-Drager disease*, and pure autonomic failure must be considered despite their rare occurrence. Transient ischemic attacks in the vertebrobasilar system or basilar migraine are conditions that rarely produce syncopal episodes. Although unilateral carotid artery disease is sometimes considered, there is no documentation of its causality. It is unusual for even bilateral critical carotid stenosis to cause syncope. The drop attacks of epileptic seizures are infrequently confused with syncope. Although these patients lose postural tone and "drop," they do not lose consciousness.

The **management of syncope** focuses on the underlying disease process, often requiring specialized medical or surgical treatments. Cardiac, neurologic, and situational mechanisms must be addressed. The therapy of reflex vasovagal syncope is problematic. Analysis of whether syncope is primarily from cardiac inhibition or hypotension is sometimes difficult because these often occur together. Education, increased salt and fluid intake, β blockers, blood volume expanders such as mineralocorticoids (fludrocortisone), α-adrenergic agonists, and SSRIs have been recommended. Antiarrhythmic agents and pacemakers are also sometimes indicated. Unfortunately, many of these treatments have not been rigorously evaluated.

REFERENCES

Bromfield EB. Seizures. In: Samuels MA, ed. *Hospitalist Neurology*. Boston, Mass: Butterworth Heinemann; 1999:79-105.

Engel J Jr, Pedley TA, eds. *Epilepsy: A Comprehensive Textbook*. Philadelphia, Pa: Lippincott-Raven; 1998.

Engel J Jr. *Seizures and Epilepsy*. Philadelphia, Pa: FA Davis Co; 1989.

Shen WK, Gersh BJ. Syncope: mechanisms, approach, and management. In: Low PA, ed. *Clinical Autonomic Disorders*. Boston, Mass: Little, Brown and Co; 1993:605-640.

Working Group on Status Epilepticus. Treatment of convulsive status epilepticus. *JAMA*. 1993;270:854-859.

Wyllie E, ed. *The Treatment of Epilepsy: Principles and Practice*. 3rd ed. Philadelphia, Pa: Lippincott Williams & Wilkins; 2001.

Chapter 26
Surgical Treatments for Epilepsy

Jeffrey E. Arle

Surgical treatment of epilepsy has a substantial history. Some of the first craniotomies on record were performed to treat refractory seizure disorders. Clinical cerebral localization techniques were used based on the specific characteristics of a seizure. Cerebral tumors causing convulsions were also removed based on these techniques. Many aspects of cortical mapping and function were derived from work related to surgery for epileptic activity.

SURGICAL CANDIDATES

Although still debated in terms of clinical severity and management style, a guide for determining the best candidates for surgical treatment of epilepsy is to consider patients with medically refractory seizures who have a desire to improve their quality of life or in whom personal safety may be enhanced. Whether patients are medically refractory is determined by a consensus among the neurologist, the patient, and the family. Statistically, if patients have not had excellent seizure control using either diphenylhydantoin, phenytoin, carbamazepine, or phenobarbital, adding a second drug has only a 15% chance of affording medical seizure control. Adding a third drug to the remaining refractory patients has only another 5% chance of seizure elimination. Considering the complicating side effects of these medications, alone or in combination, 25% to 35% of patients will be medically refractory within a few years after diagnosis. When available medications have been adequately tried, and even though newer medications are continually under development, surgical treatment remains a satisfactory option for many medically refractory seizure patients.

If timely adjustments to the medication regimen and their likelihood of achieving seizure control are unsuccessful, consideration of surgical alternatives and their various ramifications must be considered. Many factors affect the precise timing of surgery. Surgery should be pursued or rejected after preoperative psychiatric counseling and neuropsychological baseline studies are evaluated. The longer a patient has seizures, the more neurologic impairment is likely to evolve and the more refractory to all forms of management the patient may become.

PREOPERATIVE ASSESSMENTS
MRI

MRI is the critical means to identify the precise anatomical substrate responsible for the seizures, including mesial sclerosis, hippocampal atrophy, some areas of cortical dysplasia, encephalomalacia, tumors, and vascular malformations. The precise nature of the anatomical abnormality affects resection planning and seizure focus determination.

Video EEG Analysis

Video EEG analysis is one of the mainstays of preoperative evaluations. The most reliable means of localization are seizures that can be electrically recorded from the same region each time using noninvasive scalp electrodes, and correlated by video of the seizure type. Often, seizures can be localized only to one side of the brain or another or perhaps frontally, but not in a specific enough location to perform surgical resection.

Sodium Amytal Test (Wada Test)

When considering resection of mesial temporal structures, such as an amygdalohippocampectomy, it is essential to decide whether memory function will be maintained by the contralateral homologous tissue. One cannot assume that individuals have intact bilateral memory function and could routinely tolerate elective surgical extirpation of part of one temporal lobe. Sodium amobarbital or a brief-acting benzodiazepine (approximately 8 minutes) is injected into the carotid artery through a catheter to allow immediate perfusion, primarily of 1 hemisphere, leading to pharmacologic functional inactivation of that hemisphere (Figure 26-1). During the immediate post–drug perfusion time, the patient is asked to remember certain words or objects and to speak. During this period, assessments are made of language hemisphere dominance and whether adequate memory function exists on the side opposite the injection. This procedure attempts to ensure that patients are not compromised if a partial temporal lobectomy is performed. Although the information gained by this testing is useful, it is not 100% reliable. For example, parts of the hippocampus may be perfused by branches of the posterior cerebral artery supplied by the vertebrobasilar system. Therefore, some bilateral function may be maintained despite the unilateral carotid injection. An additional concern is the slight stroke risk (approximately 1%) while placing the catheter within the carotid artery, even in centers with significant experience. Despite these admonitions, the Wada test provides important adjunctive data for determining the safety of potential temporal lobe resection.

Neuropsychological Testing

Subtle dysfunction, strengths, and weaknesses in frontal, temporal, parietal, right and left, and dominant and nondominant functional brain regions may be carefully defined by a variety of discriminatory neuropsychological tests before surgery. These data can help to verify the appropriate region for resection and the safety margin of the proposed surgery. Furthermore, the baseline functional determination that is defined preoperatively can be used for postoperative comparisons.

Psychiatric Evaluation

Many patients with epilepsy, particularly those with partial complex seizures, have superimposed depression or anxiety disorders. The appreciation and, if possible, control of these problems before surgery can be extremely helpful. Concomitantly, the psychiatrist can prepare patients for potential emotional problems that are "unmasked" by the operation in approximately 25% of individuals who undergo surgery.

Invasive Electrode Placement

Invasive electrode placement is sometimes a crucial and accurate means to precisely isolate the epileptiform source within the cerebral cortex. Small openings in the skull are made or a larger craniotomy is performed, the suspected abnormal cerebral cortex is exposed, and the electrodes are placed in grids or strips over the cortical surface. The electrode wires are tunneled out through the scalp and connected to the recording system.

Patients are monitored continuously in the hospital. To increase the likelihood of capturing a typical seizure, anticonvulsants may be withheld. Individuals may be studied for up to 2 to 3 weeks; subsequently, infection risk becomes unacceptable. Most patients experience several seizures within that time. When the analysis is completed, identifying the precise epileptogenic site within the cerebral cortex, the patient is returned to surgery. The electrodes are removed, and resection of the identified seizure focus is performed, assuming the identified region can be safely removed without causing a significant neurologic deficit.

SPECT and PET

SPECT and PET are used in certain instances to provide additional data supporting or eliminating specific areas, localization of seizures, and potential surgical resection.

SPECT relies on the use of technetium Tc 99m hexamethylpropyleneamine oxime or technetium Tc 99m bicisate injected intravenously immediately after a seizure. A scan of the radiopharmaceutical uptake is performed several hours later. The agent is taken up by areas of increased blood flow, theoretically associated with an active seizure focus. An inherent problem with SPECT is the low resolution of the scan image. Additionally, certain logistic issues occur, including the need for personnel to prepare the agent and administer it with appropriate timing.

PET relies on the differential metabolic activity of various brain regions and their uptake of fluorine-18 deoxyglucose. The resolution of the re-

SURGICAL TREATMENTS FOR EPILEPSY

Figure 26-1

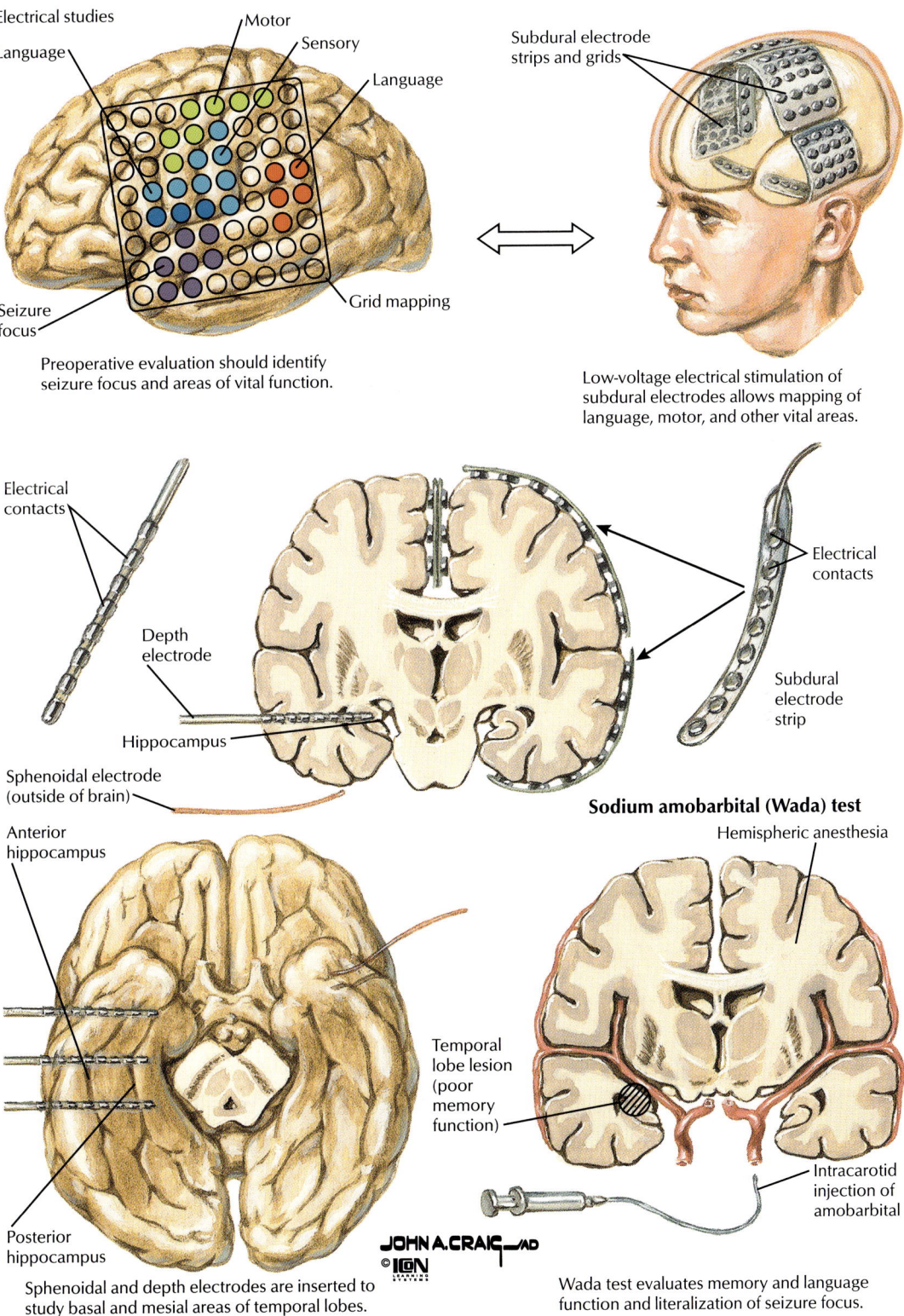

Preoperative Evaluation

EPILEPSY AND SYNCOPE

sulting image is poor but has been improving with newer technology. Similarly, the correlation between lower metabolic activity and epileptiform cerebral regions is partial. However, PET may be performed at any time between seizures, unlike SPECT, which must be used immediately after the seizure. PET thus helps to supply adjunct information in determining appropriate areas to resect.

Functional MRI

Functional MRI is rapidly developing as a means to determine the precise functional cerebral cortical areas, including the precise sites for language, motor control, and even memory function. Although it requires long scan times and sophisticated ways of repeating the testing to improve the signal-to-noise ratio, this study is noninvasive and may be performed at any time between seizures.

TYPES OF SURGERY

Temporal Lobectomy

Temporal lobectomy is the most common operation for epilepsy. It has the best prognosis (approximately 85%) for eliminating seizures when coupled with anatomical evidence of mesial temporal sclerosis. Typically, the resection includes a 3- to 6-cm section of the neocortex of the superior, middle, inferior, and basal temporal gyri and the amygdalohippocampal complex (Figure 26-2). Smaller-sized resections, usually smaller than 5 cm, should be considered on the dominant side, whereas a 6- or 7-cm segment may be removed on the nondominant temporal lobe. Larger resections risk damage to the optic radiation fibers (Meyer loop) and can result in contralateral superior quadrantanopsia.

The precise location of the resected edge in the temporal cortex is often determined by appreciating the venous anatomy of the cortical surface, some of the cortical arteries, and the sulcal pattern, when the surgeon can visually inspect the cortical surface. A hippocampal resection, often performed separately from the cortical resection, typically removes 3 to 4 cm of the hippocampus.

Focal Resection

If a relatively small area of the nontemporal cortex can be defined as a specific seizure focus (typically with subdural grid electrodes, intraoperative cortical recordings of interictal spikes, or both), its removal can successfully eliminate focal seizures. More functionally relevant brain tissue, such as the visual or language cortex, known as the "eloquent" *cortex*, must be distinguished from more "noneloquent" areas. It is important that the focus is in a relatively "noneloquent" region of cortex, such as part of the anterior frontal lobe. Also, cavernous malformations, or small tumors, may be removed similarly because they may also be epileptogenic. Intraoperative mapping of motor or language areas may be helpful during these operations.

Corpus Callosotomy

Occasionally, surgical division of this important interhemispheric connector is helpful for controlling seizures that spread quickly from one side to the other. Drop attack seizures are good examples. The appropriate extent of surgery is debatable; generally an approximate 60% to 80% resection is appropriate for the best outcome and the lowest degree of deficit. Left-handed patients with potential crossed dominance should undergo a Wada test before surgery because significant behavioral or language deficits may occur if language and handedness are entirely in opposite hemispheres.

Functional Hemispherectomy

By dividing the fiber connections between frontal, temporal, and parietal lobes, sparing deeper nuclei and structures (eg, the basal ganglia), and not performing large resections of cerebral cortex, functional isolation of specific cerebral regions within each hemisphere is possible (Figure 26-2). Typically, these patients already have widespread contralateral neurologic deficits. Although this procedure is primarily used only in extremely severe generalized seizure disorders, such as Lennox-Gastaut syndrome, some children often regain significant neurologic function as new pathways develop in the years after surgery.

SURGICAL TREATMENTS FOR EPILEPSY

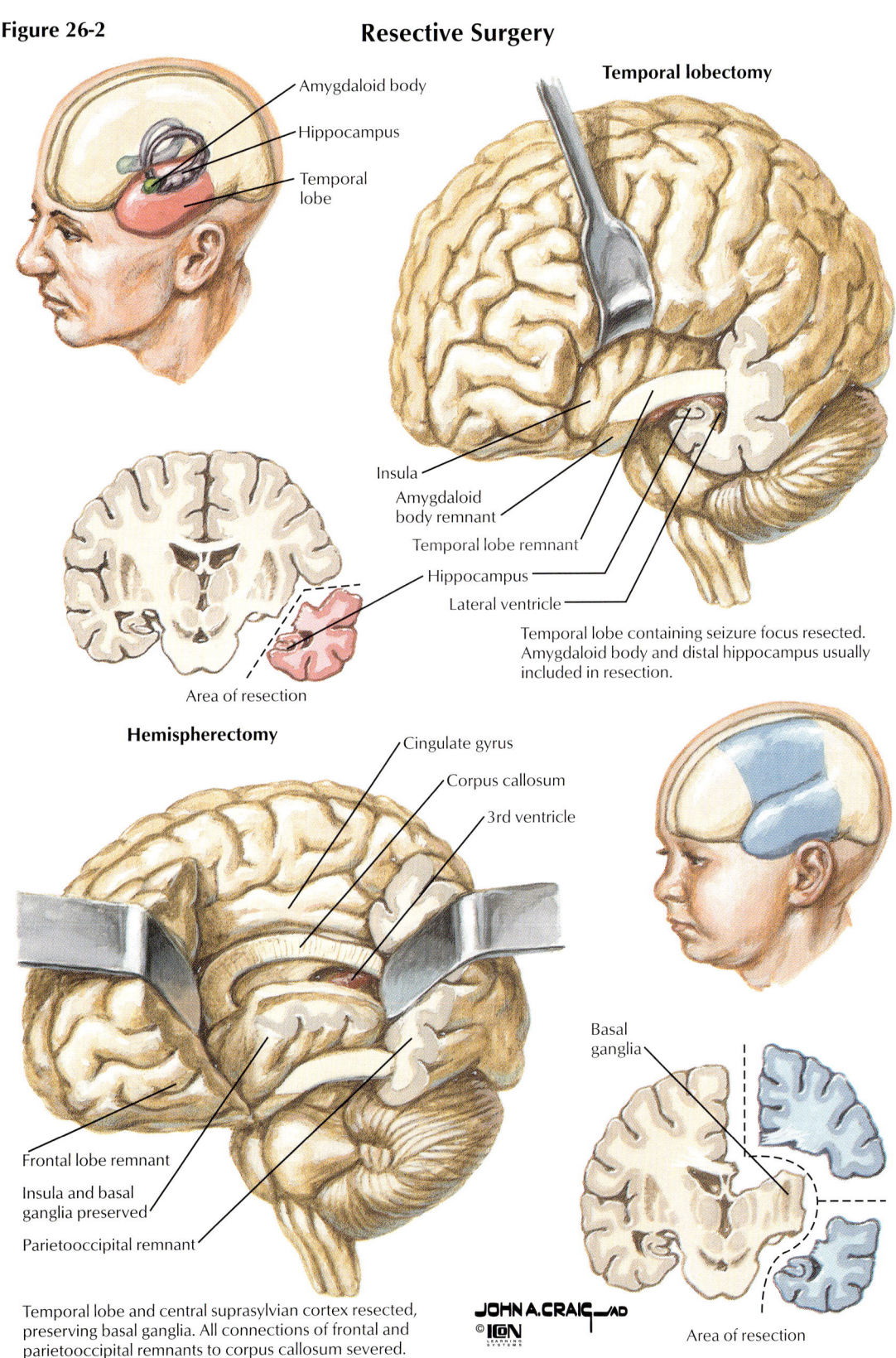

Figure 26-2

Multiple Subpial Transections

The multiple subpial transection procedure was developed to treat seizure foci localized to eloquent cortex. Surgical incisions with specially angled blades are made parallel to each other, 5 mm apart, across the cortex of interest, to section horizontally connected u-fibers while preserving many of the vertically oriented output fibers. Theoretically, it prevents spread of seizures through the cortex in this area. Although clinical outcomes vary, it may provide significant seizure control in settings where resection would be neurologically devastating. Often in the immediate postoperative period, a profound focal deficit occurs that resolves during a period of hours to weeks.

Vagus Nerve Stimulator

Stimulation of afferent fibers within the vagus nerve (performed on the left vagus nerve because it contains approximately 80% afferent fibers) can modify seizure activity. A set of 3 electrodes are coiled around the nerve after it has been dissected free within the carotid sheath in the neck. The electrodes are connected to a battery/pulse generator placed under the skin just below the clavicle. This appealing methodology does not require an intracranial procedure, although it is still prone to complications such as infection, bleeding, and occasionally hoarseness or coughing problems. Results vary, but some patients have excellent seizure control or are seizure free. This procedure warrants consideration in patients without a well-defined or accessible focus for resection.

Deep Brain Stimulator

Another procedure being evaluated places electrodes in deeper brain structures such as the thalamus, anterior internal capsule, or hippocampus to control seizures. The requisite electrodes have been successfully used for treating tremors and Parkinson disease. For patients with uncontrolled epilepsy, the electrodes may be programmed or activated automatically when seizurelike activity is recorded. Less invasive procedures such as this may become more effective than focal resective procedures.

COMMON PATHOLOGIES FOUND IN SURGICAL RESECTIONS

Mesial temporal sclerosis, appreciated histologically as a gliosis and cell loss within the mesial temporal structures, indicates previous long-term damage. There is usually no inciting event predisposing to this pathologic finding. However, it is often seen in patients who have had temporal lobe seizures for years, birth trauma, evidence of anoxic damage, or previous head injuries. Hippocampal atrophy is often seen with mesial sclerosis.

Cortical dysplasia is a general term covering many cortical developmental architectural variants. Classified by the etiology of the dysplasia (proliferation, migration, or reorganization), up to 20% to 30% of the normal population has such changes. Dysplastic abnormalities are often found microscopically in idiopathic cases in which no overt lesion is identified by MRI. Such alterations may comprise up to 40% of extramesial seizure foci.

Dysembryoplastic neuroectodermal tumor and low-grade glioma are 2 tumor types often associated with seizure generation. Typically slow-growing, they can be barely perceptible on MRI or other imaging modalities. With complete resection, patients often become seizure free.

REFERENCES

Akanuma N, Koutroumanidis M, Adachi N, Alarcon G, Binnie CD. Presurgical assessment of memory-related brain structures: the Wada test and functional neuroimaging. *Seizure*. 2003;12:346-358.

Engel J Jr, Wiebe S, French J, et al. Practice parameter: temporal lobe and localized neocortical resections for epilepsy: report of the Quality Standards Subcommittee of the American Academy of Neurology, in association with the American Epilepsy Society and the American Association of Neurological Surgeons. *Neurology*. 2003;60:538-547.

Siegel AM. Presurgical evaluation and surgical treatment of medically refractory epilepsy. *Neurosurg Rev*. 2004;27:1-18.

Section VII
SLEEP DISORDERS

Chapter 27
Sleep Disorders 288

Chapter 27
Sleep Disorders

Paul T. Gross

Primary sleep disorders, such as sleep apnea syndrome, narcolepsy, periodic limb movements, and REM sleep behavior disorder are common, presenting with varying symptomatology. They are important intrinsically and because the **circadian** (sleep-wake) **cycle** influences several medical illnesses, particularly including asthma and epilepsy. Insufficient or prolonged sleep may exacerbate migraine. From a public health perspective, many people living in western societies are sleep deprived. Excessive daytime sleepiness plays a significant role in automobile accidents and lost work productivity.

INSOMNIA

Insomnia, the most common sleep disorder, is defined as the inability to initiate or maintain sleep. Typically, adults require 7 to 9 hours of sleep daily. Disorders such as depression, musculoskeletal pain, and heart failure may significantly interfere with sleep and produce secondary insomnia. This chapter focuses on insomnia as a primary illness.

A small percentage of people with "insomnia" have a **sleep state misperception** disorder. Some individuals believe that they do not have an adequate amount of sleep but when tested do not lack appropriate sleep. Another subset of individuals sleeps reasonably well at night, but for a more limited period of time, perhaps 5 to 7 hours. Although they feel restored and function well during the day, some are inappropriately concerned that their relatively "reduced amount of sleep" is deleterious. They need reassurance that this quantity of sleep is appropriate for their health needs.

Among true sleep disorders, the most common insomnias are **primary insomnia** and **psychophysiologic insomnia**. Patients with **primary insomnia** have a history of poor sleeping since early childhood. They are unable to sleep enough to meet their needs, and this is not secondary to depression, anxiety, or an underlying illness. Good sleep hygiene, such as avoidance of stimulants and daytime naps, with adequate daily exercise and mental stimulation may help these individuals sleep. However, medication is often needed to achieve adequate sleep. Long-term hypnotic medication is usually safe in this subset of patients with sleep disorder.

Psychophysiologic insomnia is the most common cause of the inability to initiate or maintain sleep. Simply stated, it is defined as the inability to relax sufficiently to fall asleep. Multiple factors contribute to this condition including anxiety, stress, and inability to relax, resulting in a learned behavior of poor sleep. Relaxation techniques, other behavioral modification therapies, and good sleep hygiene are all important treatment modalities. Some patients sleep well when given a prescription for a hypnotic that even if never filled or taken, removes the anxiety about sleep. For others, a program of taking a hypnotic on three predetermined nights each week, such as every Sunday, Tuesday, and Thursday, allows for sleep on some nights. This relieves anxiety about sleep on other nights, helps to reestablish good sleep hygiene, and may eventually lead to reasonably good sleep without any need for medication.

SLEEP APNEA SYNDROME

Clinical Vignette

A 54-year-old plumber's wife was concerned about her husband's loud snoring. She often needed to go to another bedroom to sleep, and the children joked about the loud noise. She was also concerned that he had episodes of stopping breathing while asleep. His fishing buddies were reluctant to share a cabin with him because of his loud snoring. She noted that he fell asleep whenever he was sitting in a chair, even if guests were present. For years he was unable to stay awake at the movies. In general, he felt well, although he had some evening fatigue. He was moderately overweight and mildly hypertensive.

On examination, he appeared somewhat fatigued and modestly overweight; his blood pressure was 154/95. There was mildly reduced right nasal airflow, and his uvula was mildly enlarged.

An all-night sleep test demonstrated 200 apneas, with an apnea index (number of apneas/hour) of 34. His oxygen saturation during the apneas decreased from a baseline of 92 to 88, although occasionally it was as low as 81. Subsequently, he had a second night in the sleep laboratory for continuous positive airway pressure (CPAP) titration. A CPAP pressure of 9 nearly eliminated the apneas.

After he had been using CPAP for 1 month, he and his wife noted a distinct change in his alertness. He commented that he had not realized how sleepy he was until he saw how well he could feel under treatment.

A major group of sleep disorders causes the opposite of insomnia: excessive daytime sleepiness. These disorders are a result of either a sleep disruption at night, such as sleep apnea syndrome or periodic limb movements in sleep, or a disorder of the brain's sleep wake system, including narcolepsy or idiopathic hypersomnolence. The patient in the preceding vignette had moderately severe obstructive sleep apnea. Many similar patients underappreciate their symptoms or are totally unaware of them. Often the bed partner brings them for evaluation or the patient presents with nonspecific fatigue and weakness. When no other mechanisms are identified, a conversation with the bed partner is often particularly enlightening.

During **obstructive sleep apnea syndrome**, a common sleep disorder, the soft palate and tongue relax excessively with subsequent upper airway obstruction, which produces almost all clinically significant sleep apnea. Predisposing factors include male gender; excessive weight; abnormal structure of the palate, uvula, tongue, and jaw; increasing age; use of alcohol; use of testosterone or reduction in female hormones; and family history. Therefore, older obese male drinkers are much more likely to have sleep apnea than thin, young, premenopausal women.

Clinical Presentation

Snoring, caused by vibration in tissues of the upper airway, is the initial manifestation of sleep apnea syndrome. When the obstruction becomes complete, an apneic event occurs. Concomitantly, blood oxygen saturation decreases and carbon dioxide increases. When this develops, a sleep arousal occurs. Although the patient is usually unaware of the event, often the partner is aroused and frightened by the individual's having ceased to breathe.

The cumulative effect of hundreds of such nighttime arousals is excessive daytime sleepiness. Paradoxically, the majority of patients with obstructive sleep apnea do not report choking or gasping for breath, are unaware of their apneas, and often believe that they have had an adequate night's sleep. Loud snoring, such that it is heard in other rooms of the house, in combination with daytime sleepiness, raises the suspicion of clinically significant obstructive sleep apnea (Figure 27-1A).

Diagnosis and Treatment

An **all-night sleep study** is the best means to detect and quantitate these events. Healthy people may experience up to 10 apneas per hour of sleep at night. In contrast, patients with sleep apnea who require treatment typically have more than 20, and often 40 or more, apneas or hypopneas (episodes of partial obstruction) per hour of sleep.

Indications for treatment include sufficient sleep disruption to produce excessive daytime sleepiness or substantial time at night wherein oxygen saturation is less than 85%. An occasional dip in oxygen saturation to the 70% range during the night does not require treatment.

Most patients with sleep apnea have a good response to CPAP, providing it is well tolerated. Special attention to patient comfort in fitting and adjusting CPAP is vital to successful care. Although surgical efforts to restructure the oral pharynx are often helpful for relieving snoring, they are not as useful for obstructive sleep apnea and, therefore, are considered secondary treatment measures for the patient with sleep apnea. Respiratory stimulant medications, such as protriptyline or medroxyprogesterone, may lead to a statistical improvement in the number of

SLEEP DISORDERS

Figure 27-1

Sleep Disorders

A. Sleep Apnea

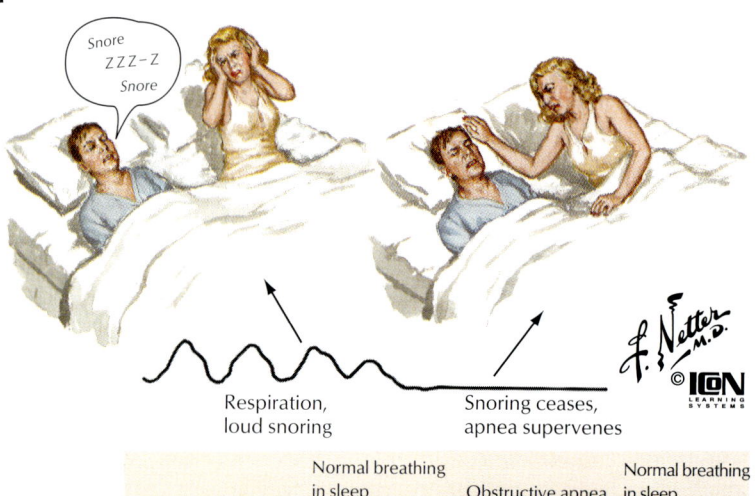

Respiration, loud snoring

Snoring ceases, apnea supervenes

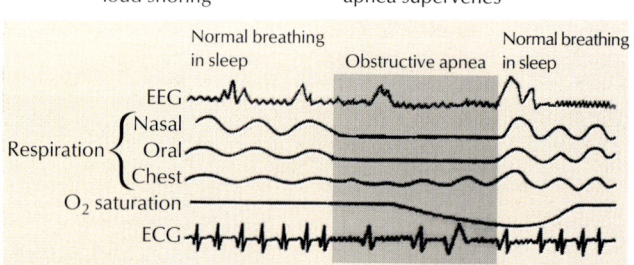

Recordings from patient with obstructive sleep apnea

B. Narcolepsy

Excessive daytime sleepiness in narcolepsy or sleep apnea

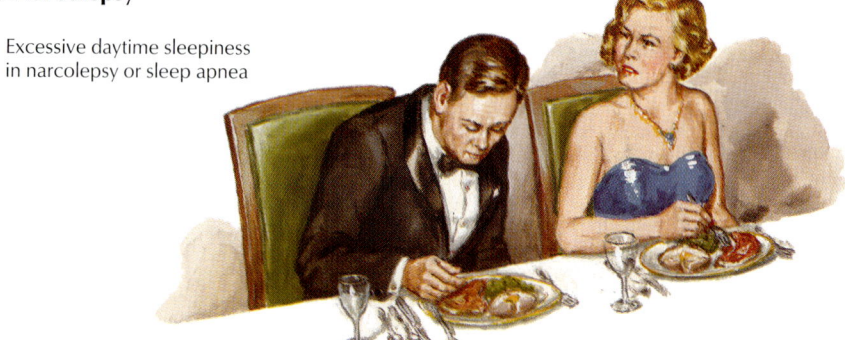

Cataplexy

Sleep paralysis

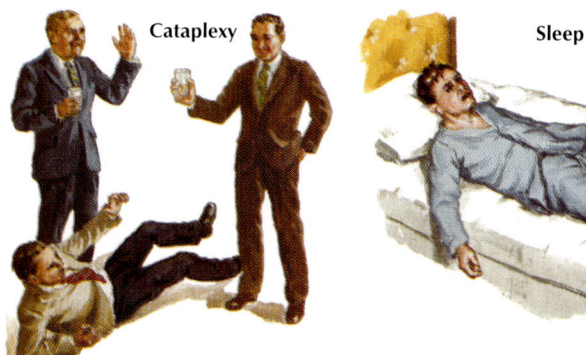

Sudden loss of muscular-postural tone with laughter or fright

Momentary paralysis on awakening lasts seconds to minutes

SLEEP DISORDERS

NARCOLEPSY

Clinical Vignette

A 24-year-old woman had begun having difficulty staying awake when she was a freshman in high school. Even with 8 to 9 hours of sleep at night, she fell asleep during class or when she was trying to study at home. After 9:00 or 10:00 PM, however, she became alert and was able to stay awake for several hours. She found that a 10-minute nap was moderately refreshing, at least for an hour or two.

A friend had commented to her that when she laughed at a joke she tended to cover her mouth. Thinking about this, the patient realized that she had difficulty keeping her jaw closed and her head up when she laughed heartily. Once, when she saw a close friend who had been overseas for a year, she was too weak to talk and also noticed weakness in her knees. On another occasion, she woke from a nap but was unable to move. She had the sense of an evil stranger peering over her and tried to scream but could not. After 30 seconds, she was able to move and talk.

Results of an all-night sleep test were normal. A multiple sleep latency test, containing 5 daytime naps, showed an average latency to sleep onset of 2.1 minutes, and 3 of the naps contained REM sleep. She was treated with modafinil, with significant improvement in her sleepiness. However, she continued to have episodes of cataplexy and sleep paralysis. The addition of fluoxetine, 10 to 20 mg daily, helped to ameliorate those symptoms.

Narcolepsy is a primary sleep disorder wherein the regulation of the brain is impaired, predominantly in REM sleep. The woman in the above vignette has all components of the narcolepsy tetrad noted below. Patients with narcolepsy tend to be much sleepier than the average person, although it is unusual for them to fall asleep under extreme circumstances, such as when crossing a street or on a first date. Depending on the severity, the external circumstances, and the patient's willpower, her or she may or may not succumb to a severe urge to sleep.

The treatment of narcolepsy includes central nervous system stimulants, such as modafinil or amphetamines, for sleepiness. Ancillary symptoms of narcolepsy are treated with SSRI drugs, such as fluoxetine.

Clinical Presentation

The symptoms of the **narcolepsy tetrad** include excessive daytime sleepiness, present in almost all patients, and various degrees of cataplexy, sleep paralysis, and hypnagogic hallucinations (Figure 27-1B). The latter three symptoms are from the inappropriate occurrence of partial episodes of REM sleep. During REM sleep, healthy individuals are often dreaming, and except for the extraocular and respiratory musculature, most muscles are paralyzed. This "paralysis" is subclinical in healthy individuals because it occurs while they are asleep.

In contrast, patients with narcolepsy retain wakefulness while they develop various episodes of brief paralysis or dreaming. Typically these paralytic events occur in two specific settings: *cataplexy*, sudden paralysis occurring in response to strong emotions such as laughter or anger, and *sleep paralysis*, occurring on awakening shortly after a dream. *Hypnagogic hallucinations* are realistic dreams that occur at sleep onset while the patient retains some degree of consciousness.

Diagnosis

Narcolepsy is diagnosed clinically by the combination of a classic history of excessive daytime sleepiness associated with one or more of the other three portions of the narcolepsy tetrad. The **multiple sleep latency test** is the best means to substantiate a clinical impression. During this study, the patient is asked to take multiple daytime naps. By measuring the average latency to sleep onset and the appearance of REM sleep during the naps, a diagnosis of narcolepsy can be supported.

Idiopathic hypersomnolence is the disorder responsible for a small percentage of patients who have excessive daytime sleepiness but do not have an REM sleep disorder. In contrast to narcolepsy, these individuals have prolonged periods of sleep at night and lapses into long sequences of daytime sleep. It is documented by a combination of all-night sleep study showing adequate sleep and no significant sleep disruption and a multiple sleep latency test demonstrating excessive daytime sleepiness but no daytime REM sleep. Similar to narcolepsy, it is treated with stimulants.

SLEEP DISORDERS

PERIODIC LIMB MOVEMENTS

Clinical Vignette

A 61-year-old woman saw her physician for excessive daytime sleepiness. She was tired much of the day but, if necessary, could stay awake. In the last several months she had become somewhat restless in the evening. If trying to sit and watch television, she needed to move her legs or get up and walk around. This provided momentary relief, but after she sat or lay down, the symptoms recurred. She has a sister with similar evening symptoms.

Findings of her general physical examination and neurologic examination were normal. Blood tests demonstrated a mild iron deficiency anemia. The possibilities of depression or hyperthyroidism were explored, but she continued to be sleepy.

An all-night sleep test showed frequent periodic limb movements of sleep associated with arousals. Correction of her iron deficiency anemia resulted in only a mild improvement.

Diagnosis of restless leg syndrome and periodic limb movements in sleep was made. Treatment with 0.25 mg pramipexole at 6:00 PM and again at 9:00 PM led to significant improvement in her restless legs and daytime sleepiness.

Periodic limb movements are another important consideration in the differential diagnosis of excessive daytime sleepiness. They consist of repeated brief episodes of movements of the lower extremities, often simply dorsiflexion of the toe. Many patients and their bed partners are unaware that they have periodic limb movements in sleep. However, a minority of these patients experience rather violent flexion and elevation of the lower extremities. These individuals present with excessive daytime sleepiness because each episode disrupts their sleep.

Many of these patients also have restless leg syndrome, an irresistible urge to move the legs while sitting or lying down. The restless leg syndrome seems to be more common in patients with iron deficiency anemia. Symptoms are best treated with L-dopa, dopamine agonists, benzodiazepines, or narcotics.

PARASOMNIAS

Clinical Vignette

A 78-year-old man was brought to the sleep specialist by his wife for episodes of disturbed sleep. His wife had recently noted him yelling or kicking in his sleep. On several occasions, he seemed to try to get out of bed. Once she had to wake him because he was punching her, completely contrary to his character and past behavior. When she woke him after this episode, he told her that he had dreamt that someone was trying to attack him. His wife reported that recently her husband had also been having difficulty with memory loss.

An all-night sleep test demonstrated abundant tonic muscle activity during REM sleep. The diagnosis of REM sleep behavior disorder was made on the basis of the wife's history and the abnormal results of the all-night sleep study. He was treated with clonazepam, 0.5 mg nightly, and the spells resolved by approximately 90%.

Parasomnias, characterized by certain unusual or unwanted symptoms occurring during nighttime sleep, are another major category of sleep disorders.

REM Sleep Behavior Disorder

The man in the vignette above has a typical history for REM sleep behavior disorder. The patient is unaware of the episodes because they occur during sleep. Treatment with clonazepam is usually successful. His wife was concerned about his memory loss and whether he had started to develop a dementia. REM sleep behavior disorder sometimes precedes Alzheimer disease or other neurodegenerative diseases.

REM sleep behavior disorder can be considered the opposite of sleep paralysis (Figure 27-2). As noted, most healthy individuals are paralyzed and dreaming during REM sleep. The characteristic paralysis, sparing both eye movements and respiratory muscles, is from activation of inhibitory reticulospinal pathways. It results in an inhibition of anterior horn cells within the spinal cord, preventing patients from acting out dreams.

However, many older males lose this ability to be paralyzed during REM sleep. Subsequently, they begin to act out their dreams by talking, yelling, kicking, or in extreme cases, attacking their bed partner. If awakened, they relate that they are in the middle of a violent dream. Although REM sleep behavior disorder is not usually associated with another neurologic disorder, it is sometimes a precursor to other neurologic degenerative disorders, particularly Parkinson or Alzheimer disease. Most patients respond positively to treatment with 0.5 mg clonazepam at bedtime.

SLEEP DISORDERS

Figure 27-2 REM Sleep Behavior Disorder

Patients who lose their ability to be paralyzed during REM sleep begin to act out their dreams and are usually unaware of these occurrences because the episodes occur during sleep. Often the first episodes are observed by the spouses of the patients.

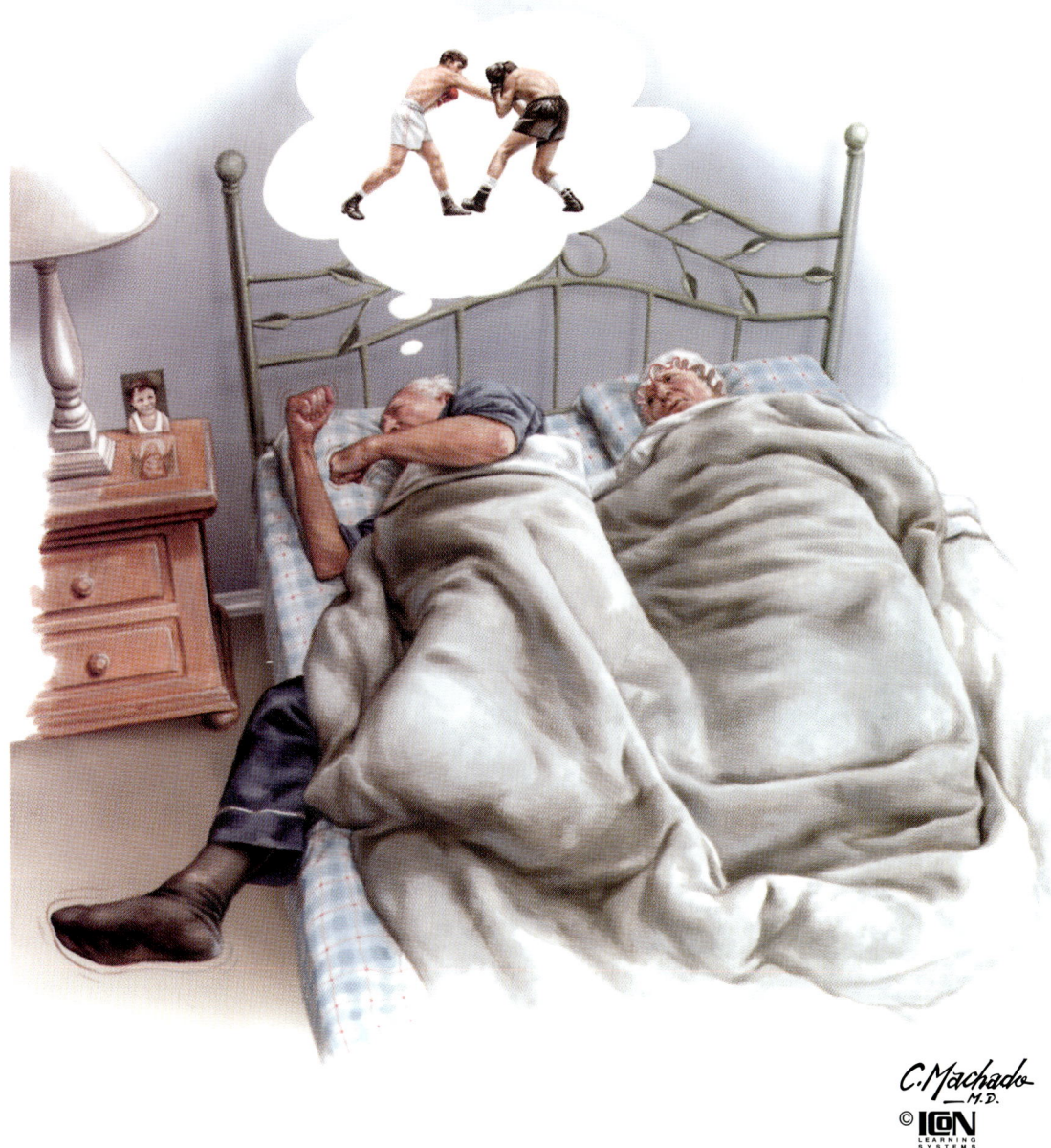

Night Terrors

Night terrors are common in small children and occasionally persist into adult life. The observer notices that the patient suddenly sits up in bed, has dilated pupils, a frightened expression, and a rapid pulse. Occasionally affected individuals dash from the bed toward the door or window. Children often return to sleep without memory of the event. If awakened, they describe a frightened feeling or image but not a complex dream because these episodes arise during stage 3 or 4 sleep, in which dreams do not usually occur. Somnambulism or sleepwalking tends to occur in the same patients, also during stage 3 or 4 sleep. Often, an explanation of the problem is sufficient; but if treatment is needed, tricyclic antidepressants or benzodiazepines may be helpful.

Delayed Sleep Phase Syndrome

Delayed sleep phase syndrome is a **circadian rhythm disorder**, differing from the other three main categories of sleep dysfunction. Individuals with this disorder are not able to adjust their circadian clock to the rest of the world. Most people can delay their sleep wake cycle 1 hour or more daily and can advance it to an earlier time by approximately a half hour daily. Therefore, it is commonly easier to sleep and awaken later, than to sleep and awaken earlier. With time, almost everyone can adjust to international travel or a new schedule.

However, some people have particular difficulty advancing to an earlier time. For example, a student with delayed sleep phase syndrome who spends 2 weeks staying up late studying for final exams, going to sleep at 3:00 AM and awakening at 11:00 AM daily, will find it impossible to learn to go to bed early and wake up early for a summer job. Depending on which symptoms are most bothersome, she will report insomnia because she cannot fall asleep at night or daytime sleepiness because she cannot awaken before 11:00 AM. The traditional treatment is to delay sleep by 3 hours every day until sleep time returns to the new desired bedtime. Hypnotic medications may also help ease this transition.

REFERENCES

Hening W, Allen R, Earley C, Kushida C, Picchietti D, Silber M. The treatment of restless legs syndrome and periodic limb movement disorder. An American Academy of Sleep Medicine Review. *Sleep.* 1999;22:970-999.

Kotagal S. Sleep disorders in childhood. *Neurol Clin.* 2003;21:961-981.

Olson EJ, Moore WR, Morgenthaler TI, Gay PC, Staats BA. Obstructive sleep apnea-hypopnea syndrome. *Mayo Clin Proc.* 2003;78:1545-1552.

Scammell TE. The neurobiology, diagnosis, and treatment of narcolepsy. *Ann Neurol.* 2003;53:154-166.

Taheri S, Mignot E. The genetics of sleep disorders. *Lancet Neurol.* 2002;1:242-250.

Verse T, Pirsig W, Stuck BA, Hormann K, Maurer JT. Recent developments in the treatment of obstructive sleep apnea. *Am J Respir Med.* 2003;2:157-168.

Section VIII
DISORDERS OF CONSCIOUSNESS

Chapter 28
Coma 296

Chapter 29
**Increased Intracranial Pressure and
Cerebral Herniation** 307

Chapter 30
Brain Death 316

Chapter 28
Coma

Gregory Allam

Clinical Vignette

A 76-year-old man was found unconscious in bed at home. His wife informed the emergency physician that he had a history of prostate cancer but no risk factors for vascular disease. She denied knowledge of any recent head injury. He was totally unresponsive to verbal and painful stimuli. Neurologic examination showed he was comatose with pinpoint pupils. Eye movements to doll's eyes maneuvers were full and conjugate, and cold caloric stimulation of the ear canals produced ipsilateral tonic deviation of the eyes without nystagmus. There were bilateral withdrawal responses of his extremities to noxious stimuli, and bilateral Babinski signs.

Intravenous administration of 0.4 mg naloxone produced dramatic change, with full awakening within a few minutes. Results of a subsequent brain CT were normal, confirming that there was no evidence of intracerebral, subarachnoid, or subdural hemorrhage, cerebral infarction, or mass lesions. When asked about narcotic use, the patient stated that he was no longer able to tolerate the pain of metastatic prostate cancer; he had taken an overdose of an opioid analgesic.

The vignette above is classic for "toxic-metabolic" induced coma (Table 28-1). Despite profound unresponsiveness and very miotic pupils, neurologic examination demonstrated retained brainstem reflexes and CT results were normal. Although pontine hemorrhage is often suspected in a comatose septuagenarian with pinpoint pupils, intact reflexive eye movement indicated a likely metabolic cause.

Consciousness is the state of awareness of internal and external stimuli coupled with the ability to react to these stimuli either by thought or by directed physical movement. Coma is the lack or disruption of awareness to stimuli reflected by a lack or disruption of response to these stimuli. The specificity of a response to a particular stimulus depends upon the degree of consciousness. Because the examining physician can only infer thought from patients' actions (eg, speech or movement), a reliable and reproducible physical examination is essential in evaluating the comatose patient.

The neurologist must make every attempt to establish the presence or absence of a directed nonreflexive response and judge its quality. For example, in a basis pontis lesion causing a "locked-in" syndrome, patients may seemingly have no directed response to stimuli, yet on close examination may blink in an exact fashion to instructions and thus indirectly answer questions appropriately. There may also be partially preserved voluntary vertical eye movements. Similarly, in patients with severe acute polyneuropathies such as Guillain-Barré syndrome, consciousness is preserved but difficult to assess and quantify.

The level of consciousness varies with the degree of general inattention to stimuli. Terms such as *stupor* or *obtundation* have been used to portray the extent of inattention. However, the most useful tool in following patients with altered mentation remains the exact description of patient behavior and reactions to specific stimuli. For example, it is more useful to indicate that a patient stays alert without stimulation but is unable to give the exact date and location or follow 2 sequential commands than to say that the patient is *confused* or *clouded*. Nevertheless, defining terms may provide uniformity in meaning when encountered in patient records. *Obtundation* describes a condition in which repeated stimuli are needed to draw patients' attention back to a task. *Stupor* is a state of extreme inattention in which wakefulness and minimal interaction with the examiner can be achieved only by repeated or constant stimulation. *Delirium* is a confusional state dominated by sympathetic nervous system overactivity with attention marred by hyperexcitabil-

COMA

Table 28-1
Stages of Coma

	Hemispheric/ Diencephalon	Mesencephalon	Pontine	Medullary
Respiratory Pattern	Cheyne-Stokes sighs and yawning	Hyperventilation; central neurogenic hyperventilation	Rapid and shallow	Irregular and shallow few gasps, then absent
Pupils				
Central	Reactive small	Irregular; midposition, poorly or nonreactive	Midposition, nonreactive	Absent response
Uncal	Ipsilateral irregular and dilated with poor reactivity	Ipsilateral pupil dilated and nonreactive; contralateral irregular, dilated, and poorly or nonreactive	Bilateral dilated and nonreactive	Bilateral dilated and nonreactive
Oculocephalogyric				
Central	Preserved; no nystagmus	Impaired/dysconjugate, internuclear ophthalmoplegia	No response	Absent
Uncal	Ipsilateral partial or complete CN-III palsy; opposite eye moves fully	Contralateral eye may move laterally only; ipsilateral eye does not move and may be abducted and downwardly deviated	Absent: eyes dysconjugate	Absent: eyes dysconjugate
Motor				
Central	Resistance to movement or paratonia, then decorticate	Decerebrate	No posturing other than Babinski signs and brief flexor knee responses	Absent or flexor responses in legs
Uncal	Contralateral paratonia and ipsilateral withdrawal; ipsilateral hemiplegia is seen in Kernohan notch phenomena	Decerebrate	As above	As above

ity. Tachycardia, perspiration, hypertension, and hallucinations may all be features of delirium.

The Glasgow Coma Scale assesses and quantifies the degree of consciousness across three measures: response to verbal commands, response of eye opening, and the nature of motor movements to verbal or physical stimuli. Those not responding to verbal commands or not opening their eyes and having a Glasgow Coma Scale score of 8 or less are defined as being in coma (Figure 28-1). The Glasgow Coma Scale is one of the primary predictors of long-term outcome, especially in cases of head trauma.

Prevalence of the different etiologies of coma varies depending on the population surveyed. For example, head trauma and intoxicants are the major causes of coma in registries based on densely populated high-crime areas. Stroke and cardiac events are the leading etiologies in suburban areas with retirement communities. Overall, trauma, stroke, diffuse anoxic-ischemic brain insult (secondary to cardiorespiratory arrest), and intoxicants are the leading mechanisms for coma. Infections, seizures, and metabolic-endocrine disorders account for the remaining cases (Figure 28-2).

DISORDERS OF CONSCIOUSNESS

COMA

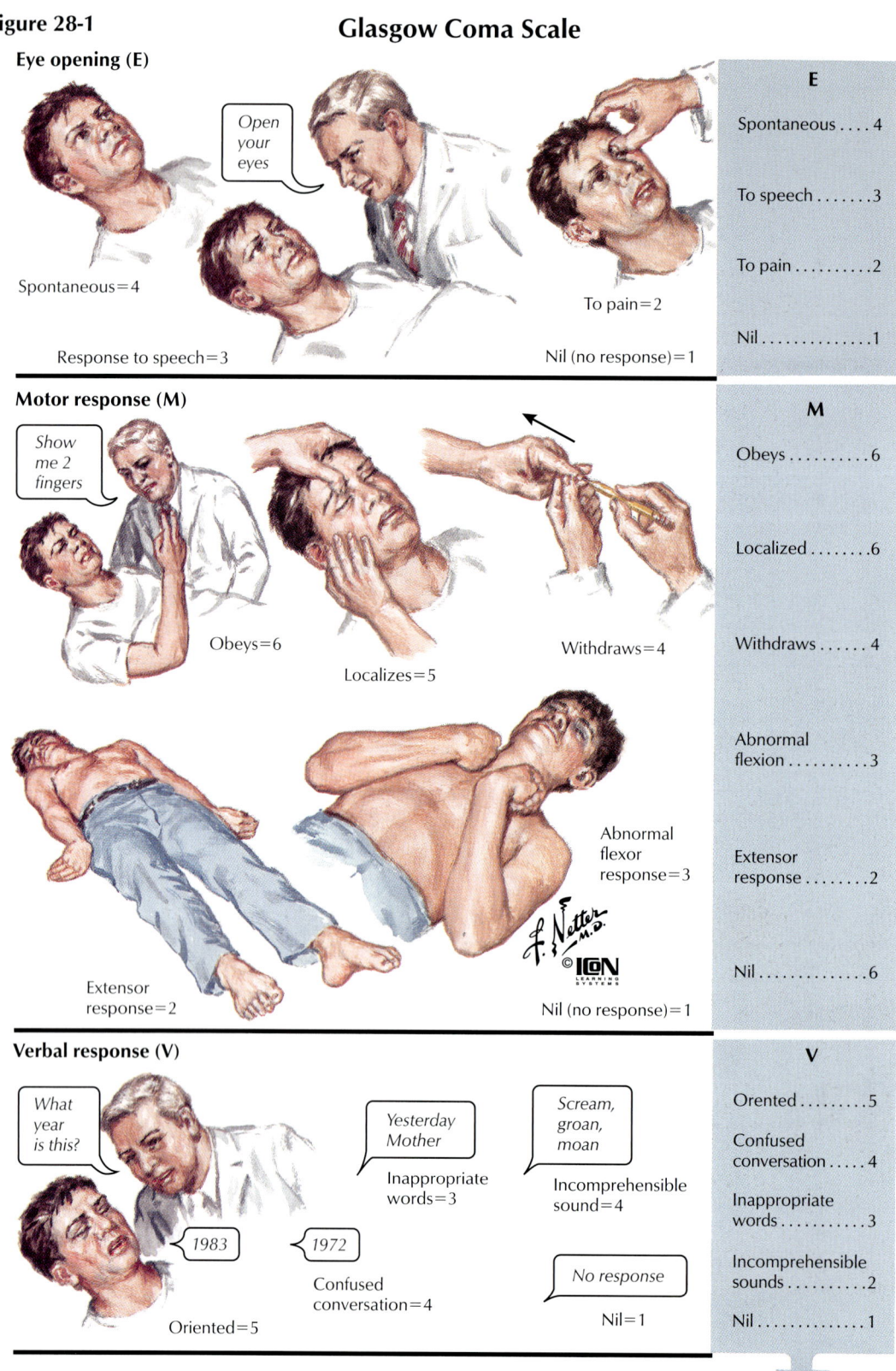

Figure 28-1. Glasgow Coma Scale

Coma score (E+M+V)=3 to 15

DISORDERS OF CONSCIOUSNESS

COMA

Figure 28-2   Differential Diagnosis of Coma

	Clinical features	Pathology (examples)	Etiologies

Bilateral cerebral hemisphere disease	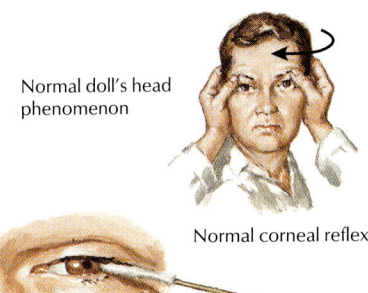
	Normal pupils (equal, reactive)
	Normal doll's head phenomenon
	Normal corneal reflex
	Absent or minor focal features (lateral paralysis, sensory or visual loss)
		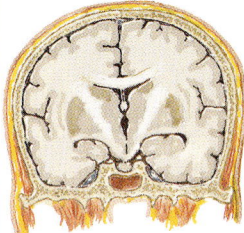
		Bilateral hemispheric swelling (small ventricles, obliterated sulci, rounded edges)
			Increased subarachnoid or extracerebral pressure
			  Meningitis
			  Subarachnoid hemorrhage
			  Bilateral subdural hematoma
			Metabolic encephalopathy
			  Liver coma
			  Kidney coma
			  Carbon dioxide narcosis
			  Hypoxia
			  Hypoglycemia
			  Hypercalcemia
			  Hyponatremia
			  Diabetic acidosis
			  Hyperosmolar coma
			Toxins or drugs
			  Barbiturates
			  Alcohol
			  Narcotics
			  Other sedative overdose
			  Lead
			Multifocal cerebral disease (usually developing sequentially
			  Infarction
			  Multiple abscesses
			  Encephalitis
			  Multiple areas of brain tumor
			  Multiple cerebral contusions

Unilateral cerebral hemisphere lesion with compression of brainstem	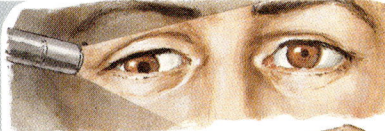
	Third cranial nerve palsy, nonreactive pupil, ptosis
	Contralateral hemiparesis
		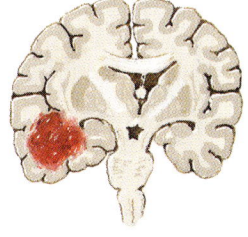
		Right temporal hemorrhage from trauma, with swelling of right hemisphere
			Cerebral
			  Tumor
			  Hemorrhage
			  Abscess
			  Infarction
			  Contusion
			Extracerebral
			  Subdural hematoma
			  Extradural hematoma

Primary brainstem lesion	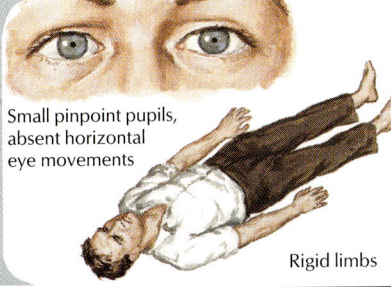 Small pinpoint pupils, absent horizontal eye movements Rigid limbs	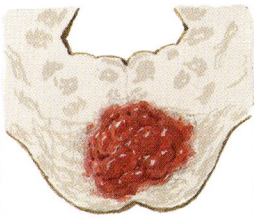 Large pontine hemorrhage	Infarction Hemorrhage Severe metabolic disturbance, sedative or phenytoin overdose Severe anoxia
Cerebellar lesion with secondary brainstem compression	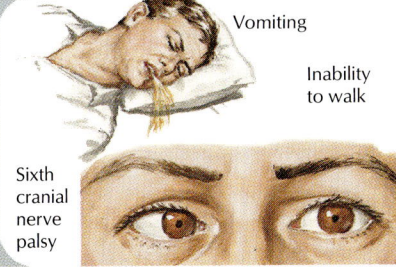 Vomiting Inability to walk Sixth cranial nerve palsy	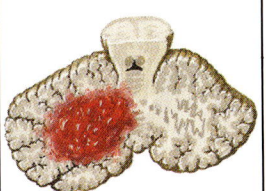 Large cerebellar hemorrhage	Infarction Hemorrhage Tumor Abscess Contusion

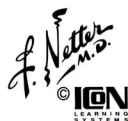

DISORDERS OF CONSCIOUSNESS

COMA

States that affect cognition and attention without affecting wakefulness such as the various degenerative dementias (characterized by progressive global cognitive deterioration) and focal brain lesions (which cause restricted cortical dysfunction) do not fit the definition of coma (section IX). Sleep is a normal patterned physiologic disconnection of the cortex from external stimuli (chapter 27).

EVALUATION AND TREATMENT OF THE COMATOSE PATIENT

The initial evaluation of a patient in coma must occur simultaneously with management of the coma. Any delay in treatment while waiting to determine the exact cause is not acceptable. Clearing or ensuring the airway and supporting breathing and oxygenation, either with a bag mask or intubation if needed, must be addressed immediately. Management of hypotension must be prompt, especially in suspected cases of increased intracranial pressure. Hemodynamic collapse should never be attributed to a primary CNS process, and cardiac or circulatory causes need to be sought. These form the "**ABCs of coma management**": airway, breathing, and circulation (Figure 28-3). Immobilizing the neck until a cervical spine injury is excluded is also important in cases of suspected trauma.

Emergent evaluation of comatose patients requires certain studies: a full blood count, glucose level, serum chemistry, toxicology screen, liver profile, thyroid function tests, arterial blood gases, and cultures. Creatine kinase and troponin measurements, in conjunction with ECG, are important for excluding myocardial infarction and transient cardiac arrest. Anticonvulsant drug levels and an EEG can help identify patients with nonconvulsive status epilepticus.

The immediately treatable causes of coma are hypoglycemia and narcotic intoxication. These can be managed promptly, once oxygenation and hemodynamic status are stable. Infusion of 100 mg thiamine must precede the infusion of 50 ml dextrose, 50%, in water as a precaution against Wernicke encephalopathy caused by postulated osmotic or metabolic damage to the mamillary bodies and the medial thalamus. When narcotics overdose is suspected, such as in comatose patients with miotic pupils, 0.4 mg IV naloxone, a central opioid antagonist, improves the level of consciousness within minutes, as in the preceding Clinical Vignette. Repeated doses may be needed to maintain wakefulness and reverse respiratory depression. Caution should be exercised for known or suspected opioid dependency, because abrupt or complete reversal of opioid effects by repeated doses may precipitate an acute withdrawal state. In such instances, only supportive care should be provided once the diagnosis is made.

Administration of flumazenil, a pure benzodiazepine antagonist (0.2 mg IV), given 3 to 4 times, can improve the mental state and reverse respiratory depression in benzodiazepine overdose. As with naloxone, it should be used cautiously in those with a history of long-term benzodiazepine use or dependency because it can precipitate seizures. It should also be avoided in patients with epilepsy and those at risk of seizures.

Urgent intravenous antibiotic coverage is indicated for febrile patients because time is crucial in treating meningitis and septicemia (chapter 64). Lumbar puncture should be performed only after brain imaging has excluded mass lesions that could lead to herniation.

Assessment of the comatose patient should include examination of the skin. Rashes may indicate *Streptococcus* or *Staphylococcus* meningitis, bacterial endocarditis, or systemic lupus erythematosus. Purpura may indicate meningococcal meningitis, a bleeding diathesis, or aspirin intoxication. Skin dryness suggests anticholinergic or barbiturate overdose, whereas excessive perspiration indicates cholinergic poisoning, hypoglycemia, and other causes of sympathetic overactivity. Dark pigmentary changes in the axillary and genital areas suggest adrenal insufficiency, whereas doughy pale skin is typical of myxedema. Renal failure may present with urea salt crystal skin condensations or "urea frost." Facial or basal skull fractures often cause ecchymosis around the eyes (raccoon eyes or panda bear sign) or in the mastoid area (Battle sign). Extremities must be examined for needle and track marks that indicate intravenous drug abuse.

The patient's breath may be uremic, fruity as in ketoacidosis, or have the musty fishy odor of hepatic failure. Fever may indicate meningitis or

COMA

Figure 28-3   **Initial Management of Severe Head Injuries**

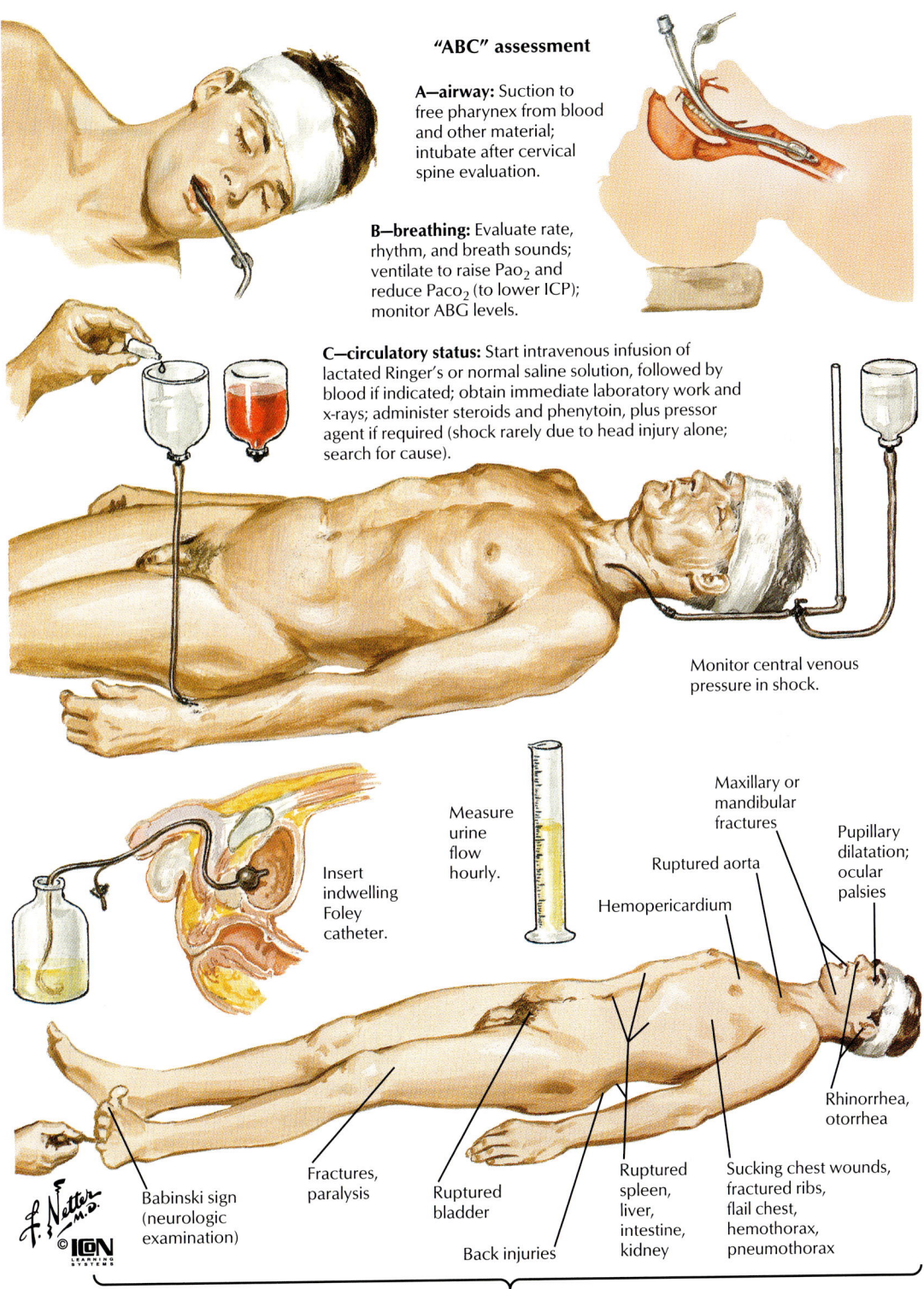

DISORDERS OF CONSCIOUSNESS

COMA

Figure 28-4   Prognosis in Coma Related to Severe Head Injuries

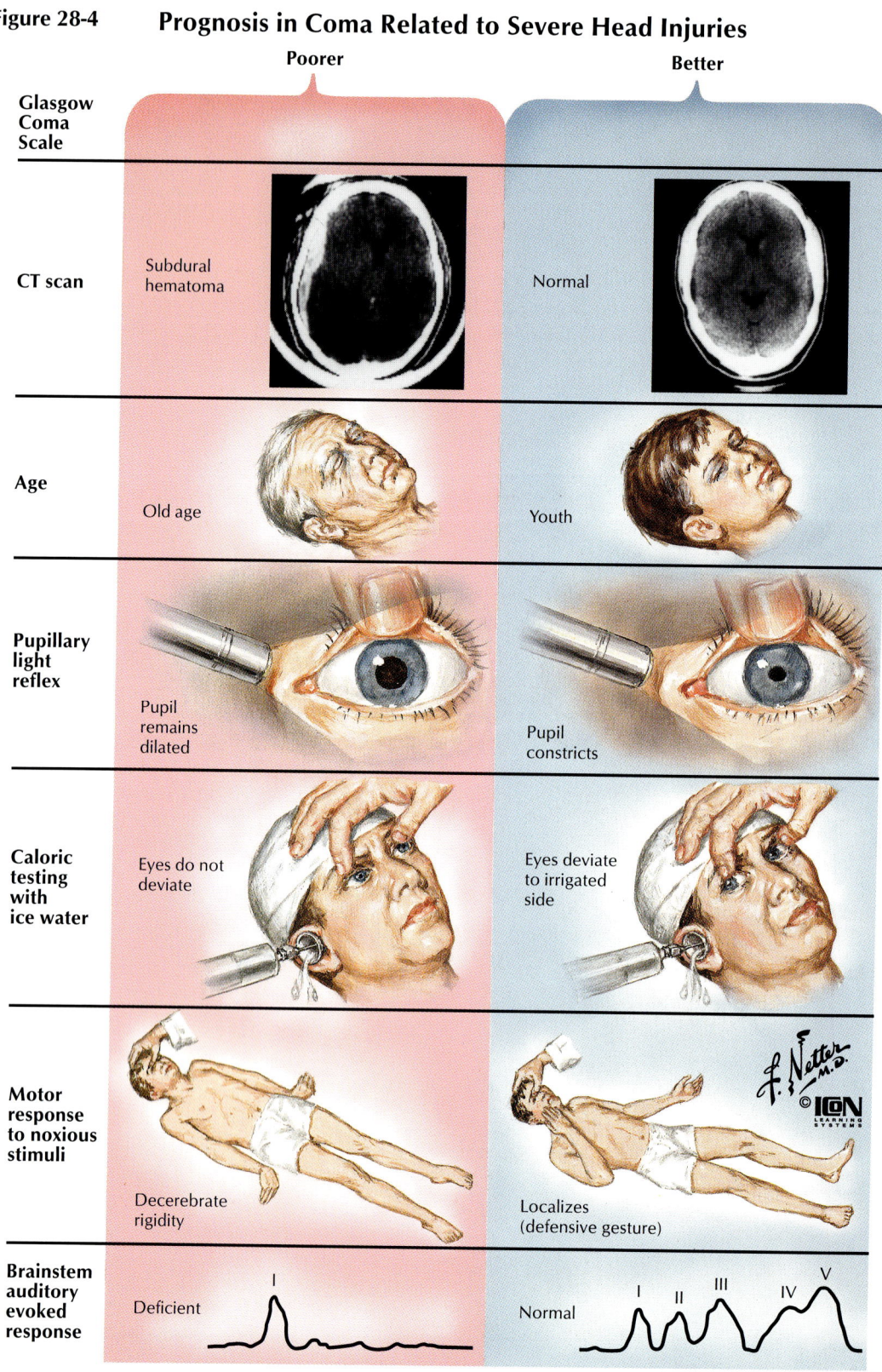

encephalitis but also occurs with sympathomimetic or tricyclic (anticholinergic) overdose and drug or alcohol withdrawal. Occasionally, a low-grade fever occurs with subarachnoid hemorrhage or brainstem lesions.

Focal neurologic signs on initial examination may implicate a structural lesion as the cause of the coma and should be followed closely for signs of evolving herniation until brain imaging can be performed. Other causes of focal presentation are compensated old brain injuries clinically reemerging as a result of seizures, toxins, or metabolic derangements. However, metabolic disorders including nonketotic hyperosmolar hyperglycemia, hypoglycemia, and hepatic coma may cause focal seizures or lateralizing neurologic signs without focal brain lesions. Evolving signs of increased intracranial pressure or herniation must be treated promptly regardless of cause; there is no use in waiting for brain CT results or other tests (chapter 29).

EEG is often helpful in evaluating patients with altered consciousness or coma. An abnormal tracing makes psychogenic coma unlikely. EEG detects nonconvulsive or absence status, which can present de novo without a history of epilepsy. Although they are nonspecific, diffuse background slowing correlates with metabolic derangements and focal slowing correlates with localized structural brain disease. Hepatic and other metabolic encephalopathies may show triphasic waves. In herpes simplex encephalitis, periodic lateralized epileptiform temporal lobe discharges may be seen. Finally, when a basis pontis lesion with the "locked-in syndrome" is suspected, a normal EEG shows that the patient is alert despite no obvious response to stimuli.

PROGNOSIS

Determining the prognosis of an individual comatose patient is a difficult task. Statistical numbers given to patients' families, as measures of outcome probability, often are difficult to apply in relation to their loved one. The focus usually shifts to the chances of recovery, no matter how unlikely, rather than the likelihood of severe disability. Each case cannot be decided by a statistical grid or flow chart alone, and numerous factors, including cause of the coma, results of the evolving neurologic examination, age, comorbidities, and the religious or philosophical beliefs of the patient and the family must be considered.

Recovery from drug intoxication is usually good, with rare mortality or instances of severe disability, barring any complications secondary to hypoxemia or circulatory collapse with superimposed ischemic brain injury. In hepatic and likely in other metabolic comas, the duration of the coma and absent localizing motor responses do not exclude recovery. Only brainstem dysfunction, with disruption of oculocephalic reflexes and loss of pupillary reactivity, increases the likelihood of poor prognosis or death.

In most instances, coma from head trauma has a better outcome than that from nontraumatic mechanisms or cardiac arrest (Figure 28-4). Although severe head trauma has a mortality of approximately 50% within the first 48 hours, few surviving patients remain in a permanent vegetative state and most progress toward some degree of functional improvement. Those who remain vegetative usually succumb within 3 to 5 years. There are rare reports of patients who awaken after a prolonged vegetative period and show some return of functionality. None, however, return to their premorbid status or even an independent state. Signs that correlate with a poor prognosis after head trauma are age older than 60, bilateral pupillary abnormalities, or absent oculocephalic reflexes at initial examination in a relatively stable patient. Large volumes of contused brain, large intra- or extra-axial hematomas, and lack of intracranial pressure response to conventional medical treatment (usually associated with compression of basal cisterns on CT) also betoken a poorer prognosis.

Other medical causes have a mortality rate of up to 60% to 70%, with generally only 10% to 15% of patients returning to a good functional status. The lack of any oculocephalic (vestibuloocular or caloric) response or the presence of pupillary abnormalities for more than 6 to 12 hours correlates highly with poor functional outcome and death. In patients who do retain or regain pupillary reactivity or oculocephalic reflexes, the absence of at least reflexive motor movements on day 1, or some withdrawal movement on day 3, also holds a poor prognosis, with a less than 10% chance of good recovery or even moderate disability. Lack of spontaneous eye opening or of localizing motor movements on day 7 holds the same grim prognostic significance. Vocalizations or any verbal response early within the first day of the causative event indicates a higher chance of functional improvement within a year.

These observations can guide families and staff toward the best course for each patient. Often the examination is changing or unclear. Consequently, further waiting and evaluation, although stressful for the family, result in more certainty in the appropriateness of the eventual actions. Those showing unfavorable prognostic signs on day 1, who show no improvement or evolution in their neurologic examination, are not likely to do well. However, for individuals who exhibit evolving neurologic function, the duration of observation needs to be extended and the final determination of outcome delayed, even if immediate examination shows no major interactive or directed function.

PERSISTENT VEGETATIVE STATE

Clinical Vignette

A 23-year-old woman was an unrestrained driver in a "head-on" automobile accident. She was ejected 30 feet through the windshield and sustained major head trauma. On arrival in the emergency department, she was totally unresponsive, hypotensive, and tachycardic. Brain CT demonstrated generalized cerebral edema and diffuse subarachnoid hemorrhage. Neurologic examination showed her to be unresponsive even to painful stimuli, other than some rare nonpurposeful right leg movements. Pupils were minimally and inconsistently reactive, and she had a dense left hemiplegia. Subsequent MRI demonstrated bilateral focal contusions of the cerebral hemispheres, shear injury of the splenium of the corpus callosum, and brainstem edema. Four months later, after no improvement in her clinical state, she was diagnosed with persistent vegetative state (PVS).

The course of the preceding vignette is typical of PVS. PVS cases frequently involve young individuals with healthy cardiovascular and pulmonary systems. Before the recognition of these patients' hopeless outcomes after a few months of no improvement, some cases were maintained in chronic care facilities or their parents' homes for many years with the unrealistic hope that they might someday regain the ability to meaningfully interact.

The *vegetative state*, *minimally conscious states*, or *post-coma unawareness* are terms that describe a state of preserved brainstem and hypothalamic functions with absent or insufficient cortical function to sustain awareness of environment and self. Wakefulness is by definition preserved, and patients may cycle through sleep stages. There is no behavioral evidence of even the simplest reproducible response. Patients may startle, look about, occasionally move a limb, shift position, or yawn, but none of these actions are consistently in response to a specific stimulus (Figure 28-5). Even the most basic voluntary actions, such as chewing and swallowing, are lost. Once reversible metabolic or exogenous causes have been eliminated, the condition is called *persistent* when it lasts without change for more than 1 month. It is considered permanent when lasting more than 12 months for traumatic brain injury and more than approximately 3 months for nontraumatic causes. After these time limits, the chance of recovery is exceedingly low and at best progresses to a severe disability level.

As with coma, individuals in a posttraumatic PVS have better chances of recovery than cases due to medical causes. Nevertheless, one third of all these patients die within the first year. Of patients with head trauma, one third regain consciousness after 3 months and approximately one half in a year. Overall, one fourth of all patients with traumatic PVS recover to a level of moderate disability, mostly those who regain awareness within 3 months.

Of patients with nontraumatic PVS, more than 50% die within a year and only approximately 10% to 15% regain consciousness by the third month. Most remain severely disabled, with rare improvement in functional status. If the condition persists longer, there is miminal chance of any significant functional recovery. Neither age nor cause seems to correlate with eventual recovery, but of those recovering, the younger patients show somewhat better outcomes than older patients, at least in locomotion and self-care. After 3 months, once PVS is considered permanent, withdrawal of nutritional support and hydration can be discussed with the family.

COMA

Figure 28-5

Persistent Vegetative State

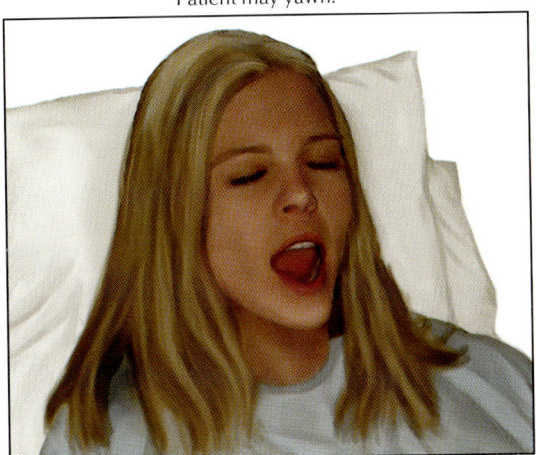

Patient may yawn.

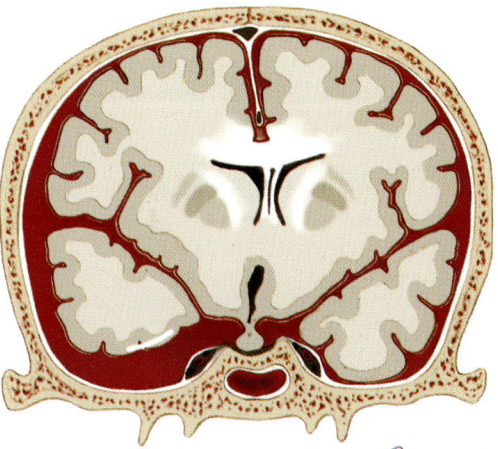

Subarachnoid hemorrhage

Condition is called *persistent* when it lasts without change for more than 1 month.

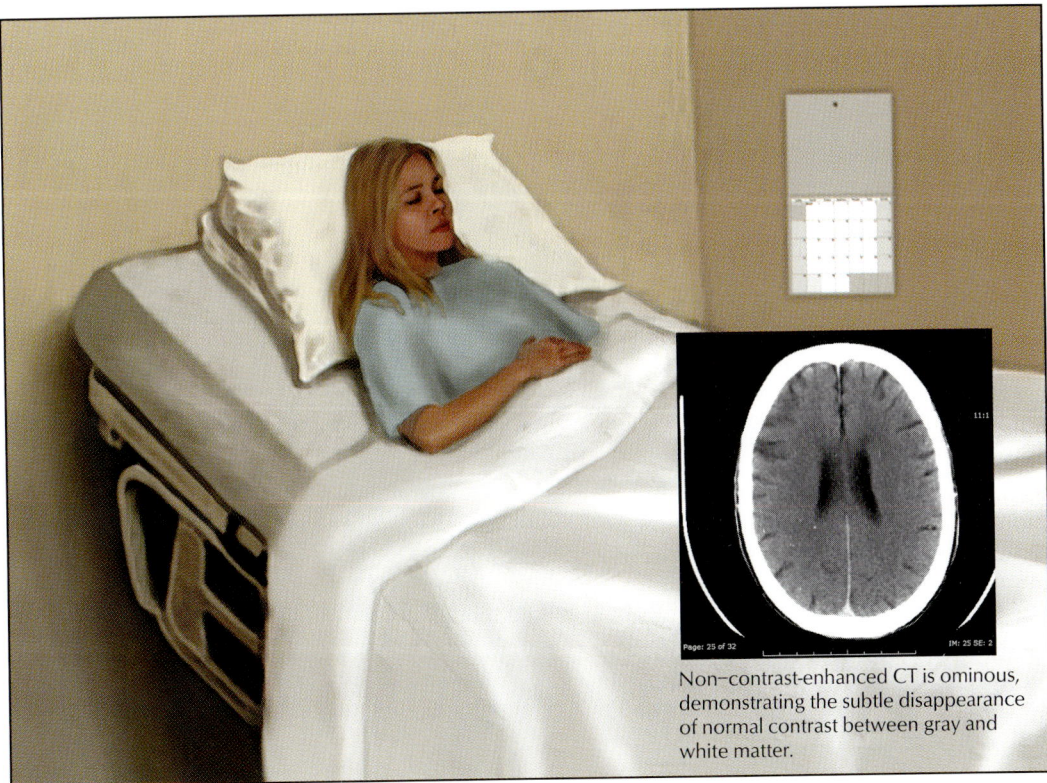

Non–contrast-enhanced CT is ominous, demonstrating the subtle disappearance of normal contrast between gray and white matter.

DISORDERS OF CONSCIOUSNESS

Many physicians consider such withdrawal acceptable, based on the contention that nutritional support in such cases constitutes medical treatment that is neither alleviating patient suffering nor improving the overall condition. When viewed as a human or legal rights issue, as in some countries, the decision becomes more complex and less applicable.

REFERENCES

Choi SC, Muizelaar JP, Barnes TY, et al. Prediction tree for severely head-injured patients. *J Neurosurg.* 1991;75:251-255.

Jennett B, Bond M. Assessment of outcome after severe brain damage. *Lancet.* 1975;1:480.

Jennett B, Teasdale B, Braakman R, et al. Prognosis of patients with severe head injury. *Neurosurgery.* 1979;4:283-288.

Levy DE, Bates D, Corona JJ, et al. Prognosis in non-traumatic coma. *Ann Intern Med.* 1981;94:293-301.

McLean SAM. Permanent vegetative state and the law. *J Neurol Neurosurg Psychiatry.* 2001;71(suppl 1):i26-i27.

Plum F, Posner JB. *The Diagnosis of Stupor and Coma.* 3rd ed. New York, NY: Oxford University Press; 1982.

Report of the Quality Standards Subcommittee of the American Academy of Neurology. 1995;1-7.

Sazbon L, Zagreba F, Ronen J, Solzi P, Costeff H. Course and outcome of patients in vegetative state of non-traumatic aetiology. *J Neurol Neurosurg Psychiatry.* 1993;56:407-409.

Teasdale G, Jennet B. Assessment of coma and impaired consciousness: a practical scale. *Lancet.* 1974;ii:81-84.

The Multi-Society Task Force on PVS. Medical aspects of the persistent vegetative state: parts I and II. *N Engl J Med.* 1994;330:1499-1508, 1572-1579.

Chapter 29
Increased Intracranial Pressure and Cerebral Herniation

Gregory Allam

Clinical Vignette

A 46-year-old man was found lying on the floor at home. Examination in the ED demonstrated a left hemiplegia, with conjugate eye deviation to the right. He was awake but had profound neglect for his left arm and limb problems. Brain CT demonstrated a large right MCA and ACA territory stroke, with incipient potential for significant brain edema and increased intracranial pressure (ICP) ("malignant brain swelling"). During the next 2 days, the patient became obtunded and progressively less responsive to external stimulation. Repeat brain CT scan showed a loss of sulcal markings and a right cerebral shift across the midline (falx) and downward, with distortion of the midbrain.

The patient underwent intubation for airway protection, and soon afterward, he could not be aroused. He had right-sided flexed arm posturing and left-sided extension, with tonic leg extension and plantar flexion. His pupils were irregular and sluggishly reactive to light. Conjugate eye movements to the "doll's eyes" maneuver were lost. He did not respond to osmotic agents or hyperventilation. A hemicraniectomy was performed, and during the following week, he awakened gradually and underwent extubation. He could eventually interact with his family and perform simple tasks, but he remained disabled, with a dense right hemiplegia, hemianopsia, and cognitive difficulties.

ANATOMICAL CONSIDERATIONS

The skull is a rigid closed cavity that serves as a basin in which the brain is suspended and protected from traumatic injury. The brain comprises approximately 90% of intracranial volume; the remaining 10% is blood and CSF. The ability to compensate for increased intracranial volume is therefore limited, and when maximum accommodation occurs, any further volume increase causes an exponential increase in ICP. Eventually, arterial and arteriolar perfusion are compromised, and ischemic tissue damage with swelling ensues, causing an even greater increase in ICP. If the exerted force on the brain is asymmetric (eg, focal brain tumor, lobar bleed, or a unilateral stroke), then shifts in brain tissue against or across fixed structures may occur. Extrusion of shifted brain across fixed intracranial structures (falx cerebri, cerebellar tentorium, and the skull) is called **herniation**. Whether brain dysfunction occurs as a result of shift without actual herniation is unclear. Shift and herniation likely represent progressive stages in an evolving continuum, starting with reversible tissue dysfunction and ending with eventual cell death.

ROSTROCAUDAL SIGNS OF BRAIN COMPROMISE

As pressure from a hemispheric lesion increases, patients gradually move from being easily roused but inattentive, to sleepy and unable to maintain wakefulness, then to coma—a state of no voluntary or directed response to external or internal stimuli.

The ascending reticular formation, excited by sensory input, mediates arousal and consciousness to the cortex via the thalamic nuclei. Coma is a clinical state that corresponds to lesions at 1 of 3 levels along the neuraxis: bilateral cerebral cortex, the thalami, or the upper brainstem. The classic concept of herniation and coma produced by a mass brain lesion pertains to a hemispheric process that ultimately causes "rostrocaudal" deterioration of function, gradually coursing down the hemispheres into the medulla. Although these stages rarely manifest bilaterally in a strict and clearly delineated se-

INCREASED INTRACRANIAL PRESSURE AND CEREBRAL HERNIATION

quential pattern, this paradigm remains useful for evaluating deteriorating patients with evolving neurologic signs. In addition to the level of consciousness, important physical examination elements are pupillary size and reactivity, eye movements, limb posturing, and breathing pattern (Figure 29-1).

Pupillary Reactivity and Eye Movements

When pressure onto or across the diencephalon exists, loss of wakefulness results, but patients may transiently continue to withdraw appropriately from uncomfortable stimuli and to resist passive limb movements. Pupils are small and retain reactivity, although blunted and subtle to detect. Although there is no visual fixation, eye movements are conjugate and full. As pressure mounts across the thalami onto the mesencephalon, pupillary and eye movement abnormalities appear. Involvement of CN-III or its nucleus initially causes irregular and poorly reactive pupils (corectopia). Eventually, eye movements are disrupted by CN-III or CN-VI lesions or from involvement of the medial longitudinal fasciculus (MLF). The MLF, a paracentral dorsally located tract, maintains conjugate eye movements initiated voluntarily in the waking state or induced reflexively from cervical or vestibular inputs in comatose patients. This pathway provides the basis of "doll's eyes" testing or caloric stimulation testing of the semicircular canals. An intact MLF system, from the vestibular nuclei to the area of the CN-III nucleus, keeps the eyes from moving passively when the examiner rolls the head to one side. The eyes remain in their primary position in relation to the examiner or seem to move to the opposite side in relation to the head rolling. With unilateral caloric stimulation of the ears, the eyes deviate conjugately to one side or another, depending on the water temperature used for ear irrigation. The direction of the convection current induced in the semicircular canals by different temperatures determines the direction of eye movement. With the head maintained in neutral, cold water causes the eye to deviate to the side of the stimulated ear; warm water causes deviation away from the stimulated ear. Disruption of the MLF system causes abnormal or absent responses of these reflexive eye movements.

Movement

If the motor pathways of the brainstem are disconnected from corticothalamic input, certain primitive tonic postures appear in succession and reflect the level of CNS damage. Depending on the area of cerebral cortex involved, patients may show unilateral signs of upper motor neuron dysfunction, with the typical triad of increased flexor tone, hyperreflexia, and paralysis. The opposite side may still show semivoluntary or directed movements, such as consistently withdrawing away from noxious stimuli or breaking the fall of a limb held against gravity. When damage progresses below the diencephalon or to the upper reticular activating system, a **decorticate posture** appears, characterized by rigid arm adduction, forearm pronation with flexion of the elbow and wrist, and leg extension at the hips and knees. With further rostrocaudal deterioration, **decerebrate rigidity** evolves, with arm extension at the elbows, hyperextension of the trunk and legs, and prominent plantar flexion of the feet. Arm adduction, wrist flexion, and forearm pronation persist. Animal models suggest that decerebrate rigidity corresponds to mesencephalic lesions at the level of the red nucleus. With ischemia to the lower pons and medulla, the body becomes flaccid, with no reactivity except occasional bilateral toe extensor responses with knee and hip flexion.

Breathing

Respiratory patterns also change with worsening levels of consciousness in coma (Figure 29-2). The earliest breathing alterations are **Cheyne-Stokes respirations**. Hemispheric forebrain structures serve to regulate breathing by mechanisms independent of CO_2 accumulation. With bilateral cerebral cortex damage, this breathing control is lost, and CO_2-driven breathing is accentuated with only modest CO_2 accumulations, thus inducing an increased rate and depth of respiration. This reactive hyperpnea leads to an eventual decrease in arterial CO_2 and, without forebrain control, loss of respiratory drive. The ensuing apnea then allows CO_2 to reaccumulate, causing the cycle to repeat, resulting in hyperpnea of a crescendo-decrescendo pattern, alternating with intervening episodes of apnea.

INCREASED INTRACRANIAL PRESSURE AND CEREBRAL HERNIATION

Figure 29-1 Eye Movements With Increased ICP

Doll's eye phenomenon

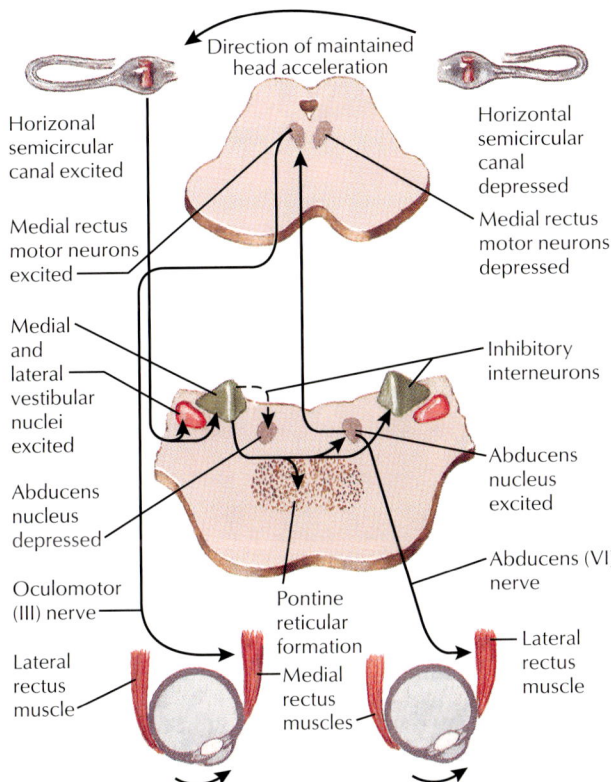

Eyes move in opposite direction to head; tend to preserve visual fixation: rate determined by degree of horizontal canal excitation

Testing for doll's head conjugate eye movement

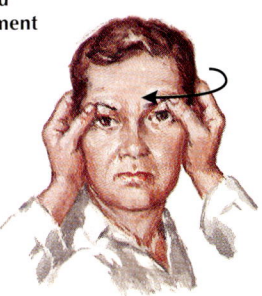

Head rotated and observed for presence and direction of eye movement; intact MLF prevents passive eye movement; with head rotation.

Normal doll's head (intact MLF)

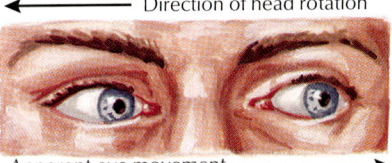

Eyes remain in primary position in relation to examiner or appear to "move opposite" to direction of head rotation.

Abnormal doll's head (disrupted MLF)

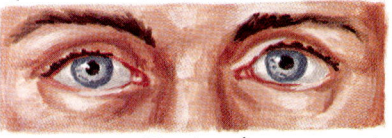

Eyes remain centered following same direction as rotation of head.

Medial longitudinal fasciculus (MLF) maintains conjugate eye movements initiated voluntarily in waking state or induced reflexively from cervical or vestibular inputs in comatose patients. MLF provides basis for doll's eye testing and caloric stimulation of semicircular canals.

Caloric testing of semicircular canals (with ice water)

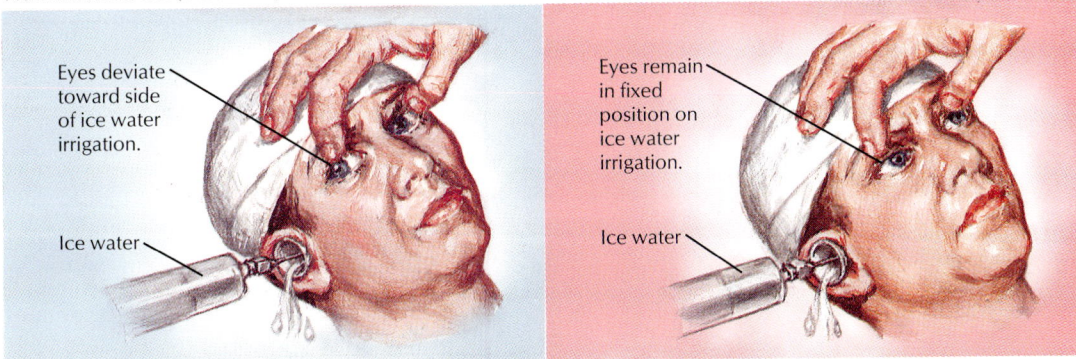

One ear irrigated with ice water solution and patient observed for presence and direction of eye movement relative to side of irrigation

Disorders of Consciousness

INCREASED INTRACRANIAL PRESSURE AND CEREBRAL HERNIATION

Figure 29-2

Respiratory Exchange in Head Injury

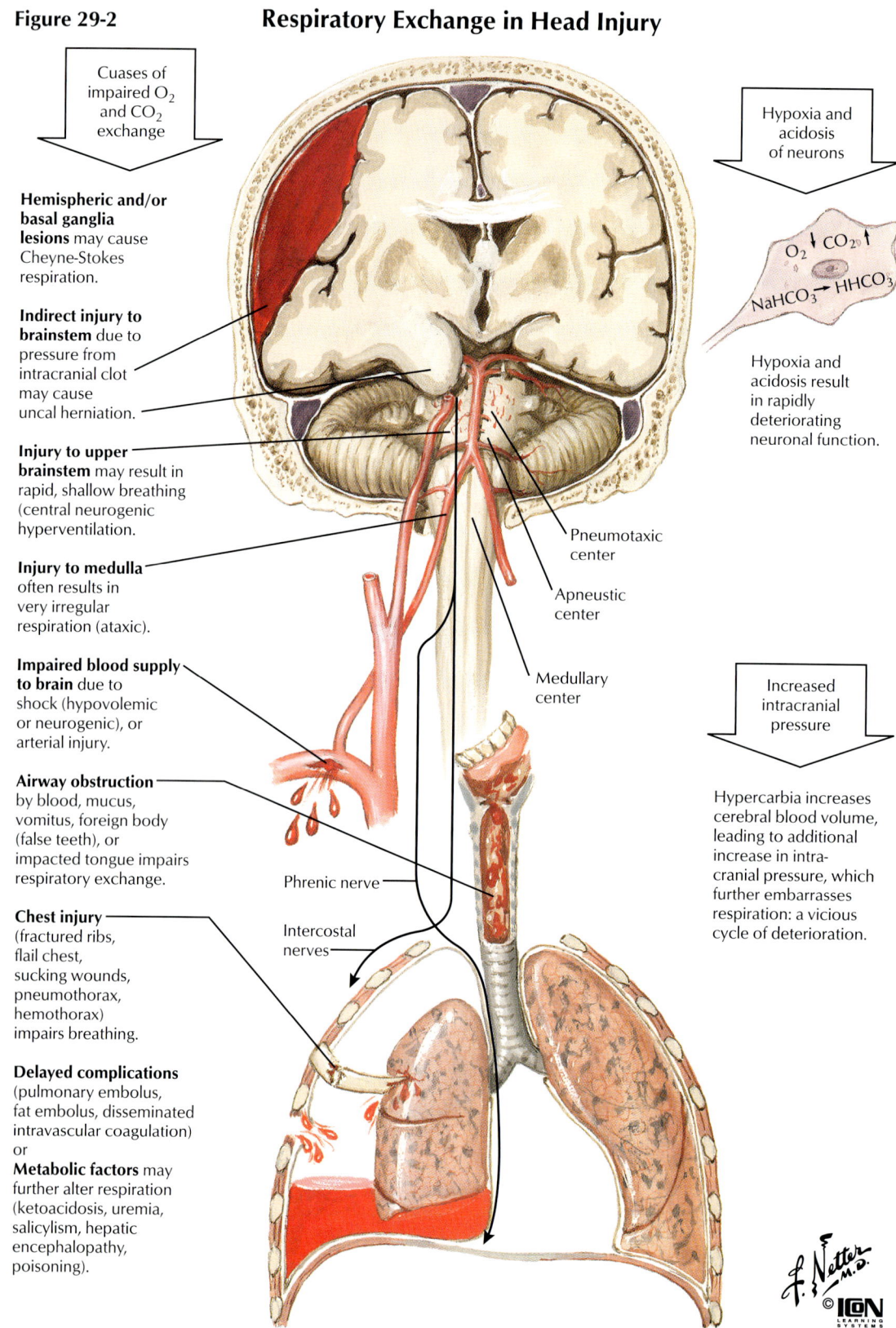

Cuases of impaired O₂ and CO₂ exchange

Hemispheric and/or basal ganglia lesions may cause Cheyne-Stokes respiration.

Indirect injury to brainstem due to pressure from intracranial clot may cause uncal herniation.

Injury to upper brainstem may result in rapid, shallow breathing (central neurogenic hyperventilation.

Injury to medulla often results in very irregular respiration (ataxic).

Impaired blood supply to brain due to shock (hypovolemic or neurogenic), or arterial injury.

Airway obstruction by blood, mucus, vomitus, foreign body (false teeth), or impacted tongue impairs respiratory exchange.

Chest injury (fractured ribs, flail chest, sucking wounds, pneumothorax, hemothorax) impairs breathing.

Delayed complications (pulmonary embolus, fat embolus, disseminated intravascular coagulation) or **Metabolic factors** may further alter respiration (ketoacidosis, uremia, salicylism, hepatic encephalopathy, poisoning).

Hypoxia and acidosis of neurons

$O_2 \downarrow\ CO_2 \uparrow$
$NaHCO_3 \rightarrow HHCO_3$

Hypoxia and acidosis result in rapidly deteriorating neuronal function.

Pneumotaxic center
Apneustic center
Medullary center

Increased intracranial pressure

Hypercarbia increases cerebral blood volume, leading to additional increase in intracranial pressure, which further embarrasses respiration: a vicious cycle of deterioration.

Phrenic nerve
Intercostal nerves

Disorders of Consciousness

INCREASED INTRACRANIAL PRESSURE AND CEREBRAL HERNIATION

Midbrain and upper pons lesions cause hyperventilation with a constant rate and amplitude, without periods of apnea. The reasons for so-called **central neurogenic hyperventilation** are unclear but are unlikely to be of purely neuronal origins. Lung congestion caused by immobility and poor airway protection likely play a major role. However, hypothalamic and midbrain lesions may engender increased sympathetic activity that promotes capillary fluid seepage, which causes worsening lung congestion and sometimes edema.

Injury to the lower half of the pons damages the respiratory control system, possibly generating **apneustic** breathing, a pattern of prolonged end inspiration pauses alternating with end expiration pauses of several seconds, without the crescendo-decrescendo pattern of Cheyne-Stokes breathing. Further damage causes this pattern to fragment into an irregular, unpredictable rhythm of varying amplitude, intermixed with pauses of variable length. Ultimately, destruction of the centrally located dorsomedial medullary respiratory center causes total cessation of breathing, even before circulatory collapse occurs.

VARIATION FROM THE CLASSIC ROSTROCAUDAL PARADIGM

Unilateral cerebral lesions can cause asymmetric pressures, leading to medial temporal lobe (**uncal**) **herniation** through the tentorial incisure, with direct compression of the midbrain. In this case, the diencephalic features described above are not seen; instead, rapid loss of consciousness is immediately follow by a decerebrate posture. This is usually heralded by compressive palsy of CN-III as it exits the ventral aspect of the midbrain and runs between the superior cerebellar and posterior cerebral arteries across the top of the tentorium. The initial sign is pupillary dilation, followed by ophthalmoplegia with ptosis and downward displacement of the abducted globe (chapter 6). Hemiplegia ipsilateral to the lesion side may result from compression of the contralateral anteriorly located pyramidal tract against the anterior edge of the tentorium (referred to as **Kernohan notch** phenomenon). A sudden worsening and increase in ICP may also result from posterior cerebral artery compression with occipital lobe infarction. Finally, the cingulate gyrus may herniate beneath the falx cerebri, compressing the ipsilateral or contralateral anterior cerebral artery and causing infarction in its distribution.

Infratentorial lesions within the brainstem tegmentum or secondary to brainstem compression, such as with cerebellar mass lesions, cause coma abruptly as a result of the almost immediate involvement of the reticular activating system. Lesions involving the midbrain result in oculomotor or infranuclear type ophthalmoplegia or both, with fixed irregular or midposition dilated pupils. If the lesion involves the pons without the midbrain, sympathetic fibers running to the CN-III nucleus are destroyed, and pupils are pinpoint in size but still reactive to light. An internuclear ophthalmoplegia occurs from bilateral MLF lesions, but vertical oculocephalic movements, controlled by the tectal midbrain, are preserved. Cerebellar mass lesions can cause forward brainstem displacement and may produce findings similar to those described for isolated pontine lesions or may cause cerebellar tissue crowding and herniation upward around the midbrain through the tentorium or downward around the medulla through the foramen magnum. Cerebellar tonsillar herniation down through the foramen magnum causes sudden respiratory and circulatory arrest, without gradual signs of evolving brainstem dysfunction.

Coma from metabolic disease rarely conforms to the typical rostrocaudal stages and often shows concurrent findings pertaining to different nervous system levels. For example, hypoglycemia can cause unconsciousness with decerebrate posturing but preserved oculocephalic responses and pupillary reactivity. In metabolic comas from opioid overdose, pupils are tiny but reactive, even though respiratory drive may be obliterated. Also, the oculocephalics are intact, despite drug-induced pinpoint pupillary changes mimicking a pontine hemorrhage, as in the vignette at the beginning of chapter 28. Finally, pupillary reactivity is resistant to metabolic effects; when other brainstem signs are absent, pupillary reactivity suggests a nonstructural metabolic or toxic cause.

INCREASED INTRACRANIAL PRESSURE AND CEREBRAL HERNIATION

TREATMENT OF INCREASED INTRACRANIAL PRESSURE

Overview

When signs of increased ICP are evident, emergent treatment is needed to halt progressive obtundation or coma and to avoid herniation and irreversible brain injury. Delaying treatment to first determine the underlying pathophysiologic mechanism is of minimal benefit. Therapeutic modalities available to acutely control increasing ICP act mainly on 3 mechanisms: vascular, osmotic, and metabolic. With induced vasoconstriction, cerebral blood flow (CBF) diminishes, reducing total cerebral blood volume, with a subsequent decrease in ICP.

Agents that create a hyperosmolar intravascular compartment in relation to brain tissue induce water movement down a gradient from cells and the interstitium into plasma, reducing total brain water content, volume, and pressure. This affects normal and damaged edematous brains. Osmotic agents may have other beneficial actions, such as preserving cerebral perfusion pressure (CPP), decreasing blood viscosity, decreasing CSF production, and scavenging free radicals.

Increased metabolic demand from injury or illness may increase blood flow and enhance the delivery of oxygen, which may cause increased free radical production and cell injury. Decreasing the metabolic drive helps limit blood flow and decreases the need for tissue oxygen delivery.

Hyperventilation

The least invasive, most effective, and fastest mechanism to decrease ICP is induced hypocapnia produced by active hyperventilation. Intact brain tissue with preserved cerebrovascular autoregulation mediates this effect. Autoregulation is abolished in damaged tissue or ischemic areas, which do not respond to hyperventilation. The goal of intact cerebrovascular autoregulation is to keep CBF stable under conditions of normal slight fluctuations in systemic pressures. Factors such as fever, hypoxemia, and ischemia induce the need for increased CBF and are mediated through the vasodilatory effect of hydrogen ions from lactic and carbonic acid accumulation. The brain is therefore sensitive to CO_2 levels, and increased CO_2 pressure produces an almost linear increase in CBF. Similarly, decreased CO_2 pressure causes vasoconstriction and a decrease in CBF. Correspondingly, intracranial blood volume and ICP decrease, provided that enough intact tissue exists to mediate this response.

The response to hyperventilation is almost immediate, with its peak effect occurring within 30 minutes. Effectiveness diminishes over the course of hours to a day, limiting the utility of hyperventilation as a long-term option to control increased ICP. Despite short-term effectiveness, cerebral vasoconstriction may eventually cause increasing ischemic brain injury, especially in vulnerable areas with previously compromised blood flow. Outcomes can worsen with its prolonged use. Therefore, hyperventilation use is confined to brief intervals to urgently control sudden increases in ICP. When more permanent treatments are instituted (ie, control of agitation, blood pressure regulation, or surgery), its use should be halted.

The relatively safe target level of P_{CO_2} is approximately 25 to 35 mm Hg; lower P_{CO_2} levels risk compromising cerebral blood perfusion with subsequent ischemia, which would eventually cause a seemingly paradoxic further increase in ICP. The usual approach is to increase respiratory rate but not tidal volume. Higher lung volumes increase intrathoracic pressure and total cerebral blood volume by compromising venous return from the brain to the heart.

Osmotic Agents and Diuretics

Mannitol (20-25%) solution is usually administered rapidly (0.75-1.0 g/kg). Its initial effect usually occurs within 20 minutes and lasts approximately 6 to 8 hours. With repeated doses of mannitol, there is diminishing effectiveness and shortening of response duration over days. Depending on the clinical response and patient status, subsequent doses of 0.25 to 0.5 g/kg are administered every 4 to 6 hours. Concomitant measurement of serum osmolality, and sometimes ICP, is indicated. Repeated mannitol use requires extreme caution to avoid hypotension or a hyperosmolar state from too frequent or brisk diuresis. Using mannitol sparingly avoids the pitfalls of hypotension and electrolyte imbalance that can seriously undermine patient care.

INCREASED INTRACRANIAL PRESSURE AND CEREBRAL HERNIATION

A staged approach in increasing the osmolarity to 295 to 300 mOsm/L initially and then gradually to 310 to 320 mOsm/L may be helpful. Osmolarities higher than 320 mOsm/L are dangerous and add little to further control ICP. Standing orders for "maintenance" doses should not be written; the clinical situation and osmolality should guide subsequent dosing. If the clinical examination and osmolarity are stable, no extra doses may be required. Serial measurement of renal function, electrolytes, and osmolarity are indicated every 4 to 6 hours. Potassium depletion is common, and frequent replacement is needed. Daily fluid balance and body weight measurements are essential to maintain the goal of a euvolemic hyperosmolar state. Only isotonic fluids should be used to replenish intravascular volume. Hypotonic fluids and free water should be avoided to avert recurrent brain edema.

Low doses of diuretics, such as furosemide (10-20 mg), may be used alone or with mannitol to enhance or hasten response, especially when transient increase in intravascular volume, such as in congestive heart failure, may be problematic. Hypertonic solutions, such as 3% saline administered over 10 to 15 minutes, can effectively reduce ICP without compromising perfusion pressure or increasing diuresis in patients already dehydrated from mannitol.

Barbiturate Anesthesia

The presumed mechanism for barbiturate anesthesia, another useful modality for reducing ICP, is its ability to reduce brain metabolic demand and therefore CBF. Evidence supporting its use is better for patients with head trauma than for those with nontraumatic injuries. It is difficult to use in a sustained fashion because of its serious adverse effects of hypotension and myocardial depression and should be reserved for recalcitrant cases of increased ICP not responsive to conservative measures and osmotic agents. A short-acting barbiturate, pentobarbital, is used at a 1 to 3 mg $\cdot$ kg^{-1} $\cdot$ h^{-1} drip after an initial loading dose of 3 to 10 mg/kg administered over at least 30 minutes and 5 mg $\cdot$ kg^{-1} $\cdot$ h^{-1} for 3 hours. The maintenance dose is adjusted to obtain a burst suppression pattern on EEG, but this is not essential if other means of assessing ICP, such as a pressure bolt or intraventricular catheter, are available. Usually, adequate treatment occurs at barbiturate levels of approximately 30 to 50 mg/dL; higher levels may produce total electrocerebral silence and are usually not necessary. Blood pressure is maintained with pressor or inotropic infusion if needed.

Other Agents

Propofol infusion (1-3 mg $\cdot$ kg^{-1} $\cdot$ h^{-1}) has been used with some benefit to control increased ICP, but it must be used with caution because of its potential to cause hypotension, adrenal suppression, and increased risk of nosocomial infections. Halogenated inhalation anesthetics and ketamine are not recommended because of their direct dilatory effect on cerebral vasculature and CBF.

General Measures

In the care of patients with or at risk for increased ICP, several other modalities help prevent escalating ICP and improve outcome.

Head Position

If blood pressure is controlled and there is no threat of compromising CPP, head position should be kept upright at approximately 30° to aid brain venous outflow and reduce total brain blood volume. The head should be kept midline and not bent to the side, which may impede jugular venous drainage. If blood pressure is fluctuating or low, the patient should remain supine to prevent decreased CPP.

Blood Pressure

The parameters of blood pressure control in treating ICP remain hard to define. Cerebral autoregulation is absent in damaged or ischemic brains, and perfusion of these areas is directly related to systemic pressure. Relatively high systemic pressures may increase edema in areas of a disrupted blood-brain barrier, whereas low systemic pressures may compromise perfusion and cause further tissue ischemia. The **Cushing response**, a reaction to increasing ICP, and a sympathetically mediated increase of systemic blood pressure with reflex bradycardia, may play a protective role in preserving CPP (ICP minus mean arterial pressure). However, if untreated, it may eventually lead to increased tissue edema in damaged areas of the brain. Conversely, overaggressive treatment may exacerbate ischemia.

The principle of preserving CPP within the range of functioning cerebral autoregulation may be the best guide, because no definite directives exist. Because the range of cerebral autoregulation shifts upward with chronic hypertension, the parameters for each patient may vary. Ideally, arterial blood pressure should be kept near its premorbid range, determined if possible from previous measurements. If arterial pressure is low, then increasing it with isotonic fluids or mild pressor agents is indicated. In cases in which ICP is stable, systemic hypertension is treated independently. If both systemic pressure and ICP are increased in conjunction, then an attempt at reducing ICP (for example, with mannitol) should be initiated first and blood pressure should be monitored closely for resolution of reflex hypertension. If there is no response within a few minutes, a gentle attempt to bring the systemic blood pressure down is made, preferably using agents with no cerebral vasodilatory effects, ie, diuretics, angiotensin-converting enzyme inhibitors, and β-sympathetic blockers. Reliance on CPP alone may not always produce favorable outcomes, and following all parameters simultaneously may provide greater benefit.

When an ICP monitor is used, the goal is to preserve CBF above the level that ensures adequate cerebral oxygen metabolic needs while keeping CPP above approximately 70 mm Hg and avoiding persistent or recurring ICP measurements of greater than 20 mm Hg.

Pathologic Stresses

Factors, such as seizures and fever, that may increase cerebral metabolic rate and blood flow require control. Seizures are emergently treated with benzodiazepines or short-acting barbiturates and long-term with other anticonvulsants. Hypoxemia must be avoided, so blood oxygenation is monitored with O_2 saturation devices or repeated arterial blood gas samples. Hyperthermia requires prompt treatment with antipyretics and with antibiotics when an infectious cause is found. Because cerebral metabolic rate is directly proportional to temperature, some authorities advocate hypothermia as a primary treatment for increased ICP. Although effective, its complications include cardiac arrhythmias, pancreatitis, infections, and rebound ICP during the rewarming process. Whether induced hypothermia improves neurologic outcome is still unknown.

It is generally accepted that steroids are not useful, and may be detrimental, in most instances of sudden increase in ICP. Other than long-term control of tumor-associated edema, they should not be used in the acute management of increased ICP.

Hemicraniectomy

In this surgical procedure, the lateral-coronal skull is removed and a dural flap is constructed without excision of necrotic brain tissue, permitting enlarging lobar lesions to expand outward without exerting pressure on deeper brainstem structures. Hemicraniectomy has been successfully used to control increased ICP when other measures have failed. Particularly used for large middle cerebral artery distribution strokes, it is clearly effective in reducing mortality. Performing it as early as possible at the first signs of deterioration yields better results and may improve outcome. However, most survivors remain with significant disability, especially if they are older than 45 years. Hemicraniectomy for difficult-to-control ICP, especially with dominant hemispheric strokes, should not be done routinely. Careful consideration of residual functional abilities, life expectancy, patient wishes if known, and input from the family of the patient should all be considered.

REFERENCES

Bullock R, Chestnut F, Clifton G, et al. Guidelines for the management of severe head injury. *J Neurotrauma*. 2000;17:471-553.

Demchuk AM. Hemicraniectomy is a promising treatment in ischemic stroke. *Can J Neurol Sci*. 200:27:274-277.

Muizelaar JP, Marmarou A, Ward JD, et al. Adverse effects of prolonged hyperventilation in patients with severe head injury: a randomized clinical trial. *J Neurosurg*. 1991;75:731-739.

North JB, Jennett S. Abnormal breathing patterns associated with acute brain damage. *Arch Neurol*. 1974;31:338-344.

Patel PM. Hyperventilation as a therapeutic intervention: do the potential benefits outweigh the known risks? *J Neurosurg Anesthesiol.* 1993;5:62-65.

Piatt J, Schiff SJ. High dose barbiturate therapy in neurosurgery and intensive care. *Neurosurgery.* 1984;15:427–444.

Plum F, Posner JB. *The Diagnosis of Stupor and Coma.* 3rd ed. New York, NY: Oxford University Press Inc; 1982.

Ropper A. A preliminary study of the geometry of brain displacement and level of consciousness with acute intracranial masses. *Neurology.* 1992;39:622-627.

Rosner MJ, Daughton S. Cerebral perfusion pressure management in head injury. *J Trauma.* 1990;30:933-941.

Shiozaki T, Sugimoto H, Taneda M, et al. Effect of mild hypothermia on uncontrollable intracranial hypertension after severe head injury. *J Neurosurg.* 1993;79:363-368.

Chapter 30
Brain Death

Gregory Allam

Clinical Vignette

A 56-year-old man suddenly collapsed at home after experiencing severe chest pain. His wife called the emergency technicians, who found him pulseless and cyanotic. ECG demonstrated ventricular fibrillation, but he was "successfully" defibrillated. After an airway was established and 100% oxygen was given, he was transported to the ED. There, results of neurologic evaluation showed that he was unresponsive to any form of communication. His pupils were dilated and fixed, and he had decerebrate posturing to noxious stimulation and bilateral Babinski signs. He eventually became flaccid, and cold caloric vestibular stimulation showed no ocular response. The next day, he developed generalized myoclonus and continued to require cardiac and full respiratory support. Three days later, there was no change in his neurologic status. An apnea test showed no respiratory response to induced hypercarbia. Although he was declared brain dead, his wife asked that further testing be performed to confirm the clinical diagnosis. An EEG demonstrated electrocerebral silence, and she agreed to have life support withdrawn.

This vignette is the classic example of a patient with an acute myocardial infarction, cardiac arrhythmia, or both with prolonged cardiorespiratory arrest. The result is devastating diffuse cerebral ischemic damage. Until a precise determination of brain death is established, there are many medical and legal issues to address in caring for individuals who have no effective residual brain function despite the return of cardiopulmonary function maintained with modern intensive care therapies.

In most medical communities, a person is considered dead once there is irreversible and total cessation of all brain function, regardless of a continuing functional circulatory system. The cause of brain damage must be clearly elucidated by history, examination, or medical tests before the diagnosis of brain death is entertained. Intoxicants, sedatives, and hypothermia may present similarly to brain death but are potentially reversible and must always be considered if the cause is not clear and well documented. In many countries, including the United States, brain death constitutes a legal definition of death, and all life support measures can be halted.

When caring for an individual, it is best to respect the family's wishes, religious or personal, regarding the timing of life support discontinuation. It is important to continue to explain the situation's finality and that circulatory collapse will invariably occur within hours to days of the onset of this clinical picture. It is paramount to broach the subject of organ donation as soon as possible because it is vital to harvest organs early. The widespread difficulty in obtaining organs for an ever-growing list of patients awaiting transplant procedures emphasizes this necessity. The physician who has an established relationship with the patient's family is perhaps the one best to initiate such discussion, before involving the transplant team.

BRAIN DEATH CRITERIA

The criteria for brain death vary among states and countries. Usually the determination is clinical, with testing used only as an ancillary or confirmatory measure. Following are the generally accepted principles of brain death determination:

1. A preceding coma of known irreversible cause must **not** be due to, or influenced by, CNS depressants, intoxicants, paralytic agents, hypothermia (less than 32°C/90°F), or endocrine or metabolic disturbances (Figure 30-1).
2. Cessation of all brain function must be documented as follows.
   a. There must be **no response to stimuli** in any way **other than** spinal **withdrawal**

BRAIN DEATH

Figure 30-1 — Differential Diagnosis of Coma

	Clinical features	Pathology (examples)	Etiologies

Bilateral cerebral hemisphere disease	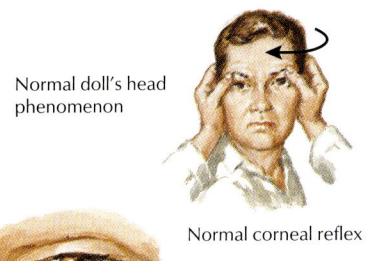 Normal pupils (equal, reactive); Normal doll's head phenomenon; Normal corneal reflex; Absent or minor focal features (lateral paralysis, sensory or visual loss)	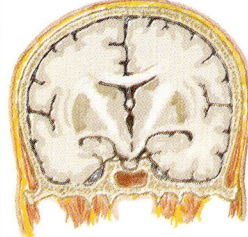 Bilateral hemispheric swelling (small ventricles, obliterated sulci, rounded edges)	Increased subarachnoid or extracerebral pressure
			  Meningitis
			  Subarachnoid hemorrhage
			  Bilateral subdural hematoma
			Metabolic encephalopathy
			  Liver coma
			  Kidney coma
			  Carbon dioxide narcosis
			  Hypoxia
			  Hypoglycemia
			  Hypercalcemia
			  Hyponatremia
			  Diabetic acidosis
			  Hyperosmolar coma
			Toxins or drugs
			  Barbiturates
			  Alcohol
			  Narcotics
			  Other sedative overdose
			  Lead
			Multifocal cerebral disease (usually developing sequentially)
			  Infarction
			  Multiple abscesses
			  Encephalitis
			  Multiple areas of brain tumor
			  Multiple cerebral contusions

Unilateral cerebral hemisphere lesion with compression of brainstem	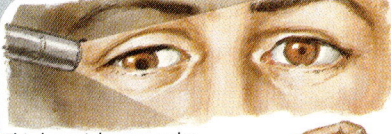 Third cranial nerve palsy, nonreactive pupil, ptosis; Contralateral hemiparesis	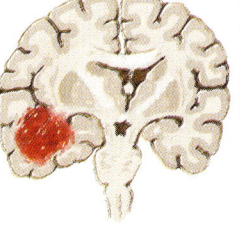 Right temporal hemorrhage from trauma, with swelling of right hemisphere	Cerebral
			  Tumor
			  Hemorrhage
			  Abscess
			  Infarction
			  Contusion
			Extracerebral
			  Subdural hematoma
			  Extradural hematoma

Primary brainstem lesion	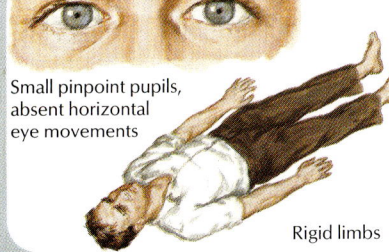 Small pinpoint pupils, absent horizontal eye movements; Rigid limbs	Large pontine hemorrhage	Infarction Hemorrhage Severe metabolic disturbance, sedative or phenytoin overdose Severe anoxia
Cerebellar lesion with secondary brainstem compression	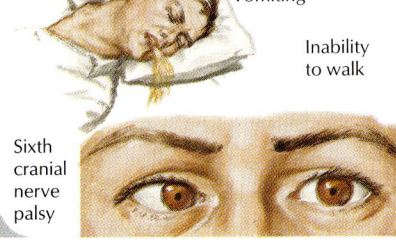 Vomiting; Inability to walk; Sixth cranial nerve palsy	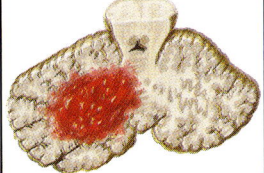 Large cerebellar hemorrhage	Infarction Hemorrhage Tumor Abscess Contusion

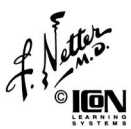

DISORDERS OF CONSCIOUSNESS

movements in the legs and arms. Spinal reflexes such as muscle stretch reflexes or extensor responses of the toes (Babinski signs) can be seen, but there must be no other spontaneous limb movements or posturing to painful stimuli, including decerebrate rigidity.
   b. **Brainstem reflexes must be absent**, including pupillary response to light (without mydriatic agents), oculocephalic reflexes by passive head turning or caloric stimulation, corneal reflexes, oropharyngeal reflexes (gag or swallowing), respiratory reflexes (spontaneous breaths or cough), and snout or jaw jerk reflex.
   c. **Apnea test must be positive**, wherein the patient exhibits no evidence of respiratory effort or change in sinus heart rate with induced hypercapnia. In this instance, the patient is ventilated with 100% O_2 for 15 minutes, then disconnected while an endotracheal catheter provides 6 L/min oxygen. Apneic oxygenation is maintained for 10 minutes or until the Pco_2 is 55 to 60 mm Hg.
3. In the presence of a clear structural brain lesion without evidence of toxic or metabolic cause, neurologic reexamination should proceed 6 hours after the initial evaluation to confirm and document the findings. Repeat examination should be performed at 12 hours if the cause is uncertain or there is no evidence of irreversible severe structural brain damage.
4. When the clinical evaluation, apnea test, or both are unclear or unfeasible, confirmatory tests to document the absence of electrical or metabolic cerebral activity are conducted. CT may support the clinical examination (Figure 30-2).
   a. A minimum 30-minute EEG isoelectric tracing (obtained with a "double" interelectrode distance bipolar montage) is sought. The first test is obtained no sooner than 8 hours after cardiac arrest and reconfirmed after 6 hours (American EEG Society Recommendations).
   b. Documentation of cessation of cerebral circulation by conventional angiography, technetium isotope study, transcranial doppler, or CT angiogram.
   c. Absent auditory evoked responses and short-latency somatosensory evoked responses may also be used to indicate absent brainstem function. However, these studies may be affected by peripheral lesions and are technically difficult to perform, especially in an intensive care unit setting, and their utility as a confirmatory test has been questioned.

MITIGATING FACTORS

When a severe cerebral insult is suspected but brain death determination cannot be confirmed due to confounding issues, the utmost should be done to correct for these specific factors before brain death assessment can proceed. For example, hypothermia is best treated with a warming blanket to bring and maintain core body temperature above 36.5°C. Fluid, and at times vasopressor agents, is administered for patients with systolic blood pressures lower than 90 mm Hg.

Patients with chronic hypercapnia secondary to lung disease such as chronic obstructive pulmonary disease have a higher respiratory center Pco_2 threshold, and a Pco_2 of approximately 60 mm Hg may not necessarily drive the chemoreceptors, even with a functioning brainstem. The CO_2 level may be allowed to climb to approximately 80 mm Hg, but such levels risks direct cardiac effect of ensuing acidosis with arrhythmias and hypotension. Therefore, it is preferable in these instances to obtain confirmatory tests to bolster the diagnosis and judge with more certainty without risking untoward and unnecessary complications.

Although most centers in the United States uphold the general outline of the principles mentioned above, there are numerous variations and differences concerning how best to ensure diagnostic certainty. Most medical centers do not require confirmatory tests. The number of evaluations and the time span between them also differs. Many institutions require a brain death evaluation by two attending neurologists at different times and their presence at the apnea test. The specific brain death criteria and protocol for

BRAIN DEATH

Figure 30-2 Hypoxic Brain Damage and Brain Death

Brain death

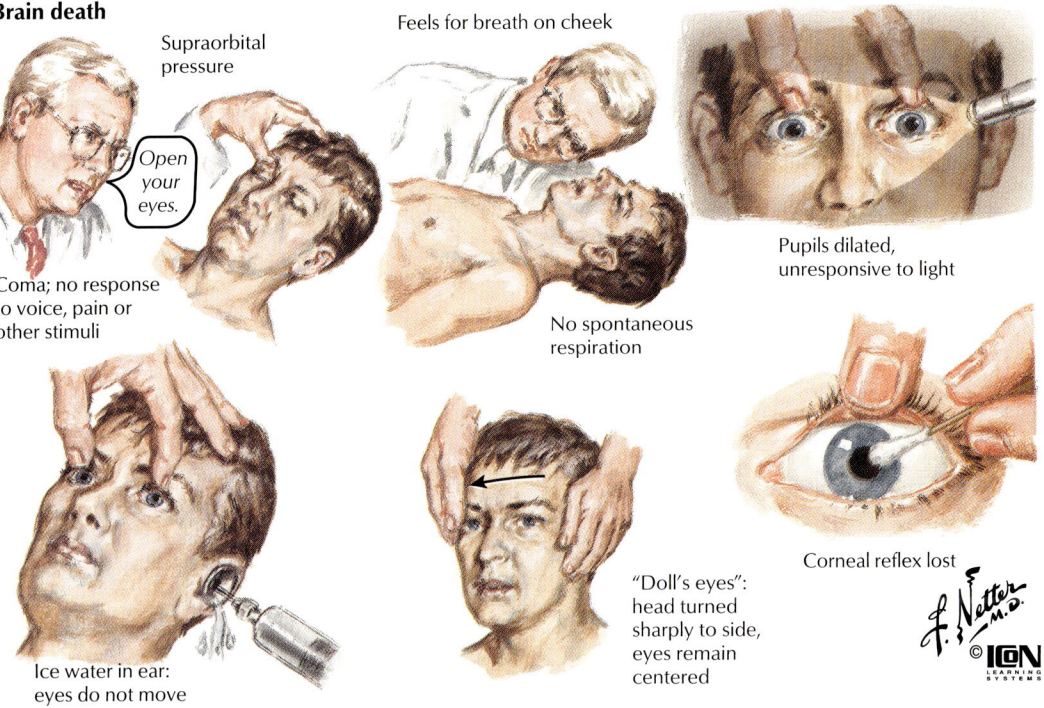

Border zone ischemia (shock, circulatory insufficiency)

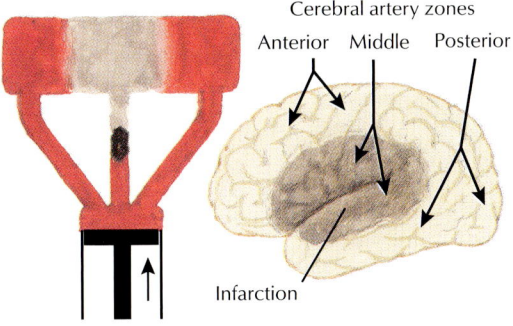
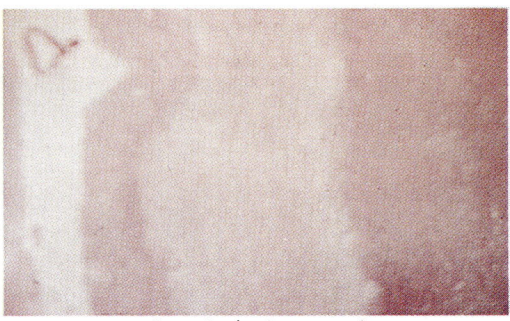

Diffuse cortical necrosis; persistent vegetative state

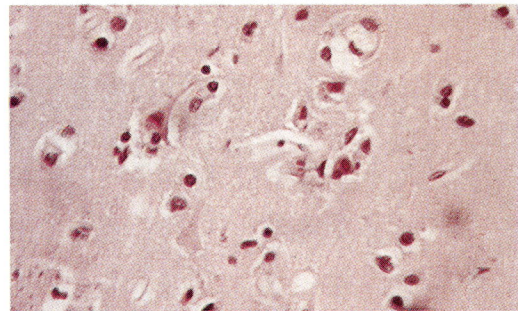

Few anoxic neurons in early anoxia

Extensive laminar necrosis

DISORDERS OF CONSCIOUSNESS

each medical center must be consulted before the evaluation is begun and a diagnosis is substantiated.

REFERENCES

Conrad GR, Sinha P. Scintigraphy as a confirmatory test of brain death. *Semin Nucl Med.* 2003;33:312-323.

Guideline three: minimum technical standards for EEG recording in suspected cerebral death. American Electroencephalographic Society. *J Clin Neurophysiol.* 1994;11:10-13.

Piatt J, Schiff SJ. High dose barbiturate therapy in neurosurgery and intensive care. *Neurosurgery.* 1984;15:427-444.

Presidents Commission on Guidelines for the Determination of Death. *Neurology.* 1982;32:395.

Plum F, Posner JB. *The Diagnosis of Stupor and Coma.* 3rd ed. New York, NY: Oxford University Press; 1982.

Qureshi AI, Kirmani JF, Xavier AR, Siddiqui AM. Computed tomographic angiography for diagnosis of brain death. *Neurology.* 2004;24;62:652-653.

Section IX
MEMORY AND COGNITIVE DISORDERS

Chapter 31
Acute Cognitive and Behavioral Disorders 322

Chapter 32
Alzheimer Disease 327

Chapter 33
Dementia With Lewy Bodies 347

Chapter 34
Frontotemporal Dementia 351

Chapter 35
Vascular Dementia 356

Chapter 36
Transmissible Spongiform Encephalopathy 360

Chapter 31
Acute Cognitive and Behavioral Disorders

Yuval Zabar

Clinical Vignette

A 48-year-old executive presented to the ED with his first generalized tonic-clonic seizure. Gradually, he awoke and became alert, without recall of the event or any focal neurologic findings. He had a sore tongue and residual generalized muscle soreness. He and his wife reported no risk factors. The results of his serum chemistry tests were unremarkable. Brain CT was normal. After 6 hours of observation, he was dismissed, with a neurologist's appointment for the following week.

Within 24 hours, the patient returned to the ED with full withdrawal syndrome with agitation, profound sympathetic release signs, tremulousness, and restlessness and began having visual hallucinations. He reported that insects were crawling all over him and that some were brightly colored and enlarging in size. He was diaphoretic, had a temperature of 39.4°C, and had a pulse rate of 126 beats/min. His neck was supple, and he had no signs of meningismus or other infectious process.

His wife asked whether he could be having **delirium tremens**. She reported for the first time that he had a long history of drinking 8 to 12 ounces of whiskey daily, sometimes with a few beers. In the past weeks, he had experienced increasing work pressure because he was not performing at his previous level. Realizing his job was in jeopardy, he became despondent, drank more, and ate little. Finally, he resolved to stop drinking; within 16 hours, he experienced the seizure.

Treatment with high doses of lorazapam brought his delirium under control. When his mental status returned to normal, intensive counseling was initiated. He agreed to join Alcoholics Anonymous and eventually overcame his alcohol addiction. He regained all of his intellectual abilities and returned to work.

This vignette exemplifies the classic setting for the development of delirium tremens after sudden alcohol withdrawal. Before confirming delirium tremens, concomitant illicit drug use and primary neurologic infectious processes must be excluded.

CLINICAL FEATURES

Delirium is a common, acquired neuropsychiatric syndrome characterized by acute cognitive and behavioral changes with resulting functional loss (Figure 31-1). Onset of symptoms is usually rapid, within hours or days. Symptoms may fluctuate diurnally, worsening at night. Cognitive impairment is characterized by poor attention span, reduced concentration, distractibility, short-term memory impairment, disorientation, and executive dysfunction. Consciousness is impaired, with either stupor or hypervigilance predominating. Fluctuations in level of consciousness are also common. Level of confusion may vary from mild disorientation to total incoherence. Delirious patients experience a reduced level of arousal; many patients with delirium are drowsy or stuporous.

Delusions and hallucinations may occur. The delusional content is typically related to disorientation, eg, the patient may believe he or she is at work, surrounded by coworkers. Many delirious patients experience persecutory delusions, which lead to agitation and combativeness. Hallucinations and sensory misperceptions (illusions) commonly occur and may affect any sensory modality. Visual and auditory hallucinations are most common. Mood disturbance, ranging from profound depression and apathy to severe fearfulness and anxiety, may also occur.

Clinical Examples

Delirium tremens is characterized by profound confusion, vivid hallucinations, delusions, agitation, restlessness, and sleeplessness. Pa-

ACUTE COGNITIVE AND BEHAVIORAL DISORDERS

Delirium

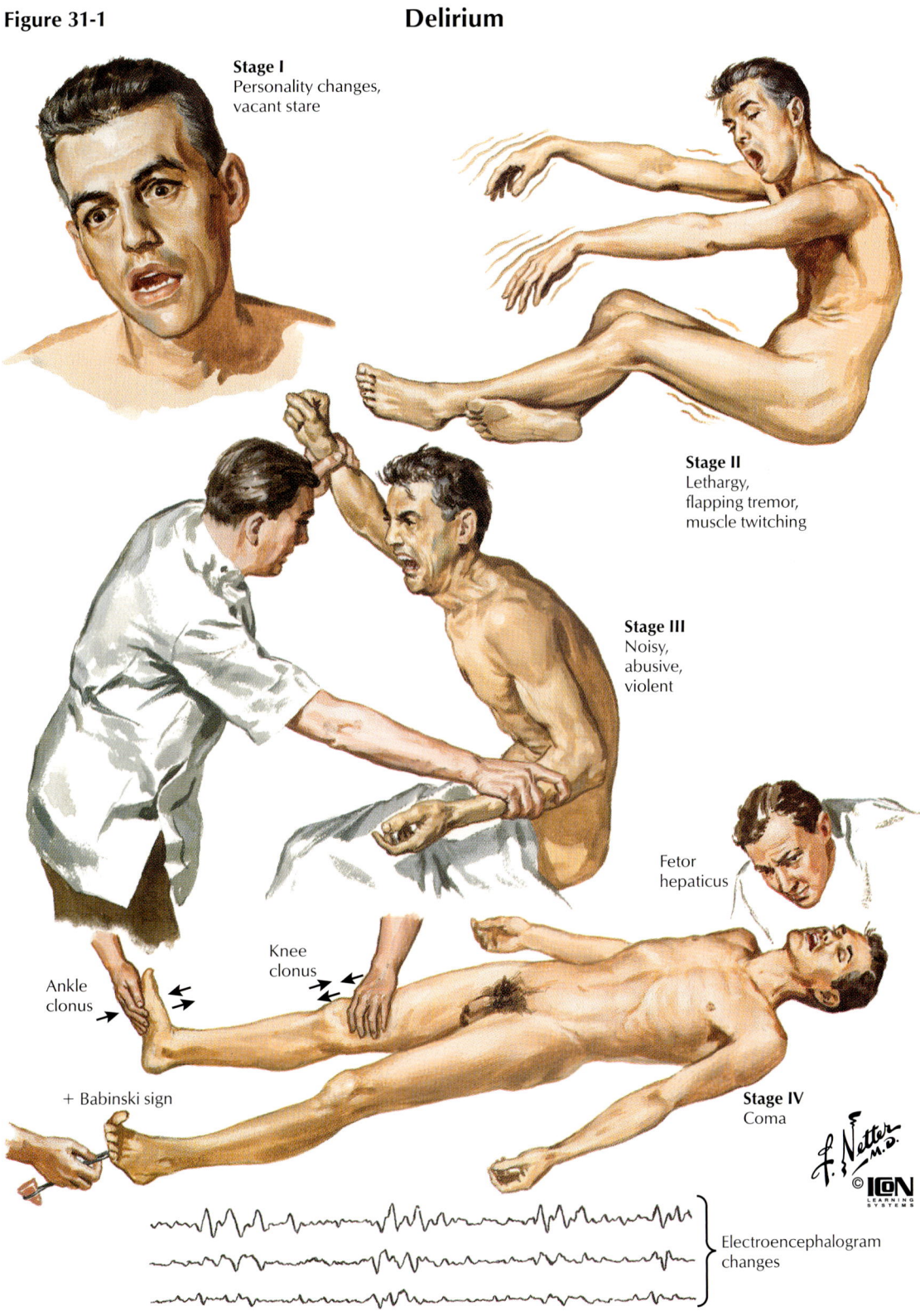

Figure 31-1

MEMORY AND COGNITIVE DISORDERS

323

tients have severe tremor and hypersympathetic activity, including dilated pupils, fever, tachycardia, hypertension, and diaphoresis. Symptoms occur in chronic alcoholics approximately 2 to 4 days after cessation of alcohol consumption. In some cases, the delirium begins 7 days later. The syndrome is typically mild and short-lived, but fulminant cases may lead to coma and death. Benzodiazepine medications are useful in reduction of morbidity and mortality of this condition.

Hepatic encephalopathy occurs in stages. Patients with liver failure experience confusion, with decreased psychomotor activity associated with increasing serum levels of NH_3. Occasionally, hyperactivity and agitation occur. During this time, patients often exhibit asterixis, which is not a sign specific to hepatic encephalopathy because it can occur in many other metabolic disturbances, such as uremic encephalopathy. Progressive stages of drowsiness, stupor, and coma follow. Significant motor abnormality develops, including rigidity, bradykinesia, brisk reflexes, and extensor plantar reflexes. Seizures may occur.

The progression of symptoms varies considerably, particularly after treatment begins. However, left untreated, coma may persist and lead to death in up to 50% of patients. In some cases, a chronic disorder of cognition and behavior occurs, with pyramidal and extrapyramidal dysfunction lasting months or years. This condition is seen in patients with repetitive bouts of hepatic encephalopathy. EEG shows generalized slowing of background rhythm with prominent triphasic waves. The purpose of treatment is to attempt to decrease NH_3 levels by reducing dietary protein, acidifying colonic contents with lactulose, and, occasionally, suppressing urease-producing colonic bacteria with antibiotics.

Wernicke encephalopathy is characterized first by ataxia, then by oculomotor abnormalities and delirium, developing during a period of days to weeks. It is caused by thiamine deficiency and commonly occurs in malnourished alcoholics. The delirium is characterized by disorientation, inattention, drowsiness, and indifference to surroundings. Conversation is sparse and tangential. Signs of alcohol withdrawal are seen in 15% of patients. Progressive stupor, coma, and death develop if the condition is left untreated. Autopsy reveals symmetric necrosis of brainstem tegmentum nuclei, superior cerebellar vermis, and mamillary bodies, resembling lesions produced by disorders of pyruvate metabolism.

Some patients have **amnesic syndrome**, also known as **Korsakoff psychosis**. This condition is a nonprogressive disorder of memory, affecting both new learning (**anterograde amnesia**) and past memory (**retrograde amnesia**). The patient cannot make new memories because of poor encoding, which is similar to the memory impairment of Alzheimer disease. The retrograde amnesia may extend back many years, rendering the patient "stuck in time." Recollection of past events is usually disorganized and erratic, sometimes suggesting deliberate confabulation. Additional cognitive impairment includes poor sequencing, arithmetic, and construction performance.

Treatment of Wernicke encephalopathy is immediate administration of large doses of thiamine, 100 mg IV, which reverses the symptoms and prevents progression of pathology. This treatment is routinely done in EDs for most patients presenting with an acute confusional state. Intravenous fluid must contain glucose to avoid precipitation of Wernicke encephalopathy. Thiamine and other B vitamins should be given to malnourished patients as supplements to replenish body stores.

EPIDEMIOLOGY

Most cases of delirium are not as well defined as the subtypes described above. The prevalence among hospitalized patients may be as high as 40%. Those at greatest risk include the elderly and postoperative patients. Comorbid illness and dementia, visual or hearing impairment, social isolation, sensory deprivation, and change in environment all predispose to delirium. Among terminally ill patients, delirium develops in 80%. Among hospitalized patients with delirium, fewer than half recover fully before discharge, according to some estimates. As many as two thirds of delirium cases go undetected and therefore may lead to significant morbidity and mortality. The epidemiology of delirium in the general community is unknown.

DIAGNOSTIC APPROACH

There are many potential causes for delirium, including, underlying medical conditions and their treatment, substance use or withdrawal, or a combination of these. Underlying medical conditions include metabolic causes (eg, hypoglycemia, electrolyte disturbances, volume depletion, renal failure, liver failure, and pulmonary insufficiency), infections, head trauma, epilepsy, neoplastic disease, and vascular disease. Prescription drugs are implicated in approximately 40% of cases. Medications with anticholinergic properties, sedatives, and narcotics are particularly likely to cause delirium.

Chronic delirium may mimic dementia (Table 31-1). Patients with so-called "reversible" dementia may represent cases of chronic delirium. Unlike delirium, dementia presents insidiously, does not affect level of consciousness until late stages, and is progressive. A firm diagnosis of dementia should never be made during an inpatient evaluation. Delirium is common in hospitalized patients, many of whom return to baseline on recovering from acute illness. Elderly patients who experience an acute confusional state while hospitalized may have unrecognized dementia, which necessitates outpatient evaluation. Cognitive impairment may be artificially amplified during hospitalization, potentially leading to inaccurate assessment and characterization of the patient's needs. Therefore, inpatients with acute confusional states (also called *change in mental status* or *delta MS*) must be assumed to have reversible or treatable conditions.

These distinctions are vital in the clinical setting, where diagnosis requires rapid determination. Evaluation should be detailed, and the examination should be thorough. There is no substitute for a careful history and review of medications and medical records. A complete physical examination is important to establish any intercurrent illness. Mental status examination, including observation of general appearance, affect, and level of consciousness, should be performed. Detailed examination of attention, orientation, language, memory, construction, praxis, and executive function is required to establish a pattern of deficits. Repeated examination over the ensuing months is often necessary to ascertain fluctuation, progression, or improvement.

Laboratory assessment for infection, metabolic disturbance, and toxin exposure are required for the delirious patient. CSF evaluation is necessary when clinical presentation suggests infectious or inflammatory problems or when systemic precipitants are not readily identified. Ancillary studies, including imaging and EEG, should be performed when clinically indicated.

TREATMENT AND COUNSELING

Management of delirium requires treatment of underlying causes, provision of environmental and supportive measures, appropriate medications for target symptoms, and regular follow-up evaluations. Identification of delirium is the first step. It is preferable to identify delirium before patients experience drastic changes in behavior or level of consciousness. At-risk patients should be identified and screened. Subtle changes in behavior, such as social withdrawal, change in mood, or anxiety, should be noted.

Table 31-1
Clinical Differences Between Delirium and Dementia

	Delirium	*Dementia*
Onset	Acute to subacute	Subacute to chronic
Level of consciousness	Impaired, fluctuates	Unaffected until late stages
Cognition	Poor attention, disorientation	Poor memory; attention and orientation affected later
Motor behavior	Variably increased or reduced	Usually normal
Psychotic features	Common and prominent	Less common and usually less prominent

When delirium is diagnosed and the underlying causes are addressed, caregivers should provide a safe environment with minimal patient demands to maximize safety. Patients may need to be placed near nursing stations for close observation. Sometimes one-to-one supervision is required. Family members should be encouraged to visit regularly and provide the patient with familiar objects. Glasses and hearing aides may facilitate the patient's sensory perception and overall orientation.

Explanation of the diagnosis to family members and caregivers is extremely important. The sudden change in a loved one's behavior may be distressing and may potentially disrupt patient care. Competency issues should always be considered and discussed.

Drug therapy should be used only when essential. Medications used to treat delirious patients often contribute to the state of delirium. Benzodiazepines reduce anxiety and sleeplessness; however, in the elderly, benzodiazepines can cause agitated delirium. Antipsychotics are effective in treating agitation, delusions, and hallucinations. Whatever medication is chosen, fixed doses are preferable to as-needed dosing. Patients should be monitored regularly for response and adverse effects.

REFERENCES

Brown TM, Boyle MF. Delirium. *BMJ.* 2002;325:644-647.

Meagher DS. Delirium: optimizing management. *BMJ.* 2001;322:144-149.

Meagher DS, O'Hanlon D, O'Mahony E, Casey PR. The use of environmental strategies and psychotropic medication in the management of delirium. *Br J Psychiatry.* 1996;168:512-515.

Chapter 32
Alzheimer Disease

Yuval Zabar

Clinical Vignette

A 66-year-old retired physicist with a history of coronary artery disease presented with progressive short-term memory problems during a 4-year period. During that time, he lost his ability to calculate his golf score. His wife had to handle the finances because he was unable to manage the bills and double-paid several times. He misplaced items at home and lost his wallet and credit cards on one occasion. He left cigarettes burning in various rooms. When his wife removed his cigarettes, he became agitated. His wife noted increasing sleeplessness and social withdrawal.

General physical examination was unremarkable. On mental status examination he registered 4 words readily. After a 10-minute delay he recalled none of them, even with verbal cues. He could not perform serial-7 calculations. He had difficulty copying the intersecting pentagon diagram of the Mini-Mental State Examination (MMSE). He could not name 3 of 6 items on the NIH stroke scale. He was disoriented with respect to date, day, and month. His MMSE score was 19 out of 30.

Brain MRI was "normal for age." During the next several years, the patient continued to decline mentally, requiring assistance with dressing and bathing. Mild parkinsonian features developed, but the patient had no falls. His speech became vague, and his comprehension was poor. Often he became agitated during assisted dressing or bathing. He was admitted to a nursing home 3 years before his death, with a total illness duration of approximately 14 years.

EPIDEMIOLOGY

The most common cause of dementia is Alzheimer disease (AD), accounting for approximately 4 million cases of dementia. Age-specific disease incidence increases exponentially with advancing age; the risk of development of AD doubles every 5 years, beginning at 65 years of age. AD affects approximately 50% of the population aged 85 years and older. Given the size of the aging population in developed countries, AD is predicted to increase fourfold through 2050.

Because dementia is a major factor in health care costs, morbidity, and mortality, the increased prevalence of AD places enormous burdens on caregivers and the health care system. Many cases are not identified until the dementia reaches an advanced stage, at which point caregiver stress is already high and treatment options are relatively limited.

The idea that dementia is a normal and inevitable consequence of aging is a long-believed myth. Moreover, diagnosis and management are often less than optimal because of the lack of recognition of the early disease stages by physicians and family members, the lack of good diagnostic screening procedures, and the fact that relatively few treatment options are available. Fewer than 50% of persons with dementia are officially diagnosed and even fewer take available medications correctly. Therefore, it is important to understand the natural history of AD, its impact on patients and primary caregivers, and the proper use of available treatment options.

PATHOGENESIS
Senile Plaques

Alzheimer disease is a neurodegenerative disorder resulting from inappropriate deposition of the protein **β amyloid** in the brain (Figure 32-1). β Amyloid is formed during processing of **amyloid precursor protein** (APP), a compound that may help regulate synaptic function and integrity, possibly by regulating excitotoxic activity of glutamate. APP is encoded on chromosome 21 and is processed at the cell membrane by secretase enzymes. Two known membrane-bound proteins called *presenilins* also contribute to APP processing: **presenilin 1** and **presenilin 2** are encoded on chromosomes 14 and 1, respectively.

β Amyloid is a short fragment of the APP protein, approximately 42 amino acids in length,

ALZHEIMER DISEASE

Figure 32-1　Amyloidogenesis in Alzheimer Disease

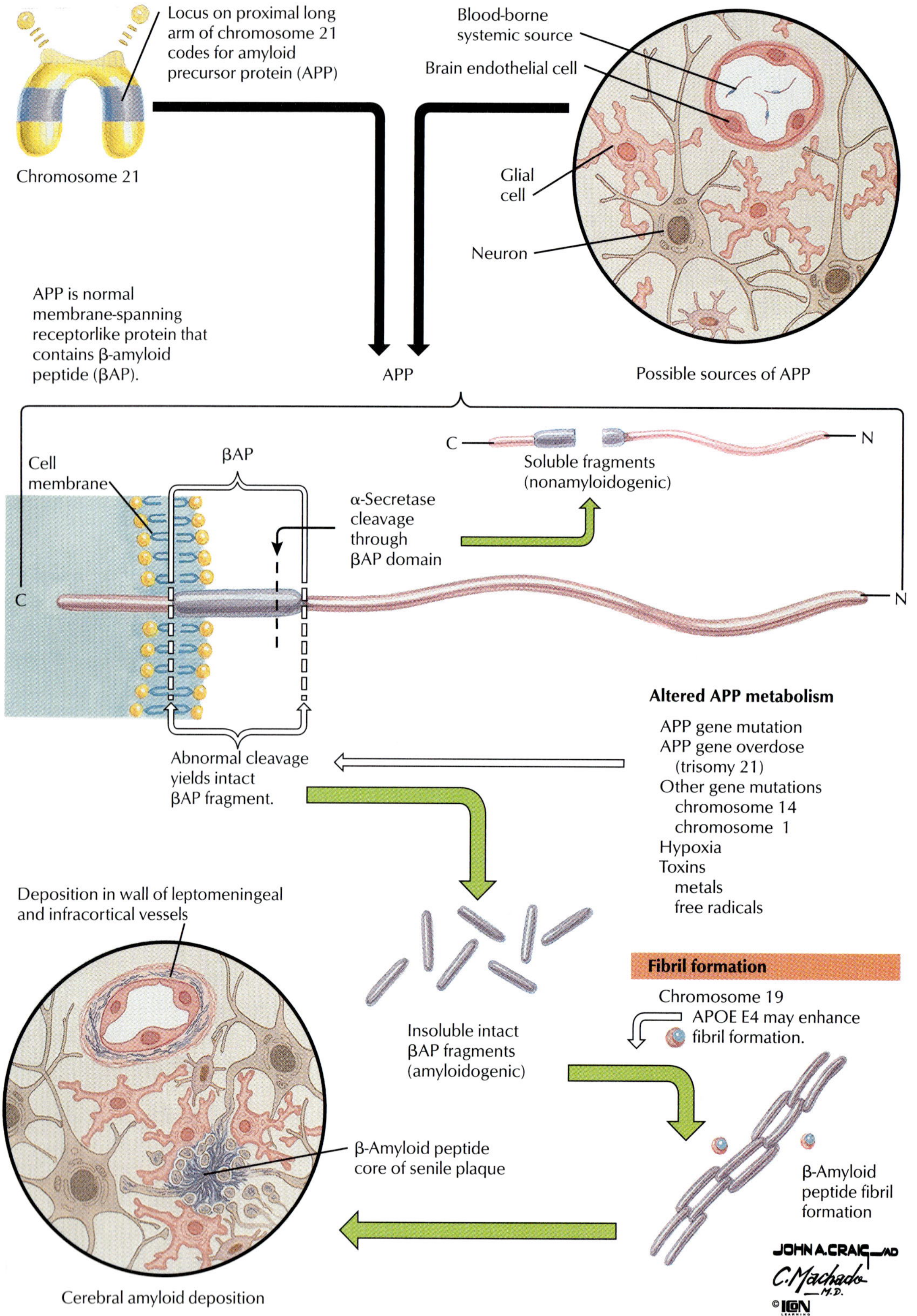

Locus on proximal long arm of chromosome 21 codes for amyloid precursor protein (APP)

Chromosome 21

Blood-borne systemic source

Brain endothelial cell

Glial cell

Neuron

Possible sources of APP

APP is normal membrane-spanning receptorlike protein that contains β-amyloid peptide (βAP).

APP

Cell membrane

βAP

α-Secretase cleavage through βAP domain

Soluble fragments (nonamyloidogenic)

Abnormal cleavage yields intact βAP fragment.

Altered APP metabolism

APP gene mutation
APP gene overdose (trisomy 21)
Other gene mutations
　chromosome 14
　chromosome 1
Hypoxia
Toxins
　metals
　free radicals

Deposition in wall of leptomeningeal and infracortical vessels

Insoluble intact βAP fragments (amyloidogenic)

Fibril formation

Chromosome 19
APOE E4 may enhance fibril formation.

β-Amyloid peptide core of senile plaque

β-Amyloid peptide fibril formation

Cerebral amyloid deposition

Memory and Cognitive Disorders

which accumulates outside the cell during APP processing. The tertiary structure of this fragment is a β-pleated sheet, which renders it insoluble. Consequently, it accumulates slowly, for many years, in the extracellular space. In vitro studies confirm that β amyloid is toxic to the surrounding synapses and neurons, causing synaptic membrane destruction and eventual cell death (Figure 32-2).

In vivo, β amyloid forms "diffuse" or immature plaques, best seen with silver-staining techniques. **Diffuse plaques**, however, are not sufficient to produce dementia; many normal elderly patients have notable brain deposition of diffuse plaques, a condition termed *pathological aging*. When these plaques mature into "senile" or neuritic plaques, dementia is more likely. **Senile plaques** consist of other substances in addition to β amyloid, including synaptic proteins, inflammatory proteins, neuritic threads, activated glial cells, and other components.

Unlike diffuse plaques, senile plaques are composed of a central core of β amyloid surrounded by a myriad of proteins and cellular debris. Senile plaques are distributed diffusely in the cortex, typically starting in the hippocampus and the basal forebrain (Figure 32-3). Gradually, the entire neocortex and subcortical gray matter become affected. Senile plaque formation correlates with increasing loss of synapses in widespread areas of the brain, which correlates with the earliest clinical sign, namely, short-term memory loss. The anatomic pattern of progression begins with the hippocampus, gradually involving neocortical and subcortical gray matter of the temporal, parietal, frontal, and, eventually, occipital cortex. Subcortical nuclei do not become involved until relatively late in the process.

Neurofibrillary Tangles

The second pathologic hallmark of AD is the **neurofibrillary tangle**. These lesions also develop and conform to an anatomical pattern that correlates with the clinical syndrome; the number and distribution of tangles is directly related to the severity of the dementia. Neurofibrillary tangles are formed intracellularly and consist of a microtubule-associated protein, **tau**, that has a vital role in the maintenance of neuronal cytoskeleton structure and function (Figure 32-4).

Tau is hyperphosphorylated in AD, causing it to dissociate from the cytoskeleton and form paired helical filaments. Consequently, the cytoskeletal structure is compromised and collapses. The most commonly used pathologic criteria for definitive AD diagnosis at autopsy require the presence of senile plaques and neurofibrillary tangles (Figures 32-5 and 32-6). Other lesions, such as **Hirano bodies**, are also seen in AD but have little diagnostic specificity.

As the basic pathologic process progresses, symptoms correlating with the specific regional pathology gradually evolve (Figures 32-7 and 32-8). For example, naming impairment occurs early, with dominant superior temporal involvement; this later progresses to more global aphasia as the dominant frontal and parietal lobes become involved. Parkinsonian syndrome develops concomitant with basal ganglia involvement.

In addition to neuronal loss, there is a gradual loss of various specific neurotransmitters. **Acetylcholine** is the earliest and most prominently affected of these vital biochemicals. Most acetylcholinergic neurons arise within the nucleus basalis of Meynert in the basal forebrain. This nucleus is affected relatively early in the process; acetylcholine levels within the brains and spinal fluid of patients with AD quickly decline with disease progression. This observation supported the cholinergic hypothesis—that acetylcholine depletion results in the cognitive decline observed in patients with AD—which led to the first limited success for treatment of AD.

RISK FACTORS

Epidemiologic studies have identified several potential risk factors for AD. The most consistent risk factors include advanced age, family history (especially in first-degree relatives), and ApoE genotype (Figure 32-9). Other risk factors include hypertension, stroke, and fasting homocysteine levels. Because vascular risk factors are modifiable, they may affect risk reduction and treatment for patients with AD and those at risk of development of AD.

Advanced age is the single most consistently identified risk factor for AD across numerous international studies. AD incidence and prevalence increase with advancing age, leading to

ALZHEIMER DISEASE

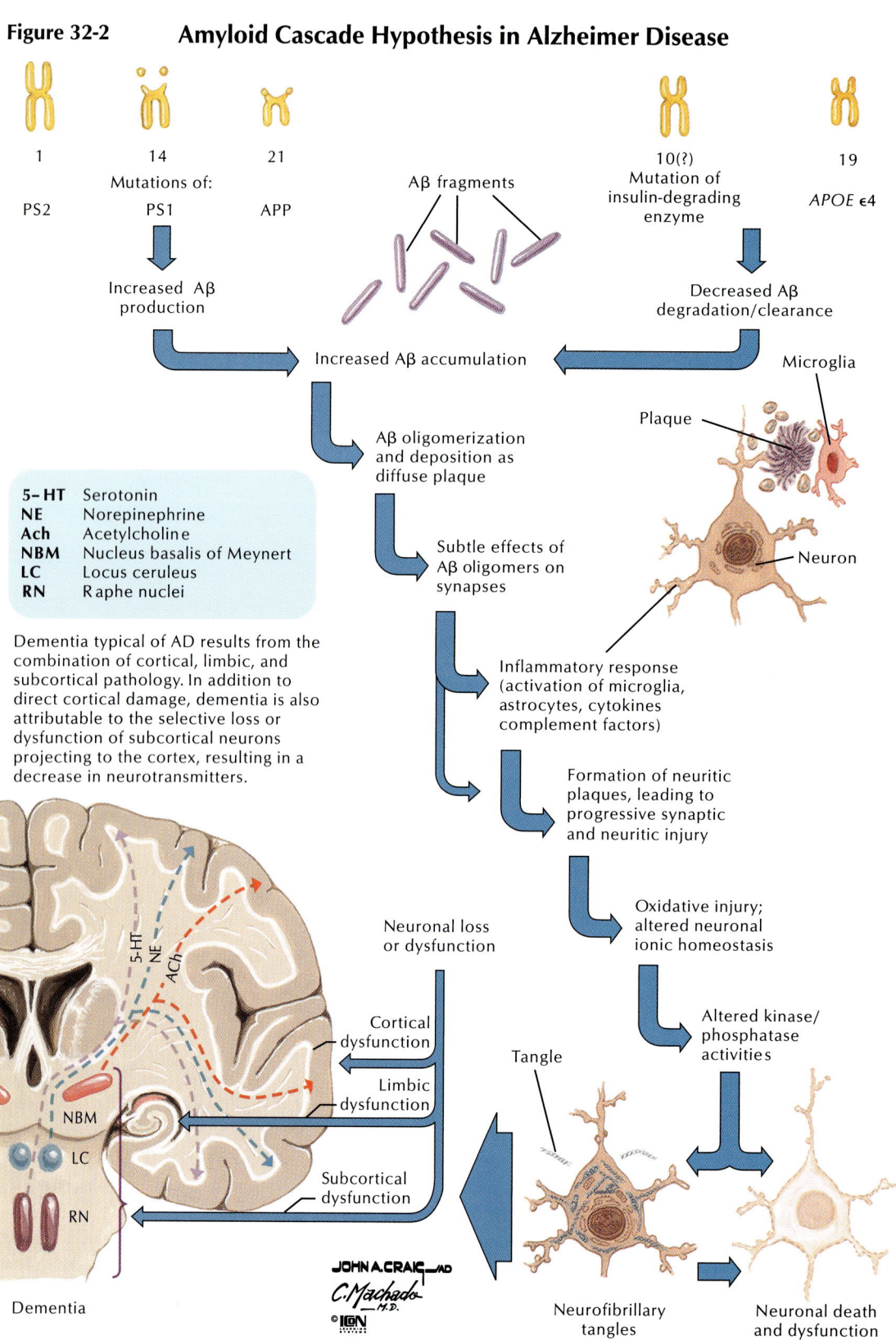

Figure 32-2 Amyloid Cascade Hypothesis in Alzheimer Disease

Memory and Cognitive Disorders

ALZHEIMER DISEASE

Figure 32-3   Distribution of Pathology in Alzheimer Disease

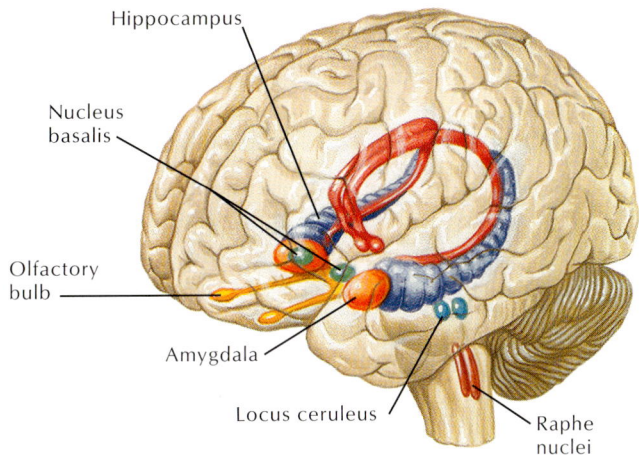

In neocortex, primary involvement of association areas (especially temporoparietal and frontal) with relative sparing of primary sensory cortices (except olfactory) and motor cortices

Pathologic involvement of limbic system and subcortical nuclei projecting to cortex

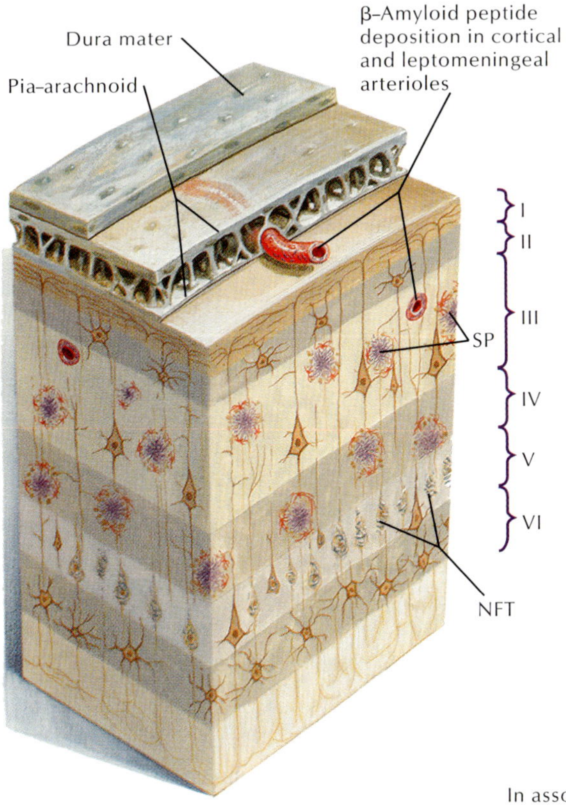

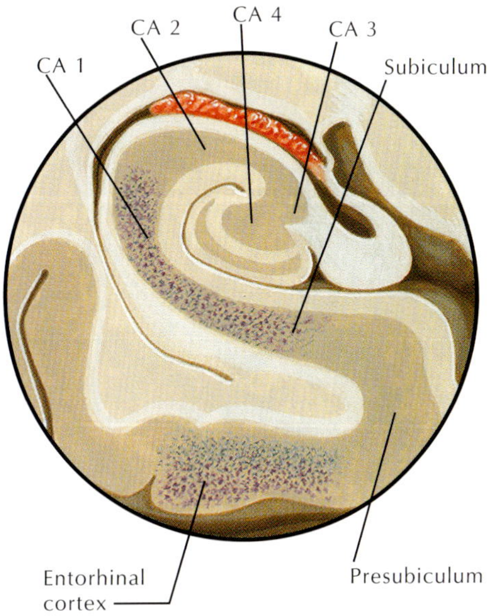

In hippocampus, neurofibrillary tangles, neuronal loss, and senile plaques primarily located in layer CA1, subiculum, and entorhinal cortex

In association cortex, neurofibrillary tangles (NFTs) and synaptic and neuronal loss predominate in layer V. Senile plaques (SPs) occur in more superficial layers.

MEMORY AND COGNITIVE DISORDERS

ALZHEIMER DISEASE

Figure 32-4   **Paired Helical Filaments (PHFs) in Alzheimer Disease**

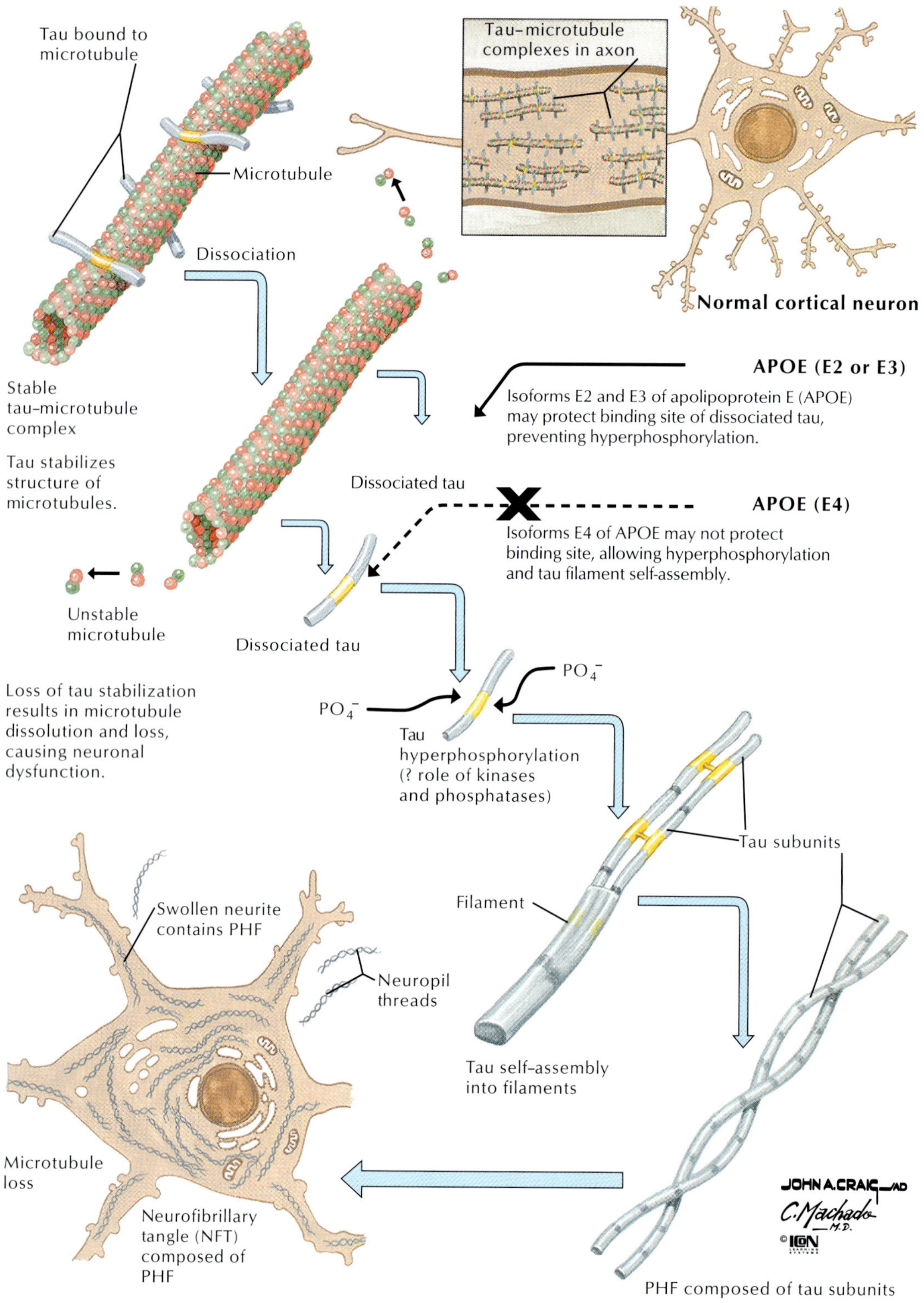

Tau bound to microtubule

Tau–microtubule complexes in axon

Microtubule

Dissociation

Normal cortical neuron

Stable tau–microtubule complex

Tau stabilizes structure of microtubules.

APOE (E2 or E3)
Isoforms E2 and E3 of apolipoprotein E (APOE) may protect binding site of dissociated tau, preventing hyperphosphorylation.

Dissociated tau

APOE (E4)
Isoforms E4 of APOE may not protect binding site, allowing hyperphosphorylation and tau filament self-assembly.

Unstable microtubule

Dissociated tau

Loss of tau stabilization results in microtubule dissolution and loss, causing neuronal dysfunction.

PO_4^- PO_4^-

Tau hyperphosphorylation (? role of kinases and phosphatases)

Tau subunits

Swollen neurite contains PHF

Neuropil threads

Filament

Tau self-assembly into filaments

Microtubule loss

Neurofibrillary tangle (NFT) composed of PHF

PHF composed of tau subunits

Cell body and neurites of neuron in Alzheimer disease

MEMORY AND COGNITIVE DISORDERS

ALZHEIMER DISEASE

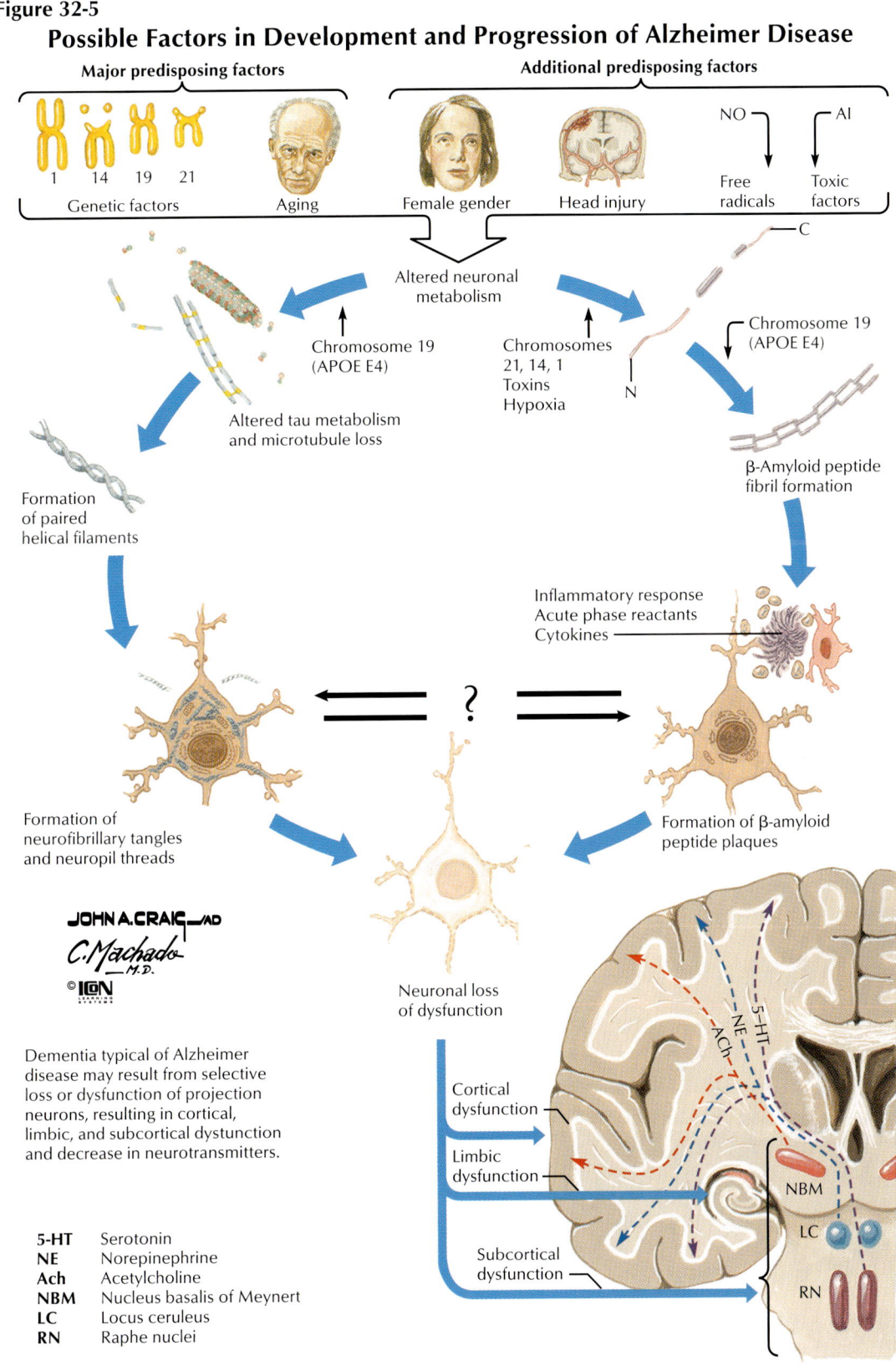

Figure 32-5
Possible Factors in Development and Progression of Alzheimer Disease

MEMORY AND COGNITIVE DISORDERS

ALZHEIMER DISEASE

Figure 32-6A Microscopic Pathology in Alzheimer Disease

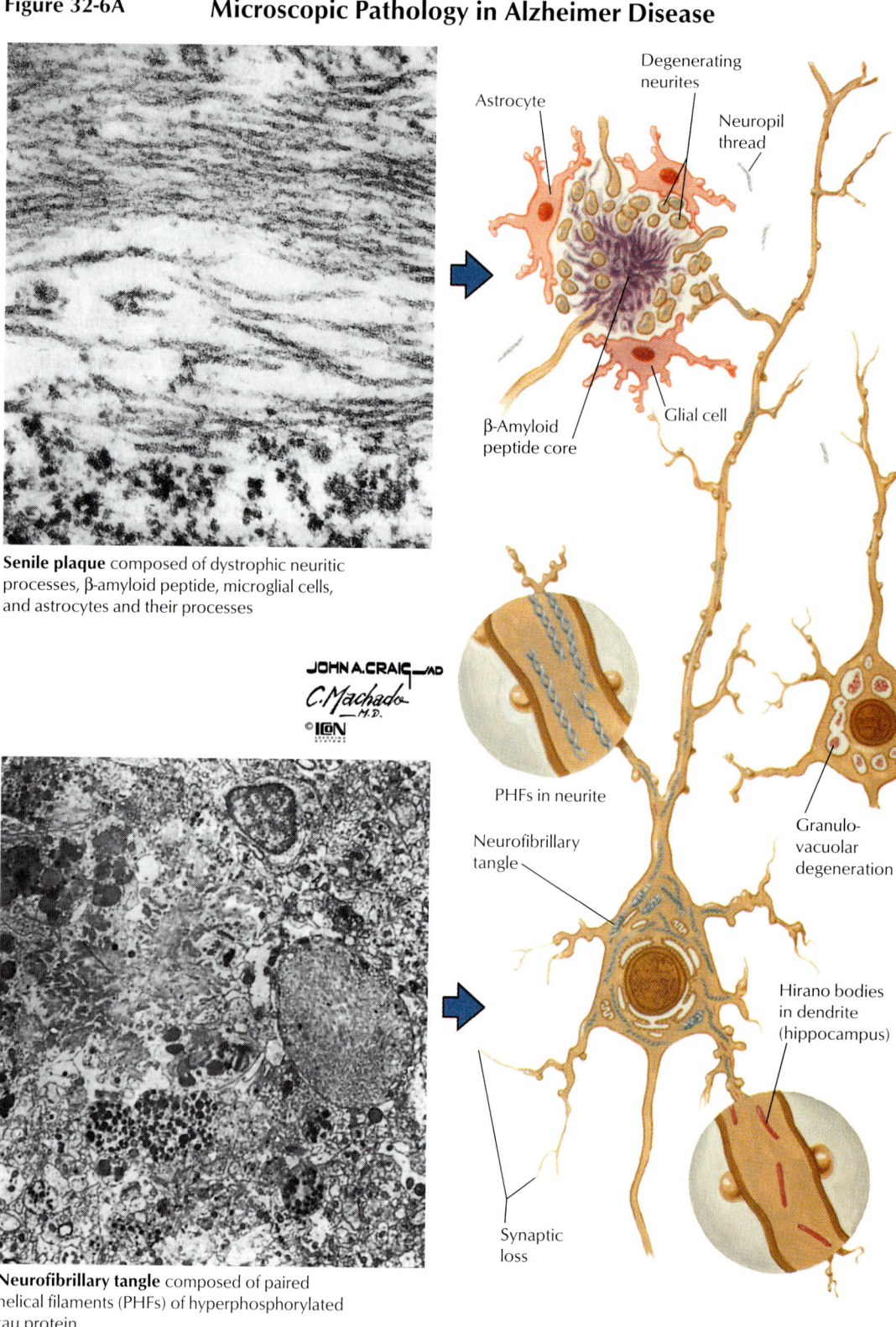

Senile plaque composed of dystrophic neuritic processes, β-amyloid peptide, microglial cells, and astrocytes and their processes

Neurofibrillary tangle composed of paired helical filaments (PHFs) of hyperphosphorylated tau protein

MEMORY AND COGNITIVE DISORDERS

ALZHEIMER DISEASE

Figure 32-6B   **Gross Pathology in Alzheimer Disease**

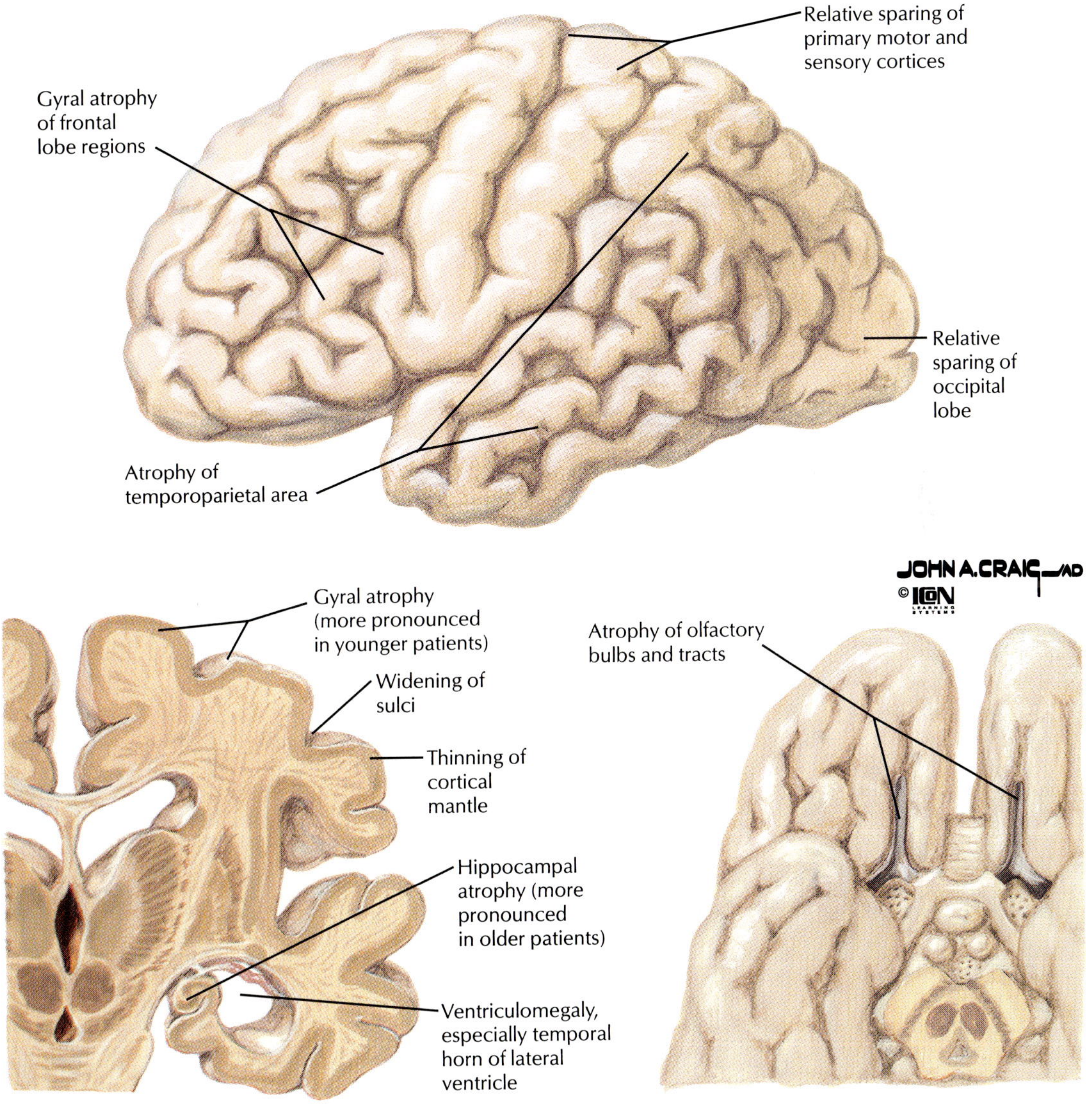

- Relative sparing of primary motor and sensory cortices
- Gyral atrophy of frontal lobe regions
- Relative sparing of occipital lobe
- Atrophy of temporoparietal area
- Gyral atrophy (more pronounced in younger patients)
- Widening of sulci
- Thinning of cortical mantle
- Atrophy of olfactory bulbs and tracts
- Hippocampal atrophy (more pronounced in older patients)
- Ventriculomegaly, especially temporal horn of lateral ventricle

the hypothesis that AD would develop in individuals who lived long enough. The true incidence in persons older than 85 years is difficult to ascertain because of this group's sharp increase in mortality. However, in many instances there is no pathologic evidence of AD at autopsy, including in persons older than 100 years.

Family history of AD is another consistent risk factor in many studies. However, the most common form of AD occurs sporadically. Establishing family history of and genetic predisposition for AD is difficult because the prevalence is greatest in persons older than 85 years. Many of these patients' relatives preceded them in death, preemptively terminating the clinical presentation of dementia.

Rare, early-onset, **presenile forms of AD** occur with an autosomal-dominant pattern of inheritance and account for less than 5% of cases worldwide. The genetic basis for many hereditary AD forms has been identified. Most mutations affect the genes that encode APP and the prese-

MEMORY AND COGNITIVE DISORDERS

ALZHEIMER DISEASE

Figure 32-7
Memory Circuits and Alzheimer Disease

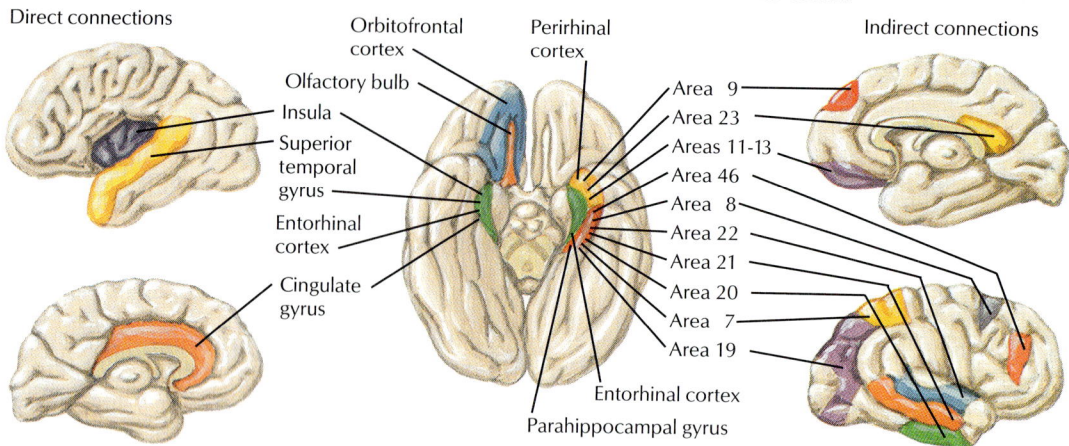

Entorhinal cortex is a major source of projections to hippocampus (major processing center for recent memory). Polysensory association cortices project directly to entorhinal cortex or indirectly via perirhinal cortex or parahippocampal gyrus. Association cortices receive reciprocal projections from entorhinal cortex.

Possible processing circuit for recent memory

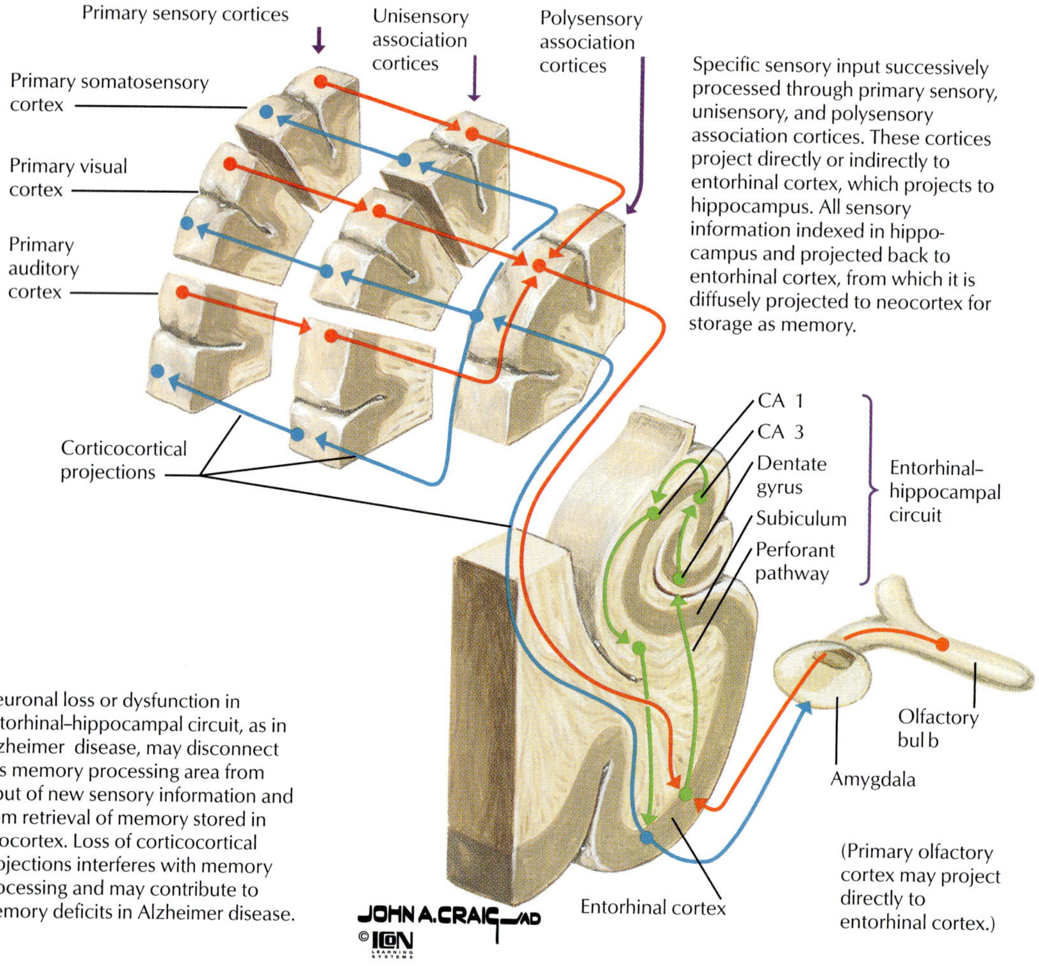

Specific sensory input successively processed through primary sensory, unisensory, and polysensory association cortices. These cortices project directly or indirectly to entorhinal cortex, which projects to hippocampus. All sensory information indexed in hippocampus and projected back to entorhinal cortex, from which it is diffusely projected to neocortex for storage as memory.

Neuronal loss or dysfunction in entorhinal–hippocampal circuit, as in Alzheimer disease, may disconnect this memory processing area from input of new sensory information and from retrieval of memory stored in neocortex. Loss of corticocortical projections interferes with memory processing and may contribute to memory deficits in Alzheimer disease.

ALZHEIMER DISEASE

Figure 32-8 Corticocortical and Subcorticocortical Projection Circuits

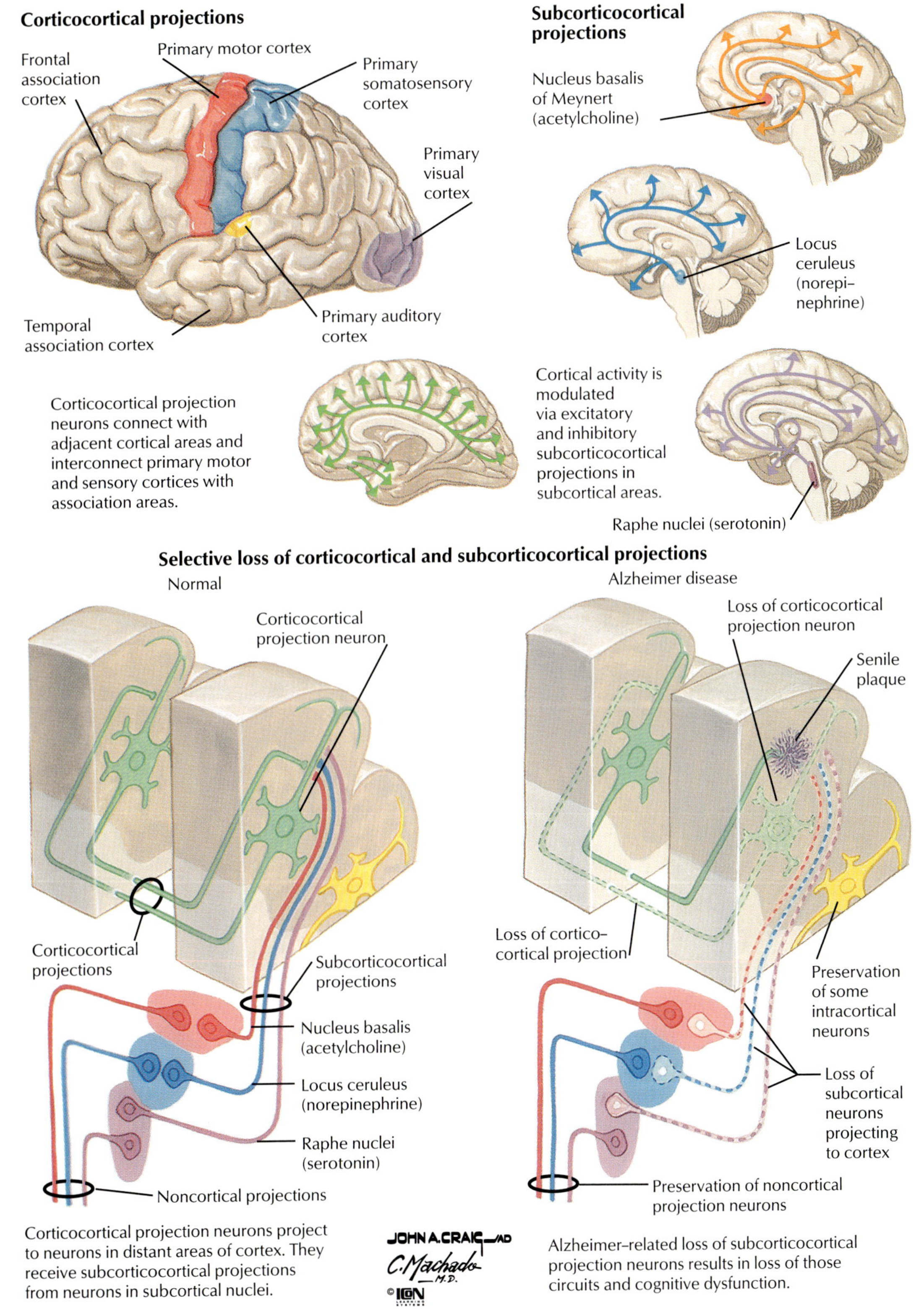

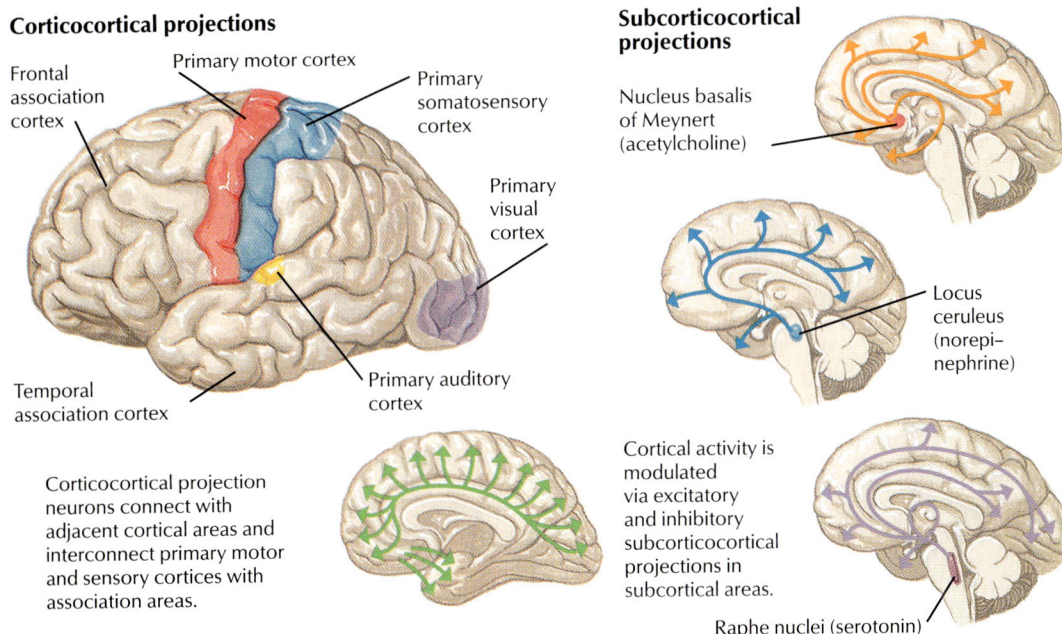

MEMORY AND COGNITIVE DISORDERS

Figure 32-9 **Risk Factors for Alzheimer Disease**

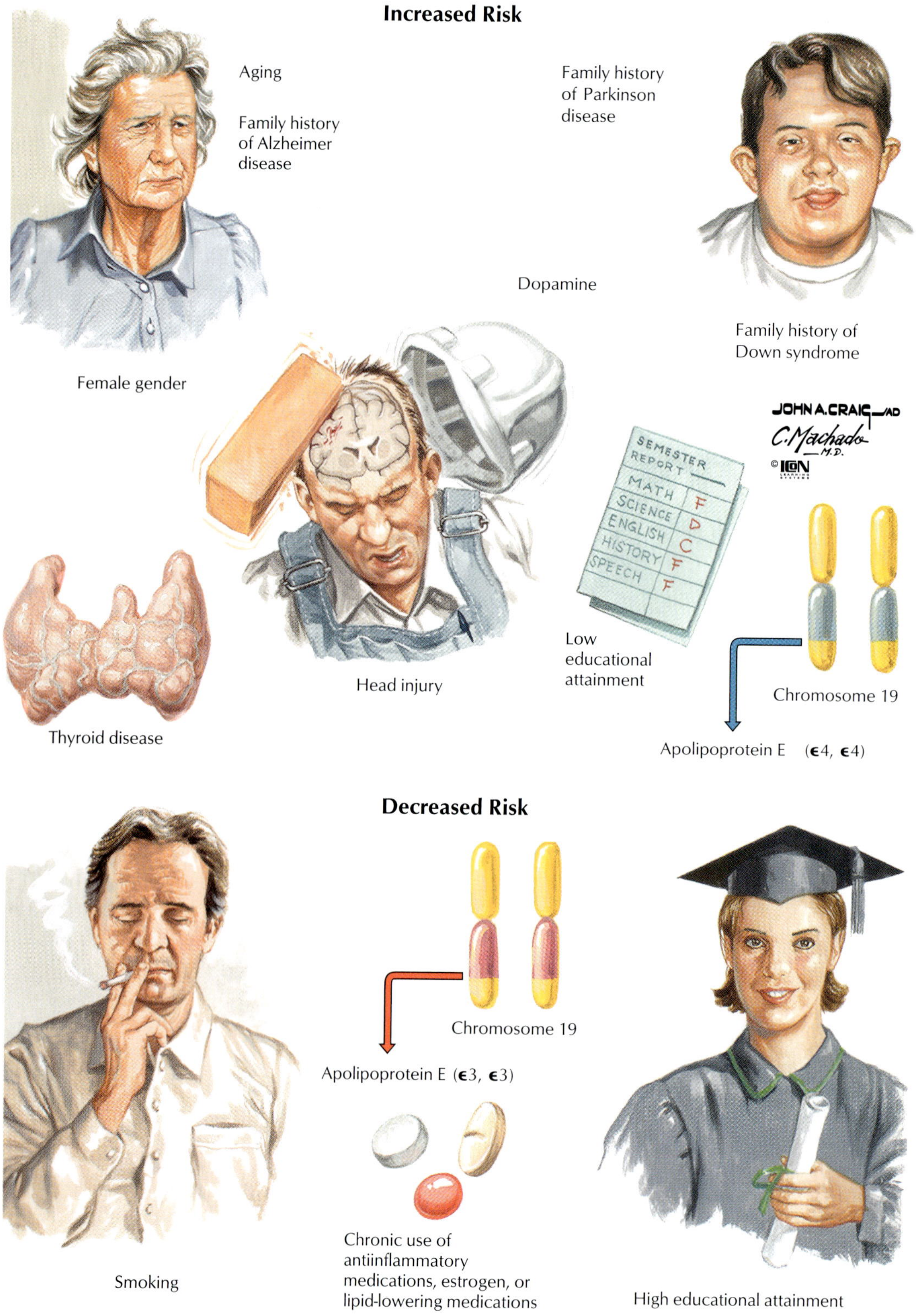
Increased Risk
Aging
Family history of Alzheimer disease
Female gender
Family history of Parkinson disease
Dopamine
Family history of Down syndrome
Head injury
Thyroid disease
SEMESTER REPORT
MATH F
SCIENCE D
ENGLISH C
HISTORY F
SPEECH F
Low educational attainment
Chromosome 19
Apolipoprotein E (ϵ4, ϵ4)
JOHN A.CRAIG AD
C.Machado M.D.
© ICON
Decreased Risk
Smoking
Chromosome 19
Apolipoprotein E (ϵ3, ϵ3)
Chronic use of antiinflammatory medications, estrogen, or lipid-lowering medications
High educational attainment

nilins. Each mutation leads to increased deposition of amyloid in affected individuals, predisposing to earlier onset. Individuals with **trisomy 21 (Down syndrome)** also have a high deposition of β amyloid. AD develops in all patients with Down syndrome by the age of 35 years.

Another genetic risk factor consistently identified for AD is the **ApoE genotype**. The 5 known allelic forms of this gene, epsilon 1 through 5, are encoded on chromosome 19. The most common ApoE allele in the gene pool is ApoE ε3, followed by ε4 and ε2; ε1 and ε5 are rare. The presence of an ε4 allele is associated with increased risk of AD and a younger age at onset. This risk is greatly increased in homozygotes. Conversely, the ε2 allele appears to impart a protective, risk-lowering effect, as replicated in numerous international, population-based studies. The association between the ApoE ε4 allele and AD seems to be disease specific. There is no clear association between ε4 and other neurodegenerative or amyloid-based diseases, with the possible exception of inclusion body myositis.

The mechanism underlying this increased risk associated with the Apo ε4 allele is not well understood but may relate to the role of ApoE in cell membrane repair. Phenotypically, the ε4 cases have greater amyloid deposition than do the non-ε4 cases. Although ApoE genotyping is available, it is not a diagnostic test for AD. Most patients with AD are non-ε4 carriers. ApoE genotyping is largely used in research, primarily as a biological marker to differentiate cases. Some studies suggest differential response to medications in cases grouped by ApoE genotypes.

CLINICAL PRESENTATION

The initial symptoms of AD are often subtle and the progression insidious (Figure 32-10). Given the preconceptions about aging, the earliest disease stages are commonly unheeded. Atypical presentations occur, but the typical case of AD begins with short-term memory loss. Often, patients have increasing forgetfulness of words and names, relying more on lists, calendars, and family members for reminders. Disorganization of appointments, bills, and medications becomes commonplace.

Family members often notice increasing repetitiveness, patients asking the same question or repeating the same conversation minutes after it was completed. Patients may forget to convey telephone messages or turn off the stove, or lose track of where they place things. Moreover, their ability to recall these incidents is impaired. They "forget that they forget." Affected individuals may become suspicious of others, and sometimes paranoid that they are being robbed of items they cannot find.

Language function gradually declines. Word-finding and name-finding difficulties are common initially. Naming impairment and gradual loss of comprehension, expression, or both are universal. Perception of temporal-events sequence is affected and disorientation eventually becomes pervasive. Geographic orientation declines, first affecting patients' ability to navigate in unfamiliar environments and later within their homes. Visuospatial skills decline and constructional apraxia occurs early. In the early stages, patients maintain their social graces. It is not uncommon when evaluating patients to discover they are good at concealing their deficits. Seasoned geriatricians can be fooled by the charms of "very pleasant" patients.

Demeanor in patients with AD is not always preserved. Agitation, combativeness, irritability, frustration, and anxiety become extremely common. Many patients seek medical attention only when family members are alarmed by behavioral changes, rather than because of their earlier progressive memory loss. Psychotic features may become prominent. Some patients also develop delusional thoughts and hallucinations, most commonly visual or auditory in nature. These may be benign, understated, hidden, or frightening, and may lead to severe agitation.

As cognitive and behavioral changes appear, patients' ability to maintain independent life declines. Altered activities that may occur early include medication mismanagement, financial disorganization, burnt pots on the stove, and driving errors. Eventually patients require assistance with activities of daily living: personal hygiene/bathing, eating, dressing, and toileting. Often, by this stage, patients exhibit signs of parkinsonism characterized by midline rigidity, symmetric bradykinesia and hypokinesia, stooped posture, and shuffling stride. The risk of falling increases. Seizures occur in up to 20% of

ALZHEIMER DISEASE

Figure 32-10 Alzheimer Disease: Clinical Manifestations, Progressive Phases

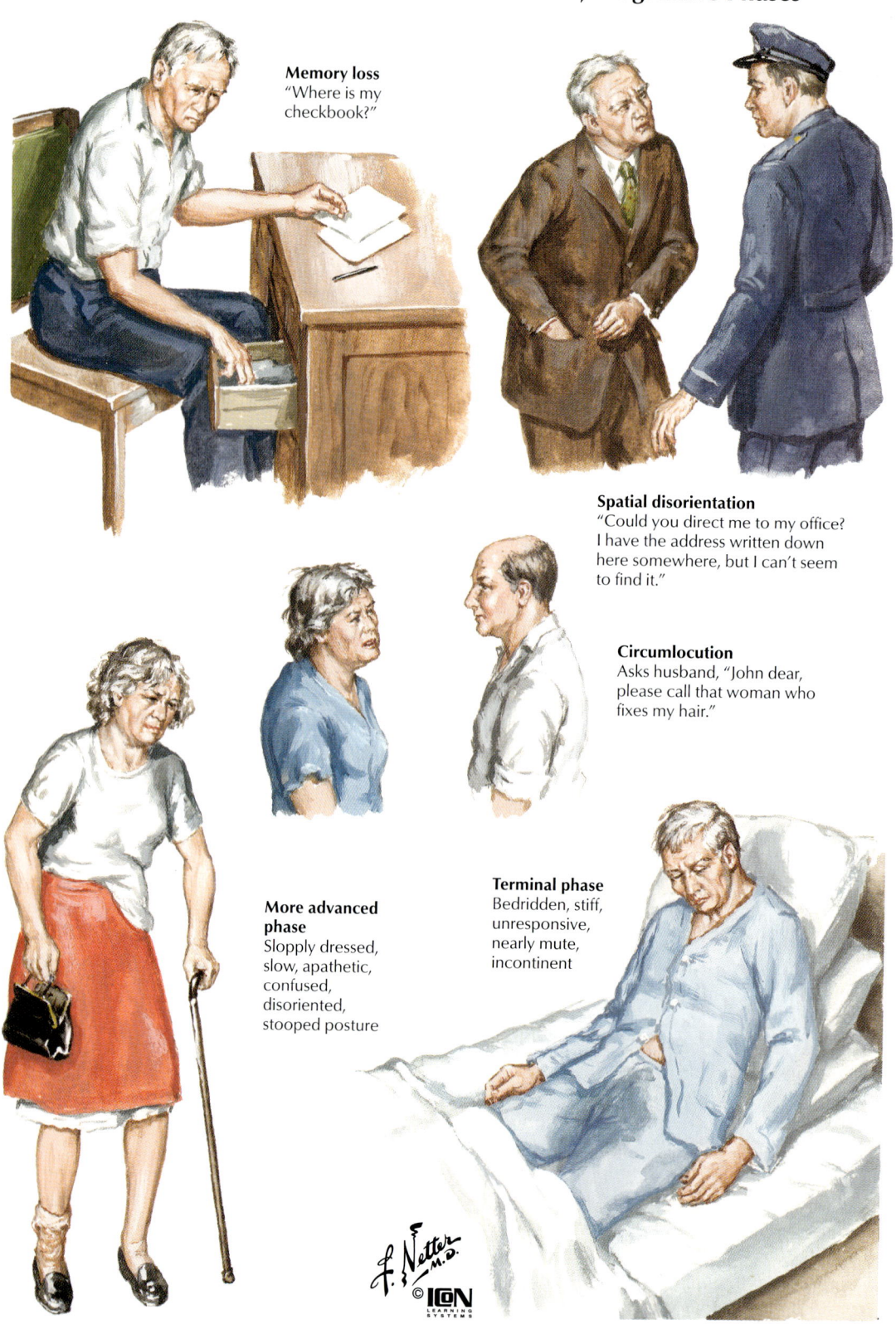

cases. Myoclonic jerks are increasingly noted in advanced stages.

Later stages of AD are characterized by loss of bladder and then bowel control, failure to recognize family members, and eventually severe akinesia, requiring total nursing care. The most common cause of death is aspiration pneumonia. On average, AD has a duration of approximately 8 years. However, this varies substantially. Some patients live 20 years or more. Nursing care marks an important end point for many patients and their caregivers. The most common causes for nursing home placement are behavioral problems, immobility, and incontinence.

DIFFERENTIAL DIAGNOSIS

The absence of motor deficits in AD differentiates it from most other dementias. Dementias without motor signs are rare and include amnestic syndrome (Korsakoff encephalopathy), Pick disease, vascular dementia, and HIV dementia complex. Depression can also produce dementia-like symptoms without motor deficits. Poor concentration and short-term memory impairment result from lack of effort, disinterest, or distractibility. "Pseudodementia" due to depression is usually not progressive, and functional loss is disproportionately severe relative to cognitive impairment.

Dementia with motor deficits is far more complex. Thyroid disease, vitamin B_{12} deficiency, and tertiary neurosyphilis are common considerations; however, these conditions usually present with characteristic sensorimotor symptoms. The presence of spastic hemiparesis or dysarthria increases suspicion of cerebrovascular disease. Parkinsonism is associated with Parkinson disease and dementia with Lewy bodies. Progressive ataxia occurs with multisystem atrophy. Chorea characterizes Huntington disease.

As AD progresses, parkinsonism becomes evident, making clinical differentiation of AD from dementia with Lewy bodies and other parkinsonian diseases more difficult. AD may also coexist with cerebrovascular or Lewy body pathology to produce dementia with motor signs.

Reversible causes of dementia without motor signs include toxic and metabolic causes of chronic delirium. Always consider chronic use of medication with anticholinergic side effects (eg, antihistamines and tricyclic antidepressants) as a possible cause of chronic delirium. β Blockers, digoxin, H_2 blockers, and various antibiotics may also contribute to chronic delirium. A detailed history and mental status examination are usually sufficient to differentiate chronic delirium from AD.

DIAGNOSTIC APPROACH
Mental Status Evaluation

Diagnosis of AD is sometimes challenging. There are no specific diagnostic tests, no adequate screening tests, nor any biologic AD markers. The subjective complaint of memory impairment is not a useful screening device because it is common in elderly individuals. Prospective studies of individuals aged 65 years who have complaints of memory loss show that dementia actually develops in fewer than 9% during a 5-year follow-up. However, dementia develops during a 5-year follow-up in 50% of patients aged 85 years who have no complaints of memory loss and are followed prospectively.

Consequently, clinicians must be proactive, particularly with patients aged 85 years or older, when assessing cognitive function. Patients may show telltale signs that raise suspicion of memory problems, including the "vague" historian, medication noncompliance, or looking to family members to answer questions in clinic. In the earliest stages, a history of functional loss may not be present; however, a profound memory deficit may exist without other significant cognitive deficits. This clinical presentation is designated *mild cognitive impairment* to differentiate it from dementia but to designate patients at high risk of development of dementia. The majority of patients with mild cognitive impairment meet the diagnostic criteria for dementia during a 5-year follow-up. Such patients require full neurologic evaluation; if it is unrevealing, these individuals require at least an annual follow-up evaluation to ascertain whether their condition is progressing.

Investigation of patients with possible dementia requires a detailed history, preferably provided by a trustworthy, knowledgeable informant. The history should describe the cognitive decline, in temporal sequence, from earliest suggestion of cognitive impairment to most recent events. Examination in early stages may reveal no neurologic deficits other than cognitive impairment. In later stages, or in patients with coexisting neuropathology, such as stroke, there may be motor deficits or other focal CNS findings on physical examination.

The mental status examination should comprehensively assess all major cognitive domains, including attention, orientation, language, memory, construction, praxis, and executive function. Standardized global measures of cognitive function, such as the MMSE, are of limited diagnostic value. The widely used MMSE is relatively insensitive to the milder stages of AD. Moreover, the MMSE depends significantly upon language ability and education level.

Impaired encoding of information, poor naming, construction impairment, and disorientation characterize memory loss in AD. The inability to encode information is identified when patients cannot recall information even with practice and when given hints or cues. The examiner may test this by presenting patients with a list of 4 unconnected words to memorize. Patients should be given ample opportunity to memorize the list, by repetition or use of cues, to assure registration of all items. Patients are asked to repeat the words after a delay of 7 to 10 minutes. If a patient cannot recall all of the items spontaneously, cues should be given to facilitate word retrieval. Cues include semantic and phonemic word descriptors; for example, "a color beginning with the letter p" could be a cue for the word *pink*. Encoding deficits exist when practice and cues do not improve delayed recall. Additional early cognitive deficits in AD include dysnomia, reduced verbal fluency (especially in word categories), orientation to time, and constructional dyspraxia.

Having the patient list as many things belonging to a category within 1 minute provides a test of verbal fluency. For example, patients are asked to list animals or words beginning with the letter *s*. Well-established norms stratified by age and education level determine abnormal performance.

Clock drawing is useful when testing construction and executive function. Patients are asked to draw a clock indicating 3:25 on a blank sheet of paper. Their performance is observed from beginning to end, including the circle shape and size, number placement, hand size placement, and so forth. The strategy (or its absence) used by patients when they attempt to draw the clock manifests itself readily and executive function can be assessed. When patients finish, they are asked to copy a clock that the examiner draws in front of them. The numbers 12, 6, 3, and 9 are placed first, and the hands drawn accurately. If construction problems exist, patients have difficulty with the copy task and probably also with the prompted task. If the copy is good, construction problems may not be a factor in cognitive impairment. Standardized scoring strategies of clock drawing enable long-term follow-up.

The 7-Minute Screen is another relatively brief cognitive tool useful for assessing patients with possible AD. It includes relatively brief, standardized tests for orientation, memory, verbal fluency, and clock drawing. These tools may provide a more sensitive means of screening for Alzheimer-type dementia than does the MMSE. When bedside tests are suggestive of AD, formal neuropsychologic testing may characterize cognitive impairment more precisely and thus improve diagnostic accuracy. Annual follow-up mental status examination testing is also useful in assessing disease progression. It is not helpful to repeat such assessments too frequently. Practice effects and fluctuations in performance on different days may result in premature medication changes.

Systemic Studies

There is no standard test panel to diagnose AD. Traditionally, levels of vitamin B_{12}, folate, TSH, and often serum RPR are measured. These tests may reveal a reversible cause of dementia and point away from a diagnosis of AD. Blood tests help determine whether metabolic or toxic processes causing chronic delirium are present.

Apolipoprotein E genotyping is not diagnostic of AD. Moreover, ApoE genotyping should not be used routinely in family members because there is no specific genetic counseling to offer. The presence of an ApoE ϵ4 genotype may only heighten anxiety unnecessarily. Fasting homocysteine levels have been linked to increased risk of AD. The effect of decreasing homocysteine on the disease course of patients diagnosed with AD is unknown. However, premorbid reduction of homocysteine levels potentially decreases the risk of development of AD.

Cerebrospinal fluid analyses for tau, β amyloid, APP, and neuritic thread proteins have shown some promise as potential diagnostic tools. However, these assays are expensive and may not improve diagnostic accuracy beyond that determined by a detailed history, physical examination, and formal neuropsychologic testing.

Imaging studies are often used to assess the presence and extent of cerebrovascular disease. Numerous autopsy series showing coexistence of stroke and AD and data linking AD with stroke risk factors mandate the use of imaging in diagnosing patients with dementia. Brain MRI, CT, or both are also important tests for excluding other potentially treatable structural brain lesions, including brain tumors and subdural hematomas. The choice between CT and MRI remains mostly discretionary, although research suggests that MRI is superior to CT in revealing "silent" infarction and small-vessel ischemic changes in white matter. Moreover, MRI may be useful in quantifying selective loss of volume, such as in the hippocampus, as an early sign of AD.

Other imaging modalities, such as PET and SPECT, have limited diagnostic value. Both demonstrate biparietal abnormalities in patients with AD. PET scanning is sensitive and shows biparietal, hypometabolic abnormalities premorbidly in patients at risk, such as in premorbid hereditary AD cases and homozygous ApoE β4 carriers. Specific labels for β-amyloid with PET imaging have emerged as another sensitive way to detect AD. However, PET scans are expensive, relatively inaccessible to most of the population and general practitioners, and primarily research tools. The utility of SPECT is questionable. SPECT may show biparietal hypoperfusion in association with AD, but it is not sensitive enough nor specific enough to be used routinely in the diagnosis of AD.

EEG may demonstrate slowing of background activity with an increased percentage of θ and sometimes even δ frequencies, especially in temporal and parietal regions; however, this tends to occur later in AD. In early stages, patients with AD have normal EEGs. Brain biopsy is not used in diagnosis, primarily because a normal biopsy may result from selection bias if the excision occurs in a cortical segment unaffected by disease. There is no substitute for a careful history, mental status examination, and neurologic examination, supplemented by neuropsychologic testing.

TREATMENT

Pharmacologic treatment of AD is only symptomatic, with more specific therapy currently unavailable (Figure 32-11). Cholinesterase inhibitors—donepezil, rivastigmine, and galantamine—reduce the decline on standardized tests better than placebo when used for 6 to 12 months, but do not slow the degenerative disease. Consequently, if medications are stopped, patients are likely to experience a precipitous decline to the severity level that they would have reached without the medication. In such cases, restarting the medication may not regain the lost ground. In addition, these medications are primarily effective at maximal doses.

Gradual titration of doses to maximal levels is required to achieve the reported results. Rivastigmine is most effective at 4.5 or 6 mg twice daily. Donepezil is effective at 5 mg/d, but maximum benefit occurs with 10 mg/d. Similarly, galantamine should always be titrated to 12 mg twice daily to maximize benefit. If patients do not tolerate these drugs at lower doses, it is prudent to try a different agent. It is unusual for patients not to tolerate all 3 drugs. Typical adverse effects that may cause discontinuation include cholinergic effects, including vomiting and persistent loose stools.

Long-term benefits of these medications may include a delay in need for nursing home placement. For example, using donepezil for 9 to 12 months may delay nursing home placement by approximately 20 months. However, functional decline continues and reasonable specific expectations for the effects of these medications must be emphasized to patients and their families. These treatments are associated with reduced behavioral problems and may reduce the need for sedatives in some patients. Determination of medication efficacy is challenging. When the maximum dosage is reached, annual follow-up examination is beneficial.

ALZHEIMER DISEASE

Figure 32-11

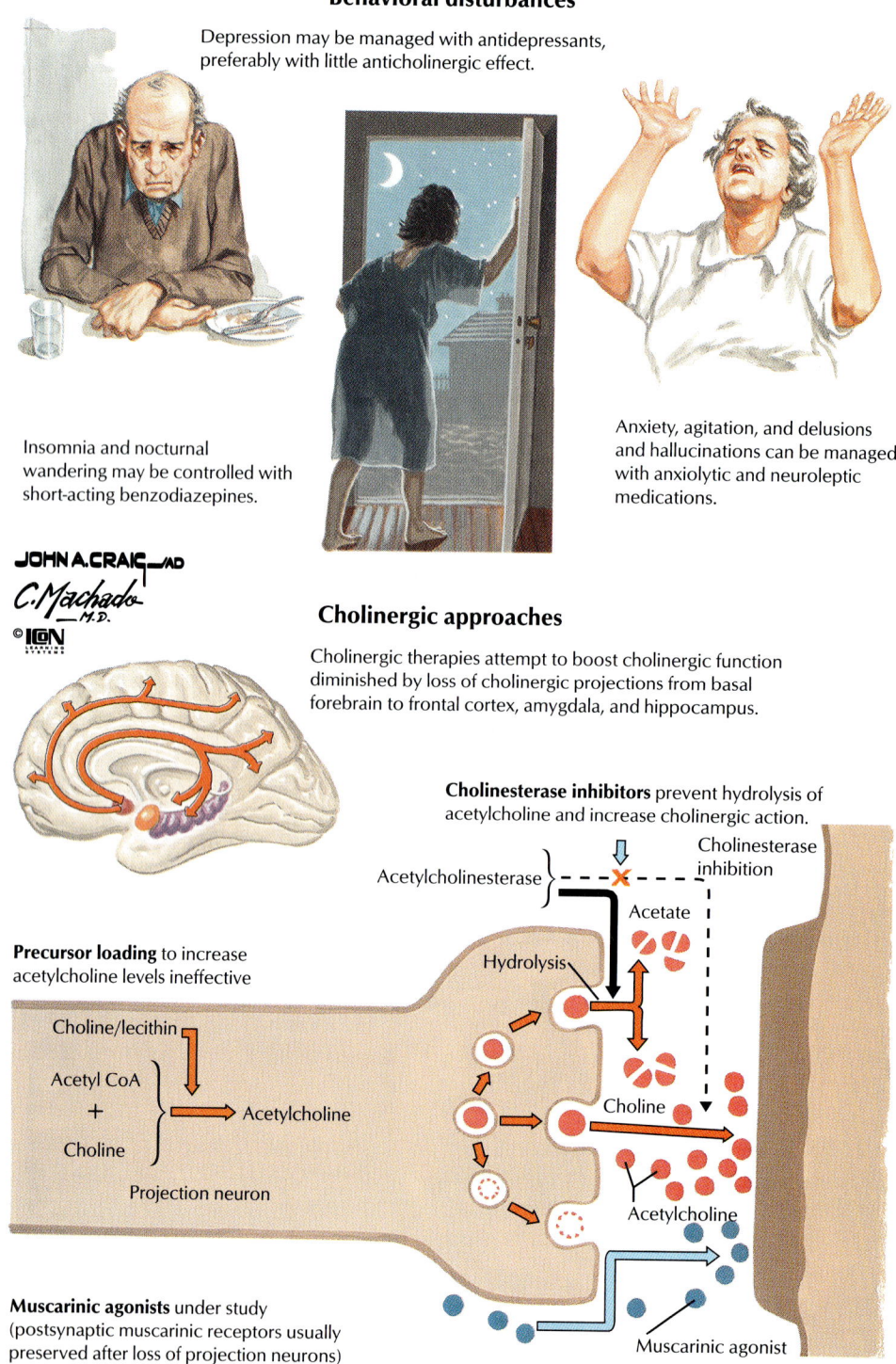

Pharmacologic Management Options in Alzheimer Disease
Behavioral disturbances

Depression may be managed with antidepressants, preferably with little anticholinergic effect.

Insomnia and nocturnal wandering may be controlled with short-acting benzodiazepines.

Anxiety, agitation, and delusions and hallucinations can be managed with anxiolytic and neuroleptic medications.

Cholinergic approaches

Cholinergic therapies attempt to boost cholinergic function diminished by loss of cholinergic projections from basal forebrain to frontal cortex, amygdala, and hippocampus.

Cholinesterase inhibitors prevent hydrolysis of acetylcholine and increase cholinergic action.

Precursor loading to increase acetylcholine levels ineffective

Muscarinic agonists under study (postsynaptic muscarinic receptors usually preserved after loss of projection neurons)

Figure 32-12

Daily Living Assessment and Nonpharmacologic Management

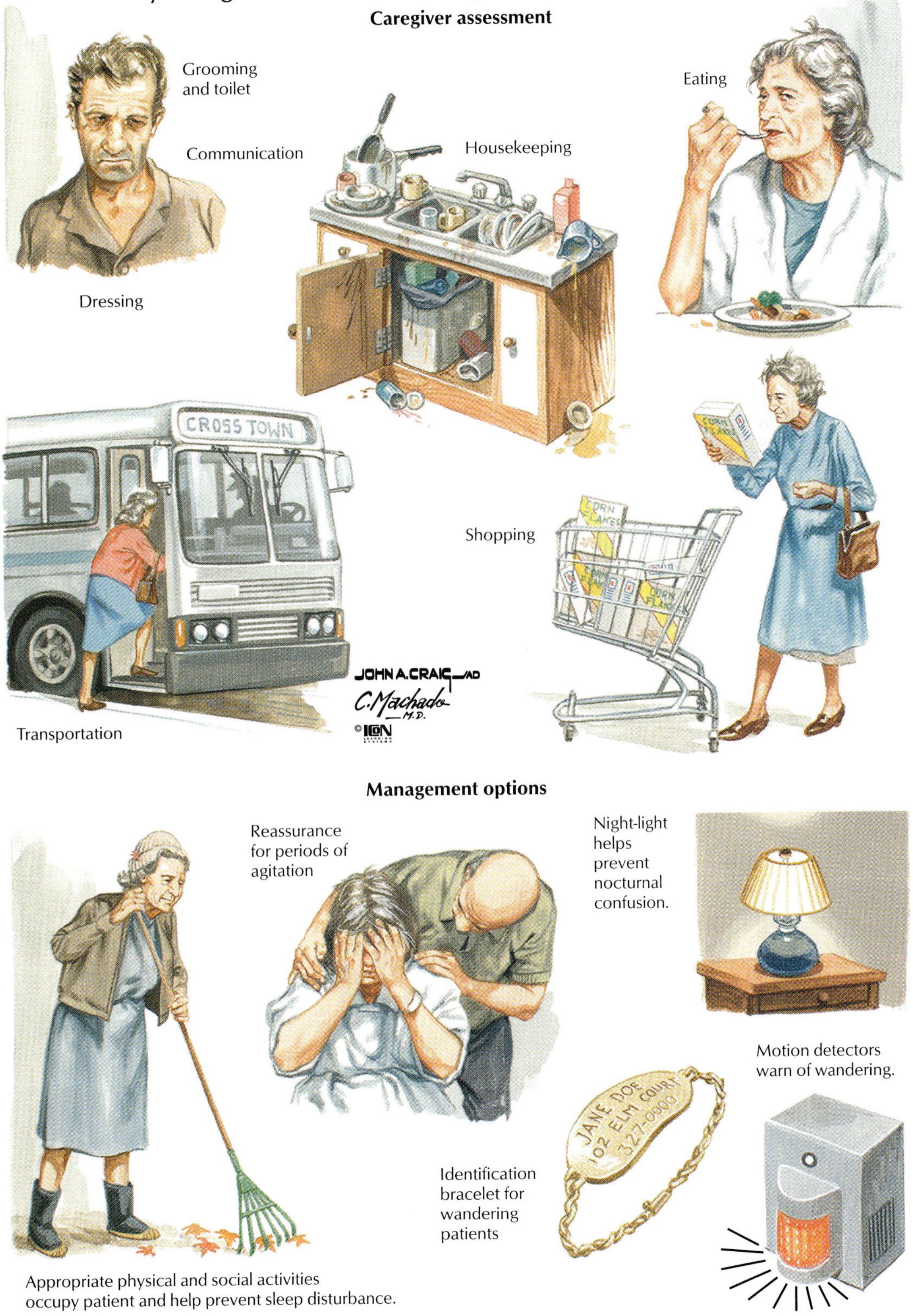

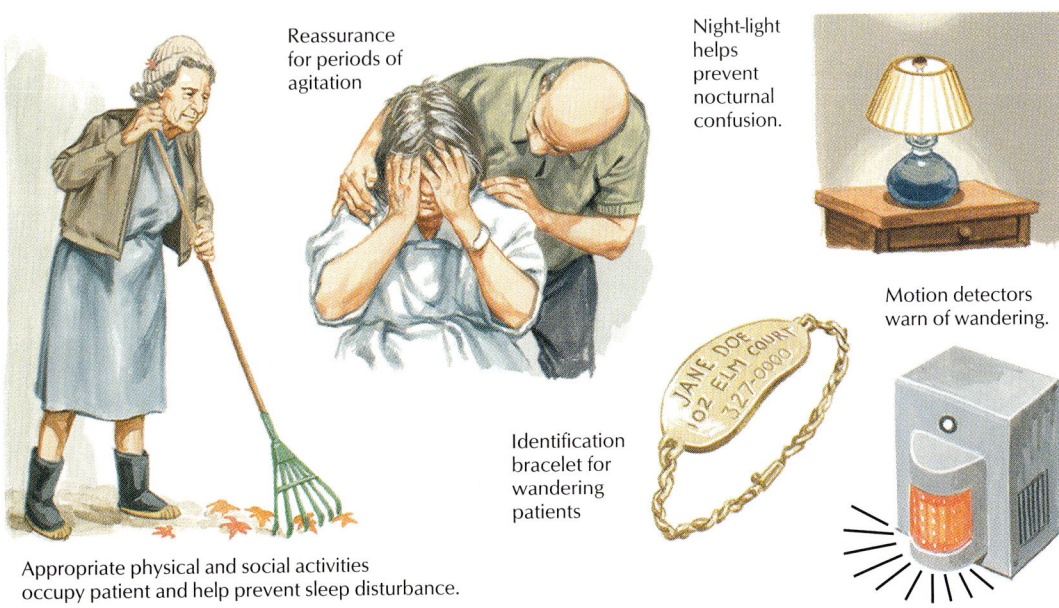

Repeated standardized mental status examinations are helpful. For example, the average rate of decline on the MMSE in AD is approximately 3 points per year. When a patient shows less than 3 points of decline, the medication may be helping. This method approximates the same measurements used in clinical trials of AD to assess medication efficacy. Such tests, in combination with the caregivers' subjective impressions, can help determine whether to continue or change medications.

Memantine, an *N*-methyl-D-aspartate receptor antagonist, is approved for use in patients with moderate to severe AD. This drug may slow disease progression, given its mode of action, and shows promise in combination with cholinesterase inhibitors.

Counseling should focus initially on safety issues: supervision of medications, finances, driving, and fire hazards. Patients often disregard recommendations to stop driving; sometimes disabling the car is the only means to discontinue a dangerous activity. Most patients are reluctant to relinquish control of these activities, leading to frustration and arguments among family members. It is important to identify these concerns as early as possible and to repeat discussion of them at follow-up visits.

Establishing power of attorney and health care proxy status should also be addressed as early as possible. Caregivers need support group referral and appropriate literature to become familiar with the disease. Placement issues should also be discussed before a crisis occurs. Often families can avoid crisis situations by anticipating needs (Figure 32-12). Patients requiring more supervision should be referred to daycare centers to reduce caregiver burden and to provide a nurturing, social environment. Most will balk at the idea, but most enjoy these centers after they arrive and become familiar with them. Those patients who are easily lost or wander should be registered with the AD Association's Safe Return program (phone number: 888-572-8566).

Nursing home placement is often a complicated and dread-filled concept. By investigating nursing homes early and choosing the most appealing facility in advance, many families and patients make the transition relatively smoothly. Some people choose to care for their loved one at home throughout the illness. This is possible, provided the patient is attended to safely and appropriately. Many services for older persons are available to assist patients who are receiving care at home.

REFERENCES

American College of Medical Genetics/American Society of Human Genetics Working Group on ApoE and Alzheimer disease. Statement on use of apolipoprotein E testing for Alzheimer disease. *JAMA*. 1995;274:1627-1629.

Blacker D, Tanzi RE. The genetics of Alzheimer disease: current status and future prospects. *Arch Neurol*. 1998;55:294-296.

Clark CM. Clinical manifestations and diagnostic evaluation of patients with Alzheimer's disease. In: Clark CM, Trojanowski JQ. *Neurodegenerative Dementias*. New York, NY: McGraw-Hill; 2000:95-114.

Clark CM, Karlawish JH. Alzheimer disease: current concepts and emerging diagnostic and therapeutic strategies. *Ann Intern Med*. 2003;138:400-410.

Joachim CL, Selkoe DJ. The seminal role of beta-amyloid in the pathogenesis of Alzheimer disease. *Alzheimer Dis Assoc Disord* 1992;6:7-34.

Seshadri S, Beiser A, Selhub J, et al. Plasma homocysteine as a risk factor for dementia and Alzheimer's disease. *N Engl J Med*. 2002;346:476-483.

Small GW, Rabins PV, Barry PP, et al. Diagnosis and treatment of Alzheimer disease and related disorders: consensus statement of the American Association for Geriatric Psychiatry, the Alzheimer's Association, and the American Geriatrics Society. *JAMA*. 1997;278:1363-1371.

Chapter 33
Dementia With Lewy Bodies

Yuval Zabar

Clinical Vignette

A 72-year-old retired engineer became acutely confused and disoriented. Symptoms resolved as mysteriously as they started. Over the next 3 years, he gradually became depressed and socially withdrawn and had progressive short-term memory impairment and repetitiveness. During this time, he would occasionally have visual hallucinations associated with periodic confusional states. His gait deteriorated, and he developed postural instability with retropulsion and stooping. There was no response to a trial of carbidopa/levodopa (Sinemet).

Examination was notable for symmetric parkinsonian features, masked facial expression, and postural tremor in his hands. Mental status examination revealed profound impairment in delayed recall, with no benefit from cues or practice trials.

Brain MRI demonstrated atrophy; EEG showed diffuse slowing. Trials of various SSRI agents, H2 blockers for reflux, and neuroleptics caused delirium. The patient continued this downward, fluctuating course until his death in a nursing home 7 years later.

Dementia is a recognized clinical manifestation of Parkinson disease (PD) and other parkinsonian syndromes, particularly multiple system atrophy. The pathologic substrate of dementia in these disorders includes the hallmark histopathology of Alzheimer disease (AD) and possibly cerebrovascular disease. However, careful observation at autopsy and advances in staining techniques, including immunohistochemistry, suggest that another pathologic lesion commonly occurs. Lewy bodies (LBs), originally described at the turn of the 20th century, also occur in widespread areas of the cortex and other subcortical nuclei in many cases of parkinsonism with dementia. Neurodegenerative changes with LB formation were first linked with dementia in the 1960s.

Early case descriptions noted LBs distributed diffusely within the cerebral cortex and brainstem and were termed *diffuse Lewy body disease*. Subsequent neuropathologic studies found a surprisingly high frequency of LB pathology in the brains of patients with AD. These cases showed coexisting lesions characteristic of AD and LBs and were classified *Lewy body variant of AD*. In general, "variant" cases showed relatively less AD pathology than pure AD cases matched for clinical dementia severity. Reports of *Lewy neuritis* located in the CA2 region of the hippocampus suggest that dementia with Lewy bodies (DLB) is a unique neurodegenerative cause of dementia distinct from AD. However, LBs are also found in the brains of patients with hereditary AD, suggesting a possible pathophysiologic link between these diseases. Few familial cases of DLB are described, and there are no known mutations associated with hereditary DLB.

A definitive diagnosis of DLB requires only the presence of cortical LB pathology, regardless of coexisting AD pathology. Many of these cases also fulfill pathologic criteria for a definitive diagnosis of AD. Consequently, controversy surrounds this diagnosis, and no agreement exists on a single disease classification of cases with mixed LB and AD pathology. Dementia autopsy series show DLB as the second most common cause of elderly dementia after AD. Clinical epidemiologic studies are pending.

PATHOGENESIS

Lewy bodies are intracytoplasmic inclusion bodies and hallmark histopathologic lesions of PD. They occur within neurons of the substantia nigra and other brainstem nuclei in PD cases. Spherical shape and eosinophilic staining properties characterize LBs morphologically. The center stains densely, and a pale halo surrounds

DEMENTIA WITH LEWY BODIES

it. In cases of PD with dementia, LBs occur in cortical neurons and other nonbrainstem locations. Cortical LBs are characterized by irregular shapes and do not have the characteristic pale halo seen with PD.

Hence, cortical LBs can easily be missed when routine neuropathologic staining techniques are used. Moreover, LBs do not stain with silver-based stains often used to identify neuropathologic lesions in AD. A synaptic protein called a *synuclein* is the major LB component. Specific immunohistochemical stains for a synuclein greatly improve LB detection throughout the brain. Ubiquitin staining also detects these lesions well. The function of a synuclein is not completely understood. It may have a role in presynaptic, nerve-terminal vesicular function. Mutations in the a synuclein gene produce a mixed phenotype within members of affected kindred. Symptoms are predominantly PD-like, with cases of dementia occurring less frequently.

CLINICAL PRESENTATION AND DIFFERENTIAL DIAGNOSIS

Clinical manifestations of DLB include cognitive decline, behavioral change, and motor dysfunction. The most crucial component for this clinical diagnosis is dementia, although the initial manifestations of DLB may be characteristic motor or behavioral impairment.

A critical clinical feature of DLB is **fluctuating mental status**, which may be dramatic, ranging from relatively lucid to severe confusion. Episode duration and frequency vary greatly, lasting minutes, days, or weeks. Awareness and arousal levels may vary and include periodic somnolence and unresponsiveness. Transient neurologic symptoms (ie, dysarthria, dizziness, or unexplained falls) may occur. Such episodes may suggest complex partial seizures, delirium, or TIAs. Although patients with AD have "good and bad days," the fluctuations of patients with DLB are more pronounced. Clinical assessments

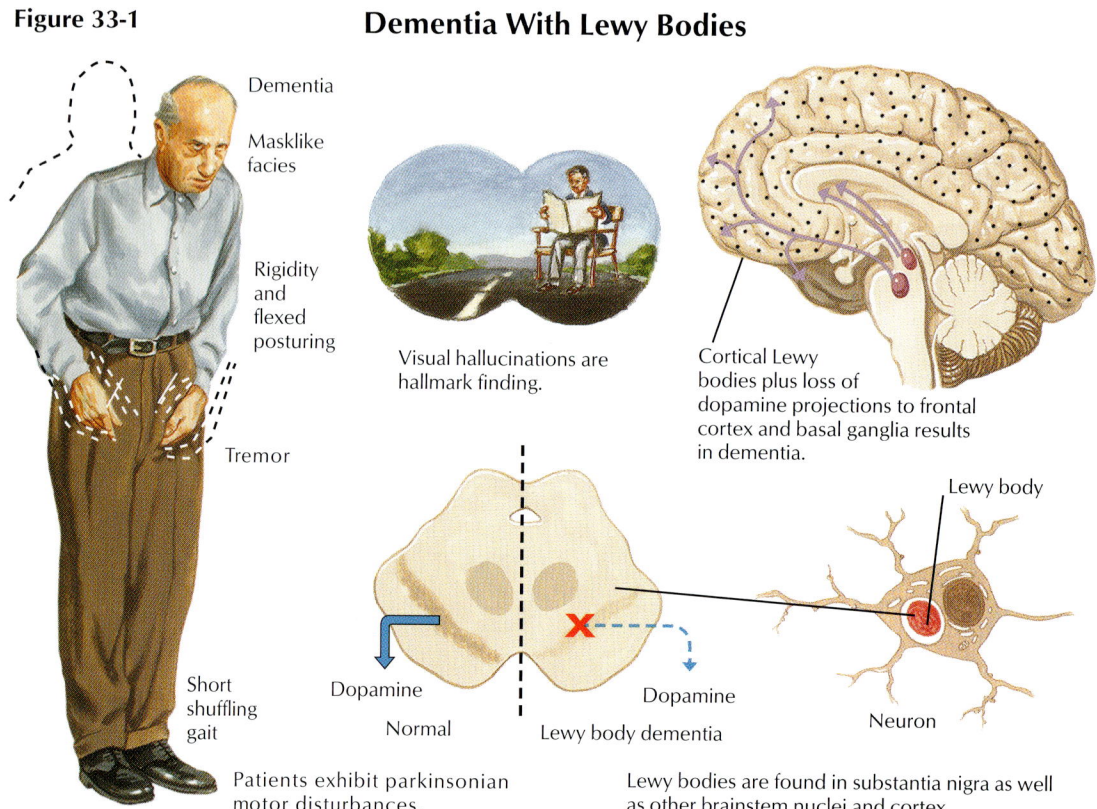

Figure 33-1 **Dementia With Lewy Bodies**

may vary significantly from visit to visit. Caregivers often become stressed by the unpredictability of symptoms.

The **cognitive impairment** in DLB can be **similar to that in AD**, although there are some **important differences**. The memory loss in DLB tends to be less severe than in AD, and retrieval deficits are more pronounced than encoding deficits. Therefore, patients with DLB have a **greater problem retrieving previously learned information** and show a greater benefit with cueing than do patients with AD.

In AD, encoding difficulty predominates, and consequently, patients do not benefit as much from practice or from cueing. In DLB, visuospatial and construction skills may be impaired earlier than in AD. Patients with DLB may present with geographic disorientation in familiar neighborhoods or even in their own homes while their memory is mildly impaired. Executive function is also impaired significantly earlier in DLB than in AD, manifested as impaired problem solving, inability to complete tasks, and marked disorganization of daily activities. Formal neuropsychological tests help to differentiate AD from DLB, particularly in early disease stages.

Prominent psychotic features, including hallucinations and delusions, also develop in patients with DLB (Figure 33-1), although such symptoms are not typically seen early in the disease course. In DLB, psychosis can be an early and severely disabling feature, sometimes heralding the onset of dementia. **Recurrent vivid and detailed visual hallucinations** are particularly prevalent in DLB. The emotional response to these hallucinations ranges from relative indifference to severe agitation and combativeness. Agitation typically occurs when the patient has little insight or the hallucinations are perceived as threatening. Hallucinations in other senses also occur but are less specific for DLB. **Delusions** are frequently **bizarre**, **complex**, and unrelated to cognitive impairment. In contrast, delusions in patients with AD often occur from misinterpretation secondary to forgetfulness. For example, patients with AD may accuse people of stealing when they cannot find things they misplaced. Other behavioral problems such as depression and anxiety also occur frequently but are not unique to DLB (Table 33-1).

Motor signs include all the typical features of PD. However, in DLB **bradykinesia and rigidity** are more **characteristic**, whereas tremor is relatively uncommon. **Signs** tend to be **distributed** more **symmetrically** and axially than they are in PD. Unexplained falls occur early and often in patients with DLB, unlike postural instability in PD, which tends to mark more advanced dis-

Table 33-1
Comparison of DLB and AD Manifestations*

Manifestation	DLB	AD
Memory loss	Less pronounced, poor retrieval	Characteristic, poor encoding
Visuospatial and construction skills	Severely impaired early	Mildly impaired early
Executive function	Impaired earlier	Impaired later
Fluctuating mental status	Pronounced	Less pronounced
Psychotic features	Can be prominent early	Not typical early
Delusions	Bizarre, unrelated to impaired cognitive function	Often related to memory loss
Depression and anxiety	Common	Common
Parkinsonism	Within 1 to 2 years of dementia	Later in disease course

*AD indicates Alzheimer disease; DLB, dementia with Lewy bodies.

ease. Response to dopaminergic medications is limited or absent in DLB, although they may exacerbate hallucinations. Parkinsonism is also seen in advanced AD and in frontotemporal dementia. If parkinsonism occurs within 1 to 2 years of dementia, either before or after the onset of cognitive decline, DLB should be considered in the differential diagnosis.

DIAGNOSTIC APPROACH

The workup for DLB is similar to that for AD. Formal neuropsychological tests can be useful early in the course to differentiate DLB from AD or other dementing illnesses. There are no specific findings on blood tests or spinal fluid analysis. Brain MRI and CT do not reveal any specific abnormalities. Volumetric MRI studies suggest there is relative sparing of hippocampal volumes in DLB cases. EEG shows nonspecific abnormalities, including focal or diffuse brain wave slowing. PET imaging may be helpful in the future, particularly in highlighting affected dopaminergic systems.

TREATMENT

Cholinergic CNS deficits occur in DLB as they do in AD. Some studies suggest that DLB is associated with greater cholinergic deficit than is AD. In theory, cholinesterase inhibitors—donepezil, rivastigmine, and galantamine—should be effective, and small, controlled clinical trials show that these medications have a favorable effect on cognitive outcome measures in DLB. The benefit duration is not known but may be similar to that in AD. Cholinesterase inhibitors offer only symptomatic benefits, having no known effect on the degenerative process. Drug discontinuation results in decline to the level of cognitive impairment congruent with pathologic burden at any given disease stage. These drugs may reduce the extent and severity of cognitive fluctuations and behavioral problems.

When psychotic features are disabling, use of atypical neuroleptic agents is common, based on their proven efficacy in cases of PD with psychotic features. Efficacy of these drugs for DLB has not been studied in controlled clinical trials. Atypical neuroleptics produce fewer extrapyramidal adverse effects than "typical" neuroleptics, an important consideration in DLB.

However, patients with DLB often exhibit sensitivity to various centrally acting drugs, most prominently to neuroleptic medications, and may become completely incapacitated by severe akinesia, dystonia, or delirium. The incidence of neuroleptic malignant syndrome in DLB is unknown. Good clinical judgment and conservative dosing strategies should be used in every case. The treatment of psychotic features in DLB is arguably the most challenging management aspect. Neuroleptic medication should be avoided if possible. Often, psychotic symptoms distress caregivers more than patients, but this should not prompt initiation of such medications. Treatment of motor symptoms is based largely on anecdotal reports. Dopaminergic drugs may be tried with caution in selected cases; however, psychosis may be exacerbated, and efficacy is often minimal.

As in AD, caregiver counseling about the disease course and realistic treatment expectations is paramount for successful monitoring, intervention, and improved quality of life. The most common causes for nursing home placement in the demented population include psychosis with behavioral problems and parkinsonism. Patients with DLB are therefore at high risk for early nursing home placement. As in AD, use of cholinesterase inhibitors may help to delay nursing home placement.

REFERENCES

Leverenz JB, McKeith IG. Dementia with Lewy bodies. *Med Clin North Am.* 2002;86:519-535.

Luis CA, Mittenberg W, Gass CS, Duara R. Diffuse Lewy body disease: clinical, pathological, and neuropsychological review. *Neuropsychol Rev.* 1999;9:137-150.

McKeith IG. Dementia with Lewy bodies. *Br J Psychiatry.* 2002;180:144-147.

McKeith IG, Perry EK, Perry RH. Report of the second dementia with Lewy body international workshop: diagnosis and treatment. Consortium on Dementia with Lewy Bodies. *Neurology.* 1999;53:902-905.

McKeith IG. Spectrum of Parkinson's disease, Parkinson's dementia, and Lewy body dementia. *Neurol Clin.* 2000;18:865-902.

Chapter 34
Frontotemporal Dementia

Yuval Zabar

Clinical Vignette

A 55-year-old man, premorbidly described by family as "thoughtful, accomplished, and intelligent," began neglecting his home and work responsibilities over a 2-year period. He became increasingly inflexible and uncaring. At work he missed several deadlines, and clients complained that he "forgot" about them. Consequently, he stopped working. He became more impulsive, driving late at night without reason. He obsessively checked his furnace numerous times each day and night, unconcerned about this safety risk.

His wife became increasingly tearful and anxious, whereas he seemed unaware of her turmoil and his change in personality. The patient's personal hygiene declined; he stopped shaving and dressed sloppily. At social functions, he interrupted conversations, touched people inappropriately, and spoke in a tasteless and loud fashion, often embarrassing his wife. Despite these changes, he continued to garden and perform other favored activities, albeit with less attention to detail.

Examination results revealed a malodorous and unshaven man with disheveled clothes. He spoke out of turn and was repetitive, stating, "I have to go." At times he attempted to leave the examination room but returned with gentle coaxing. His affect was otherwise flat. He gave concrete, terse responses to questions, mostly affirmative, negative, or stating, "I don't know." Naming was impaired. He followed some simple commands, but more complex sequences were incomplete or disorganized. His memory was relatively intact, although retrieval of relatives' names was impaired. He listed only 5 animals in 1 minute, a significant impairment given his postgraduate education level. Other than motor impersistence and a mild rooting reflex bilaterally, the results of the neurologic examination were relatively unremarkable. Over the next 2 years, the patient became increasingly withdrawn, spoke less, and required prompting for virtually every activity.

Brain MRI showed atrophy of the frontal lobes, affecting the left side slightly more than the right. Blood work, CSF studies, and EEG results were unremarkable.

This vignette exemplifies evolving dementia related to a degenerative process primarily confined to the frontal and temporal lobes. A previously accomplished individual initially demonstrated signs of intellectual decline, diminished sense of responsibility, and loss of social graces manifested by a disinhibited personality. More than a century ago, Arnold Pick originally described behavioral and personality changes associated with frontotemporal atrophy. He subsequently described progressive aphasia and progressive apraxia syndromes on the basis of focal lobar atrophy. Around the same time, Alois Alzheimer described the histopathology of so-called **Pick disease**.

The pathologic changes of **Pick disease** were later found in other clinically dissimilar disease processes, including **corticobasal degeneration** (chapter 48), **motor neuron disease (MND)–type dementia**, **primary progressive aphasia (PPA)**, and **dementia lacking distinctive histology**. Subcortical regions are often affected, characterized by extrapyramidal features, including akinesia and rigidity. In other cases, similar pathologic features appear in cortical regions other than the frontal or temporal lobes. For example, in PPA, parietal cortical involvement predominates, with pathologic changes correlating with clinical features. The term **frontotemporal dementia** (FTD) does not account for the spectrum linking pathology and clinical phenomenology. As the disease progresses, lobar degeneration occurs, often asymmetrically and bilaterally. The term **Pick complex** has been suggested instead of *FTD* to provide a more inclusive diagnostic entity that defines the pathologic and clinical features of these diseases inclusively.

PATHOGENESIS

The pathology of FTD is characterized by gliosis, neuronal loss, and spongiform degeneration in the superficial layers of the frontal and temporal neocortex. The formation of Pick bodies and Pick cells occurs in less than 25% of cases. **Pick bodies** are round, argyrophilic intracytoplasmic inclusions, easily detected by most silver-staining techniques and mildly eosinophilic on standard hematoxylin and eosin staining. Cortical Pick bodies form in small neurons; they are pathognomonic for Pick disease when they occur in the dentate gyrus. **Pick cells** are large, ballooned neurons that affect superficial cortical cells. In many cases, evidence exists of complement and microglial activation, suggesting that inflammatory mechanisms may play a role in pathogenesis. However, this pathologic profile is not unique to FTD. Various syndromes arise, depending on the precise neurodegeneration distribution. In Pick disease, degeneration is restricted to frontal and temporal lobes, producing a characteristic "knife-edge" atrophy of sulci.

A positive labeling for **pathologic tau protein** within neuronal inclusions, astrocytes, and oligodendrocytes is another common thread in the pathogenesis of these disorders, termed **tauopathies**. However, some cases demonstrate no significant tau labeling, and some investigators suggest a deficiency of tau in those cases. **Tau** is involved in the pathogenesis of Alzheimer disease. However, the mechanism by which tau is affected in Alzheimer disease and Pick disease differs. A range of mechanisms may transform tau, determining the final pathologic and clinical picture.

CLINICAL PRESENTATION

Frontotemporal dementia/Pick disease accounts for approximately 15% to 20% of all degenerative dementias. The typical age of onset is broad, ranging from 21 to 75 years, usually affecting persons aged 45 to 60 years. Men and women are equally affected. The median illness duration is 8 years, although this ranges from 2 to 20 years. Family history is present in more than 50% of cases.

The distinguishing clinical features of FTD are striking behavioral and personality changes (Figure 34-1). Most patients are unaware of their problem. There is often a major breakdown in social behavior, personal hygiene, and affect. Mental processes become concrete and perseverative. Three major behavioral subtypes include disinhibition, apathy, and stereotypic behavior.

Disinhibited patients exhibit overactivity, restlessness, inattention and distractibility, impulsivity, lack of application, and impersistence. There is mental disorganization and frequent set shifting, moving unproductively from one activity or conversation topic to the next. Demeanor is often inappropriately jocular and socially inappropriate. Some exhibit signs of the Klüver-Bucy syndrome, namely hyperorality, hypersexuality, and utilization behavior. These patients frequently gain weight rapidly. They may impulsively touch or pick up objects within sight or within reach. In extreme cases, incontinence of stool and urine may be associated with coprophagia, sometimes in an otherwise oriented patient.

Apathetic patients are amotivational and pseudodepressed. Left alone, they spend the day sitting or lying in bed. They stop bathing and grooming and dress sloppily. Behavior is "economical," with minimal expenditure of energy or mental effort. These patients often have prolonged response latency to questions, although the eventual answer is often accurate. There is economy of speech, with many responses characterized by single words or short phrases with no attempt at elaboration. Speech prosody may be lost. Perseveration of verbal and motor activity is common. There may be a loss of concern for self and others because patients become emotionally shallow. Apathetic states are commonly mistaken for depression, and treatment with antidepressants is typically not effective.

Stereotypic patients exhibit repetitive, ritualistic, and idiosyncratic behaviors. These individuals require a rigid daily routine, becoming agitated when their routine is interrupted. They may repeat the same story verbatim and with the same prosodic inflection numerous times during a single clinic visit. They evidence mental inflexibility and difficulty shifting mind-set. Ritualistic behaviors, picking lint from the floor, rearranging the silverware drawer, rewriting a letter, etc, have a compulsive quality lacking the anxiety associated with obsessive-compulsive disorder. Clinical FTD features often overlap during the course of illness. Patients may present with predominant apathetic features only to later de-

FRONTOTEMPORAL DEMENTIA

Lobar Dementias

Figure 34-1

Frontotemporal dementias (FTDs)

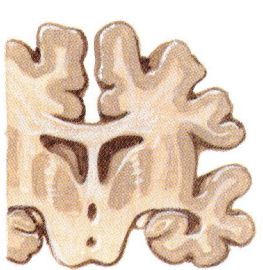

Atrophy of frontal and/or temporal areas

Clinical features of frontal lobe variant

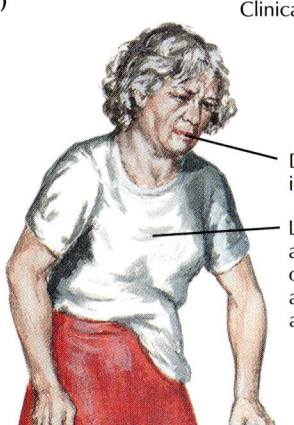

Decrease in speech

Loss of awareness of personal appearance and hygiene

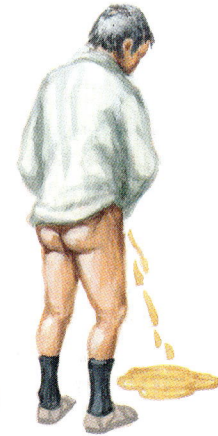

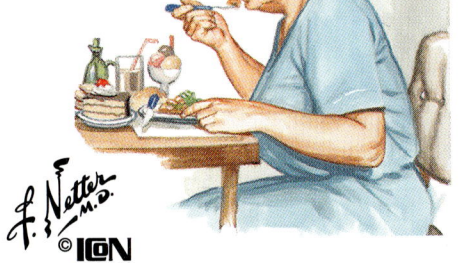

Oral fixation: increased eating causes weight gain.

Bizarre, uninhibited socially inappropriate behavior

Decreased concern and empathy for others

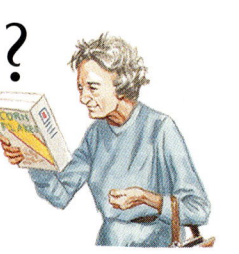

Temporal lobe variant may exhibit severe naming and word comprehension deficit.

Corticobasal degeneration

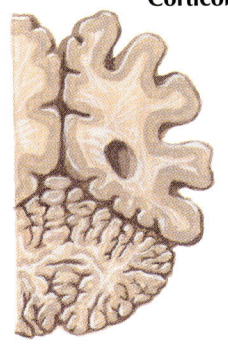

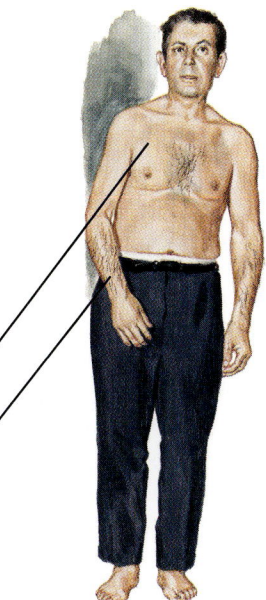

Contralateral assymetric atrophy of parietal lobe

Apraxia may inhibit everyday activities such as dressing.

Stiff, jerky limb posturing

Patient may exhibit "alien limb" phenomenon in limb contralateral to cortical atrophy.

Primary progressive aphasia

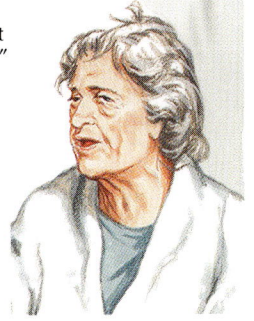

"I have went to dat town."

Patients show grammatical and phonological deficit as well as deficits in reading and writing.

MEMORY AND COGNITIVE DISORDERS

velop increasingly disinhibited or stereotypic behavior or both. As symptoms progress, most patients experience akinesia, progressive rigidity, mutism, and incontinence, requiring total nursing care. Features of disinhibition are associated with degeneration within the orbital frontal and adjacent temporal lobes. Apathetic features correlate with degenerative changes within the dorsolateral frontal lobes. Stereotypic behavior type seems to correlate with more widespread involvement of frontal and temporal lobes, although greater emphasis may exist in the region of the cingulate gyrus.

Cognitive function is initially relatively spared, so that neuropsychologic testing may be notable only for distractibility, inattentiveness, or perseveration rather than clear impairment of memory or constructional apraxia. One of the more striking cognitive features of FTD is executive dysfunction seen on sorting and sequencing tasks, loss of verbal fluency, and impairment in general problem-solving skills.

Clinical Subtypes

Frontotemporal lobar degeneration with motor neuron disease (FTD/MND) presents most often in men aged younger than 65 years. Characteristic FTD typically precedes onset of motor neuron symptoms, and disinhibited-type behaviors predominate. The motor neuron component leads to a more rapid decline and death in these cases. Consequently, akinesia and mutism are not often seen. The duration of illness is typically 2 to 3 years. A family history of disease is only occasionally found.

Primary progressive aphasia is divided into fluent and nonfluent types. In both conditions, progressive aphasia is the predominant clinical feature, often remaining the only feature throughout the illness. Fluent PPA is also called *semantic dementia*. Typically women, patients with fluent PPA usually present between the ages of 50 and 65 years. Illness duration ranges from 3 to 15 years. There is gradual loss of comprehension and naming, with relatively less impairment in reading and writing. Behavioral features include mental rigidity, stereotypic behaviors, self-centeredness, and disregard for personal safety. Many patients are easily agitated. Memory, calculations, and constructional skills are relatively spared, whereas visual agnosia and prosopagnosia may occur relatively early.

Nonfluent PPA patients typically present at the same ages. Men and women are affected equally. Illness duration is between 4 and 12 years. There is overall good comprehension, with impaired verbal expression. Patients have effortful, agrammatic, stuttering speech, with impaired repetition and word retrieval. Reading and writing are also affected, but less so than speech. These individuals are aware of their impairment and become frustrated and depressed easily. Behavioral problems develop later in the disease and may include any FTD symptoms. Nevertheless, the focal characteristic of PPA clinically differentiates it from classic FTD.

DIAGNOSTIC APPROACH

The use of appropriate tests in patient evaluation must be emphasized. MRI, important for excluding other mechanisms for frontal lobe syndromes such as tumor or infection, demonstrates atrophy predominating within frontal and temporal lobes. Brain imaging may show focal left temporal or asymmetric atrophy of the left

Figure 34-2

Frontal Temporal Atrophy

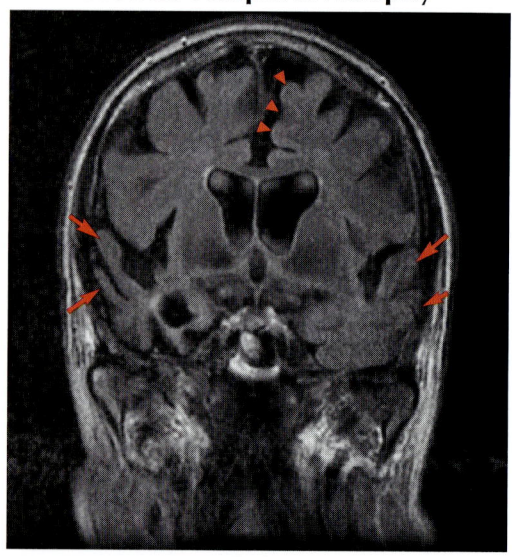

Coronal FLAIR MR image demonstrates ventricular enlargement especially of the right temporal horn, atrophy of superior and middle temporal gyri (arrow), and prominence of frontal sulci. Notice prominent widening of the interhemispheric fissure (arrowheads).
Courtesy of Richard Caselli, MD.

hemisphere in PPA cases. EMG in cases of FTD/MND may be diagnostic. SPECT may show deficits in a similar distribution, although it does not have a sensitivity that provides a definitive diagnosis. EEG is normal, especially early in the disease course. Blood work and CSF studies are not helpful.

TREATMENT

The clinical and pathologic overlap of tauopathies and Pick complex has led to complicated and ineffective nomenclature for these disorders. Given the heterogeneity of these conditions, a single set of diagnostic criteria has been virtually impossible to develop. Consequently, controlled clinical trials have been limited, and treatment protocols for FTD are unavailable. Treatment of FTD is, therefore, supportive.

In FTD, there is no known role for the cholinesterase inhibitors commonly used in Alzheimer disease. Caregiver education and reduction of caregiver stress are essential in successful management of agitation and other behavioral problems. When patients become aggressive and combative, caregivers tend to oppose their behavior. Distraction and redirection are more effective than verbal instruction in these instances. Unfortunately, sedatives are often used excessively to quell such behavior. Conservative approaches should be emphasized to limit sedative use as much as possible. Benzodiazepines may, paradoxically, exacerbate agitation. Use of SSRIs may help some patients with depression or anxiety. Other drugs, including atypical neuroleptics, mood stabilizers, and atypical anxiolytics (eg, trazodone, buspirone), sometimes help with problematic behavior when used as monotherapy or in combination.

REFERENCES

Kertesz A, Munoz DG. Frontotemporal dementia. *Med Clin North Am.* 2002;86:501-518, vi.

Morris JC. Frontotemporal dementias. In: Clark CM, Trojanowski JQ. *Neurodegenerative Dementias.* New York, NY: McGraw-Hill; 2000:279-290.

Snowden JS, Neary D, Mann DMA. *Fronto-Temporal Lobar Degeneration: Fronto-Temporal Dementia, Progressive Aphasia, Semantic Dementia.* New York, NY: Churchill Livingstone; 1996.

Chapter 35
Vascular Dementia

Yuval Zabar

Clinical Vignette

A 67-year-old man with a history of hypertension and coronary artery disease, who had lived alone since his wife's death 3 years previously, came to the clinic at his daughter's insistence because he had become increasingly complacent and inactive. The daughter noted that he had stopped fixing his own meals and might not eat unless she brought something to him. He tended to eat junk food and sweets. She was unsure whether he was taking his antihypertensive medications regularly. He had neglected housework and the yard, stopped balancing his checkbook, and decreased participation in social activities.

The patient reported dizziness, and his ability to walk had gradually deteriorated. Although he had not fallen, he felt that his legs might give way. He also reported urinary frequency and occasional incontinence. He did not report a depressed mood but was not particularly happy. He gave up previous interests because they were "too much to keep track of."

Five years previously, the patient had experienced a stroke with no residual deficit. Approximately 1 year previously, he had stayed in the hospital for a transient ischemic attack characterized by transient right-sided weakness and dysarthria. MRI then showed extensive subcortical and periventricular white matter changes and numerous microvascular infarcts in the basal ganglia.

His affect was flat; he was slow to respond. Mental status examination results showed impaired motor sequencing, executive dysfunction, and memory impairment. He could not spell WORLD backward. He was able to register 4 words but recalled only 1 of 4 spontaneously. With cueing, he recalled all 4 items. He could not draw a clock to command but copied a clock, drawn by the examiner, well. He had evidence of a wide-based, spastic gait, with bilateral Babinski signs. Stride and arm-swing amplitudes were reduced. Muscle stretch reflexes were brisk throughout. His blood pressure was 190/100 mm Hg.

Repeated MRI demonstrated more extensive subcortical and periventricular changes. Blood test results revealed normal cell counts, a normal B_{12} level, and a normal TSH level. Serum RPR was nonreactive. The fasting serum homocysteine level was slightly increased, at 17 mol/L.

The association between cerebrovascular disease and dementia has been recognized for years. Vascular mechanisms were postulated to be the main cause of senile dementia until Alzheimer disease (AD) was recognized as the most common cause in the 1960s. Subsequently, the concept of vascular dementia (VD) underwent several revisions. Given the array of clinical syndromes possible with stroke, VD presentation varies considerably. Renewed interest in AD initially prompted disproportionate emphasis on AD as a dementia prototype, leading to the development of diagnostic criteria for dementia biased toward identification of AD that deemphasized vascular mechanisms.

Clinical differentiation of vascular disease as a pure cause of dementia versus a cause of "mixed" dementia poses a challenge. The heterogeneity of stroke complicates defining VD as a single clinical entity with specific diagnostic criteria when vascular mechanisms are the only cause of dementia, so-called pure VD. Further, autopsy series show cerebrovascular disease coexisting with AD, influencing clinical dementia in approximately 20% of cases. These cases seem clinically much like AD and often meet universally accepted diagnostic AD criteria. Some authors propose using the term *vascular cognitive impairment*, instead of *VD*, to describe the contribution of cerebrovascular disease in dementia syndromes, whether purely from vascular disease or mixed with another dementing disorder.

EPIDEMIOLOGY

Although pure VD is often cited as the second most common cause of dementia, its prevalence and incidence may be less than previously thought because its measurement varies widely based on selected diagnostic criteria. Given the inherent bias in criteria toward AD, many AD cases may be misclassified and not identified as pure VD. Concomitantly, many true VD cases are missed because they do not fit the AD bias.

The risk of VD increases with age just as the risk of stroke increases with age. Most epidemiologic studies of dementia do not differentiate among AD, VD, and mixed dementia. The prevalence of VD as a pure cause of dementia is probably less than 10% of dementia cases, according to autopsy series. However, the prevalence of vascular cognitive impairment may be much greater.

CLINICAL PRESENTATION AND DIFFERENTIAL DIAGNOSIS

The potential for intervention to prevent or slow VD highlights the importance of recognizing vascular causes of dementia. Cardinal dementia features are early and prominent memory loss and progression, irreversibility, and impairment in daily activities. *Diagnostic and Statistical Manual* diagnostic criteria and research criteria "specific" for VD emphasize these "cardinal" features as diagnostic requisites. However, because stroke is not usually associated specifically with memory impairment, these criteria are misleading. Stroke more commonly causes aphasia or apraxia. Progression of cerebrovascular disease varies greatly. Residual symptoms may seem to improve acutely but then contribute to future cognitive decline. Moreover, several mechanisms of stroke—hemorrhagic or ischemic, occlusive or embolic—affect differently sized vessels in different locations, cortical and subcortical regions, gray and white matter, with marked variability in clinical presentation.

Typically, modern diagnostic criteria require imaging studies demonstrating evidence of stroke or ischemia to establish a diagnosis of VD. However, VD does not have a characteristic appearance on imaging studies, although absence of lesions strongly argues against this diagnosis. MRI is more sensitive than CT in showing subcortical and periventricular white matter changes consistent with small-vessel disease, and smaller infarcts. Therefore, diagnosis requires recognition of various syndromic features commensurate with findings on imaging studies.

Clinical presentation is somewhat arbitrarily divided into large-vessel and small-vessel disease, which are not mutually exclusive (Figure 35-1). **Large-vessel disease** tends to affect large vascular territories, producing well-known clinical syndromes. For example, frontal lobe involvement may produce aphasia, apraxia, disinhibition, or apathy. Mesial temporal involvement produces amnesia, angular gyrus lesions result in constructional apraxia, and parietal lesions produce alexia or apraxia. The clinical syndrome of multiinfarct dementia typically proceeds in a stepwise fashion with clear-cut stroke events leading to successive, cumulative impairment of various cognitive domains. **Small-vessel disease** results in subcortical infarcts, sometimes localized within strategic locations such as the thalamus or basal ganglia, and involving white matter tracts such as frontosubcortical and thalamocortical tracts. Moreover, small-vessel pathology is often seen in the context of "normal" aging, where the smallest branches become increasingly tortuous, producing twists and loops along paths deep in the brain. Morphologic changes are amplified by hypertension and diabetes. The result is diffuse myelin loss in deep vascular territories such as periventricular and subcortical white matter regions.

Clinical correlates of small-vessel disease include executive dysfunction, apathy, inattentiveness, and personality changes typical of frontal lobe syndromes as occur with hydrocephalus and primary **frontotemporal dementia**. Involvement of specific circuits correlates with recognized clinical manifestations. **Dorsolateral prefrontal circuit** dysfunction correlates with executive dysfunction, decreased verbal fluency, poor performance on sequencing tasks, impersistence, set shifting, and perseveration. **Subcortical orbitofrontal circuits** are associated with disinhibition, manic behavior, and compulsive behavior. **Medial frontal circuits** produce apathy, psychomotor retardation, and mood lability.

Binswanger disease may be representative of dementia due to small-vessel disease. Characteristically, patients are aged between 50 and 70 years; more than 80% have a history of hypertension, diabetes, or both. Initial symptoms vary but often include behavioral changes such as depression, emotional lability, or abulia. Gait dis-

VASCULAR DEMENTIA

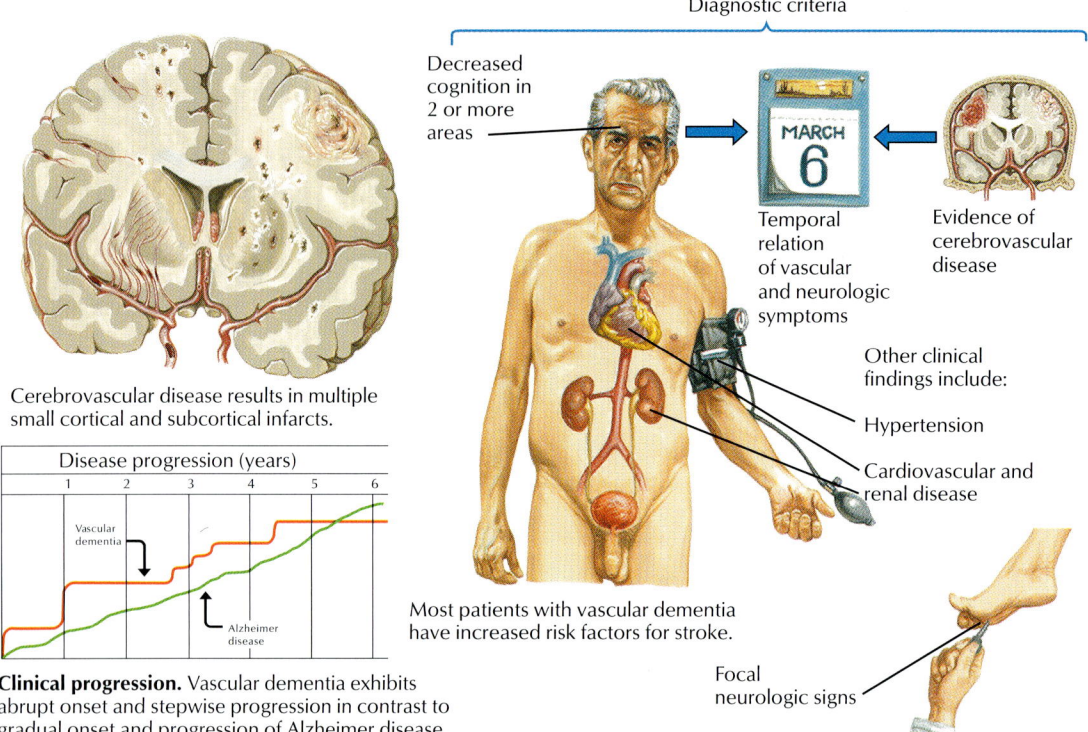

Figure 35-1

Vascular (Multi-infarct) Dementia

Cerebrovascular disease results in multiple small cortical and subcortical infarcts.

Clinical progression. Vascular dementia exhibits abrupt onset and stepwise progression in contrast to gradual onset and progression of Alzheimer disease.

Most patients with vascular dementia have increased risk factors for stroke.

Diagnostic criteria: Decreased cognition in 2 or more areas; Temporal relation of vascular and neurologic symptoms; Evidence of cerebrovascular disease; Other clinical findings include: Hypertension, Cardiovascular and renal disease, Focal neurologic signs.

turbances are characterized by parkinsonism, ataxia, or spasticity. Dysarthria and other focal motor signs may be present. Urinary incontinence is common. Patients often have histories of dizziness or syncope. Progressive executive dysfunction, slow mental processing, and memory impairment affecting information retrieval rather than encoding characterize cognitive impairment. The course of Binswanger disease is intermittently progressive, typically over 3 to 10 years, often without clear strokelike events. Pathologically, numerous subcortical and periventricular infarcts spare cortical u-fibers. When patients present with the clinical picture typical for Binswanger disease but do not have hypertension or diabetes, a diagnosis of cerebral autosomal-dominant arteriopathy with subcortical infarcts and leukoariosis (CADASIL) should be considered. It is one of the few hereditary causes of VD.

In the elderly, the possibility of mixed dementia exists when patients exhibit clinical features of AD and VD and imaging studies reveal evidence of infarct, widespread leukoariosis, or both. Silent brain infarction, especially in basal ganglia and thalamic regions, and significant ischemic white matter changes enhance the clinical presentation and progression of AD. Moreover, various vascular risk factors, such as hypertension, hypercholesterolemia, and hyperhomocysteinemia (levels >14 μmol/L), also increase the risk of AD. Brains with mixed pathologies, matched for dementia severity, reveal fewer AD lesions compared with pure AD cases. Clearly clinical presentation is influenced by cerebrovascular disease in these cases. Finally, the risk of developing poststroke dementia increases with advancing age, recurrent stroke, and larger periventricular white matter lesions on MRI. Hypoxic and ischemic stroke complications, such as pneumonia or seizure, also increase the risk of poststroke dementia.

PREVENTION AND TREATMENT

Primary prevention should be aggressively pursued. When at-risk patients are identified, treatment of arterial hypertension, cardiac disease, lipid abnormality, and diabetes are important in reducing dementia risk. Secondary prevention, treatment when cerebrovascular disease is recognized, begins with appropriate acute management of stroke and its complications. Prevention of stroke recurrence by appropriate antiplatelet or anticoagulant therapy and addressing primary risk factors are also important. Use of Ca^{2+} channel blockers for hypertension treatment may be more effective in dementia prevention than other antihypertensive medications. Dietary supplementation with folic acid and vitamins B_6 and B_{12} reduces levels of homocysteine. The role of "neuroprotective agents" in prevention of poststroke dementia is unknown.

When dementia develops, cholinesterase inhibitors may be helpful. As in AD, titration of these medications to maximum doses is recommended; their long-term efficacy in VD is unknown. Their potential value may be partly from the relatively high coexistence of AD and VD in elderly patients. However, subcortical vascular disease also interrupts major cholinergic pathways from the basal forebrain to widespread regions of the cerebral cortex. Deficits of CSF acetylcholine levels are found in VD cases when compared with healthy controls. As in all dementia cases, caregiver education and support are essential to long-term success and quality of patient life.

REFERENCES

Forette F, Seux ML, Staessen JA, et al. Prevention of dementia in randomised double-blind placebo-controlled Systolic Hypertension in Europe (Syst-Eur) trial. *Lancet.* 1998;352:1347-1351.

Forette F, Seux ML, Staessen JA, et al. The prevention of dementia with antihypertensive treatment: new evidence from the Systolic Hypertension in Europe (Syst-Eur) study. *Arch Intern Med.* 2002;162:2046-2052.

Pohjasvaara T, Erkinjuntti T, Vataja R, Kaste M. Dementia three months after stroke. Baseline frequency and effect of different definitions of dementia in the Helsinki Stroke Aging Memory Study (SAM) cohort. Stroke. 1997;28:785-792.

Roman GC. Vascular dementia revisited: diagnosis, pathogenesis, treatment, and prevention. *Med Clin North Am.* 2002;86:477-499.

Selden NR, Gitelman DR, Salamon-Murayama N, Parrish TB, Mesulam MM. Trajectories of cholinergic pathways within the cerebral hemispheres of the human brain. *Brain.* 1998;121(pt 12):2249-2257.

Seshadri S, Beiser A, Selhub J, et al. Plasma homocysteine as a risk factor for dementia and Alzheimer's disease. *N Engl J Med.* 2002;346:476-483.

Snowdon DA, Greiner LH, Mortimer JA, Riley KP, Greiner PA, Markesbery WR. Brain infarction and the clinical expression of Alzheimer disease. The Nun Study. *JAMA.* 1997;277:813-817.

Vermeer SE, Prins ND, den Heijer T, Hofman A, Koudstaal PJ, Breteler MM. Silent brain infarcts and the risk of dementia and cognitive decline. *N Engl J Med.* 2003;348:1215-1222.

Chapter 36
Transmissible Spongiform Encephalopathy

Yuval Zabar

Clinical Vignette

A 56-year-old man with a history of smoking noted that he was increasingly clumsy when writing. A tremor developed in his right hand, and he soon noted slurred speech. Initial neurologic evaluation demonstrated an action tremor in the right hand and some reduction in fine dexterity. Brain MRI and EEG results were normal. During the next 2 months, the patient's wife believed that her husband seemed confused. He called her by his sister's name. She reported that he had trouble initiating and maintaining sleep. His driving became erratic and dangerous. He was pulled over for driving too slowly and his license was revoked. On follow-up examination, he was disoriented. He spoke slowly and gave inappropriate responses. His dysarthria was more pronounced.

The results of repeated MRI and EEG were normal, as were CSF study results, including protein 14-3-3. Over the next 6 months, the patient's motor function declined precipitously. His gait became progressively ataxic, and he fell numerous times. He lost proper use of his hands and legs, requiring assistance with eating, dressing, and bathing. Occasionally, his limbs would jerk suddenly, and he appeared startled and anxious. Speech output became largely unintelligible and palilalic. He would shout occasionally but mostly stayed quiet and passive.

Repeated EEG showed generalized slowing and intermittent periodic sharp waves, approximately 1 per second. Right frontal lobe biopsy showed vacuolar encephalopathy consistent with a transmissible spongiform encephalopathy (TSE). The final stages were characterized by increasing stupor and aspiration pneumonia. The patient died 14 months after onset. Autopsy confirmed the diagnosis.

EPIDEMIOLOGY

Transmissible spongiform encephalopathy includes rare, subacute, universally fatal neurodegenerative diseases affecting humans and animals. Clinical presentation and distribution of pathologic lesions vary widely, complicating classification of these diseases. Classification focuses on **pathogenic mechanisms** rather than clinical and pathologic features. Currently, human TSE is classified into 3 categories: sporadic, familial, and infectious. Most animal TSE cases fall into the infectious category, including scrapie (sheep); bovine spongiform encephalopathy, also known as *mad cow disease* (cattle); and chronic wasting disease (deer and elk).

The **sporadic** form of human TSE, Creutzfeldt-Jakob disease (CJD), accounts for 85% of cases of this disorder. Sporadic fatal insomnia cases are also described.

The **inherited** form of human TSE, accounting for 15% of cases, includes familial CJD, fatal familial insomnia, Gerstmann-Straussler-Scheinker disease, and other less well-defined clinical syndromes.

The so-called **infectious** forms of TSE, comprising less than 1% of cases, include iatrogenic cases of CJD (exposure via dural grafts, infected surgical instruments, and growth hormone injections), kuru (cannibalism), and variant CJD (vCJD, via ingestion of beef contaminated with bovine spongiform encephalopathy).

Given concerns regarding potential transmission of bovine spongiform encephalopathy causing vCJD in humans who ate contaminated beef, a controversy regarding monitoring of blood products has emerged. The Centers for Disease Control in the United States are under congressional mandate to track donated blood to possible human cases of prion disease and to discard any blood or blood products originating from patients with confirmed CJD. Of course, in many instances, the blood is already used by the time CJD is diagnosed in the donor. In theory, transfusion of any blood product may pose a risk; however, to date there are no confirmed cases of infectious TSE secondary to blood transfusion. There seems to be increased risk of CJD among venison eaters. The incidence of human TSE is approximately 1.5/1 million people per year. This rate has remained stable over the past decades.

However, vCJD, probably transmitted by ingestion of beef with mad cow disease, may produce a significant increase in the overall incidence of human TSE in the near future. The appearance of symptoms after exposure to "infected" tissue varies widely, and incubation periods lasting several decades are described. Nearly 100 vCJD cases have been reported in Europe since 1996. These were predominantly in the United Kingdom, where most cases of mad cow disease occurred. No instances of vCJD have been diagnosed in the United States. With the potentially long incubation period of vCJD, all cases of TSE are reported and monitored by several European surveillance centers. A similar laboratory, the National Prion Diseases Pathology Surveillance Center, operates in the United States.

PATHOGENESIS

The histopathologic hallmarks of TSE include severe neuronal loss, spongiform vacuolization, and astrocytosis. There is no associated inflammatory response, and some disease forms have an accumulation of amyloid plaques. However, TSE amyloid differs from β amyloid typically found in Alzheimer disease. The agent responsible for TSE is a "proteinaceous infectious particle," termed *prion protein* (PrP^C). PrP^C is a normally occurring cell-surface glycoprotein, encoded on chromosome 20, which is highly conserved in mammals. Its normal function is not well defined, but it may have importance in response to oxidative stress.

All 3 TSE forms are thought to result from conversion of PrP^C into PrP^{Sc}, also known as *scrapie protein*. PrP^{Sc} is a self-replicating and infectious agent lacking nucleic acid. The mechanisms by which PrP^{Sc} leads to neurodegeneration remain largely unknown. It is questionable whether the prion is the sole pathogenic mechanism of TSE. The disease can be experimentally transmitted between various animals, with some variability, by inoculation of infected nervous tissue. However, inoculation with pure PrP^{Sc} has not led to transmission of disease. Therefore, PrP^{Sc} alone does not account for horizontal transmission.

More than 20 pathogenetic mutations of the prion gene are identified, accounting for 15% of inherited human TSE. Mutations of the PrP gene predispose mutant PrP to transform into the PrP^{Sc} tertiary structure. A difference in just 1 amino acid can drastically affect the disease phenotype. With infectious TSE, PrP^{Sc} enters the CNS via ingestion or iatrogenically and precipitates the conversion of PrP^C into PrP^{Sc}. In sporadic cases, the conversion may occur via rare stochastic changes of the normal protein. Individual susceptibility to conversion of PrP^C also may be determined by genetic polymorphisms, some of which are identified and associated with varying phenotypic expression.

For example, patients who are homozygous for methionine at residue 129 tend to present with cognitive loss, aphasia, myoclonus, or insomnia and tend not to have plaquelike lesions at autopsy. Patients who are homozygous for valine at residue 129 present primarily with cognitive loss or insomnia but not aphasia or myoclonus, and all have plaquelike lesions at autopsy. Moreover, individuals who are homozygous for methionine at residue 129 are more susceptible to vCJD than individuals with other polymorphisms at the same residue.

CLINICAL PRESENTATION

The initial symptomatology depends on which anatomical substrate TSE initially involves. Cognitive impairment is often the first sign and may be recognized by attentive patients who note subtle changes in their intellectual capacities that are sometimes difficult for the examining physician to define. Intellectual impairment may affect any cognitive domain, depending on the cortical regions involved. Behavioral and personality disturbances such as impulsivity, disinhibition, or apathy often occur concomitantly. Progressive dementia eventually develops in all individuals, often with significant psychiatric and behavioral disturbance.

Various motor deficits occur and sometimes are the presenting signs of TSE with subacute progressive dementia following. Cerebellar ataxia develops in some patients and myoclonus

TRANSMISSIBLE SPONGIFORM ENCEPHALOPATHY

Figure 36-1   Transmissible Spongiform Encephalopathy

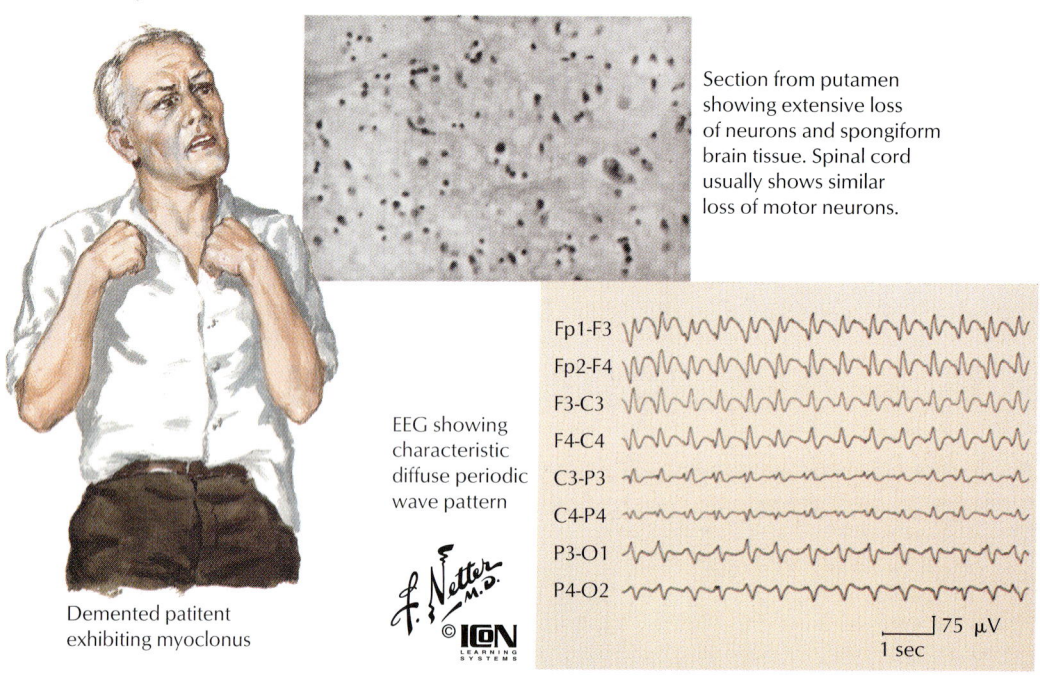

Creutzfeldt-Jakob disease

Section from putamen showing extensive loss of neurons and spongiform brain tissue. Spinal cord usually shows similar loss of motor neurons.

EEG showing characteristic diffuse periodic wave pattern

Demented patitent exhibiting myoclonus

Spongiform Encephalopathy: Early Cortical Involvement

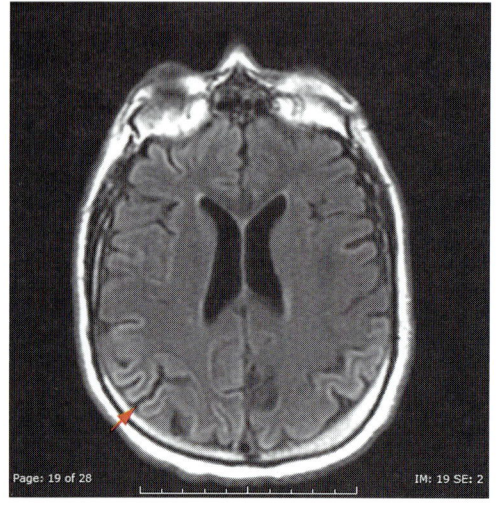
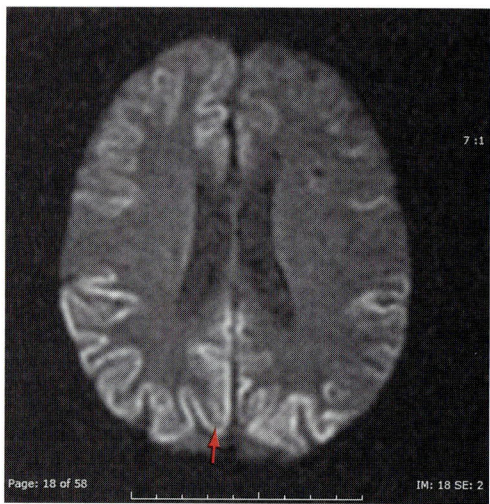

(**A**) FLAIR image shows increased intensity in frontal and parietal cortical gray matter. (**B**) Diffusion mimics the subtle restriction of diffusion in similar cortical regions.

develops in others; progressive parkinsonism, weakness and neurogenic muscle atrophy, and bulbar dysfunction also may occur. Motor signs may be unilateral or asymmetric, reflecting focal or multifocal disease, respectively. As symptoms progress, a multifocal pattern emerges with global cognitive impairment, severe loss of motor control, and marked behavioral changes. Many individuals experience myoclonus, some with a hyperactive startle response (Figure 36-1).

Terminal TSE stages are characterized by progressive stupor leading to coma and aspiration. Sporadic CJD cases usually present between the fifth and seventh decade of life, but vCJD occurs in younger adults and teenagers. The mean survival time for patients with sporadic disease is approximately 5 months; most die within 12 months. Inherited forms of the disease and vCJD have younger onset ages and more protracted courses than do sporadic cases.

DIAGNOSTIC APPROACH

The results of routine laboratory studies are normal. Identification of pathogenic mutations in **hereditary** cases is available via rapid screening tests that can be performed on non-CNS tissue, including peripheral blood. **Sporadic** disease remains a diagnostic challenge. A family of proteins called *14-3-3* is increased in the CSF of affected patients. Although initially reported to have greater than 90% sensitivity and specificity for TSE, it is likely overestimated because 14-3-3 proteins are essentially markers for any brain parenchymal damage. Nevertheless, CSF assays for protein 14-3-3 are useful when TSE is suspected. False-positives do occur, so positive results should not be considered diagnostic of TSE.

MRI has also begun to show some utility in TSE diagnosis. In some cases of vCJD, bright lesions on T2-weighted and FLAIR imaging occur within the pulvinar, the so-called pulvinar sign. In CJD, focal hyperintense lesions may be found in the basal ganglia on T2-weighted images or multifocally within the cortex on diffusion-weighted images (Figure 35-1). MRI abnormalities are supportive, like 14-3-3, but are not diagnostic of TSE. EEG may demonstrate 0.5- to 1-Hz periodic sharp waves focally or diffusely at some stage of the disease (Figure 36-1). Brain wave slowing is more common but less specific than periodic sharp waves.

Brain biopsy should be considered in every case, particularly when the results of other studies are negative. Although biopsy is susceptible to sampling error, examining tissue from areas initially demonstrating clinical symptomatology and findings can increase the likelihood of a positive biopsy result. Frontal lobe and cerebellar biopsies can be particularly successful. CSF samples and brain tissue should be sent to the national surveillance center for analysis and monitoring. Autopsy should be discussed well in advance of death because it is essential in diagnosis, and confirmation allows epidemiologic surveillance of disease activity.

TREATMENT

Treatment is at best supportive. No anti-PrP^{Sc} prion therapies are available. For individuals presenting primarily with cerebellar or striatal forms of these disorders, whose intellect is maintained, it is important to include them in discussion of end-of-life issues. Hospice care should be pursued where available.

Given the possibility of epidemic TSE, a simple, rapid diagnostic test is greatly needed. Means of preventing TSE transmission must be clearly defined. This endeavor would require significant regulatory and legislative measures to assure appropriate standards in the meat packing industry, as well as a public education effort. Consistent case ascertainment and reporting to the National Prion Disease Pathology Surveillance Center are imperative for the development of diagnostic and preventive strategies.

REFERENCES

Mastrianni JA, Roos RP. The prion diseases. *Semin Neurol.* 2000;20:337-352.

Spencer MD, Knight RS, Will RG, et al. First hundred cases of variant Creutzfeldt-Jakob disease: retrospective case note review of early psychiatric and neurological features. *BMJ.* 2002;324:1479-1482.

Shiga Y, Miyazawa K, Sato S, et al. Diffusion weighted MRI abnormalities as an early diagnostic marker for Creutzfeldt-Jakob disease. *Neurology.* 2004;63:443-449.

Sy MS, Gambetti P, Wong BS, et al. Human prion diseases. *Med Clin North Am.* 2002;86:551-571, vi-vii.

Section X
PSYCHIATRIC DISORDERS

Chapter 37
Major Depression 366

Chapter 38
Bipolar Disorder 369

Chapter 39
Schizophrenia 372

Chapter 40
Obsessive-Compulsive Disorder 375

Chapter 41
Panic Disorder 378

Chapter 42
Dysthymia 381

Chapter 43
Borderline Personality Disorder 384

Chapter 44
Attention Deficit Disorder 387

Chapter 45
Drug and Alcohol Abuse 390

Chapter 46
Delirium 399

Chapter 37
Major Depression
Kenneth Lakritz

Clinical Vignette

A 34-year-old woman was admitted to an inpatient psychiatric service after telling her internist that she had had thoughts of killing herself and her 3 small children. The patient described herself as a failed parent who had "ruined" her children and needed to be punished. Feelings of hopelessness, intense anxiety, difficulty concentrating, severe insomnia, and a spontaneous 20-lb weight loss had developed gradually over a 6-month period.

This vignette is a classic example of severe depression. Depression is the most common serious psychiatric disorder; practicing physicians encounter it frequently. In morbidity and economic loss, it ranks second only to cardiovascular disease. Up to 20% of people have at least 1 major depressive episode. Women have a higher incidence of depression between menarche and menopause, with an especially high postpartum risk. However, men have a higher risk of suicide.

Depression usually begins in adolescence or early adulthood. It is a chronic illness with a propensity for recurrence. One common clinical pattern, called *double depression*, is characterized by repeated episodes of depression with eventual remission to a milder "dysthymic" state (see chapter 42). Familial clustering is apparent, although specific genes have not been identified. Depression beginning after the age of 60 years is probably a different disorder. It is usually not associated with a significant family history but is often associated with cerebrovascular disease.

CLINICAL PRESENTATION

The primary symptoms of major depression include a sad or anxious mood, anhedonia (loss of pleasure from normally enjoyable experiences), insomnia (often with early morning wakening), loss of appetite, excessive guilt, and impaired energy and concentration (Figure 37-1). Diurnal mood fluctuation—feeling worse in the morning—is almost pathognomonic. Many patients have subtle endocrine disturbances, especially hypercortisolism. It is not uncommon to find disturbed sleep architecture with shortened REM latency.

Suicide ideation and attempts are common in more severely depressed patients. Although attempts are notoriously difficult to predict, physicians must try to assess suicide risk and intervene when necessary. Risk factors for suicide include male sex, psychosis, intense anxiety or agitation, history of suicide attempts, advanced age, and alcohol abuse.

Many medical conditions provoke or mimic major depression, most commonly hypothyroidism, alcohol abuse, and corticosteroid use. Depressed alcoholics and drug abusers are unlikely to recover unless they maintain sobriety.

Severely depressed patients sometimes become psychotic. If so, they have "affect consonant" delusions, eg, delusions of poverty, moral depravity, or life-threatening illness. Among physical complaints, bowel delusions are especially common. The recognition of psychosis in depressed patients is important because this subgroup does not respond to standard antidepressant medications. For psychotically depressed patients, there are 2 therapeutic options: electroconvulsive therapy or combined antidepressant and antipsychotic medication.

At least 10% of individuals who present with depression are in the depressed phase of bipolar disorder. A single episode of mania establishes this diagnosis. Suspicion is raised by a family history of bipolar disorder, childhood onset of depressive illness, and a sudden response to antidepressant medication ("switching") rather than

MAJOR DEPRESSION

Figure 37-1 Major Depression

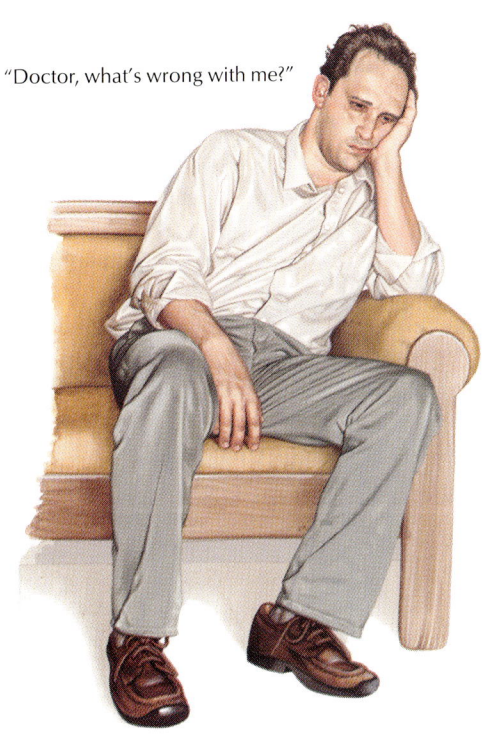
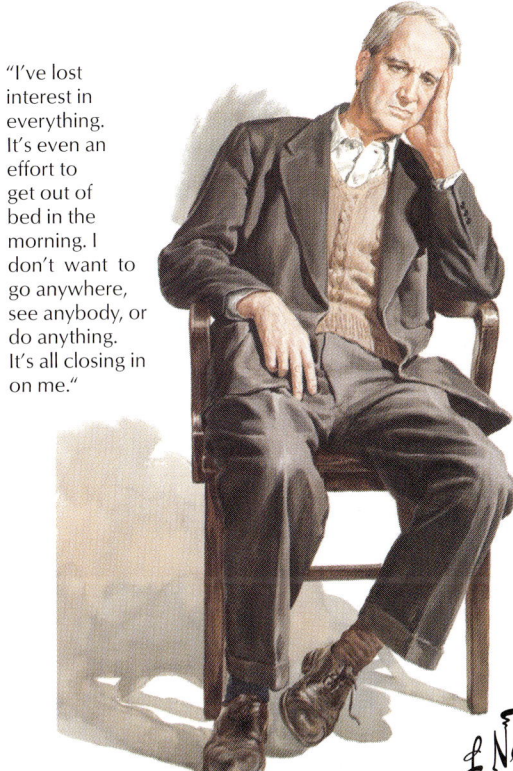

"Doctor, what's wrong with me?"

"I've lost interest in everything. It's even an effort to get out of bed in the morning. I don't want to go anywhere, see anybody, or do anything. It's all closing in on me."

the usual delayed response. Efforts should be made to limit the exposure of patients with known or suspected bipolar disorder to antidepressant medications (see chapter 38).

TREATMENT

Treatment of major depression combines medications with psychotherapy; the two are synergistic. Depressed patients have characteristically distorted thinking even when well. They are overly passive, feel powerless, and evaluate problems in "all-or-none" terms. Cognitive therapies that target these patterns are the best-validated psychotherapeutic interventions.

Most antidepressant medications are equally effective, producing significant improvement in 60% to 70% of patients and full remission in 30% to 40%. SSRIs are preferred for initial treatment. They have milder side effects and de-creased lethality in overdose compared with tricyclic antidepressants. However, controversy exists about whether SSRIs are as effective as tricyclics in severely ill patients. Monoamine oxidase inhibitors are often effective for depression. Unfortunately, monoamine oxidase inhibitors have the unique potential to precipitate a hypertensive crisis when patients are exposed to tyramine-containing foods or various other medications, particularly meperidine and SSRIs.

Patients with only a partial response to treatment may respond to an antidepressant from a different class or to addition of an augmenting agent. The best documented of these are lithium and triiodothyronine. Atypical antipsychotic agents are also promising.

Electroconvulsive therapy is indicated for severely depressed individuals who fail medication trials. It has a response rate of more than 90% in well-selected populations. Electroconvulsive therapy is also the first-line treatment for psychotic depression, intense suicidal ideation, and medically ill patients. It is underutilized, possibly because of public misunderstanding. Unilateral electrode placement significantly diminishes post–electroconvulsive therapy confusion. With modern anesthetics, other complications, such as spinal compression fractures, are rare.

Because depression is usually a chronic illness, maintenance and prophylactic treatment should be considered at diagnosis. Active treatment for first episodes should last at least 6 months, preferably 1 year. After 3 episodes, indefinite prophylaxis with full-dose antidepressant medication is indicated.

Because the treatment of depression is sometimes unsatisfactory, novel and experimental treatments abound. Sleep deprivation, especially REM sleep deprivation, often yields prompt improvement in mood, although the effect is hard to sustain. Patients who get depressed in the winter (seasonal affective disorder) often respond to bright light therapy, although standard antidepressant treatment is also effective. Transcranial magnetic stimulation and vagus nerve stimulation are potential but unproven alternatives to electroconvulsive therapy. Dietary supplementation with amine precursors (tryptophan, phenylalanine) may help. Inhibitors of substance P or corticosteroid-releasing hormone will probably be available in the future.

REFERENCES

Beck AT, Rush AJ, Shaw BF, Emery G. *Cognitive Therapy of Depression*. New York, NY: Guilford Press; 1987.

Carroll BJ, et al. A specific laboratory test for the diagnosis of melancholia. *Arch Gen Psychiatry*. 1981;38:15-22.

Mann JJ. The neurobiology of suicide. *Nat Med*. 1998;4:25-30.

Solomon A. *The Noonday Demon: An Atlas of Depression*. Scribner; 2002.

Chapter 38
Bipolar Disorder

Kenneth Lakritz

Clinical Vignette

Police arrested a 44-year-old man for fighting in a bar and brought him to the ED. He told the arresting officer that he was a wealthy state senator and offered to buy him a sports car.

The patient gave an address 1000 miles away, stating he had just arrived by airplane. Although unemployed, he was staying at an expensive hotel, and told hospital staff that he was "the richest man in North America" and an English prince. He was restless, euphoric, and irritable but also friendly and overly flirtatious with female staff.

One month earlier, he had been hospitalized for the third time for depression with suicidal ideation. He had responded rapidly to an antidepressant and was discharged after 3 days. He had a history of alcohol and cocaine abuse. His family history was positive for depression in 3 of 5 first-degree relatives and "manic-depressive psychosis" in his maternal grandmother.

This clinical vignette illustrates bipolar disorder manifesting as a "switch" from depression to mania after initiation of antidepressant therapy. The finding of a strong family history of similar illness is typical.

Classic mania has a unique presentation. The patient, often colorfully dressed and wearing a large amount of jewelry, is excessively cheerful, overly familiar, and brimming with schemes and ideas (Figure 38-1). The patient often talks incessantly; the surest sign of mania is needing to interrupt the patient. In the extreme, manic patients lose touch with reality; they may declare themselves emperor, suddenly relocate to another state, or flirt dangerously with strangers. They stop sleeping and become irritable and aggressive. In contrast to schizophrenic patients, who seem odd and distant, manic patients are engaging and often likeable.

Nevertheless, bipolar disorder is not benign. Almost all manic patients eventually have serious depressions. (In contrast to unipolar depression, unipolar mania is uncommon.) With time, episodes of bipolar illness become more frequent, more autonomous—less clearly tied to external stresses—and more difficult to treat. Patients are at high risk for repeated hospitalizations, suicide, and drug and alcohol abuse.

CLINICAL PRESENTATION

The first episode of illness is usually in the teens or 20s, but childhood onset is not rare. Half of the patients with childhood depression are eventually found to be bipolar. Males and females are equally affected.

Patients do not always present with classic mania. Their first episodes of illness may be depression. Previous high episodes may be of mild or "hypomanic" intensity, not easily recognized as illness. Although mania and depression seem like opposites (happy-sad, accelerated-slowed, etc), at a neurobiologic level, the 2 states are more alike than different, and patients often present with features of mania and depression simultaneously. In these "atypical" mood states, variously described as *mixed states, dysphoric mania,* and *agitated depression,* patients are excited and restless but also sad or irritable, or rapidly oscillating between elation and sadness. Atypical states may actually be more common than classic mania.

Complex presentations make a careful history the diagnostic key. Patients' reluctance to see or acknowledge their mania mandates gathering information from reliable third parties, particularly family members, past caregivers, and others.

BIPOLAR DISORDER

Figure 38-1

Bipolar Affective Disorder: Manic Episode

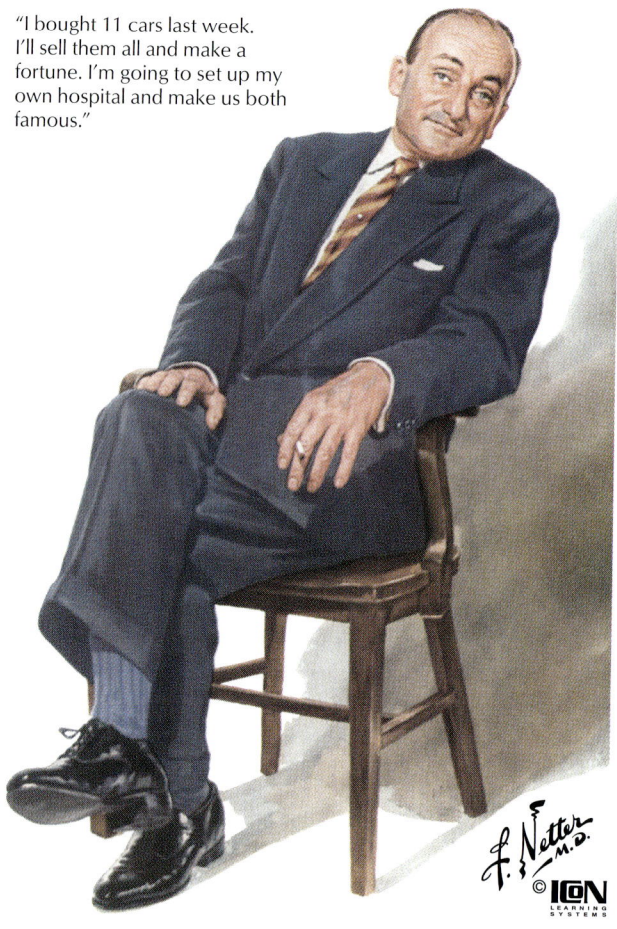

"I bought 11 cars last week. I'll sell them all and make a fortune. I'm going to set up my own hospital and make us both famous."

Bipolar disorder is the most heritable of all the major psychiatric illnesses. Most patients with bipolar disorder have at least 1 affected relative. Conversely, anyone with a first-degree bipolar relative has at least a 10% chance of developing bipolar disorder. When such patients present with a complaint of depression or alcohol abuse, suspicion of bipolar disorder must be high.

TREATMENT

Mood stabilizing medications are the main treatment. Given the natural history of bipolar disorder, when the diagnosis is established, patients must be treated indefinitely.

Lithium, the first specific treatment for bipolar disorder, is effective for the manic and depressed phases and for prophylaxis. It remains the only medication clearly shown to reduce suicide rates in bipolar disorder. However, it has a narrow therapeutic index and many annoying side effects, requires frequent blood level monitoring, and causes renal and thyroid dysfunction.

Anticonvulsants are more effective than lithium in mixed or atypical cases, especially for patients with "rapid cycling"—more than 4 episodes of illness per year. Valproic acid and carbamazepine are demonstrably effective; other anticonvulsants may also be effective. Atypical antipsychotics seem to have mood-stabilizing properties. Clozapine is sometimes considered as a treatment of last resort.

Treatment of bipolar depression is especially challenging. Antidepressants promote mood instability and rapid mood **cycling**. Any antidepressant can cause a "switch" to mania. Nevertheless, judicious use of antidepressants is often required because most mood stabilizers have only weak antidepressant effects. Among anticonvulsants, lamotrigine may be specifically effective for bipolar depression. Electroconvulsive therapy is highly effective in both phases of bipolar disorder. Supraphysiologic doses of thyroid hormone often help to stabilize mood. Conversely, subclinical hypothyroidism is associated with rapid cycling, and poor treatment response and should be sought, especially in patients treated with lithium.

Most successfully treated bipolar patients eventually miss their high moods. Hence, noncompliance is almost universal. When it occurs, a strong interpersonal and educational relationship between the psychiatrist, the patient, and the family is beneficial. All must learn to recognize and report early signs of relapse. Among these signs, many researchers consider sleep loss to be the final common pathway to decompensation; in bipolar patients insomnia requires aggressive treatment.

Bipolar disorder seems to be less common in populations that consume large quantities of fatty fish. The fatty acids found in these fish—ω-3 unsaturated fatty acids—seem to play an important role in the secondary messenger systems activated by amine neurotransmitters. (Lithium is thought to affect the same pathways.) Dietary augmentation with ω-3 fatty acids seems to decrease relapse rates among bipolar patients. Because these supplements seem harmless and even beneficial for cardiovascular health, they can be widely recommended.

REFERENCES

Goodwin FK, Jamison KR. *Manic-Depressive Illness*. New York, NY: Oxford University Press; 1990.

Jamison KR. *An Unquiet Mind: A Memoir of Moods and Madness*. New York, NY: Vintage; 1997.

Manji HK, Bowden CL, Belmaker RH, eds. *Bipolar Medications: Mechanisms of Action*. Washington, DC: American Psychiatric Publishing; 2000.

Chapter 39
Schizophrenia

Kenneth Lakritz

Clinical Vignette

A 20-year-old college junior was brought to the student health service after repetitively accosting his physics professors at the library. He repeatedly requested advice on the design of "shielding" from radio signals that were "emanating from outer space." He asserted that the signals were an attempt to control his thoughts, take over his body, and turn him into a woman. When one professor refused to help, the patient described him as an "invader."

The patient had no history of psychiatric treatment. He had done well in school through his freshman year in college, but his grades had recently declined and he was in danger of failing. His roommates described him as increasingly irritable and isolated, rarely leaving his room. On examination, he appeared tense and fearful. He wore a hat stuffed with aluminum foil to prevent "messages from reaching [his] brain." He had delusional beliefs about an invasion from space, auditory hallucinations, delusions of passivity (feelings of being controlled by outside forces), and thought insertion. The results of physical examination, cranial MRI, and routine laboratory testing, including drug screening, were unremarkable. He was hospitalized involuntarily, and his anxiety improved with an atypical antipsychotic drug. His delusions continued but seemed to bother him less. He was unable to continue school and returned to live with his parents.

In the 1880s, Emil Kraepelin delineated *schizophrenia* as a syndrome of global impairment of psychic functioning distinguished from the dementias by its early onset and from the affective psychoses by its unremitting course. The onset of schizophrenia typically occurs in late adolescence and early adulthood. Patients with this syndrome, who are often initially odd or unsociable, become progressively more isolated and eccentric, commonly failing to care for themselves and sometimes creating a public nuisance. Late-onset cases are uncommon, occur overwhelmingly in females, and usually present with prominent paranoid symptoms.

On examination, patients are found to have hallucinations (usually of voices), disordered thinking, and delusional beliefs. Untreated, patients exhibit declining cognitive function, especially in the first decade of the illness, although remissions and long-term improvement are possible. Still, only a minority of patients with schizophrenia achieve functional recovery. Most are chronically disabled and account for a large proportion of nursing home and some prison populations. The suicide rate is as high as 10%.

Schizophrenia affects 0.5% to 1% of the population; a milder form of the illness, schizotypal personality disorder, is more common. The cause is unknown. Familial clustering is obvious, but identical twins have disease concordance of only approximately 50%, excluding purely genetic explanations. Twin studies have refuted theories about defective parenting and "schizophrenogenic mothers." There are weak associations with winter birth, maternal malnutrition, and prenatal viral exposures, suggesting a "stress-diathesis" model, combining genetic vulnerability with early environmental insults. Schizophrenia is strongly associated with increased paternal but not maternal age, indicating that new germ-line mutations are involved in up to 25% of cases.

CLINICAL PRESENTATION

Schizophrenic symptoms can be categorized into 3 large clusters, with only weak associations between the clusters: positive symptoms, negative symptoms, and cognitive disturbance.

Compared with affective psychosis, **positive symptoms**, including schizophrenic delusions and hallucinations, are often more bizarre and illogical. Many experts consider certain "first-rank" symptoms (eg, delusions of passivity or

SCHIZOPHRENIA

Figure 39-1

Schizophrenic Disorder

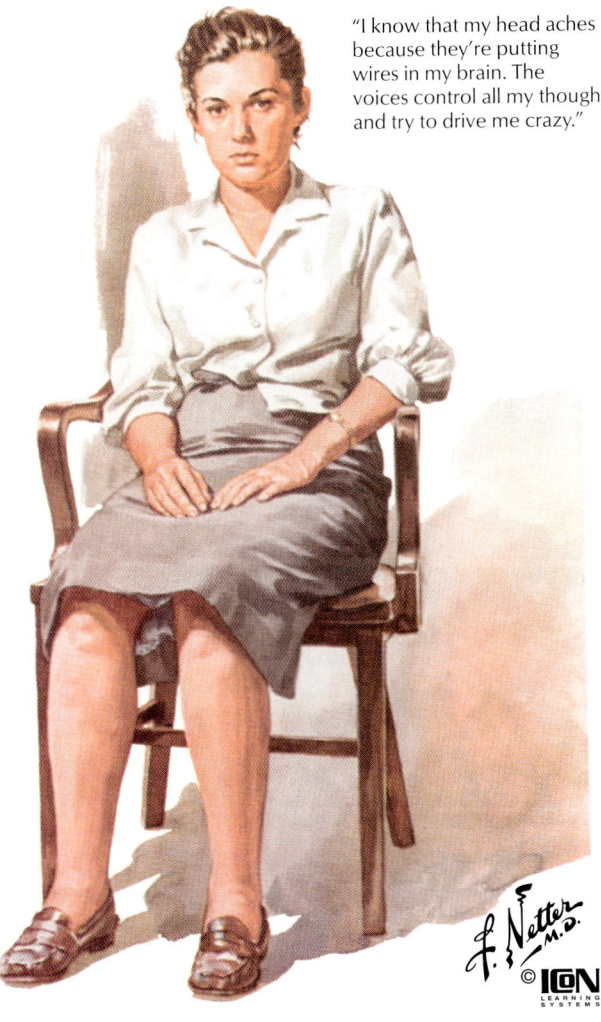

"I know that my head aches because they're putting wires in my brain. The voices control all my thoughts and try to drive me crazy."

outside control, thoughts being withdrawn from the patient's brain, thoughts being broadcast by the patient to others) as pathognomonic for schizophrenia. Others maintain that only the long-term course of the illness reveals the diagnosis. **Negative symptoms** include emotional flatness, social withdrawal, and lack of initiative and self-care (Figure 39-1). Patients with schizophrenia usually show **cognitive disturbance**, with deficits in many areas of reasoning, such as working memory and abstract reasoning.

Patients with schizophrenia have more than the expected number of neurologic "soft signs." Specific findings include abnormalities of smooth pursuit eye movement, auditory evoked potentials, and olfactory deficits. At least 50% of patients with schizophrenia have gross CNS pathology visible on CT or MRI, including ventricular enlargement and decreased temporal and frontal lobe volume. Cerebellar abnormalities are also common. Ventricular enlargement seems to correlate with negative symptoms and treatment resistance.

TREATMENT

Therapy of patients with schizophrenia is challenging. Until neuroleptic medications were introduced in 1953, no effective biologic treat-

PSYCHIATRIC DISORDERS

ments existed. The classic neuroleptic agents, which work by blocking dopamine receptors, are often effective against positive symptoms but do not help and may exacerbate negative symptoms. The "atypical neuroleptics," beginning with clozapine, are more broadly effective.

Patients with schizophrenia respond poorly to stress. Those living in rural or less industrialized settings tend to have better outcomes. Episodes of relapse correlate with expressed emotion, a measure of interpersonal turbulence, in patients' households. Psychotherapy and educational measures focus on preventing these and other stressors.

REFERENCES

Green MF. *Schizophrenia Revealed: From Neurons to Social Interactions.* New York, NY: WW Norton; 2003.

Pearlson GD. Neurobiology of schizophrenia. *Ann Neurol.* 2000;48:556-566.

Torrey EF. *Surviving Schizophrenia: A Manual for Families.* Consumers and Providers, Quill; 2001.

Chapter 40
Obsessive-Compulsive Disorder

Kenneth Lakritz

Clinical Vignette

A 44-year-old electrical engineer consulted a psychiatrist at the request of his wife, who complained about his unwillingness to discard old newspapers and journals. The patient acknowledged that his wife's complaint was accurate. He subscribed to 8 technical journals that he never actually read; old issues filled 3 rooms in his house. He worried that if he discarded them, he would miss an important development in his field. He also admitted that he had to check the appliances and faucets 4 times before leaving the house to ensure they had been turned off. He had a 1-hour ritual of washing and shaving that he had to perform in strict order every morning.

Despite these time-wasting habits and rituals, the patient had a successful career. He was well liked by friends and family, who worked around his eccentricities. His symptoms gradually diminished with combined treatment with a serotonergic antidepressant and a behavioral program of exposure and response prevention.

Patients with obsessive-compulsive disorder (OCD) report unwelcome, intrusive, and repetitive thoughts or urges to act in ways they find meaningless or inappropriate. The thoughts or urges are ego-dystonic, unwelcome and seemingly imposed on the patient. Someone who hoards newspapers and bits of string or spends hours every day polishing a new car but does so happily does not have OCD, however odd the behavior is. People with OCD are tormented by their thoughts and behaviors, usually struggling with them for years before seeking help.

CLINICAL PRESENTATION

Patients with OCD usually fit into one of a few categories. Some clean obsessively and worry about germs or contamination (Figure 40-1). Others repeatedly check that they have turned off their appliances or locked their doors. Some are obsessed with symmetry or arranging their possessions in exactly the right order. Another group hoards what most would call junk. Often, patients with OCD are troubled by thoughts of violence; they may fear that they will run someone over while driving or that, as they eat, a knife will slip from their hands and cut someone. Inexperienced clinicians sometimes err by seeing these obsessions as real threats, thereby exacerbating patients' fears. In fact, patients with OCD are terrified of these thoughts and do not act on them.

Most diagnostic classifications use a category of *obsessive-compulsive personality disorder*, or something similar, to describe individuals who are highly controlled, formal, emotionally distant, parsimonious, perfectionist, resistant to change, and intolerant of ambiguity. Despite the similarity in names, this personality constellation and OCD are unrelated.

Several other disorders of impulse control seem superficially related to OCD. Pathologic gamblers and "sex addicts" seem obsessed and compulsive, as do those who have trichotillomania, the compulsion to pull out body hairs. However, these apparently similar patients share neither the unique pathophysiology of OCD described below nor the same pattern of response to treatment.

Patients with OCD typically have no structural brain abnormalities. In contrast, functional brain imaging (PET or functional MRI) reliably shows excess metabolic activity in caudate and frontal regions; OCD is the first neuropsychiatric disorder that can be detected by brain scan. Although this pattern is not required to diagnose OCD and its significance is unknown, the findings themselves are robust.

TREATMENT

Patients with OCD share a unique pattern of response to medications. They improve when given antidepressants that block reuptake of

OBSESSIVE-COMPULSIVE DISORDER

Figure 40-1

Obsessive Compulsive Disorder

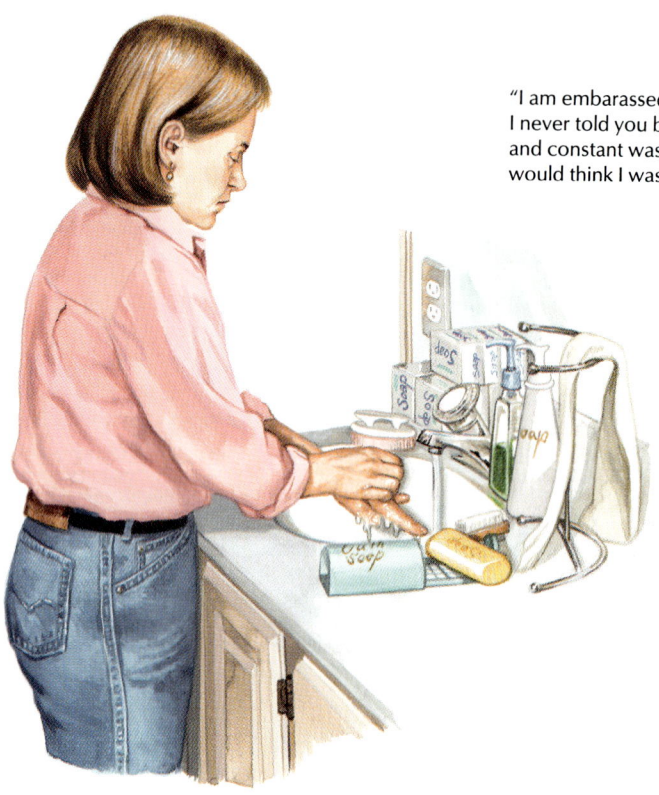

"I am embarassed that my hands are so chapped. I never told you before about my fear of germs and constant washing because I was afraid you would think I was crazy."

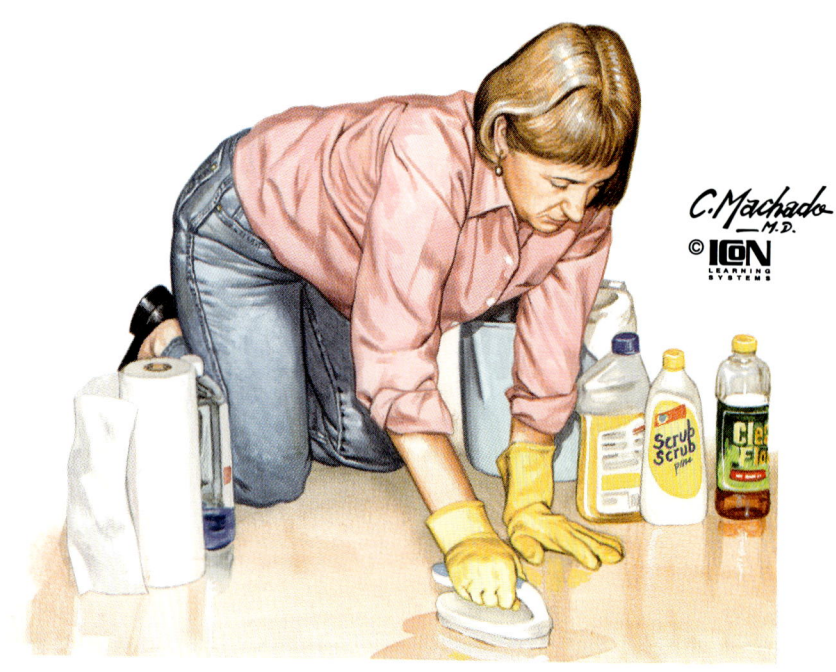

PSYCHIATRIC DISORDERS

serotonin. Antidepressants that block reuptake of norepinephrine, and which are as effective for treating depression as the serotonergic antidepressants, are ineffective for OCD. Curiously, a canine model for OCD, acral paw lick syndrome, shows the same pattern of medication response.

At a clinical level, OCD responds less well to serotonergic antidepressants than does depression. Typically, higher doses of medication are required to treat OCD, the response is slower, and full remissions with medication alone are uncommon.

Some form of behavioral therapy is almost always also required. The most effective of these is exposure and response prevention. If a patient has a compulsion to wash his hands, the quickest way to cure him is to get dirt on his hands and prevent him from washing them. Naturally, patients need support and encouragement to try this method. The metabolic abnormalities resolve whether patients improve through medication or behavioral treatment.

Some cases of childhood-onset OCD, especially those with abrupt onset or associated movement disorders, are caused by *Streptococcus* infections and subsequent reactivity of anti-streptococcal antibodies with basal ganglia. Antibiotic treatment and plasmapheresis to remove the antibodies help these patients.

REFERENCES

Clark DA. *Cognitive-Behavioral Therapy for OCD*. New York, NY: Guilford; 2004.

Rapoport JL. *The Boy Who Couldn't Stop Washing: The Experience and Treatment of Obsessive-Compulsive Disorder*. New York, NY: Signet; 1997.

Swedo SE, Leonard HL, Garvey M, et al. Pediatric autoimmune neuropsychiatric disorders associated with streptococcal infections: clinical description of the first 50 cases. *Am J Psychiatry*. 1998;155:264-271.

Chapter 41
Panic Disorder

Kenneth Lakritz

Clinical Vignette

A 23-year-old woman was referred to a psychiatric clinic after presenting to a hospital ED on 4 consecutive nights, reporting chest pain, dyspnea, and faintness. Each time, the results of a careful cardiac and pulmonary examination were unremarkable, and the patient was sent home with a benzodiazepine prescription and reassurance from the ED staff that she was not ill.

She had reported similar attacks since childhood, but not as frequently as recently. She felt a desperate need to have help available if an attack occurred and rarely left home unaccompanied. She worried that she would lose consciousness during an attack or lose control of her bowels but admitted that neither had ever happened.

The patient had given up driving and air travel. She worked at an undemanding job near home and had little or no social life, which troubled her, but she felt helpless about socializing more. She avoided caffeine, which made her feel "wired," and presented the psychiatrist with a long list of medications to which she was "allergic." She acknowledged occasional excess alcohol consumption to lessen her anxiety.

ED staff frequently encounter patients with and diagnose panic disorder. These individuals experience unpredictable and sudden bouts of intense anxiety and frightening physical symptoms, leading them to fear they are experiencing a heart attack, stroke, or other medical emergency. The vignette in this chapter is classic for panic disorder. Typically, patients require a combination of anxiolytic pharmacologic agents and behavior psychotherapy.

CLINICAL PRESENTATION

Patients with panic disorder are invariably focused on the details of their bodily sensations and tend to reach catastrophic conclusions based on minor aches, palpitations, and shortness of breath (Figure 41-1). They may present repeatedly in the ED with dyspnea, chest pain, tachycardia, and faintness. Extremity numbness or paresthesias suggest that patients are vasoconstricted from hyperventilation-induced respiratory alkalosis. Typically, patients are not reassured by negative examination results and may present again a few days later with the same complaints. They may feel entirely well between episodes but more commonly remain anxious and vigilant for signs of the next attack.

Many individuals with panic attacks have agoraphobia. (Probably all agoraphobic patients have had panic attacks.) Agoraphobia is not a fear of open spaces but a fear of being isolated from help and support. Patients with agoraphobia avoid novel places and circumstances and may also avoid driving on familiar highways, fearing isolation in a traffic jam. Eventually, patients may become so fearful that they cannot leave home without accompaniment or at all.

DIAGNOSIS

Intravenous lactic acid infusion, which mimics respiratory acidosis but has no subjective effects in controls, reproduces the panic attacks in many patients. This and other evidence has suggested the "suffocation alarm" theory of panic disorder, which asserts that affected individuals are overly sensitive to minor changes in blood pH and P_{CO_2}. Hence, severe asthma, chronic obstructive pulmonary disorder, and pulmonary embolus are some of the respiratory disorders that must be excluded in panicky patients. Other considerations include cardiac arrhythmias, myocardial infarction, ingestion of sympathomimetics (particularly cocaine), excess caffeine, alcohol and sedative-hypnotic withdrawal, hypoglycemia, partial complex seizures, and, rarely, pheochromocytoma or carcinoid tumors. Some of these are eliminated by the chronicity of the illness, eg, no one survives daily pulmonary emboli.

PANIC DISORDER

Figure 41-1

Panic Disorder

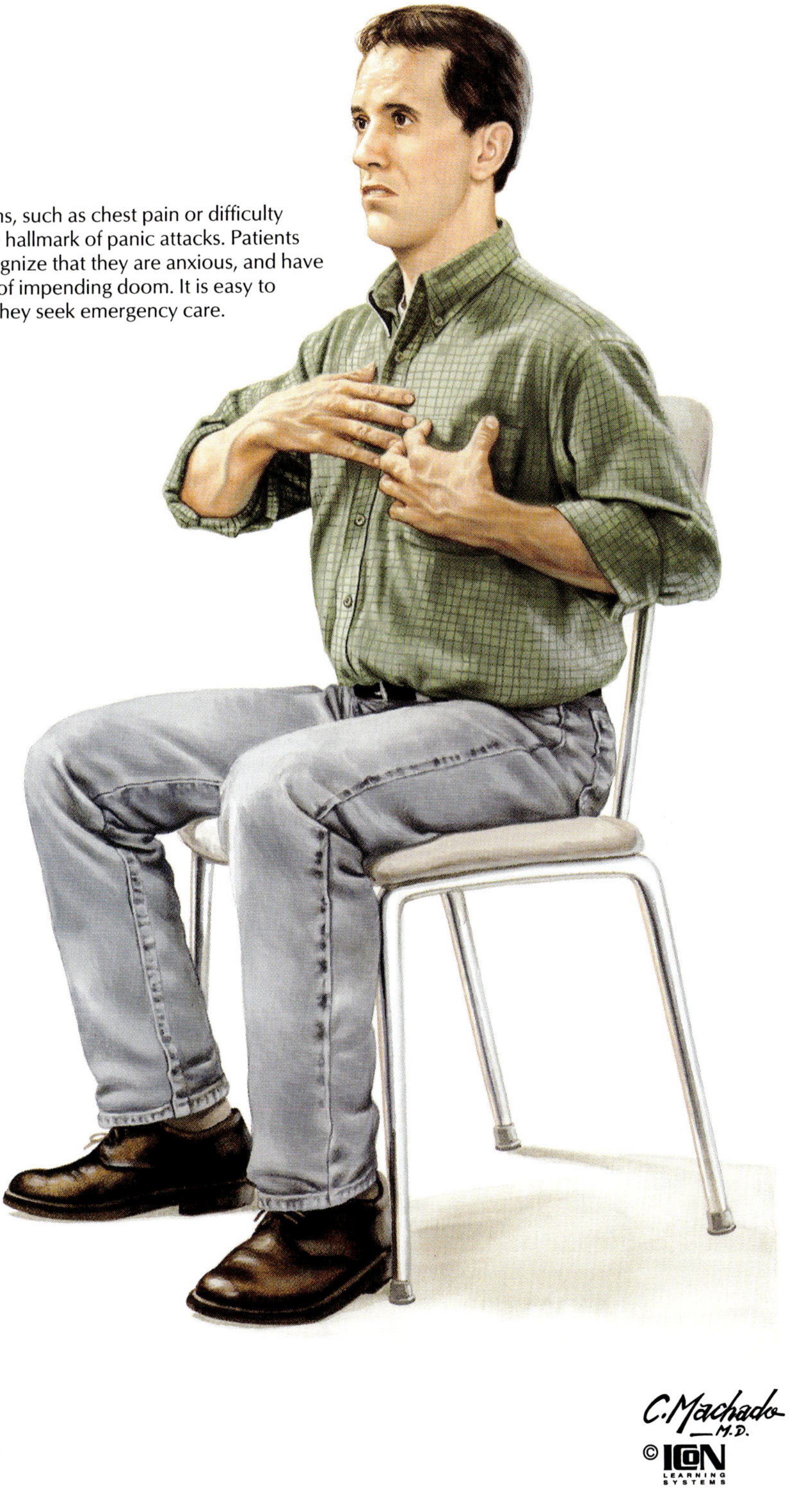

Somatic symptoms, such as chest pain or difficulty breathing, are the hallmark of panic attacks. Patients often do not recognize that they are anxious, and have a very real sense of impending doom. It is easy to understand why they seek emergency care.

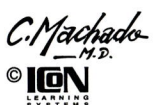

PSYCHIATRIC DISORDERS

PANIC DISORDER

TREATMENT

Psychotherapeutic approaches to panic disorder include patient education about the medically benign natural history of the syndrome and remediation of patients' catastrophic thinking and overgeneralizations. For some, this is sufficient, although most phobic patients also need a course of graded exposure to feared situations.

Many patients require pharmacologic treatment. Benzodiazepines abort panic attacks quickly and can be used as needed if attacks are infrequent. Most antidepressant medications (possibly excepting bupropion) have antipanic efficacy; they are the first choice for extended treatment. Anxious patients are sensitive to the initial activating or anxiogenic effects of antidepressants and need to begin with lower-than-usual doses. Monoamine oxidase inhibitors may work when other antidepressants are ineffective. However, caution is needed with monoamine oxidase inhibitors because of their potential for serious adverse effects.

REFERENCES

Barlow D. *Anxiety and Its Disorders: The Nature and Treatment of Anxiety and Panic.* New York, NY: Guilford; 2002.

Gorman JM, ed. *Fear and Anxiety: The Benefits of Translational Research.* Washington, DC: American Psychiatric Publishing; 2004.

Klein DF. False suffocation alarms, spontaneous panics, and related conditions: an integrative hypothesis. *Arch Gen Psych.* 1993;50:280-285.

Chapter 42
Dysthymia

Kenneth Lakritz

Clinical Vignette

A 47-year-old woman was referred by her internist, who was uncertain of a diagnosis but wondered whether she was depressed. The patient resented the referral but agreed to a single consultation. Her primary symptoms were chronic fatigue and diffuse achiness. She admitted inadequate and poor-quality sleep, impaired concentration, migratory chest pain, and migraine headaches.

She had been clearly depressed at the age of 19 years after her father's death and at the age of 26 years after the birth of her first child but did not report current feelings of sadness, guilt, or hopelessness. She described herself as overworked, justifiably pessimistic, socially isolated, and burdened with an unappreciative and unsympathetic husband. She wondered whether she had chronic fatigue syndrome, fibromyalgia, or multiple chemical sensitivities, but she had no obvious delusions about her health. An extensive medical workup had revealed iron deficiency anemia and hypothyroidism, both now corrected. She was sedentary, and her physician had recommended aerobic exercise, but she felt too tired to try it.

She reluctantly acknowledged that her pessimism and low mood might be contributing to her problems. She agreed to a trial of cognitive behavioral therapy, which she found helpful and which induced her to exercise more and change jobs. She also convinced her husband to start marriage counseling.

Mood disorders are extremely common and diverse in their presentation and clinical course. Previously called *minor depression* and *subsyndromal depression*, dysthymia is among the most common and easily overlooked.

CLINICAL PRESENTATION

Patients with dysthymia have fewer and less intense depressive symptoms than patients with major depression. To establish the diagnosis, the *Diagnostic and Statistical Manual of Mental Disorders, Fourth Edition*, requires at least a 2-year course of predominantly depressed mood, while noting that chronic low mood may be such a fixture of the patient's life as to be unrecognized by the patient. Two other symptoms must also be present from a list including sleep disturbance, appetite disturbance, fatigue, hopelessness, low self-esteem, and impaired concentration (Figure 42-1). Dysthymia usually has an early and insidious onset and a chronic course. Family history of mood disorder is common.

Although dysthymic patients do not meet the criteria for a diagnosis of major depression, dysthymia is not a benign illness. As a chronic disease, it causes immense suffering and loss of human potential. Dysthymic patients do less well than they should at school, at work, and in personal relationships. They overuse medical resources and substances, both legal and illegal. They are at high risk for the development of more severe affective disorders, one of the most common being "double depression," a pattern of repeated major depressive episodes with partial recovery to a state of dysthymia.

Most physicians follow patients with poorly characterized pain or other vague but persistent physical complaints. Even after excluding appropriate medical diagnoses, hypochondriasis, malingering, and delusional disorder, puzzling cases remain and are best understood as disguised presentations of dysthymia. Rheumatologists, gastroenterologists, and neurologists see large numbers of dysthymic patients. Patients and clinicians are usually frustrated and resentful.

TREATMENT

Patients with dysthymia deserve careful evaluation and intensive treatment. They often re-

DYSTHYMIA

Figure 42-1

Dysthymia
Some of the common complaints of dysthymic patients may include:

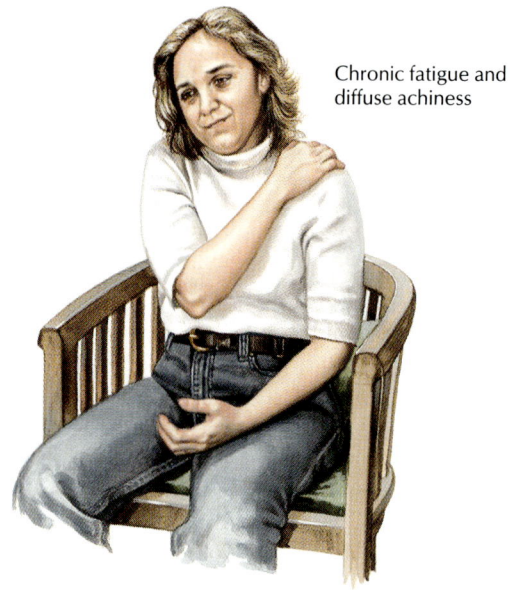

Chronic fatigue and diffuse achiness

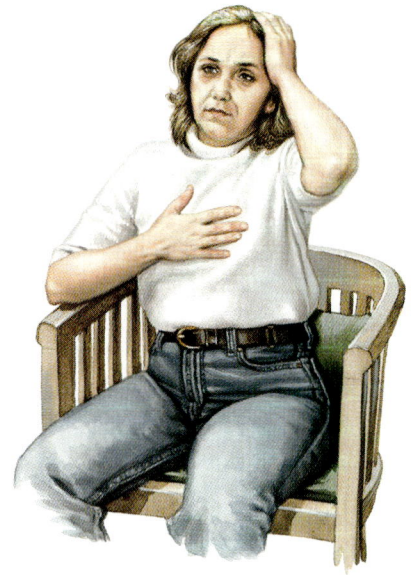

Headache and poorly localized chest or abdominal pain without positive physical findings

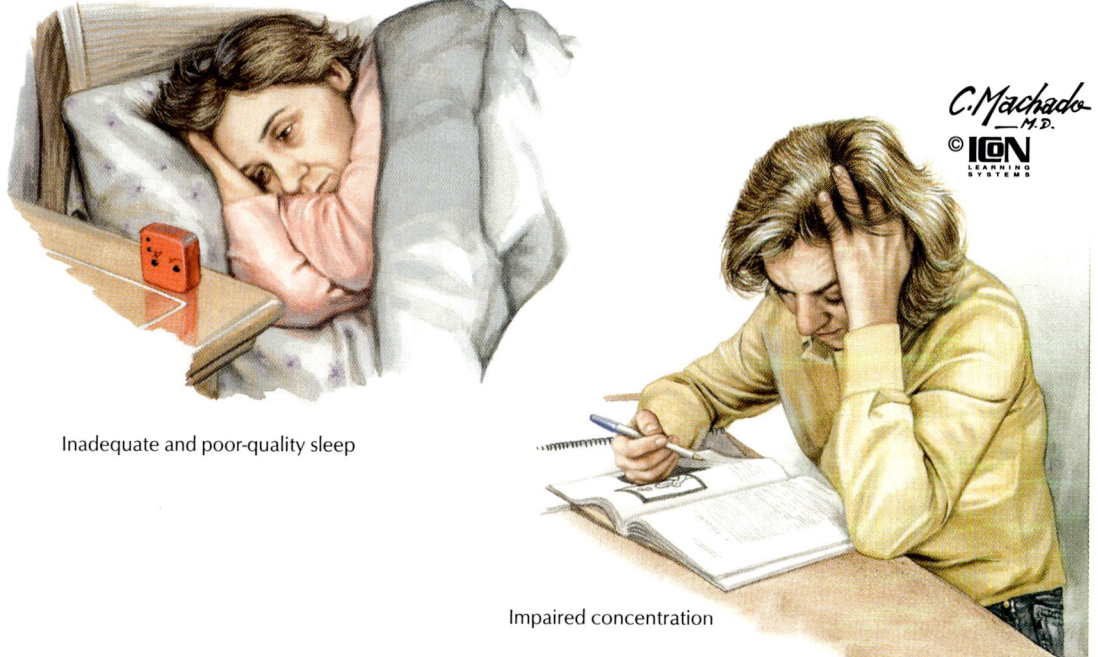

Inadequate and poor-quality sleep

Impaired concentration

PSYCHIATRIC DISORDERS

spond well to specific counseling techniques, such as cognitive-behavioral therapy or interpersonal therapy. Often, a combination of psychotherapy and antidepressant medication produces the best outcome.

REFERENCES

American Psychiatric Association. *Diagnostic and Statistical Manual of Mental Disorders*. 4th ed. Washington, DC: American Psychiatric Press; 1994.

Ratey J, Johnson K. *Shadow Syndromes: The Mild Forms of Major Mental Disorders That Sabotage Us*. New York, NY: Pantheon Books; 1997.

Chapter 43
Borderline Personality Disorder

Kenneth Lakritz

Clinical Vignette

A 24-year-old woman was brought to the ED by her parents after cutting her wrists, apparently in response to the loss of a 6-week romance. Her injuries were superficial, but she remained suicidal and would not reassure staff about another attempt. When committed for inpatient treatment, however, she attempted to flee and threatened to file a lawsuit.

This was the patient's fifth psychiatric hospitalization in 3 years; all but 1 had been preceded by a suicide gesture or attempt. The patient lived with her parents and sporadically took adult education courses with a vague ambition to direct films. Despite high intelligence, she had failed 3 tries at college; in 1 instance, she was dismissed for selling drugs. She had seen 4 therapists but derided them as "only being in it for the money."

Her arms showed multiple burn marks, and she admitted burning herself with cigarettes "to relieve tension." Her dentition was poor, and she acknowledged binge eating and purging.

She quickly established an alliance with a psychotic male patient and announced plans to move in with him when she was discharged. She was angry and sarcastic with some staff members but pleasant with others, leading to disagreements over her treatment and disposition.

Psychoanalysts of the 1920s and 1930s described patients who appeared superficially healthy but could not be analyzed because of their inability to establish a stable therapeutic relationship. These patients tended to have tumultuous life histories, poor social and vocational adjustment, and occasional brief regressions to psychosis. They were called *ambulatory schizophrenics, pseudoneurotic schizophrenics,* or *borderline schizophrenics*. The term *borderline* stuck.

CLINICAL PRESENTATION

In the 1950s, one subgroup of borderline patients was identified, patients with persistent odd or flat affect, mild but stable thought disorder, and family history of schizophrenia. These patients have a *forme fruste* of schizophrenia and are now diagnosed with schizotypal personality disorder.

The remaining borderline patients, those with *Diagnostic and Statistical Manual of Mental Disorders, Fourth Edition*, borderline personality disorder, are described as "the stably unstable." They have rapid mood fluctuations, are often strikingly angry, and react disastrously to minor slights and disappointments (Figure 43-1). Their interpersonal relationships are intense and stormy. They do not establish consistent vocational identities, frequently abuse drugs, injure themselves, and become briefly paranoid or disorganized.

Developmental psychologists and psychoanalysts speculate that this syndrome originates with a disordered parent-child relationship in the second and third years of life. Because of either parental inconsistency or the child's innate mood lability and aggression, borderline children are unable to integrate disparate experiences of parental love and hostility into a stable, "internalized" parent, leaving the child oscillating between extremes of idealization and devaluation in self-image and perception of others. This scheme receives support from documented high rates of childhood neglect and sexual abuse reported in hospitalized borderline patients.

TREATMENT

Borderline patients are frightening and exhausting to treat because frequent crises and their simultaneous neediness and hostility extend into the therapeutic relationship. Dialectical behavioral therapy, a comprehensive system of treatment with extensive institutional support

BORDERLINE PERSONALITY DISORDER

Figure 43-1   **Borderline Personality Disorder**

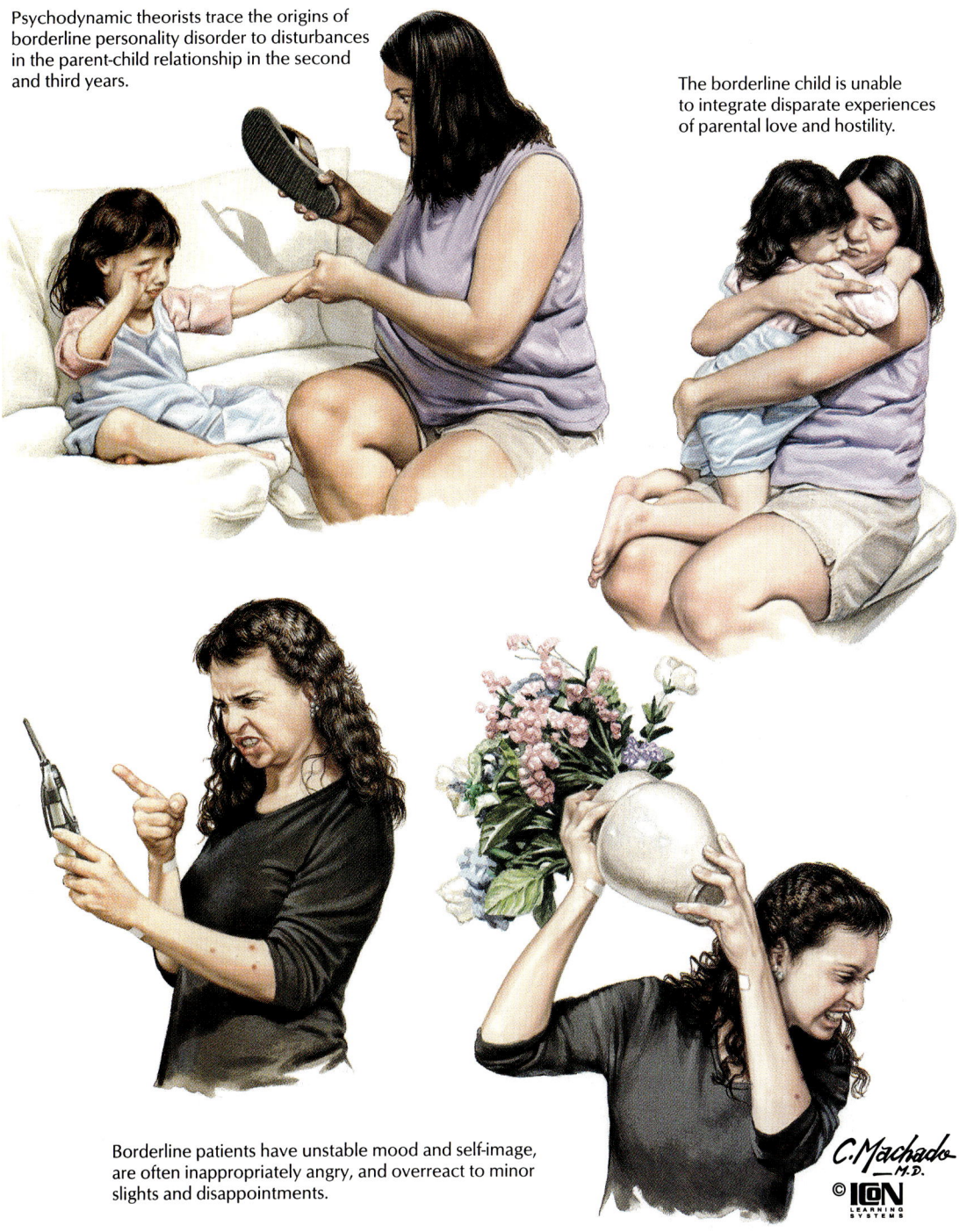

Psychodynamic theorists trace the origins of borderline personality disorder to disturbances in the parent-child relationship in the second and third years.

The borderline child is unable to integrate disparate experiences of parental love and hostility.

Borderline patients have unstable mood and self-image, are often inappropriately angry, and overreact to minor slights and disappointments.

BORDERLINE PERSONALITY DISORDER

for patients and therapists and a persistent emphasis on diminishing suicidal thinking and behavior, has shown great promise.

No clear medication guidelines are available. Low-dose antipsychotic medications are probably the most helpful. Lithium and other mood stabilizers sometimes help. By contrast, benzodiazepines may disinhibit borderline patients and are likely to be abused.

REFERENCE

American Psychiatric Association. *Diagnostic and Statistical Manual of Mental Disorders.* 4th ed. Washington, DC: American Psychiatric Press; 1994.

Chapter 44
Attention Deficit Disorder

Kenneth Lakritz

Clinical Vignette

A 26-year-old draftsman consulted a psychiatrist for help with anxiety. He had begun a job 3 months earlier and had just been placed on probation for slowness and inattention to detail. This was his third job in the 3 years since completing vocational education.

The patient reported falling behind at work but was unsure why. He admitted a tendency to procrastinate and was behind on his taxes and mortgage, despite having adequate funds. He described initial enthusiasm for his work that quickly faded and difficulty maintaining focus when work became "boring." He reported sporadic abuse of cocaine and alcohol.

He had been diagnosed with attention deficit disorder, hyperactive type, at the age of 8 years and was treated with methylphenidate, with good response, and maintained adequate academic progress. After high school graduation at the age of 18 years, the methylphenidate prescription was stopped, and the patient's hyperactivity had not reappeared.

The man in this vignette exemplifies an individual whose hyperactivity was successfully treated during childhood and later tolerated discontinuation of stimulant treatment but whose other cognitive limitations continued. He needs a retrial of medication.

CLINICAL PRESENTATION

Attention deficit hyperactivity disorder (ADHD) is a common, well-characterized, highly treatable neuropsychiatric disorder surrounded by social and political controversy. It is diagnosable in 3% to 9% of school-age children and is highly heritable. Some studies find higher prevalence in boys than in girls, but others dispute this, claiming that the sex disparity is an artifact of the more manifest hyperactivity and behavioral disturbance in boys. ADHD can present with or without hyperactivity. The core symptoms are distractibility and difficulty sustaining attention (Figure 44-1).

Imaging studies demonstrate anatomical abnormalities, usually size reduction or loss of symmetry, in the prefrontal cortex, striatum, and cerebellum. Functional imaging shows decreased frontal and striatal perfusion, especially on tests of sustained attention. Affected children are at increased risk for school failure, antisocial personality disorder, and substance abuse.

DIAGNOSIS

It had been thought that ADHD resolved spontaneously in adulthood. Hyperactivity does improve, but 50% of patients maintain their cognitive disabilities and need continued treatment. However, these patients must be distinguished from adults with new reports of restlessness, boredom, or impaired attention. ADHD is diagnosable by the age of 8 years and never starts in adulthood.

Attention deficit hyperactivity disorder must be distinguished from childhood mania. Both groups of patients are hyperactive and inattentive, but manic children are also irritable and usually overtalkative. This distinction can be difficult, in part because of comorbidity between the disorders; most patients with childhood-onset bipolar disorder also have ADHD. These children's mood symptoms should be treated first with mood stabilizers. A stimulant can then be added.

TREATMENT

Objections to current approaches to diagnosis and treatment of ADHD stem from its high prevalence and the fear that children are being inappropriately drugged, rather than having their educational needs carefully assessed and met. Although improper use of medication can occur, individual assessment and medical treatment are

ATTENTION DEFICIT DISORDER

Figure 44-1   ## Attention Deficit Disorder

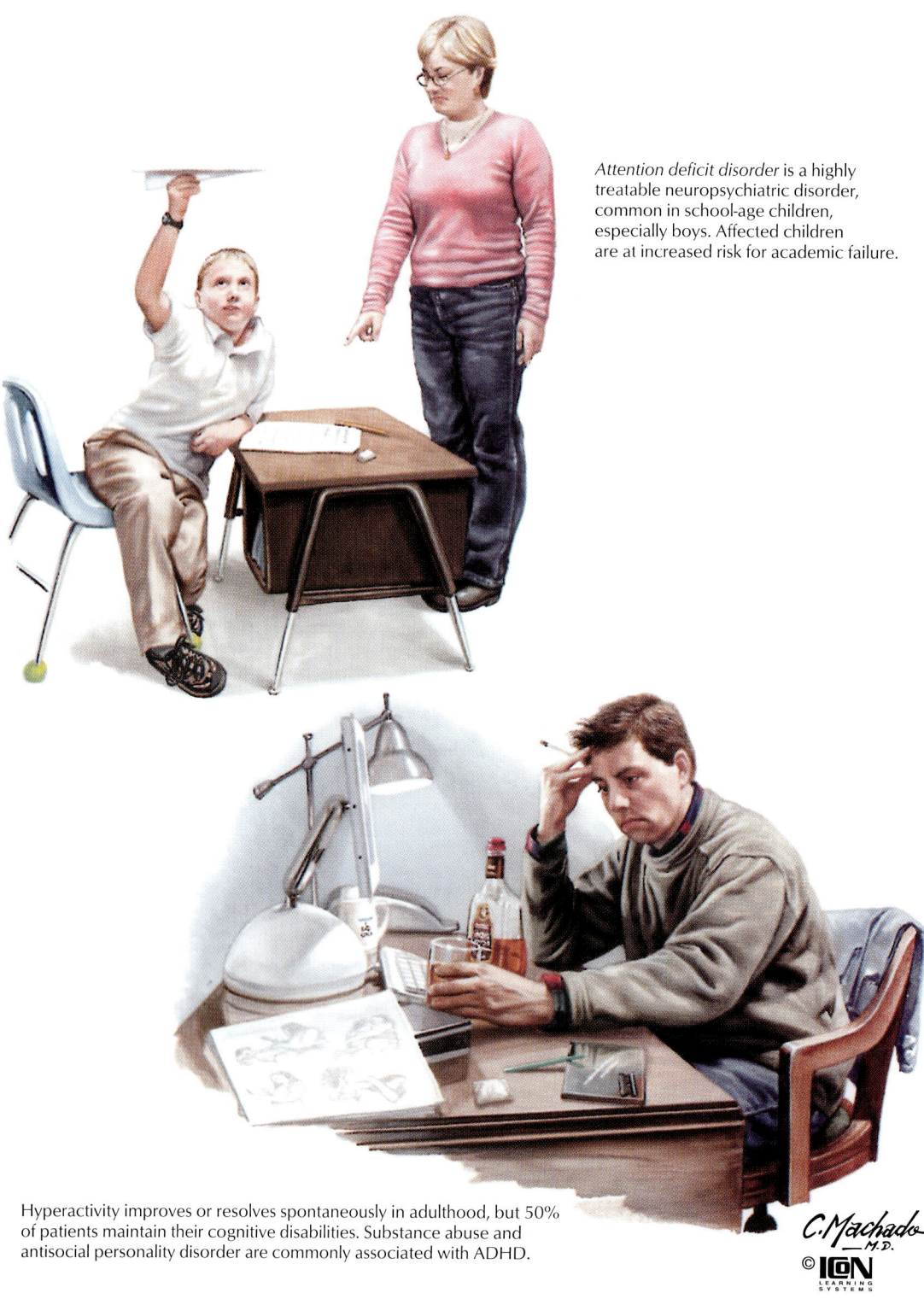

Attention deficit disorder is a highly treatable neuropsychiatric disorder, common in school-age children, especially boys. Affected children are at increased risk for academic failure.

Hyperactivity improves or resolves spontaneously in adulthood, but 50% of patients maintain their cognitive disabilities. Substance abuse and antisocial personality disorder are commonly associated with ADHD.

PSYCHIATRIC DISORDERS

not mutually exclusive, and failure to diagnose and treat a real illness is as undesirable as overtreatment.

Stimulant medications, the principal treatment, are highly effective and free of adverse effects. Fears that stimulants would promote illicit drug use have been dispelled by studies showing that appropriate treatment actually decreases future risk of drug abuse.

REFERENCE

American Psychiatric Association. *Diagnostic and Statistical Manual of Mental Disorders*. 4th ed. Washington, DC: American Psychiatric Press; 1994.

Chapter 45
Drug and Alcohol Abuse
Kenneth Lakritz

Clinical Vignette

A 57-year-old bank president was admitted to the hospital for elective hip replacement. Surgery was uncomplicated, but on the second postoperative day, the patient was anxious and diaphoretic and had a low-grade fever. Broad-spectrum antibiotic treatment was begun after a surgical site culture. That night, the patient seemed to have hallucinations of family members and hardly slept. The next morning, he had an observed grand mal seizure.

A neurologic consultant noted agitation, disorientation, impaired recall, visual hallucinations, tremor, and tachycardia. The patient had described his drinking as "2 per day," but his wife described those drinks as tumblers of scotch and estimated his intake at a pint of whiskey daily. He had no history of liver disease, gastrointestinal bleeding, blackouts, withdrawal symptoms, or occupational impairment.

The patient was started on high-dose benzodiazepines, thiamine, and fluid and electrolyte replacement. His autonomic signs rapidly stabilized, and he had no further seizures, but he remained confused and agitated for the next 2 weeks.

ALCOHOL ABUSE AND DEPENDENCE

Most physicians are intimately familiar with the protean manifestations of alcohol abuse (Figure 45-1) and dependence (Figure 45-2). Incidence rates vary widely between cultural groups (alcoholism is almost unheard of in traditional Muslim communities), but lifetime rates of 5% to 10% are the rule in North America and Europe. Therefore, doctors who never see alcoholism may be missing the diagnosis. The diagnosis can be missed easily, in part because of patient denial. This denial has several sources. Admitting to a problem with alcohol or other drugs may be humiliating for patients, and alcohol use, even at dangerous levels, is a culturally embedded and approved, often pleasurable part of social life.

Etiology

Liability to alcohol abuse and dependence, especially early-onset abuse, runs in families, but the mechanism of inheritance is not understood. Findings of a link between alcoholism and a particular dopamine DR-2 receptor allele remain controversial. Some Asian populations are relatively protected from alcoholism because they possess a variant form of the enzyme alcohol dehydrogenase and metabolize alcohol poorly. This causes them to become flushed and nauseated with minimal doses. Conversely, young adults with a high alcohol tolerance, evaluated on measures of incoordination or subjectively, are at increased risk for later alcoholism. Young adults often assume they are not getting into difficulties with drinking because of their tolerance. Physicians must convince them that this is wrong.

Alcohol is a CNS depressant with cross-tolerance to benzodiazepines, barbiturates, and some other sedatives. It is distinguished within this group by its ease of manufacture, legal status, wide availability, rapid absorption, and exceptionally low therapeutic index. The lethal dose of alcohol is only a few times the intoxicating dose; 1 bottle of whiskey can be lethal to an individual who has not acquired tolerance. The dose at which tissue damage occurs is lower and falls within the range of commonly ingested doses. In most adults, chemical signs of hepatic injury are detectable after consumption of 3 or more drinks within 24 hours. Alcohol is a potent fetal teratogen with no threshold dose; it is absolutely contraindicated in pregnancy.

Clinical Presentation

Acute alcohol intoxication at moderate doses causes disinhibition and incoordination. Even at

DRUG AND ALCOHOL ABUSE

Figure 45-1

Alcohol Abuse

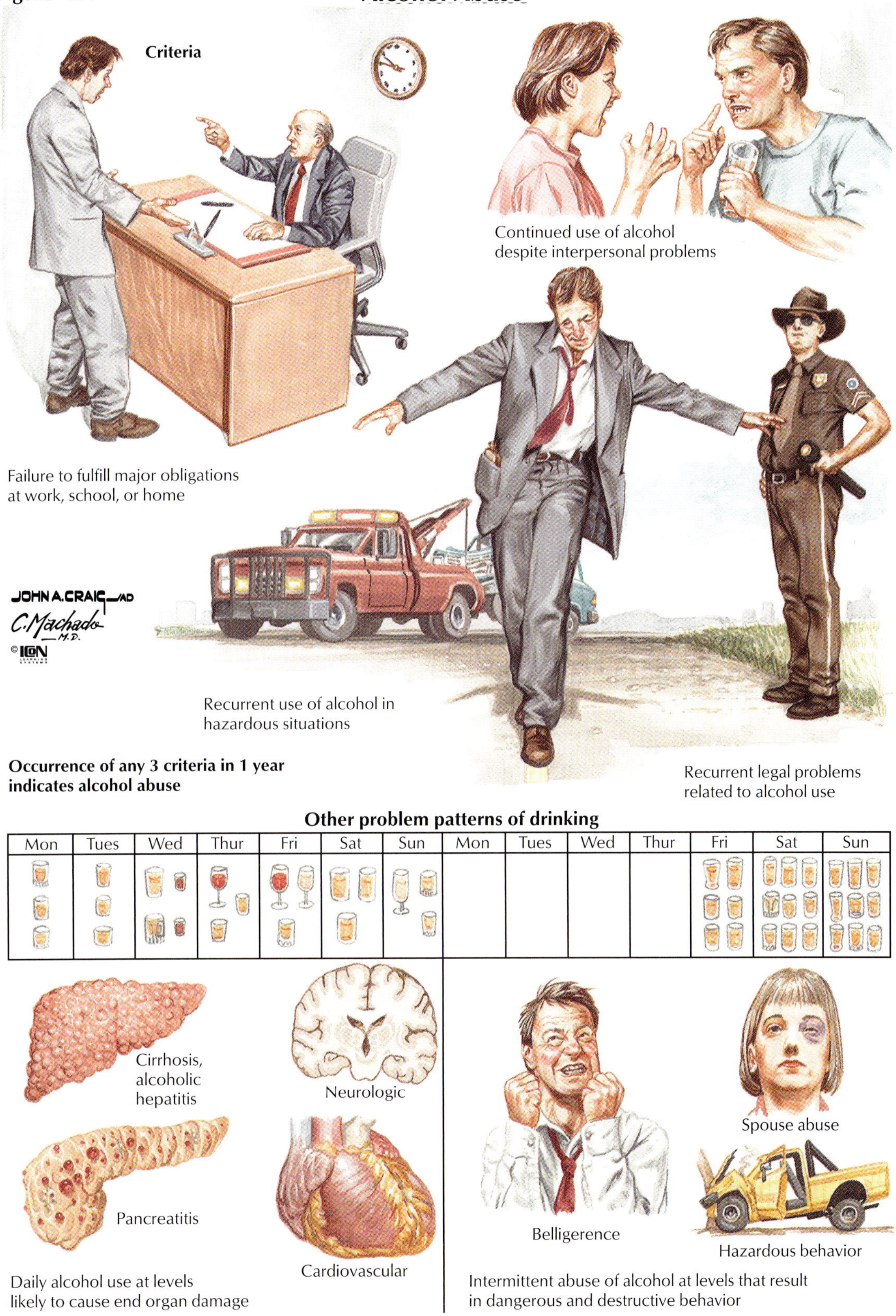

Criteria

Failure to fulfill major obligations at work, school, or home

Continued use of alcohol despite interpersonal problems

Recurrent use of alcohol in hazardous situations

Recurrent legal problems related to alcohol use

Occurrence of any 3 criteria in 1 year indicates alcohol abuse

Other problem patterns of drinking

Mon	Tues	Wed	Thur	Fri	Sat	Sun	Mon	Tues	Wed	Thur	Fri	Sat	Sun

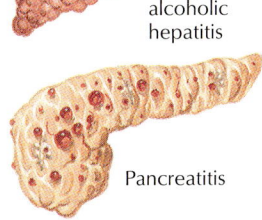

Cirrhosis, alcoholic hepatitis

Pancreatitis

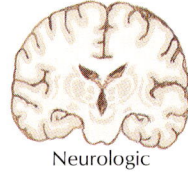
Neurologic

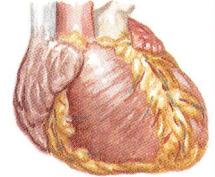
Cardiovascular

Daily alcohol use at levels likely to cause end organ damage

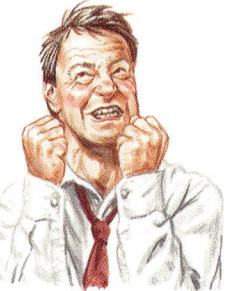
Belligerence

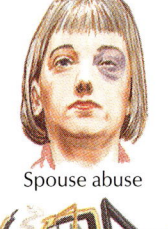
Spouse abuse

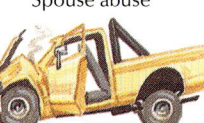
Hazardous behavior

Intermittent abuse of alcohol at levels that result in dangerous and destructive behavior

PSYCHIATRIC DISORDERS

391

DRUG AND ALCOHOL ABUSE

Figure 45-2

Alcohol Dependence

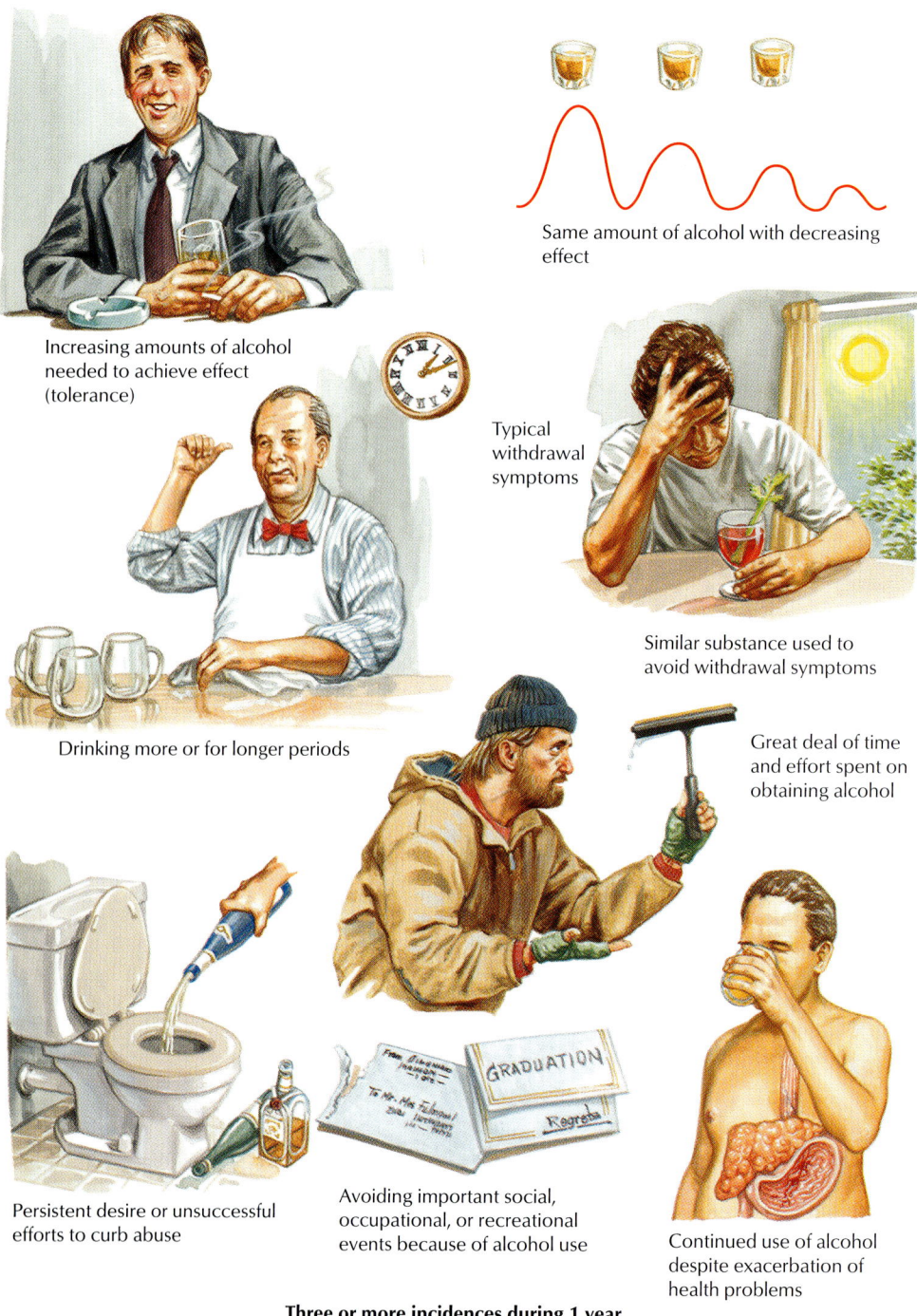

DRUG AND ALCOHOL ABUSE

Figure 45-3 Signs Suggestive of Alcohol Abuse

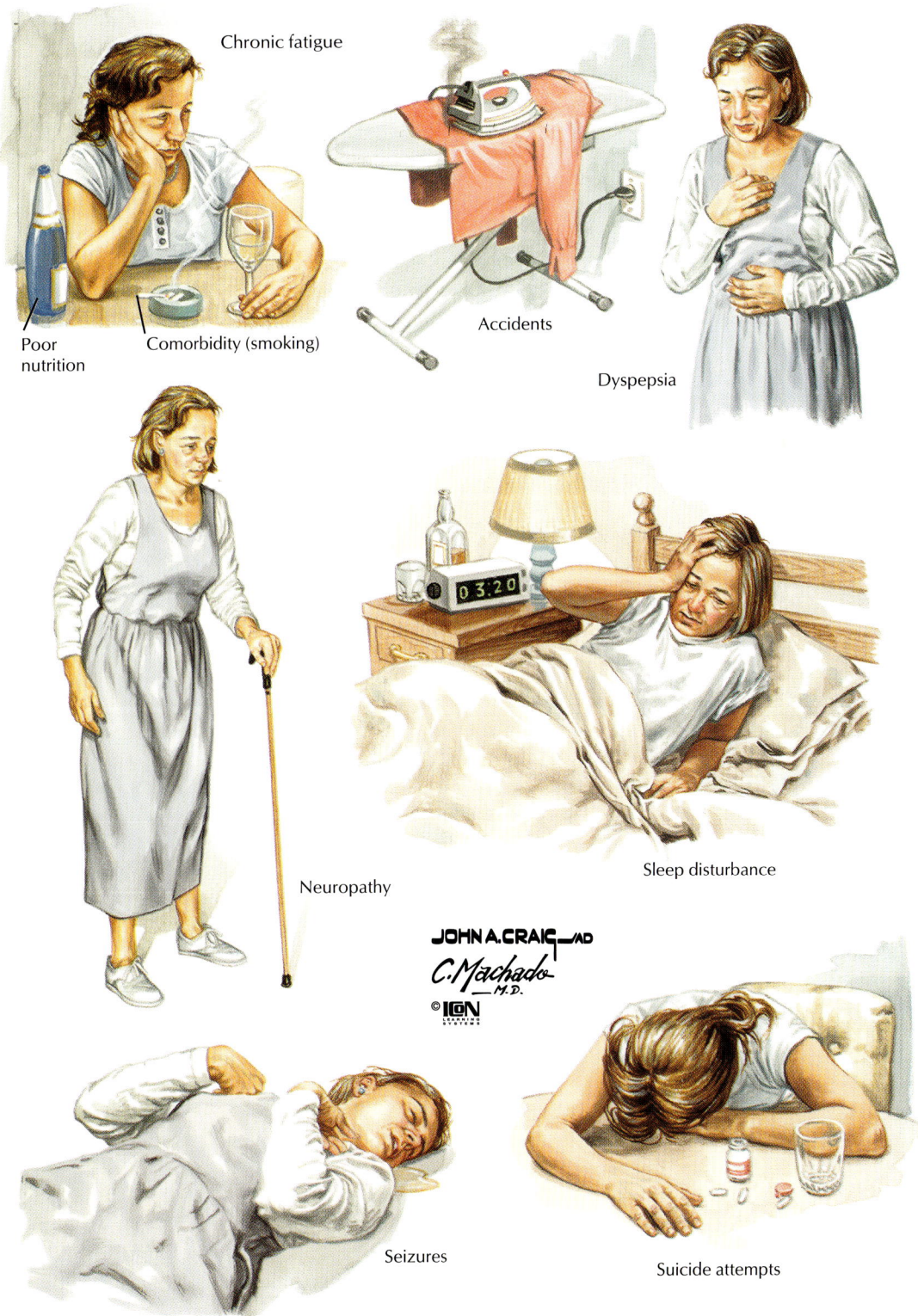

PSYCHIATRIC DISORDERS

DRUG AND ALCOHOL ABUSE

socially acceptable doses, it impairs driving and is implicated in approximately half of all highway accidents and deaths. It is linked to a similar proportion of sexual assaults.

Alcohol interacts with psychiatric illnesses and treatments. Patients with most major psychiatric illnesses have increased rates of alcohol abuse. Many patients use alcohol to treat mood disorders, anxiety, or insomnia, but it is not a safe or effective treatment for any medical disorder. The toxicity and short duration of action of alcohol make it useless as an anxiolytic, and it disrupts sleep architecture and decreases sleep efficiency. The combination of alcohol abuse and depression is especially lethal. Alcohol use makes patients who are depressed more depressed and interferes with antidepressant response. Drinkers who are depressed experience an approximately 10-fold increase in suicide rate compared with nondrinkers who are depressed.

Alcohol has direct toxic effects on multiple tissues, including the liver, the pancreas, and the heart, and the CNS. Patients may present with acute or chronic hepatitis, cirrhosis, esophageal varices, cardiomyopathy, and dementia. Wernicke syndrome, a neurologic emergency resulting from acute thiamine and other B-vitamin depletion, is seen almost exclusively in alcoholics and presents with confusion, ophthalmoplegia, and ataxia. Without immediate repletion of thiamine, Wernicke syndrome may progress to Korsakoff psychosis, which is a devastating inability to form and consolidate long-term memories and another syndrome mostly confined to alcoholics.

Diagnosis

To avoid missing diagnoses of alcohol abuse or dependence, physicians must maintain a high index of suspicion and make alcoholism screening a part of their routine (Figure 45-3). Asking about average levels and patterns of alcohol use should be part of every examination. Because patients underestimate their consumption, a useful rule of thumb is to double the amount reported by the patient. Patients should also be questioned about binge drinking, withdrawal signs, blackouts, and excessive tolerance. The 4-question CAGE questionnaire is a good screening instrument (Table 45-1). One positive answer to a CAGE question is cause for concern; 2 positive answers corresponds to a 50% risk of alcoholism.

Patients with even 1 drunk-driving conviction can be safely assumed to have a problem with alcohol, as can the occasional patient who presents in an intoxicated state for his appointment. In the latter case, the physician must take whatever steps necessary to prevent the patient from driving away from the office.

When diagnostic uncertainty persists, interviewing family or friends is often decisive; typically, they present a more accurate picture of the patient's drinking. Laboratory test results that reveal increased GGTP or transaminase levels, mild macrocytic anemia, or both can add confirmatory evidence. Asking the patient to stop drinking for 6 months is helpful as both a diagnostic and a therapeutic maneuver. Heavy drinkers who achieve a few months of sobriety may feel so much better that they stay sober, and patients who refuse are obviously in trouble.

Treatment

Successful long-term treatment of alcoholism and other addictions demands a reorientation of the patient's life and a commitment to sobriety. Inpatient treatment is often required at the outset and may be necessary for relapses. Patients must be educated in relapse prevention principles. They need to learn how to recognize and avoid the cues that set off their drinking. Patients who return to their favorite bar armed only with a determination to stick to soft drinks will fail. Alcoholics Anonymous and other therapeutic communities can be lifesaving.

Table 45-1
CAGE Questionnaire

Ask patients whether
- they have felt a need to **C**ut down their intake.
- others have **A**nnoyed them by criticizing their drinking.
- they have felt **G**uilty about their drinking.
- they have ever needed an **E**ye-opener (a morning drink) to calm their nerves or treat a hangover.

DRUG AND ALCOHOL ABUSE

Figure 45-4 Alcohol Withdrawal

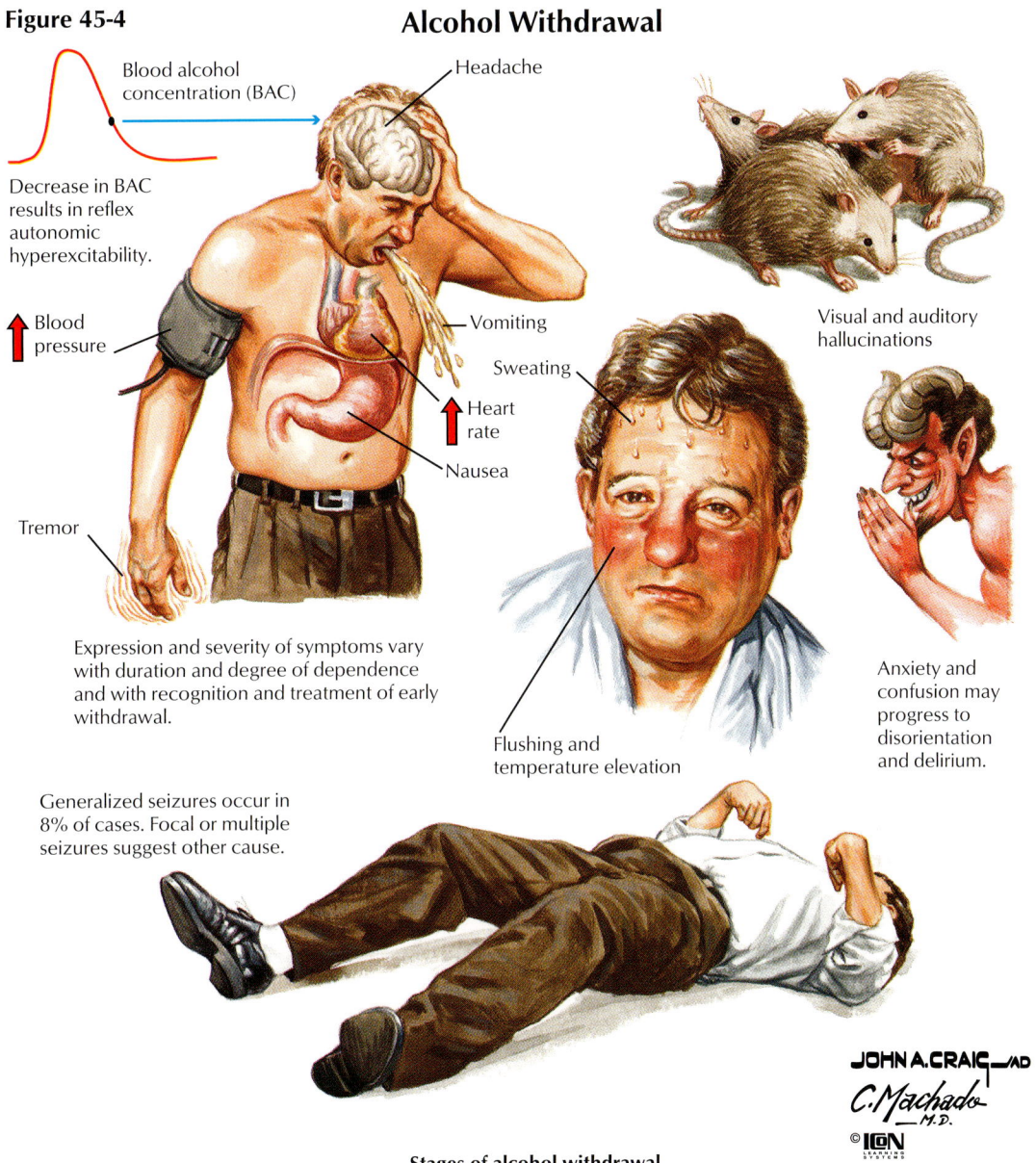

Stages of alcohol withdrawal

	Stage 1	Stage 2	Stage 3
Hours after alcohol consumption	24 36 (peak) 48	(48-72)	(72-105)
Symptoms	Mild-to-moderate anxiety, tremor, nausea, vomiting, sweating, elevation of heart rate and blood pressure, sleep disturbance, hallucinations, illusions, seizures	Aggravated forms of stage 1 symptoms with severe tremors, agitation, and hallucinations	Acute organic psychosis (delirium), confusion, and disorientation with severe autonomic symptoms

Stage 1 withdrawal usually self-limited. Only small percentage of cases progress to stages 2 and 3. Progression prevented by prompt and adequate treatment.

PSYCHIATRIC DISORDERS

DRUG AND ALCOHOL ABUSE

Figure 45-5

Opioid Withdrawal
Signs and Symptoms

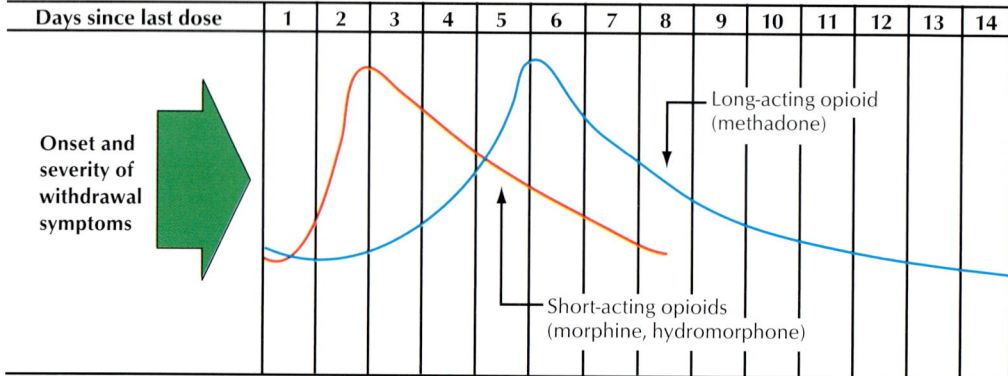

Sweating
Dilated pupils
Lacrimation
Rhinorrhea
Yawning

Nausea and vomiting
Diarrhea

Locus ceruleus

Noradrenergic effects of withdrawal (mediated via locus ceruleus) increase heart rate and blood pressure.

Noradrenergic effects may be blocked by α_2 agonists.

↑ Blood pressure
Heart rate

Insomnia and muscle aches are mediated via μ receptors and relieved by μ agonists.

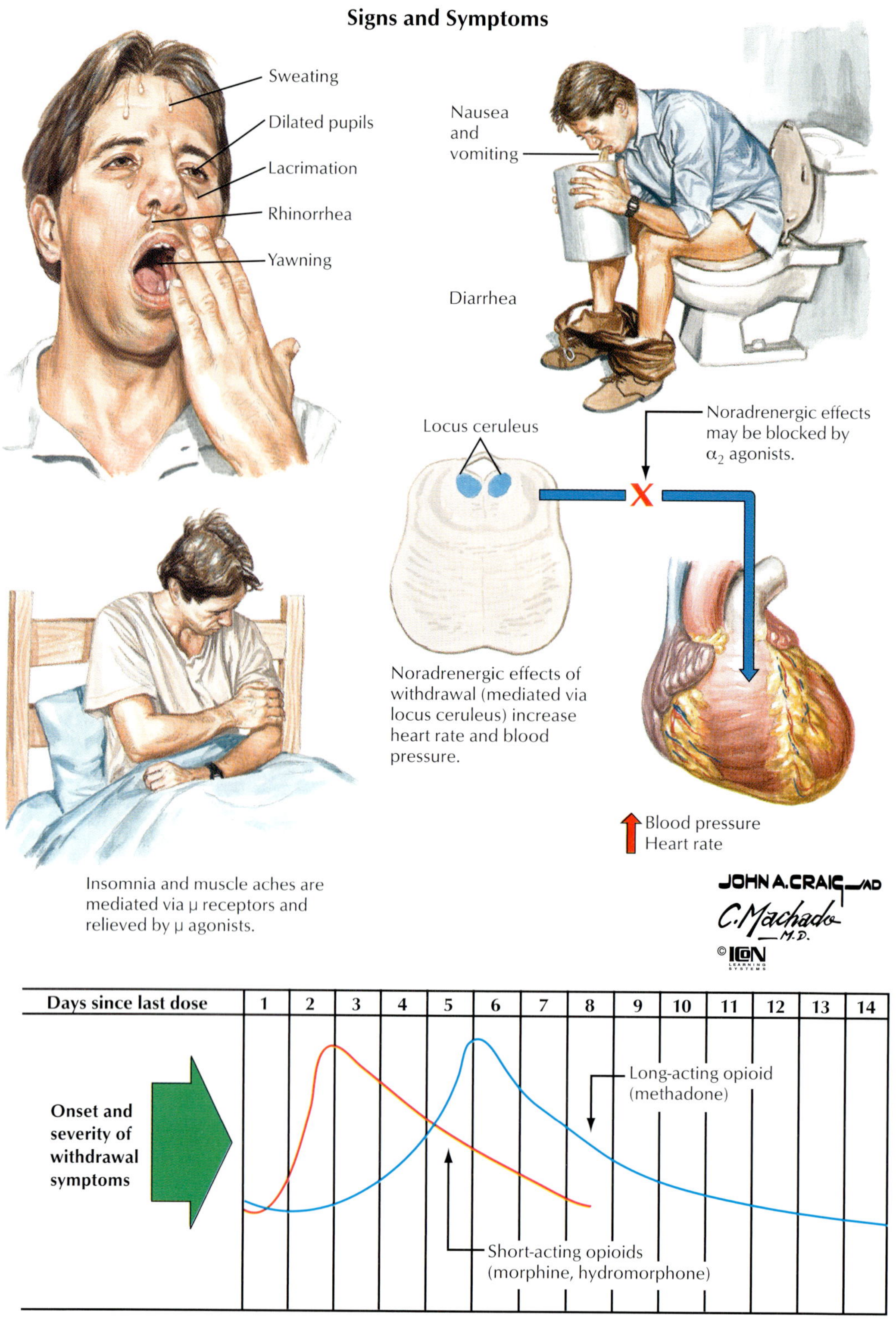

Severity of opioid withdrawal varies with dose and duration of opioid use. Onset and duration of symptoms after last drug dose depend on half-life of particular drug.

PSYCHIATRIC DISORDERS

DRUG AND ALCOHOL ABUSE

Figure 45-6 Benzodiazepine Withdrawal

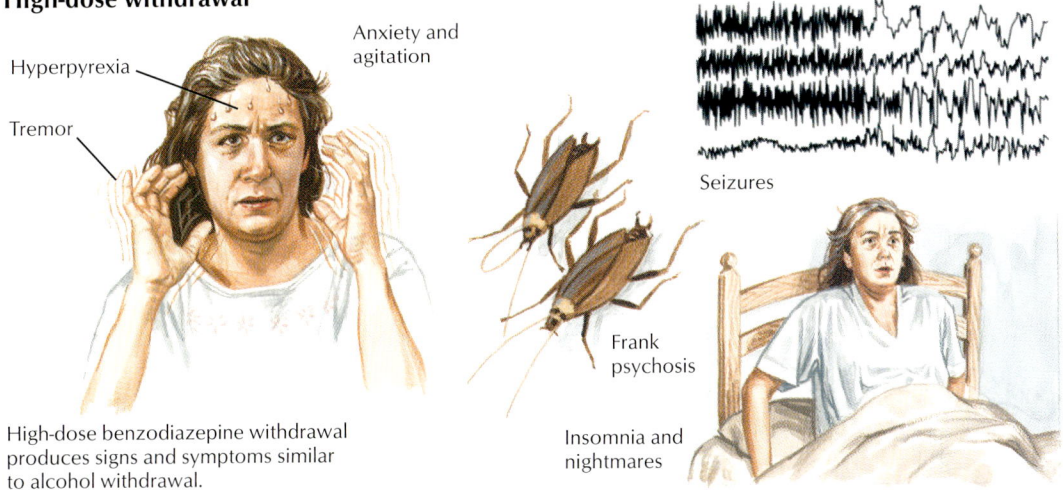

High-dose benzodiazepine withdrawal produces signs and symptoms similar to alcohol withdrawal.

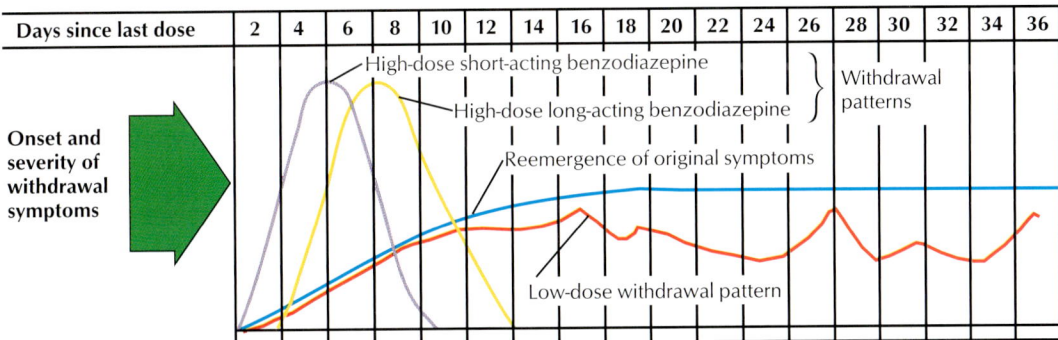

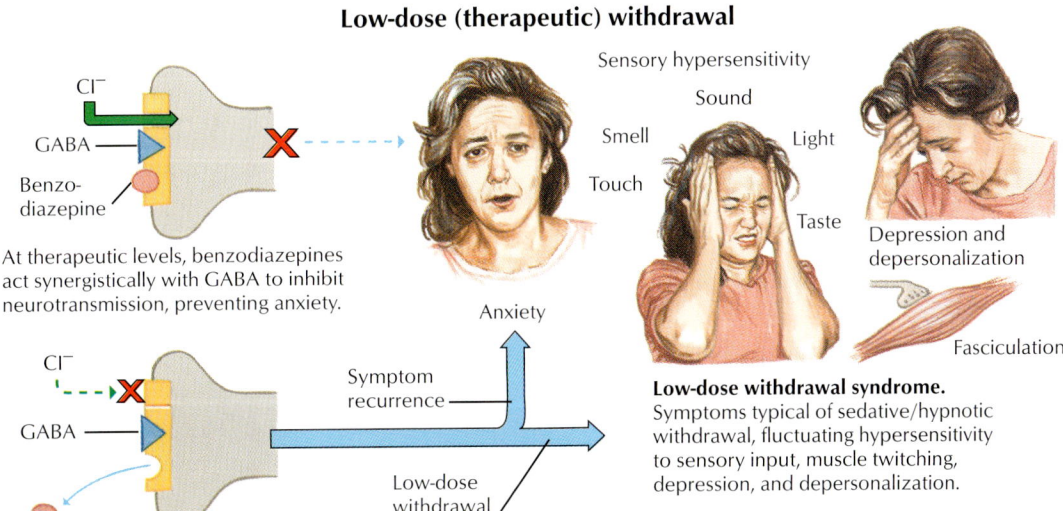

Low-dose withdrawal syndrome. Symptoms typical of sedative/hypnotic withdrawal, fluctuating hypersensitivity to sensory input, muscle twitching, depression, and depersonalization.

Withdrawing long-term benzodiazepine causes loss of synergism with GABA inhibition, resulting in recurrence of original symptoms and low-dose withdrawal syndrome.

PSYCHIATRIC DISORDERS

DRUG AND ALCOHOL ABUSE

The pharmacologic treatment of alcoholism remains limited. Disufiram discourages drinking by producing a painful and potentially dangerous syndrome when taken in combination with alcohol. However, it is appropriate only for the minority with intact hepatic function, generally reliable judgment, and a pattern of binge drinking. Naltrexone, an opiate antagonist, discourages drinking by blunting the euphoric response to alcohol. It may be more effective when combined with acamprosate, an investigational agent.

Delirium Tremens

As in the vignette at the beginning of this chapter, withdrawal symptoms may come as a surprise and can be deadly (Figure 45-4). Without prompt diagnosis and appropriate treatment, delirium tremens, a major medical emergency that can occur in any social group, is associated with a 15% mortality rate. Withdrawal syndromes are treated with B vitamins and benzodiazepines or other cross-tolerant anticonvulsants, and the doses required can be exceptionally high. Patients who are acutely ill are at risk for seizures, fluid and electrolyte imbalances, and infections.

DRUG ABUSE AND DEPENDENCE

The rubric of drug abuse subsumes dozens of syndromes, but a few useful generalizations can be offered. Most drugs have safe and unsafe uses. Physicians routinely use opiates, sedative-hypnotics, psychostimulants, and dissociative anesthetics, all of which have abuse and addiction potential. Even over-the-counter drugs can be abused. Conversely, illegal or widely abused substances such as cannabinoids and nicotine have, or are likely to have, future medical uses.

Potentially abusable drugs cause dopamine release in several forebrain structures. Beyond this, dosage, route of administration, and social context are the factors that make drugs dangerous. High doses, routes of administration that rapidly deliver drug to the brain, and use outside a stable social or religious context all predispose substances to abuse and addiction. These factors, not the pharmacology, explain why the Peruvian practice of chewing coca leaves is safe but smoking freebase cocaine is not.

Liability to other addictions, like liability to alcoholism, may be partially inherited. Physiologic and epidemiologic evidence suggests that the adolescent brain is especially vulnerable to addiction, particularly to nicotine. Few smoking habits begin after the age of 18 years.

Treatment

The goal of treatment is abstinence. Therapies incorporating a return to controlled use have been proposed and are always unsuccessful. Patients who are addicted must remove themselves from the environments where drugs are available and where their use is permitted. Pharmacologic replacement of illicit opiates with methadone (Figure 45-5) or buprenorphine can be effective, as is substituting transdermal nicotine for cigarettes. Other medication treatments are only mildly helpful, and none work without a commitment to sobriety.

Persons with psychiatric illnesses, especially bipolar disorder, attention deficit hyperactivity disorder, and personality disorders are at heightened risk for drug abuse and dependence (Figure 45-6). Patients with a dual diagnosis are the rule rather than the exception and need simultaneous treatment for both disorders.

REFERENCE

American Psychiatric Association. *Diagnostic and Statistical Manual of Mental Disorders, 4th ed.* Washington, DC: American Psychiatric Press; 1994.

Chapter 46
Delirium

Kenneth Lakritz

Clinical Vignette

A 78-year-old retired teacher was brought to the ED by her daughter, who had found her confused. Usually gregarious, the patient had not been outside her house in 4 days. A concerned neighbor found her house in disarray, with the patient sitting quietly in her bedclothes in midafternoon. She did not recognize her visitor.

The patient had been in excellent health until 1 month previously, when thoracic shingles had developed. Although her rash had faded, she still had intense burning and stinging pain. Her primary physician had prescribed oxycodone, amitriptyline, and gabapentin.

Neurologic examination revealed her to be quiet, polite, and healthy appearing but disheveled. She was oriented to person but disoriented to date and place. Her short-term memory was profoundly impaired. There were no focal neurologic signs. CSF test results were normal. Cranial MRI showed mild and diffuse atrophy. EEG results demonstrated nonspecific slowing.

The patient's new medications were withheld; her confusion resolved within 72 hours, and her postherpetic pain was managed with topical capsaicin, NSAIDs, and a low-dose oral narcotic. She was discharged in good condition but declined cognitively and was diagnosed with Alzheimer disease 2 years after her admission.

This vignette demonstrates the potential for well-meaning physicians to cause delirium by overmedicating a patient. Patients can also make themselves delirious by hoarding and abusing appropriately prescribed medications. Therefore, suspicion of overmedication or drug abuse is warranted in any patient presenting with delirium. Like the woman in the above vignette, some individuals have an underlying chronic neurologic condition that is "uncovered" by overmedication.

CLINICAL PRESENTATION

Because delirium is easily mistaken for psychosis or oppositional behavior, it is frequently encountered by neurologic and psychiatric consultants. Delirium is a medical emergency; therefore, correcting misdiagnoses is crucial.

Delirious patients can be quietly confused or agitated (Figure 46-1). Characteristically, their mental state fluctuates by the hour, often causing disagreements among clinicians. Many patients are worse at night—sundowning—presumably because of diminished sensory input and social interaction. Whatever the presentation, the core of the syndrome is a subtly diminished level of consciousness, resulting in disorientation, distractibility, and impaired short-term memory.

Additional signs may suggest specific diagnoses. Tremor, restlessness, diaphoresis, and tachycardia suggest alcohol or sedative withdrawal. Mydriasis, flushing, and dry mucous membranes imply anticholinergic toxicity. However, the clinical state of delirium is nonspecific and has diverse causes, including other withdrawal states and intoxications, CNS infections, respiratory insufficiency, liver failure, and endocrine disturbances. A careful history and review of systems can often identify the cause and lead to appropriate therapy.

Although anyone can become delirious, the elderly, the demented, and others with limited cognitive reserve are most vulnerable. While delirium is, in principle, distinguishable from dementia by its more rapid onset and reversibility, in practice, the 2 conditions often coexist. Mildly impaired elders who become confused taking the wrong sleeping pill or painkiller for an otherwise asymptomatic urinary tract infection are familiar to most physicians.

REFERENCE

American Psychiatric Association. *Diagnostic and Statistical Manual of Mental Disorders.* 4th ed. Washington, DC: American Psychiatric Press; 1994.

DELIRIUM

Figure 46-1
Delirium

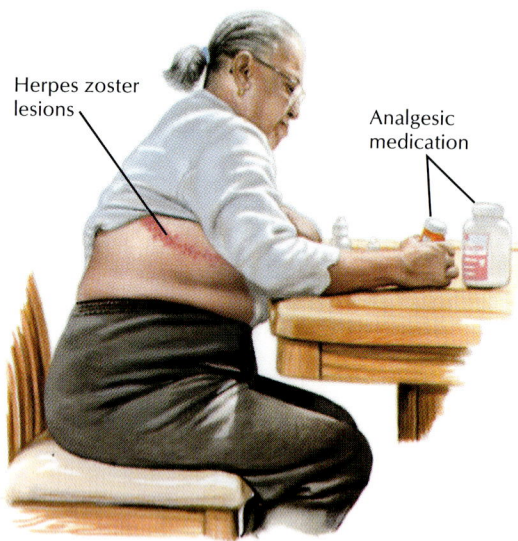

Use of analgesics and sedatives can precipitate delirium in patients with limited cognitive reserve, especially the elderly and the demented.

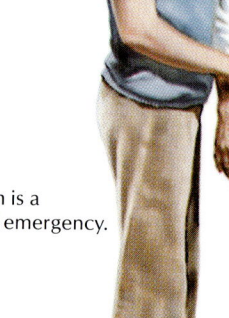

Delirium is a medical emergency.

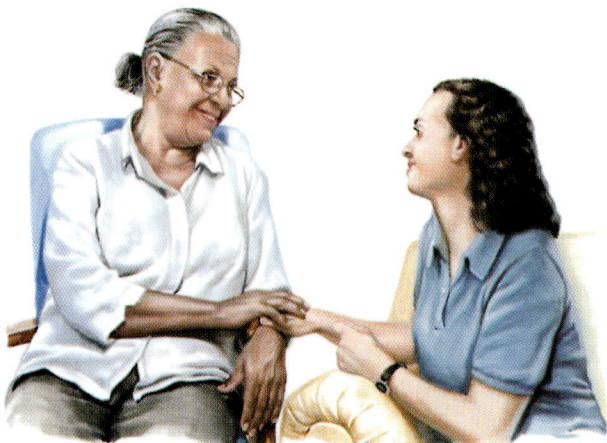

The mental state of delirious patients often changes from hour to hour.

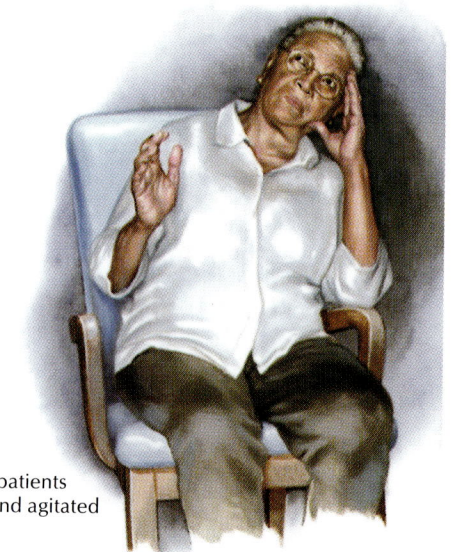

"Sundowning." Delirious patients are often more confused and agitated at night.

PSYCHIATRIC DISORDERS

Section XI
MOVEMENT DISORDERS

Chapter 47
Parkinson Disease 402

Chapter 48
Atypical Parkinsonian Syndromes 414

Chapter 49
Tremors 422

Chapter 50
Medication-Induced Movement Disorders 432

Chapter 51
Dystonia 438

Chapter 52
Myoclonus 447

Chapter 53
Chorea 453

Chapter 54
Tic Disorders 460

Chapter 55
Wilson Disease 466

Chapter 56
Psychogenic Movement Disorders 472

Chapter 57
Surgical Treatments for Movement Disorders 475

Chapter 47
Parkinson Disease

Diana Apetauerova

Clinical Vignette

A 79-year-old, right-handed, retired teacher presented with a 5-year history of generalized slowness of movement, especially walking; increasingly smaller handwriting (micrographia); and difficulty dressing and performing other fine motor tasks with his right hand. His speech had become slow and soft; occasionally, it was difficult to understand. Two years previously, a resting tremor of his right hand developed. Stress worsened the symptoms. He was not taking any medications that could lead to parkinsonism.

On neurologic examination, his facial expression was nonanimated or masklike, and he tended to drool. His BP was normal, with no orthostasis. He had slight problems with memory recall. His speech was hypophonic and slow. There was mild cogwheel rigidity of all extremities, more prominent on the right, and axial rigidity. He had a 6-Hz resting tremor of both hands, again more prominent on the right. Rapid alternating movements and foot tapping were slow and irregular, more so on the right than on the left. His muscle strength was normal. Initiation of all movements was slow. His gait was shuffling, with a forward flexed posture. While walking, the usual arm swing was absent, and his hand tremors were prominent. When he attempted to turn, he was hesitant and required a few extra small steps. Retropulsion was observed when pulling him backward to test his postural stability.

Head CT scan was normal. No other investigations were indicated because the diagnosis of Parkinson disease (PD) is clinical. Because of the patient's moderate functional impairment and his age, levodopa/carbidopa was initiated. Within 4 weeks, he demonstrated marked improvement. He was able to move faster, and his fine motor activities and tremor were significantly improved. This excellent response suggested idiopathic PD as the likely diagnosis.

Idiopathic *PD*, named by James Parkinson's 1817 description, is a neurodegenerative disorder characterized by bradykinesia, resting tremor, cogwheel rigidity, and postural reflex impairment. PD is one of the most common neurological disorders, affecting at least 1,000,000 persons in the United States. Typical onset is between 40 and 70 years of age, with peaks in the sixth decade of life. Usually, clinical status progresses from a relatively modest limitation at diagnosis to an ever-increasing disability over 10 to 20 years. The primary neuropathologic features are the loss of pigmented dopaminergic neurons mainly in the substantia nigra (SN) and the presence of Lewy bodies, eosinophilic, cytoplasmic inclusions found within the pigmented neurons (Figures 47-1 and 47-2). The cause of PD is unknown; its treatment remains symptomatic.

ETIOLOGY

Despite intensive research, the etiology of PD remains elusive. One conceptualization is that an unknown environmental toxin acts on genetically susceptible individuals to cause PD. The principal link between PD and an environmental toxin is the chemical MPTP that caused PD in drug abusers and laboratory models. MPTP interferes with the function of nerve cell mitochondria; investigators conjectured that impairment in mitochondrial DNA may cause PD. Evidence exists for a disturbance in oxidative phosphorylation, particularly reduced activity of complex I of the mitochondrial electron transport chain. Additionally, there are increased levels of free iron that may enhance toxic free radical formation. Of patients with PD, 15% have a family history of PD; a small percentage has at least 3 affected generations. It is unknown whether this is from a defective gene, a shared environmental injury, or both. Several causative genes, specific to young-onset PD, are identified. The most common defect affects the gene for the protein **parkin (PARK2)** on chromosome 6. Mutations here result in **autosomal recessive**, slowly progressive PD with onset before the age of 40 years. Another gene is that for the chromosome 4 protein, α-**synuclein (PARK1)**, where

PARKINSON DISEASE

Figure 47-1 Parkinson Disease: Anatomy With Biochemical Pathways

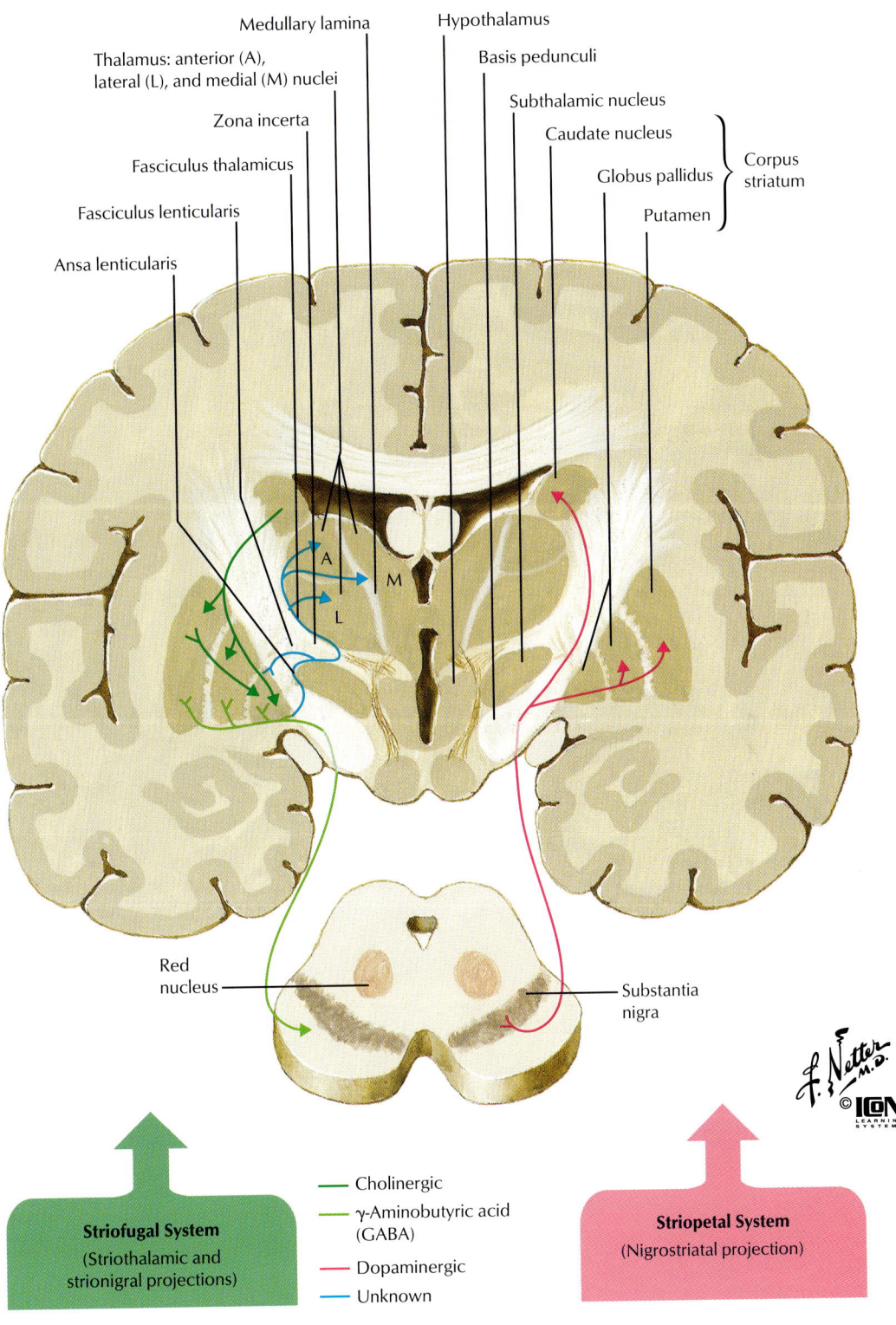

MOVEMENT DISORDERS

PARKINSON DISEASE

Figure 47-2   Neuropathy of Parkinson Disease

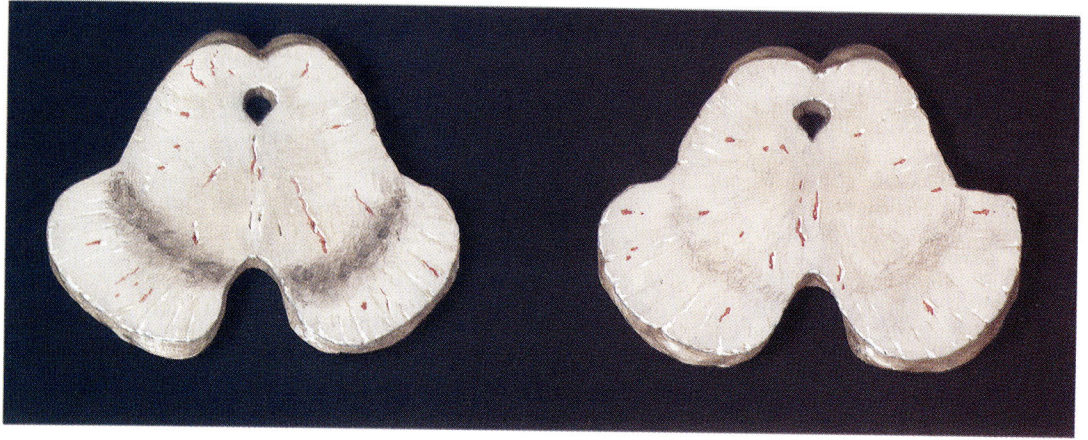

Normal: section through cerebral peduncles and substantia nigra

Parkinson disease: substantia nigra depigmented

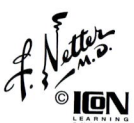

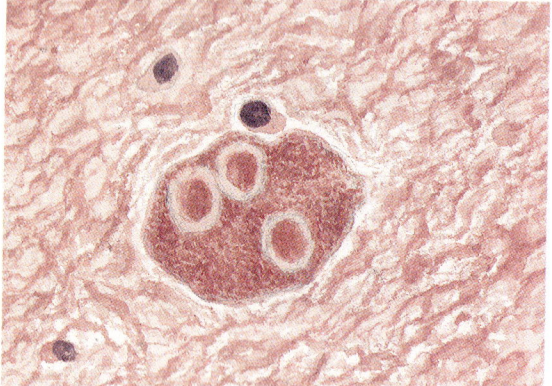

Lewy inclusion bodies in cell of substantia nigra in Parkinson disease; may also appear in locus ceruleus and tegmentum, cranial motor nerve nuclei, and peripheral autonomic ganglia

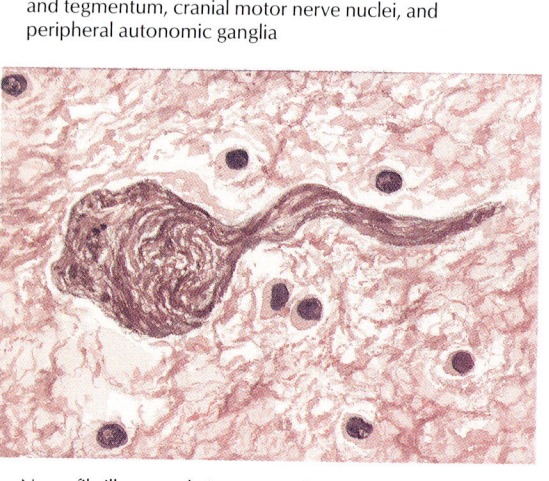

Neurofibrillary tangle in nerve cell of substantia nigra as seen in postencephalitic parkinsonism, progressive supranuclear palsy, and parkinsonism-dementia complex

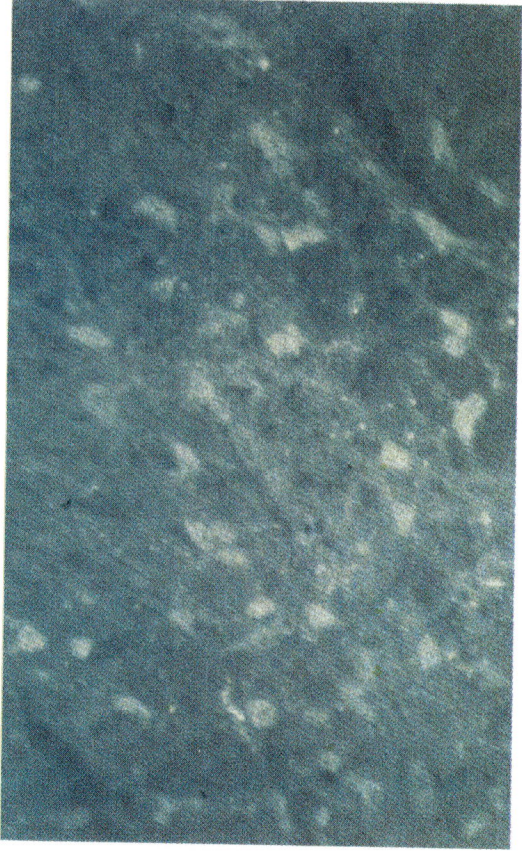

Section of substantia nigra of normal animal: treatment of section with formaldehyde vapor causes formation of polymers with monoamines (dopa and norepinephrine) which fluoresce to bright green under ultraviolet light

MOVEMENT DISORDERS

mutations result in an **autosomal dominant** PD and finally ubiquitin-C-hydrolase-L1 (PARK5).

PATHOPHYSIOLOGY

The pathologic sites responsible for the parkinsonian disorders reside in a group of brain gray matter structures called the extrapyramidal system or basal ganglia. The basal ganglia include the striatum (caudate nucleus and putamen), the globus pallidus interna and externa, the subthalamic nucleus, the substantia nigra pars reticulata and pars compacta, and the ventral nuclei of the thalamus.

In PD, degeneration of the substantia nigra pars compacta is the major pathologic finding (Figure 47-3). The nerve cells of the SN make the neurotransmitter dopamine and contain a dark pigment called *neuromelanin*. When approximately 60% of these cells die, PD symptoms develop. Concomitantly, analysis of the SN demonstrates abnormal pallor compared with normal coloration.

Direct SN dopaminergic projections influence basal ganglia motor processing; they facilitate movement execution and help to suppress unwanted movement. When SN dopaminergic neuron cell death occurs, the number of dopamine nerve terminals in the striatum decreases, leading to rigidity and akinesia, the classic PD symptoms. The basal ganglia function seems to extend beyond simple motor control concepts. The cortico-striato-pallido-thalamo-cortical circuit comprises several distinct and segregated loops, each having a different agonistic function. Within each loop are parallel pathways having antagonistic effects on this circuit outflow. The loss of dopamine provokes a less active direct pathway and a more active indirect pathway. Disinhibition of the major output nuclei and increased inhibition of the thalamo-cortical system result in abnormal movement.

The **direct pathway** arises from neurons that connect the striatum with the output nuclei, including the globus pallidum internum (Gpi) and the substantia nigra pars reticularis (SNr). Direct pathway neurons contain GABA, the inhibitory neurotransmitter, and substance P and express the excitatory D1 dopamine receptor. Direct pathway neurons receive glutamatergic projection from the cortex to the striatum. They also send GABAergic projections from the SNr/Gpi to the ventral anterior and ventral lateral thalamic nuclei, completing the loop by sending glutamatergic fibers back to the cortex. The direct striatopallidal influence inhibits the Gpi neurons. These neurons inhibit the thalamic outflow to the cortex. The net effect of direct pathway activity is excitatory by stimulating cortical activity.

The **indirect pathway** includes intermediate synapses in the globus pallidum externum (Gpe) and the subthalamic nucleus. Neurons within this pathway contain enkephalins and express the inhibitory D_2 dopamine receptor. This pathway consists of 3 glutamatergic and 3 GABAergic-type neurons. Glutamatergic neurons in the cortex project to the striatum; striatal GABAergic neurons project to the Gpe. From the Gpe, a second set of GABAergic neurons projects to a second set of glutamatergic neurons in the subthalamic nucleus that project to the Gpi/SNr. The neurons from the Gpi/SNr send GABAergic neurons to the thalamus. The final thalamocortical projection is glutamatergic. By contrast, increased indirect pathway activity excites the Gpi neurons, ultimately inhibiting cortical activity.

Decreased dopaminergic neurons in PD affect the direct pathway by reducing activity at the Gpi and the SNr, leading to increased inhibitory output of the Gpi and the SNr. In the indirect pathway, dopamine deficiency disinhibits striatopallidal neurons synapsing in the Gpe, reducing activity in the inhibitory pallidosubthalamic neurons. Dopamine loss increases the striatal activity via the projections to GABAergic neurons that increase actions on the Gpe. Furthermore, dopamine loss causes a disinhibition of the subthalamic nucleus through the indirect pathway.

CLINICAL PRESENTATION

The 4 **primary signs** of PD are bradykinesia, rigidity, tremor, and gait disturbance (Figure 47-4). The primary criteria for PD diagnosis require the patient to have at least 2 of these 4 features. Other features suggestive of idiopathic PD, in contrast to some of the atypical parkinsonism syndromes, include an asymmetric or unilateral onset and a clear response to levodopa treat-

PARKINSON DISEASE

Figure 47-3   Parkinsonism: Hypothesized Role of Dopa

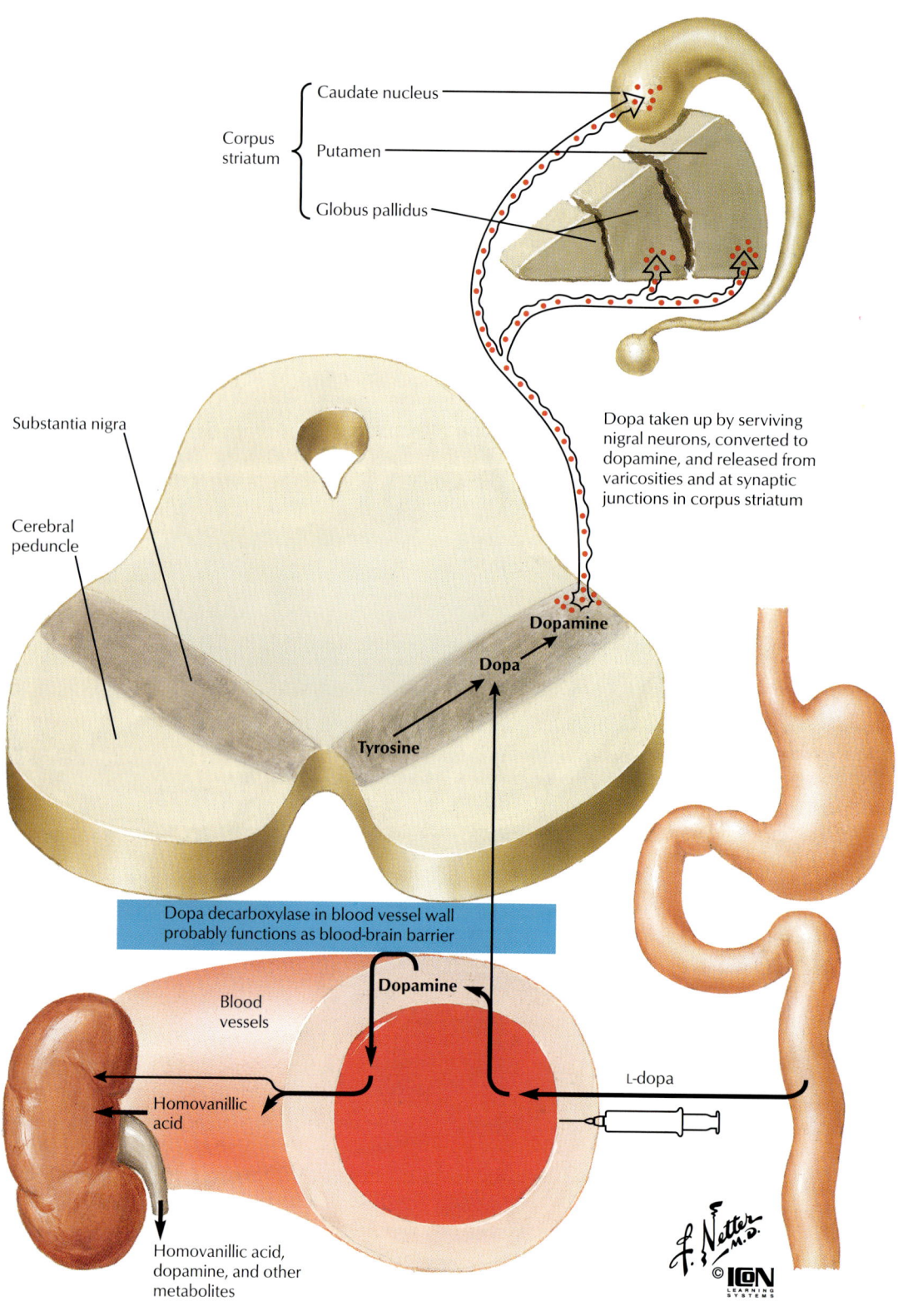

MOVEMENT DISORDERS

PARKINSON DISEASE

Figure 47-4 Clinical Signs of Parkinson Disease

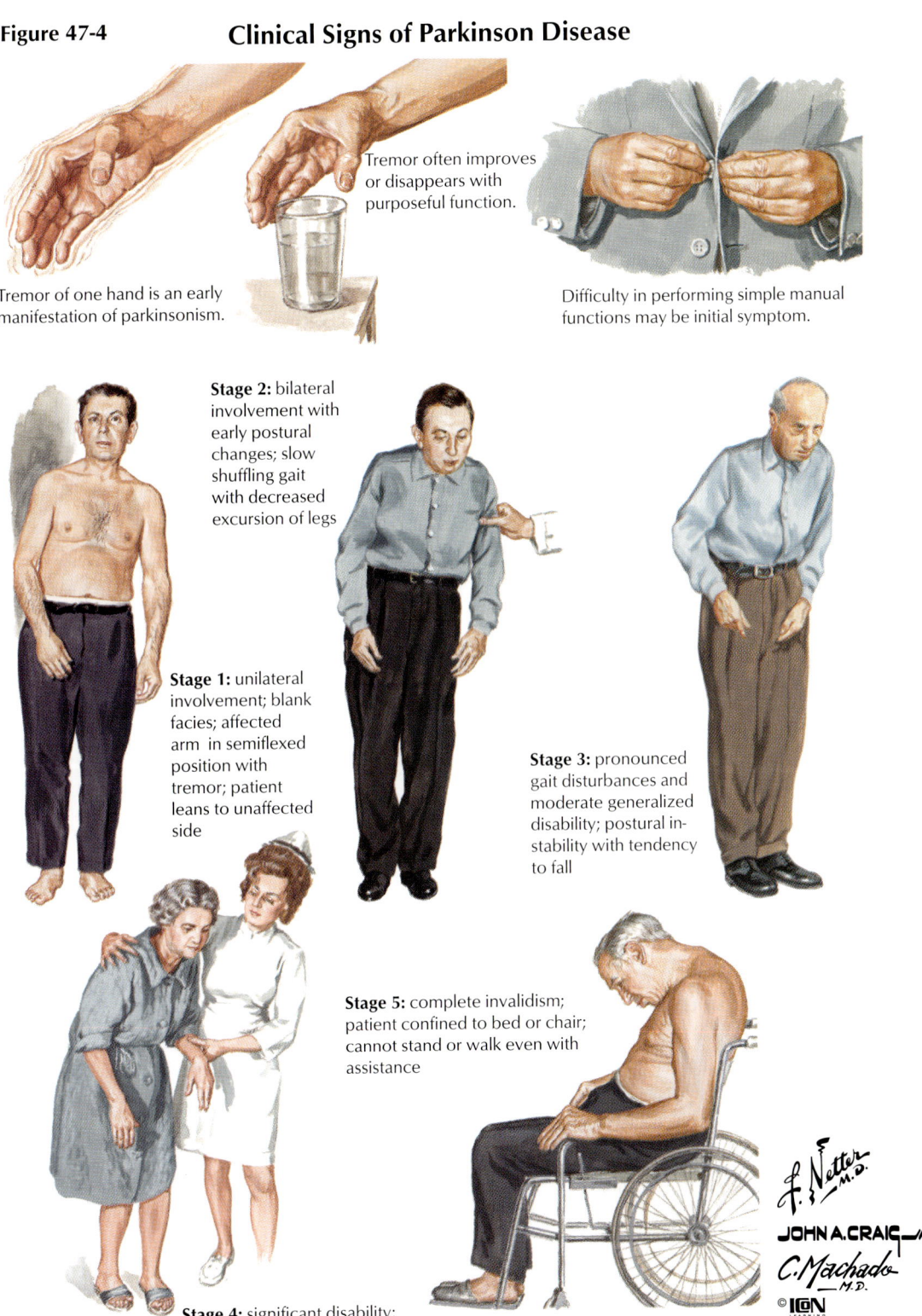

PARKINSON DISEASE

ment. **Bradykinesia**, the most disabling PD symptom, is a decreased ability to initiate movement (akinesia is the extreme manifestation). This may affect multiple functions, particularly fine motor tasks such as buttoning a shirt or handwriting, the latter becoming micrographic. Other individuals may present with masked facies, decreased blink frequency, muted speech, and slowed swallowing. Typically, the gait is shuffling, with decreased arm swing, stooped posture, and en bloc turning, not unlike a wooden figure.

Rigidity is a resistance to passive movement throughout the entire range of motion occurring in flexor and extensor muscles. The classic cogwheel quality (stop-and-go effect) is from a tremor superimposed on the altered muscle tone. Patients are often concerned about stiffness, weakness, or fatigue, representing the combination of bradykinesia with rigidity.

Tremor occurs in 75% of patients. Typically, it is prominent at rest, having a frequency of 3 to 7 Hz. Occasionally, a PD tremor has a significant postural or action component, complicating distinction from the more benign essential tremor.

Gait disturbance, **postural instability**, or both usually present in later stages of PD and are characterized by a change in the center of gravity typified by falling forward (propulsion) or backward (retropulsion) and a festinating (shuffling, slowly propulsive) gait. When these symptoms are found early in PD, evaluation for other causes of parkinsonism, including progressive supranuclear palsy and multiple system atrophy, is required.

Many patients, even early in the disease course, can present with **seborrheic dermatitis**. Some patients experience **hyposmia**. Later in the course of PD, certain secondary features can be observed. Patients experience difficulties with sleep initiation and maintenance. This **sleep disturbance** can be from early morning dystonia or tremor, restless leg syndrome, or REM behavior disorder. Approximately 30% of patients also experience periodic leg movement during sleep. **Autonomic dysfunction** is seen commonly, manifested as orthostatic hypotension, impaired gastrointestinal motility, urinary bladder dysfunction, disorders in thermoregulation, and sexual dysfunction. **Dysphagia** is usually present late in PD from oropharyngeal and esophageal motility disorders.

Psychiatric and cognitive symptomatologies also frequently accompany or even precede the diagnosis of PD in some patients. Approximately 40% experience a major **depression** that may precede the diagnosis of the movement disorder; **anxiety** occurs in up to 40% of patients; **hallucinations** (visual, most likely nonthreathening), psychosis, and vivid nocturnal dreams are common later in the disease; and **cognitive dysfunction** usually presents as a subcortical dementia, typically as a later manifestation.

The course of PD is variable, although usually the disease progresses slowly but inexorably. Typically, the illness begins unilaterally with focal tremor or difficulty using 1 limb. Eventually, the symptoms become more generalized and occur on the contralateral side, interfering with activities of daily living. Several secondary signs of parkinsonism also develop.

Certain characteristics serve as red flags suggesting some of the "Parkinson plus" syndromes, including progressive supranuclear palsy, cortical basal degeneration, and multiple system atrophy (Table 47-1). If possible, it is useful to exclude these early in the disease course because they may change the treatment and prognosis.

Table 47-1
Exclusion Criteria for Diagnosis of Parkinson Disease

Parkinsonism due to identifiable causes, such as stroke, head injury, encephalitis, neuroleptic exposure, hydrocephalus, or brain tumor
Oculogyric crises
Sustained remissions
Supranuclear gaze palsy
Cerebellar signs
Early severe autonomic insufficiency, particularly orthostatic hypotension
Early severe dementia
Poor response to large doses of levodopa

Table 47-2
Differential Diagnoses of Parkinson Disease

1. Drug induced
2. Familial
3. Toxic
4. Young onset
5. Metabolic
6. Parkinsonism diagnosable by imaging studies
7. Infectious or postinfectious
8. Miscellaneous causes
9. Degenerative diseases causing parkinsonism

DIFFERENTIAL DIAGNOSES

Although there is a broad differential diagnosis for PD in most patients presenting with akinesia, rigidity, and tremor, there is a relatively limited set of conditions to consider (Table 47-2).

Dopamine receptor-blocking agents used in psychiatry and, for gastrointestinal symptoms, are the most common drugs causing parkinsonism, creating the most important category of secondary parkinsonism. Of patients taking neuroleptic agents on a long-term basis, parkinsonism develops in approximately 15%. Recovery after withdrawal of the offending agent may take weeks to months. If antiparkinsonian medication is required, the drugs of choice are anticholinergic.

Some infectious diseases can cause parkinsonism. Postencephalitic parkinsonism (von Economo disease, encephalitis lethargica, sleeping sickness) has the most prominent features. Other rare associations include AIDS, cryptococcal meningoencephalitis, cysticercosis, fungal abscesses in the striata, herpes simplex encephalitis, Japanese B encephalitis, malaria, mycoplasma infection, postvaccinal parkinsonism, prion diseases (Creutzfeldt-Jakob disease), St Louis encephalitis, subacute sclerosing panencephalitis, syphilis, tuberculosis, and Whipple disease.

Postencephalitis Parkinsonism occurred in a pandemic in Europe and North America from 1916 to 1927. The precise infectious agent is not identified, although DNA studies are under way. Typically, parkinsonism symptoms occurred immediately after the acute infectious process; however, in some patients, prominent symptoms were not evident for up to 20 years. Clinically, patients had parkinsonism with other distinctive features: behavioral and mental disturbances in the acute illness; changes in sleep patterns; and ocular motor dysfunction, particularly oculogyric crisis (ie, spasms of conjugate eye muscles, deviating eyes upward, downward, or to one side for minutes or hours). Other neurologic deficit pro-

Table 47-3
Degenerative Causes of Parkinsonism*

α-Synuclein Deposition	Tau Deposition	Polyglutamine Tract Deposition
Parkinson disease	Progressive supranuclear palsy	Juvenile Huntington disease
Multiple system atrophy	Corticobasal ganglionic degeneration	Autosomal dominant cerebellar ataxia (SCA-3)
	Parkinsonism dementia complex of Guam	Dentato-rubro-pallido-luysian atrophy
	Postencephalitic Parkinson syndrome	Sporadic neuronal intranuclear inclusion disease
	Frontotemporal dementia with parkinsonism linked to chromosome 17	
	Posttraumatic parkinsonism	

*SCA indicates spinocerebellar atrophy.

PARKINSON DISEASE

gression was extremely slow and included forms of other movement disorders. Levodopa was not as well tolerated as in idiopathic PD; high doses of anticholinergic medications were better tolerated.

Exposure to numerous toxins is associated with rare forms of parkinsonism. Around 1980, the substance **MPTP** inadvertently led to a series of acute PD cases in California. These individuals illicitly manufactured and used designer drugs. MPTP is highly toxic to the SN neurons and is used to produce animal models mimicking PD. The symptoms of MPTP parkinsonism respond well to levodopa. The globus pallidus is another target for parkinsonism toxins, such as **carbon monoxide**, *cyanide*, and **manganese**. Manganese toxicity is seen in miners and industrial workers.

Hypothyroidism, easily identified and treatable, is a metabolic condition that can cause parkinsonism. Other rare conditions include acquired chronic hepatocerebral degeneration, hemochromatosis, ceroid lipofuscinosis, folate deficiency, Niemann-Pick type C disease, and postanoxic parkinsonism.

Few patients have familial parkinsonism. The most common inheritance is autosomal dominant. Frontotemporal dementia with parkinsonism is linked to chromosome 17.

When parkinsonism develops before the age of 40 years, Wilson disease is in the differential diagnosis, necessitating tests for copper metabolism and slit lamp examination.

Characterized by a poor levodopa response, arteriosclerotic parkinsonism (ie, lower body parkinsonism) is the PD variant most likely to be associated with head CT or MRI abnormalities. They are primarily visible as periventricular white matter changes. Normal pressure hydrocephalus, also in the PD differential diagnosis, typically presents with a gait disorder different from that of idiopathic PD. Cognitive decline may occur earlier in this syndrome. Mass lesions, such as tumors, are exceedingly rare causes of parkinsonism.

Multiple head trauma, as seen in boxers, can cause parkinsonism. Degenerative diseases causing parkinsonism are best classified by the type of abnormal degree of neurochemical deposition (Table 47-3 and chapter 48).

DIAGNOSTIC EVALUATION

Key diagnostic elements are the presence of 2 of the 4 cardinal signs. However, it is unusual for a patient to present initially with the full-blown disease, and characteristic signs may not be present. Reexamination in several month intervals is often needed to confirm PD. Signs of another degenerative process sometimes become evident.

Although approaches to preclinical detection of PD have been investigated, a practical, inexpensive, sensitive, specific screening test is not available. Use of CT and MRI helps to distinguish idiopathic PD from other forms, particularly when findings are purely unilateral. Imaging studies may show atherosclerotic brain disease or normal pressure hydrocephalus and rarely demonstrate a structural lesion. MRI sometimes shows signs typical for multiple system atrophy (putaminal atrophy, a hyperintense putaminal rim, and infratentorial signal changes). When the PD diagnosis is confirmed, it is useful to measure severity qualitatively (Table 47-4).

Table 47-4
Parkinson Disease Rating Scales

Hoehn and Yahr
Stage I: unilateral disease
Stage II: bilateral disease with preservation of postural reflexes
Stage III: bilateral disease with impaired postural reflexes but preserved ability to ambulate independently
Stage IV: severe disease necessitating considerable assistance
Stage V: end stage disease, confinement to bed or chair

United Parkinson Disease Rating Scale

Four major subsets
  Cognitive
  Activities of daily living
  Motor examination
  Complications of treatment

Scale: 0 to 4 (0 = normal, 4 = most severe)

TREATMENT

Treatment for PD remains symptomatic; no neuroprotective therapy is available. Patient treatment requires careful consideration of the patient's symptoms and signs, stage of disease, degree of functional disability, and levels of activity and productivity. Treatment can be classified into nonpharmacologic, pharmacologic, and surgical. Most patients with idiopathic PD have a significant therapeutic response to levodopa. Complete absence of response to a dose of 1000 to 1500 mg/d strongly suggests that the original diagnosis was incorrect and should prompt a search for other causes of parkinsonism.

Pharmacologic therapy for PD consists of 5 types of medication (Table 47-5). There is no simple approach to treating PD; guidelines depend on functional impairment and response to therapy. Later in the illness, there are a number of support groups for patients, families, and caregivers.

Dopaminergic

Levodopa

Levodopa, the most commonly used, most potent antiparkinsonian medication, is equally beneficial for all symptoms. Levodopa is the immediate natural precursor of dopamine and is converted to dopamine by an enzyme aromatic amino acid decarboxylase. Initially, levodopa was associated with a high rate of adverse effects, particularly nausea and vomiting, from peripheral dopamine receptor stimulation. The addition of the peripheral decarboxylase inhibitor carbidopa decreased the incidence of peripheral adverse effects, permitted more levodopa to cross the blood-brain barrier, and allowed reduction of the total levodopa dose. Carbidopa-levodopa is available in immediate-release and controlled-release formulations.

Adverse effects are numerous. Early adverse effects, including nausea and orthostatic hypotension, are more easily managed than the late motor complications. Late adverse effects include involuntary movements (dyskinesias) resulting from excessive dopaminergic stimulation; motor fluctuations; and psychosis, typically hallucinations and delusions.

Dopamine Agonists

Dopamine agonists (DAs) directly stimulate dopaminergic receptors. They are particularly indicated for monotherapy in younger patients, who are more prone to the early development of levodopa-related clinical fluctuations and who require long-term treatment. At least 2 general classes of DAs exist: one coupled to adenylate cyclases (D_1) and another not so linked (D_2). Most effective antiparkinsonian DAs stimulate predominantly D_2 receptors. DAs are used mainly early in the illness because they reduce the need for levodopa. Although not as effective as levodopa, DAs often provide satisfactory relief of mild symptoms. In those instances when severe symptoms interfere with the patient's social or occupational activities, early symptomatic treatment with levodopa, later combined with a DA, may be necessary. Commonly used preparations include pramipexole, ropinirole, bromocriptine, and pergolide (Table 47-6).

Anticholinergic Agents

Anticholinergic agents are the oldest drug class used for PD. They act as muscarinic receptor blockers by penetrating the CNS to antagonize acetylcholine transmission by striatal interneurons. They are most effective for tremor but, because of adverse effects, must be used with caution in the elderly. Usually used as monotherapy or as an adjunct to dopaminergic therapy, the most commonly used anticholinergic agents include benztropine, procyclidine, and trihexyphenidyl. Adverse effects, resulting

Table 47-5
Pharmacologic Therapy for Parkinson Disease*

1. Dopaminergic
  A. Levodopa
  B. Dopamine agonist

2. Anticholinergics
3. MAOIs
4. COMT inhibitors
5. Amantadine

*COMT indicates catechol-O-methyltransferase; MAOI, monoamine oxidase inhibitor.

PARKINSON DISEASE

Table 47-6
Advantages and Disadvantages of Dopamine Agonists*

Advantages

Some antiparkinson effect
Reduced incidence of levodopa-related adverse events (dyskinesia and motor fluctuations)
Selective stimulation of dopamine receptor subtypes and longer duration of action
Do not generate oxidative metabolites
Levodopa-sparing effect

Disadvantages

Limited antiparkinson efficacy, always require levodopa adjunctive therapy
Specific adverse effects (nausea, vomiting, postural hypotension, drowsiness, constipation, psychiatric reactions: hallucinations, confusion)
Do not completely prevent development of levodopa-related adverse events; after dyskinesias have developed, DAs exacerbate them
Do not treat all features of PD, such as freezing, postural instability, autonomic dysfunction, dementia
Do not stop disease progression

*DA indicates dopamine agonist; PD, Parkinson disease.

from both peripheral and central cholinergic blockade, include dry mouth, narrow-angle glaucoma, constipation, urinary retention, memory impairment, and confusion with hallucinations.

COMT Inhibitors

Inhibition of the enzyme catechol-O-methyltransferase (COMT) blocks dopamine metabolism. COMT inhibitors prolong the benefits of levodopa by extending the life span of the dopamine to which it is converted. There are 2 major COMT inhibitors. Entacapone is generally used adjunctively to levodopa. Tolcapone can cause severe hepatotoxicity, requires regular laboratory monitoring, and therefore is used less frequently.

Monoamine Oxidase B Inhibitors

Selegiline is a selective inhibitor of monoamine oxidase B. Its primary mechanism of action is blockade of central dopamine metabolism. It may improve response to levodopa, especially in patients with mild dose-related fluctuations. Selegiline has been studied as a neuroprotective agent because it can block free radical formation from the oxidative metabolism of dopamine. A large, prospective, double-blind, placebo-controlled, multicenter study (DATATOP) found that it delayed the progression of parkinsonian signs in previously untreated patients by 9 months. However, no persistent, long-term benefit in slowing the progression of PD has been demonstrated.

Amantadine

Amantadine is an antiviral agent that was serendipitously found to have an antiparkinsonian effect. Its mechanism of action, thought to include blocking an N-methyl-D-aspartate receptor, is controversial. Amantadine has a mild beneficial effect on tremor, bradykinesia, and rigidity. It is the only antiparkinsonian medication that can decrease the severity of levodopa-induced dyskinesias. Common adverse effects include livedo reticularis and lower extremity edema.

FUTURE DIRECTIONS

Because PD is more common with increasing age, its prevalence is expected to triple over the next 50 years because of the aging US population. The most promising research is focused on the function and anatomy of the motor system, ways of controlling neurodegeneration, location of possible environmental factors, identification of a gene causing PD, and new medical and surgical therapies.

The isolation of at least 5 individual brain receptors for dopamine is likely to help in discovery of more effective PD medications. Information about the unique effects of each dopamine receptor on different brain areas has led to treatment theories and clinical trials. Other research includes studying brain areas distinct from the SN that may be involved in the disease, evaluating the consequences of dopamine cell degeneration in the basal ganglia and malfunction

analysis of dopamine transporters that carry dopamine in and out of the synapse.

Animal models are used for studying methods for delivering dopamine to critical brain areas by implanting tiny dopamine-containing particles into brain regions affected by the disease. Such implants could partially ameliorate the movement problems exhibited by these animals. Also under investigation are implantable pumps that can produce a continuous supply of levodopa and help to prevent fluctuations. Another promising method involves implanting capsules containing dopamine-producing cells into the brain. Neural grafting, or transplantation of nerve cells, is a proposed technique. Animal models show that damaged nerve cells can regenerate after fetal brain tissue from the SN is implanted. Other therapeutic attempts are directed to replace the lost dopamine-producing neurons with healthy, fetal neurons and thereby improve movement and response to medications. A promising approach is the use of genetically engineered cells (eg, modified skin cells grown in tissue culture) that could have the same beneficial effects. Skin cells would be much easier to harvest, and patients could serve as their own donors.

REFERENCES

Effects of tocopherol and deprenyl on the progression of disability in early Parkinson's disease. The Parkinson Study Group. *N Engl J Med.* 1993;328:176-183.

Fahn S, Przedborski S. Parkinsonism. In: Rowland LP, ed. *Meritt's Neurology.* 10th ed. New York, NY: Lippincott; 2000:679-693.

Jankovic J, Tolosa E. *Parkinson's Disease and Movement Disorders.* Philadelphia, Pa: Lippincott Williams & Wilkins; 2002:67-220.

Jellinger K. Pathology of parkinsonism. In: Fahn et al, eds. *Recent Development in Parkinson's Disease.* New York, NY: Raven Press, 1986.

Management of Parkinson's disease: an evidence-based review. *Mov Disord.* 2002;17(suppl 4):1-166.

Obeso J, Olanow C, Nutt J. Levodopa motor complications in Parkinson's disease. *Trends Neurosci.* 2000;23:S2-S7.

Olanow C, Tatton W. Etiology and pathogenesis of Parkinson's disease. *Annu Rev Neurosci.* 1999;22:123-144.

Olanow CW, Watts RL, Koller WC. An algorithm (decision tree) for the management of Parkinson's disease (2001): treatment guidelines. *Neurology.* 2001;56(suppl 5):S1-S88.

Parkinson Study Group. Entacapone improves motor fluctuations in levodopa-treated Parkinson's disease patients. *Ann Neurol.* 1997;42:747-755.

Chapter 48
Atypical Parkinsonian Syndromes

Diana Apetauerova

Atypical parkinsonian syndromes (Table 48-1), previously called Parkinson plus syndromes, are chronic, progressive neurodegenerative disorders characterized by rapidly evolving parkinsonism in association with other signs of neurologic dysfunction outside the spectrum of idiopathic Parkinson disease (PD). These include early postural instability, supranuclear gaze palsy, early autonomic failure, and pyramidal, cerebellar, or cortical signs. The most common disorders are corticobasal degeneration (CBD), progressive supranuclear palsy (PSP), and multiple system atrophy (MSA). Unlike idiopathic PD, they have poor or transient responses to dopaminergic therapy and are associated with a worse prognosis. They are classified as tauopathies and synucleinopathies based on accumulation of the abnormal proteins tau and a-synuclein in certain brain areas within neurons and glial cells in various anatomical distribution and forms of the filaments.

Tau is found in a hyperphosphorylated form in PSP and CBD. It functions in a healthy human brain as a microtubule binding protein and a stabilizer of the neuronal cytoskeleton. In a diseased brain, tau is found in glial cells and neurons and produces a special cluster of fibrils called a *neurofibrillary tangle*. Generally, there are 6 isoforms of tau made by alternative splicing from the tau gene. Tau also accumulates in the less common tauopathy, frontotemporal dementia with parkinsonism linked to chromosome 17 (FTPD-17).

α-Synuclein is a highly soluble synaptic protein found in the healthy human brain. Typically, in MSA, it accumulates as insoluble aggregates in white matter oligodendrocytes called *glial cytoplasmic inclusions*.

There are no effective therapies for these syndromes. Therapeutic trials with free radical scavengers and a better understanding of the role of the abnormal protein within the brain may help to improve understanding of these uncommon disorders.

CORTICOBASAL DEGENERATION

Clinical Vignette

A 64-year-old woman started to fall and noted difficulties with fine motor activities of the right hand 4 years previously. Her hand felt stiff and uncoordinated. An abnormal posture of her right arm developed wherein she often kept it abducted and elevated with a closed hand. She noted difficulty letting go of objects with her sometimes hyperemic and swollen right hand. Clumsiness of the right leg developed. Treatment with high doses of levodopa (up to 1500 mg) was ineffective.

The patient's neurologic examination demonstrated mild difficulty generating vertical more than horizontal saccadic eye movements, reduced blink frequency, apraxia (using a body part as an object), mild arm levitation, dystonic posture of the right arm, striking rigidity and bradykinesia on the right side, brisker right muscle stretch reflexes, and a right Babinski sign. Her gait was stiff, with inability to walk without the assistance of 2 people.

Corticobasal degeneration is a rare sporadic neurodegenerative tauopathy. It occurs mainly after the age of 60 years and shows no population clusters; its incidence, prevalence, and etiology are unknown. The typical presentation is an asymmetric progressive akinetic-rigid syndrome, cortical signs, dystonia, and alien hand phenomenon, all poorly responsive to levodopa therapy.

Pathophysiology

Corticobasal degeneration primarily affects the cerebral cortex. Clinical presentation correlates with asymmetric cortical atrophy contralateral to the involved limb. The frontoparietal cortex is the most involved with major changes in the perirolandic area. Macroscopically prominent cortical atrophy with reduction of cerebral white matter is also apparent in the cerebral peduncles and the corpus callosum. Additionally, there is neuronal loss in the substantia nigra and the locus ceruleus.

Table 48-1
Atypical Parkinsonian Syndromes*

Syndrome	Abnormal	Clinical Features	Age at Onset, y	Genetic	Pathology	Therapy
CBD	Tau	Akinetic-rigid asymmetric parkinsonism Cortical signs Dystonia Action/postural tremor Myoclonus Alien limb phenomenon	60	Sporadic	Atrophy in FP cortex Tau-positive neurons in cortex Swollen and achromatic neurons (ballooned neurons)	Poor response to dopaminergic medication Botox for blepharospasm Supportive therapy
PSP	Tau	Gait disorder, falls Symmetric axially predominant parkinsonism Abnormal eye movements Dysarthria and dysphagia Frontal lobe abnormalities Cognitive impairment	55-70	Sporadic ? Familial	Atrophy of BG and brainstem regions Normal cerebral cortex Globose, NFT	Poor response to dopaminergic medication Botox for blepharospasm Supportive therapy
FTDP-17	Tau	Highly variable: behavioral disturbance Cognitive impairment Motor disturbance (later in the disease) Positive family history	50	Autosomal dominant	Atrophy in FT cortex, BG, SN, LC Neuronal loss Argentophilic neuronal inclusions	Poor response to dopaminergic therapy
MSA	α-Synuclein	Parkinsonism Cerebellar signs Autonomic features Pyramidal features	60	Sporadic	Glial and neuronal cytoplasmic inclusions Absence of Lewy bodies	Poor or marginal response to dopaminergic therapy Fludrocortisone or midodrine for orthostatic hypotension

*BG indicates basal ganglia; CBD, corticobasal degeneration; FP, frontoparietal; FT, frontotemporal; FTDP-17, frontotemporal dementia with parkinsonism linked to chromosome 17; LC, locus ceruleus; MSA, multiple system atrophy; NFT, neurofibrillary tangle; PSP, progressive supranuclear palsy.

Typical microscopic features include neuronal loss (cortex, subcortical regions, substantia nigra), astrocytic gliosis, ballooned (achromatic) neurons, and neurofibrillary tangle and tau-positive glial inclusions. The microscopic hallmarks of CBD are the ballooned, swollen, or achromatic neurons lacking Nissl substance.

Clinical Presentation

An asymmetric akinetic-rigid parkinsonism, primarily affecting the arm and hand, is often the major feature. Patients usually present with limb clumsiness, awkward, slow voluntary movements of one arm, with dystonic posturing and tremor. Cortical signs include apraxia, cortical sensory disturbance, and finger myoclonus. The alien limb phenomenon, failure to recognize ownership of a limb without visual cues, is also common. Gradually, a gait disorder with limb rigidity and impaired position sense develops. Dementia usually develops late in CBD, but it can be the predominant feature. Less common features include eye movement abnormalities also seen in PSP. Slowed speech production, dysarthria, swallowing difficulties, and cognitive deficit occur later in this disease. Less common CBD presentations include dementia, aphasia, and altered behavior.

Diagnosis

Corticobasal degeneration is relatively easy to diagnose because of its stereotypic clinical presentation. Some conditions clinically mimic CBD, including PSP, Pick disease, Alzheimer disease, some vascular lesions, and rare leukodystrophies. Neuropathologic evaluation is necessary to confirm the diagnosis. Imaging studies are not diagnostic. MRI and CT can show asymmetric cortical atrophy in the frontoparietal region, maximal on the side contralateral to the involved limb. The asymmetrically reduced pattern in frontoparietal cerebral cortical metabolism, CBF, or both, coupled with bilateral reduction of fluorodopa uptake in the caudate and putamen on PET scanning, provide strong evidence for CBD.

Treatment

There is no definitive treatment; dopaminergic therapy is of limited benefit, clonazepam can be used for myoclonus, and botulinum toxin improves dystonia. Occupational, physical, and speech therapy may also help. The average survival from symptom onset to death is 5 to 6 years.

PROGRESSIVE SUPRANUCLEAR PALSY

Progressive supranuclear palsy is another sporadic tauopathy. A progressive illness characterized by parkinsonism with supranuclear gaze palsy, early postural instability, falls, bradykinesia, and dysarthria, PSP has a poor response to dopaminergic therapy. Its prognosis is poor, with a median survival of 5 to 7 years.

The etiology of PSP, like that of CBD, is unknown. Observations of a large cohort demonstrated that 31 of 87 consecutive patients with parkinsonism referred to 1 neurology department had PSP. More patients with PSP consumed herbal teas and tropical fruits possibly representing exogenous environmental toxins. A genetic susceptibility may also be invoked.

Pathophysiology

Unlike CBD or FTPD-17, PSP is primarily a subcortical neurodegenerative tauopathy. Macroscopic substantia nigra and locus ceruleus depigmentation and atrophy of the pons, the midbrain, and the globus pallidus are visible. Microscopically, the most affected regions are brainstem nuclei III, IV, IX, and X, the red nucleus, the locus ceruleus, the substantia nigra, the globus pallidus, and the cerebellar dentate nucleus. Tau protein accumulates within neurons as neurofibrillary tangle and in glia as spherical neuropil threads.

Clinical Presentation

Progressive supranuclear palsy typically occurs between the sixth and seventh decades of life. Onset before the age of 40 years is rare. Prevalence varies between 1 and 6.4 in 100,000. PSP is sporadic in most individuals, but rarely, an autosomal dominant inheritance is suggested.

The typical clinical presentation is gait instability and early falls backward; both are rare early in PD. The parkinsonism is typically axial and symmetric, unlike the asymmetric presentation of PD. Patients with PSP have an erect posture in contrast to the flexed PD stance (Figure 48-1). Often, they lack the typical PD tremor. Dystonia is common.

Abnormal eye movements, characteristically vertical and later horizontal supranuclear gaze palsy, are the hallmark of PSP. The patient usually perceives these as blurry vision and difficulties with reading and walking down stairs. Dysarthria and dysphagia are common, often early in the disease course. Cognitive dysfunction develops later.

Diagnosis

Progressive supranuclear palsy and other atypical parkinsonian syndromes, including CBD, MSA, and dementia with Lewy bodies, are often misdiagnosed as PD or as cerebrovascular disease (atherosclerotic parkinsonism). The most important diagnostic clues are the results of a careful clinical evaluation and a poor response to dopaminergic therapy. CT and MRI may show generalized or brainstem (dorsal midbrain) atrophy. Other studies are not commonly available. Metabolic PET studies have demonstrated global reduction in cerebral metabolism; fluorodopa F 18 PET uptake studies have revealed reduced caudate and putamen uptake. SPECT has revealed bifrontal hypometabolism.

Treatment

There is no effective treatment for PSP. Although some patients with slowness, stiffness, and balance problems respond to antiparkinsonian therapies such as levodopa, or levodopa combined with anticholinergic agents, the effect is usually temporary. Speech, vision, and swallowing difficulties are usually unresponsive to any pharmacotherapy.

Antidepressant drugs have had modest success in PSP; fluoxetine, amitryptyline, and imipramine are the most commonly used, although their benefit seems to be unrelated to their ability to relieve depression. Botulinum toxin injections are used for blepharospasm. Physical and occupational therapy are the most important patient treatment aspects.

Progressive supranuclear palsy is progressive, with an average survival from symptom onset to death of 5 to 6 years. Head injury and fractures from falls are common. Because of dysphagia, patients with PSP are predisposed to other serious complications, such as choking and pneumonia, the most common cause of death.

FRONTOTEMPORAL DEMENTIA PARKINSONISM–CHROMOSOME 17

Frontotemporal dementia with parkinsonism linked to chromosome 17 is an autosomal dominant tauopathy caused by a tau gene mutation located on chromosome 17q21. Many different mutations located in the microtubule-binding region of the tau gene have been identified. FTDP-17 has clinical and neuropathologic variability. Behavioral changes and parkinsonism are the most common features.

Pathophysiology

Pathologically, the neocortex is degenerated with marked frontal and temporal lobe atrophy. The subcortical basal ganglia and brainstem nuclei are also involved.

Clinical Presentation

Frontotemporal dementia with parkinsonism linked to chromosome 17 is a highly variable neurodegenerative disease. The first symptoms typically occur in the fifth decade of life but range from the third to the sixth decade, although onset is insidious. Often, multiple family members have a positive family history. Behavioral disturbances are often the initial and typical features, including disinhibition, inappropriate behavior, and poor impulse control (see Figure 34-1). Other individuals present with apathetic, socially withdrawn behavior and often neglect personal hygiene. A prominent psychosis, similar to schizophrenia with auditory hallucination, delusion, and paranoia, is sometimes apparent.

Cognitive impairment affecting executive function, judgment, planning, and reasoning may be the initial sign of FTDP-17. Surprisingly, patients with this variant do have preservation of memory, orientation, and visuospatial functions.

Motor disturbance is usually not noted early in the disease. Later, patients have bradykinesia with axial and limb rigidity and postural instability. Resting tremor is uncommon.

In the typical patient, disinhibited behavior develops in the fifth decade of life, without impair-

ATYPICAL PARKINSONIAN SYNDROMES

ment of memory or orientation. However, there is progressive worsening over several years, associated with severe dementia, bradykinesia, rigidity, and evidence of frontal or temporal atrophy or both.

Diagnosis and Treatment

Other conditions that present with parkinsonism and dementia include Pick disease, CBD, PSP, and Alzheimer disease. The prominent family history of FTDP-17 is usually lacking in these other disorders. Careful attention to the family history and the clinical presentation are key. DNA genetic testing demonstrates the chromosome 17 gene mutation. PET scanning, used infrequently, shows a reduction of caudate and putamen fluorodopa uptake.

There is no therapy for FTDP-17. As with other tauopathies, the response to dopaminergic therapy is poor. The disease duration averages 10 to 12 years.

MULTIPLE SYSTEM ATROPHY

Clinical Vignette

A 58-year-old woman noted right hand clumsiness during her job as a hairdresser. During the subsequent 2 years, facial masking, generalized bradykinesia, right-sided rigidity, and mild gait disturbance developed. There was no tremor, autonomic disturbance, or cognitive impairment. Although levodopa initially produced improvement in all motor symptoms, prominent orofacial, cervical, and lower extremity dyskinesia and shorter duration levodopa responses occurred within 1 year. Tolcapone aggravated the patient's dyskinesia. Despite continued response of her upper extremity akinesia to levodopa, gait and balance difficulty progressed. She became wheelchair bound, hypophonia increased, and she showed deterioration on neurologic examination. Bilateral Babinski signs, hyperreflexia, and cerebellar signs were then elicited. MRI showed lateral putamen and pontine cruciate patterns of T2 hyperintensity.

Multiple system atrophy is a sporadic, degenerative CNS disease classified as a synucleinopathy. It presents with a combination of extrapyramidal, pyramidal, cerebellar, and autonomic symptoms and signs. Its clinical manifestations may change as it evolves.

Multiple system atrophy comprises 3 clinical conditions previously called *striatonigral degen-*

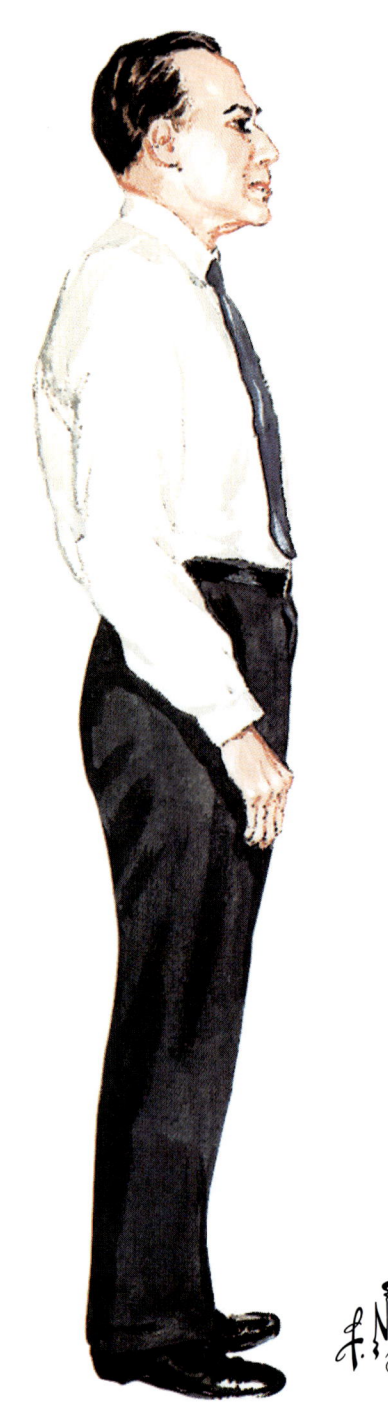

Figure 48-1A

Typical Posture of Patient With Progressive Supranuclear Palsy

Patient stands in modified hyperextension in contrast to flexed position in Parkinson disease.

MOVEMENT DISORDERS

ATYPICAL PARKINSONIAN SYNDROMES

Figure 48-1B Tumors of Pineal Region

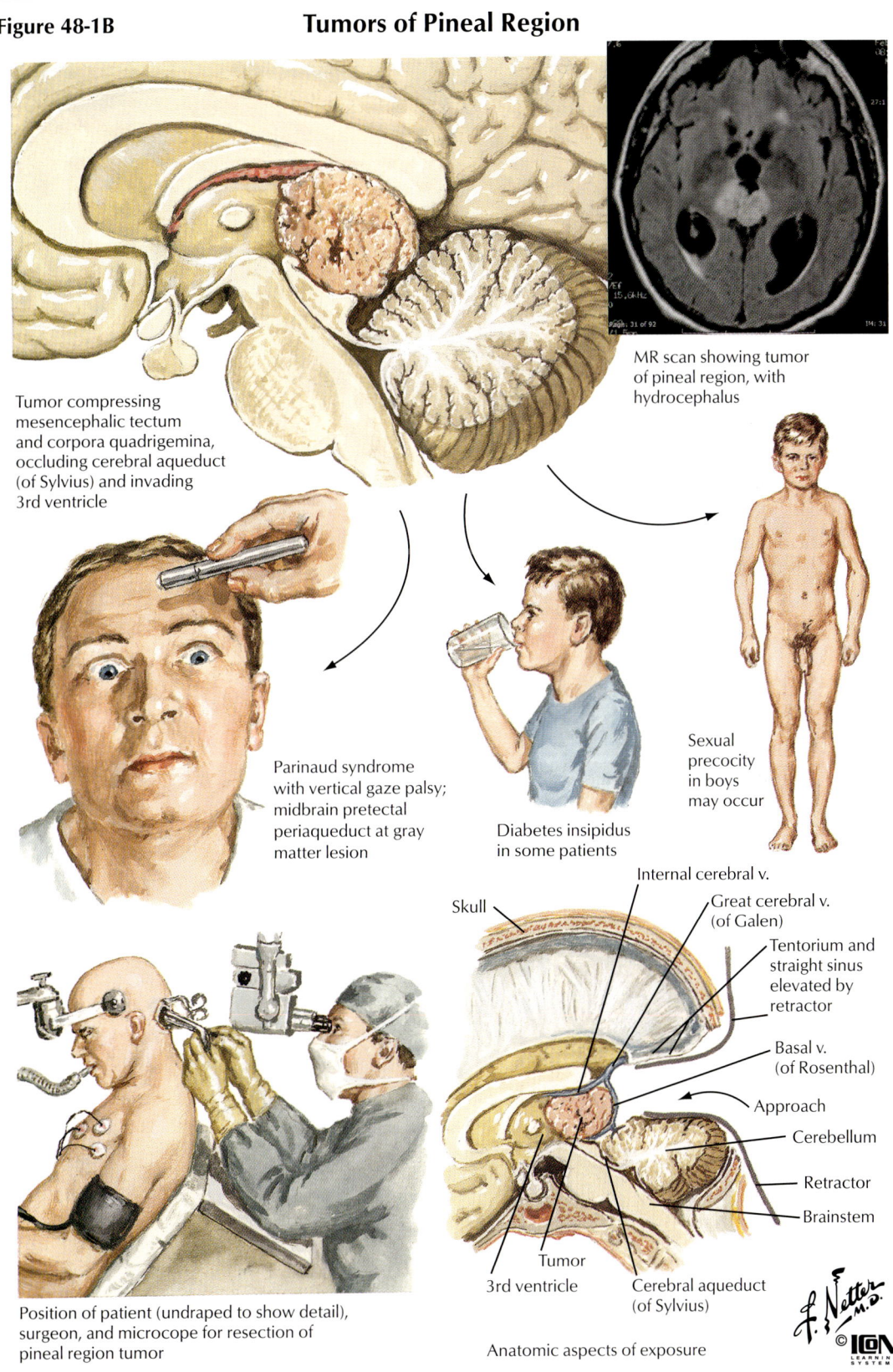

MOVEMENT DISORDERS

eration with predominant parkinsonism and a poor response to levodopa; *Shy-Drager syndrome, parkinsonism* or *cerebellar syndrome*, or both with predominant autonomic dysfunction; and sporadic *olivopontocerebellar atrophy* with predominant cerebellar dysfunction. MSA is a specific condition with a specific pathology, regardless of previous striatonigral degeneration, Shy-Drager syndrome, or olivopontocerebellar atrophy labels. It is characterized by oligodendroglial cytoplasmic inclusions that stain for a-synuclein and therefore is one of the synucleinopathies. Its etiology is unknown.

Pathophysiology

Macroscopically, neuronal loss and gliosis are primarily seen in many subcortical areas such as the substantia nigra, the locus ceruleus, the putamen, the globus pallidus, the inferior olive nucleus, the pons, the cerebellar cortex, the autonomic nuclei of the brainstem, and the intermediolateral columns of the spinal cord. A major microscopic finding, characteristic of but not specific for MSA, is glial cytoplasmic inclusions, the accumulation of the protein a-synuclein in oligodendrocytes. They are distributed selectively in the basal ganglia, the motor cortex, the reticular formation, the middle cerebellar peduncle, and the cerebellar white matter.

Clinical Presentation

Multiple system atrophy affects a slightly younger age group than does PD, with peak onset in the sixth decade of life. The clinical syndromes corresponding to the previously named striatonigral degeneration, olivopontocerebellar atrophy, and Shy-Drager syndrome are parkinsonism, cerebellar dysfunction, and autonomic failure, any of which may be the most prominent.

The parkinsonism of striatonigral degeneration tends to be more symmetric, rest tremor is less common, and postural instability develops earlier than in classic PD. However, early stages can be identical to idiopathic PD presentation, with a similar response to levodopa, including fluctuations and dyskinesias. Red flags suggesting MSA, including orthostatic hypotension, urinary retention or incontinence, ataxia, falls, stimulus sensitive myoclonus, antecollis, slurred speech, stridor, and corticospinal tract signs, should be sought.

Multiple system atrophy is a chronically progressive disorder characterized by gradual onset of symptoms. Patients who present initially with extrapyramidal features commonly progress to experience autonomic disturbances, cerebellar disorders, or both. Conversely, patients whose first symptoms are cerebellar dysfunction often later have extrapyramidal or autonomic disorders or both.

Diagnosis

Distinguishing MSA from idiopathic PD and PSP is challenging. Some features, such as autonomic dysfunction, poor or marginal response to levodopa with early clinical fluctuations, and dyskinesia, can help in differentiating MSA from early PD. Dementia and psychiatric features are more common in PD than MSA. Autonomic failure is common in MSA and rare in early PD.

CT can show cerebellar atrophy. Characteristic MRI abnormalities include hypointensity on T1 or hyperintensities on T2 in the lateral border of the putamen or putaminal atrophy. Cerebellar and pontine atrophy with the "hot cross bun" sign in the pons are seen; however, MRI results are not specific and are often normal.

Other tests used in diagnosis of MSA include autonomic testing, external anal or urethral sphincter EMG, and dopamine transporter scan.

Treatment

Only symptomatic therapy is available. Parkinsonism is treated with levodopa despite its inconsistent efficacy. Orthostatic hypotension may respond to conservative measures such as raising the head of the bed, binding stockings, and liberal salt intake. Medications such as fludrocortisone or midodrine are commonly required. Urinary dysfunction can be treated with antispasmodics such as oxybutynin and self-catheterization. The typical disease duration is 3 to 10 years. Breathing problems such as aspiration and cardiopulmonary arrest are common causes of death.

REFERENCES

Bennett P, Bonifati V, Bonuccelli U, et al. Direct genetic evidence for involvement of tau in progressive supranuclear palsy. *Neurology.* 1998;51:982-985.

Buee L, Delacourte A. Comparative biochemistry of tau in progressive supranuclear palsy, corticobasal degeneration, FTDP-17 and Pick's disease. *Brain Pathol.* 1999;9:681-693.

Gibb RG, Luthert PJ, Marsden CD. Corticobasal degeneration. *Brain.* 1989;112:1171-1192.

Gilman S. Multiple system atrophy. In: Jankovic J, Tolosa E, eds. *Parkinson's Disease and Movement Disorders.* Baltimore, Md: Williams & Wilkins; 1998:245-295.

Litvan I, Cummings JL, Mega M. Neuropsychiatric features of corticobasal degeneration. *J Neurol Neurosurg Psychiatry.* 1998;65:717-721.

Litvan I, Agid Y, Calne D, et al. Clinical research criteria for the diagnosis of progressive supranuclear palsy (Steel-Richardson-Olszewski syndrome). *Neurology.* 1996;47:1-9.

Rebeiz JJ, Edwin MD, Kolodny H, Richardson EP Jr. Cortico-dentatonigral degeneration with neuronal achromasia. *Arch Neurol.* 1968;18:20-33.

Savoiardo M, Grisoli M, Girotti F. Magnetic resonance imaging in CBD, related atypical Parkinsonian disorders, and dementias. *Adv Neurol.* 2000;82:197-208.

Chapter 49
Tremors

E. Prather Palmer

Clinical Vignette

A 31-year-old woman with no family history of neurologic disease and no history of trauma or drug abuse had the spontaneous onset of a horizontal ("no-no") head tremor. Initially, it was mild and asymptomatic, but as it increased in severity, the patient noted that turning her head to the right seemed to increase the tremor, whereas turning her head to the left decreased the tremor. Her neurologic examination results were otherwise normal, as was her brain MRI. β Blockers, primidone, and alcohol had little effect on the tremor. Eighteen months later, the patient returned, reporting that driving had become difficult because of a tendency for her head to turn involuntarily to the left, and her attempts to hold her head in the neutral position markedly increased the tremor and caused discomfort in her neck. Stress also caused similar problems. Over time, the involuntary movements were present almost continuously. Mild finger pressure on her left chin dampened the tremor and the involuntary movements of her head.

Neurologic examination demonstrated hypertrophy of the right sternocleidomastoid muscle. A trial of anticholinergic medication increased the tremor and precipitated a psychotic reaction. Eventually, the patient was treated with botulinum toxin in the right sternocleidomastoid muscle and some of the left paracervical muscles. This treatment controlled the involuntary movements and dampened the involuntary tremor.

Tremors are involuntary, rhythmic, and stereotyped oscillatory movements of a body part. They result from alternating or irregularly synchronous contractions of reciprocally innervated skeletal muscles. Tremors are the most prevalent movement disorders and are usually distinguishable from other abnormal involuntary movements by their rhythmic quality and the concomitant involvement of agonist and antagonist muscle groups.

The pathogenesis of tremor is unclear. Bursts of EMG activity separated by relative silence occur in all tremors, with the exception of low-amplitude physiologic tremor. EMG bursts in agonist-antagonist muscle pairs are not characteristic of tremors; the recorded pattern of any tremor can vary over a short period (ie, co-contraction of the muscles, alternation of contraction, or contraction of the antigravity muscles alone). More complex relations between the agonist-antagonist muscles also occur. Hence, no universal method exists of definitively rating, measuring, or classifying tremors. The clinical examination is therefore the most important step in tremor evaluation.

PHYSIOLOGIC TREMOR

Physiologic tremor is normally present in everyone because of many factors. Peripheral components include muscle mass and stiffness, long and short loop reflexes, grouped motor neuron firing rates, and the inertia of muscles and other structures. The central component of a physiologic tremor, the **central generator**, contributes weak 8- to 12-Hz low-amplitude movement not affected by inertial loading or physical manipulation. Other components, including the heartbeat (cardioballistics), may contribute. This normal tremor is best seen by holding an arm straight in front of the body and placing a sheet of paper across the outstretched fingers. With entrainment of the motor units (discharged in groups), the tremor can become more pronounced, called an *exaggerated physiologic tremor*, as seen during muscular fatigue, fear, excitement, or emotional distress and in certain medical conditions, including thyrotoxicosis, pheochromocytoma, catecholamine intake, methylxanthine use, drug withdrawal, and alcohol intoxication.

Exaggerated physiologic tremors have the same peripheral and central components as

Table 49-1
Approximate Frequencies of Tremors*

Frequency Range, Hz	Tremor Type
1-5	Holmes cerebellar tremor
2-10	Multiple sclerosis
2-12	Drug-induced tremor
2-12	Neuropathic tremor
3-10	Parkinsonian tremor
3-10	Task- and position-specific tremor
3-12	Dystonic tremor
4-10	Psychogenic tremor
4-8	Essential tremor
7-12	Physiologic and enhanced physiologic tremor
16-25	Orthostatic tremor

*After Bain PG. The management of tremor. *J Neurol Neurosurg Psychiatry.* 2002;72(suppl 1):i3-i16.

physiologic tremors but with greater stretch reflex and central oscillator participation. When exaggerated physiologic tremors become clinically symptomatic with postural changes or movement without provoking factors, they are similar or identical to **essential tremors**. Early in their course, essential tremors are difficult to separate from exaggerated physiologic tremors. Exaggerated physiologic tremors are reversible with cause identification and correction. β-Receptor agonists enhance physiologic tremor, and β-receptor blocker and β$_2$-receptor antagonists effectively decrease it. Physiologic tremor frequency is 8 to 12 Hz in young adults and decreases to 6 to 7 Hz in persons older than 60 years (Table 49-1).

PATHOPHYSIOLOGY

The cause of many tremors is unknown. Lesions in Parkinson disease predominate in the substantia nigra. However, experimental lesions of the substantia nigra in animals do not cause tremor, and not all patients with lesions at this level have a tremor. Moreover, a tremor develops in only half of patients poisoned with the analog of meperidine that destroys part of the substantia nigra (MPTP), and those tremors have more characteristics of action or postural tremors than of the classic resting tremor.

Ventromedial tegmentum lesions in monkey midbrain produce a resting-type tremor, presumably by interrupting the descending fibers releasing the oscillating mechanism of the lower brainstem. Pathologic tremors such as essential tremor, dystonic tremor, and the Parkinson disease tremors are thought to have multiple central generators, resulting in variable frequencies from approximately 1 to 26 Hz. With the exception of rare neuropathic tremors primarily associated with chronic inflammatory demyelinating polyneuropathy, pathologic tremors usually overwhelm any peripheral contribution to the tremor.

PATHOLOGIC TREMOR

The most common and clinically most useful classification of pathologic (nonphysiologic) tremors is based on their clinical features, especially distribution (proximal or distal, body part involved), symmetry, and the conditions that best activate them (Table 49-2). Tremors of a body part completely supported against gravity and at rest are called **rest tremors** (Figure 49-1). Tremors during voluntary muscular contraction are called **action tremors**. Action tremors are further classified as **postural** (occur in a body part maintained in position against gravity), **kinetic** (occur during voluntary movement), or **isometric** (occur within a muscle contracting against a stationary object).

Essential Tremor

Essential tremor is neither "essential" (an inherent characteristic of the individual) nor "benign." This acquired tremor usually worsens with age and may greatly interfere with normal activities. It is an action tremor with a lower frequency (4-8 Hz) than the physiologic tremor (7-12 Hz) and may be the only neurologic disability. If several family members are affected, it is called **familial** or **hereditary tremor**. Of those with an essential tremor, approximately 50% have a positive family history, usually involving an auto-

TREMORS

Table 49-2
Classification of Tremors

Type of Tremor	Clinical Features	Common Examples
Action		
Postural	A posture is maintained against gravity	Physiologic tremor Essential tremor Drug-induced tremor
Kinetic	With voluntary movements	Parkinson disease Cerebellar lesions (intention tremor) Writing tremor Holmes tremor
Isometric	With voluntary muscle contraction against a rigid, stationary object	Orthostatic tremor
Orthostatic tremor	Tremor of lower limbs on standing and remits on walking or sitting	Orthostatic tremor Head trauma Neuropathic tremor
Dystonic tremor	Tremor in body part affected by dystonia	Spasmodic torticollis
Resting tremor	Limb fully supported against gravity; improves with voluntary movement	Parkinson disease
Psychogenic tremor	Acute onset, inconsistent, fatigues, decreases amplitude with distraction	Somatoform disorders Malingering Depression
Asterixis	Arrhythmic lapses of sustained postures	Toxic and metabolic encephalopathies

somal dominant trait with virtually complete penetrance. If the essential tremor occurs late in life, it may be called a **senile tremor**. Whether familial or spontaneous, it has a bimodal onset peak in the fourth to sixth decades of life. Although the familial forms tend to begin earlier, they rarely occur during infancy or after the sixth decade. Essential tremor is 20 times more frequent (prevalence, 0.2-33%) than Parkinson disease. Although many adult patients who experience essential tremors fear they have Parkinson disease, an essential tremor is not an indication that Parkinson disease is present or will result.

Typical essential tremors are mild, symmetric postural tremors of the upper limbs, accentuated by voluntary movements. They commonly consist of pronation-supination and extension-flexion movements, and in severe or advanced cases, they may have a resting or kinetic component. They may spread to the head, face, lips, voice, jaw, tongue, chin, or occasionally the legs. Head tremors may be horizontal ("no-no") or vertical ("yes-yes"). Although essential tremor is a monosymptomatic illness, abnormalities in tandem gait are seen in nearly 50% of patients. Mild parkinsonian features (ie, rest tremor, cogwheeling, and breakdown in rapid alternating movements) may also be present. Some instances of "no-no" tremor may be from spasmodic torticollis (dystonia) in patients with minimal abnormal posturing. These tremors increase when the head is turned opposite to the direction of the pull.

Treatment of essential tremor can be frustrating. Up to 66% of patients with essential tremor experience a dramatic reduction after alcohol intake. Alcohol reduces the overactivity of the cerebellum that is seen in PET scans of patients with essential tremor. However, over time, larger amounts of alcohol are needed to produce this effect and alcoholism may result. Some studies suggest that more than 75% of patients respond

TREMORS

Figure 49-1

Tremor

Rest tremor

Usually called parkinsonian tremor, occurs in a limb that is not voluntarily activated. It is suppressed with voluntary movement. It may appear as "pill rolling."

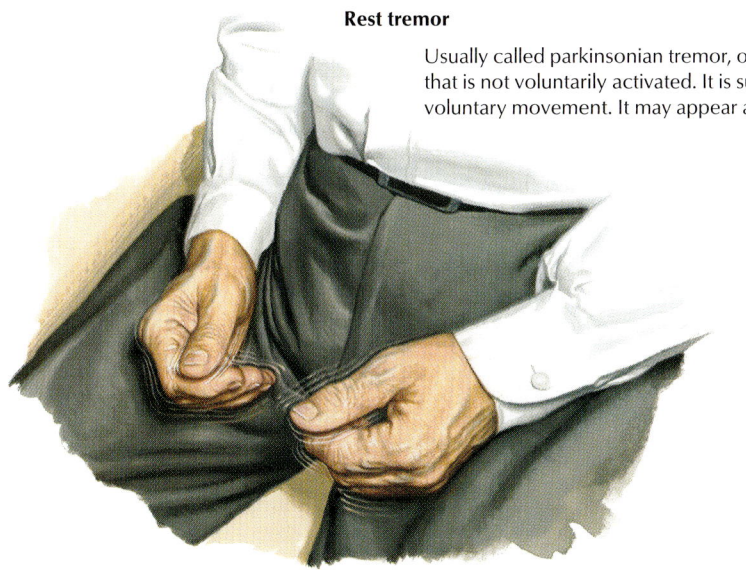

Action tremor (example: essential tremor)

Typically bilateral, this movement disorder is the most common. It may be accentuated with goal-directed movement of the limbs. Essential tremor affects the hands and facial musculature (in this order of prevalence). Most common presentation is the association of hand tremor and tremor in cranial musculature.

However considered benign, it can become incapacitating. In the severe forms the patient may not be able to perform essential daily activities, such as drinking from a cup or dressing.

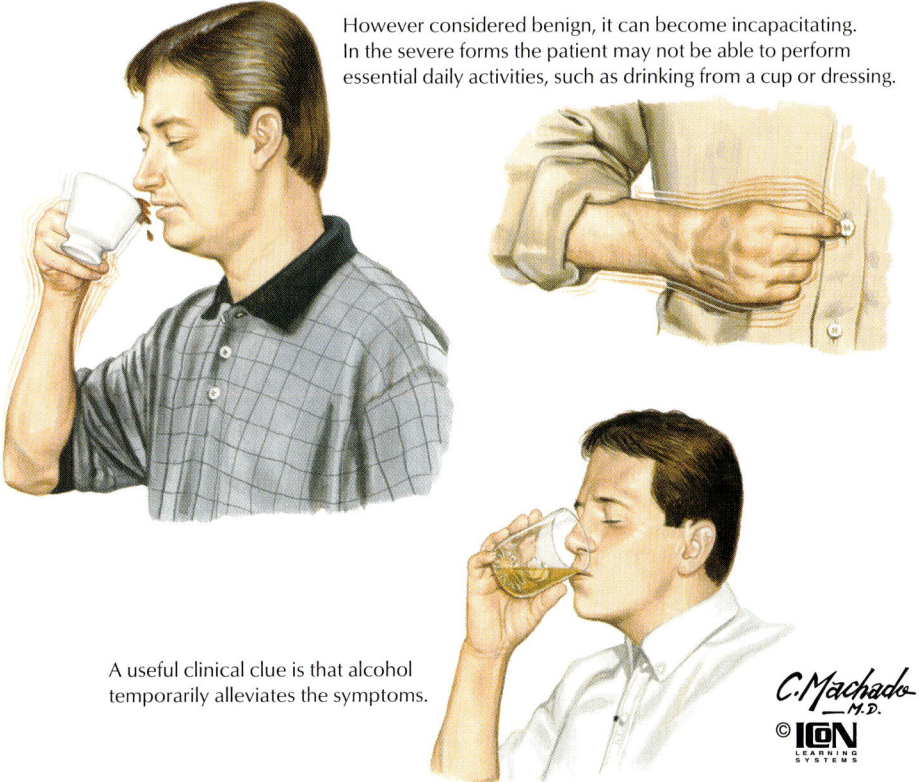

A useful clinical clue is that alcohol temporarily alleviates the symptoms.

MOVEMENT DISORDERS

TREMORS

Table 49-3
Pharmacologic Options for Essential Tremor

Drug	Dosage	Precautions	Comment
β Blockers*			
Propranolol	30-240 mg/d	Avoid in patients with asthma, bradycardia, heart failure, or diabetes; may cause memory difficulties and confusion in the elderly	50% patients may benefit and benefit may extend beyond 1 year, but escalation of the dose may be needed. Best tolerated by the young.
Metoprolol (Lopressor, Toprol)	50-200 mg/d	As above	Alternative to propanolol
Anticonvulsants*§			
Primidone*§ (Mysoline)	50-1000 mg/d	May cause ataxia, flulike symptoms, and drowsiness	Effective in up to 50% of patients; may be effective in patients who are unresponsive to β blockers
Gabapentin†§ (Neurontin)	100-2400 mg/d	May cause mild drowsiness, headache, and abdominal discomfort	Studies show inconsistent improvement, well tolerated.
Topiramate* (Topamax)	25-300 mg/d	May cause weight loss, paresthesiae, lethargy, or memory difficulties	Need to start with low doses and increase slowly
Benzodiazepines†			
Clonazepam (Klonopin)	0.25-4 mg/d	May cause confusion, drowsiness, ataxia, hypotension, and apnea	Good for intermittent use; loss of effectiveness with long-term use
Diazepam (Valium)	1-10 mg/d	Same as above	Same as above
Calcium channel blockers‡			
Nimodipin (Nimotop)	30-80 mg/d	May cause hypotension	Option if other drugs unsuccessful
Carbonic anhydrase inhibitors‡			
Methazolamide (Glauc Tabs, Neptazane)	100-200 mg/d	May cause paresthesiae, abdominal discomfort, and drowsiness	Adverse effects limit usefulness-may help with voice and head tremors
Botulinum toxin‡			
Botox	Varies with injected muscles	Causes weakness of injected muscles	May be useful for voice or head tremors

*First-line drugs.
†Second-line drugs.
‡Drugs that may be helpful if others fail.
§Drugs better tolerated by the elderly.
‖Hart after Evidente VGH. Understanding essential tremor: differential diagnosis and options for treatment. *Postgrad Med.* 200;108:138-149.

to medication; however, adverse effects often limit the doses that patients tolerate (Table 49-3). Treatment is not indicated for mild tremors that do not interfere with patients' quality of life. Surgical treatment (thalamotomy and deep brain stimulation) is effective in severely disabling, drug-resistant, or intolerant cases.

Resting Tremor

Most resting tremors are associated with Parkinson disease or its variants (chapters 47 and 48). Parkinsonian tremors can be flexion-extension or abduction-adduction of the fingers or hand and pronation-supination of the hand and forearm. A combination of these movements gives the classic "pill-rolling" tremor. The tremor is often initially asymmetric and may remain so for years, but it is slowly progressive. It usually affects the hand but can include the feet, mandible, and lips. It is somewhat suppressed by anticholinergic drugs and, less consistently but occasionally impressively, by levodopa and other dopamine agonist drugs. Monosymptomatic resting tremors, without other parkinsonian features, may occur and are often refractory to treatment. Occasionally, other features of Parkinson disease occur years later.

With the increased understanding of the pathogenesis and treatment of Parkinson disease, many patients mistakenly assume that most tremors are related to it. The physician must be able to differentiate the more common, postural essential tremor from the serious resting tremor of Parkinson disease (Table 49-4).

Orthostatic Tremor and Other Action Tremors

Clinical Vignette

A 72-year-old man reported that in the past 6 months he had experienced difficulty playing golf. He noted that when he stepped to the tee, he had increasing problems maintaining his balance because his legs became very tremulous. Although he could walk all 18 holes without difficulty, he was unable to maintain his balance when he tried to stand still to make his shots. To compensate, he assumed an ever-widening posture, but this became increasingly less helpful. Similarly, he had routinely begun to sit down when he urinated. In contrast, he found that he could still walk well, but when he stopped, he had to sit down because he was unable to maintain his balance while standing.

Table 49-4
Essential Tremor Versus Parkinson Tremor

Characteristic	Essential Tremor	Parkinson Tremor
Type	Action/postural	Resting, "pill rolling"
Frequency	4-10 Hz	3-5 Hz
Age at onset	All ages	Middle age or elderly
Family history	First-degree relative often	None affected
Body part	Hands, head, voice	Hands, legs
Symmetry	Usually symmetric onset	Asymmetric onset, slowly
Course	Stable or slowly progressive	Progressive proximal as it generalizes to both sides
Other symptoms	Usually monosymptomatic	Rigidity, bradykinesia, flexed posture, balance problems
Origin	Olivocerebellar and other midbrain circuitry	Multiple generators within corticobasal ganglia and corticocerebellar circuitry
Other	Often transmitted as autosomal dominant, classically diminished by alcohol	May exhibit many types of tremors, including a postural one at the wrist at 5-8 Hz that may be difficult to distinguish from an essential tremor

TREMORS

Neurologic examination demonstrated an alert, pleasant man with normal facial expression. He arose from his chair without difficulty, walking with a normal gait, including a good arm swing. However, when he stopped and tried to stand still, he stood with an abnormally wide base, soon with development of an 18- to 20-Hz tremor of both of his legs. It was necessary for him to hold on to someone to keep from falling. He had no tremor while seated at rest, there was no cogwheeling or rigidity, and his strength was normal in all four extremities, with normal muscle stretch reflexes and sensation, particularly position sense.

Brain MRI and EMG were normal. Various medications were tried, including primidone, but no effective remedies were found.

Orthostatic tremor is a rare and often misdiagnosed problem of late middle age that is characterized by a 16- to 25-Hz tremor affecting the lower extremities, typically with weight bearing. Isometric limb muscle contraction, the critical generation factor, induces the tremor. No other tremors have a frequency greater than 16 Hz. Often, if patients cannot sit down or resume walking, they become distressed and sometimes fall. Patients stand with a wide base but can walk normally as the tremor abates in the non–weight-bearing extremity. Among individuals who have orthostatic tremor, 30% also have an essential leg tremor that does not attenuate with walking.

The limited differential diagnosis for patients with orthostatic tremor includes aqueduct stenosis, head trauma, pontine lesions, and chronic inflammatory demyelinating polyneuropathy. Therefore, brain MRI is important, as is EMG if the MRI is normal. Treatment with toparimate, benzodiazepines, or valproic acid may help. Although anxiety often accompanies orthostatic tremors and may require treatment, patient and family may need reassurance of the nonpsychiatric nature of the tremor (Table 49-5).

Table 49-5
Other Action-Type Tremors

Type	Description
Isolated chin tremors	Familial syndrome with onset in infancy or childhood; often intermittent and stress-induced
Dystonic tremor	A postural or kinetic tremor in an extremity or body part affected by dystonia; may at times be more obvious than the dystonic movement it accompanies.
Isolated voice tremor	May be a variant of essential tremor or dystonic tremor accompanying focal dystonia of the vocal cords (spasmodic dystonia)
Alcohol withdrawal tremor	An action/postural tremor is a prominent feature of the alcohol withdrawal syndrome; after recovery from the withdrawal state, some individuals have a persistent essential-type tremor; withdrawal of other sedative-type drugs (barbiturates, benzodiazepines) after prolonged use may also produce the same type of tremor
Task-specific tremors	May occur primarily during the performance of specific tasks or postures; primary writing tremor is the most common, but similar task specific tremors have been described in typists, musicians, and sportsmen
Neuropathic tremor	Irregular, asymmetric, usually distal tremor, with frequencies of 3-12 Hz; may occur at rest, with posture or with movement, and is associated with peripheral nerve disease; usually subsides with treatment of the underlying neuropathy or with β blockers

Ataxic Intention Tremor

These tremors could be classified as an action or kinetic tremor; however, its characteristics and similarities to cerebellar disorders make it a separate clinical entity. The tremor is not intentional but occurs primarily during the demanding phase of active volitional movement. It is absent when the limbs are inactive and during the beginning of a voluntary movement. As the action continues and fine adjustments are demanded (eg, finger-to-nose task), 2- to 4-Hz side-to-side oscillations interrupt the movement and may continue for several beats after the target has been reached. Ataxic intention tremor always occurs in combination with cerebellar ataxia and may seriously interfere with performance of skilled acts.

Another more violent form of an intention tremor, **Holmes tremor**, is associated with cerebellar ataxia, wherein slight lifting of the arms or maintenance of a static posture (eg, arms abducted at the shoulders) results in a wide-range, rhythmic, 2- to 5-Hz "wing-beating" movement, often sufficiently forceful to throw patients off balance. The lesion is usually in the midbrain near the red nucleus (the tremor was formally called a *rubral tremor*). There is no treatment for these tremors. In severe cases, surgery (usually a thalamotomy) may help.

Palatal Tremor

Palatal tremors are rare, rapid, rhythmic, and involuntary movements of the soft palate. Previously considered to be a form of myoclonus (hence the term *palatal myoclonus* or *palatal nystagmus*), palatal tremor has 2 forms: essential or symptomatic. Essential palatal tremor has no pathologic basis. It is associated with rhythmic activation of the tensor veli palatini, often recognized by the patient noting an audible click that ceases with sleep. MRI demonstrates no specific abnormalities in essential palatal tremor.

Symptomatic palatal tremor is often associated with pendular vertical nystagmus, oscillopsia, and cerebellar signs and continues during sleep. Unlike essential palatal tremor, it involves the levator veli palatini muscles. Symptomatic palatal tremor is associated with vascular disorders, multiple sclerosis, encephalitis, trauma, and neurodegenerative diseases. MRI shows tegmental lesions and inferior olivary nucleus enlargement, unilateral or bilateral, in the symptomatic form.

Asterixis

Asterixis is typically a series of arrhythmic interruptions in a sustained posture (ie, sustained muscular contractions). A lapse in postural muscles is associated with EMG silence for a period of 35 to 300 milliseconds. During this silence, gravity or the inherent elasticity of muscles produces the movement. Asterixis, therefore, differs physiologically from tremors and myoclonus. It is easily demonstrated by asking patients to hold their arms outstretched with hands dorsiflexed and fingers extended. Flexion hand movements may occur several times each minute. Asterixis can be produced by persistent contraction of any muscle group (eg, sustained protrusion of the tongue). It can occur in normal persons in the neck and arms with drowsiness.

Asterixis is usually seen in hepatic or uremic encephalopathy and sometimes in other metabolic and toxic states, including those iatrogenically induced by phenytoin and other anticonvulsants. Unilateral asterixis is sometimes observed with contralateral thalamic or brainstem lesions. Clonazepam, sodium valproate, tetrabenazine, and haloperidol sometimes help to alleviate the symptoms of asterixis.

Drug-Induced (Iatrogenic) Tremor

Many pharmacologic agents can induce tremors, depending on the individual and the underlying illness. Some drugs, such as lithium, can cause several types of tremor, depending on the dose or treatment duration. The most common drug-induced tremor is an enhanced physiologic tremor related to sympathomimetics or antidepressants (especially the tricyclics and serotonin reuptake inhibitors). Although specific predisposing risk factors are not well defined, patients with an essential tremor, older patients, and women are thought to have a higher risk for drug-induced tremors.

A parkinsonianlike tremor (resting tremor) may occur after ingestion of neuroleptic, antidopaminergic drugs (including dopamine-

TREMORS

depleting drugs). Unlike the tremor of Parkinson disease, the resting, pharmacologically induced tremor is initially bilateral and symmetric. Intention tremor may occur with lithium intoxication or chronic alcoholism. A **tardive tremor** is associated with long-term neuroleptic use. The anticonvulsants phenytoin and sodium valproate can cause various action tremors. An action tremor resembling an enhanced physiologic tremor is also produced by substances such as calcium channel blockers, amiodarone, theophylline, adrenaline, amphetamine, lithium, caffeine, cocaine, marijuana, and drug or alcohol withdrawal (Table 49-6).

Psychogenic Tremor

Psychogenic tremors present as manifestations of underlying psychiatric disorders, particularly in patients with somatoform disturbances, malingering, or depression. Clinical presentations vary and are usually bizarre combinations of resting, postural, or intention tremors. Diagnosis is often by exclusion and is frequently difficult but is best confirmed when psychotherapy leads to remission.

Recognized diagnostic criteria include acute onset and spontaneous remission; decreased tremor with distraction; variation of frequency and amplitude during movements; history of

Table 49-6
Drug-Induced Tremors

Drug	Type of Tremor
Alcohol withdrawal	Postural, intention
Drug withdrawal	Postural
Insulin (by inducing hypoglycemia)	Postural
CNS acting	
Neuroleptics	Resting, postural
Reserpine	Resting, postural
Metoclopramide	Resting, postural
Antidepressants	Resting
Lithium	Resting, postural, intention
Cocaine	Postural
Alcohol	Postural, intention
Sympathomimetics	
Bronchodilators (β_2 agonist)	Postural, intention
Theophylline	Postural
Caffeine	Postural
Dopamine	Postural
Cyclosporine	Postural
Lithium	Postural, action
Thyroxine	Postural
Methylzanthines	Postural, action
Steroids	Postural, resting, intention
Miscellaneous	
Valproate	Postural, action
Phenytoin	Postural, action
Antiarrhythmics (amiodarone)	Postural
Antidopaminergic drugs (eg, metoclopramide)	Postural, rest
Mexiletine	Postural
Thyroid hormones	Postural
Cytostatics (vincristine, cytosine)	Postural, intention
Immunosuppressants	
Cyclosporine	Postural

somatization; coactivation of antagonist muscles during passive flexion or extension and tremor cessation as the increased resistance to passive movements stops; and lack of responsiveness to acceptable treatment, placebo, or both. In very few patients, the whole body shakes, and the tremor may cease spontaneously or during examination as the movements exhaust the patient. More difficult cases involve predominately extremity tremors, often without finger involvement. The prognosis in psychogenic tremors is poor without prompt recognition and treatment.

REFERENCES

Bain PG. The management of tremor. *J Neurol Neurosurg Psychiatry*. 2002;72(suppl 1):i3-i16.

Evidente VGH. Understanding essential tremor: differential diagnosis and options for treatment. *Postgrad Med*. 2000;108:138-149.

Habib-ur-Rehman. Diagnosis and management of tremor. *Arch Intern Med*. 2000;160:2438-2444.

Zesiewicz TA, Hauser RA. Phenomenology and treatment of tremor disorders. *Neurol Clin*. 2001;19:651-680.

Chapter 50
Medication-Induced Movement Disorders

Diana Apetauerova

Clinical Vignette

A 22-year-old woman with a history of Tourette syndrome (TS) and depression presented with recent onset of tongue-protruding movements, lip puckering, and lip smacking. She said that she had no urge to perform these movements. She had restarted the neuroleptic pimozide 4 months earlier because of increasing TS symptomatology. The orofacial movements occurred while the primary TS symptoms improved. Because tardive dyskinesia (TD) was suspected, the pimozide dose was decreased, with some symptom alleviation. She had never before experienced any adverse effects of other neuroleptics. The family history was significant for TS in her father and depression in her mother. She was currently taking no other medication.

Cranial nerve examination results were significant for nearly constant chewing, tongue protrusion, vermicular tongue motion, lip smacking, puckering, and pursing. The patient had multiple episodes of vocal tics in the form of grunting and complex motor tics in the form of touching her arm with right hand and turning around while walking. The rest of her mental status, motor, sensory, cerebellar, and general physical examinations were normal.

That her orofacial movements were dyskinesia rather than a form of complex motor tic was suggested by their occurrence during neuroleptic therapy and her denial of an urge for her other motor and vocal tics. Because the neuroleptic was the most likely cause of her TD, it was discontinued. Subsequently, the orofacial dyskinesias decreased significantly, although they were still present in a mild form at follow-up 6 weeks later.

Many drugs with different mechanisms of action cause movement disorders (Table 50-1). Most interfere with dopaminergic transmission within the basal ganglia (levodopa, dopamine agonists, dopamine receptor–blocking agents [DRBs]); however, the mechanisms of action of many other drugs are not well understood (eg, CNS stimulants, anticonvulsants, tricyclic antidepressants, estrogens). Clinically, the drugs most commonly causing movement disorders are neuroleptics and pharmacologic agents that block or stimulate dopamine receptors.

The onset of drug-induced movement disorders can be acute, subacute, or chronic. Acute syndromes include dystonia, choreoathetosis, akathisia, and tics. Subacute syndromes include drug-induced parkinsonism and tremor. Chronic syndromes include levodopa-induced dyskinesias in Parkinson disease and TD.

No direct evidence exists of CNS pathology to explain drug-induced movement disorders. Therefore, because no anatomical correlation or model has been developed, this supports the concept that these are purely biochemical in nature.

CLINICAL SYNDROMES
Acute Dystonic Reactions

Acute dystonic reactions usually occur within 5 days after initiation of neuroleptic medication, making them one of the earliest onset drug-induced movement disorders. The craniocervical region is the most commonly affected site. Pathophysiologically related to a sudden imbalance between the striatal dopamine and cholinergic systems, acute dystonia resolves spontaneously on drug withdrawal. Standard treatment is parenteral anticholinergics or antihistamines such as diphenhydramine.

Medication-Induced Parkinsonism

All dopamine-blocking agents and drugs interfering with the synthesis, storage, and release of dopamine may precipitate an akinetic-rigid syndrome nearly indistinguishable from idiopathic Parkinson disease (Figure 50-1). Substituted ben-

Table 50-1
Types of Drug-Induced Movement Disorders and Responsible Medications

Syndrome	Responsible Medication
Postural tremor	Sympathomimetics Levodopa Amphetamines Bronchodilators Tricyclic antidepressants Lithium carbonate Caffeine Thyroid hormone Sodium valproate Antipsychotics Hypoglycemic agents Adrenocorticosteroids Alcohol withdrawal Amiodarone Cyclosporin A Others
Acute dystonic reactions	Antipsychotics Metoclopramide Antimalarial agents Tetrabenazine Diphenhydramine Mefenamic acid Oxatomide Flunarizine and cinnarizine
Akathisia	Antipsychotics Metoclopramide Reserpine Tetrabenazine Levodopa and dopamine agonists Flunarizine and cinnarizine Ethosuximide Methysergide
Parkinsonism	Antipsychotics Metoclopramide Reserpine Tetrabenazine Methyldopa Flunarizine and cinnarizine Lithium Phenytoin Captopril Alcohol withdrawal MPTP Other toxins (manganese, carbon disulfide, cyanide) Cytosine arabinoside

(continued)

zamides (metoclopramide) used to treat gastrointestinal disorders and calcium channel blockers can also cause parkinsonism. The pathophysiologic mechanism allowing parkinsonism induction may be a predominant presynaptic effect on dopamine and serotonin neurons.

Therapeutic drug-induced parkinsonism is often characterized by a symmetric presentation, unlike the more focal onset of Parkinson disease. Bradykinesia predominates over typical rigidity and resting tremor. When a tremor is present, it is usually postural instead of resting. Drug-

MEDICATION-INDUCED MOVEMENT DISORDERS

Table 50-1
Types of Drug-Induced Disorders and Responsible Medications (continued)

Syndrome	Responsible Medication
Chorea, including tarditive and orofacial dyskinesia	Antipsychotics Metoclopramide Levodopa Direct dopamine agonists Indirect dopamine agonists and other catecholaminergic drugs Anticholinergics Antihistaminics Oral contraceptives Phenytoin Carbamazepine Ethosuximide Phenobarbital Lithium carbonate Methadone Benzodiazepines Monoamine oxidase inhibitors Tricyclic antidepressants Methyldopa Digoxin Alcohol withdrawal Toluene sniffing Flunarizine and cinnarizine
Dystonia, including tarditive dystonia (excluding acute dystonic reactions)	Antipsychotics Metoclopramide Levodopa Direct dopamine agonists Phenytoin Carbamazepine Flunarizine and cinnarizine
Neuroleptic malignant syndrome	Antipsychotics Tetrabenazine with α methyl paratyrosine
Tics	Withdrawal of antiparkinsonian drugs in Parkinson disease Levodopa Direct dopamine agonists Antipsychotics Carbamazepine
Myoclonus	Levodopa Anticonvulsants Tricyclic antidepressants Antipsychotics
Asterixis	Anticonvulsants Levodopa Hepatotoxins Respiratory depressants

MEDICATION-INDUCED MOVEMENT DISORDERS

Figure 50-1
Medication-Induced Parkinsonism

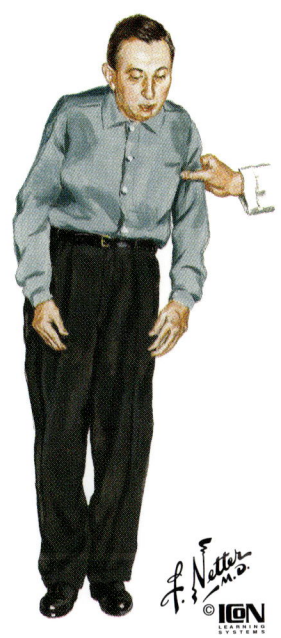

induced parkinsonism may persist long after withdrawal of the offending drug. Therapeutic interventions are seldom necessary if use of the drug can be stopped.

Akathisia

Akathisia is characterized by an inability to keep still; subjectively, it is often accompanied by feelings of restlessness, primarily resulting from the initiation of neuroleptic therapy. Akathisia is the most poorly understood, acute drug-induced syndrome; no neuroanatomical correlates explain it. Dose reduction or withdrawal of the offending drug is the most effective treatment. Other drugs, such as propranolol and clonidine, can be used in treatment; however, neuroleptics have little or no direct effect on β-adrenergic receptors.

Neuroleptic Malignant Syndrome

An unusual complication, neuroleptic malignant syndrome is one of the most severe reactions to neuroleptic therapy. Its incidence is 0.5% to 1% of patients taking neuroleptic medication. Symptoms occur after institution of neuroleptic therapy or with increased dosage. Clinical characteristics—acute onset of a severe movement disorder with rigidity, tremor, and dystonia—are often associated with autonomic disturbances including fever, diaphoresis, and cardiovascular and pulmonary disorders. Often, a concomitant myonecrosis significantly increases serum creatine kinase. Certain complications, including dehydration, cardiac arrhythmias, pulmonary embolism, and stupor associated with leukocytosis lead to death in up to 20% of cases. Young men are at higher risk than the general population. Pathogenesis is thought to involve both central and peripheral effects of dopamine receptor blockade. Medications that are frequently useful include levodopa, dopamine agonists, and the antispastic agent dantrolene.

Tardive Dyskinesia Syndromes

Tardive dyskinesia syndromes have a latent onset, occurring at least 3 months after—or, more commonly, 1 to 2 years after—initiation of the responsible medication. They can occur during treatment, after dose reduction, or subsequent to medication withdrawal and are sometimes irreversible. The offending drugs are usually DRBs and most commonly neuroleptics. The prevalence of TD varies between 0.5% and 65%, making it the most feared complication of long-term neuroleptic therapy.

Clinically, TD usually manifests with hyperkinesias, including chorea, athetosis, dystonia, and tics most commonly affecting the orofacial region (chewing, tongue protrusion, vermicular tongue motion, lip smacking, puckering, and pursing), limb and truncal regions, or paroxysms of rapid eye blinking (Figure 50-2). Older patients, female sex, and therapy duration and dosage are proposed risk factors. If the TD abates, it may take months.

The pathophysiology of TD is partly understood. The primary theory is that striatal dopamine receptors are chronically blocked by DRBs. Subsequently, these receptors develop a supersensitivity to dopamine such that amounts normally too small to induce dyskinesia in an otherwise healthy individual do so. The persistence of TD after drug withdrawal also suggests underactivity of GABA-mediated inhibition of

MEDICATION-INDUCED MOVEMENT DISORDERS

Figure 50-2A Chorea

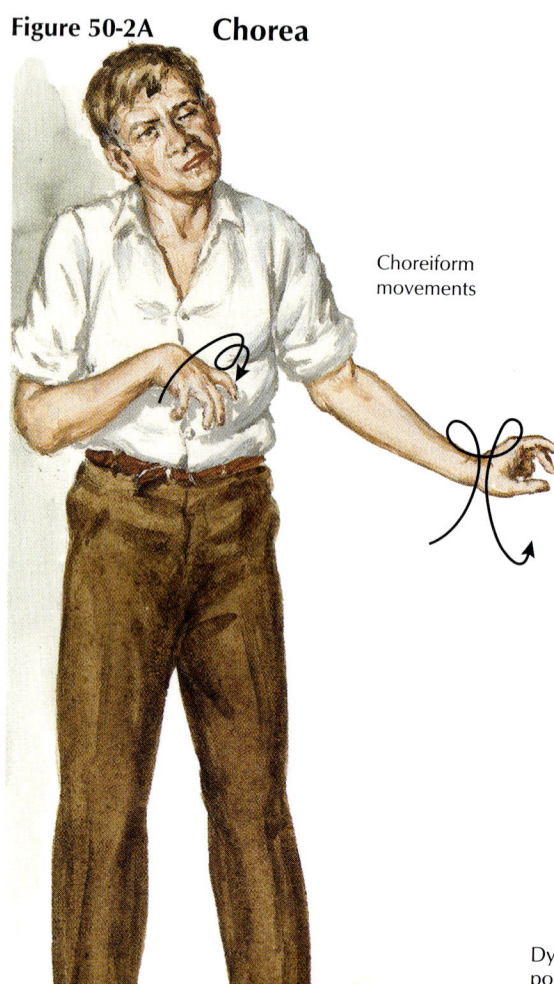

Choreiform movements

tial diagnosis. Also, some systemic illnesses are associated with various dyskinesias; hyperthyroidism, hypoparathyroidism, hyperglycemia, chorea of pregnancy, Sydenham chorea, and inflammatory or space-occupying brain lesions rarely cause a pseudo-TD.

No single therapeutic strategy is significantly effective for TD. The best methods are prevention and early recognition. Reduction or withdrawal of medication, when possible, is advisable. Drugs used in its treatment include dopamine-depleting agents (reserpine, tetrabenazine), benzodiazepines, GABA mimetics

Figure 50-2B Tardive Dyskinesia

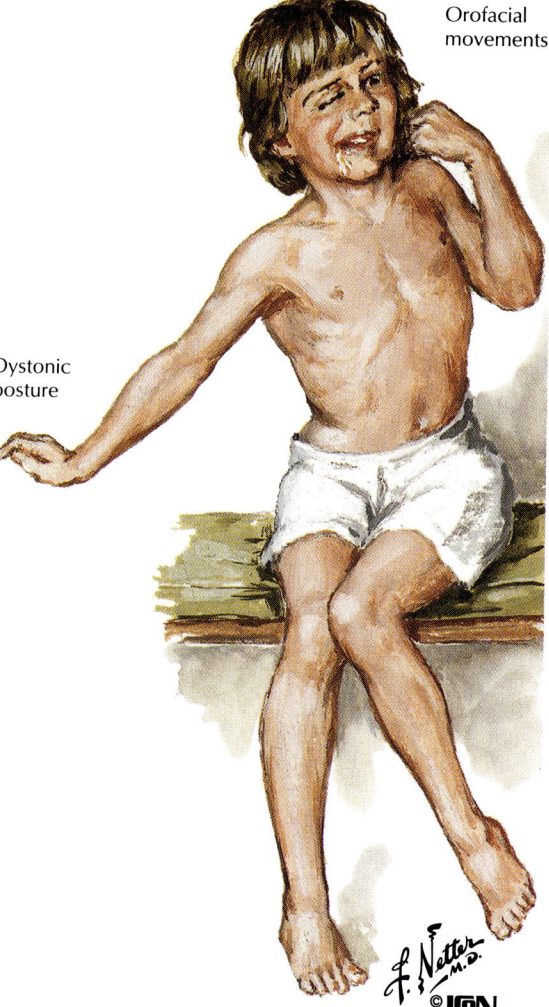

Orofacial movements

Dystonic posture

the thalamocortical pathway and an excitotoxic DRB mechanism.

The differential diagnosis of TD includes idiopathic movement disorders such as stereotypic behavior in psychotic patients, TS, simple or complex motor tics, and dental problems. Other drug-induced dyskinesias deserve consideration, particularly antiemetics such as chlorpromazine. Inheritable disorders including Huntington disease, Wilson disease, and Hallervorden-Spatz neurodegeneration with brain iron accumulation type 1 disease are in the differen-

MOVEMENT DISORDERS

(valproate sodium and baclofen), and dopamine agonists in low doses. Use of antioxidants such as vitamin E has been proposed, but study results conflict.

DIAGNOSIS

Careful clinical observation and review of the patient's medication history are key to the diagnosis of drug-induced movement disorders. When the possibility of other etiologic mechanisms exists, studies to exclude hereditary or systemic illness or the rare structural basal ganglia lesion should be performed.

Medication-induced movement disorders have primarily been studied in case reports. Solid epidemiologic data are lacking. Prospective, multicenter studies are needed to elucidate the specifics of individual susceptibility for these syndromes.

REFERENCES

Gershanik OS. Drug-induced dyskinesia. In: Anodic J, Tolosa E, eds. *Parkinson's disease and Movement Disorders*. Baltimore, Md: Williams & Wilkins; 1998:579-600.

Kiriakakis V, Bhatia K, Quinn NP, Marsden CD. The natural history of tardive dystonia: a long-term follow-up study of 107 cases. *Brain*. 1998;121:2053-2066.

Woerner MG, Alvir JMJ, Saltz BL, Lieberman JA, Kane JM. Prospective study of tardive dyskinesia in the elderly: rates and risk factors. *Am J Psychiatry*. 1998;155:1521-1528.

Chapter 51
Dystonia

E. Prather Palmer

Clinical Vignette

An 18-year-old man was seen for a 3-year history of progressive, painful weakness and stiffness of his legs. Formerly very active, he was no longer able to play tennis or walk more than several blocks. The patient volunteered that he was able to ambulate much better and without pain during the morning hours. On examination, he walked stiffly on painful legs. There was sustained clonus at the ankles and bilateral Babinski signs. The tone in his arms was increased, and rapid alternating movements of his fingers was slowed.

Dopa-responsive dystonia was considered as a diagnosis. PET showed normal basal ganglia uptake of labeled fluorodopa (unlike Parkinson disease). Treatment with levodopa gave immediate symptom relief, and the patient was able to return to an active life. On the next visit, the patient was accompanied by his brother, who had been treated for several years, unsuccessfully, with high-dose anticholinergic medications for a painful torticollis. He also improved significantly with levodopa therapy. A genetic cause for the familial syndrome was not found. Treatment with tetrahydrobiopterin was not helpful. Both brothers remained active after 10 years of treatment.

Involuntary writhing twisting movements that may initially occur during voluntary actions are the principle characteristics of dystonia. They are often repetitive, sometimes leading to abnormal and bizarre postures. Both agonist and antagonist muscles contract simultaneously to cause the dystonic movements. The movements may be intermittent or sustained, rapid or slow, rhythmic or unpatterned, tremulous or jerky. **Brief shocklike contractions (<1 second) may be called *dystonic spasms* or *myoclonic dystonia*. Sustained** (several seconds) postures are called *dystonic movements* or *athetoid dystonia*. If the movements last **several minutes or hours**, they are classified as *dystonic postures*. When the contractions are present for **weeks or longer**, the postures can lead to **permanent fixed** contractures. Dystonic movements sometimes increase during attempted purposeful activities, nervousness, and emotional stress; they also may be task specific and quite painful. However, these types of movement disorders diminish during relaxation and completely resolve during sleep. Dystonia involving only 1 body part is recognized in approximately 30/100,000 population, and that affecting multiple body parts has a prevalence of 2 to 7/100,000 population.

No satisfactory classification for dystonia exists, partly because of the wide variety of disorders in which dystonia is a feature. Standard classifications use age of onset, symptom distribution, and etiology (Table 51-1). The discovery of genetic defects responsible for some hereditary dystonias may improve classification.

Focal dystonia is the most common and involves a single body part (eg, task-specific dystonia, cervical dystonia or torticollis) (Figure 51-1).

Table 51-1
Classification of Dystonia

Age at Onset

Early onset (age <25 years)
Late onset (age >25 years)

Distribution

Focal
Segmental
Multifocal
Generalized
Hemidystonia

Etiology

Primary
Dystonia plus
Secondary
Paroxysmal dystonia
Heredodegenerative
Psychogenic

DYSTONIA

Figure 51-1

Torticollis

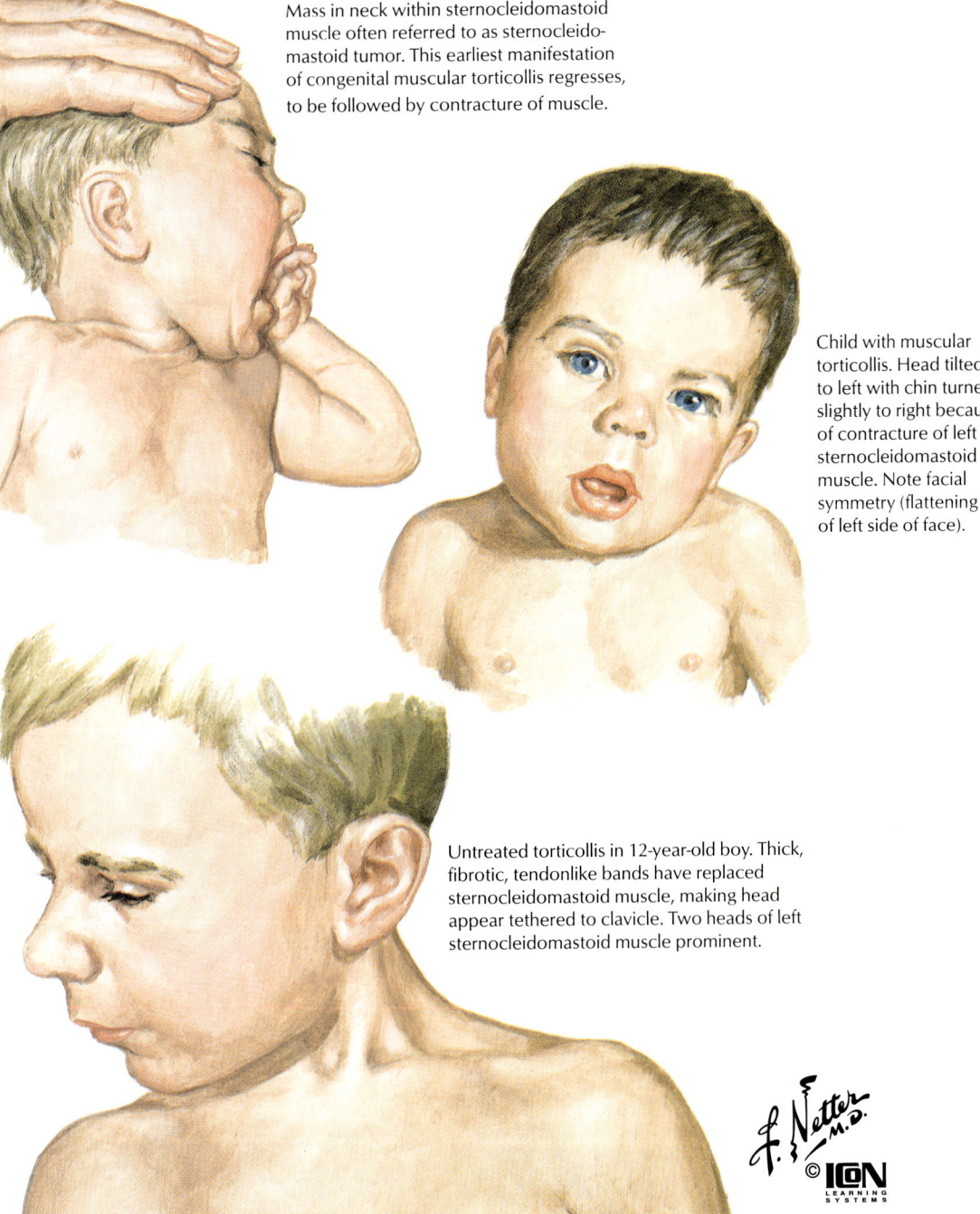

Mass in neck within sternocleidomastoid muscle often referred to as sternocleidomastoid tumor. This earliest manifestation of congenital muscular torticollis regresses, to be followed by contracture of muscle.

Child with muscular torticollis. Head tilted to left with chin turned slightly to right because of contracture of left sternocleidomastoid muscle. Note facial symmetry (flattening of left side of face).

Untreated torticollis in 12-year-old boy. Thick, fibrotic, tendonlike bands have replaced sternocleidomastoid muscle, making head appear tethered to clavicle. Two heads of left sternocleidomastoid muscle prominent.

MOVEMENT DISORDERS

DYSTONIA

Restricted or **fragmentary** forms of dystonia (dyskinesias) are commonly encountered. **Segmental** dystonia involves 2 or more contiguous body parts, whereas **multifocal** dystonia involves 2 or more noncontiguous body regions. **Generalized** dystonia involves both legs and at least 1 other body part (Figure 51-2). Dystonia restricted to 1 side of the body (hemidystonia) is distinct because a structural brain lesion is usually the cause. Other than hemidystonia, these disorders are usually hereditary or drug induced.

Focal or multifocal dystonias are more often sporadic than genetic in origin. Childhood-onset dystonia (age <12 years) is often hereditary, beginning in a limb (leg > arm) and progressing to a more generalized distribution. Adolescent-on-

Figure 51-2

Cerebral Palsy

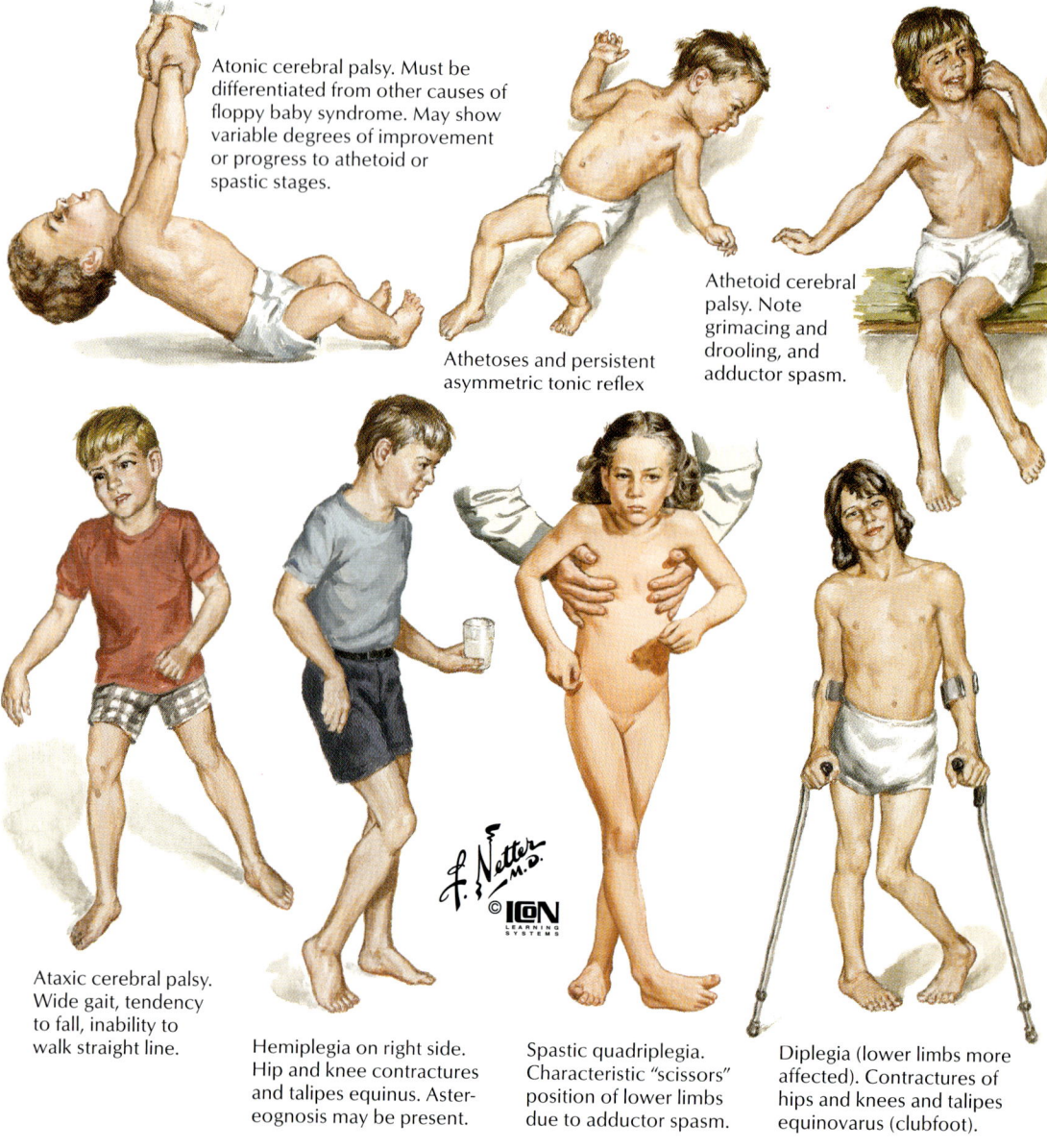

Atonic cerebral palsy. Must be differentiated from other causes of floppy baby syndrome. May show variable degrees of improvement or progress to athetoid or spastic stages.

Athetoses and persistent asymmetric tonic reflex

Athetoid cerebral palsy. Note grimacing and drooling, and adductor spasm.

Ataxic cerebral palsy. Wide gait, tendency to fall, inability to walk straight line.

Hemiplegia on right side. Hip and knee contractures and talipes equinus. Astereognosis may be present.

Spastic quadriplegia. Characteristic "scissors" position of lower limbs due to adductor spasm.

Diplegia (lower limbs more affected). Contractures of hips and knees and talipes equinovarus (clubfoot).

set dystonia often involves the arm or neck initially and is less likely to progress. Adult-onset dystonia (age >26 years) is usually sporadic in origin and begins and remains focal or multifocal.

PATHOPHYSIOLOGY

There is no adequate animal model mimicking dystonia. Although certain centrally active medications may cause "dystonic reactions," the primary pathophysiologic mechanism is unknown. Strong clinical support upholds dystonia as a CNS disorder, not a musculoskeletal system disorder. For example, when a patient with dystonia receives chemical denervation with botulinum toxin injections into the overactive muscles, abnormal postures often appear in additional muscle groups, implying that the lesion is not in the muscle cells but in the CNS representation of normal postures. Conversely, when dystonia occurs after peripheral nervous system injury, sensory input or "tricks" (see below) can diminish the severity of some patients' abnormal movement. Hence, the peripheral nervous system can be an important, if poorly understood, part of dystonia.

No clear brain abnormalities exist in patients with secondary dystonia. However, evidence shows that dystonia can result from abnormal dopaminergic transmission in the basal ganglia. Acute dystonic reactions are often observed in patients treated with dopamine D2-receptor antagonists, such as phenothiazines. Patients with dystonia secondary to strokes usually have a lesion in the putamen or globus pallidus, the targets of dopaminergic neurons. Some dystonic syndromes result from biochemical abnormalities in dopamine synthesis pathways (ie, DYT5 dopa-responsive dystonia). PET and functional MRI demonstrate the associations of dystonia with abnormalities in multiple brain areas, including the motor cortex, supplementary areas, cerebellum, and basal ganglia.

CLINICAL PRESENTATION
Sporadic Primary Dystonia

Idiopathic or sporadic primary dystonia is the most common dystonia. Although most cases of focal dystonia are classified as sporadic, 25% have similarly affected relatives. Common forms of focal dystonia include those of the neck (torticollis), craniofacial muscles (Meige syndrome), eyelids (blepharospasm), vocal cords (spasmodic dysphonia), or isolated muscles of the hand or foot. Some dystonias are task specific (eg, writer's cramp, musical instruments). Sporadic primary generalized dystonia occurs but is less common and likely to have an underlying genetic predisposition. Patients with primary sporadic focal dystonia often report that certain postures or sensory "tricks" transiently suppress their involuntary movements. For example, a gentle counterpressure by a hand against the chin or resting the back of the head against a wall or a chair back may transiently attenuate a cervical dystonia, whereas using a large-barrel pen or writing on a blackboard may relieve writer's cramp. Many patients with dystonia have an associated postural/action type tremor (dysgenic tremor) in addition to contorted posture.

Genetic Primary Dystonia

More than a dozen different forms of dystonia have a genetic origin. They have been assigned numerical designations, beginning with the abbreviation *DYT* (Table 51-2). For some, the specific gene defect has been identified. However, a particular clinical phenotype may be related to more than 1 genetic defect. Three of the more common syndromes are reviewed here.

Predominantly Generalized

DYT1 dystonia, formerly called *dystonia musculorum deformans*, has a chromosome 9 mutation that accounts for approximately 90% of early-onset limb dystonia in those of Ashkenazi Jewish descent and approximately 50% of early-onset dystonia in the non-Jewish population. The pattern of penetrance is only approximately 30%; a majority of gene carriers never exhibit overt symptoms. Torsin A is identified as a mutated protein, although its function is unknown. Initial symptoms, usually in the legs, may be seen only during activity and are often mistaken for a mannerism or hysteria. Later, as the dystonia generalizes, postural abnormalities become more persistent, especially toward the middle and end of the day, although they may cease when the body is in repose. Severe cases lead to grotesque body movements and distorted pos-

DYSTONIA

Table 51-2
Classification of Genetic Primary Dystonias*

Designation	Type	Chromosome	Inheritance
Predominantly generalized			
DYT1	Early-onset generalized torsion dystonia	9	AD
DYT2	Autosomal recessive dystonia	?	AR
DYT4	Autosomal dominant dystonia	?	AD
Predominantly focal or segmental			
DYT6	Adolescent-onset torsion dystonia	8	AD
DYT13	Focal dystonia with cranial-cervical features	1	AD, incom.
Dystonia plus			
DYT3	X-linked dystonia-parkinsonism (Lubag)	X	X
DYT5	Dopa-responsive dystonia (Segsawa)	14	AD, incom.
DYT7	Adult-onset focal dystonia	18	AD, incom.
DYT11	Myoclonic dystonia	7	AD, incom.
DYT12	Rapid-onset dystonia with parkinsonism	19	AD, incom.
Paroxysmal dystonia			
DYT8	Nonkinesigenic dystonic choreoathetosis	2	AD, incom.
DYT9	Choreoathetosis, spasticity, and episodic ataxia	1	AD
DYT10	Kinesigenic choreoathetosis	16	AD, incom.

*AD indicates autosomal dominant; AR, autosomal recessive; incom., incomplete penetrance.

tures; sometimes the whole musculature seems to be thrown into spasm by an effort to move an arm or to speak. The average age of patients at onset is approximately 12 years; it rarely begins after the age of 30 years. There is some evidence that environmental factors, such as trauma, may interact with the abnormal gene to precipitate or worsen symptoms.

Predominantly Focal

Most cases of *DYT 7* **adult-onset focal dystonia** are sporadic, but 25% of these patients have similarly affected relatives, suggesting that a genetic basis for focal dystonia may be significant. In one German family, a gene localized to chromosome 18, also implicated in several other families, was responsible. However, most cases of focal dystonia are not caused by mutations of this chromosome. The average age of patients at onset is approximately 43 years. Family members have presented with a variety of forms, including spasmodic dysphonia, writer's cramp, and torticollis.

Dystonia Plus

Many of the dystonia-plus disorders are genetic; several arise from genetic mutations that change biochemical synthesis or release of dopamine. Other neurologic signs and symptoms without structural brain abnormalities characterize these disorders.

DYT5 dopa-responsive dystonia (**Segawa syndrome**) with diurnal fluctuation is characterized by childhood onset with a dramatic and sustained response to relatively low doses of levodopa. Many of the dystonia-plus disorders are genetic. Several arise from mutations that change the biochemical synthesis or release of dopamine.

Patients with Segawa syndrome usually present with a dystonic gait abnormality, and parkinsonian features develop subsequently. However, wide phenotypic variability exists in the clinical picture. Other neurologic signs and symptoms and the absence of neurodegenerative or other structural brain abnormalities characterize these disorders (Table 51-3). The average age of patients at onset is 6 years but ranges from infancy to adulthood. Symptoms are most severe later in the day and are improved or absent in the morning (diurnal fluctuation) or after a nap.

A chromosome 14 genetic defect for the enzyme GTP cyclohydrolase is identified in 50% of these dopa-responsive dystonia patients. This enzyme is required for the biosynthesis of tetrahydrobiopterin, an essential cofactor in the production of dopamine, serotonin, and other catecholamines (Figure 51-3). Administration of levodopa bypasses the defect in dopamine synthesis, providing long-lasting treatment. Therefore, all patients with a clinical picture suggestive of this syndrome require a clinical trial of levodopa.

Secondary Dystonia

Known to produce a short-term dystonic reaction from a single dose or a tardive dystonia with long-term use, dopamine receptor-blocking medications include neuroleptics and phenothiazine-based antiemetics. *Wilson disease* is a rare disorder of copper metabolism (chapter 55) that may produce dystonia and other movement disorders. Other secondary causes of dystonia include hypoxic encephalopathy, neurotoxins (ie, carbon monoxide, methanol, manganese), head trauma, stroke, cerebral malformations, encephalitis, HIV and other infections, metabolic disorders, drugs (ie, dopamine antagonist, anticonvulsant, serotonin reuptake inhibitors, cocaine), and mitochondrial disorders. Dystonia may also occur subsequent to spinal cord trauma or even after injury to the peripheral nerves.

Table 51-3
Clinical Features of Dopa-Responsive Dystonia*

Dystonic

- Limb dystonia
- Generalized dystonia
- Blepharospasm
- Oromandibular dystonia
- Cervical dystonia (torticollis)
- Writer's cramp
- Hand tremor
- Truncal dystonia

Other Features

- Response to low-dose levodopa
- Response to low-dose anticholinergics
- Developmental delay
- Abnormal gait
- Parkinsonism
- Diurnal fluctuation
- Spastic paraparesis
- Scoliosis
- Stiffness

*From Nemeth AH. The genetics of primary dystonias and related disorders. *Brain.* 2002;125:695-721.

DIFFERENTIAL DIAGNOSIS

In **primary** dystonia, abnormal posture is the only symptom and neurologic finding; there is no clinical evidence of an underlying neurologic disorder (Table 50-4). Primary dystonia includes sporadic and genetic disorders. **Dystonia-plus** patients have dystonia and additional symptoms, such as parkinsonism, myoclonus, or a paroxysmal course, including sporadic cases and cases with genetic deficits, such as dopa-responsive dystonia. **Secondary dystonias** occur within a wide variety of nervous system injuries that are usually static but may develop after the injury and become progressive. **Paroxysmal dystonia** presents as discrete episodes of abnormal movements lasting minutes to hours, with intervening periods of normalcy. Episodes may be precipitated by exercise (paroxysmal **kinesigenic** dystonia) or occur at rest (paroxysmal **nonkinesigenic** dystonia).

Psychogenic dystonia is a diagnosis of exclusion, supported by well-defined clinical features: an abrupt onset, a consistent inconsistency in

DYSTONIA

Figure 51-3

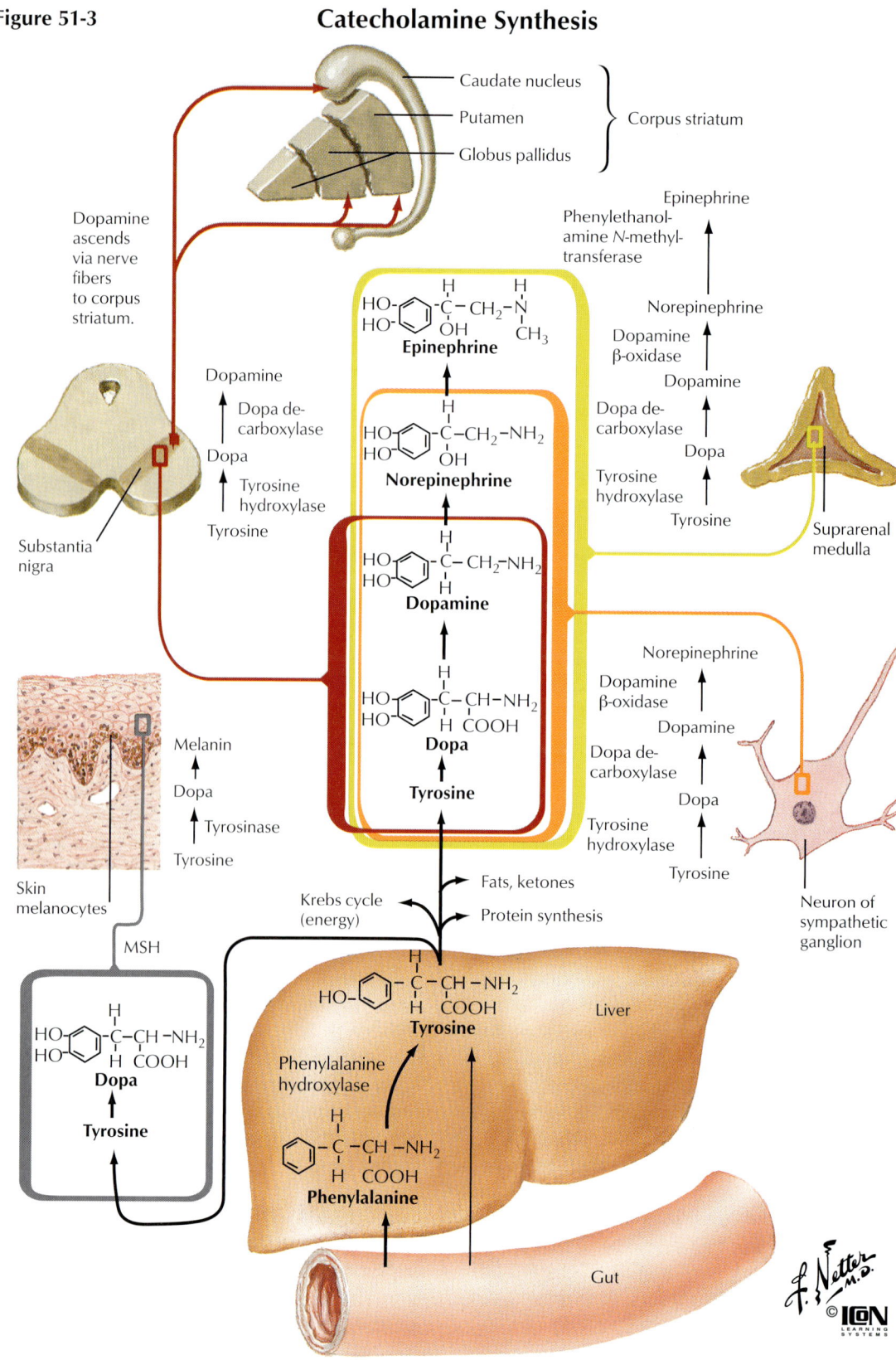

Catecholamine Synthesis

Table 51-4
Characteristics of Dystonia as Seen at a Movement Disorders Clinic*

Focal	44%
Oromandibular	7%
Cervical (torticollis)	19%
Isolated limb	12%
Craniofacial	4%
Blepharospasm	1%
Segmental	10%
Hemidystonia	9%
Multifocal	4%
Generalized	7%
Paroxysmal	2%
Tardive Dystonia	9%
Psychogenic	13%

*From Scott BL. Evaluation and treatment of dystonia. *South Med J.* 2000;93:746-751.

the character of movements, a decrease in degree of the movements with distraction, and intervening periods of normalcy.

Heredodegenerative dystonias are part of widespread neurodegenerative syndromes that often have known inheritance patterns. The most common example is Parkinson disease, in which focal dystonias may be seen in treated and untreated patients. Wilson disease, Huntington disease, lysosomal storage disorders, and certain mitochondrial disorders must also be considered in the differential diagnosis of dystonia.

DIAGNOSTIC APPROACH

As with most neurologic disorders, the history and physical examination are critical to providing an adequate evaluation of patients presenting with dystonia. Most instances of primary and secondary hereditary dystonias have a gradual onset, whereas cases of acquired secondary dystonia are often acute or subacute. The patient's medication history is vital, particularly to exclude use of antidopaminergic agents (such as neuroleptics and metoclopramide). A careful family history must be obtained to find family members who may have histories suggestive of movement disorders. If possible, these family members should be examined for subtle and unrecognized signs of a movement disorders. The patient examination must establish the distribution of the dystonia, the presence of other movement disorders, and evidence of other neurologic problems (eg, hyperreflexia, paresis, sensory defects). Individuals with early-onset or generalized dystonia, hemidystonia, and other neurologic signs on examination may need a neuroimaging study of the brain or spinal cord.

Children with torticollis must be evaluated for signs of concomitant oculomotor palsies to exclude intrinsic brainstem lesions. Laboratory testing in children should include a CBC (with smear to look for acanthocytes), metabolic panel (liver disease), serum ceruloplasmin or copper (Wilson disease) in blood and urine, and testing for hereditary metabolic disorders, including serum amino acid and urine organic acids or copper. Genetic testing for the DYT1 gene on chromosome 9 in patients with onset before the age of 26 years is reasonable. A neuro-ophthalmologic examination for Kayser-Fleischer rings to exclude Wilson disease should be considered in patients with dystonia onset before the age of 50 years.

Patients with adult-onset focal dystonia require little workup. Neuroimaging may be considered for torticollis or limb dystonia if seen soon after onset but is usually not required for patients with spasmodic dysphonia, blepharospasm, or lower facial dystonia.

TREATMENT

No medication for dystonia is curative, and the use of oral medications is based on trial and error. All dystonia medications have potential adverse effects that usually resolve when the therapy is discontinued. Drug treatment is therefore worth a trial. The general guideline is to start with low doses and increase slowly to toxicity, stopping at the lowest effective dose.

A trial of **dopaminergic therapy** merits consideration in all patients with dystonia, especially in early-onset dystonia that may be dopa-responsive (such as DYT5 dystonia or other dopamine synthesis abnormalities). Dopaminergic treatment may also be partially effective in patients without identified biochemical defects.

DYSTONIA

In patients with a partial response to levodopa, trials of a direct-acting dopamine agonist, such as pergolide, pramipexole, or ropinirole, may be useful. Dopaminergic therapy usually does not help with adult-onset blepharospasm, torticollis, or spasmodic dysphonia.

Anticholinergic drugs, such as trihexyphenidyl or benztropine, may be the most effective medications for dystonia, but they work only in a minority of patients. They should be initiated in low doses and increased slowly (15-20 mg trihexyphenidyl daily as the maximum dosage). At these doses, adults, especially the elderly, often experience intolerable side effects, including sedation, confusion, depression, dry mouth, and prostatism. When anticholinergic treatment is ineffective, additional medications may help: baclofen, as an oral or intrathecal agent; clonazepam; anticonvulsants; lithium; or the dopamine antagonist tetrabenazine (not available in the United States).

Botulinum toxin injection is effective therapy for focal dystonia and is the treatment of choice for cervical dystonia, blepharospasm, and spasmodic dysphonia. Botulism toxins block the release of acetylcholine at the neuromuscular junction, resulting in a flaccid paralysis of the injected muscles. For patients with involvement of large muscles or with multifocal or generalized dystonia, botulinum injections may be less effective because of the large amount of toxin necessary to relieve symptoms. The effect lasts only 3 to 6 months, and the involuntary activity gradually returns, necessitating repeated injections.

Numerous peripheral surgical procedures have been used for dystonia that is unresponsive to medications or botulinum toxins. Myectomy may help with blepharospasm. However, selective peripheral denervation of cervical muscles for torticollis has not generally been satisfactory over time. Direct cerebral interventions in the form of thalamotomy, pallidotomy, or deep brain stimulation are yielding promising results. Stimulation of the globus pallidus is effective in patients with DYT1 dystonia.

REFERENCES

Friedman J, Standaert DG. Dystonia and its disorders. *Neurol Clin.* 2001;19:681-705.

Nemeth AH. The genetics of primary dystonia and related disorders. *Brain.* 2002;125:695-721.

Scott BL. Evaluation and treatment of dystonia. *South Med J.* 2000;93:746-751.

Chapter 52
Myoclonus

Diana Apetauerova

Clinical Vignette

A 59-year-old, right-handed woman presented with a 1-year history of jerking movements that she described as fast and somewhat irregular, affecting various regions of the trunk, arms, and legs. She noted that they occurred more frequently later in the afternoon, when she felt fatigued. She was unaware of any other triggering factors. Alcohol alleviated these symptoms. Her medical history only included several years of restless leg syndrome treated with carbidopa/levodopa (Sinemet). She had no seizures or decline in memory. Essential tremor in her mother was the only familial neurologic disorder.

The patient was an obese, otherwise healthy woman. Neurologic examination, during late afternoon hours, demonstrated multiple, brief, shocklike movements in her trunk, arms, and legs. These movements occurred randomly and were observed with the patient at rest. Many movements were stimulus sensitive and could not be voluntarily controlled. Her neurologic examination results were otherwise normal.

Brain MRI and EEG were unremarkable. A diagnosis of essential myoclonus was made. A low dose of clonazepam yielded some improvement.

Myoclonus is characterized by sudden, abrupt, brief, involuntary, jerklike contractions of a single muscle or muscle group. They are related to involuntary muscle contractions (**positive myoclonus**) or sudden inhibition of voluntary muscular contraction, with lapses of sustained posture (**negative myoclonus or asterixis**). Myoclonus may affect any bodily region, multiple bodily regions, or the entire body, interfering with normal movements and posture.

Numerous classifications of myoclonus use etiology, affected body region, provocative factors, and nervous system origin of the abnormal neuronal discharges (Table 52-1). One classification categorizes myoclonus into focal, segmental, multifocal, or generalized forms. Another system uses the presence or absence of specific provocative factors. **Spontaneous myoclonus** has no clinically identifiable mechanism. **Reflex myoclonus** occurs in response to specific external sensory stimuli. Voluntary movement or attempts to perform specific movements induce **action** or **intention myoclonus**.

Neurophysiologic classification relates myoclonus to the abnormal neuronal discharge site within the CNS. **Cortical myoclonus** arises from the cerebral cortex and is considered epileptic, often being associated with other seizure types. **Subcortical myoclonus** usually arises from the brainstem. **Spinal myoclonus** originates within the spinal cord. Clinically, differentiation is often impossible, but electromyography may help.

Another classification, based on etiology, categorizes myoclonus into physiologic or pathologic forms. Common examples of "normal," nonpathologic, **physiologic myoclonus** include hiccups or "sleep starts" occurring as one drifts into sleep. In **pathologic myoclonus**, the brief muscle jerks may occur infrequently or repeatedly. Examples include essential myoclonus, myoclonic epilepsy, and secondary myoclonus. Postanoxic encephalopathy and spongiform encephalopathy, ie, Creutzfeldt-Jakob disease, are the best-known examples of **pathologic myoclonus**. Additional rare forms include palatal myoclonus (chapter 18), periodic limb movements of sleep, and psychogenic myoclonus. Although **pathologic myoclonus** is always a sign of CNS dysfunction, its pathophysiologic mechanism often remains unknown.

Myoclonus may be an important clinical indicator in determining the proper diagnosis. It is also sometimes a nonspecific feature within more widespread neurologic abnormalities.

MYOCLONUS

Table 52-1
Classification of Myoclonus

Classification Bases	Classifications
Affected body part	Focal Segmental Multifocal Generalized
Provoking symptom	Spontaneous Reflex Action
Neurophysiology	Cortical Subcortical Spinal
Etiology	Physiological Essential Myoclonic epilepsy Secondary
Additional forms	Palatal myoclonus Periodic limb movements of sleep Psychogenic myoclonus

PATHOPHYSIOLOGY

The pathophysiologic mechanism leading to myoclonus is not well understood, thus complicating anatomical correlation. Cortical myoclonus is possibly a disorder of decreased cortical inhibition, although the reason for the reduced inhibition is unknown. Its frequent association with seizure disorders suggests a common pathophysiologic mechanism for myoclonus and some forms of epilepsy. Mechanisms for subcortical and spinal myoclonus are even less well appreciated.

CLINICAL PRESENTATION
Physiologic Nonpathologic

Shocklike contractions of the arms or legs during sleep or as individuals drift off to sleep are a common form of physiologic myoclonus, sometimes described as ***physiologic sleep myoclonus***.

Pathologic

It is essential to distinguish the various forms of presumed pathologic myoclonus (Table 52-2). **Essential myoclonus** is an isolated neurologic finding that has no association with seizures, dementia, or ataxia. It is nonprogressive, usually multifocal in distribution, typically induced by voluntary movements (action myoclonus), and usually responds to alcohol (Figure 52-1).

Although often familial, essential myoclonus can occur sporadically. **Familial essential myoclonus** seems to be an autosomal dominant trait with reduced penetrance and variable expressivity. Symptoms typically begin before the age of 20 years. Essential myoclonus often occurs in association with other movement disorders, particularly tremor and dystonia.

Various forms of epilepsy may be accompanied by myoclonus. For example, in forms of idiopathic epilepsy, such as **juvenile myoclonic epilepsy** and **benign myoclonus of infancy**, myoclonus may be a primary finding.

Any underlying disease process or cause of CNS dysfunction may lead to **secondary myoclonus** (Figure 52-2).

Additional Forms of Myoclonus

Palatal myoclonus has rapid, rhythmic jerking of muscle of one or both sides of the soft palate. It is more appropriately classified as a form of tremor despite continued use of the term *palatal myoclonus*.

Periodic limb movements of sleep differ from physiologic sleep myoclonus in that they typically consist of repeated, stereotypic, upward extension of the great toe and foot, possibly followed by flexion of the hip, knee, or ankle. They usually involve both legs, tend to occur in repeated episodes lasting a few minutes to several hours, and occur during non-REM sleep. An association with restless legs syndrome is common.

In **psychogenic myoclonus**, symptoms have a mental or emotional basis rather than an organic origin. In most patients, the condition worsens with stress or anxiety. The myoclonus can be segmental or generalized.

DIFFERENTIAL DIAGNOSES

Myoclonus must be differentiated from other movement disorders, including tics, tremors, ataxia, and chorea. When the jerks are single or repetitive but arrhythmic, a **tic** diagnosis should be considered. Myoclonus is usually briefer and less coordinated or patterned than tics. A history of an urge associated with tics is helpful in the diagnosis.

MYOCLONUS

Table 52-2
Etiologies of Pathologic Myoclonus

Type of Myoclonus	Etiologies
Essential	Autosomal dominant trait with reduced penetrance and variable expressivity
Myoclonic epilepsy	Juvenile myoclonic epilepsy, benign myoclonus of infancy
Secondary	Brain trauma, infection, inflammation (encephalitis), tumors (neoplasms), or cerebral hypoxia due to temporary lack of oxygen (ie, posthypoxic myoclonus or Lance-Adams syndrome)
Spinal	Spinal cord trauma, infection, inflammation, or lesions may produce segmental myoclonus
Inborn biochemical errors	Inborn errors of metabolism (lysosomal storage diseases: Tay-Sachs disease, Sandhoff disease, sialidosis)
Neurodegenerative	Creutzfeldt-Jakob disease, parkinsonism, Huntington disease, Alzheimer disease, corticobasal degeneration, progressive supranuclear palsy, or olivopontocerebellar atrophy
Metabolic	Metabolic conditions, such as kidney, liver, or respiratory failure, hypokalemia, hyperglycemia, etc
Mitochondrial	Mitochondrial encephalomyopathy, particularly MERFF syndrome (myoclonus epilepsy with ragged-red fibers), or other progressive myoclonic encephalopathies, including those characterized by epilepsy and dementia (eg, Lafora disease) or epilepsy and ataxia (eg, Unverricht-Lundborg disease)
Medications	Drug-induced myoclonus; selective serotonin receptor inhibitors, toxic levels of anticonvulsants, levodopa, and certain antipsychotic agents (tardive myoclonus)
Toxins	Exposure to toxic agents, such as bismuth or other metals

Rhythmic forms of myoclonus may be confused with **tremors**. The pattern of myoclonus is more repetitive, abrupt-onset, square-wave movements, unlike the smoother sinusoidal activity of tremor. Rhythmic myoclonus usually ranges from 1 to 4 Hz, differing from faster tremor frequencies.

Myoclonus, particularly action (intention) myoclonus, is often confused with cerebellar ataxia. Myoclonic jerking occurs during voluntary motor activity, especially when patients attempt to perform a fine motor task, such as reaching for a target.

DIAGNOSTIC EVALUATION

A diagnosis of myoclonus is based on a thorough clinical assessment, evaluation of the nature of the myoclonus (eg, electrophysiologic characteristics), bodily distribution, provocative factors, and a careful family history. Examination and observation of patients with myoclonus are important diagnostic steps. However, patients with myoclonus can have entirely normal examination results, particularly with physiologic and essential myoclonus. When myoclonus is present during examination, characterization of its rhythm, repetitiveness, onset, and frequency is important. Because myoclonus may occur with other movement disorders, it is important to look for evidence of dystonia, tremor, ataxia, or spasticity.

The clinical distribution of the myoclonus is also helpful. Focal myoclonus is more commonly associated with CNS lesions. **Segmental** involvement may suggest brainstem or spinal cord lesions. **Multifocal** or **generalized** myoclonus suggests a more diffuse disorder, particularly involving the reticular substance of the brainstem. **Precipitating factors** are important for stimulus-sensitive myoclonus. Therefore, somes-

MYOCLONUS

Figure 52-1

Essential Myoclonus

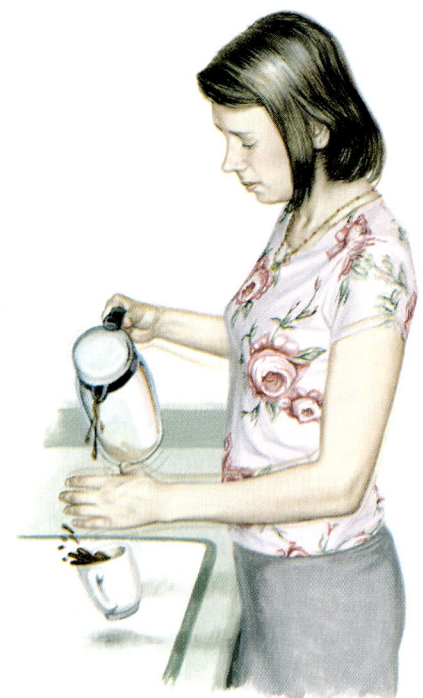

Usually multifocal in distribution, often familial, typically induced by voluntary movements causing a single jerk of the extremity (action myoclonus). Symptoms begin before age 20 and frequently occur associated with tremor, dystonia, and other movement disorders.

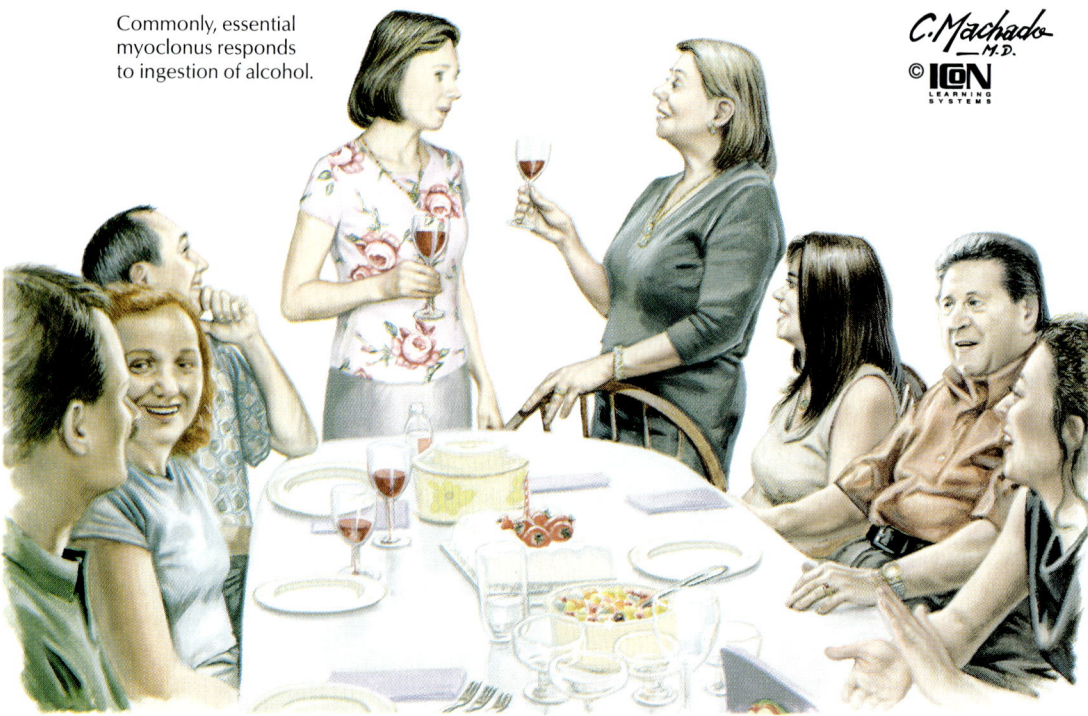

Commonly, essential myoclonus responds to ingestion of alcohol.

MOVEMENT DISORDERS

MYOCLONUS

Figure 52-2   Lancet-Adams Syndrome (Posthypoxic Myoclonus)

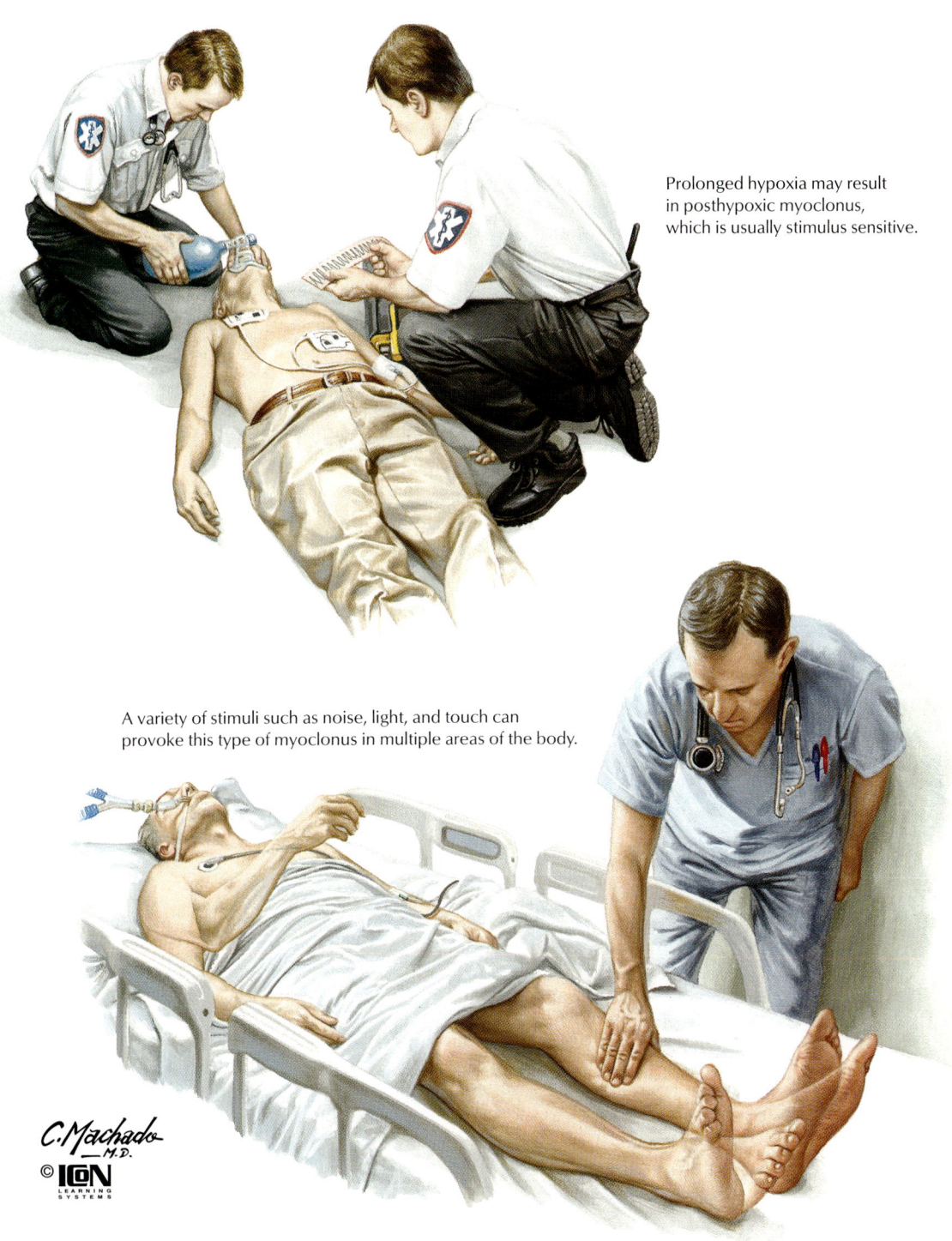

Prolonged hypoxia may result in posthypoxic myoclonus, which is usually stimulus sensitive.

A variety of stimuli such as noise, light, and touch can provoke this type of myoclonus in multiple areas of the body.

MOVEMENT DISORDERS

thetic sensory input testing is needed. It is important to determine whether the myoclonus occurs spontaneously and whether symptoms improve or worsen with voluntary activity.

During testing for negative myoclonus (asterixis), patients are asked to extend their arms with the wrists back or to perform another movement that requires holding the limb against gravity. In this way, a sudden loss of muscle contraction causes the hand or the arm to fall downward.

Specialized testing can be used to determine the site of the abnormal neuronal discharge within the CNS (eg, cerebral cortex, brainstem, or spinal cord) and establish the underlying cause. These studies typically include EMG, EEG, or somatosensory evoked potential testing. Neuroimaging studies such as MRI or CT can reveal structural lesions. Other specialized diagnostic tests may help to exclude particular conditions such as hereditary, metabolic, mitochondrial, infectious, vascular, neoplastic, toxic, or neurodegenerative processes.

TREATMENT AND PROGNOSIS

The treatment of myoclonus varies depending on the type. If a specific cause is found, myoclonus usually resolves with effective treatment of the underlying disease. Symptomatic treatment typically includes medications to reduce the severity of the myoclonus, such as benzodiazepines. Cortical myoclonus may respond to valproate, piracetam, levetiracetam, or lamotrigine. Myoclonus from a hypoxic event may respond to 5-hydroxy-tryptophan, and this may help in other causes. Carbamazepine may worsen myoclonus and should be avoided. Juvenile myoclonus epilepsy usually responds to valproate and may require lifelong treatment.

Prognosis depends on the form of myoclonus. Generally, although myoclonus is not a life-threatening condition, it may be secondary to serious, debilitating impairments. The worst outcome occurs with postanoxic myoclonus, which is associated with a poor prognosis.

Researchers are attempting to clarify the genetic and molecular aspects of myoclonus. Newer physiologic techniques, such as magnetoencephalography, are being used to study cortical activity in cortical reflex myoclonus.

REFERENCES

Gordon MF. Toxin and drug-induced myoclonus. *Adv Neurol.* 2002;89:49-76.

Hallet M. Neurophysiology of brainstem myoclonus. *Adv Neurol.* 2002;89:99-102.

Obeso JA. Therapy of myoclonus. *Clin Neurosci.* 1995-1996;3:253-257.

Shafiq M, Lang AE. Myoclonus in parkinsonian disorders. *Adv Neurol.* 2002;89:77-83.

Watts RL, Koller WC, eds. *Movement Disorders: Neurologic Principles and Practice.* New York, NY: McGraw-Hill Companies, Inc; 1997.

Chapter 53
Chorea

Diana Apetauerova

Clinical Vignette

Jane, a 7-year-old girl, came to the ED, reporting clumsiness of the right hand. She was previously healthy. Three weeks earlier, her mother had had a febrile illness with a positive Streptococcus throat culture. Soon, Jane also developed fever and sore throat but did not see a doctor. Three weeks later, she began to drop things from her right hand frequently. Her handwriting became illegible. Involuntary movements of her right hand occurred mainly during motor tasks; they were absent during sleep. She became irritable. Her medical history and family medical history had been unremarkable.

On general physical examination, Jane appeared well; the only abnormality was a 2/6-holosystolic murmur revealed by her cardiac examination. Neurologically, she was awake and cooperative. Her behavior seemed appropriate. Motor examination demonstrated right-sided choreiform movements primarily visible during motor tasks such as eating, writing (she was unable to hold a pen), and walking. Coordination was affected by hemichorea on the right side but was normal on the left. She had no weakness. Sensory examination results were normal. Gait revealed right-sided hemichorea.

Jane was admitted to the hospital. ASLO titer was 400:800. She had a positive Streptococcus throat culture. ESR was 63 mm/h. Echocardiogram and brain MRI were normal. Jane was diagnosed with Sydenham chorea, and treatment with a prolonged course of penicillin was initiated. Her involuntary movements did not require any medication because they subsided spontaneously within 2 weeks of the initial visit.

Chorea (from Latin *choreus*, dance) is an abnormal involuntary movement usually distal in location, brief, nonrhythmic, abrupt, and irregular, that seems to flow from one body part to another. The movements are random, unpredictable in timing, direction, and distribution. Chorea can be partially suppressed; some patients can incorporate these into semipurposeful movements called *parakinesia*. Typical of chorea is its motor impersistence, the inability to maintain a sustained contraction.

Athetosis and **ballism** are sometimes confused with chorea. *Athetosis* is a slow, writhing, continuous set of involuntary movements, usually affecting limbs distally, but it can involve the axial musculature (neck, face, and tongue). If athetosis becomes faster, it sometimes blends with chorea, ie, *choreoathetosis*. Ballism is large-amplitude, involuntary movements affecting the proximal limbs, causing flinging and flailing limb movements. It has a higher incidence than chorea.

Patients with chorea are often initially unaware of these involuntary movements. Usually, chorea is first interpreted by observers as fidgetiness. Subjectively, patients usually note incoordination or clumsiness.

ETIOLOGY

Of the numerous causes of chorea, all disrupt the basal ganglia's modulation of thalamocortical motor pathways: structural lesions, neuronal degeneration in selective regions, neurotransmitter receptor blockade, or other metabolic factors within the basal ganglia. Chorea is classified into inherited (primarily Huntington disease [HD]), immunologic (Sydenham chorea), drug-related, structural, and miscellaneous causes (Table 53-1).

PATHOPHYSIOLOGY

The putamen, globus pallidus, and subthalamic nuclei are the key pathologic sites underlying the development of chorea. Balance is critical between the direct and indirect motor pathways to produce normal movement patterns and avoid the various movement disorders. In normal individuals, the **excitatory glutamate pathway** from the subthalamic nucleus excites the globus pallidus interior and the substantia ni-

CHOREA

Table 53-1
Causes of Chorea

Type of Chorea	
Inherited	Huntington disease Neuroacanthocytosis Wilson disease Benign hereditary chorea OPCA Ataxia telangiectasia Idiopathic torsion dystonia Tic disorder Myoclonic epilepsy Dentatorubropallidoluysian degeneration Gerstmann-Strussler-Scheinker syndrome
Metabolic	Amino acid disorders (glutaric academia) Leigh disease Lesch-Nyhan disease Lipid disorders (gangliosidoses) Mitochondrial myopathy Nonketotic hyperglycemia Disorders of calcium, magnesium, glucose
Immunologic	Sydenham chorea Systemic lupus erythematosus Antiphospholipid antibody syndrome Chorea gravidarum Reaction to immunization
Drug related	Tardive dyskinesia (neuroleptics, serotonin reuptake inhibitors, others) Withdrawal emergent syndrome Sympathomimetics Cocaine Anticonvulsants Contraceptives Lithium Tricyclic antidepressants Levodopa Amantadine Dopamine agonist Theophylline and β-adrenergic agents Ethanol Carbon monoxide Gasoline inhalation
Structural	Traumatic brain injury Anoxic encephalopathy Multiple sclerosis Cerebrovascular disease Pseudochoreoathetosis (spinal cord injury, peripheral nerve injury) Delayed onset following perinatal injury
Miscellaneous	Encephalitis (herpes simplex, HIV, Lyme disease) Endocrine dysfunction (eg, hyperthyroidism) Metabolic disturbance (eg, hypocalcaemia, hypoglycemia, hyperglycemia) Kernicterus Nutritional (eg, B_{12} deficiency) Postpump chorea (cardiac bypass) Normal maturation

gra. These areas then signal the **GABA inhibitory pathway** into the thalamus. In the simplified model, the excitatory action of the subthalamic nucleus is reduced or lost, and this produces disinhibition of the pallidothalamic pathway.

In Huntington disease, neurodegenerative changes occur primarily within the caudate nuclei and the putamen (striatum), but associated neuronal degeneration also occurs within the temporal and frontal lobes of the cerebral cortex. These changes primarily affect nerve cells of the striatum called *medium-sized "spiny" neurons*, which project into the globus pallidus and substantia nigra and secrete the inhibitory neurotransmitter GABA. Selective loss of these specialized cells theoretically may result in decreased thalamic inhibition (ie, increased activity) that causes increased output to regions of the cerebral cortex of the brain, causing the disorganized, excessive (hyperkinetic) movement patterns of chorea.

With Sydenham chorea, various streptococcal proteins or antigens (streptococcal M proteins) induce the body's production of antineuronal antibodies. These cross-react against the body's own cells in certain brain regions. These antibodies, IgG in children, interact with specific cellular proteins (ie, neuronal antigens) in the basal ganglia, such as the caudate nuclei and subthalamic nucleus.

CLINICAL PRESENTATION

The spectrum of clinical findings in chorea varies, presenting in isolation or with other involuntary movements. At the simplest level, chorea appears as semipurposeful movement resembling fidgetiness exemplified by flitting movements of the fingers, wrists, toes, and ankles. The movements can be focal, as in tardive dyskinesia, where they are more repetitive and stereotypical. They may present as lip pouting or pursing, cheek puffing, lateral or forward jaw movements, or tongue rolling or protruding. Asymmetric chorea in hemichorea primarily affects the limbs on 1 side of the body. Sometimes chorea, such as respiratory chorea, affects only specific functional muscle groups. Chorea is often accompanied by parkinsonism, tics, and dystonia if more diffuse basal ganglia disease is present. Later, chorea can interfere with activities of daily living; eg, limb chorea can cause falls. Chorea of the face, jaw, larynx, and respiratory muscles may produce inability to communicate verbally, as well as other manifestations.

On neurologic examination, the performance of various tasks is altered. Finger-to-nose testing and rapid alternating movements are executed with a jerky and interrupted performance. When patients grasp examiners' fingers, a squeezing motion called *milkmaid's grip*, a sign of motor impersistence is sometimes noted. Chorea is frequently aggravated while walking. Oculomotor abnormalities include slow and hypometric saccades and saccadic pursuit, convergence paresis, and gaze impersistence. Parkinsonian features, particularly bradykinesia and dystonia, can be seen later in the disease.

Huntington Disease

This hereditary, progressive neurodegenerative disorder is the most common cause of chorea. The classic signs of HD include the development of chorea, neurobehavioral changes, and gradual dementia (Figure 53-1). Symptoms typically become evident during the fourth or fifth decades of life, although onset varies from early childhood (juvenile form has onset in patients younger than 20 years) to late adulthood. However, the symptoms of HD vary among patients in range and severity, by age at onset, and in clinical progression rate. Early onset is associated with increased severity and more rapid progression. For example, adult-onset HD typically lasts approximately 15 to 20 years, whereas the course of juvenile HD tends to last approximately 8 to 10 years.

The initial characteristic signs may be neurologic or psychiatric. Typical early clinical presentation includes slight personality changes, forgetfulness, clumsiness, and gradual development of fidgeting movement of the fingers or toes (chorea). Neurobehavioral changes include the gradual onset of emotional or behavioral disturbance. Patients present with increased irritability, suspiciousness, impulsiveness, lack of self-control, and anhedonia. Sometimes anxiety, depression, mania, obsessive-compulsive behaviors, and agitation are seen early in the disease. Later, a severe distortion in thinking and occasionally hallucinations (such as the perception of sounds,

CHOREA

Figure 53-1

Chorea

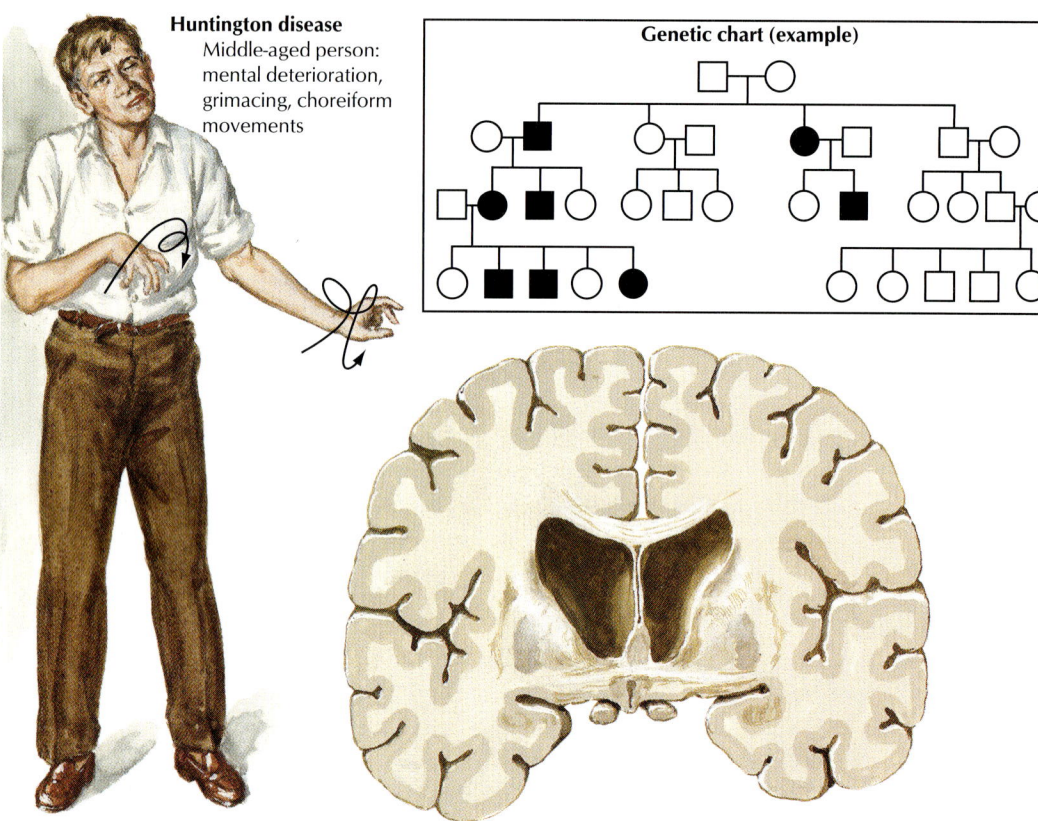

Huntington disease
Middle-aged person: mental deterioration, grimacing, choreiform movements

Genetic chart (example)

Degeneration and atrophy of caudate nucleus and cerebral cortex, with resulting enlargement of ventricles

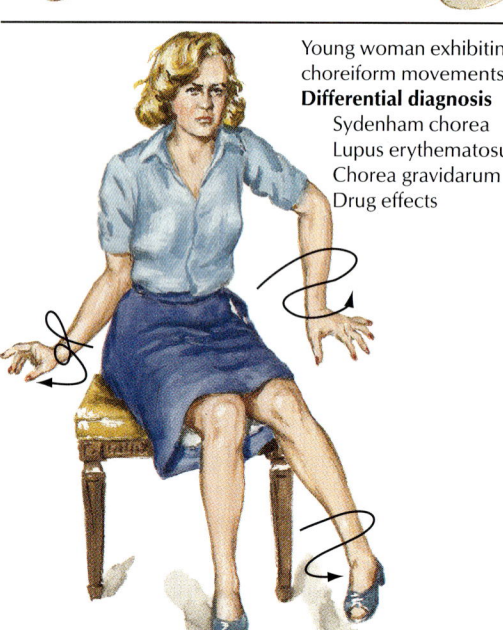

Young woman exhibiting choreiform movements:
Differential diagnosis
  Sydenham chorea
  Lupus erythematosus
  Chorea gravidarum
  Drug effects

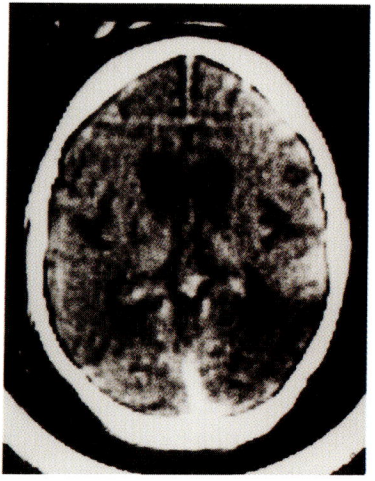

CT scan of brain: atrophy of caudate nucleus and enlargement of ventricles

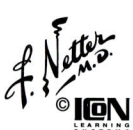

MOVEMENT DISORDERS

sights, or other sensations without external stimuli) may develop.

Cognitive decline is characterized by progressive dementia or gradual impairment of the mental processes involved in comprehension, reasoning, judgment, and memory. Typical early signs include forgetfulness, inattention, and increased difficulty in concentrating. Communication difficulties develop, including problems expressing thoughts in words, initiating conversations, or comprehending others' words and responding appropriately.

Motor disturbances are characterized by the gradual onset of clumsiness, balance difficulties, and fidgeting movements. Early chorea may be limited to the fingers and toes, later extending to the arms, legs, face, and trunk. Eventually, chorea tends to become widespread or generalized. Parkinsonism and dystonia are sometimes seen later in the disease. Many patients with HD develop a distinctive manner of walking that may be unsteady, disjointed, lurching, and dancelike. Eventually, postural instability, dysphagia, and dysarthria appear.

Later disease stages are characterized by severe dementia and progressive motor dysfunction; patients usually become unable to walk, have poor dietary intake, become unable to care for themselves, and eventually cease to talk. Life-threatening complications may result from serious falls, poor nutrition, infection, choking, aspiration pneumonia, or heart failure.

Sydenham Chorea

The other most recognized form of chorea, Sydenham chorea, seems to result from an autoimmune response following infection with group A beta-hemolytic streptococci. With the widespread availability of antibiotics for *Streptococcus* A infection, rheumatic chorea has become rare in developed countries.

The initial illness is usually characterized by pharyngitis, followed within approximately 1 to 5 weeks by the sudden onset of acute rheumatic fever (ARF). Chorea usually occurs only in patients between the ages of 5 and 15 years, usually 1 to 6 months after the onset of the sore throat. It may occur as an isolated condition or subsequent to other characteristic features of ARF. The distribution of chorea is usually generalized, and choreic movements consist of relatively fast or rapid, irregular, uncontrollable, jerky motions that disappear with sleep and may increase with stress, fatigue, and excitement (Figure 53-2). When movements are severe, they become ballistic. Occasional additional findings include emotional and behavioral disturbances. Affected children are often described as unusually restless, aggressive, or "excessively emotional."

In some patients, Sydenham chorea is a self-limited condition, resolving spontaneously within approximately 9 months (average duration) to 2 years. In others, residual signs of chorea and behavioral abnormalities wax and wane over a year or more. In approximately 20% of patients, Sydenham chorea may recur, usually within approximately 2 years of the initial occurrence. Recurrences are also reported during pregnancy and in association with certain medications in women who had ARF during childhood.

DIFFERENTIAL DIAGNOSES

The differential in chorea is broad (Table 53-1). HD, the most common cause of chorea, is usually easily diagnosed when an adult has the typical triad of chorea, dementia, and family history. Sydenham chorea has an earlier onset, lacks the characteristic mental disturbance, and is usually self-limiting. Chorea and mental disturbances occurring as manifestations of lupus erythematosus are usually more acute in onset, with more localized chorea, and with characteristic clinical and serologic abnormalities (history of recurrent vascular thromboses or spontaneous abortions and disappearance after therapy with prednisone).

Involuntary movements in psychiatric patients on long-term treatment with neuroleptic agents (tardive dyskinesia) occasionally pose a diagnostic problem. Usually repetitive, these movements contrast the nonrepetitive and flowing nature of chorea. There is usually an oral-lingual-buccal dyskinesia predominance. Unlike HD, gait is usually normal in individuals with tardive dyskinesia. With some dementing disorders

CHOREA

Figure 53-2
Choreiform Movements

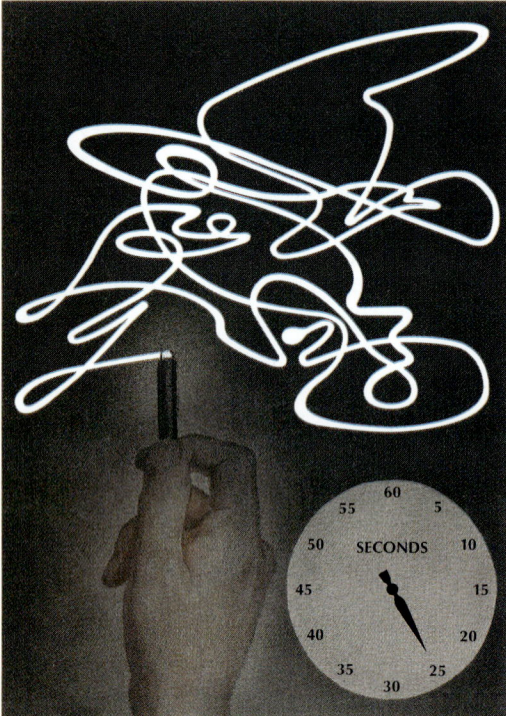

Sydenham chorea: spontaneous uncoordinated movements demonstrated by electric penlight held in patient's hand

DIAGNOSTIC EVALUATION

The evaluation of patients with chorea includes detailed family history and other tests to exclude possible causes (Table 53-2). Genetic testing is the most accurate test for HD. Available for presymptomatic individuals at risk for HD, it requires careful pretest and posttest counseling to guard against suicidal risk in individuals who request the study and find out they have the illness. Other investigations are less important, but MRI or CT are commonly done. Head MRI is preferable to CT for better delineation of the affected subcortical tissue. Atrophy of the caudate nucleus may be demonstrated. PET typically shows glucose hypometabolism in the striatum.

In Sydenham chorea, the diagnosis primarily relies on recognition of acute chorea in the presence of typical findings of rheumatic fever, which strongly support the diagnosis. Other manifestations of ARF are not mandatory for the diagnosis. Less helpful, because of the latency between the infection and the onset of the movement disorder, are tests of acute-phase reactions: ESR, C-reactive protein, leukocytosis, other blood tests including rheumatoid factor, mucoproteins, and supporting evidence of preceding streptococcal infections (increased antisterptolysin-O or other antistreptococcal antibodies, positive throat culture for group A *Streptococcus*). Brain CT usually fails to display abnormalities. Head MRI is often normal but occasionally shows reversible hyper-

(Alzheimer or Pick disease), although there are similar mental dysfunctions, language is more involved. In this setting, myoclonus is more typical than chorea, especially with spongiform encephalopathies. Structural lesions need consideration: basal ganglia infarction or hemorrhage or, rarely, polycythemia rubra vera.

If the onset of chorea occurs during childhood, other hereditable disorders such as leukodystrophies and gangliosidosis require differentiation. The hereditary disorder called **neuroacanthocytosis** is manifested by mild chorea, tics, parkinsonism, and dystonia. Laboratory findings include increased serum creatine phosphokinase and red cell acanthocytes. In all age groups, possible reactions to drugs or toxins must always be investigated.

Table 53-2
Initial Laboratory Investigation of Chorea*

Huntington disease gene testing
Electrolyte panel
Complete blood count (look for acanthocytes)
Antinuclear antibody test (SLE)
Urine toxicological screen for illicit drugs
Thyroid hormone assay
Brain MRI/PET

*SLE indicates systemic lupus erythematosus.

intensity in the basal ganglia. PET and SPECT show reversible striatal hypermetabolism.

TREATMENT

Chorea is treated with dopamine-blocking or dopamine-depleting medications. Therapy depends on the severity of symptoms; mild chorea does not usually require any treatment. Dopamine antagonists haloperidol and pimozide are the drugs of choice after eliminating readily reversible causes of chorea. Nonspecific suppression with benzodiazepine drugs is another possible modality. With severe chorea, dopamine-depleting agents such as reserpine or tetrabenazine are sometimes considered.

The treatment of patients with HD requires an integrated, multidisciplinary approach including symptomatic and supportive medical management; psychosocial support; physical, occupational, or speech therapy; genetic counseling; and additional supportive services needed by patients or their families. No treatment is available that slows, alters, or reverses HD progression.

Sydenham chorea is usually not disabling, but patients requiring treatment may respond to dopamine antagonists or valproic acid. Severely affected patients may improve with immunosuppressants, plasmapheresis, or intravenous immunoglobulin. Drug treatment should be withdrawn after a short period because remission invariably occurs. Penicillin prophylaxis for ARF is advisable.

Prognosis depends on the cause of chorea. Drug-induced chorea is usually transient. Patients with a past history of rheumatic chorea are more susceptible to developing chorea during pregnancy or drug-induced chorea, eg, from phenytoin or oral contraceptives.

FUTURE DIRECTIONS

Research is ongoing to examine the inheritance patterns, pathophysiology, symptoms, and progression of HD and to develop new and improved therapies. Investigators are evaluating whether excessive activation of glutamate may be reduced by blocking receptors of *N*-methyl-D-aspartate, a similar neurotransmitter, possibly helping to halt abnormal nerve cell death. Studies are being conducted to assess the potential symptomatic and neuroprotective effects of riluzole, an agent thought to moderate the effects of glutamate. Other possible disease-modifying therapies, such as antioxidants (eg, coenzyme Q10) or certain growth factors that may have a protective effect on striatal nerve cells (neurotrophic growth factors), are under investigation. Experimental animal studies and clinical investigations are evaluating the safety and potential effectiveness of certain surgical techniques for HD, including replacement of degenerated neuronal tissue through transplantation of human or pig fetal cells.

REFERENCES

Brooks DJ. Functional imaging of movement disorders. In: Marsden CD, Fahn S, eds. *Movement Disorders 3*. Oxford, England: Butterworth-Heinemann Ltd; 1996:79-81.

Harding AE. Movement disorders: genetic aspects. In: Marsden CD, Fahn S, eds. *Movement Disorders 3*. Oxford, England: Butterworth-Heinemann Ltd; 1996:51-57.

Huntington's disease and other choreas. In: Fahn S, Greene PE, Ford B, Bressman SB, eds. *Handbook of Movement Disorders*. Philadelphia, Pa: Current Medicine, Inc; 1998:75-95.

Jankovic J, Beach J. Long-term effects of tetrabenazine in hyperkinetic movement disorders. *Neurology*. 1997;48:358-362.

O'Brien CH. Chorea. In: Jankovic J, Tolosa E, eds. *Parkinson's Disease and Movement Disorders*. Baltimore, Md: Williams & Wilkins; 1998:357-364.

Chapter 54
Tic Disorders

E. Prather Palmer

Clinical Vignette

An 8-year-old child's teacher reported to the child's mother that she had noticed repetitive facial grimacing movements that were increasing in frequency. The movements increased with stress but were also present when the child was sitting quietly. Soon, the family also noted these involuntary movements at home. The mother took the child to a pediatric neurologist and requested treatment. There was no family history of neurologic disease and no history of trauma or medication use. The boy was a well-adjusted, bright child.

Neurologic examination results were normal. The neurologist counseled against any drug treatment and advised the family not to upset the child about the tics. Later, when the paternal grandmother learned about the tics, she recounted how the father had made repetitive mildly disruptive grunting sounds during his ninth year of life and that for several years he had also had a "habit" of twitching his left shoulder. Within 11 months, the facial grimacing spontaneously ceased without any treatment.

Tics are rapid, usually repetitive movements that erupt suddenly from a background of normal motor activity, often with premonitory feelings or sensations and temporal suppressibility. These movements are classified as motor (muscle) or phonemic (abnormal sounds). *Phonemic* is preferred over *vocal tics* because abnormal sound production may be produced at multiple sites including the vocal cords but also by respiratory, pharyngeal, oral, or nasal movements. Tics are further classified as complex or simple and as clonic, dystonic, or tonic (Table 54-1).

Generally, tics are insuppressible, but sometimes, they can be suppressed over varying periods—hence the rationale for why tics are often not observed in the doctor's office. However, forced suppression is often associated with mounting tension in the patient, "**psychic tension**," not relieved until the tic is performed. The patient may sometimes feel an urge to repeat the tic until it is done in "just the right way." Premovement sensations that may be localized, or vague "**psychic sensation**," such as rage, anger, or anxiety, may precede involuntary tics.

Differentiating tics from other movement disorders is surprisingly difficult in certain settings. Although some coordinated movements resemble **complex motor tics**, these may actually represent attempts to conceal the tic by incorporating it into seemingly purposeful acts (**parakinesias**) such as adjusting one's hair during a head-jerk tic. Distinguishing complex motor tics from compulsions (**compulsive tics**) requires knowledge of the motivating factors. The latter is often associated with an irresistible urge to perform the movement or sound and a fear that if the movement is not performed promptly and properly, something "bad" might happen. Self-injurious behavior, such as scratching, itching, or picking, frequently suggests a compulsive tic disorder. The distinction may be impossible if the patient is unable to express such feelings.

Simple motor tics can also resemble myoclonus, but their association with other complex motor and phonemic tics often provides a diagnostic clue. These tics are frequently repetitive but may lack rhythmicity while varying in their intensity. Unlike myoclonus, these tics may involve eye movements. Dystonic tics are usually differentiated from primary dystonia because of the presence of other tics, the relatively short duration of the sustained posture, and onset during childhood. Chorea is characterized by its flow of continuous movement (Table 54-2).

Stereotyped motor behavior, as opposed to tics, can occur in healthy persons throughout their lives. However, it is also observed in other primary neurodegenerative disorders. **Stereotypy** is a coordinated, purposeless movement of a body part performed repetitively at the ex-

Table 54-1
Classification of Tics*

A. Simple motor: isolated, simple, or repetitive movement of just 1 muscle group
  1. Clonic: brief (<100 milliseconds) jerklike movement, ie, blinking, head jerk, tongue protrusion, facial grimace, or shoulder shrug
  2. Dystonic: (>300 milliseconds) a more sustained twisting or squeezing movement, ie, blepharospasm, oculogyric crisis, bruxism, torticollis, or mouth opening
  3. Tonic: (>500 milliseconds) sustained isometric contraction usually without overt movement, ie, tension of muscles of leg, arm, shoulder or abdomen

B. Complex motor: coordinated or sequential contraction of muscles that may resemble a normal movement or gesture but is usually inappropriate in intensity and timing; these are occasionally repetitive, ie, trunk bending, head shaking, touching, throwing, hitting, kicking, obscene gestures, grabbing or exposing one's genitalia, copropraxia, or imitation of gestures (echopraxia)

C. Simple phonemic: meaningless sounds or noises, ie, clearing throat, snuffling, squeaking, blowing, or sucking

D. Complex phonemic: meaningful utterances and vocalizations: obscenities (**corprolalia**), repetition of someone else's words or phrases (**echolalia**), or the repetition of ones own words or phrases (**palilia**)

E. Blocking: cessation of all motor activity (head bobbing [clonic], interruption of ongoing motor activity such as speech [dystonic], or inability to initiate motor activity [tonic])

F. Compulsive: movements in response to the thought that it will prevent harm from coming to the individual; the premonitory symptom distinguishes a complex tic from a compulsion

G. Sensory: sudden, brief sensory symptoms (feeling in throat, itching sensation, need to scratch) that are followed by overt movements

H. Secondary: tics occurring in association with an underlying acquired or congenital neurologic disorder

*After Jankovic J. Tourette syndrome: phenomenology and classification of tics. *Neurol Clin.* 1997;15:267-275.

pense of other activities and often for long periods. Examples include head nodding, head banging, body rocking, thumb sucking, and chewing of the lips or tongue. Some persons have compulsive, self-gratifying, often socially offensive, coordinated, voluntary body movements (habitual movements or spasms) when they are anxious, bored, fatigued, or self-conscious, eg, nail biting, hair twirling, eye rubbing, nose picking, ear touching, manipulation of genitalia, and aerophagy. The individual often feels compelled to make the movements to relieve perceived tension.

Table 54-2
Tic Characteristics for Differentiation From Other Movement Disorders

1. Childhood onset
2. Premonitory feelings or sensations
3. Temporary suppressibility
4. Repetitive and stereotyped
5. Increase with stress and during subsequent relaxation
6. Waxing and waning, transient remissions
7. Usually persist during all stages of sleep
8. Suggestibility
9. Both motor and phonemic component

PATHOPHYSIOLOGY

The pathophysiologic mechanisms causing tics are unknown. Evidence suggests an organic rather than a physiologic origin. Even though some tics may be partially voluntary, studies suggest that tics are not mediated through the normal motor pathways of willed movements. Subjects who voluntarily make **ticlike** movements have a premovement potential, **bereitschaftspotential**, recorded in the motor area of the cerebral cortex. Patients with a **true tic** disorder do not have this premonitory potential associated with their tics, suggesting that tics are involuntary in response to an external cue. Although

MRI and CT scans are normal in patients with tics, recent volumetric MRI studies demonstrate abnormalities in cerebral lateralization, especially in the basal ganglia. PET and SPECT identify abnormal perfusion in the basal ganglia, the thalamus, and the frontotemporal areas. The dopamine receptor hypersensitivity hypothesis of the underlying pathophysiologic abnormality has been questioned because dopaminergic drugs may not worsen the tic disorder, and the dopamine agonist, pergolide, may dramatically decrease tic severity. The cause of tics is likely to involve both the basal ganglia and the frontotemporal circuits.

TIC SYNDROMES

Tic disorders are generally childhood disorders. With the exception of secondary tic syndromes, adult onset of tics is rare, and most adult patients with tics have a similar childhood history. The **transient tic disorder (TTD) of childhood** is the most common and mildest form of an idiopathic tic disorder. TDD occurs in up to 24% of school-age children. It is usually a simple motor tic lasting less than 1 year. **Chronic multiple tic disorder** is similar to **Tourette syndrome**, (TS) but these patients have only **chronic motor tics** or, more unusually, only **phonemic tics** that last more than 1 year. Separation of tic disorders into transient tic disorder of childhood, chronic multiple tic disorder, chronic motor tics, chronic phonemic tics, or TS is probably inappropriate because they can all occur in the same family and likely reflect variable expression of the same genetic defect.

Tourette Syndrome

Chronic, simple, complex, and dystonic motor tics and simple and complex phonemic tics are the clinical hallmarks of TS, although it may be one end of a continuous tic disorder spectrum (Figure 54-1). TS affects all cultures and racial groups and has a prevalence of 5 in 10,000 persons, with a 4:1 male:female ratio.

The onset of TS usually occurs around the age of 7 years (range, 2-18 years), usually with simple tics around the eyes (eg, blinking), followed by more complex movements (licking, spitting, jumping, kicking, etc). Phonemic tics usually start 1 to 2 years later, although in approximately 15%, vocalizations are the initial symptom. Less than 30% have coprolalia, the most infamous feature. Other common features in full-blown cases include copropraxia, echolalia, echopraxia, and palilalia. These symptoms are not necessary for the diagnosis (Table 54-3). Although involuntary, these tics are suppressible for varying periods at the cost of increasing inner tensions. Anxiety, fatigue, excitement, and stimulants exacerbate the tics, whereas relaxation and alcohol may temporally suppress the tics completely. During sleep, the tics can continue in an attenuated form, confirming their involuntary nature. TS may be a lifelong illness but has a variable presence as symptoms wax and wane, with an eventual gradual reduction in severity. Only 25% of patients may need medications during adulthood, and more than 40% may become symptom free. Surprisingly, tic severity during childhood has little predictive value for the future course.

Tourette syndrome is often associated with other conditions. An exaggerated startle response that does not habituate with repetition is seen in 20% of cases. **Attention deficit hyperactivity disorder** (ADHD) afflicts 50% of patients with TS. Symptoms include impulsively, inattention, restlessness, fidgeting, poor concentration, poor school, or work performance. ADHD can be a major problem because severely hyperactive children, especially those with severe phonic tics or coprolalia, often disrupt other children in the classroom. **Obsessive-compulsive disorder** (OCD), with symptoms of repetitive, stereotyped, involuntary, senseless thought or behaviors that protrude into the patient's consciousness, occurs in 30% to 50% of patients with TS. OCD significantly increases these patients' social impairment and emotional distress. Other behaviors including exhibitionism, aggression, self-injury, and discipline problems occur in approximately 20%. All of these behavioral symptoms can lead to a misdiagnosis of TS when more serious neurologic or psychiatric conditions, including schizophrenia, are present.

Genetics

Analysis of large kindreds unequivocally demonstrates that TS is genetically determined; however, the results of genetic linkage studies are inconclusive. Most researchers believe that

TIC DISORDERS

Figure 54-1

Tourette Syndrome

Tics around the eyes is the most common sign of the onset of Tourette syndrome. It is usually followed by more complex movements such as spitting, facial grimacing movements, jumping, kicking, and then vocalization (coprolalia, echolalia, and others).

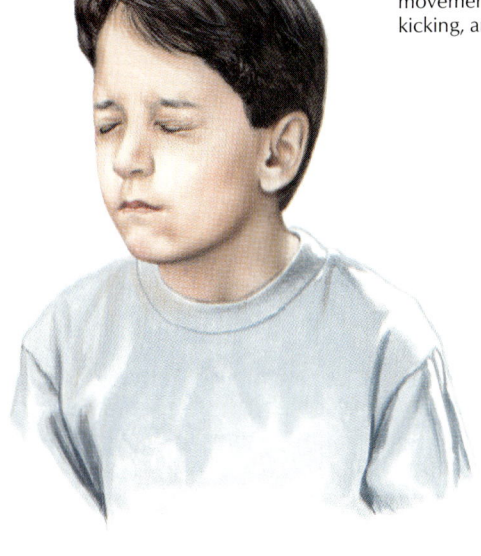
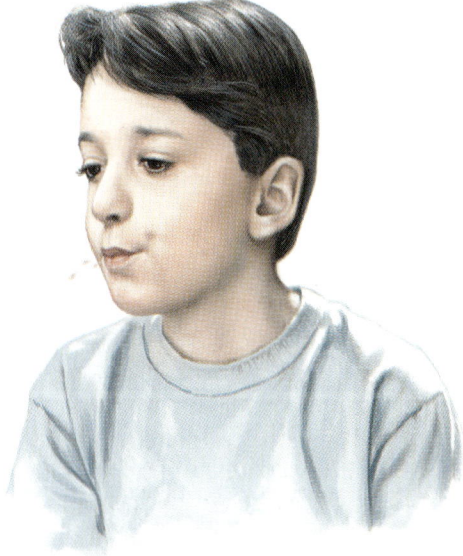
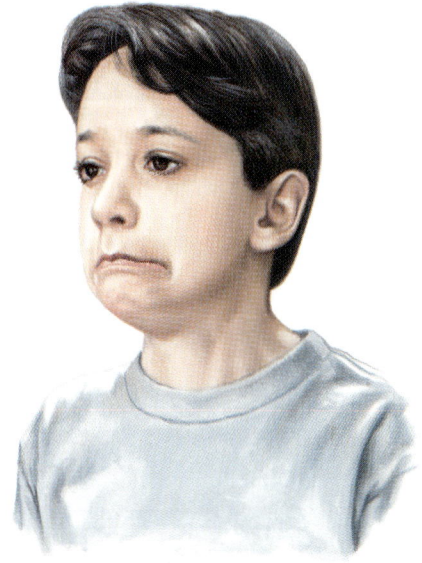
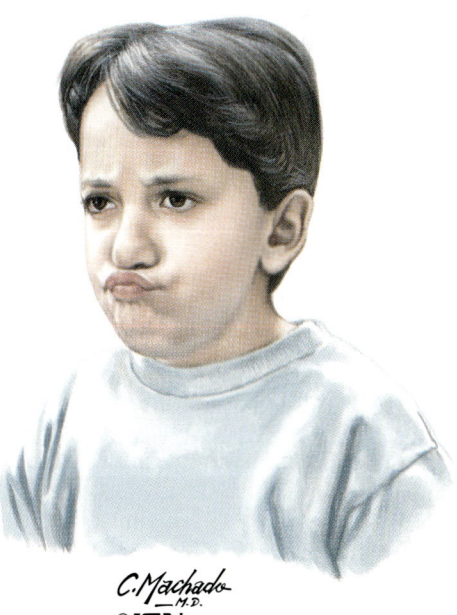

MOVEMENT DISORDERS

TIC DISORDERS

Table 54-3
Criteria for Diagnosis of Tourette Syndrome

1. Both multiple motor and 1 or more phonemic tics present sometime during the illness, although not necessarily concurrently.
2. The tics occur many times a day, nearly every day, or intermittently for more than a year, with symptom-free intervals not exceeding 3 months.
3. Onset occurs before the age of 18 years.
4. Variations occur in anatomical location, number, frequency, complexity, and severity of the tics over time.
5. Involuntary movements and noises cannot be explained by any other medical condition.
6. A reliable examiner must directly witness motor and/or phonemic tics.
7. Symptoms often cause significant impairment of social, academic, and occupational functioning.

an individual may inherit a vulnerability to a **spectrum disorder** that includes TS, OCD, and ADHD. Family genetic data show that OCD may represent an alternative expression of the TS genetic trait. Although ADHD may not be a variant expression of TS, the 2 conditions may be etiologically related in some individuals. Twin studies in TS show a concordance of 53% for monozygotic and 8% for dizygotic twins. However, if all primary tic disorders are included, the concordance rates increase to nearly 80% and 25%, respectively. Of the probands, one third have a family history of full TS, whereas another one third have a positive family history of simple tics. Often, the father has a history of tics that may or may not persist through adulthood, whereas the mother may have features of OCD. Therefore, TS may represent part of a spectrum of which TTD is the mildest manifestation and the most severe is the full-blown TS syndrome that includes the behavioral features.

Secondary Tic Syndromes

Tics occur in association with numerous different acquired and congenital neurologic and neuropsychiatric disorders. They may develop with exposure to many medications or drugs. The terms **secondary tics** or **tourettism** describe these disorders (Table 54-4). Many of these disorders and drugs affect basal function, and many

Table 54-4
Secondary Tic Disorders*

Acquired	Genetic	Drugs
Trauma	Huntington disease	Cocaine
Encephalitis	Neuroacanthocytosis	Amphetamines
Stroke	Idiopathic dystonia	Pemoline
Sydenham chorea	Tuberous sclerosis	Antipsychotics
Creutzfeld-Jakob disease	Chromosomal disorders	Antidepressants
Neurosyphilis	Asperger syndrome	Antiepileptic
Hypoxic head injury		L-Dopa
Carbon monoxide		Anticholinergics
PANDAS syndrome		Lithium
Mental retardation		Opioids

*PANDAS indicates pediatric autoimmune neuropsychiatric disorders associated with streptococcal infections.

basal ganglia lesions may result in obsessive-compulsive symptomatology, which commonly coexists with TS.

TREATMENT

Tics and their associated conditions can be difficult to manage. Fortunately, most patients have a mild syndrome requiring no specific pharmacologic therapy. After adolescence, 85% of children with TS experience significant clinical improvement or remission. Tics continuing beyond adolescence or starting in adult life often persist. Patient and family education are key to appropriate therapy. Reassurance is achieved by discussing the normal waxing and waning of TS symptomatology and the tendency for symptoms to improve with age. This may be all that is necessary. Some patients with TS require short-term therapy during periods of exacerbation. It is also critical to distinguish between tics, ADHD, and OCD.

The primary treatment choices for tics usually include **α-adrenergic agents** because of their effectiveness and fewer long-term adverse effects. Although clonidine is usually the first drug used, guanfacine may cause less drowsiness and can often be given once daily. Clonidine is available as a transdermal 1-week patch, which is advantageous for small children. Second-line therapy usually requires an **atypical antipsychotic** such as risperidone or olanzapine. These are preferred over the classic neuroleptic antipsychotic medications because of their better adverse effect profile, especially their lower tendency to cause extrapyramidal effects, including acute dystonia, tardive dyskinesia, and parkinsonism, complications that may be particularly prevalent in patients with TS. **Traditional neuroleptic antipsychotic** medications, such as haloperidol and pimozide, remain the most predictable tic-suppressing drugs. Because of their tendency to cause extrapyramidal syndromes, sedation, weight gain, irritability, and various phobias, they remain third-line medications. Other drugs may be tried if these are not effective. Tetrabenazine (not readily available in the United States), baclofen, clonazepam, and calcium channel blockers have demonstrated some effectiveness. In severe cases, intramuscular botulinum toxin and thalamic stimulation may be effective for the most severely impaired patients with TS.

Patients with TS and OCD often respond to a serotonin reuptake inhibitor or to the tricyclic antidepressant clomipramine. Clonidine, guanfacine, and the stimulants methylphenidate, pemoline, or dextroamphetamines are helpful in patients with ADHD. These stimulant drugs have usually not been associated with an increased frequency of the tics. Lithium carbonate or carbamazepines are sometimes helpful for patients with severe mood changes and poor impulse control.

REFERENCES

Burd L, Kerbeshian PJ, Barth A, Klug MG, Avery PK, Benz B. Long-term follow-up on an epidemiologically defined cohort of patients with Tourette syndrome. *J Child Neurol.* 2001;16:431-437.

Evidente, VG. Is it a tic or Tourette's? *Postgrad Med.* 2000;108:175-182.

Marcus D, Kurlan R. Tic and its disorders. *Neurol Clin.* 2001;19:735-758.

Robertson MM. Tourette syndrome, associated conditions and the complexities of treatment. *Brain.* 2000;123:425-462.

Chapter 55
Wilson Disease

E. Prather Palmer

Clinical Vignette

A 31-year-old man was referred to a neurologist for evaluation of dysarthric speech. Recently, the patient's internist had diagnosed viral hepatitis based on increased serum transaminases. The patient had a recent history of IV drug abuse. His speech problem began more than a year previously and had been progressive. His wife noted that his speech had become soft and slurred, making comprehension difficult at times. She had also noted a concomitant change in his personality. Her husband had become irritable with marked mood swings. Sometimes he seemed depressed, and at other times he was belligerent. This personality change caused problems at his work.

The patient's neurologic examination results were normal except for the presence of microsaccades on smooth horizontal pursuit of the eyes. Head CT demonstrated hypodensity of the putamen and the globus pallidus extending into the pons. Slit-lamp examination of the eyes showed a gold/brown-pigmented ring at the limbus of the cornea. The serum ceruloplasmin level was low, and a 24-hour urine copper excretion level was increased. A diagnosis of Wilson disease was made; the patient was started on penicillamine. Within 6 weeks, bradykinesia, rigidity, and mutism developed. Twelve months later, the patient's speech had returned to normal, and his behavior had improved, although he still showed some depressive symptoms. Zinc acetate was started as a long-term therapy.

Wilson disease is a rare hereditary disorder of copper metabolism, biochemically characterized by abnormal accumulation of this essential trace metal in the liver and the brain, leading to cirrhosis and neuronal degeneration. Excess copper accumulation in the liver was reported in 1913 and later in the basal ganglia. A reduced serum ceruloplasmin level was recognized in 1952. Treatment with dimercaprol (British antilewisite) was reported in 1951; penicillamine treatment was introduced in 1956. Wilson disease thus became the first inherited metabolic disorder with specific treatments.

Wilson disease has an autosomal recessive inheritance found in all known ethnic groups. Its worldwide distribution has an estimated frequency of 1 in 30,000 and a carrier rate of 1 in 90. Presentations vary and include hepatic dysfunction, neurologic impairment, or psychiatric disturbance; less common are acute hemolytic crisis, arthralgias, renal stones, pancreatic disease, cardiomyopathy, or hypothyroidism.

CLINICAL PRESENTATION

Neurologic symptoms are the initial presentation in approximately 60% of patients, usually in the third or fourth decade of life. Although Wilson disease is usually thought to present as an involuntary movement disorder, the most common initial neurologic signs are dysarthria, dysphagia, bradykinesia, and behavioral disturbance. Speech manifestations vary from rapid speech to hypophonia and slurred speech. Speech involvement is a constant feature with neurologic involvement. All patients with unexplained speech impairment should be evaluated for Wilson disease.

Parkinson disease symptoms may predominate with reduced facial expression, bradykinesia, and tremors. Tremors range from subtle in the outstretched fingers to severe, coarse, proximal tremors of the arms and legs, unlike that of Parkinson disease. An upper extremity coarse tremor is common and usually positionally dependent, especially when the arms are elevated and flexed at the elbow, giving the appearance of "wing beating" or "chest beating." Dystonia, hypertonicity, and choreoathetosis are also seen. Dystonia occurs with equal frequency to tremor, sometimes coexisting with it. The dystonia is more typically generalized, involving the extremities, neck (torticollis), and face (grimacing), but may be focal, such as involving a hand. Ultimately, patients may become severely rigid with a pseudobulbar palsy. Usually, no evidence exists of cerebellar, peripheral, or cranial nerve, or skeletal muscle involvement.

Psychiatric disturbances are the presenting feature in 25% to 65% of patients, although no particular behavioral syndrome is characteristic. Usually, it is an insidiously progressive change in personality. Irritability and aggression are typical; affective changes include depression and emotional lability. Cognitive changes, anxiety, catatonia, and psychosis are uncommon. Transient psychosis may occur during treatment.

Ophthalmologic manifestations are common in Wilson disease and are often crucial to diagnosis. The classic and best-known finding is the dull, yellow-brown pigment at the limbus of the cornea called **Kayser-Fleischer rings** (Figure 55-1). Most dense at the upper and lower poles of the cornea, Kayser-Fleischer rings result from copper deposition in the Descemet membrane at the limbus. Kayser-Fleischer rings are present in nearly all patients with Wilson disease who have neurologic or psychiatric symptoms, but the rings may be missed on casual examination, particularly in patients with brown irises. Commonly, slit-lamp examination is required for detection and verification. Kayser-Fleischer rings are often absent in asymptomatic individuals and in up to 50% of individuals with a hepatic presentation. Other signs include reduced saccadic velocity, interruption of smooth pursuit by saccadic intrusions, and sunflower cataracts (15-20% of patients).

Hepatic dysfunction manifests in the early teens to the early 20s, although it may present in earlier childhood or late adulthood. Symptoms of hepatocellular disease vary from a mild increase of serum transaminases in asymptomatic individuals to chronic active hepatitis and cirrhosis with episodes of jaundice, chronic malaise, and vomiting. More severe acute hepatic failure may be associated with episodes of hemolytic anemia from the sudden release of excess copper into the circulation. Irrespective of the initial symptoms, almost all patients have some evidence of cirrhosis on liver biopsy, reflecting the clinically occult injury after years of hepatic copper accumulation. Histopathology demonstrates chronic hepatitis with nodular regeneration (nodular cirrhosis) and copper deposition. Hepatocellular carcinoma is a rare complication.

HEPATIC COPPER METABOLISM

Copper facilitates electron transfer in critical metabolic pathways involving cellular respiration, iron homeostasis, pigment formation, neurotransmitter production, peptide biosynthesis, connective tissue biosynthesis, and antioxidant defense. Within the brain, copper is found in high concentrations in catecholamine-containing neurons. It is a component of the dopamine β-hydroxylase enzyme complex. Copper balance is maintained entirely by gastrointestinal absorption and biliary excretion. Urinary copper excretion cannot adequately compensate for reduced biliary excretion.

Dietary copper is absorbed in the proximal small intestine, where, inside the mucosal cells, a portion is irreversibly bound to metallothionein, a family of complex proteins that are poorly understood. Some copper is lost with cell desquamation into the intestine. Most dietary copper enters the hepatoportal circulation, where it rapidly enters the hepatocytes. Hepatocytes "sense" this cytoplasmic copper accumulation and regulate copper excretion into the bile, depending on the concentration. A copper-transporting adenosine triphosphatase located on the trans-Golgi network and the cytoplasmic vesicular compartment near the canalicular membrane provides rapid and responsive intracellular copper homeostasis and facilitates rapid excretion of excess copper.

Copper bound within ceruloplasmin represents 95% of plasma copper. Synthesized in the hepatocytes, this glycoprotein is secreted as the holoprotein with 6 atoms of copper incorporated during transit through the secretory pathway. Copper has no effect on the rate of synthesis or secretion of ceruloplasmin, but failure to incorporate copper causes secretion of an apoprotein that is rapidly degraded in the plasma.

GENETICS

An autosomal recessive disorder, the Wilson disease gene is located on chromosome 13. Carrier frequency among whites is estimated as 1%. The risk to any child of an affected individual

WILSON DISEASE

who marries an unrelated spouse is 0.5%. The gene encodes for a copper-transporting adenosine triphosphatase that shows considerable homology to an X-linked, copper-transporting gene responsible for Menke syndrome in children. DNA analysis from patients with Wilson disease shows more than 100 mutations, complicating DNA diagnosis and the correlation between the various mutations and clinical features. Only a few patients are homozygous for the same mutation. DNA testing can identify asymptomatic affected subjects when Wilson disease has been diagnosed within a family.

The gene for ceruloplasmin is located on chromosome 3 and is distinct from the gene for Wilson disease. The degree of incorporation of copper into ceruloplasmin is a reflection of the relative abundance of the protein and does not suggest a role for it in normal copper transport. Copper homeostasis is normal in patients with aceruloplasminemia. In Wilson disease, the adenosine triphosphatase defect influences plasma secretion and biliary excretion of ceruloplasmin. The apoprotein of ceruloplasmin without copper that is secreted into the plasma is rapidly degraded, so plasma ceruloplasmin levels are usually low in patients who have Wilson disease.

DIAGNOSIS

Devastating neurologic and hepatic deterioration may be prevented with early diagnosis and treatment. Early diagnosis of Wilson disease depends on clinical suspicion regarding signs and symptoms (Table 55-1 and Figure 55-1).

Hepatic dysfunction is the most common initial manifestation in childhood, with patients presenting at an average age of 10 to 13 years, a decade or more earlier than those who present with neurologic or psychiatric symptoms. Hepatic copper measurement (the accepted standard laboratory test) is not usually necessary to make a diagnosis.

Ceruloplasmin levels are reduced in 95% of patients with Wilson disease. In contrast, as an acute-phase reactant, ceruloplasmin levels may be increased in patients with inflammation, pregnant patients, or patients taking birth control pills. Gene carriers often have reduced plasma ceruloplasmin levels. However, ceruloplasmin levels are not reduced in all patients, especially those presenting with liver disease. Therefore, ceruloplasmin concentration is not an absolute diagnostic test, but its measurement influences clinical suspicion of Wilson disease. Patients with aceruloplasminemia may present with neurologic symptoms but have normal hepatic copper levels and marked increases of parenchymal iron.

Deposition of copper in tissues other than liver may help with the diagnosis. Asymptomatic copper deposition is clinically best detected in the limbus of the cornea by slit lamp examination (Kayser-Fleischer rings) (Figure 55-1). Although present in nearly every patient with neurologic involvement, Kayser-Fleischer rings may be absent in asymptomatic patients or those who primarily have hepatic involvement. They are not pathognomonic for Wilson disease and may be seen in other chronic, severe liver diseases, such as primary biliary cirrhosis.

Patients with Wilson disease have increased urinary copper excretion because the nonceruloplasmin component of plasma copper is increased, filtered by the glomerulus, and incompletely reabsorbed by the renal tubules. The

Table 55-1
Consideration of the Diagnosis of Wilson Disease

Primary

- **Speech impairment** that is progressive and unexplained
- **Extrapyramidal dysfunction** that is progressive and unexplained
- **Psychiatric disturbances** of new onset in patients younger than 30 years, especially if associated with dysarthria, extrapyramidal dysfunction, or cognitive impairment
- **Chronic**, unexplained **liver disease**
- **Acute hepatitis**, especially **if** prolonged, recurrent, or associated with hemolysis
- Siblings of patients with Wilson disease

Secondary

- Hemolytic anemia
- Fanconi syndrome with aminoaciduria and nephrolithiasis
- Arthritis or arthralgias with early onset

WILSON DISEASE

Figure 55-1

Wilson Disease

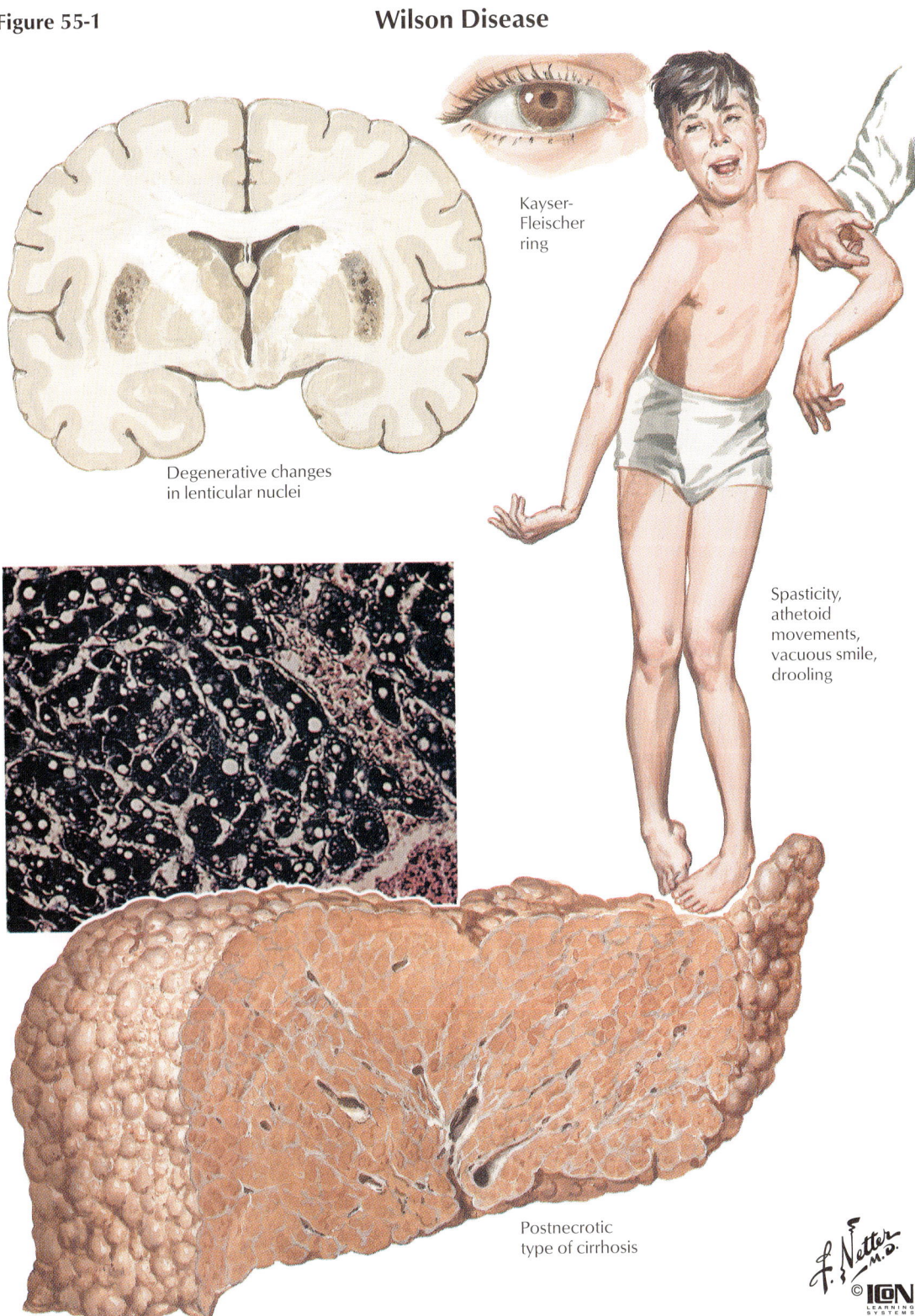

Degenerative changes in lenticular nuclei

Kayser-Fleischer ring

Spasticity, athetoid movements, vacuous smile, drooling

Postnecrotic type of cirrhosis

MOVEMENT DISORDERS

WILSON DISEASE

Table 55-2
Laboratory Testing in Wilson Disease*

1. Liver biopsy with measurement of liver copper†
2. 24-hour urine for copper (in patients not using penicillamine)†
3. Slit lamp examination for Kayser-Fleischer rings†
4. Plasma ceruloplasmin†
5. Total serum copper
6. Assay of Cu^{64} uptake into the plasma
7. Genetic testing

*In order of accuracy.
†In practice, only the first 4 items are useful in diagnosis.

increased renal copper excretion does not adequately compensate for the reduced biliary copper excretion. Measurement of 24-hour copper excretion (more accurate before initiating penicillamine therapy) is a standardized and reliable diagnostic test (Table 55-2). Plasma copper concentration is not diagnostic because total plasma copper (ceruloplasmin bound plus non-ceruloplasmin bound) may be reduced, normal, or increased. Although assaying Cu^{64} uptake into plasma has been suggested as a diagnostic test, the results have not proven particularly useful.

Neurologic features mirror the underlying pathologic changes of cavitary degeneration within the basal ganglia, including extensive gliosis and neuronal loss in association with a marked increase in copper content. MRI detects underlying structural changes, seen in virtually all patients with neurologic symptoms. In general, brain MRI correlates with the presence or absence of neurologic impairment. The changes may improve with chelation therapy.

The molecular heterogeneity in Wilson disease precludes diagnostic DNA testing in most cases. Using the combination of clinical history, physical examination, slit lamp examination, and supplementary laboratory data, the diagnosis of Wilson disease can usually be made with great accuracy.

TREATMENT AND PROGNOSIS

Restoration of hepatic homeostasis by systemic chelation therapy is the treatment of choice. Clinical improvement is accompanied by marked decrease in hepatic copper content. Penicillamine, the preferred chelator, binds copper in the plasma and organs, promotes urinary copper excretion, and prevents copper accumulation in presymptomatic individuals. Its usefulness is often limited by adverse effects (commonly fever, skin rash, thrombocytopenia, nephrotic syndrome, and acute arthritis) seen in up to 20% of patients. Late immune complex–mediated nephropathy, systemic lupus erythematosis, Goodpasture syndrome, oral ulcers, pseudoxanthoma, and autoimmune-mediated myasthenia gravis may occur. Therefore, patients must be carefully monitored for these toxicities.

The most significant adverse effect of penicillamine treatment is the paradoxic worsening or new appearance of neurologic deficits. Estimated to occur in up to 50% of patients, the mechanism is thought to be deposition of mobilized liver copper within the basal ganglia. Triethylamine tetramine (trientine) has an efficacy similar to that of penicillamine and is approved for initial therapy and patients who do not tolerate penicillamine. Although less toxic, triethylamine tetramine has the same spectrum of toxicity as penicillamine and requires similar monitoring. Ammonium tetrathiolmolybdate (TM) binds with dietary copper and food protein and prevents copper absorption. When taken between meals, TM is absorbed and binds to nonceruloplasmin copper, preventing copper uptake into tissues. TM-complexed copper is excreted in urine and bile. TM has a greater binding affinity for copper than does penicillamine and has fewer tendencies to redistribute copper from the liver to the brain. Hence, TM therapy is not associated with worsening of existing neurologic signs. TM is only available as an investigational drug.

Orally administered zinc acetate is a safe and effective maintenance therapy. Zinc acetate blocks copper absorption and induces intestinal mucosal cell production of metallothionien, which irreversibly binds with dietary copper preventing entrance into the hepatoportal circulation. Dietary consumption of liver and shellfish, both high in copper, should be avoided or eliminated. Other dietary modifications are seldom necessary with proper maintenance therapy. Liver transplantation is sometimes necessary for patients with advanced liver disease, especially those with fulminate hepatic failure. This heroic therapy may reduce neurologic symptoms in some patients.

Neurologic and psychiatric impairment is preventable if therapy is instituted in the early stages of disease, making early diagnosis a challenge. Clinical improvement usually occurs 6 to 24 months after adequate therapy is instituted. Not all patients improve to the same extent. However, improvements in neurologic and psychiatric symptoms can be sustained over long periods; patients have been followed up for more than 10 years. Death may occur from neurologic (eg, dysphagia) or hepatic complications.

REFERENCES

Fink JK, Hedera P, Brewer GJ. Hepatolenticular degeneration (Wilson's disease). *Neurologist.* 1999;5:171-185.

Loudianos G, Gitlin JD. Wilson's disease. *Semin Liver Dis.* 2000;20:353-364.

Chapter 56
Psychogenic Movement Disorders

Diana Apetauerova

Clinical Vignette

A 20-year-old man with a medical history of anxiety and depression presented with a 2-week history of intermittent right hand tremor. He first noticed the tremor while taking a college examination when he was unable to hold a pencil in his right hand because of the severe tremor. The second episode occurred after a disagreement with his mother; at that time, the tremor occurred in both hands. Subsequently, he noticed an intermittent tremor mainly in the right hand, both during activities and at rest. He said that he had no other associated symptoms. The tremor did not affect other parts of his body; alcoholic beverages were ineffective in lessening the tremor.

His family history was unremarkable; however, he had an older friend with history of Parkinson disease (PD). This contributed to his concern about the diagnosis of PD. He was not using any medications and had no drug allergies.

He appeared anxious; however general physical examination was unremarkable. Neurologic examination demonstrated an intermittent resting tremor in both hands, present during action and posture and seeming more prominent in the right hand. This tremor became enhanced during direct observation of the patient's hands. When holding his hands in front of him, the tremor amplitude increased in the right hand, and he was unable to hold a cup. However, on several occasions while he was distracted, the tremor disappeared. When asked to alternately pronate and supinate his hands, the tremor also disappeared. The same effect was produced after he was asked to count backward from 50 and during walking. He was unable to write and lost control of his pen during several occasions. One of the major characteristics of this tremor was its irregularity: it varied in amplitude and frequency during posture, action, or rest; it was suppressed with distraction; and it was voluntarily, intermittently suppressed for a short period of time.

The results of testing for Wilson disease and head MRI were normal. The diagnosis of psychogenic tremor was suspected. Several treatment options were tried, including propranolol, anxiolytics, and antidepressants, without subjective improvement. Later, after undergoing psychotherapy, he had sudden remission of these symptoms.

Psychogenic, hysterical, or functional movement disorders are conditions related to underlying psychiatric illness where no evidence of an organic etiology exists. There is a major inherent difficulty in making this diagnosis because up to 30% of patients diagnosed with psychogenic disorders eventually are found to have an organic illness, often neurologic, accounting for their symptoms. Other diagnostic caveats include that idiopathic movement disorders are diagnosed by history and physical examination, and most commonly there is no specific diagnostic laboratory test or neuroimaging finding available. It is often important to carefully follow patients for a period of time, to monitor them for signs of an evolving neurologic process or to become more comfortable with the importance of psychogenic factors in an individual's illness.

Among the psychiatric diagnoses reported in patients with psychogenic neurologic disorder are somatoform and factitious disorders, malingering, depression, anxiety, and histrionic personality disorders. In some cases, despite a high suspicion of psychogenicity of the motor symptoms, a psychiatric diagnosis is not confirmed. This does not preclude such a diagnosis, but caution is advised.

The most common types of psychogenic movement disorders are psychogenic dystonia, tremor, myoclonus, and parkinsonism. These emotionally based movement disorders are more common in women than in men. Patients usually reveal multiplicity and variability of symptoms. These patients often have a psychiatric background, and the examination reveals signs not commonly described with organic movement disorders, namely that the movements are consistently inconsistent often changing or decreasing during distraction. Frequently, patients with psychogenic movement disorders display

PSYCHOGENIC MOVEMENT DISORDERS

uneconomic postures and have exaggerated effort during examination, producing fatigue. They may demonstrate marked slowness when asked to do certain tasks such as rapid alternating movements.

Therapeutically, psychogenic movement disorders often respond to placebo or suggestion.

ETIOLOGY

Because the etiologies of psychogenic movement disorders are unknown, no anatomical correlation can be made. Whether any neurochemical interplay exists between the effect of the presumed underlying psychiatric condition and the patient's clinical presentation is a matter of future conjecture.

CLINICAL PRESENTATION
Psychogenic Dystonia

Dystonia is an involuntary, sustained muscle contraction causing repetitive twisting and abnormal postures. Most patients with dystonia have no identified mechanism, although some have a genetic basis. Because no specific test for organic dystonia exists, the diagnosis of psychogenic dystonia is difficult. The clinical breadth of organic dystonia must be appreciated before making a diagnosis of a psychogenic lesion. Patients with psychogenic dystonia may present with foot or leg involvement, which would not occur in organic adult-onset idiopathic dystonia. Often, patients with a psychogenic dystonia have symptoms at rest; this differs from organic dystonia, which is often action specific.

Psychogenic Tremor

Tremors are rhythmic, bidirectional, oscillating movements resulting from contraction of agonist and antagonistic muscles. Tremors can be resting, postural, or action.

Psychogenic tremor usually varies in frequency and amplitude, is complex, occurs with rest, posture, and action, and has amplitudes unlike that of midbrain tremor. Psychogenic tremor lessens with distraction.

Psychogenic Myoclonus

Myoclonus is defined as brief, shocklike movements caused by muscle contraction or lapses in posture. The frequency, amplitude, body distribution, symmetry, and course differ with various etiologies. Psychogenic myoclonus decreases in amplitude during distraction and often occurs at rest, in contrast to organic myoclonus, which decreases at rest.

Psychogenic Parkinsonism

Parkinsonism is a symptom complex consisting of resting tremor, rigidity, bradykinesia, and impaired postural reflexes. Psychogenic tremor varies in frequency and rhythmicity, remitting with distraction. Rigidity related to psychiatric problems consists of voluntary resistance without any evidence of cogwheeling. As with other psychogenic movement disorders, the symptoms of psychogenic parkinsonism lessen with distraction. Gait is atypical, with extreme or bizarre postural instability.

DIFFERENTIAL DIAGNOSES

The distinction between these clinical presentations and those of organic movement disorders must be made and often is challenging, delaying diagnosis sometimes several years after the onset of symptoms. Psychogenic movement disorders have certain common characteristics, such as acute onset, static course, spontaneous remissions, inconsistent character of movements (amplitude, frequency, distribution, selective disability), unresponsiveness to appropriate medications, response to placebo, movements increasing with attention, movements decreasing with distraction, remission with psychotherapy, and diagnosed psychopathology.

Other factors supporting the possibility of a psychogenic movement disorder include multiple poorly defined, somatic complaints within the patient's history. On physical examination, nonanatomical sensory findings, consistently inconsistent weakness, and a seemingly deliberate slowness of movement are also typical. Questions regarding possible secondary gain are important, especially pending litigation. A negative family history is common; however, sometimes psychiatrically ill patients have used a family member or friend with an organic movement disorder as a subconscious model for their own adventitious movements.

PSYCHOGENIC MOVEMENT DISORDERS

DIAGNOSTIC EVALUATION

The diagnosis of psychogenic movement disorder usually requires both a neurologist and a psychiatrist. The first step is a detailed clinical history and examination, review of current and previous medications, and subsequent exclusion of a true organic movement disorder. Diagnostic tests follow clinical assessment and may include brain MRI, serum ceruloplasmin and urine copper excretion, thyroid functions, and other tests based on clinical suspicion. The diagnostic evaluation may also include an appropriate trial of specific medications typically used for various organic movement disorders and tailored to the patient's clinical picture. After these steps are taken, and certain suggestions of psychogenicity exist, a diagnostic psychiatric evaluation is needed. However, the definition of a psychiatric illness does not prove that the movement disorder has a psychogenic basis.

TREATMENT AND PROGNOSIS

Treatment of psychogenic movement disorders is difficult. Usually, periodic neurologic evaluation of the patient with the same neurologist in conjunction with psychotherapy may be necessary to alleviate excessive concerns about the possibility of the presence of an organic illness and to maintain a reduction or remission of motor symptoms. Ongoing psychotherapy and physical therapy are important, as is treatment of the underlying psychiatric conditions (antidepressants, anxiolytics, etc). Finally, the use of placebo is debatable. Some physicians and patients interpret this as confrontational. Unfortunately, some patients may be more resistant to the diagnosis and psychiatric treatment.

Prognosis depends on the psychodynamic specifics underlying the movement disorder. Generally good prognostic signs include acute onset, short duration of symptoms, healthy premorbid functioning, absence of coexisting organic and psychogenic disease, and presence of an identifiable stressor.

FUTURE DIRECTIONS

When specific laboratory tests, possibly neurochemical or autoimmune in type, become available for the diagnosis of organic movement disorders, psychogenic movement disorders will be easier to confirm. More research in the field of neurotransmitters, more specific brain studies, such as functional MRI, and genetic testing will probably aid the understanding of this complex and difficult therapeutic problem.

REFERENCES

Fahn S, Williams D. Psychogenic dystonia. *Adv Neurol.* 1988;50:431-455.

Koller WC, Marjama J, Troster A. Psychogenic movement disorders. In: Jankovic J, Tolosa E, eds. *Parkinson's Disease and Movement Disorders.* Baltimore, Md: Williams & Wilkins; 1998;859-868.

Chapter 57
Surgical Treatments for Movement Disorders

Jeffrey E. Arle

Surgical therapies for certain movement disorders are important treatment modalities, particularly in medically refractory patients who have become increasingly and significantly disabled (Table 57-1 and Figure 57-1). Although thousands of surgically placed brain lesions were performed from 1950 through 1970 for various problems, including movement disorders, the understanding of the physiology of movement disorders and the ability to assess baseline and outcome data in these patients has markedly improved since then. A predominantly different subset of disease etiology exists with regard to Parkinson disease. Most Parkinson disease cases are idiopathic, compared with a significant percentage of postencephalitic patients treated in the mid-20th century. In general, several operations are currently performed for movement disorders.

The operations are performed stereotactically, typically with the help of a frame affixed to the patient's head. The frame creates a space with x, y, and z coordinates within which the head, and therefore the brain, lies. Thus, any location within that space can be targeted using devices to place and hold a probe tip, recording electrode, or stimulating electrode at the desired coordinates. The accuracy of such systems is often less than 1 mm, reliable enough to target precise regions in deep brain structures. Specific neuroanatomical sites are selected with the help of stereotactic targeting software using common brain locations as initial reference points, such as the anterior and posterior commissures.

Intraoperatively, the patients are typically kept awake. The specifically selected neurons are verified physiologically by microelectrode recordings taken along the trajectory into the brain, proceeding toward the intended target. Cells in certain areas have reproducible firing rates and patterns. Using these physiologic techniques, neurosurgeons are able to validate the exact electrode location. Of the major risks associated with these stereotactic procedures, the most significant include debilitating or fatal cerebral hemorrhage. These occur in approximately 0.5% to 3% of cases.

OPERATIONS PERFORMED FOR MOVEMENT DISORDERS
Pallidotomy

Definitive lesions of the posteroventrolateral region of the globus pallidus pars interna are made after a test "lesion," wherein the probe is heated to a lower temperature for a shorter time to test for adverse effects. Care must be taken to avoid producing lesions that are damaging to the

Table 57-1
Summary of Current Best Procedures for Movement Disorders*

Essential (Familial) Tremor
Vim thalamic DBS
Thalamotomy (unilateral)
Parkinson Disease
STN DBS
Gpi DBS
Pallidotomy (unilateral)
Dystonia
Gpi DBS

*DBS indicates deep brain stimulation; Gpi, globus pallidus pars interna; STN, subthalamic nucleus; Vim, ventralis intermedius.

SURGICAL TREATMENTS FOR MOVEMENT DISORDERS

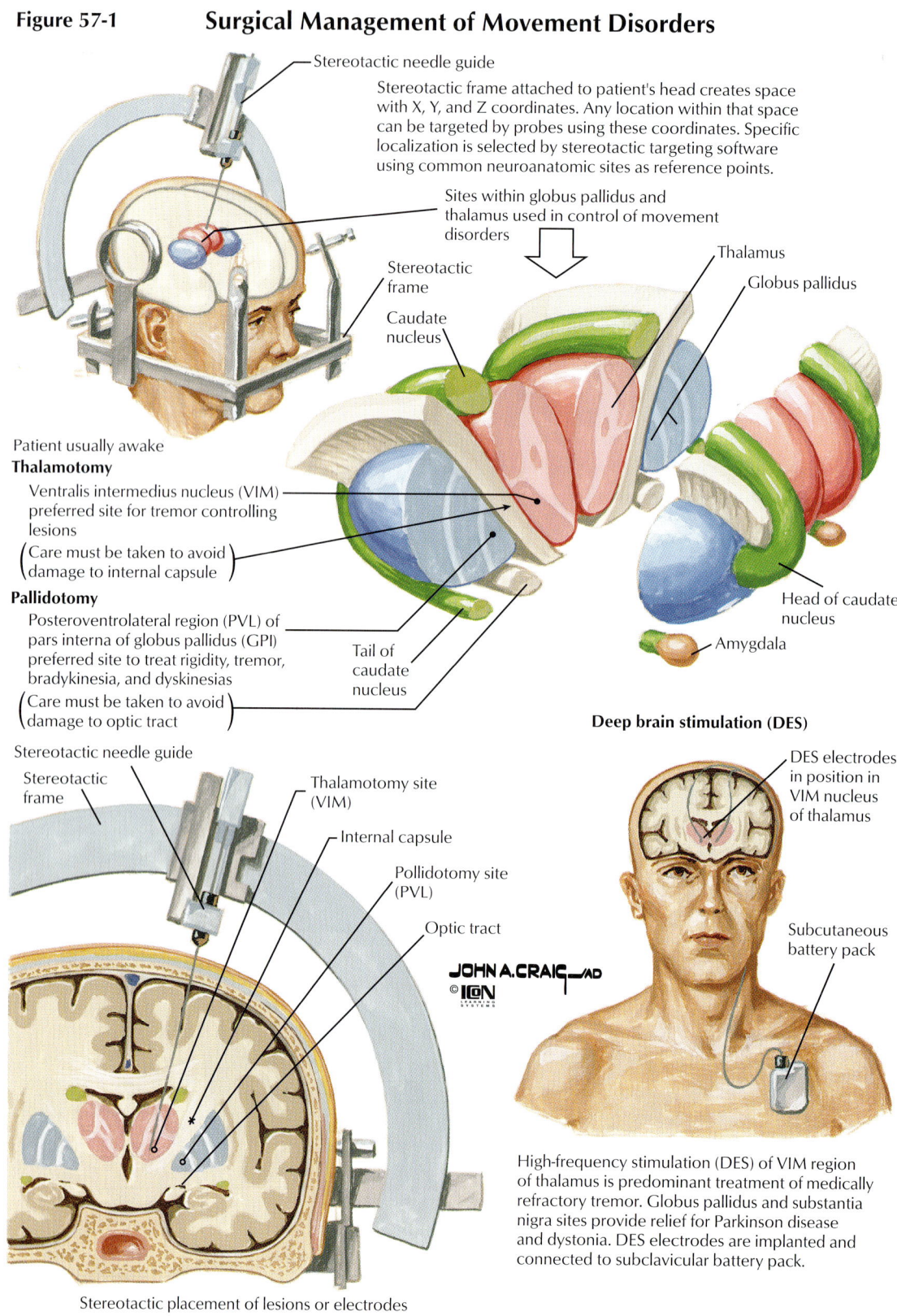

Figure 57-1

nearby optic tract. Thousands of pallidotomies have been performed, with generally good results, in the treatment of rigidity, tremor, bradykinesia, and various dyskinesias. However, bilateral posteroventrolateral lesions have produced a high percentage of significant cognitive impairments. Therefore, bilateral ablations are only performed under rare circumstances.

Thalamotomy

The ventralis intermedius nucleus seems to be the best area to make tremor-controlling lesions. The thalamic lesions are generally produced in the same manner as pallidotomies. Care must be taken to avoid damage to the internal capsule, laterally, or to nearby regions of the thalamus that manage sensory processing. Bilateral thalamic lesions are associated with dysarthria or poor cognitive outcomes and, like bilateral pallidotomies, are now typically avoided.

Deep Brain Stimulation

High-frequency deep brain stimulation (DBS) of the ventralis intermedius region of the thalamus is the predominant treatment for medically refractory tremor. This typically is helpful for benign essential tremor and tremor-predominant **Parkinson disease**.

Globus pallidus and subthalamic nucleus stimulation have also been reported in large numbers. DBS has also been tried in other brain areas. However, most experience continues to focus on stimulation in the globus pallidus and the subthalamic nucleus for treatment of Parkinson disease and dystonia. Excellent relief of major parkinsonian symptoms including rigidity, bradykinesia, tremor, and akinesia, can be achieved in most patients with classic Parkinson disease. Primary or secondary dystonia is also treated using DBS, with usually very good results.

In all cases, DBS 4-contact electrodes may be placed bilaterally if indicated. This is true even when there have been previous thalamotomies or pallidotomies (although not in those lesioned areas). When the electrodes are placed deep within the selected DBS sites, they are brought out through the brain and secured at the skull edge. A battery is placed in a small subcutaneous pocket just under the clavicle and tunneled to the electrode with a connecting wire.

Only relatively small series of patients with **dystonia** have been reported. Globus pallidus DBS seems to have the best chance for success, especially in patients found to have the DYT-1 gene, a marker for some types of primary dystonia. Also useful for some secondary dystonias, this treatment modality has the potential to relieve most dystonic posturing, particularly in all 4 limbs and, in some cases, in the neck and speech muscles.

Disadvantages of DBS include the somewhat higher risk of infection, the need for battery changes in the future, and the need to reprogram the stimulation parameters, often within the immediate several months after the postoperative period.

Future directions in surgical treatment of movement disorders may involve the implantation of genetically engineered stem cells that can make natural connections within the patient's own brain circuitry and replace cells that have degenerated or been damaged. This approach has had with mixed results so far. In addition, the DBS approach may be refined by using rechargeable batteries and eliminating both connection wires as well as the need for invasive surgery using externally applied transmitters to modify brain activity in a beneficial way.

REFERENCES

Gildenberg PL, Tasker RR, eds. *Textbook of Stereotactic and Functional Neurosurgery*. New York, NY: McGraw Hill; 1998:995-1220.

Arle JE, Alterman R. Surgical options in Parkinson's disease. *Med Clin North Am.* 1999;83:483-498.

Section XII
GAIT DISORDERS AND DIZZINESS

Chapter 58
Gait Disorders 480

Chapter 58
Gait Disorders

Kinan K. Hreib

Clinical Vignette

An 85-year-old man presented to the neurology clinic with a 3-year history of dizziness. He stated that, as a result, he had restricted his activity and started using a cane. He had fallen once while leaning forward to pick up his keys from the floor. Although he did not believe that he had any other problems, his wife thought that over the past few years he had "slowed down." He had become more reliant on her for basic directions while driving, and she noted that he had become more forgetful. She also commented that, although a retired accountant, he seemed to be having problems with numbers. His dizziness never occurred when he was sitting or in bed and was most prominent when he walked. He denied any illusion of movement or light-headedness.

This vignette describes a typical history for a senior citizen who has multidimensional mechanisms, including vestibular, visual, and often mental aging, leading to decline in gait stability. However, it is often impossible to find one specific mechanism that when treated will improve the patient's stability when walking.

Patients with gait disorders often present to their physician with "dizziness," but when their history is clarified, they are seen not to have vertigo. Extracting detailed information regarding the symptoms is sometimes difficult. The symptom acuity, overall temporal profile, and associated symptoms are essential for determining the possible etiology of the gait disturbance. When patients with vestibular dysfunction have a gait disturbance, it is often secondary to the impairment in their vestibular-ocular response. However, brainstem and cerebellar disorders, particularly when acute, may have an associated vertiginous component secondary to a disruption of input from vestibular nuclei into the cerebellum, via the inferior cerebellar peduncle (see also chapter 12).

In contrast, gait ataxia is a true disturbance of balance secondary to disruption of cerebellar processing. Whether there is ischemic disease in the posterior circulation or a mass lesion causing brain compression, usually within the posterior fossa, examination findings often help to determine the extent of brainstem and cerebellar involvement. With more indolent gait disorders, the evolution of the clinical profile is important, as is determination of whether other associated peripheral or CNS symptoms exist. The concomitant presence of behavioral changes or cognitive dysfunction often suggests a neurodegenerative process. In contrast, recent-onset headaches, particularly if posturally related, may point to an intracranial structural lesion.

The CNS control of gait involves a complex, constantly monitored and adjusted sequence of events. The use of multiple inputs depends on the integrity of information received, various feedback mechanisms, and the capability of the processor. Although many musculoskeletal conditions interfere with appropriate execution of coordinated movements, this chapter focuses on the primary neuroanatomical elements. These include lesions at many neuroaxis levels, beginning with the large myelinated peripheral nerve fibers carrying proprioceptive inputs via the posterior columns, the cerebellum, and feedback inputs from spinal reflexes. The cerebellum and the corticospinal tracts provide the elemental pieces to achieve well-coordinated and programmed gait output. Equally important are connections including information processed in association cortical areas, especially from the frontal lobe, although their precise physiology is not as well understood.

An intact nervous system can often adjust to one improper input such as toxic vestibular damage. When multiple inputs, such as failing eye sight, diminished levels of awareness, and a peripheral neuropathy, fail, though, as so often occurs with aging, the patient is no longer able to accommodate. Concomitantly, when CNS integrity is also in question, as occurs with neurodegenerative or destructive brain processes, then inputs cannot be appropriately processed.

FRONTAL GAIT DISORDERS

Clinical Vignette

A 62-year-old woman presented with a 2-year history of increasing gait unsteadiness with routine walking. Subsequently, she would spontaneously lose bladder control without warning. On neurologic examination, she had a broad-based, somewhat apraxic gait, as if her feet were glued in cement, and slight difficulty with heel-knee testing. Her mentation, Romberg sign, muscle strength, muscle stretch reflexes, and remaining complete neurologic examination results were all normal.

*Brain MRI demonstrated greatly enlarged ventricles with well-preserved cerebral gray matter and sulci and no signs of intraventricular obstruction (Figure 58-1). Clinical course and MRI findings were compatible with the diagnosis of **normal pressure hydrocephalus (NPH)** (Figure 58-1). A ventriculoperitoneal shunt was placed; shortly thereafter, the patient's gait returned to normal.*

The clinical picture of an insidiously progressive broad-based gait disorder, without any other signs to suggest a cerebellar lesion or a myelopathy, and concomitant loss of bladder control fit the typical picture of **NPH**. Most commonly seen with patients in their 60s and older, this eventually leads to a classic frontal gait disorder. If the diagnosis is unrecognized at this stage, some individuals develop a dementia. Although often no predisposing cause is identified, this syndrome may occur subsequent to a purulent meningitis or subarachnoid hemorrhage. The above patient's presentation and MRI were typical of classic NPH, as was her fine response to treatment.

Frontal Ataxia

The main features of frontal ataxia are those of unsteady gait without any associated focal neurologic abnormalities. Although the etiology is variable, the most common is presumed related to subcortical frontal infarcts. Less commonly, other processes, including a frontal lobe meningioma or glioma, subdural hematomas, and NPH, may present with difficulty walking. The exact mechanism of the gait disturbance is thought to be related to disruption of the frontopontocerebellar tracts (Arnold bundle) originating in Brodmann area 10 of the frontal lobe. In general, a frontal ataxia develops only when there is bilateral frontal-lobe pathology. NPH, with increasing ventricular pressure directed against the descending subcortical periventricular fibers adjacent to the most lateral edge of the frontal horns, may also disrupt these frontal pathways, causing a gait and associated bladder disturbance as in the preceding vignette.

Magnetic Gait

Common in the elderly, magnetic gait is a problem of gate initiation. After the gait is initiated, these patients tend to walk fast, with a slight flexion of the torso. Stopping and turning may be challenging and often lead to falls. Symptoms may be interpreted as a cautious or parkinsonian gait. Although the anatomical substrate is unknown, damage to associated motor cortex is likely to explain this phenomenon. The lack of rigidity and other parkinsonian features helps exclude a primary basal ganglia disease.

Hysterical Gait

Hysterical gait takes several forms. Some patients may report unsteadiness, whereas others report severe weakness in 1 or more limbs that prevents them from walking. On examination, these individuals may drag the affected limb but when asked to perform other motor tasks while seated or in bed, no motor incoordination or weakness is defined (astasia-abasia), ie, they are consistently inconsistent. When attempting to walk, the patient's feet are often positioned properly, ie, no wide separation. However, walking is usually abnormal in other respects, including swaying of the torso and extension of the arms to the side as if to brace against a fall, and in most instances patients lurch into the wall, seemingly avoiding disaster each time. Rarely, in the most dramatic cases, a patient may fall, but they do not usually sustain any significant trauma. This relatively rare condition is most common in young women. The examining physician must give the patient the benefit of the doubt and always search for an organic process.

GAIT DISORDERS

Figure 58-1

Normal Pressure Hydrocephalus

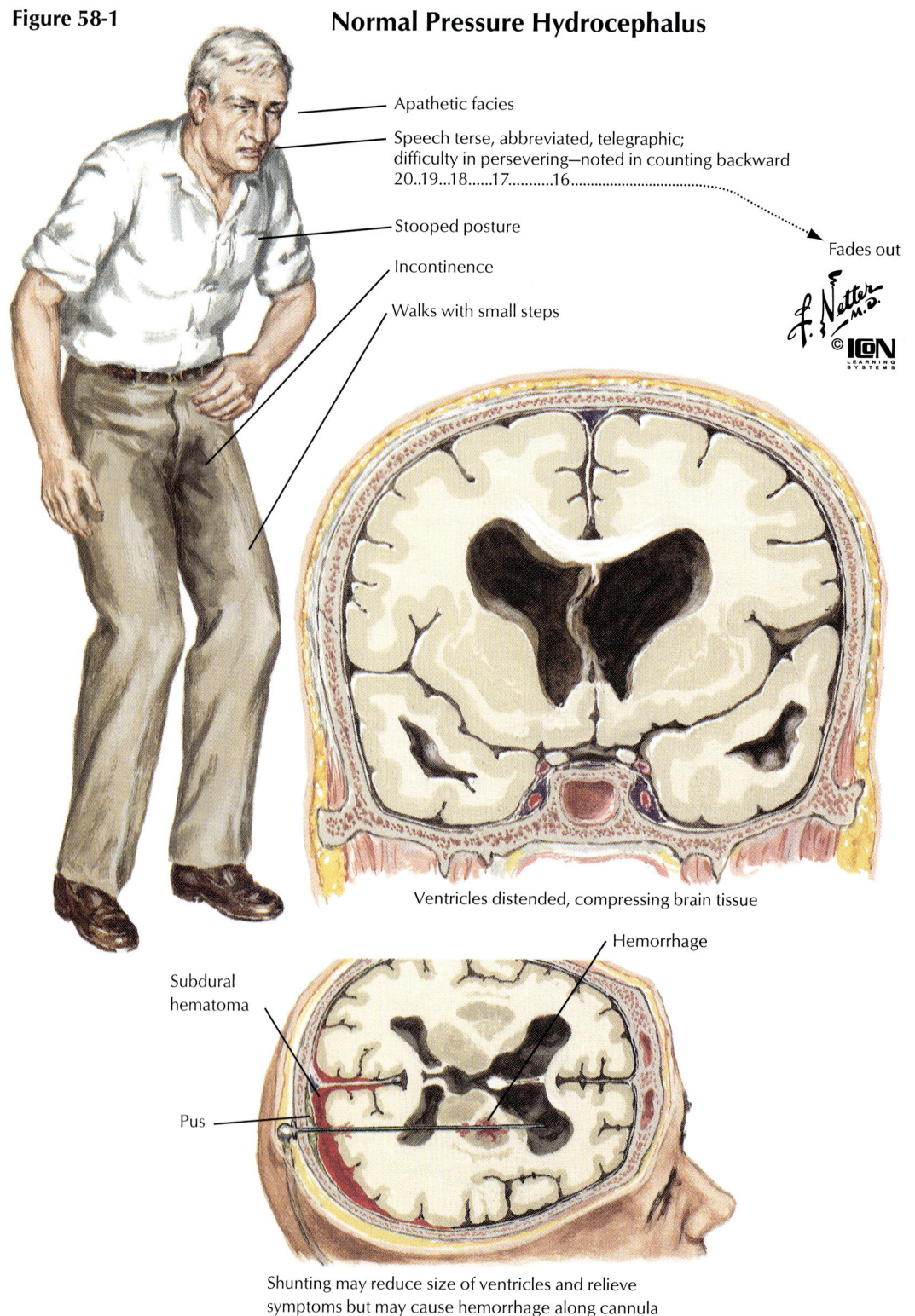

Ventricles distended, compressing brain tissue

Shunting may reduce size of ventricles and relieve symptoms but may cause hemorrhage along cannula tract, brain edema, subdural hematoma, and infection.

GAIT DISORDERS

Figure 58-1   Normal Pressure Hydrocephalus (continued)

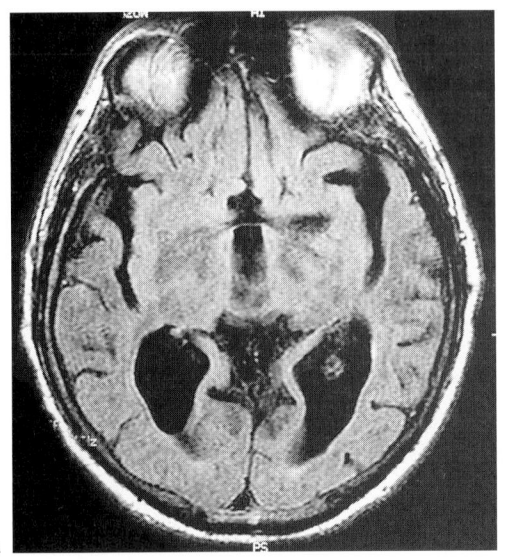
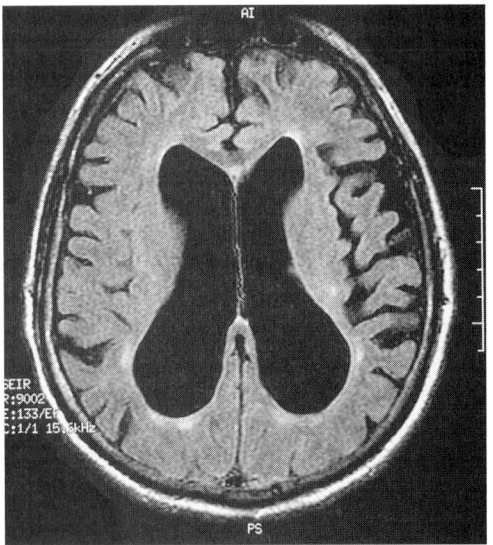

(**A** and **B**) Axial FLAIR images demonstrate moderate enlargement of the third and lateral ventricles, more normal sulcal pattern, and patchy periventricular increased T2 changes.

With the availability of MRI, organic disorders can be excluded with a high level of confidence.

STRIATAL, BASAL GANGLIA, GAIT DISORDERS
Parkinson Gait

In this classic gait disorder, the patient is typically stooped, moving forward with a petit pas shuffling gait, absent arm swing and a concomitant pill-rolling tremor (Figure 58-2). Initially, Parkinson disease presents with a small portion of these features (chapter 47). The parkinsonian syndromes do not usually have the classic tremors but often have other features, such as orthostasis, limited vertical eye movements, cognitive changes, and, rarely, myoclonus.

The neurologic examination should focus on determining the anatomical source of the lesion: brain, basal ganglia, cerebellar, myelopathic, or peripheral motor unit. Rigidity, akinesia, and cogwheeling without weakness are typically related to basal ganglia dysfunction. Rigidity impairs patients' ability to maintain proper posture, necessitating a shift in the center of gravity. To compensate for this increased rigidity, particularly in the lower extremities, patients often develop a flexed torso.

CEREBELLAR DISORDERS

Cerebrovascular disease is the most common cerebellar disorder leading to ataxia (Table 58-1). Infarcts in various arterial territories of the cerebellum cause different types of ataxia with variable potentials for recovery (Figure 58-3). Forunately, there is often full recovery in patients with an infarct or resection of part of the cerebellar hemisphere, possibly from redundancy of certain circuits or the presence of compensatory connections. In contrast, lesions that affect the deep nuclei of the cerebellum from **invasive tumors** or large resections seem to cause more enduring disabilities. Indolent cerebellar disorders, particularly the various **neurodegenerative processes**, such as olivoponto-cerebellar degeneration, progress over years and are often accompanied by other symptoms or findings.

Creutzfeldt-Jakob disease, a spongioform encephalopathy, is a fatal infectious disease caused by a prion that sometimes presents with a progressive cerebellar syndrome. In contrast to that

GAIT DISORDERS

Figure 58-2

Parkinsonism: Successive Clinical Stages

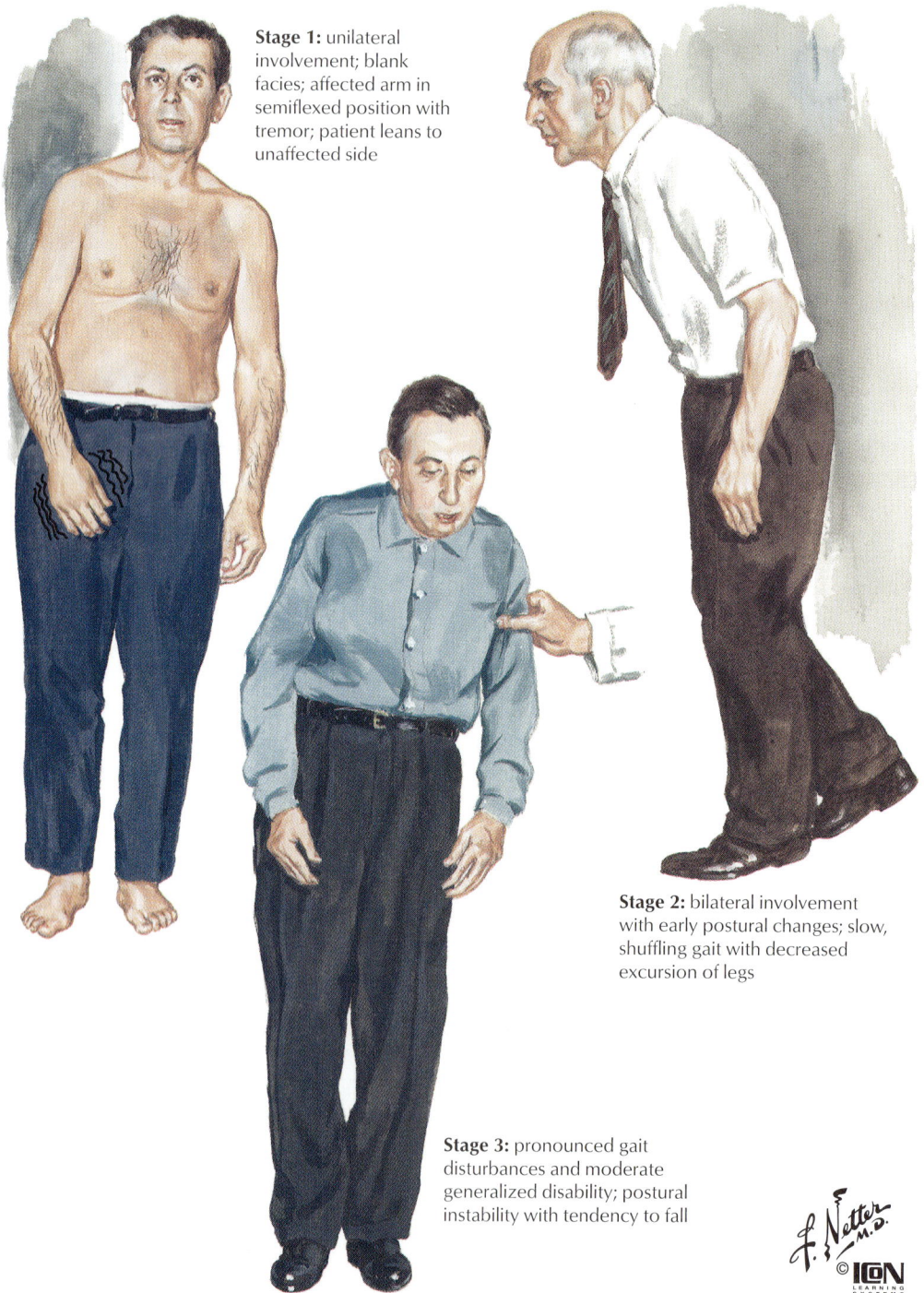

Stage 1: unilateral involvement; blank facies; affected arm in semiflexed position with tremor; patient leans to unaffected side

Stage 2: bilateral involvement with early postural changes; slow, shuffling gait with decreased excursion of legs

Stage 3: pronounced gait disturbances and moderate generalized disability; postural instability with tendency to fall

GAIT DISORDERS AND DIZZINESS

GAIT DISORDERS

Table 58-1
Acquired Processes Affecting the Cerebellum

Cerebral vascular disease
Tumors
Abscesses
Demyelinating, ie, multiple sclerosis, progressive multifocal leukoencephalopathy
Viral
Prion disease
Metabolic diseases: hypothyroidism, thiamine deficiency, vitamin E deficiency, hyperpyruvic acidemia of childhood, Leigh syndrome, Refsum disease
Paraneoplastic

in **progressive multifocal leukoencephalopathy** (PML), the MRI in Creutzfeldt-Jakob disease may have only subtle signs early on. As with progressive multifocal leukoencephalopathy, an open cerebellar biopsy may be indicated to make the diagnosis if other methodologies are unsuccessful.

The rare **paraneoplastic cerebellar degenerations** usually evolve over months until the neoplasm takes its typical course. These paraneoplastic processes can be associated with different types of cancer, usually lung, ovarian, or uterine, and Hodgkin lymphoma. They can also affect other parts of the nervous system, causing optic neuritis, limbic encephalitis, necrotizing myelopathy, sensory neuropathy, autonomic neuropathy, neuromuscular junction abnormalities, and cerebellar degeneration, the best-characterized of the paraneoplastic syndromes. Most patients present with ataxia and limb incoordination before the diagnosis of cancer is documented, often predating the diagnosis by several years. A rapid progression over weeks or a few months may precede the stabilization of the disease. Although location and treatment of the malignancy is the only hope, lung cancer is the most common cause, and even after identified, the ataxia progresses inexorably.

Classification of the **neurodegenerative disorders** relies on symptom identification and mode of inheritance (Table 58-2 and Figure 58-4). Often a significant overlap exists among these

Table 58-2
Degenerative and Inherited Disorders

Name	Age at Onset, y	Symptoms/Findings	Mode of Inheritance	Pathology
Cortical cerebellar atrophy of Holmes	40	Ataxia, tremor, dysarthria	Familial and sporadic	Vermis
Olivopontocerebellar degeneration	28-50	Athetosis, ptosis Retinal degeneration Dementia Ataxia Dysarthria Parkinsonism	Autosomal dominant Autosomal recessive	SC, cerebellum Pons
Machado-Joseph-Azorean disease	16	Ataxia, parkinsonism Distal weakness Ophthalmoplegia Fasciculations Areflexia, extensor Plantar response	Autosomal dominant variable expression	Dentate nucleus Anterior horn cells Pons Substantia nigra
Ataxia telangiectasia	1-2	Ataxia Chorea Dysarthria, ocular Apraxia	Autosomal recessive	Cerebellum Posterior columns Peripheral nerves

GAIT DISORDERS

Figure 58-3 **Ischemia in Vertebrobasilar Territory: Clinical Manifestations**

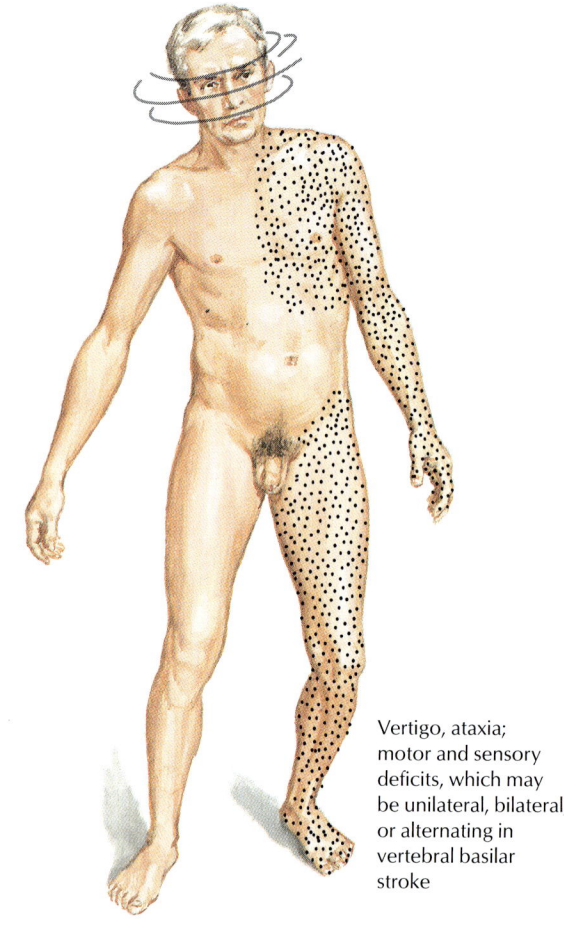

Vertigo, ataxia; motor and sensory deficits, which may be unilateral, bilateral, or alternating in vertebral basilar stroke

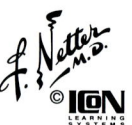

Intracerebral hemorrhage: clinical manifestations related to site

Pathology	CT scan	Pupils	Eye movement	Motor and sensory deficits	Other
Cerebellum		Slight constriction on side of lesion	Slight deviation to opposite side; movements toward side of lesion impaired, or sixth cranial nerve palsy	Ipsilateral limb ataxia; no hemiparesis	Gait ataxia, vomiting

processes. DNA testing can provide logical classification of this seemingly variable group of gait disorders.

An **infectious** or **postinfectious cerebellitis** most commonly occurs in children after a febrile illness, particularly those with chicken pox, measles, mumps, or Epstein-Barr virus infections. It has also been seen in patients after measles vaccination. **Prion diseases** such as the spongioform encephalopathies often present with gait unsteadiness before other cognitive or behavioral changes manifest. **Gerstmann-Sträussler-**

GAIT DISORDERS AND DIZZINESS

GAIT DISORDERS

Figure 58-4

Neurodegenerative Disorders

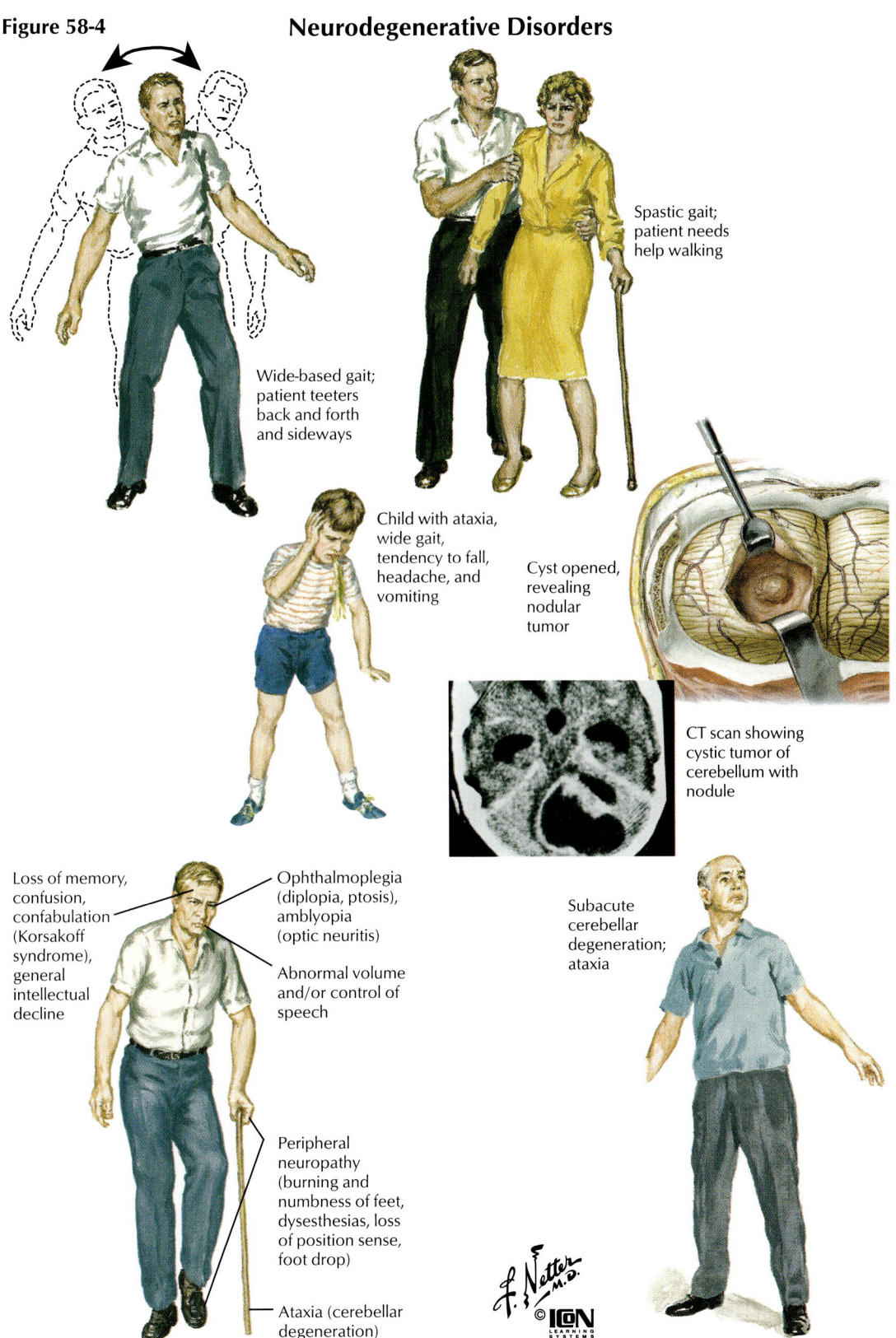

GAIT DISORDERS

Scheinker syndrome is another form of prion disease presenting with ataxia. Many patients with prion disease have ataxia, myoclonic jerks, cognitive and behavioral changes, and EEG abnormalities. Although most of the occurrence of prion disease is sporadic, approximately 12% clusters in families. **Whipple disease** may present with ataxia in addition to ocular abnormalities and dementia.

Wernicke disease is another consideration in patients with recent gait ataxia. Typically related to poor nutrition in patients with excessive alcohol use, it results from thiamine deficiency. The usual manifestations include ataxia, nystagmus, weakness of conjugate gaze and abduction of the eyes, confusion, altered consciousness, and, in the most severe cases, amnesia with confabulation. Early recognition and supplementation with thiamine is crucial to reversing some if not all symptoms, albeit the improvement may be delayed for up to a year.

SPINAL CORD DISORDERS

Lesions that affect the posterior columns, most commonly **multiple sclerosis** and **vitamin B_{12} deficiency**, myelopathies with **cervical spinal spondylosis**, and spinal canal or cord tumors, can also present with gait difficulties. (Previously, tabes dorsalis associated with tertiary syphilis was one of the most common causes of a gait disorder associated with a myelopathy.) Less common processes seen today include the myelopathy from **HTLV-1** (tropical spastic paraparesis) or **primary lateral sclerosis**. HIV and AIDS also need to be considered in the differential diagnosis.

Inherited disorders, such as **Friedreich ataxia**, that primarily affect the spinal cord often have associated cerebellar abnormalities. Although this is the most common inherited ataxia, myriad similar disorders exist, with significant overlap and different inheritance modes. Friedreich ataxia may occasionally start suddenly but usually progresses insidiously over several years, later accompanied by dysarthria and tremors. Some patients with Friedreich ataxia phenotype have a combination of degenerative processes, including retinitis pigmentosa and cardiac abnormalities. The early-onset form has autosomal recessive inheritance, and symptoms begin by the age of 12 years. The late-onset form begins at 20 years of age and has an autosomal dominant inheritance. Unlike other processes affecting the spinal cord, wherein spasticity predominates, in Friedreich ataxia the limbs have decreased tone and are areflexic but do have positive Babinski signs.

EVALUATION OF GAIT DISORDERS

A thorough understanding of the patient's history is essential, including his or her report of symptoms and results of neurologic, diagnostic, and vestibular testing. Patients often use the nonspecific term of *dizziness* to describe symptoms more consistent with dysequilibrium, as seen in certain cerebellar lesions, or feelings of unsteadiness, often more consistent with gait disorders. More specific questions may lead to the patient stating, "I look like I'm drunk when I walk." Other patients may inappropriately use the term *vertigo* to describe a variety of symptoms. Strictly speaking, vertigo refers to a subjective or objective illusion of rapid personal or environmental rotary movement or spinning. This complaint must be carefully probed by defining the onset and duration of vertigo and performing positional testing similar to that described in reference to benign paroxysmal positional vertigo. Patients may also describe vague symptoms of light-headedness or a floating feeling.

The investigation of patients with gait disorders requires a full neurologic examination to define the relative contribution of the central and peripheral nervous system elements to the problem, documenting the precise type and level of functional disability by history. The underlying site of pathology needs to be identified by whether there are solitary or concomitant findings of cognitive impairment; various apraxias; or basal ganglia, cerebellar, spinal cord, peripheral nerve, or musculoskeletal involvement. These findings lead to selection of the appropriate clinical studies for defining the precise pathophysiologic mechanism.

TREATMENT

Once the diagnosis of a gait disorder is established, the first step is to identify the presence of any disorders that have specific treatment strategies. For example, the individual with vitamin B_{12}

deficiency can receive supplementation, the neurosurgeon may help the patient with NPH by placing a ventriculoperitoneal shunt, patients with cervical spondylosis will benefit from a laminectomy, and patients with a meningioma will be greatly aided by resection of these benign tumors. However, many degenerative disorders such as Friedreich ataxia, HTLV-I, and HIV myelopathy will not benefit from any specific therapy.

A carefully designed rehabilitation program can help individuals with potentially remediable gait disorders. When identifying means to help patients compensate for their physical challenges, it is sometimes useful to observe the techniques developed by patients to compensate for their imbalance. For example, those individuals who compensate by adjusting their feet when they also suffer from a severe peripheral neuropathy, may be using the wrong strategy to correct the imbalance.

Certain tests in balance centers can provide help analyzing gait disturbances. During posturography, for example, the patient is challenged to maintain balance during different controlled circumstances, including use of a tilting platform. Although the value of posturography is unresolved, it does seem to aid in designing rehabilitation strategies. Some data help differentiate among possible causes for imbalance (chapter 12).

REFERENCES

Fregley AR, Graybiel A, Smith MJ. Walk on floor eyes closed (WOFEC): a new addition to an ataxia test battery. *Aerospace Med.* 1972;43:395-399.

Horak FB. Clinical measurement of postural control in adults. *Phys Ther.* 1987;67:1881-1885.

Horak FB, Jones-Rycewiccz C, Black FO, Shumway-Cook A. Effects of vestibular rehabilitation on dizziness and imbalance. *Otolaryngol Head Neck Surg.* 1992;106:175-180.

Mathias S, Nayak U, Issacs B. Balance in elderly patients: the "Get Up & Go" test. *Arch Phys Med Rehabil.* 1986;67:387-389.

Norrving B, Magnusson M, Holtas S. Isolated acute vertigo in the elderly: vestibular or vascular disease? *Acta Neurol Scand.* 1995;91:43-48.

Shumway-Cook A, Brauer S, Woollacott M. Predicting the probability for falls in community-dwelling older adults using the timed up and go test. *Phys Ther.* 2000;80:896-903.

Section XIII
MYELOPATHIES

Chapter 59
Anatomical Aspects of Myelopathies 492

Chapter 60
Acute Myelopathies 503

Chapter 61
Chronic Myelopathies 514

Chapter 59
Anatomical Aspects of Myelopathies

Ann Camac and H. Royden Jones, Jr

A *myelopathy* is defined as any disorder that impairs spinal cord function. Myelopathies can develop acutely or gradually and have numerous causes. The clinical syndrome depends on the process and the site and extent of cord damage, categorized as **intramedullary**, ie, intrinsic to the cord, or **extramedullary**, occurring secondary to disorders extrinsic to the cord. Extramedullary processes are either **intradural** or **extradural**, each leading to mass effects on the spinal cord. The diseases can be primary and specific to the spinal cord region or part of a systemic process, such as metastatic tumors, granulomatous processes, or various infections.

Detailed neuroanatomy knowledge is crucial to providing appropriate care to patients having potential myelopathies. Spinal cord lesions cause degeneration of ascending tracts above and descending tracts below the lesions. The key to localizing the site of spinal cord involvement is identification of the exact distribution of the various motor, reflex, and sensory deficits. Loss of spinal function results distal to an acute lesion, the best example being traumatic injuries.

A variable to complete paralysis usually occurs, typically affecting all muscles subserved by both the adjacent corticospinal tracts and the segmental anterior horn cells at the precise spinal lesion site. Acutely, there may be a stage of **spinal shock**, where the muscle stretch reflexes are hypoactive or absent, but subsequently these reflexes become exaggerated and brisk. More indolent lesions may not initially be evident on examination, even though a patient is symptomatic and reports subtle changes in performance.

Sensory evaluation is also key to appropriate assessment of myelopathies. Testing of pain and temperature sensation often provide evidence of a distinct "spinal level" of sensory loss when the pathology affects the spinothalamic tract. Often a "cord level" is a dramatic and easy-to-elicit finding. It is vital to examine sensation in the extremities and the patient's trunk anteriorly and posteriorly to attempt to define the most subtle sensory level. With incomplete lesions, such as the **Brown-Séquard syndrome**, pain and temperature loss are confined to one side of the body. The converse may occur with a different modality, such as position sense. These various combinations often provide the clinical confirmation of a myelopathy (chapter 60). Sometimes in a rapidly evolving subacute myelopathy, the precise definition of a spinal level suggests an impending spinal disaster. Similarly, the dorsal columns may be affected, with loss of proprioceptive, position, and sometimes vibration and touch modalities.

Certain classic spinal cord lesion presentations prove clinically and diagnostically useful. Initial determination of lesion location is necessary: outside the dura, ie, **extradural extramedullary**; within the dura and outside of the cord, **intradural extramedullary**; or intrinsic within the parenchyma of the spinal cord, ie, **intradural intramedullary**. Intradural intramedullary (intra-axial) lesions typically present with 1 of 4 clinically identifiable syndromes.

Extramedullary processes are intradural or extradural, each leading to spinal cord mass effect. The primary disease is localized to the spinal cord region or is part of a systemic process such as metastases. Although MRI often expeditiously demonstrates the site and type of spinal cord abnormality, an appreciation of the anatomy and clinical profile of the spinal cord disorder is

ANATOMICAL ASPECTS OF MYELOPATHIES

fundamental to the care of patients with myelopathies.

SPINAL CORD ANATOMY
Gross Anatomy

The spinal cord has major functional importance although representing 2% of the total CNS volume. It is elongated (42-45 cm long) and cylindrical, but flattened dorsoventrally lying within the vertebral canal and extending from the atlas (continuous with the medulla through the foramen magnum) to the first or second lumbar vertebra, where it tapers into the conus medullaris and terminates (Figure 59-1). Its cervical and lumbar enlargements supply nerve roots that innervate upper and lower limbs.

The position of the cord changes with movement. The spinal canal dimensions are larger than the cord, allowing it to move freely during neck and back flexion and extension.

Three protective membranes ie, the **meninges**, surround the cord. These are the **dura mater** being the outer, then the **arachnoid** and **pia** (Figure 59-2). CSF flows between the arachnoid and pia. Epidural fat is present in the epidural space between the spinal canal and dura mater.

Internal Structure

White matter, consisting of myelinated fibers, surrounds the butterfly or H-shaped gray matter that contains cell bodies and their processes within the center of the cord (Figure 59-3). Longitudinal furrows on the surface of the cord divide the white matter into columns, or funiculi, that are large bundles of nerve fibers having diverse functions. The anterior median fissure, posterior median, posterior intermediate, and the anterolateral sulci divide the dorsal or posterior, lateral, and anterior columns. The posterior columns are further divided into 2 fasciculi, gracilis medially (present at all spinal levels) and cuneatus (T6 and above) laterally.

Spinal Nerves

Thirty-one pairs of spinal nerves with dorsal sensory roots and ventral motor roots exit the cord (8 cervical, 12 thoracic, 5 lumbar, 5 sacral, 1 coccygeal). Although there are 7 cervical vertebrae, there are 8 cervical nerve roots (Figure 59-4). The C1 through C7 roots exit above their respective vertebrae, whereas C8, thoracic, lumbar, and sacral roots exit below their specific vertebrae.

Tracts

Ascending and descending tracts within the cord are interrupted at sites of cord damage (Figure 59-5). Clinical sequelae develop based on which tracts are affected (Figure 1-14).

Ascending Sensory Tracts

Posterior columns subserving **touch**, **pressure**, **position**, and **movement** sensation arise from dorsal root fibers and ascend posteriorly. Their fibers do not decussate until within the medulla. They then travel to the ventral posterolateral (VPL) thalamic nuclei.

Anterior spinothalamic tracts arise from dorsal horn neurons within the spinal cord, cross in the anterior commissure, and ascend anterolaterally to the posterior thalamic and ventral posterolateral thalamic nuclei. The anterior spinothalamic tract provides **light touch** sensation.

Lateral spinothalamic tracts arise from secondary **pain** and **temperature** neurons within the spinal cord, cross into the anterior commissure, and ascend in the lateral funiculus to the reticular formation and ventral posterolateral thalamic nuclei.

The **dorsal spinocerebellar tract** is uncrossed, ascending in the lateral funiculus to the cerebellar vermis. At subconscious levels, it provides fine coordination of posture and limb muscle movement. The **ventral spinocerebellar tract**, dedicated to lower-extremity movement and posture, initially crosses and then ascends the lateral funiculus to the cerebellum. The **cuneocerebellar tract**, concerned with upper-extremity coordination and movement, is uncrossed and ascends to the cerebellum.

Descending Motor Tracts

The **corticospinal tract** is responsible for **voluntary, skilled movement** (Figures 59-6 and 59-7). Originating in the motor cortex (precentral and premotor areas 4 and 6), postcentral gyrus, and adjacent parietal cortex, fibers descend via the corona radiata, posterior limb of internal capsule, pons, and through the medulla. They then

MYELOPATHIES

ANATOMICAL ASPECTS OF MYELOPATHIES

Figure 59-1   Spinal Cord and Ventral Rami In Situ

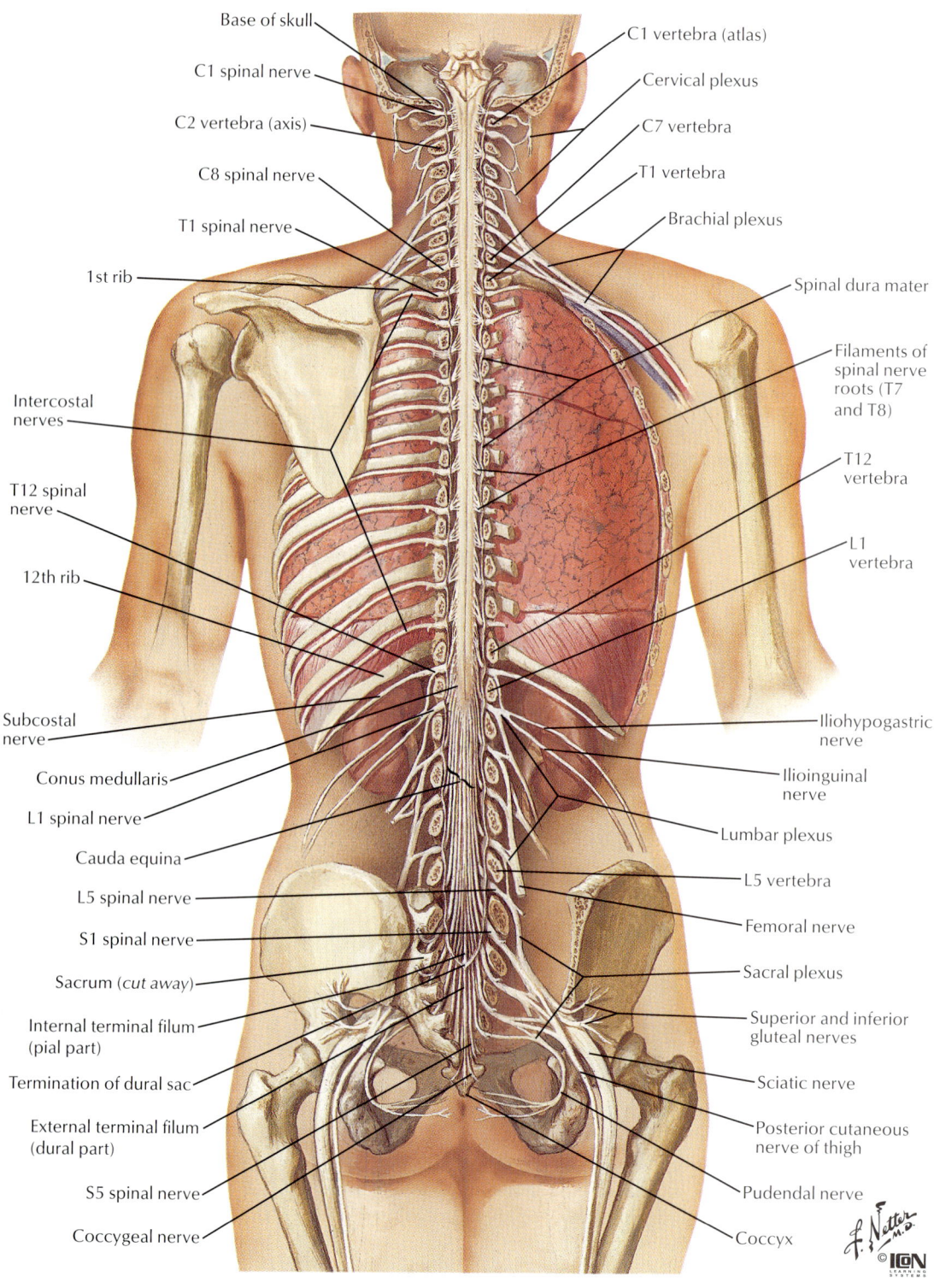

MYELOPATHIES

ANATOMICAL ASPECTS OF MYELOPATHIES

Figure 59-2 — **Spinal Membranes and Nerve Roots**

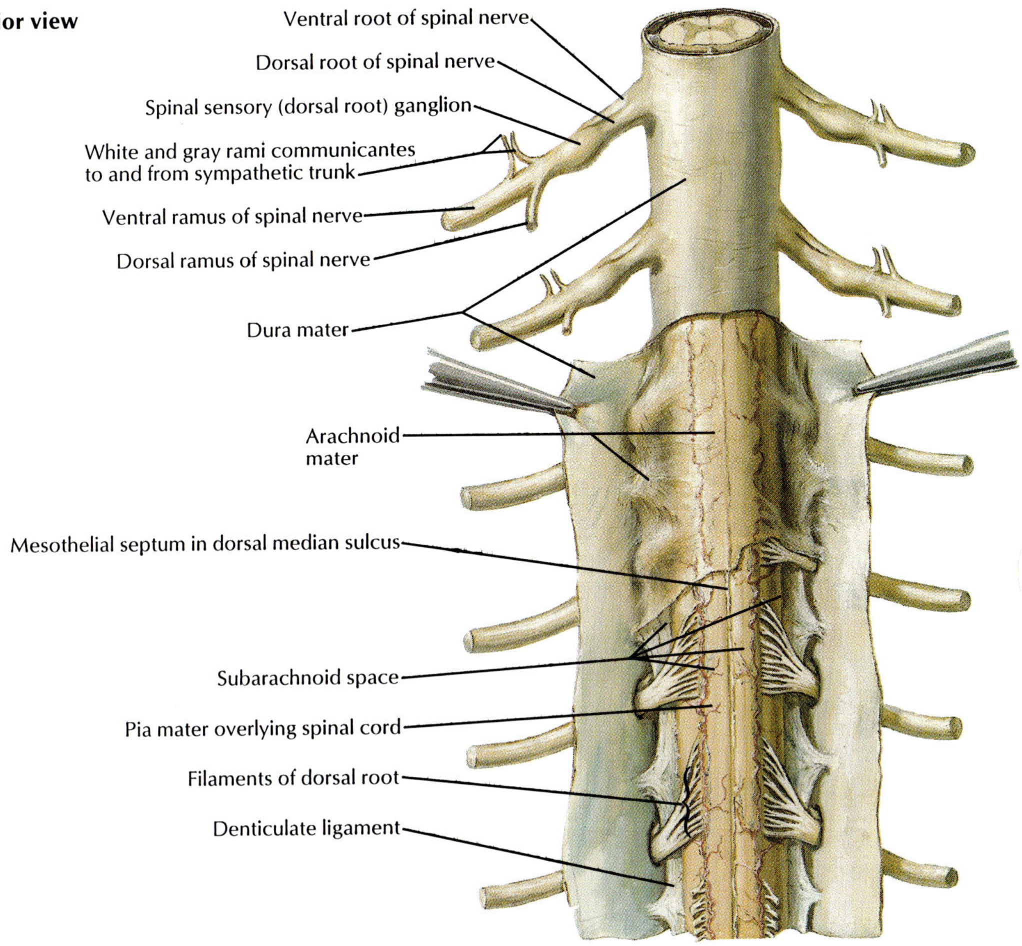

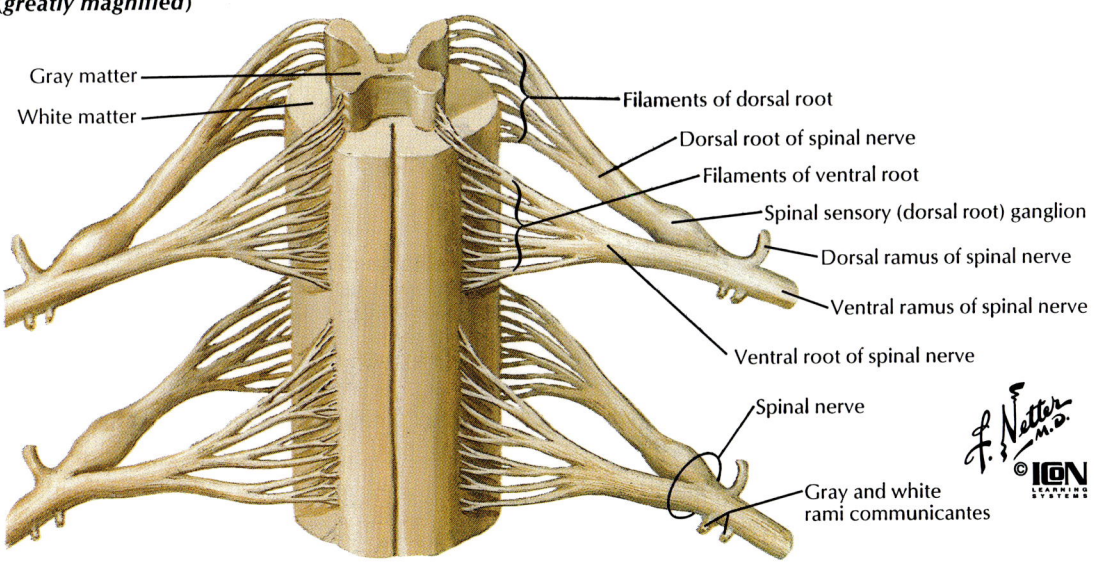

MYELOPATHIES

495

ANATOMICAL ASPECTS OF MYELOPATHIES

Figure 59-3 — Spinal Nerve Origin: Cross Sections

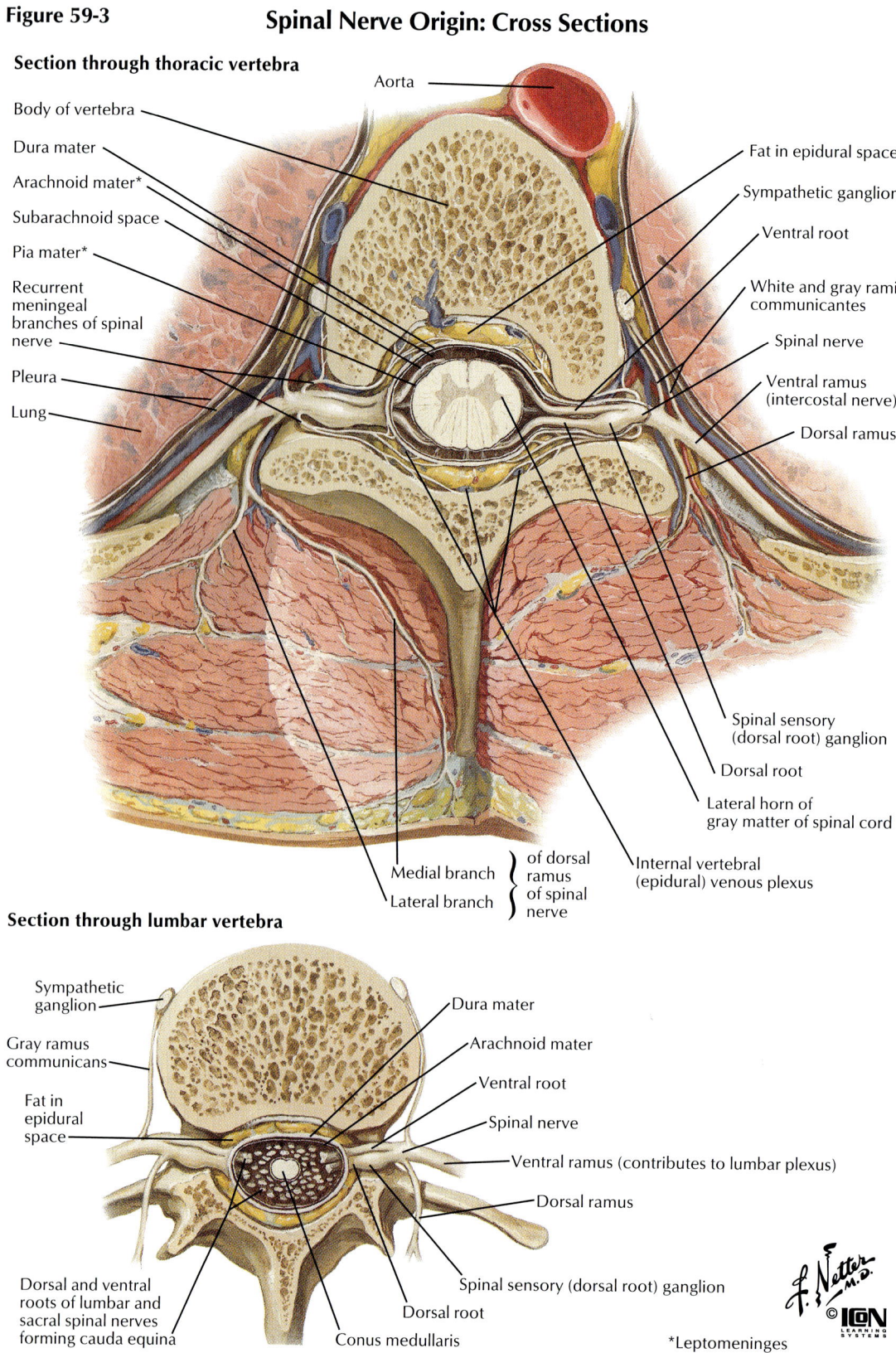

*Leptomeninges

ANATOMICAL ASPECTS OF MYELOPATHIES

Figure 59-4   **Relation of Spinal Nerve Roots to Vertebrae**

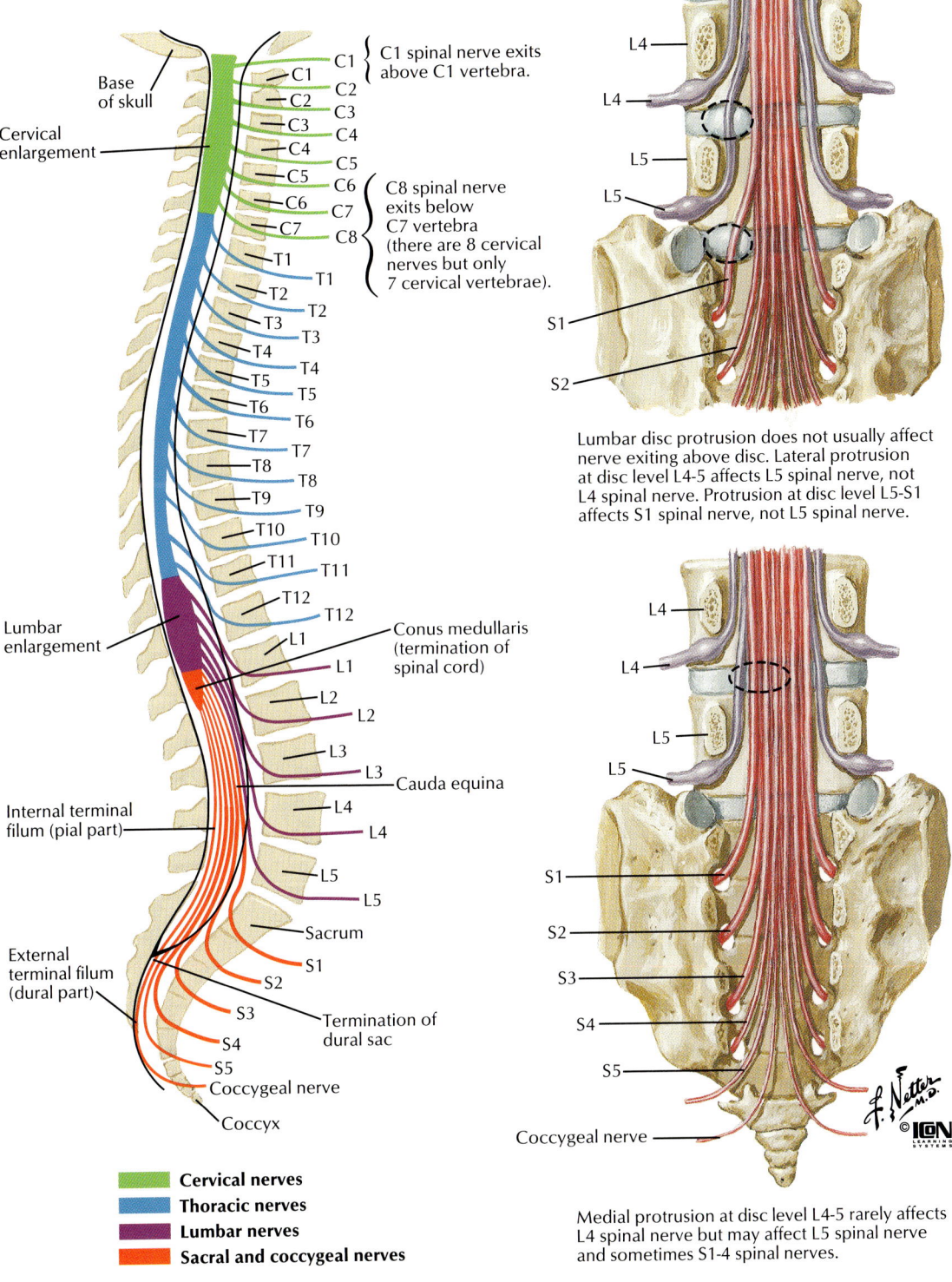

MYELOPATHIES

ANATOMICAL ASPECTS OF MYELOPATHIES

Figure 59-5 — Spinal Cord Cross Sections: Fiber Tracts

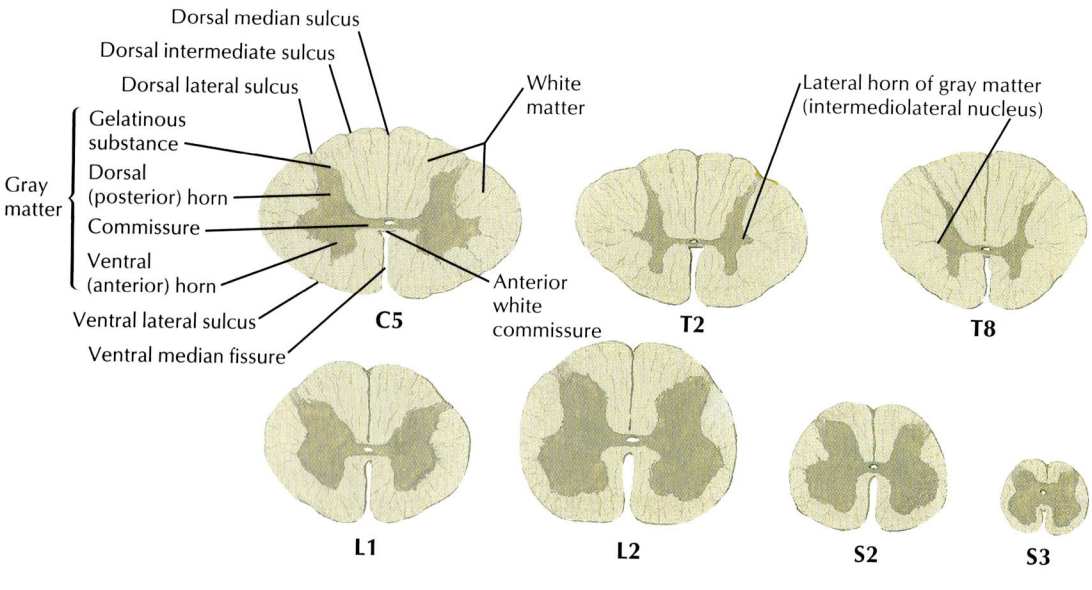

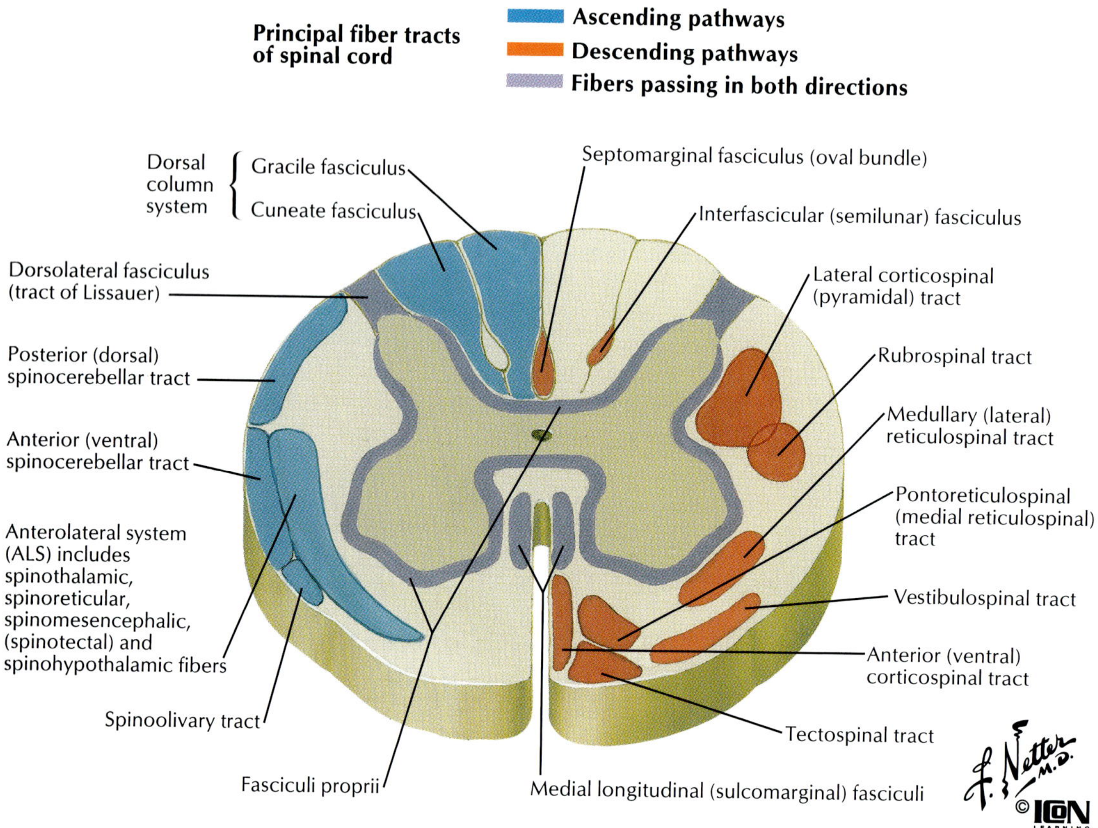

ANATOMICAL ASPECTS OF MYELOPATHIES

Figure 59-6 **Major Descending Tracts and Ascending Pathways**
Termination of Major Descending Tracts

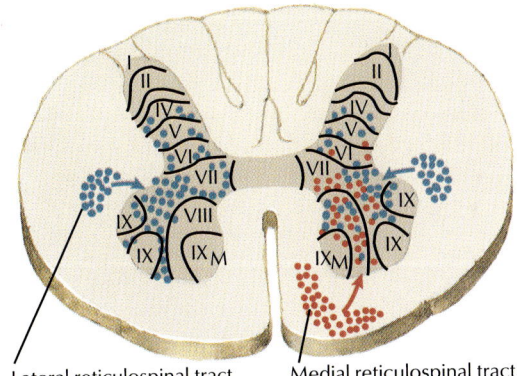

Afferent Connections to Ascending Pathways

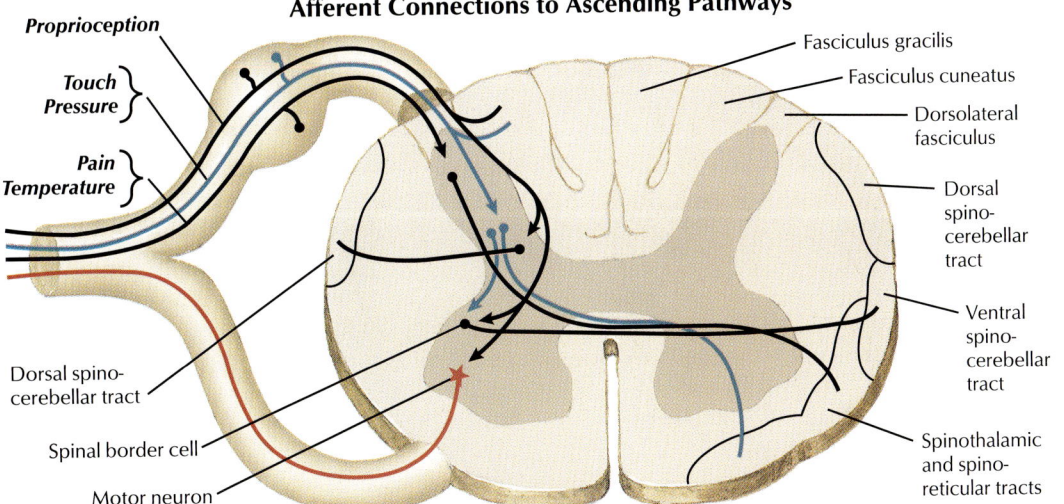

MYELOPATHIES

ANATOMICAL ASPECTS OF MYELOPATHIES

Figure 59-7

Cerebral Cortex: Efferent Pathways

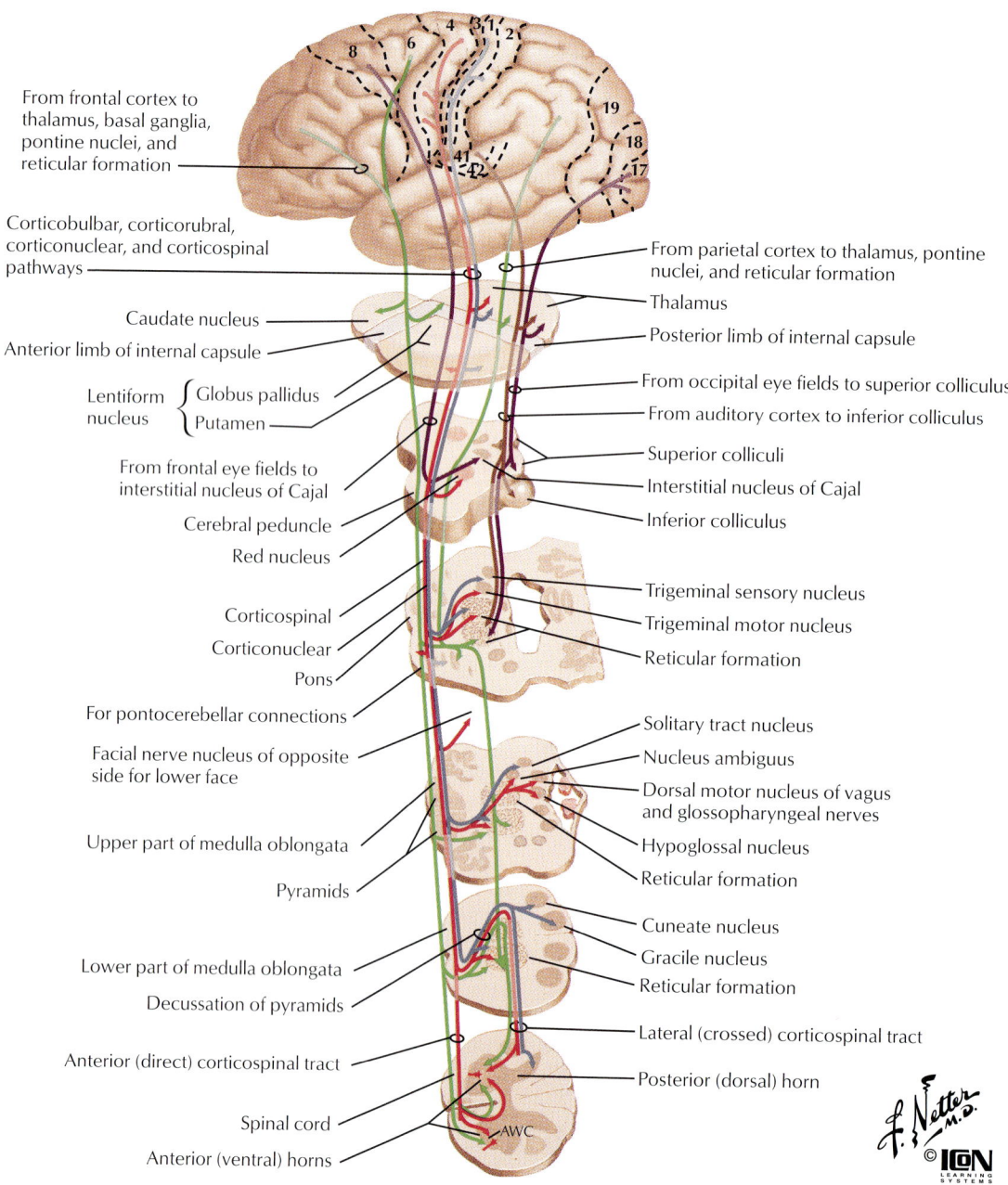

divide into 3 tracts; up to 90% of the fibers descend in the lateral funiculus as the **lateral corticospinal tract**. Most decussate within the distal medulla; the uncrossed lateral corticospinal tract is much smaller. The **anterior corticospinal tract** travels in the anterior funiculus, crossing within the cord.

The **tectospinal, rubrospinal,** and **vestibulospinal tracts** originate in the superior colliculus, red nucleus, and the lateral vestibular nucleus, respectively. They variously affect reflex postural movements and tone in flexor muscles and facilitate antigravity and extensor muscles.

Vascular Supply
Arterial

One **anterior** and 2 **posterior spinal arteries** course the length of the cord, supplying the anterior two thirds and posterior one third of the cord, respectively. Sulcal or central branches of the anterior spinal artery supply the central cord, whereas coronal or circumferential branches supply the ventral and lateral columns. Hence, the anterior spinal artery supplies the anterior horn, spinothalamic tract, and corticospinal tract, whereas the posterior spinal artery supplies the dorsal column, dorsal gray matter, and superficial dorsal aspect of lateral columns. Medullary branches off the vertebral arteries join the anterior and posterior spinal arteries to supply the cervical cord.

Segmental arteries from the aorta supply the remainder of the cord by branching into dural arteries that supply the dura and nerve root sleeve, radicular branches that supply the anterior and posterior nerve roots, and medullary branches that join the anterior and posterior spinal arteries to supply the cord. Adamkiewicz artery, at the lumbar enlargement, usually arises from the left side between T6 and L4. It provides the major arterial supply to the lower cord. C1 to T2 levels and T9 caudally have excellent vascular supplies. In contrast, the T3-8 vasculature is more limited and usually considered a watershed area.

Venous

The anteromedial cord (anterior horns and white matter) is drained by the central or sulcal veins into the anterior median spinal vein that extends the length of the cord. The anterolateral, peripheral, and dorsal cord capillary plexus drains into the radial veins. The radial veins subsequently drain into the coronal venous plexus on the spinal cord surface. This plexus, with superficial spinal cord veins (anterior median, anterolateral, posterior median, posterior intermediate), drains into medullary veins, which travel with nerve roots to the intervertebral foramen and form the epidural venous plexus. Subsequent drainage is to the inferior vena cava, azygous, and hemizygous veins.

CORRELATIVE ANATOMICAL SYNDROMES
Extradural Extramedullary

Pain is one of the hallmarks of lesions at this anatomical level. Often these lesions affect the meninges, adjacent sensory nerve roots, or the concomitant bone, as with metastatic cancers. Each of these structures has significant clinical pain potential. As the size of the lesion increases, it puts direct pressure on the adjacent spinal cord, compromises the primary vascular supply predominantly affecting the anterior two thirds of the cord, or both. Subsequently, these expand or displace cord tissue acutely, essentially leading to pathophysiologic cord transection. Therefore, the final clinical picture may mimic a traumatic myelopathy; thus, it is mandatory to expeditiously evaluate these patients.

Intradural Extramedullary

External pressure on the cord can cause gradual onset spasticity if the corticospinal tracts are involved. If the spinothalamic tract is also compromised, the individual may note decreased pain, temperature sensation, or both in the opposite leg, as exemplified by one patient who did not recognize that she had cut herself while shaving the leg opposite to the one that affected her gait. She was developing a **hemicord lesion** known as the ***Brown-Séquard syndrome***. A meningioma, particularly in the thoracic spine, is the archetypical lesion presenting this way.

Intramedullary

There are 4 classic patterns of intra-axial spinal cord pathologies (Figure 61-3).

Transverse Cord

With **complete transverse cord lesion**, all sensory and motor functions are interrupted below the damaged level. An acute injury causes flaccid paralysis and areflexia secondary to spinal shock; subsequently, spasticity and hyperreflexia develop, as in more ingravescent lesions. These chronic lesions are associated with a slowly evolving weakness. If the anterior horn cells, ventral roots, or both are also involved, lower motor neuron signs, including fasciculations, atrophy, areflexia, and weakness, occur at the lesion level. An extensive cord injury is necessary to completely lose touch sensation because both the posterior columns and spinothalamic tracts provide touch. The demonstration of a sensory level, assessed by testing pain (spinothalamic tract) and joint position (dorsal column), segmental paresthesia, or radicular pain, often helps localize the spinal cord level.

Anterior Cord

The primary damage involves those spinal cord areas in the distribution of the **anterior spinal artery**, leading to damage to the corticospinal, lateral spinothalamic, and anterior spinothalamic tracts and the anterior horn cells. Therefore, typically patients are paraparetic or paraplegic or, less commonly, have weakness in all 4 extremities, and have complete sensory loss below the lesion level except for the posterior column proprioception modalities that remain intact; therefore, a transverse anterior two-thirds lesion.

Posterolateral Column

The **posterolateral column** predominantly affects the dorsal columns and corticospinal tracts as seen with cervical spondylosis, multiple sclerosis, vitamin B_{12} (cyanocobalamin) deficiency, and HIV-associated vacuolar myelopathy. Vibration and proprioception are impaired in the lower extremities. Paresthesias may be more pronounced in the feet, although the hands are often earlier affected with cyanocobalamin deficiency. Classically, sensory ataxia, spasticity, and hyperreflexia develop, whereas pain and temperature sensations are preserved. This is, therefore, a posterior one-third myelopathy.

Central Cord

Cord damage begins centrally, as classically seen with syringomyelia or intramedullary cord tumors. Decussating fibers of the spinothalamic tracts are initially affected. Patients typically experience thermoanesthesia and analgesia in a cape pattern over the shoulders. Light touch and proprioception are preserved. Extension to anterior horn cells leads to segmental neurogenic atrophy, paresis, and areflexia. As the corticospinal tracts become involved, spastic paralysis below the lesion level develops. In the extreme, dorsal columns may become affected much later.

REFERENCES

Brazis PW, Masdeu JC, Biller J. *Localization in Clinical Neurology.* Boston, Mass: Little, Brown & Co; 1990:69-92.

Carpenter MB. *Core Text of Neurology.* Baltimore, Md: Williams & Wilkins; 1985:52-101, 392-395.

Patten J. *Neurological Differential Diagnosis.* New York, NY: Springer-Verlag; 1987:139-171.

Chapter 60
Acute Myelopathies

Ann Camac and H. Royden Jones, Jr

An acute myelopathy is one of the most significant neurologic emergencies, demanding rapid and careful patient evaluation followed immediately by MRI. An expeditious evaluation can reverse a potentially disastrous clinical outcome. Although relatively uncommon, disorders of the spinal cord challenge the physician to first localize the lesion, define its pathophysiologic mechanism, and, finally, consider the potential for treatment (Figure 60-1). The 2 most common causes of acute myelopathy are spinal fracture or dislocation (chapter 76) and metastatic tumors (chapter 74).

ACUTE EXTRADURAL SPINAL LESIONS

Trauma

Acute spinal cord injuries, with subsequent paraplegia or quadriplegia, are among the most dreaded sequelae to a serious bodily injury (Table 60-1). Their propensity to occur among vigorous and healthy young persons is tragic. Automobile and motorcycle accidents and sports injuries commonly involve the spinal cord. Gunshot wounds, whether resulting from war, accident, or assault, are another source of traumatic spinal cord injury. Acute spinal damage also occurs in the elderly, particularly in those prone to sudden falls due to diminished gait stability of neurologic or orthopedic origin, cardiac arrhythmias leading to syncope, or epileptic seizure.

Typically, in acute conditions, spinal shock results, with complete paralysis, loss of sensation, and areflexia distal to the trauma site.

A fracture dislocation with resultant ligamentous tear allowing bony fragments to directly tear or transect the spinal cord is the common denominator in this setting. Sometimes a concomitant compromise of the spinal arteries causes an associated spinal cord infarction, hematomyelia, or both.

Although these neurologic/neurosurgical emergencies are relatively rare, some are occasionally amenable to surgical correction. Emergent medical treatment requires intervention with dexamethasone to immediately decrease spinal cord edema. Spinal stabilization is attempted with external traction, surgery, or both.

Respiratory support is often needed for those with lesions at C4 and above. Prognosis is always guarded with clinical evidence of a complete spinal cord transection. When emergent management is completed, these patients are candidates for special spinal rehabilitation centers. Although electronic technologies allow increased mobilization of these physically limited patients and treatment of autonomic and sphincter dysfunction have greatly improved the long-term survival for many patients, spinal cord repair, leading to functional recovery, is one of the

Table 60-1
Acute Extradural Myelopathy

Trauma

Metastatic bone tumors with secondary invasion of the epidural space
    Breast
    Lung
    Prostate
    Kidney
    Colon
    Thyroid
    Myeloma
    Plasmacytoma

Lymphoma
Abscess
Disc herniation affecting central cord
Arteriovenous malformation
Hematoma

ACUTE MYELOPATHIES

Figure 60-1A Acute Spinal Cord Syndromes: Evolution of Symptoms

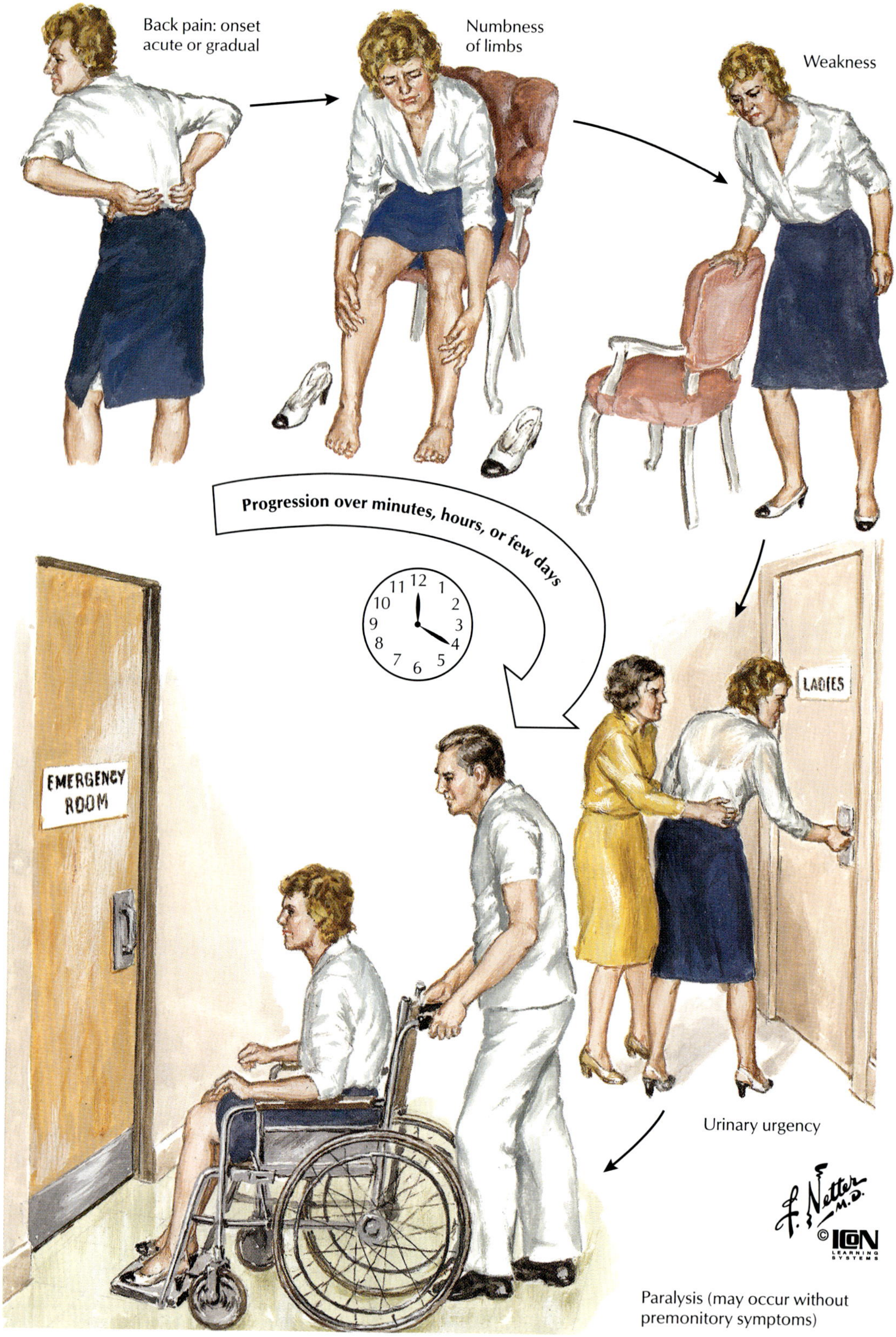

Back pain: onset acute or gradual

Numbness of limbs

Weakness

Progression over minutes, hours, or few days

Urinary urgency

Paralysis (may occur without premonitory symptoms)

MYELOPATHIES

ACUTE MYELOPATHIES

Figure 60-1B
Acute Spinal Cord Syndromes: Pathology, Etiology and Diagnosis

A. Metastatic lesion

Common primary sites, noted on history or examination

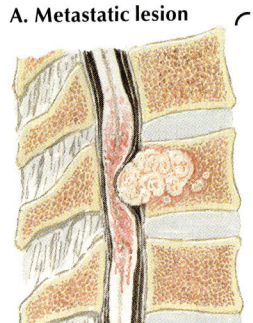
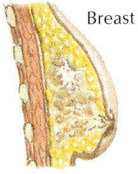
Breast
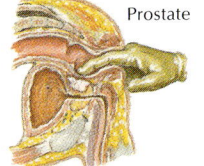
Prostate
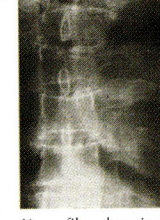
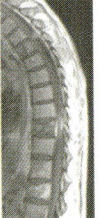

Lung

Melanoma (skin or mucous membrane)

Lymphoma (may be primary)

X-ray film showing destruction of pedicle and vertebral body by metastatic carcinoma

Enhanced MRI showing spinal cord compression

B. Trauma

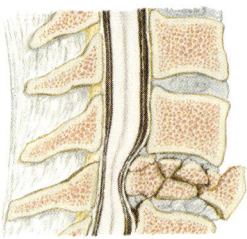
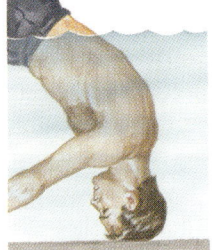
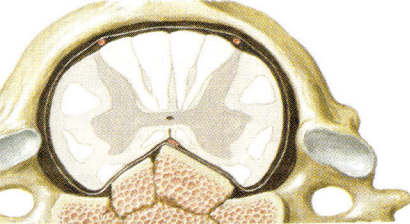

"Burst" fracture: entire vertebral body crushed, with intraspinal bone fragments

Mechanism: vertical blow on the head as in diving or surfing accident, being thrown from car, or football injury

Dislocated bone fragments compressing spinal cord and spinal artery: blood supply to anterior two thirds of spinal cord is impaired

C. Infarction

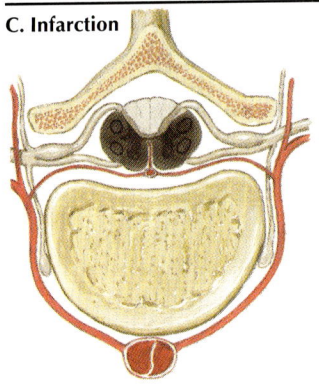
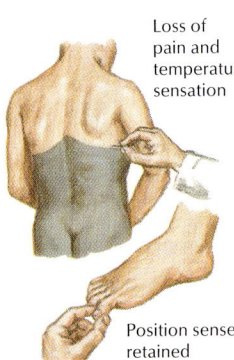

Loss of pain and temperature sensation

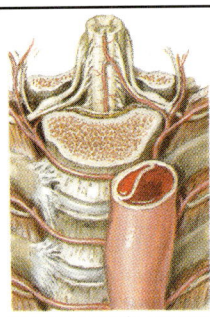
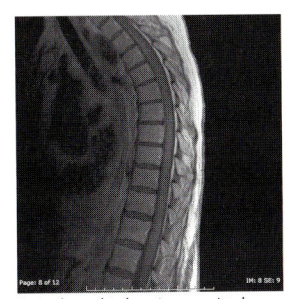

Position sense retained

Dissecting aortic aneurysm obstructing artery of Adamkiewicz by blocking intercostal artery

Spinal cord infarction: sagittal T2-weighted image with increased T2 signal throughout spinal cord representing edema

D. Epidural abscess

Sources of infection

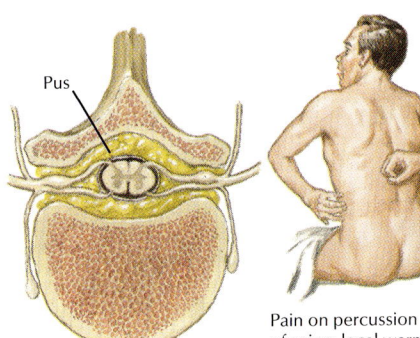

Pus

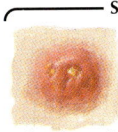
Skin: furuncle, carbuncle

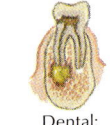
Dental: abscess

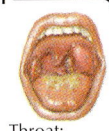
Throat: pharyngitis, tonsillitis, abscess

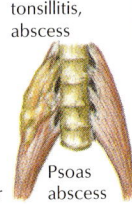
Psoas abscess

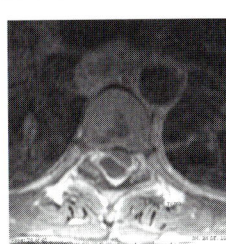

Pain on percussion of spine; local warmth may be noted

Lung: pneumonia, abscess, bronchiectasis

Urinary tract: renal, perirenal, or prostatic abscess; pyelonephritis

Axial T1-weighted gadolinium-enhanced image shows epidural enhancement especially around posterior nonenhancing pus. The spinal cord is compressed and is placed forward and to the left.

MYELOPATHIES

ACUTE MYELOPATHIES

greatest challenges for neurology in the 21st century.

Acute Central Disc

Clinical Vignette

A 65-year-old, part-time musician suddenly fell as he was reaching for his morning newspaper. He called for help. His wife found him unable to move his arms and legs, and he noted numbness in all extremities. He recalled a brief, involuntary ballistic movement of his right arm; a diagnosis of a brainstem stroke was made at the local hospital. It was initially presumed that he fell because of the stroke. Brain CT was normal. Within a few days, he recovered right-sided motor function. The family sought a second opinion.

On arrival at the clinic, the patient had a left hemiparesis, bilaterally brisk muscle stretch reflexes, Babinski signs, and a right-sided subjective C5-6 sensory level to pain and temperature with preserved position sense particularly to the midcervical spine. MRI demonstrated a herniated nucleus pulposus at C34 with spinal cord compression and contusion and a severe stenotic lesion at that level. Surgical decompression was performed emergently. The patient had a gradual increase in function; within 1 year he could perform most activities of daily living independently, although his finger dexterity for clarinet playing was not back to his preinjury level.

Although a brainstem stroke is the most common mechanism leading to quadriparesis in a patient in his seventh decade, a thorough neurologic examination is essential. Initially the patient in the preceding vignette was thought to have an untreatable brainstem stroke, ie, a lesion in an entirely different area within the neuroaxis. Patients with brainstem stroke do not have total loss of sensory function in a spinal cord level distribution (Figure 60-2) as determined above, and they do not have an incomplete anterior spinal artery syndrome as seen on examination 5 days later. Once the syndrome was clearly defined, emergency studies and surgery led to an almost complete functional recovery. Falls at home may lead to an acute central-disc protrusion. As they are eminently treatable with acute neurosurgical intervention, consideration of these less common lesions is vital in patients who have sudden unexplained falls and findings of a cord lesion.

Anatomically, the extruded disc arising from between 2 adjacent vertebral bodies produces acute compression of the anterior cord. Although generally an acutely extruded central disc can lead to an acute myelopathy, occasionally these lesions present subacutely or chronically. Chronic cases lead to the appearance of incomplete spinal cord processes such as Brown-Séquard syndrome.

Because associated bony pain or tenderness may be present, these lesions often mimic metastatic or primary tumors. However, if the patient does not have a history of malignancy, a benign mechanism, such as a central disc, must be sought. Rarely, a dural AVM or spinal epidural hematoma mimics this clinical picture.

MRI is the study of choice unless a medical contraindication, such as a pacemaker, exists. Then a combined spinal myelogram/CT scan is appropriate.

Neurosurgery is the primary treatment. Prognosis depends on the degree of cord compromise before surgery, the general health status of the patient, and the disc location. Cervical lesions are treated by a neurosurgeon, although a combined approach with an orthopedic surgeon is sometimes indicated. When the central disc is in the thoracic cord area, a combined neurologic and thoracic surgical approach is required.

Metastatic malignancies are the other most common pathophysiologic etiology of an acute or subacute extradural myelopathy. Typically, spinal pain secondary to bony metastases from a known systemic malignancy develops in these patients initially, although occasionally the metastasis may be the presenting sign of a previously undiagnosed primary tumor, particularly in the lung, breast, and prostate. Treatment of metastatic extradural tumors includes radiation and sometimes surgery, chemotherapy, or both. Primary intrinsic spinal cord tumors usually have an intradural extramedullary origin or are primarily intramedullary.

Epidural Abscess

Clinical Vignette

A 52-year-old man with diabetes presented with "the flu," followed by left-hip and leg pain 2 days previously. On the evening before coming to the hospital, the pain moved to the patient's upper thoracic spine. He

Figure 60-2 Sensory Impairment Related to Level of Spinal Cord Injury

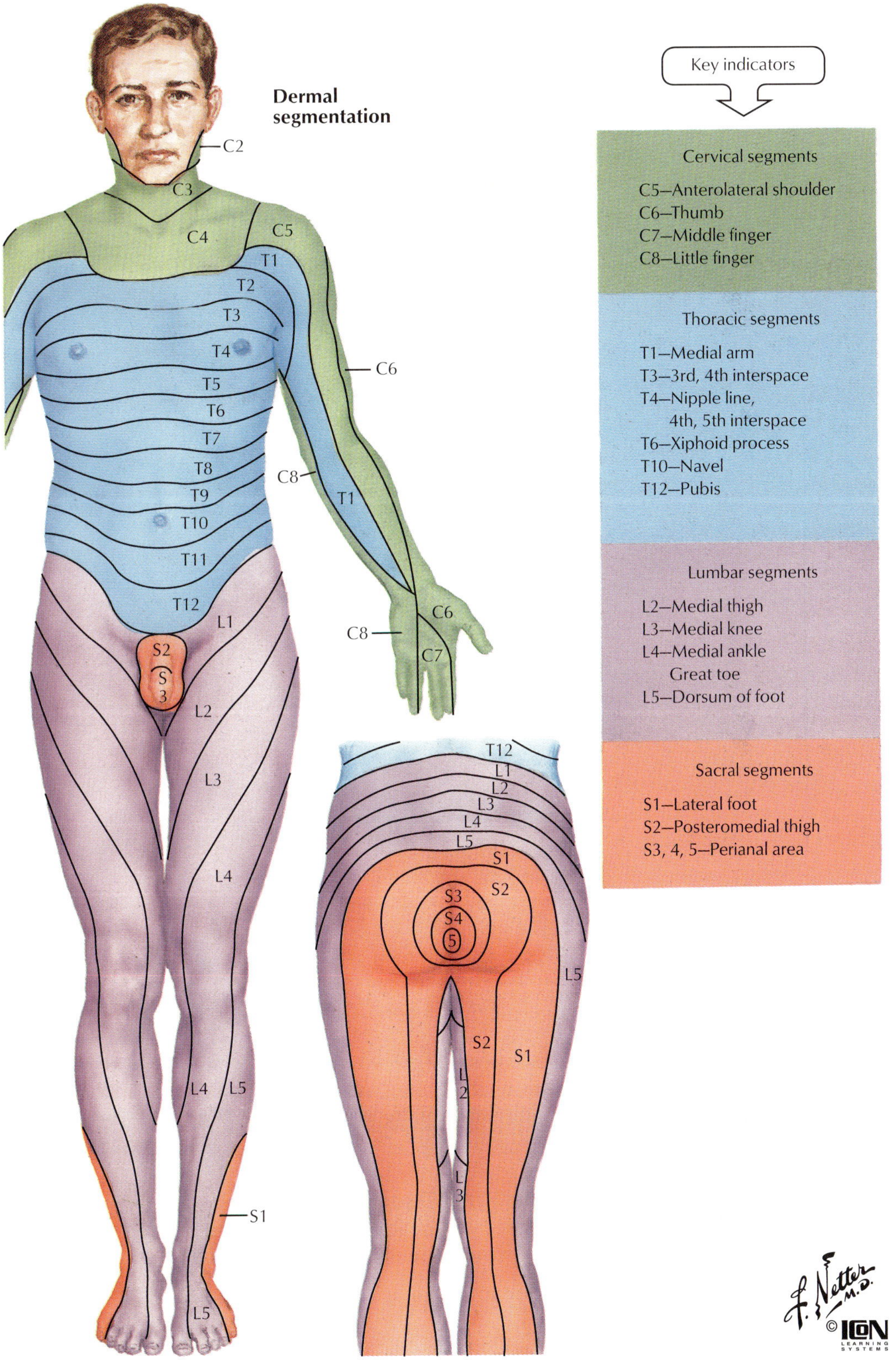
Dermal segmentation
C2
C3
C4
C5
T1
T2
T3
T4
T5
T6
T7
T8
T9
T10
T11
T12
C6
C8
T1
C6
C8
C7
L1
S2
S3
L2
L3
L4
L4
L5
S1
L5
T12
L1
L2
L3
L4
L5
S1
S2
S3
S4
5
L5
S2
S1
L2
L3
Key indicators
Cervical segments
C5—Anterolateral shoulder
C6—Thumb
C7—Middle finger
C8—Little finger
Thoracic segments
T1—Medial arm
T3—3rd, 4th interspace
T4—Nipple line, 4th, 5th interspace
T6—Xiphoid process
T10—Navel
T12—Pubis
Lumbar segments
L2—Medial thigh
L3—Medial knee
L4—Medial ankle Great toe
L5—Dorsum of foot
Sacral segments
S1—Lateral foot
S2—Posteromedial thigh
S3, 4, 5—Perianal area
F. Netter M.D.
© ICON LEARNING SYSTEMS

sought outpatient medical care and was treated with meperidine. Later that evening he began to have trouble walking and had to crawl on one occasion. Overnight, his difficulties rapidly worsened. He lost some sensation in his legs and then discovered he was unable to walk or urinate.

Neurologic examination demonstrated a febrile, acutely ill individual with a flaccid paraplegia, brisk muscle stretch reflexes at the knees, bilateral Babinski signs, loss of position sense in the feet, and a cord level to both pin and temperature sensation at approximately T6. He had percussion tenderness over his upper thoracic spinous processes.

MRI demonstrated an extensive epidural collection extending from C6 to T10. Emergency laminectomy was performed, which demonstrated a purulent epidural abscess. Although the patient underwent surgery shortly after the MRI, he is still significantly limited by residual paraplegia.

Epidural spinal abscess is a rare clinical process occurring in 2 to 20 cases per 100,000 hospital admissions (Figures 60-1B and D). The incidence and/or recognition appears to be increasing. Spinal epidural abscess is usually seen in middle-aged adults, more often men. Despite its rarity, its potential to cause permanent paraplegia makes it one of the most urgent spinal cord emergencies, mandating careful consideration of every patient presenting with acute and increasing back pain. The epidural space in the posterior thoracic cord is the primary development site for an epidural spinal abscess, which may extend to the cervical cord and, rarely, into the lumbar spine. Experimental studies suggest that the abscess' mass effect leading to cord compression is a more important clinicopathologic mechanism than anterior spinal artery infarction.

Staphylococcus aureus is the predominant microorganism identified in epidural spinal abscesses. Usually a distant septic focus provides bacterial seeding via the blood stream, eg, skin furuncles, dental abscesses, simple pharyngitis, or a recently infected traumatic site. Often there is a history of diabetes mellitus, alcoholism, drug abuse, or recent spinal or extraspinal trauma. Less commonly, epidural spinal abscesses develop subsequent to vertebral osteomyelitis, pulmonary or urinary infection, sepsis or, rarely, bacterial endocarditis. Invasive procedures, including epidural anesthesia, spinal surgery, vascular access lines, and paravertebral injections, also provide potential mechanisms for bacterial sources. A history of corticosteroid therapy contributes to immune suppression and the possibility of secondary nosocomial infections.

Typically, these patients are middle-aged, previously healthy individuals who recently became at risk for epidural spinal abscess. Any patient presenting with back pain, particularly when assessed to be severe, is at risk for an epidural spinal abscess, despite the ubiquitous and usually benign nature of back pain. The potential for disastrous neurologic sequelae mandates consideration of epidural spinal abscess in the differential diagnosis.

Percussion tenderness over the posterior spinal process is an important finding. Kernig sign or similar signs of meningeal irritation soon develop in patients having an epidural spinal abscess. Soon thereafter a rapidly developing combination of motor, sensory, and sphincter dysfunction occurs. At the abscess' maximum, the patient becomes paraplegic at a particular cord level.

Other acute space-occupying lesions within the spinal canal deserve consideration in the differential diagnosis. These include acute disc, epidural metastasis, acute pathologic fracture, and hematoma.

A highly elevated erythrocyte sedimentation rate, often greater than 70 mm/h, with a modestly increased WBC count, provides initial support to the classic picture for ordering emergency MRI.

Emergency surgical decompression is the treatment of choice. Occasionally, when no significant neurologic compromise exists, antibiotics can be the primary treatment, with the caveat that if presentation evolves to indicate intra-axial cord involvement, the patient requires another MRI and probably surgical intervention.

Prognosis depends entirely on the clinician's level of suspicion and ability to diagnose epidural spinal abscess early in its temporal evolution. If treatment is not initiated until after the patient becomes paraplegic, prognosis is extremely guarded.

ACUTE MYELOPATHIES

Table 60-2
Acute Intradural Intramedullary Spinal Cord Lesions

Inflammatory	Transverse myelitis
	Multiple sclerosis
	Neuromyelitis optica
	Systemic lupus erythematosus
	Sjögren syndrome
	Sarcoidosis
Vascular	Infarction
Infectious	HTLV-I
	HIV
	Syphilis
	Tuberculosis
	Other bacteria, viruses, fungi, and parasites, ie, schistosomiasis
Trauma	Hematomyelia

ACUTE INTRADURAL INTRAMEDULLARY SPINAL LESIONS
Transverse Myelitis

Clinical Vignette

A 30-year-old woman had a 3-month history of right-arm numbness, and weakness of that arm developed recently. Sixteen months previously, she had experienced intermittent dizziness, with blurred vision in her right eye, and Lhermitte sign, wherein forward bending of her neck produced a momentary, electric-shock, lightninglike sensation going down to her buttocks. She reported fatigue and worsening symptoms in heat. Medical history was significant for irritable bowel syndrome and migraine. Family history was noncontributory.

Neurologic examination demonstrated a slightly spastic gait on the left, increased muscle stretch reflexes of the left leg with a left Babinski sign, poor position sense on the left, and reduced pin and temperature sensation over right arm and thigh.

Cervical spine MRI showed an area of increased signal with ill-defined enhancement located posteriorly and on the left side of the cord from C2 to C4. Brain MRI with and without gadolinium was normal. Her CSF was significant for 10 WBCs/µL (99% lymphocytes, 1% monocytes), 17.4 mg IgG/total protein (reference range, 6.0-13.0), and the presence of oligoclonal bands.

This vignette presents a classic clinical picture of early multiple sclerosis (MS). The patient has an incomplete demyelinating myelitis consistent with classic hemicord syndrome, affecting crossed sensory fibers, called *Brown-Séquard syndrome* (Figure 61-3). Other mechanisms to consider are outlined in Table 60-2.

Clinical Vignette

A 41-year-old woman presented with a 3-day history of bilateral pain at the level of her lower ribs. Simultaneously, she experienced numbness from her waist down, leg weakness, urinary urgency, and lack of pressure sensation in her rectum, with reduced ability to push out stool.

Her neurologic evaluation demonstrated grade 4/5 weakness confined to the iliopsoas, dysmetric heel-to-shin testing, and a broad-based gait. Muscle stretch reflexes were hyperactive and plantar stimulation was flexor. Vibratory sensation was reduced at feet, ankles, and knees. She had a definite sensory level to pinprick at T8. Results of clinical investigations are summarized in Table 60-3.

She responded to a course of IV methylprednisolone, although she had persistent leg symptoms.

Table 60-3
Laboratory Results for Clinical Vignette*

Data	Initial	2½ Years Later
CSF	5 WBCs (80% lymphocytes, 20% monocytes)/cc	23 WBCs (100% lymphocytes)/cc
	Glucose 54 mg/dL	Glucose 83 mg/dL
	Protein 21 mg/dL	Protein 33 mg/dL
MRI	Brain, cervical, thoracic, and lumbar sacral spine—normal	↑ Signal thoracic cord
ANA	1:1280	1:2560

*Lyme, B_{12}, HIV, HTLV-I, VDRL, TSH, ESR, RF, oligoclonal bands were either negative or normal.

ACUTE MYELOPATHIES

She presented with worsening leg numbness and weakness, and urinary incontinence 2½ years later. Lower-extremity strength ranged from 0/5 to 4/5: iliopsoas 0/5, quadriceps 4/5, anterior tibialis 0/5, gastrocnemius 3/5, hamstrings 4/5, adductors 4/5. Muscle stretch reflexes were hyperactive in her legs. She had bilateral Babinski signs. Vibratory sensation was absent at feet and reduced elsewhere. Response to pinprick was reduced only in the right leg.

A diagnosis of systemic lupus erythematosus (SLE) was made in the above vignette. Often with a transverse myelitis, no underlying pathology is identified. Sometimes a transverse myelitis is preceded by or associated with optic neuritis. Known as **neuromyelitis optica**, this combination is thought to represent an uncommon form of MS. Occasionally, it responds to intensive methylprednisolone therapy (1 g IV per day for 5-10 days) and does not recur. However, most uncomplicated instances of transverse myelitis are related to more classic MS.

Acute transverse myelitis encompasses a group of disorders causing focal spinal cord inflammation leading to significant intradural intramedullary spinal injury and dysfunction. Commonly, there is an isolated or partial multifocal CNS lesion or sometimes a multisystemic process. The primary identifiable causes of transverse myelitis are MS and a "viral infection." Other etiologies may exist; however, it is thought that most instances of acute transverse myelitis represent an autoimmune CNS disorder. Commonly, when MS is not identified, no precise etiologic mechanism is found.

Transverse myelitis, if complete, interrupts all ascending tracts from below the lesion and concomitantly all descending tracts at the pathologic site. Interruption of the corticospinal tracts causes a flaccid paraplegia or tetraplegia, depending on the lesion level. Over time, spasticity develops. Light touch, temperature, pain, position, and vibration are lost below the lesion if the anterior and lateral spinothalamic tracts and dorsal columns are completely interrupted. Pinprick is the most easily localized, with loss 1 to 2 levels below the lesion. Bladder and bowel functions are also impaired. The degree of motor and sensory dysfunction depends on the extent of the lesion, ranging from none to mild paresis to quadriplegia and from minimal sensory disturbance to complete loss.

Transverse myelitis occurs with MS, acute disseminated encephalomyelitis, SLE (1% of lupus patients), vasculitis, sarcoidosis, Sjogren syndrome, antiphospholipid antibody syndrome, and *Schistosoma mansoni* parasitic infection. Transverse myelitis is sometimes associated with a recent viral or bacterial infection and may occur subsequent to immunization. Viruses that may precipitate a transverse myelitis include coxsackie, ECHO, cytomegalovirus, varicella zoster, herpes simplex, polio, HIV, Epstein-Barr, mumps, enterovirus, and others. There can be a concomitant encephalitis, ie, encephalomyelitis. Bacterial causes include *Mycoplasma* and *Borrelia burgdorferi*. Hepatitis B, smallpox, measles, and influenza vaccines are rarely associated with subsequent transverse myelitis.

Direct infection, immune-mediated response to infection, or an autoimmune response to the nervous system cause neuronal injury by different mechanisms. Pathologic findings vary depending on the process. Perivascular lymphocyte cuffing and parenchymal mononuclear cell infiltrate are seen in MS. Inflammatory demyelinating lesions, with demyelinated axons and some axonal loss, occurs. Vasculitic or granulomatous changes are seen with SLE, primary CNS vasculitis, and sarcoidosis. Inflammatory cell infiltration with demyelination is found in postvaccinal myelitis or encephalomyelitis and in idiopathic transverse myelitis.

Motor, sensory, and sphincter disturbances vary in degree if the process begins subacutely. However, with an acute onset, a lesion can develop rapidly, mimicking a traumatic lesion with paraplegia or quadriplegia, total sensory loss, and absence of bladder and rectal sphincter function. In neuromyelitis optica syndrome, myelitis and optic neuritis occur simultaneously or are temporally proximate. In MS, motor and sensory deficits tend to be less symmetric, the initial symptoms are often sensory, and the motor component may be less severe.

Differential diagnosis includes cord infarct, arteriovenous malformation, radiation myelopathy, metastatic or intrinsic tumors, and spondylosis.

MRI with gadolinium is the procedure of choice to exclude compressive lesions, especially when history and examination suggest a specific level of spinal cord dysfunction. Transverse myelitis appears with T2 signal hyperintensity on MRI. The area of signal abnormality may be focal or extensive in cross section and length. Gadolinium enhancement is frequent. Cord swelling varies. In MS, the lesions tend to be smaller, usually involving only 1 to 2 segments, lateral, posterior, and multifocal. Large cross-sectional area, multisegment length, cord expansion, and peripheral enhancement are less consistent with MS. SLE typically affects the middle to lower thoracic cord.

Evaluation for infection and systemic inflammatory disease includes lumbar puncture for CSF analysis (cell count, protein, oligoclonal bands, culture, glucose, and viral PCRs), viral titers or specific PCR, and serologies. Blood work should include ESR, antinuclear antibodies, anti-DNA antibodies, SSA, SSB, anticardiolipin antibodies, lupus anticoagulant, complement, and angiotensin-converting enzyme. Viral and bacterial screen might include varicella zoster, enterovirus, coxsackie virus, Epstein-Barr virus, cytomegalovirus, herpes simplex, hepatitis, HIV, and Lyme titers.

Brain MRI with gadolinium and visual evoked potentials help determine the extent of the demyelinating disease. Associated cerebral white-matter lesions and oligoclonal bands in CSF increase the later probability of developing unequivocal MS.

Methylprednisolone, 1 g IV per day for 3 to 10 days, is used, with variable responses. Additional immunosuppressive agents such as cyclophosphamide, 1-2 mg · kg^{-1} · d^{-1}, are sometimes necessary for SLE. They can improve the clinical course, especially if initiated early. Anticoagulants are sometimes indicated in patients positive for antiphospholipid antibody.

The degree of recovery depends on the rapidity of development and severity of deficit. Relapsing transverse myelitis is rare. However, this temporal profile is seen with MS, SLE, antiphospholipid antibody syndrome, and vascular malformations of the cord. Incomplete lesions, associated white-matter lesions, and CSF oligoclonal bands each increase the risk of MS.

Spinal Cord Infarction/Ischemic Myelopathy

Clinical Vignette

A vigorous 56-year-old policeman was found to have an extensive thoracoabdominal aneurysm requiring heroic surgical repair. Although the primary surgical procedure appeared to be successful, when the patient awakened he was unable to move his legs or empty his bladder, and he had numbness distal to T8-10. Neurologic examination demonstrated the patient to be paraplegic, with excellent strength in his arms and upper body, loss of temperature and pain sensation with a vague numbness from his upper abdomen to the tips of his toes, and preserved position and vibratory sensation.

Thoracic and cervical MRI performed within a few hours after the patient awoke were normal. His clinical course was otherwise stable. When there was no improvement in his neurologic status, he was transferred to a spinal rehabilitation unit.

The clinical picture of paralysis and sensory change secondary to loss of corticospinal tract and lateral and anterior spinothalamic function, with preserved posterior column function, is classic for an anterior spinal artery distribution spinal cord infarction (Figures 60-1B and C). Spinal ischemia is significantly less common than cerebral ischemia, but spinal cord infarction and transient ischemic attacks rarely occur. This diagnosis must be considered in patients who present with sudden onset of nontraumatic weakness, a sensory loss with a definable level, and bladder dysfunction. Recent aortic surgery, concomitant chest or abdominal pain, limb ischemia, or loss of peripheral pulses suggesting a possible aortic dissection add support to this diagnosis.

Spinal cord infarction is typically secondary to inadequate arterial flow through the anterior spinal artery, which supplies the anterior funiculi, anterior horns, base of the dorsal horns, and anteromedial aspects of the lateral funiculi. Therefore, the corticospinal and spinothalamic tracts are affected bilaterally. The upper to midthoracic spinal cord is poorly vascularized, and these watershed zones are more susceptible to infarction. Interruption of blood supply from the aorta to the intramedullary spinal vasculature can cause infarction. In contrast, a posterior spinal artery infarction is rare because of well-developed collaterals.

Spontaneous aortic dissection, atherosclerosis of the aorta and its branches, and iatrogenic ischemia from surgical procedures are the usual pathophysiologic mechanisms underlying spinal cord ischemia. Rarely, emboli or arteritis may be responsible for an intramedullary cord infarction.

Dissecting aneurysms of the descending thoracic or upper abdominal aorta can occlude the ostia of segmental spinal arteries. Atherosclerosis of the aorta and its branches is a gradual process and, unlike aortic dissection, can allow development of collateral flow. Surgical aortic repair for aneurysm, dissection, or coarctation can reduce vascular supply to the radicular and spinal arteries. Procedures such as thoracotomy and nephrectomy sometimes compromise intercostal or lumbar artery flow, which give rise to radicular arteries.

Emboli to the anterior spinal artery may be derived from atheromatous, septic, fibrocartilaginous, and air (decompression illness/caisson disease) sources. Vascular angiitis with subsequent thrombosis from primary CNS vasculitis, syphilis, tuberculosis, sarcoidosis, and schistosomiasis can all cause cord infarction.

CLINICAL PRESENTATION
Anterior Spinal Artery Syndrome

Onset of anterior spinal artery syndrome, although usually sudden, may be gradual over hours or days. A bilateral flaccid paraplegia or quadriplegia, depending on the occlusive level, develops in patients. At the cervical level, the arms are flaccid and eventually atrophic because of anterior horn involvement, although the legs become spastic. Thoracic cord infarcts lead to a spastic paraplegia. Initial areflexia changes to hyperreflexia with Babinski signs present. Paresthesiae or radicular pain can occur at the infarct level.

Typically, there is dissociated sensory loss. Pain and temperature are affected, whereas vibration, position, and partial touch sensation are preserved due to intact blood supply to the dorsal columns. Bladder and bowel function are impaired. When spinal cord infarction occurs secondary to an aortic dissection, the patient usually experiences intense tearing chest or abdominal pains.

Posterior Spinal Artery Syndrome

A rare form of spinal stroke, posterior spinal artery syndrome presents with ataxia; loss of position, vibration, and fine tactile sensation; and bladder and bowel disturbance. Well-developed arterial collaterals on the posterior cord account for its rarity.

DIAGNOSIS AND TREATMENT

Any condition that leads to a rapid onset of a partial transverse spinal cord lesion must be considered: trauma, metastatic cancer, dural arteriovenous malformations, acute transverse myelitis, MS, and intramedullary tumors. Spinal claudication alternatively presents as exercise-induced painless lower-extremity weakness.

MRI can exclude cord compression, arteriovenous malformation, tumor, syrinx, hemorrhage, and demyelinating disease. Infarction appears isointense on T1 and eventually hyperintense on T2. A CT/myelogram can exclude spinal cord compression but provides less information regarding the cord. Spinal fluid evaluation can help detect infection, demyelinating disease, and subarachnoid hemorrhage. Acutely, the possibility of a dissecting aortic aneurysm should be pursued with appropriate body imaging. If negative, studies to search for a cardiac source of embolism, vasculitis, hypercoagulable states, and aortic atherosclerosis are indicated.

With the exception of an aortic dissection where surgery may be indicated to preserve life, treatment is supportive. Aneurysmal repair will not affect spinal cord damage. Underlying etiologic factors must be corrected, as possible, if discovered.

Prognosis depends on the level of anterior spinal artery occlusion, which determines whether the patient is paraplegic or quadriplegic. Once the infarction occurs, recovery is rare, although it is possible. Less commonly, the arterial occlusion is farther from the cord, so the chance for collateral arterial supply is greater. Slow, gradual occlusion is offset by collateral development. Anatomic variations are also important; damage to a particular intercostal artery can be of variable importance. Hypoxia and low perfusion pressure aggravate damage caused by ischemia.

REFERENCES

Anderson O. Myelitis. *Curr Opin Neurol.* 2000;13:1311-1316.

Chan KF, Boey ML. Transverse myelopathy in SLE: clinical features and functional outcomes. *Lupus.* 1996;5:294-299.

de Seze J, Stojkovic T, Breteau G, et al. Acute myelopathies: clinical, laboratory and outcome profiles in 79 cases. *Brain.* 2001;124:1509-1521.

El-Toraei I, Juler G. Ischemic myelopathy. *Angiology.* 1979;30:81-94.

Kerr DA, Ayetey H. Immunopathogenesis of acute transverse myelitis. *Curr Opin Neurol.* 2002;15:339-347.

Kovacs B, Lafferty TL, Brent LH, DeHoratius RJ. Transverse myelopathy in systemic lupus erythematosus: an analysis of 14 cases and review of the literature. *Ann Rheum Dis.* 2000;59:120-124.

Sandson TA, Friedman JH. Spinal cord infarction report of 8 cases and review of the literature. *Medicine.* 1989;68:282-292.

Scotti G, Gerevini S. Diagnosis and differential diagnosis of acute transverse myelopathy: the role of neuroradiological investigations and review of the literature. *Neurol Sci.* 2001;22:S69-S73.

Yasargil MG, Symon L, Teddy PJ. Arteriovenous malformations of the spinal cord. *Adv Tech Stand Neurosurg.* 1984;7:62-102.

Chapter 61
Chronic Myelopathies
Ann Camac and H. Royden Jones, Jr

EXTRADURAL MYELOPATHIES
Cervical Spondylosis

Clinical Vignette

A 62-year-old man presented with a 2-month history of progressive leg weakness and neck discomfort. He had recently experienced arm weakness with bilateral hand pain. At first, he required a cane for balance, and later, he required a walker. His medical history included diabetic polyneuropathy, myocardial infarction, and obesity.

Abnormalities on neurologic examination included atrophic and weak deltoid and biceps, with scattered fasciculations, as well as weakness of the triceps, abductor pollicis brevis, and iliopsoas, right greater than left. His gait was broad based and spastic. Muscle stretch reflexes were brisk. He had a right Babinski sign. Pinprick sensation was reduced in a glove and stocking distribution. Position sense was absent at the toes, and vibratory sense was lost at the ankles. There was no cord level.

MRI revealed spinal stenosis and cord edema at C3-4 secondary to a combination of a diffuse disc protrusion, end plate osteophytes, and neural foraminal stenosis. A C3-6 posterior laminectomy was performed. The patient improved gradually.

Spondylosis, a normal aging process, is the most common cause of a cervical myelopathy (Table 61-1). It results from disc degeneration followed by reactive osteophyte formation, fibrocartilaginous bars, spondylotic transverse bars, articular facet hypertrophy, and thickening of the ligamentum flavum causing spinal canal narrowing. Subsequently, gradual spinal cord compression may occur; it is particularly likely in patients with congenitally narrowed spinal canals. In its simplest form, a herniated nucleus pulposus in patients with congenital stenosis can produce cervical myelopathy. Although many individuals have radiographic signs of cervical spondylosis (perhaps 90% by the age of 70 years), most are asymptomatic. When a myelopathy develops, clinical findings can present acutely, subacutely, or over many years. Cervical myelopathy and radiculopathy may occur in the same spondylotic patient.

Pathophysiology and Etiology
Typically, the spinal canal is 17 to 18 mm in diameter between C3 and C7. A narrower cervical spinal canal may range from 9 to 15 mm; however, myelopathy is rare if the canal diameter is greater than 13 mm. Cervical cord diameter ranges from 8.5 to 11.5 mm, averaging approximately 10 mm. Disc protrusion and other reactive and degenerative processes further reduce canal dimension. Direct cord compression, compromised blood supply to the cord or venous stasis, and mechanical factors can in combination or independently cause irreversible damage. Normally, the spinal cord moves cephalad

Table 61-1
Extradural Causes of Chronic Myelopathy

Disc osteophyte complex with chronic disc protrusion
Primary bone tumors with secondary invasion of the epidural space: chondrosarcoma, osteogenic sarcoma, hemangioma
Lymphoma
Arteriovenous malformation
Lipoma
Miscellaneous disorders sometimes affecting spinal cord: Paget disease, rheumatoid arthritis, Pott disease (tuberculosis)

and posteriorly within the canal during neck flexion and caudally and anteriorly during neck extension. If osteophytes, discs, and hypertrophied ligaments make contact with the cord, the cord sustains additive trauma leading to development of a clinical myelopathy. The disc levels most frequently affected are C5-6, C6-7 and C3-4, in order of clinical relevance.

Pathologically, the spinal cord may become grossly flattened, distorted, or indented. Demyelination of the lateral columns occurs at the lesion site with consequent lateral columns degeneration below the lesion. Concomitant dorsal column degeneration occurs at and above the damaged segments. There may also be damage and loss of nerve cells in gray matter. Ischemic changes, gliosis, demyelination, and even cavitation necrosis sometimes also result.

Clinical Presentation

Gait difficulties, secondary to asymmetric spastic paraparesis, and numb, clumsy hands are the usual initial symptoms and findings (Figure 60-1), primarily related to lateral cord compression. Initially, 1 leg may drag, or the person may have difficulty climbing stairs. When upper extremity weakness develops, it varies in degree and is typically less pronounced than in the lower extremities. Other upper motor neuron corticospinal tract findings include hyperreflexia with exaggerated muscle stretch reflexes and sometimes Babinski signs. Bowel and bladder disturbances are usually late findings.

If there is concomitant ventral cord compression, the anterior horn cells within the gray matter may be damaged, characterized by muscle fasciculations, atrophy, and weakness appropriate to the specific nerve roots.

Limb paresthesias can range from mild dysesthesias to severe paresthesias. The ability to grasp objects may be difficult because of impaired proprioception and dexterity secondary to posterior column involvement. Sensory ataxia sometimes also results when position and vibratory sensations are compromised.

Neck pain varies. The Lhermitte sign may occur, characterized by recurrent lightninglike paresthesias traversing down the back with neck flexion. When the syndrome is purely spinal, a myelopathy without root signs or symptoms occurs. However, a radicular syndrome can also present with radicular pain, sensory or motor deficit or both, localized to the area innervated by the specific nerve root.

The clinical course varies among patients. Although some individuals have a mild protracted insidious course, even over decades, others have subacute temporal profiles progressing over a few weeks to a severe disability. Acute cord compression occurs infrequently, secondary to trauma, sometimes mimicking a stroke. Search for a cervical spinal sensory level can be diagnostic. Rarely, sudden neck hyperextension leads to a temporary "person in the barrel" syndrome in which acute anterior cord compression transiently renders the segmental anterior horn cells of the arms nonfunctional while preserving lateral column function, so the legs are unaffected.

Diagnosis

Amyotrophic lateral sclerosis, multiple sclerosis, vitamin B_{12} deficiency, HTLV-I myelopathy, adrenoleukodystrophy, syringomyelia, and spinal cord tumors always require consideration. Hand or leg paresthesias, Lhermitte sign, prominent neck pain, or significant sensory loss provides historic and examination means to distinguish cervical spondylosis with myelopathy from motor neuron disease/amyotrophic lateral sclerosis. MRI is the diagnostic procedure of choice, providing longitudinal segmental views of the cord, dural space, and relations to bony and ligamentous structures. CT/myelography is an alternative when MRI is contraindicated because of cardiac pacemakers or severe claustrophobia. CT can provide additional information regarding the foramen, facets, and uncovertebral joints. Electromyography/nerve conduction can help to identify anterior horn cell disease, concomitant peripheral nerve dysfunction, or nerve root compression.

Treatment

Epidemiologic data regarding the natural history of cervical spondylosis are lacking. In patients with mild deficits from cervical myelopathy, it is unclear whether surgical decompression is superior to conservative management. Some patients remain stable or improve without treat-

CHRONIC MYELOPATHIES

Figure 61-1

Cervical Spondylosis

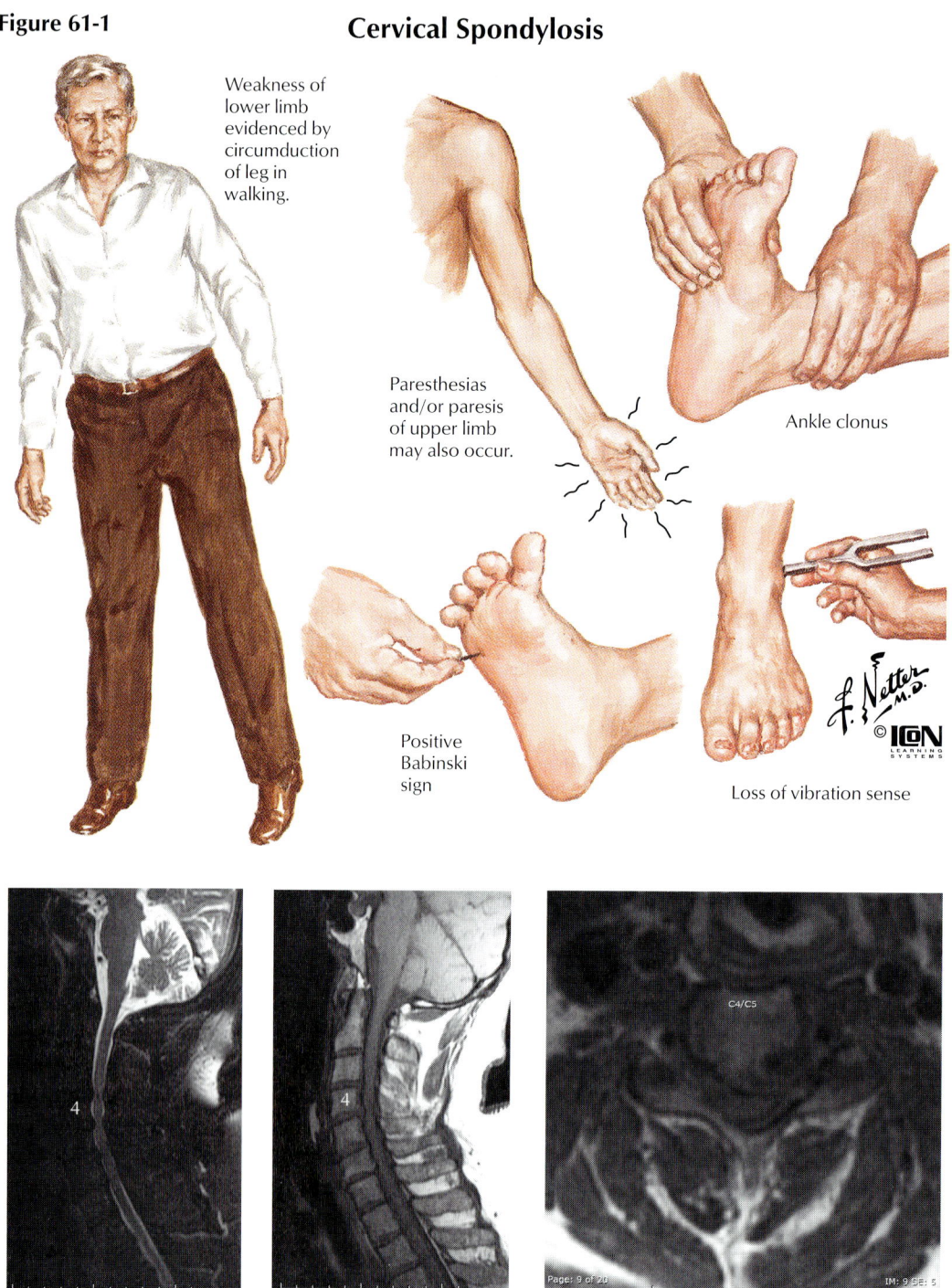

Degenerative disease with spinal cord compression. Idiopathic spinal stenosis with disk protrusion anteriorly and hypertrophy of ligamentum flavum posteriorly, most extreme at C4-5.

ment. For patients with worsening symptoms and deficits, surgical decompression is the treatment of choice to arrest myelopathy progression. Functional recovery may not occur if the deficit is already severe, possibly because of chronic ischemic cord damage from spinal artery compression.

Surgical exposures include the posterior approach, which allows for generous decompressive laminectomies, and the anterior approach, which enables operation on bars and spurs anterior to the cord and fusion when instability or subluxation is present. Discectomy, corpectomy, laminectomy, and laminoplasty are other surgical options. Significant variations exist in the degree of postsurgical clinical improvement. Duration and severity of the myelopathy before surgery are key determinants for clinical outcome. Cord atrophy, irreversible signal change within the cord on T2-weighted MRI (gliosis rather than cord edema), superimposed trauma, and advanced age are negative prognostic factors. Maintaining spinal stability and treating anterior compression improve outcome.

Spinal Cord Arteriovenous Malformations

Clinical Vignette

A 45-year-old woman with no medical history presented with intermittent lower extremity paresthesias and heaviness for 1 year. She had an episode of difficulty walking that lasted for a few hours and then resolved. Two months later, she experienced low back pain, constipation, and problems voiding. She had a second episode of inability to walk, lasting for several hours.

Her upper extremity strength, sensation, and coordination were normal. Her lower extremity strength was 3/5 proximally; the distal muscles were normal. Pinprick was reduced in a patchy distribution in her legs. Her gait was broad based and unsteady, and she was unable to walk on her heels or toes. Increased lower extremity muscle stretch reflexes and a right Babinski were present.

MRI demonstrated a swollen conus and possible abnormal vasculature. A selective intercostal angiogram revealed a dural AVM with feeder and nidus at T11 on the left, not involving the artery of Adamkiewicz.

The patient had a T10-11 laminectomy to remove the AVM. Large arterialized vessels were found medial to the nerve roots filling the dorsal subarachnoid space. These epidural vessels and large feeders at T10-11 were coagulated. The patient's strength improved after the procedure, returning to normal within 1 year. Bladder dysfunction was minimal.

Spinal AVMs are a group of vascular disorders that can cause acute, subacute, or chronic spinal cord dysfunction. The most common type is the dural AVM (80-85%), although intradural AVMs, combination intradural and extradural AVMs, and cavernous angiomas (cavernous malformations) also occur. A high index of suspicion is needed so as not to miss the diagnosis in patients with unexplained myelopathy. Spinal AVMs can cause problems associated with venous hypertension or bleeding. Complete spinal angiography and obliteration of the AVM is usually indicated.

Pathophysiology and Etiology

Many **dural AVMs** are AV fistulas, essentially a single hole in an artery connected to a vein. Radicular or dural branches from the segmental arteries supply the AVM, usually within the dura of an intervertebral foramen. The AVM nidus is typically a low-flow shunt drained by a single vein that joins the coronal plexus on the dorsal cord surface. The coronal plexus is arterialized by the AVM fistula and becomes dilated, coiled, and elongated. Blood flow through this vessel is slow, leading to venous congestion. Increased venous pressure is transmitted to the cord. The majority of dural AVMs occur in the mid to lower thoracic and lumbar spine (Figure 61-2).

Venous hypertension occurs with dural AVMs. The increased venous pressure is transmitted in an intramedullary manner, reducing the arteriovenous pressure gradient. Cord perfusion decreases. Prolonged ischemia/hypoxia due to venous congestion causes a progressive myelopathy. The effects of hypoxia, initially reversible, become irreversible with degenerative cord necrosis. The corticospinal tracts, lateral white matter, and dorsal columns are especially involved. Later, the spinothalamic and spinocerebellar tracts and anterior gray can be affected. The anteromedian cord tends to be spared. Dural AVMs present in later adulthood and may be acquired.

Medullary arteries from the anterior spinal artery supply **intradural AVMs**. The nidus can be

CHRONIC MYELOPATHIES

Figure 61-2 Spinal Arteriovenous Malformations (AVMs)

Normal Spinal Segment

The spinal cord is supplied via the radicular arteries (branches of intercostal arteries), which give off dural branches as well as forming the anterior spinal and posterolateral spinal arteries. The latter vessels supply the cord with medullary branches.

Dural Arteriovenous Malformation

In dural AVM the nidus is usually a low-flow AV shunt located within dura of intervertebral foramen. Supplied by the dural artery and drained via a single vein into the coronal plexus on dorsal surface of cord. Coronal plexus is "arterialized" and becomes coiled, dilated, and elongated. Multiple segments from T3 to L3 involved.

Intradural Arteriovenous Malformation

Intradural AVMs are high-pressure malformations located within cord (intramedullary) or dura (extramedullary) or both. Supply is via medullary branches of anterior spinal artery. They are often congenital and may occur anywhere throughout length of cord.

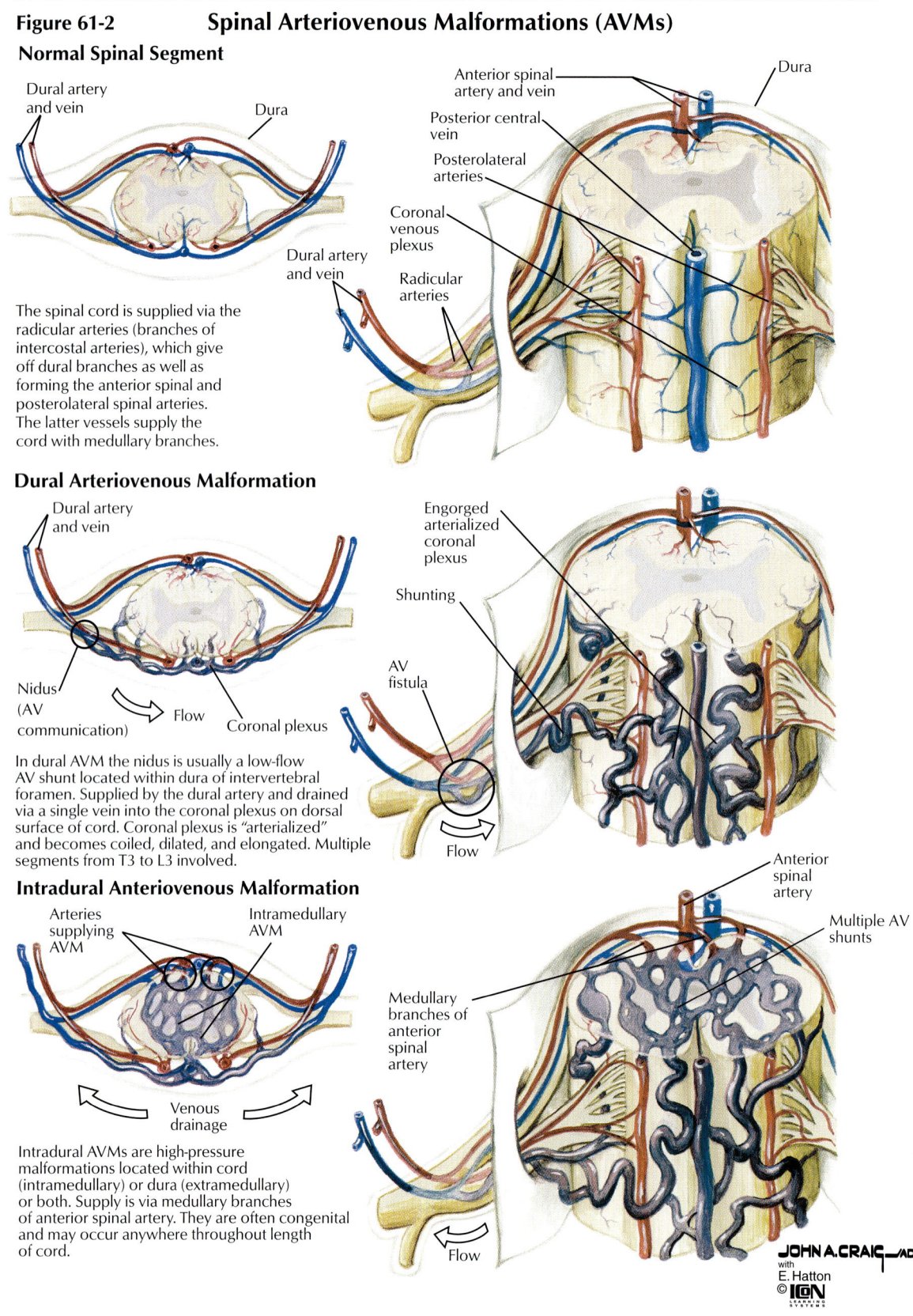

MYELOPATHIES

CHRONIC MYELOPATHIES

Figure 61-2
Spinal Arteriovenous Malformations (AVMs) (continued)
Spinal Dural AVM

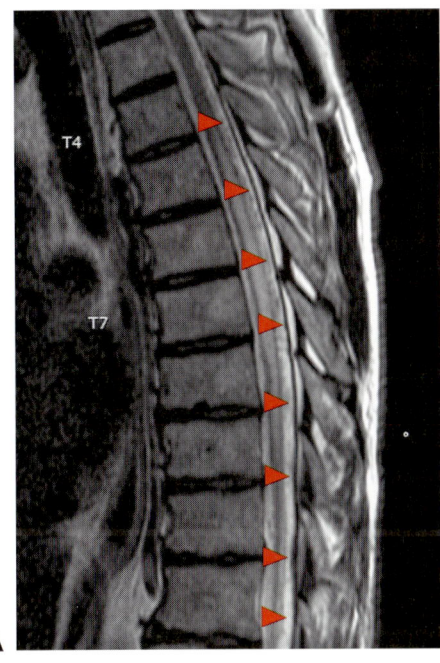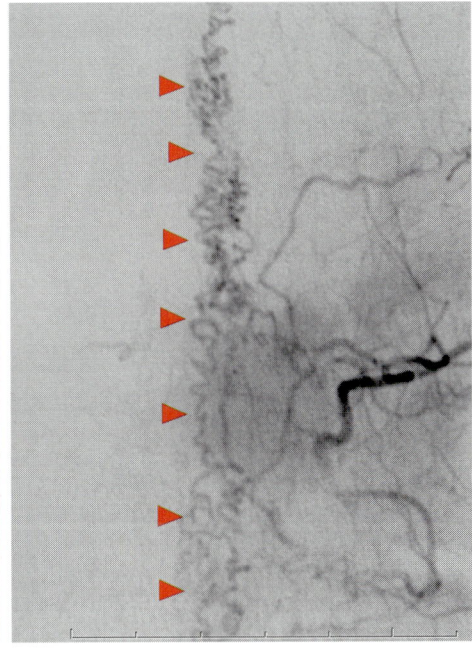

(**A**) Sagittal T2 image shows increased T2 signal in the central cord representing edema and/or gliosis. Multiple signal voids behind the spinal cord are secondary to tortuous vessels from the malformation (arrowheads). (**B**) Spinal angiogram of radicular artery, left T6, with arteriovenous fistula filling multiple draining veins at the dural level. These join to form a complex medullary venous plexus.

in the cord (intramedullary), can be in the pia on cord surface (extramedullary), or can be a combination of intramedullary and extramedullary. These AVMs are high-pressure systems that can contain arterial aneurysms. They can spontaneously hemorrhage within the cord or into the subarachnoid space. Unlike dural AVMs, intradural AVMs occur throughout the length of the cord.

Intradural AVMs affect younger patients and may be congenital. Recurrent subarachnoid and intramedullary hemorrhage is the main cord injury mechanism. Blood flow is rapid, and aneurysms may be present.

Cavernous angiomas or **malformations** are rare, isolated or multiple lesions, more common in the cerebral hemispheres than in the cord. These low flow lesions can spontaneously hemorrhage and are best shown by MRI (spinal arteriography is normal).

Clinical Presentation

Men have **dural AVMs** more commonly than women do. Symptoms can begin throughout adulthood but typically emerge after the age of 40 years, peaking at 50 to 70 years. The thoracolumbar region is more frequently involved (T3-L3, especially T6-L1). Symptoms are gradual in onset and slowly progressive. Pain is the most frequent presenting symptom, localized to the back or radicular distribution. In most patients, a combination of motor, sensory, and sphincter disturbance slowly develops. Leg weakness can progress from abnormal stance or gait to needing an assistive walking device to wheelchair or bed dependence. Patients often have a combination of upper and lower motor neuron findings with spasticity, weakness, fasciculations, atrophy, hyperreflexia, hyporeflexia, and Babinski signs. Sensory loss is attributable to dorsal column and spinothalamic tract injury, manifested by impaired joint position, vibration, pain, and temperature sensation. A discrete or vague sensory level is sometimes present. Various degrees of bladder, bowel, and sexual dysfunction develop. Auscultation over the spine demonstrating a bruit can rarely help to diagnose a high-flow AVM. Certain activities or postures may precipitate or exacerbate symptoms. Dural AVMs rarely hemorrhage.

Intradural AVMs affect men and women more evenly. They present at an early age, usually before the age of 40 years, sometimes during childhood. The AVM nidus is distributed evenly along the cord from the foramen magnum to the conus medullaris. Early symptoms are usually from intramedullary or subarachnoid hemorrhage leading to neurologic deficit. Patients can have progressive weakness, numbness, and sphincter dysfunction. Because the intradural AVM may be located in the upper cord, the upper and lower extremities are sometimes affected. Typically, recurrent hemorrhage leads to clinical deterioration.

Diagnosis

Entities in the differential diagnosis include multiple sclerosis, spinal pseudoclaudication associated with spinal stenosis, disc disease, acute or chronic infection, tumor, syringomyelia, and subarachnoid hemorrhage. All of these conditions can have acute or slowly ingravescent courses.

In **dural AVMs**, MRI demonstrates serpentine filling defects of reduced signal in the subarachnoid space corresponding to blood flow in the dilated, tortuous coronal venous plexus. Sometimes, cord signal is increased from edema or venous congestion. Rarely, MRI misses a dural AVM.

With **intradural AVMs**, the spinal cord may have low signal corresponding to an intradural AVM nidus. A target sign may be seen at the site of previous hemorrhage.

Myelography may demonstrate serpentine linear defects. However, this medium is less helpful in distinguishing intramedullary from extramedullary lesions. Selective spinal arteriography offers more precise information regarding AVM anatomy.

Treatment and Prognosis

Treatment depends on the location, size, source of arterial supply, and site of the shunt. Surgical removal, endovascular embolization, or both are often helpful.

For **dural AVMs**, goals are to eliminate the dural nidus and interrupt the AV fistula between the nidus and coronal venous plexus, resolving the venous hypertension and congestion, subsequently improving the myelopathy. Elimination of the fistula/nidus at the intervertebral foramen can be curative. The dilated veins of the coronal plexus can remain; their removal can be damaging and unnecessary.

Intramedullary AVMs are often inoperable. Embolization can occlude feeding vessels and the nidus, reducing flow and allowing lesion thrombosis. Collateral spinal vascular supply is needed to prevent cord damage from the subsequent ischemia. If the treated vessels recanalize, subsequent embolization may be required.

Early detection and treatment can improve gait disturbances, sometimes bladder dysfunction, and other myelopathy signs, especially if they are less severe. A previously progressive course can be arrested by surgery.

Epidural Lipomatosis

Clinical Vignette

A 64-year-old man, hospitalized for an acute myocardial infarction, was dyspneic with worsening heart failure. He reported weakness and inability to ambulate. Additional medical history included obstructive pulmonary disease and low back pain, for which he received intermittent steroids, including epidural injections.

Neurologic examination demonstrated that his iliopsoas strength was 3/5 right and 2/5 left, with no movement of the left foot. Muscle stretch reflexes were 2+ for the upper extremities and knees and absent at the ankles. The right toe was up-going. Within 5 days, the patient's legs became plegic. Vibratory sensation was absent in lower extremities. There was no sensory level to pinprick. The thoracic spine was tender to palpation. Rectal tone was decreased.

The patient was febrile. Sputum and blood cultures grew pseudomonas. A pacemaker precluded MRI. CT/myelography demonstrated an epidural process extending dorsally from T4 to T10, and severe stenosis especially at T8 and T9. The spinal cord was displaced anteriorly, with marked compression. The patient was taken to the operating room for decompression and possible abscess drainage. Epidural lipomatosis was diagnosed.

Epidural lipomatosis is defined as excess adipose tissue deposition posterior to the spinal cord. Rarely described in children, it occurs primarily in a thoracic (61%) and sometimes lumbar (39%) distribution but not within the cervical spine. Men are affected more than women, with an average age of 44 years (range, 18-64 years).

Pathophysiology and Etiology

Epidural fat accumulation leads to cord compression with corticospinal tract and dorsal column compromise. Venous thrombosis can be a significant part of the pathology.

Epidural lipomatosis is sometimes a rare consequence of therapeutic corticosteroids, ie, iatrogenic Cushing syndrome. The correlation between duration and dosage of steroid treatment is unknown. It can occur with prednisone dosages ranging from 5 to 180 mg/d (average, 30-100 mg/d). Epidural lipomatosis is also seen in patients who use steroid inhalers or have had epidural steroid injections. It can occur as early as 6 months or more than 10 years after initiation of steroid treatment.

Idiopathic epidural lipomatosis rarely occurs in obese patients who may or may not have concurrent hypercortisolism. An abundance of epidural fat and congenitally narrowed spinal canal are predisposing factors.

Clinical Presentation

Weakness is the most frequent (72%) symptom and finding. Progressive paraparesis sometimes develops over months. Acute irreversible paraplegia rarely occurs. Other common manifestations include low back pain (66%), radicular pain (50%), numbness/dysesthesias (50%), and changes in muscle stretch reflexes (50%). Lumbar radiculopathy, cauda equina syndrome, and neurogenic claudication are other manifestations.

Diagnosis and Treatment

Extraaxial tumors, epidural abscess, epidural hematoma, and other rare extrinsic compressive processes should be considered.

MRI is the study of choice, especially noting the unique signal characteristics of fat. When MRI cannot be performed, CT/myelogram demonstrates complete block in 69% of patients.

Weight loss and discontinuation or reduction of steroid dose are the primary medical modalities. Sometimes, a multilevel laminectomy with debulking of lipid tissue is the operative mainstay. The choice of medical versus surgical management is based on the severity of the clinical picture, possibility for reversing the causative mechanism, and the potential for surgical complications. Surgical intervention is associated with high morbidity and mortality.

INTRADURAL EXTRAMEDULLARY SPINAL CORD LESIONS
Meningioma

Clinical Vignette

A 43-year-old woman had a history of numbness and cold sensation in her right leg for several months. She did not perceive pain in her right leg when she cut it while shaving. She believed that her tennis game was slipping. Her medical history was otherwise unremarkable.

Initial neurologic examination results were normal. At follow-up 6 weeks later, the patient's examination demonstrated reduced light touch, pin, and temperature sensation to a level of T12 on the right side. Her position and vibration senses were intact. Her strength, gait, and reflexes were normal.

MRI demonstrated a thoracic meningioma on the left at T5-6 that was intradural and extramedullary. The spinal cord was markedly thinned. Surgical resection of the meningioma led to rapid and full recovery.

Spinal cord meningiomas comprise more than 25% of primary spinal cord tumors, although they are less common than intracranial meningiomas (Table 61-2). Most are intradural. They can be located ventrally, dorsally, or laterally to the cord.

Pathophysiology and Etiology

Typically, corticospinal tract dysfunction is the most prominent feature of cord compression secondary to tumor. As the tumor enlarges, spinothalamic tract and dorsal column compromise become evident. Localized radicular pain can occur secondary to mass effect with resul-

CHRONIC MYELOPATHIES

Table 61-2
Chronic Intradural Extramedullary Spinal Cord Lesions

Meningioma
Schwannoma
Neurofibroma
Arteriovenous malformation

tant traction on the nerve roots adjacent to the meningioma.

Spinal cord meningiomas have the same histologic classification as intracranial meningiomas and can become densely calcific. Meningothelial (syncytial), psammomatous, transitional, and fibroblastic meningiomas are seen; meningotheliomatous meningiomas are the most frequent.

Clinical Presentation

Individuals in their fourth to seventh decades of life are most commonly affected by meningiomas, although meningiomas can occur at any age. Their incidence in women is greater than in men. The thoracic cord is the most frequent site (approximately 80% of cases). Occasionally the cervical cord is involved, sometimes at the level of the foramen magnum. Meningiomas rarely occur at the lumbar level. Localized radicular pain may antedate other symptoms. Weakness, sensory loss, bladder and bowel dysfunction, and gait difficulty occur.

Spasticity, hyperreflexia, and Babinski signs ipsilateral to the lesion characterize corticospinal tract involvement. Ipsilateral loss of proprioception may occur from dorsal column involvement. When the spinothalamic tract is affected, contralateral pain and temperature loss are produced. If all these modalities are affected, it is called *Brown-Sequard syndrome*, indicating a hemicord lesion (Figure 61-3).

Diagnosis

Intradural extramedullary spinal tumors include meningiomas, schwannomas, and neurofibromas. Ependymomas can affect the filum terminale. Other spinal cord tumor categories include extradural and intradural intramedullary lesions (Table 61-3 and Figure 61-4). Additional diagnoses in the differential are multiple sclerosis, spinal dural AVMs, B_{12} deficiency, central disc herniation (Figure 61-5), and syringomyelia.

MRI provides an excellent means to diagnose intradural extramedullary lesions. Meningiomas enhance homogeneously with gadolinium. Axial MRI can determine whether the tumor is circumferential. MRI should be performed to the foramen magnum because initial false sensory localizing signs and apparent low thoracic le-

Table 61-3
Intradural Intramedullary Chronic Spinal Cord Lesions

Type	Examples
Congenital or acquired	Syringomyelia Hydromyelia
Genetic	Hereditary spastic paraparesis Friedreich ataxia Adrenomyeloneuropathy
Neurodegenerative	Amyotrophic lateral sclerosis Primary lateral sclerosis
Infectious	HTLV-I HIV Syphilis Tuberculosis Schistosomiasis Other bacteria, viruses, and fungi
Inflammatory	Multiple sclerosis Sjögren syndrome Sarcoidosis Systemic lupus erythematosus
Neoplasms	Ependymoma Astrocytoma Hemangioblastoma Metastasis
Vascular	Cavernous malformation
Nutritional	Vitamin B_{12}, cobalamin deficiency (subacute combined degeneration)
Toxic	Lathyrism Konzo Radiation Intrathecal chemotherapy

CHRONIC MYELOPATHIES

Figure 61-3 **Incomplete Spinal Cord Syndromes**

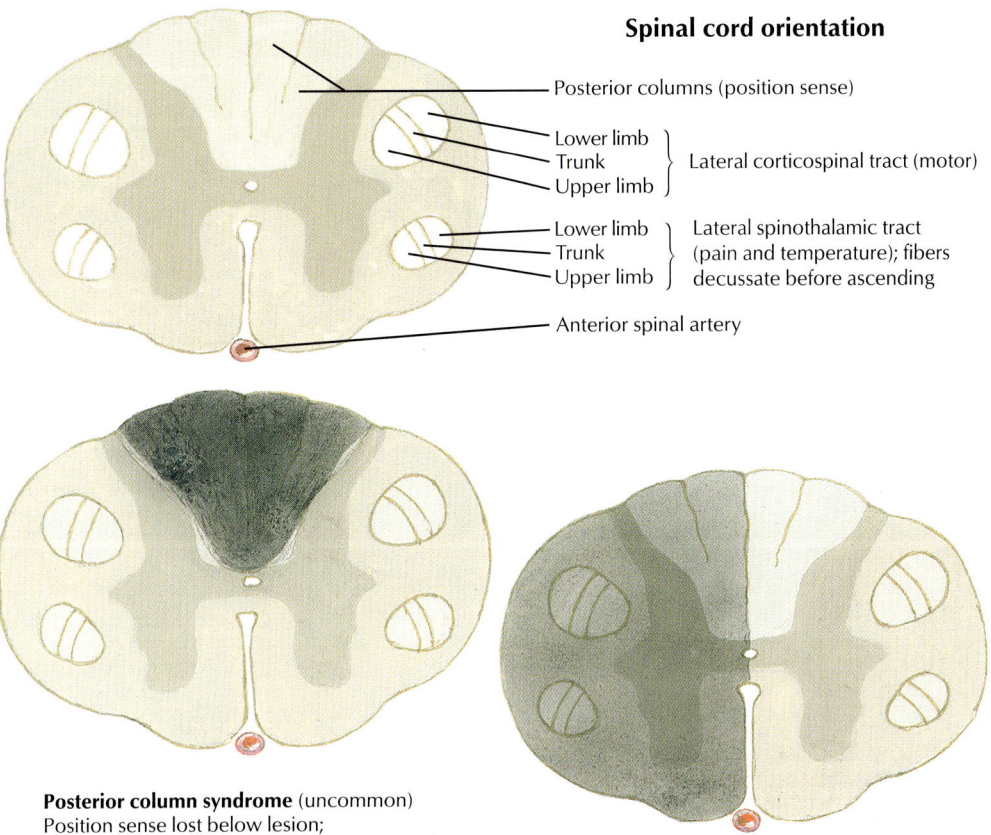

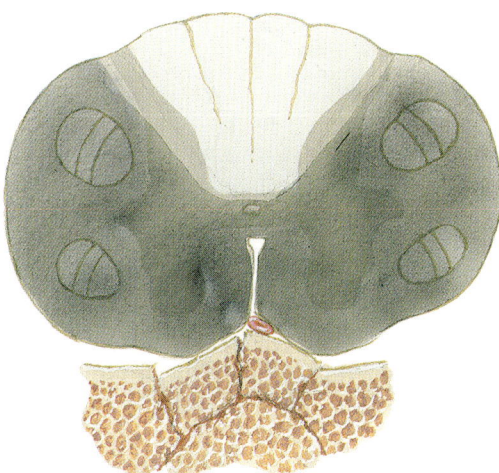

Anterior spinal artery syndrome
Artery damaged by bone or cartilage spicules (shaded area affected); bilateral loss of motor function and pain sensation below injured segment; position sense preserved

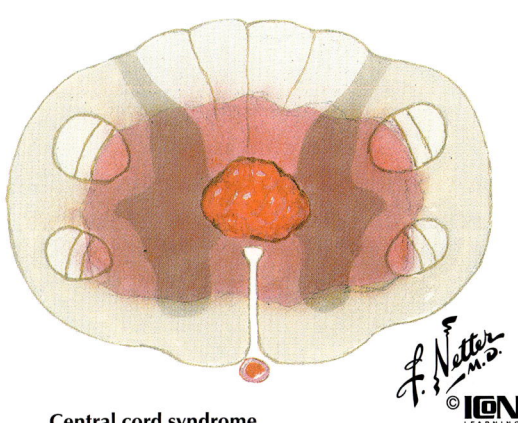

Central cord syndrome
Central cord hemorrhage and edema; parts of 3 main tracts involved on both sides; upper limbs more affected than lower limbs

MYELOPATHIES

CHRONIC MYELOPATHIES

Figure 61-4 Myelographic and CT Characteristics of Spinal Tumors

Extradural tumors

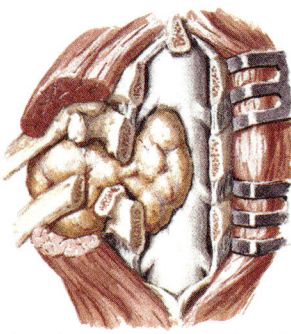

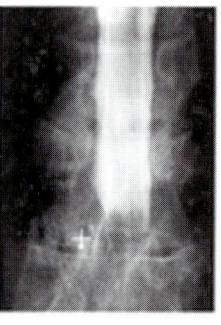

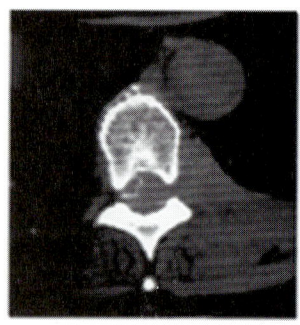

Lymphoma invading spinal canal via intervertebral foramen, compressing dura mater and spinal cord

Frontal (left) and lateral (right) metrizamide myelograms show complete obstruction just above T6-7. Spinal cord displaced forward and to right, with similar displacement of arachnoid, which suggests that mass is extradural.

CT scan more graphically displays left and posteriorly situated soft-tissue mass within spinal canal and its extension through left intervertebral foramen. Absence of bony involvement confirmed.

Intradural extramedullary tumors

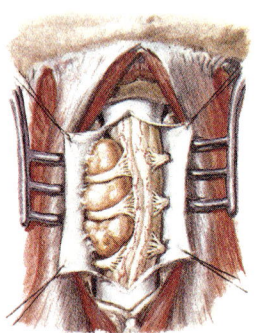

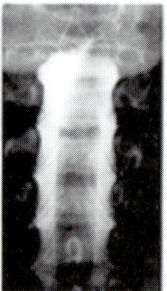

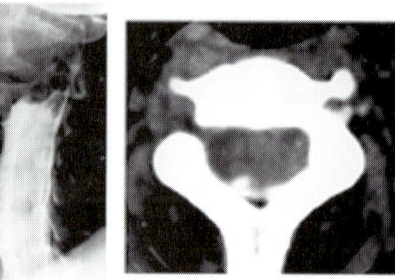

Meningioma compressing spinal cord and distorting nerve roots

Frontal (left), lateral (center), and oblique (right) metrizamide myelograms show right lateral displacement of spinal cord and complete obstruction. Frontal view shows injection from above; lateral and oblique views show inferior margin of intradural mass, separate from spinal cord, defined by injection from below.

CT scan at C2 shows only small amount of contrast medium posteriorly. Tumor is more dense than spinal cord, which is displaced to right and severely deformed and compressed.

Intramedullary tumors

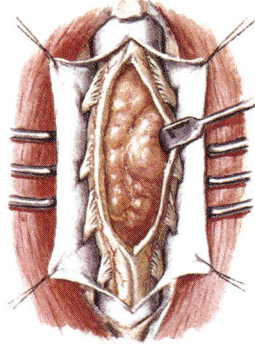

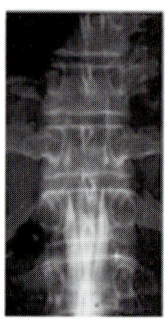

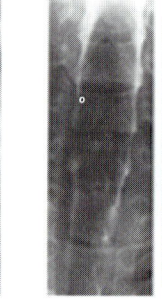

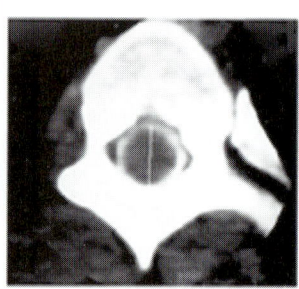

Astrocytoma exposed by longitudinal incision in bulging spinal cord

Frontal (left) and lateral (right) metrizamide myelograms with injection from below show high-grade stenosis caused by nearly symmetric expansion of spinal cord beginning at T12.

Myelogram with injection from above shows extension of tumor to upper cervical level.

CT scan of lower thoracic region showing rounded, expanded spinal cord that is nearly twice normal sagittal diameter

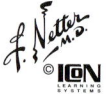

CHRONIC MYELOPATHIES

Figure 61-5 — Cervical Disc Herniation

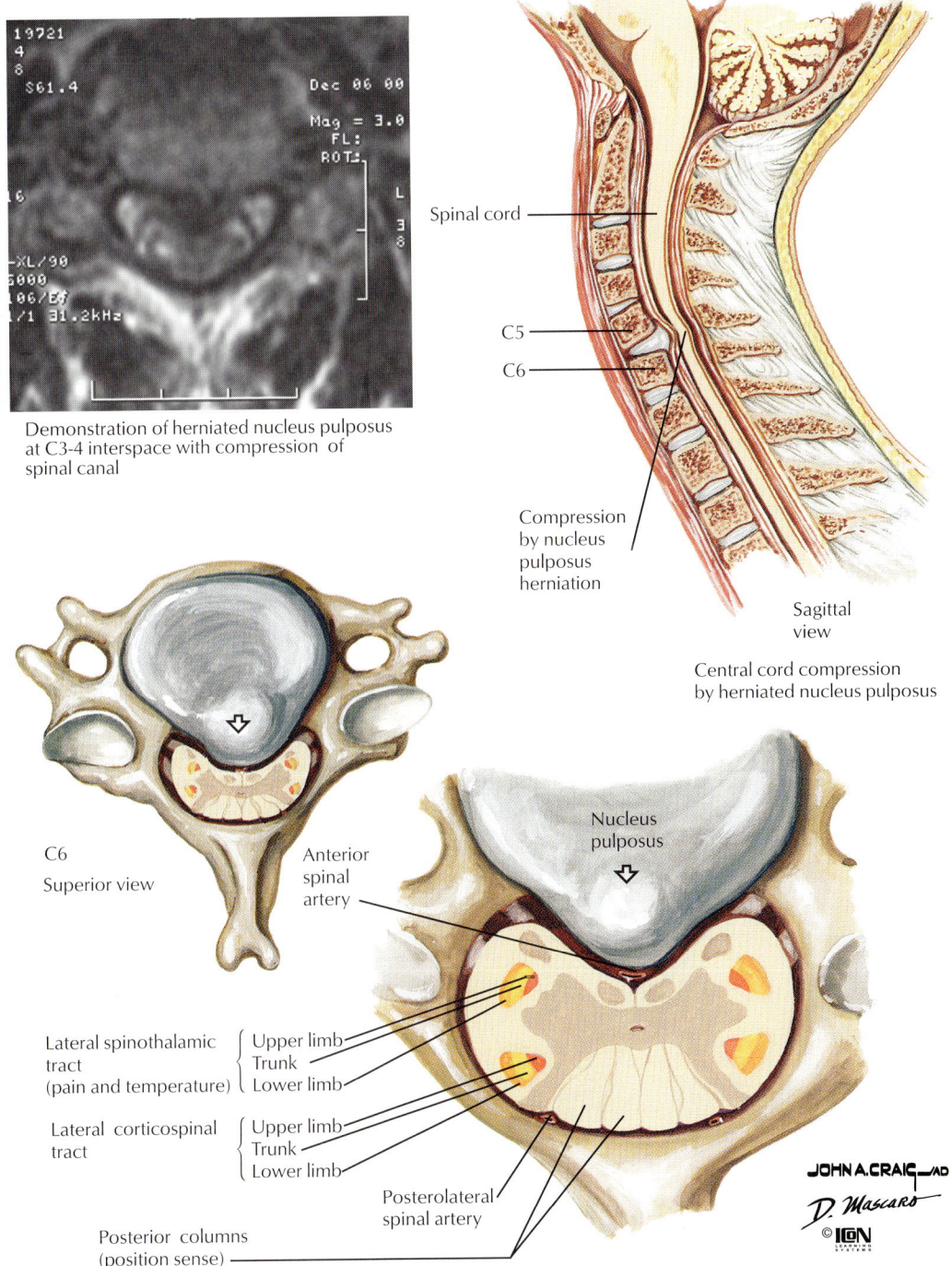

MYELOPATHIES

sions may later be found situated higher in the canal. CT/myelography helps to evaluate for partial or complete block and assess tumor calcification, but is not commonly used. Plain spine films may demonstrate erosion of a pedicle or articular process by the meningioma and intraspinal calcification.

Treatment and Prognosis

The majority of meningiomas can be successfully resected surgically. Radiation therapy may be administered in cases of early recurrence or limited surgical resection.

Prognosis is often good with surgery, particularly when the lesion is diagnosed at an early stage. Most meningiomas are benign, slow growing, and well circumscribed. Patients have particularly good functional results with improved motor and sensory deficits and variable bladder function. Postoperative mortality is low. CSF leakage is a potential complication. The tumor recurs in a minority of patients. Negative prognostic factors include old age, severe neurologic deficits, long duration of symptoms before diagnosis, subtotal tumor resection, and extradural extension.

INTRADURAL INTRAMEDULLARY SPINAL CORD LESIONS
Syringomyelia

Clinical Vignette

A 43-year-old man noted a 5-year history of numbness beginning in the left upper quadrant of his abdomen with a patch of sensory loss under his rib. Thereafter, he noted diminished ability to discern degrees of temperature when he put his left foot into the bathtub, which, over the next 8 months, gradually spread up his entire left side, then to his right arm, and finally to his right foot. He could only safely discern water temperature by sticking his head under the shower spray.

One year before evaluation, he had a paroxysm of coughing. Suddenly, he had a peculiar feeling in his neck; concomitantly, he lost sensation in his right third to fifth fingers and his medial forearm. His wife noted that he tended to trip on his right leg when jogging. A 50-pack-year smoker, he intermittently burned his fingers with cigarettes but was not aware when this initially occurred. Previous orthopedic evaluations suggested that he had a cervical disk lesion. He used a fair amount of alcohol. There was a strong family history of diabetes mellitus.

Neurologic examination demonstrated hypoactive biceps and brachioradialis stretch reflexes, modestly brisk triceps, and very brisk knee jerks. Bilateral Babinski signs were present. Sensory examination demonstrated a dissociated pattern of loss of temperature and pain sensation on the right from C5 to T7, on the left from T5 to S5, and of both hands, the right arm and shoulder, and a "cape" over the chest and back from C5 to T2. Touch, vibration, and position sensation were normal, as were the remainder of results of a complete neurologic examination.

MRI demonstrated an intramedullary lesion with a pathologically enlarged central canal. Six years later, when the patient experienced significant weakness in his left hand and gait difficulties, a shunt was placed. His course remained stable during the next 5 years.

Syringomyelia is a rare neurologic disorder with clinical findings specific to a central cord syndrome and an incidence of 8 per 100,000 population. The clinical presentation of this vignette is characteristic of an intramedullary central canal syndrome. Insidious onset of sensory and motor symptoms predominantly affecting one or both hands is common. Subsequently, some individuals have a sudden worsening or change in symptomatology with straining or Valsalva maneuver. Clinical diagnosis is assisted by the dissociated sensory loss with loss of pain and temperature but preservation of touch, vibration, and position sense. Usually the syrinx is clinically maximal at the cervical spinal cord level; thus, the "cape" distribution is present (Figure 61-6). These findings are secondary to the expanding intramedullary lesion interrupting the crossing pain and temperature fibers before they join the contralateral spinothalamic tract.

Pathophysiology and Etiology

Typically there is a tubular cavity, ie, a syrinx, within the central spinal canal. It is thought to arise from a diverticulum directly communicating with the central canal. The syrinx maximally affects the cervical cord but often extends rostrally into the brainstem (syringobulbia) and distally sometimes almost to the lower end of the thoracic cord. As it enlarges transversely within the cord, it gradually puts pressure on the decussating pain and temperature fibers as they cross through the central gray matter and the anterior horn gray matter. Eventually, the enlarging size

CHRONIC MYELOPATHIES

Figure 61-6   ## Syringomyelia

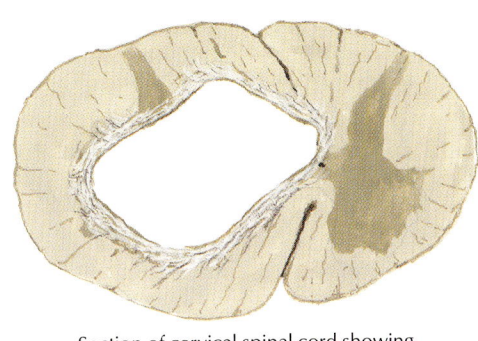

Section of cervical spinal cord showing cavity of syrinx surrounded by gliosis

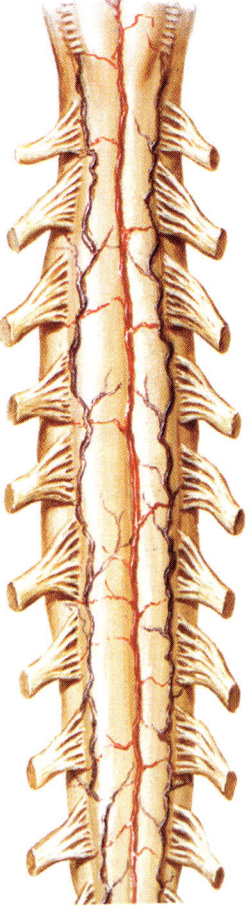

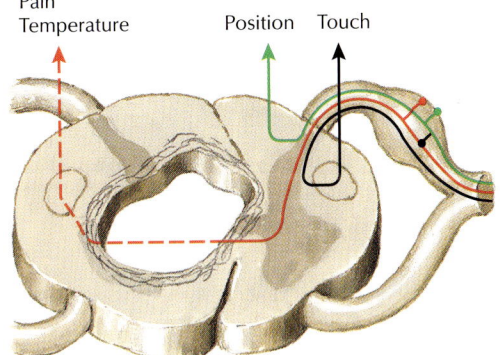

Diagram demonstrating interruption of crossed pain and temperature fibers by syrinx; uncrossed light touch and proprioception fibers preserved

Bulging of spinal cord due to syrinx

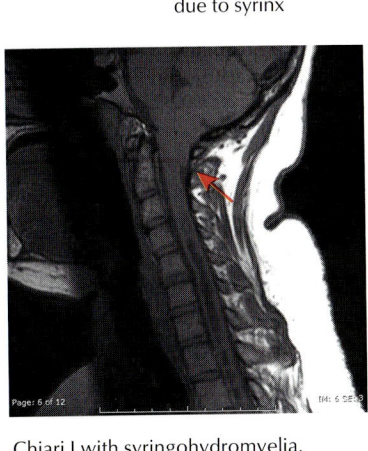

Chiari I with syringohydromyelia. Sagittal T1-weighted image shows deformity of the cerebellar tonsils, which extend below the posterior arch of C1 (thin arrow), and irregular central cord cavity extends from C3-4 into the thoracic region.

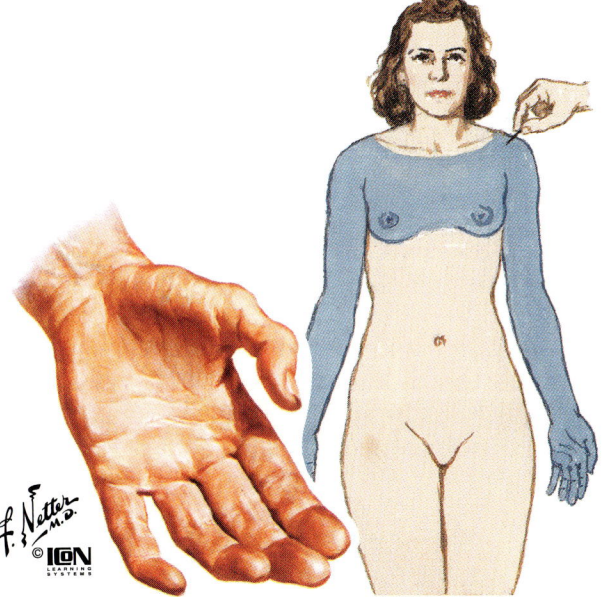

Atrophy of hand muscles due to neurotrophic deficit

Capelike distribution of pain and temperature sensation loss

MYELOPATHIES

of the syrinx also affects the corticospinal tracts in the lateral funiculus and posterior columns, modifying proprioception function.

Although no specific pathophysiologic mechanism is recognized, certain concomitant findings suggest a congenital origin. For example, the Arnold-Chiari malformation frequently accompanies a syrinx, typically with an extension of the cerebellar tonsils below the foramen magnum. Rarely, a syrinx develops after spinal trauma, possibly by creation of a central hematomyelia. Rare intramedullary neoplasms such as ependymomas or astrocytomas may lead to central canal obstruction and the development of a secondary syrinx.

Clinical Presentation

Classic symptoms and findings include dissociated sensory loss, preferentially affecting pain, and temperature modalities in a cape distribution at the cervical level, concomitant with distal upper extremity muscle weakness and atrophy. Eventually, with cavity enlargement, corticospinal and dorsal column function is affected.

Temporal profile of clinical progression varies from an insidiously evolving lesion to episodes of sudden worsening. Occasionally, the loss of pain sensation leads to a Charcot joint in the shoulder or arm. Another unusual complication is the development of a severe cervical kyphoscoliosis secondary to anterior horn cell damage affecting the appendicular musculature and paraspinal muscles.

Diagnosis

Differential diagnoses include amyotrophic lateral sclerosis, ulnar or median neuropathy or both, a medial brachial plexus lesion such as occurs secondary to a Pancoast tumor, and a primary spinal intramedullary neoplasm. When intrinsic hand muscle atrophy is an early sign, an anterior horn cell process or a specific peripheral mononeuropathy should be considered.

MRI is the diagnostic modality of choice. CT/myelography is also useful when MRI is contraindicated. EMG is indicated if the MRI is normal.

Treatment and Prognosis

Decompression of the frequently accompanying cerebellar tonsillar herniation may sometimes be sufficient. If there is no Arnold-Chiari lesion, sometimes a syringotomy is performed, providing a communication to drain fluid from the self-contained central canal/syrinx to the subarachnoid space.

Within 2 decades, approximately 50% of patients become wheelchair bound. Some patients have a rapidly evolving course and become quadriplegic within 10 years. Factors explaining the disparity in clinical progression are not well appreciated, increasing the difficulty of counseling recently diagnosed patients with relatively mild compromise.

Hereditary Spastic Paraplegia

Clinical Vignette

A 25-year-old man who jogged short distances daily began to trip over pavement and uneven surfaces. His jogging became slower and more labored over the course of a year. Eventually, he stopped running completely. On examination, he had a slightly broad-based, spastic gait, hyperreflexia with ankle clonus, and bilateral Babinski signs. He was adopted and had no knowledge of family medical history.

Hereditary spastic paraplegia is a genetically and clinically heterogeneous condition characterized by progressive lower extremity spastic weakness. Additional neurologic or nonneurologic features can be associated. Commonly, patients notice physical limitations secondary to these hereditary processes. Sometimes, patients note spontaneous clonus.

Pathophysiology and Etiology

Axonal degeneration of the distal ends of long axons in the spinal cord occurs. Corticospinal tract and dorsal column involvement cause motor and sensory findings, respectively.

The condition is genetically heterogeneous with autosomal dominant, autosomal recessive, and X-linked inheritance. Multiple genes and loci have been identified. The SPG4 gene encodes spastin. Mutations in SPG4 account for approximately 40% of autosomal dominant hereditary spastic paraplegia cases. This is the most common form of hereditary spastic paraplegia and is linked to chromosome 2p. It is thought that spastin located within the cytoplasm interacts with microtubules. Another gene, SPG3, encodes atlastin. The genetic basis for this disease entity continues to expand as more kinds are identified and new loci and genes are discovered for other autosomal dominant, recessive, and X-linked forms.

Clinical Presentation

Progressive lower extremity weakness and spasticity are the main findings of hereditary spastic paraplegia. The age at onset and the severity of symptoms may vary widely within a given family. The pure or uncomplicated form is more common than the complicated form. The pure form is characterized by spastic gait, increased muscle tone in the lower extremities, increased muscle stretch reflexes, and Babinski signs. Vibratory sensation and sphincter disturbances are sometimes mildly decreased. The complicated form can include other neurologic and nonneurologic impairments: cognitive impairment, mental retardation, aphasia, dysarthria, dysphagia, optic disk pallor, nystagmus, cataracts, upper extremity weakness, motor neuronopathy, amyotrophy, cerebellar or cerebral atrophy, hydrocephalus, white matter changes, thin corpus callosum, bladder and bowel dysfunction, and gastroesophageal reflux.

Diagnosis and Treatment

The differential diagnosis includes multiple sclerosis, primary lateral sclerosis, HTLV-I myelopathy, B_{12} deficiency, intrinsic or extrinsic cord tumor, dural AVM, and leukodystrophies. Positive family history is the most important diagnostic clue. Genetic screening is possible for some forms. Other laboratory studies such as the C26:C22 long-chain fatty acid analysis for X-linked adrenoleukodystrophy may be useful, especially when the mother may be the carrier.

MRI may demonstrate severe spinal atrophy. Other causes of spastic paraparesis are excluded by performing brain and spinal MRI and a CSF examination, especially in the absence of a family history.

Treatment is supportive. No treatment prevents, reverses, or slows the underlying disease process.

HTLV-I Myelopathy

Clinical Vignette

A 52-year-old man had a 6-year history of low back pain. Four years previously, right leg weakness and bilateral leg spasms had developed. The next year, he became impotent, experienced nocturnal incontinence, and required catheterization for a neurogenic bladder. He underwent an L5-S1 laminectomy for a degenerative disc. Subsequently, his right leg weakness worsened, and right leg numbness developed. He reported his right leg dragging when he walked, difficulty with stairs, and recent numbness in both hands.

Abnormalities on neurologic examination included bilateral iliopsoas weakness, spastic gait, inability to perform tandem gait, and reduced vibratory and pinprick sensation with a sensory level at T6. Muscle stretch reflexes were brisk, more in the lower extremities, and he had a left Babinski sign.

MRI of the patient's entire neuroaxis was normal except for signs of the L5-S1 laminectomy. Routine laboratory values, including serum HTLV-I, were unremarkable. However, CSF studies showed HTLV-I antibodies by enzyme-linked immunosorbent assay and Western blot analysis. It also showed oligoclonal bands; normal cell count, glucose, protein, and IgG/total protein ratio; and negative culture, cytology, and VDRL results.

First described in 1956, a syndrome of chronic progressive myelopathy with spastic paraparesis and sensory and bladder disturbance was renamed *tropical spastic paraparesis/HTLV-I myelopathy* with the 1985 discovery of antibodies to HTLV-I. The preceding vignette is characteristic of patients with HTLV-I myelopathy, although symptoms were initially attributed to disc disease. Because of its subtle onset, the diagnosis may not be considered. Travel history is essential because many patients acquire this sexually transmitted disease while in the Caribbean, where HTLV-I is endemic.

Pathophysiology and Etiology

The mid to lower thoracic cord is most severely affected. Loss of myelin and axons occurs predominantly in the lateral columns and the corticospinal tracts, although the posterior and anterior columns are also affected. Relevant inflammatory changes can extend, involving the entire cord. Milder lesions are scattered in the brain. Generally, areas of slow blood flow are preferentially involved. The cord may become atrophic, and the meninges may become fibrous and thick.

HTLV-I is a type C oncovirus in the Retroviridae family. It occurs in geographic clusters throughout the world. It is endemic in the Caribbean, eastern South America, equatorial Africa, and southern Japan. Transmission is via semen, blood or blood products, breast milk, and shared needles of parenteral drug abusers. Blood transfusion is the most effective mode of transmission, with 40% to 60% seroconversion within 2 months.

Of HTLV-I carriers, approximately 5% are at lifetime risk for development of the disease. Those with a higher proviral load are at greatest risk. Typically, the time from infection to disease development is years to decades, although it is shorter in children and recipients of HTLV-I–infected blood products.

HTLV-I proviral DNA integrates into $CD4^+$ T lymphocytes, its target cells. $CD8^+$ HTLV-I–specific cytotoxic T lymphocytes develop in affected patients. These $CD4^+$ and $CD8^+$ T lymphocytes infiltrate the parenchyma and perivascular regions. Perivascular cuffing, demyelination, astrocytic and microglial proliferation, leptomeningeal fibrosis, and neuronal loss occur by an unknown mechanism. Various inflammatory cytokines in the spinal cord tissue include increased tumor necrosis factor a, granulocyte-macrophage colony-stimulating factor, IFN-γ, and IL-β. HLA type affects risk of disease: HLA-DR1 increases risk, whereas HLA-A2 lowers risk. Over time, the initially inflammatory response becomes less inflammatory and more degenerative.

Clinical Presentation

Estimates suggest that 10 to 20 million people worldwide are infected, but most are asymptomatic carriers. Onset is usually between the ages of 35 and 45 years but can occur at much younger or older ages. Women are affected more than men.

The course is slowly progressive. Affected individuals develop a spastic paraparesis that can progress to paraplegia. Hyperreflexia, clonus, and Babinski signs are present. Numbness and paresthesias of the lower extremities and trunk as well as low back pain may occur. Vibratory and position senses can be affected. Bladder disturbance (frequency, urgency, incontinence), impotence, and later constipation develop. Rarely, optic atrophy, deafness, ataxia, hand tremor, or nystagmus occurs.

HTLV-I also causes a broad clinical spectrum of other neurologic disease, including meningitis, encephalopathy, cranial and peripheral neuropathies, and polymyositis. Associated systemic disorders include adult T-cell leukemia/lymphoma, uveitis, infective dermatitis, sicca syndrome, alveolitis, arthritis, and thyroiditis.

Diagnosis

Differential considerations are broad, including any process leading to thoracic myelopathy. Multiple sclerosis and vitamin B_{12} deficiency are frequent considerations. A history of living many years ago in an endemic area where sexual contact with an HTLV-I–infected person may have occurred can be helpful.

Most affected individuals are seropositive for HTLV-I antibodies in the serum and CSF. Enzyme-linked immunosorbent assay test results are then confirmed by recombinant Western blot. CSF may include a mild pleocytosis, increased protein, and increased IgG, with oligoclonal band positivity. MRI sometimes reveals an atrophic cord, and brain MRI sometimes shows white matter lesions, similar to those in multiple sclerosis.

Treatment and Prognosis

No effective treatment exists for HTLV-I–related tropical spastic paraparesis/HTLV-I myelopathy. Response to glucocorticoids varies and may occur early in the disease. Treatment is primarily symptomatic with antispasticity agents, physical therapy, and bladder catheterization. HTLV-I carriers who are asymptomatic can transmit the virus. Screening blood products, adjusting sexual practices, and using formula rather than breast milk for infants of infected mothers can reduce transmission.

The disease is insidious and progresses slowly over decades. Eventually, affected individuals become wheelchair bound with paraplegia and neurogenic bladder. Hand function may also eventually become impaired.

AIDS-Associated Vacuolar Myelopathy

Vacuolar myelopathy associated with AIDS occurs late in the course of HIV infection. Earlier onset of coexistent neurologic conditions including dementia and peripheral neuropathy may detract from the diagnosis. The incidence in patients with AIDS is unknown.

Pathophysiology and Etiology

Thoracic cord white matter is primarily involved. There is vacuolization of the lateral and posterior columns; the anterior and anterolateral columns are less affected. Wallerian degeneration of the corticospinal tracts and posterior columns also occurs. Vacuolization increases over time, and more cord segments become involved, although the process is confined to white matter.

The etiology is unknown. Macrophage secretion of cytokines that damage the cord and a metabolic disorder of the B_{12}-dependent transmethylation pathway are among the theories postulated.

Clinical Presentation

HIV-associated vacuolar myelopathy occurs in the later stages of this systemic illness. Patients usually present with slowly progressive leg weakness, spasticity, gait disorder, and painless sensory changes, including vibratory and position sense impairment and sensory ataxia. If paresthesias are present, patients may have a coexistent peripheral neuropathy. Additionally, bladder and bowel dysfunction and impotence in men can develop. Arms and hands are usually uninvolved or minimally affected because the thoracic cord is the primary pathologic site. Rarely, an acute transverse myelitis occurs at the time of HIV seroconversion but is a different entity.

Diagnosis

Intrinsic cord disease and extramedullary lesion with compression are the main differential considerations. Infectious causes of cord disease, some of them opportunistic, include cytomegalovirus, herpes simplex virus, varicella-zoster virus, toxoplasmosis, tuberculosis, syphilis, and HTLV-I. Neoplasms, particularly lymphoma and B_{12} or folate deficiency, should also be considered.

HIV vacuolar myelopathy is a diagnosis of exclusion. MRI cord imaging with and without gadolinium help to exclude a mass, focal enhancement, abnormal cord signal, cord enlargement, or atrophy. Focal cord enlargement suggests lymphoma or toxoplasmosis. The cord may appear normal or mildly atrophic. The cord signal may or may not be increased.

Brain imaging augments cord imaging information. Serologies and CSF studies help to exclude other causes of myelopathy. CSF may have slight pleocytosis and protein increases. Vacuolar myelopathy may be difficult to distinguish from HIV myelitis. Myelitis is less common and is usually seen concomitant with HIV encephalitis.

Treatment and Prognosis

Treatment is supportive. Antispasticity agents, treatment of sphincter dysfunction, and physical therapy are the treatment mainstays. Antiretroviral drugs do not clearly improve symptoms or slow myelopathy.

AIDS-associated vacuolar myelopathy is slowly progressive. Patients sometimes progress to wheelchair dependence and double incontinence.

Vitamin B_{12} Deficiency

Clinical Vignette

A 72-year-old man presented with distal paresthesias, more pronounced in his hands than in his feet, unsteady gait, and frequent falls. His family noted some memory loss of unclear duration.

On examination, he was oriented to self and place but not to month or year. He immediately registered 3 items, but recalled only 1 item at 5 minutes with clues provided. Visual acuity was poor. On motor examination, he had 4/5 lower extremity strength. His gait was broad based, spastic, and ataxic. Romberg sign was positive. He had loss of vibratory sense in the legs, absent position sense in toes, and hyperesthesia to pinprick in distal extremities. Muscle stretch reflexes were normoactive. Babinski signs were present. The patient's hematocrit was 29%, with a mean corpuscular volume of 112 μm^3. Vitamin B_{12} level was 34 (reference range, >190 pg/mL).

Vitamin B_{12}, or cobalamin, deficiency causes neurologic and hematologic difficulties. Megaloblastic anemia, myelopathy, and peripheral neuropathy are cardinal features; rarely, there is cognitive impairment. The degrees of neurologic and hematologic abnormalities do not always correlate.

Pathophysiology and Etiology

Vitamin B_{12} deficiency is called *subacute combined degeneration of the spinal cord* or *combined system disease*. White matter degeneration of the cord is characteristic and occasionally affects the brain. Symmetric loss of myelin, particularly in the posterior and lateral columns, exceeds the coexistent axonal damage. Typically, the process begins in the posterior columns at the cervical thoracic junction, spreading laterally, anteriorly, inferiorly, and superiorly. Peripheral nerve involvement with myelin loss also occurs, although cord involvement is the more significant component. Vitamin B_{12} deficiency causes these pathologic changes.

Appropriate laboratory testing makes earlier diagnosis common, so clinical evidence of demyelination in the cerebral white matter and optic nerves is unusual.

Impaired vitamin B_{12} absorption most commonly results from the autoimmune-mediated pernicious anemia. Rarely, B_{12} deficiency is a component of a postgastrectomy syndrome or a deficient diet (vegetarians).

Clinical Presentation

Although most patients with pernicious anemia do not have signs of neurologic sequelae, some occasionally present with a neurologic syndrome and minimal hematologic abnormalities. Distal paresthesias from peripheral nerve damage are often presenting symptoms, particularly in the hands. Loss of vibratory sensation, abnormal joint position sense, sensory ataxia, and a positive Romberg sign correlate with posterior column damage (Figure 61-7). Lower extremity weakness and spasticity, with later upper extremity involvement, reflect corticospinal tract damage. Muscle stretch reflexes can be increased or decreased depending on whether a peripheral neuropathy coexists with the myelopathy. Memory loss, confusion, paranoia, irritability, and hallucinations rarely occur.

Diagnosis

Carpal tunnel syndrome may be the initial diagnosis because of hand paresthesias. HIV vacuolar myelopathy also requires consideration because the posterolateral cord is the main involved site. Peripheral neuropathy and dementia may also be comorbid AIDS complications.

Megaloblastic anemia is an important clue to the diagnosis. However, because some patients have few or no hematologic abnormalities, awareness of the clinical syndrome is important. Diagnosis is straightforward when vitamin B_{12} levels are low. When B_{12} levels are normal or only slightly abnormal, increases of methylmalonic acid and homocysteine are important indicators of cobalamin deficiency.

Treatment and Prognosis

Replenishment of vitamin B_{12} (parenteral 1000 μg monthly) can reverse the disorder. Oral supplementation is insufficient. Hematologic abnormalities improve more rapidly than neurologic ones, although clinical changes can be dramatic over weeks to months.

Prognosis for neurologic recovery is best with early diagnosis. The course is progressive and can be fatal without treatment.

FRIEDREICH ATAXIA

Clinical Vignette

A 12-year-old girl presented with difficulty running and standing stationary and frequent stumbling. General examination demonstrated scoliosis and pes cavus. On neurologic examination, the patient had truncal and gait ataxia, a positive Romberg sign, areflexia, and extensor plantar responses. EMG demonstrated absent sensory nerve action potentials (SNAPs) but was otherwise normal.

Friedreich ataxia is an autosomal recessive neurodegenerative condition characterized by progressive ataxia. The disease affects the posterior columns, lateral corticospinal tracts, dorsal and ventral spinocerebellar tracts, dorsal roots and ganglia, and peripheral nerves, causing a combination sensory and cerebellar ataxia.

CHRONIC MYELOPATHIES

Figure 61-7

Subacute Combined Degeneration

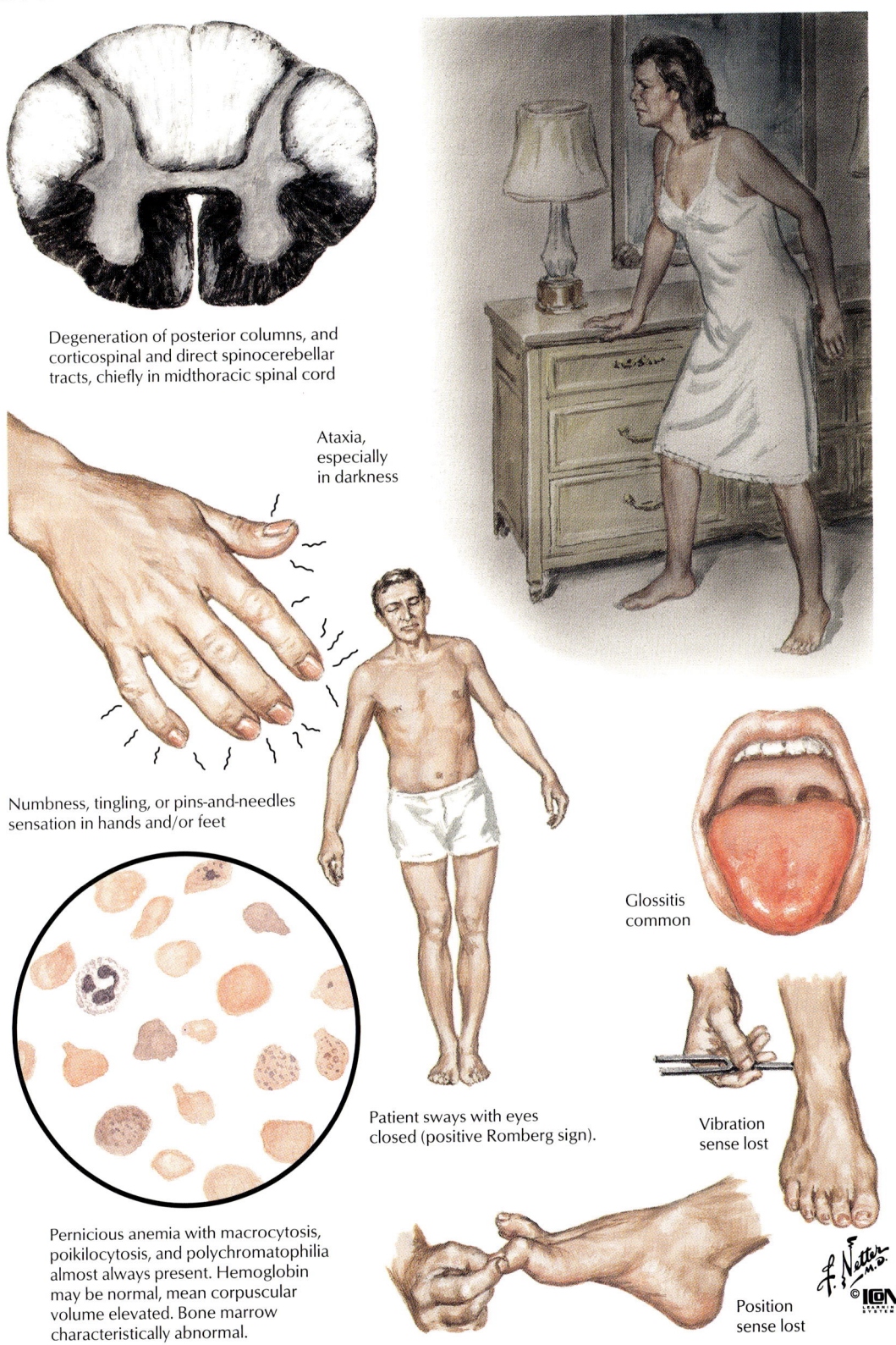

Degeneration of posterior columns, and corticospinal and direct spinocerebellar tracts, chiefly in midthoracic spinal cord

Ataxia, especially in darkness

Numbness, tingling, or pins-and-needles sensation in hands and/or feet

Glossitis common

Patient sways with eyes closed (positive Romberg sign).

Vibration sense lost

Position sense lost

Pernicious anemia with macrocytosis, poikilocytosis, and polychromatophilia almost always present. Hemoglobin may be normal, mean corpuscular volume elevated. Bone marrow characteristically abnormal.

MYELOPATHIES

533

CHRONIC MYELOPATHIES

Pathophysiology and Etiology

The spinal cord is small from fiber loss in the corticospinal and spinocerebellar tracts. Neuronal loss also occurs in the Clarke column, the dorsal root ganglia, and especially the dentate nuclei. Compensatory gliosis follows axonal degeneration and demyelination. The heart is affected, with myocardial muscle fibers replaced by myophages and fibroblasts.

Hyperexpansion of GAA triplet repeat in the first intron of the frataxin gene interferes with gene transcription. This leads to deficiency of frataxin, a nuclear encoded mitochondrial protein, and is responsible for Friedreich ataxia in most patients. The size of the expanded repeat correlates with the severity of the phenotype. Longer repeats are associated with earlier onset and more severe disease.

Frataxin plays a role in iron homeostasis. Its deficiency leads to increased mitochondrial iron accumulation, sensitivity to oxidative stress, and free radical–mediated cell death—particularly to neurons and cardiomyocytes.

Clinical Presentation

Childhood or adolescent onset is typical in Friedreich ataxia, but onset can range from infancy far into adulthood. The earliest symptom is gait ataxia. Vibration and position sense are also compromised early. Affected individuals may stumble and have difficulty standing steadily or running. The ataxia is progressive. Hand clumsiness and dysarthria may occur months or years later. Areflexia results from peripheral nerve damage, although plantar responses are extensor because of corticospinal tract damage. Nys-

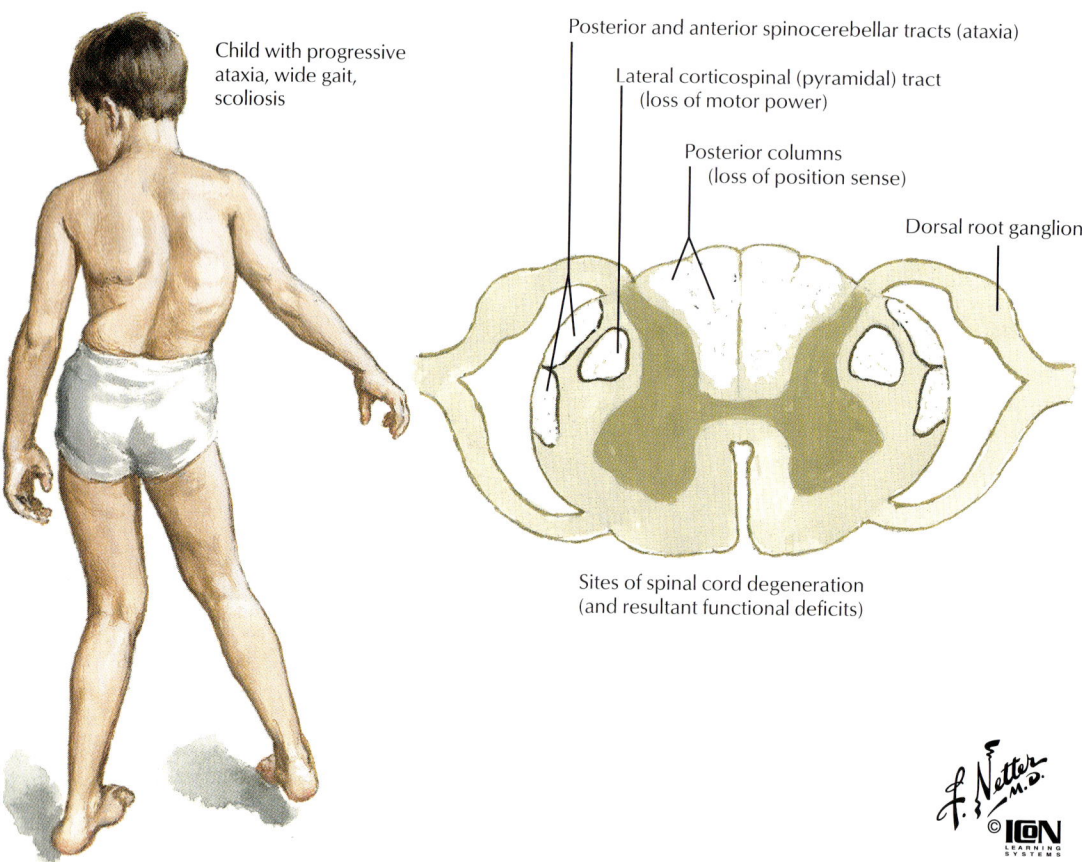

Figure 61-8   Friedreich Ataxia

tagmus, tremor, athetoid and choreiform movements, and visual and hearing loss can occur.

High-arched feet (pes cavus) and hammertoes may present at birth or later or can be a forme fruste in individuals who do not progress to full-blown disease. Scoliosis and cardiomyopathy with arrhythmia develop in most affected individuals (Figure 61-8).

Diagnosis

Diagnosis was formerly made on clinical grounds, with progressive ataxia, skeletal deformities, and cardiomyopathy being the cardinal features. The degree of scoliosis and cardiomyopathy varies in patients who present later. Genetic testing shows most affected individuals to be homozygous.

Differential diagnosis includes multiple sclerosis, hereditary spastic paraplegia, peroneal muscular atrophy, olivopontocerebellar and spinocerebellar degeneration, as well as tabes dorsalis and ataxia telangiectasia. Most of these diagnoses can be readily distinguished clinically.

Treatment and Prognosis

Affected individuals should maintain activity as long as possible. Balance training and muscle strengthening can be helpful. If bracing is inadequate, orthopedic surgery for scoliosis may be necessary. Regular orthopedic and cardiology follow-up is key. Scoliosis and cardiomyopathy treatment can prolong life. Over time, individuals may become wheelchair dependent or bed bound. Death is secondary to cardiac arrhythmia, infection, or restrictive pulmonary disease.

Antioxidants to enhance respiratory chain function and free radical scavengers are being studied. Idebenone, a short-chain analog of coenzyme Q10 with antioxidant properties has been used to treat Friedreich ataxia. Its long-term effects are yet to be determined.

REFERENCES

Bohlman HH. Cervical spondylosis and myelopathy. *Instr Course Lect.* 1995; 44:81-97.

Ferguson RJL, Caplan LR. Cervical spondylitic myelopathy. *Neurol Clin.* 1985;3:373-382.

Fink JK. The hereditary spastic paraplegias: nine genes and counting. *Arch Neurol.* 2003;60:1045-1049.

Lestini WF, Wiesel SW. The pathogenesis of cervical spondylosis. *Clin Orthop.* 1989;239:69-93.

Levin MC, Jacobson S. HTLV-1 associated myelopathy/tropical spastic paraparesis (HAM/TSP): a chronic progressive neurologic disease associated with immunologically mediated damage to the central nervous system. *J Neurovirology.* 1997;3:126-140.

Muraszko KM, Oldfield EH. Vascular malformations of the spinal cord and dura. *Neurosurg Clin North Am.* 1990;1:631–652.

Pandolfo M. Friedreich ataxia. *Semin Pediatr Neurol.* 2003;10:163-172.

Quencer RM, Donovan Post MJ. Spinal cord lesions in patients with AIDS. *Neuroimaging Clin North Am.* 1997;7:359-373.

Yasargil MG, Symon L, Teddy PJ. Arteriovenous malformations of the spinal cord. *Adv Tech Stand Neurosurg.* 1984;7:6-102.

Section XIV
MULTIPLE SCLEROSIS AND OTHER DEMYELINATING DISORDERS

Chapter 62
Multiple Sclerosis and Acute Disseminated Encephalomyelitis 538

Chapter 62
Multiple Sclerosis and Acute Disseminated Encephalomyelitis

Mary Anne Muriello, H. Royden Jones, Jr, and Claudia J. Chaves

MULTIPLE SCLEROSIS

Multiple sclerosis (MS) is one of the most common etiologies for chronic neurologic dysfunction in young and middle-aged adults. Advances in other areas of science have generated diagnostic tools and treatments that have revealed detailed data about the nature of MS. MRI technology is probably responsible for the greatest change in patterns of diagnosis. The study of immunomodulatory interventions has improved treatment and understanding of MS pathogenesis. Despite intensive research, MS remains an enigma.

Epidemiologic studies suggest that MS is more prevalent in northern latitudes, more common in women, and most often recognized during the third and fourth decades of life. Prevalence in women is almost twice that in men. In the US, whites are twice as likely as nonwhites to acquire MS. Genetic factors alone cannot account for this variability, because genetically comparable populations vary in MS prevalence depending on place of birth and age of migration. Race- and age-matched individuals born in a northern region assume the risk of equatorial regions if they move there before the age of 15 years. Persons who do not move north to south until after 15 years of age retain the higher risk of the northern region. These observations are consistent; nevertheless, genetic factors undoubtedly also exert some influence on susceptibility.

Genetic Factors

Although heritability of MS does not conform to any straightforward pattern, disease clusters occur within families. The risk of MS in a first-degree relative of an affected individual (estimated at 1 in 500-1000) is approximately 20 times that in the general population. Of patients with MS, 10% to 15% have at least 1 affected first-degree relative, but the risk is not much different for parent-child relationships than for sibling relationships, thus negating typical dominant, recessive, or sex-linked inheritance. The risk of MS in first-degree relatives is never greater than 5%, except in monozygotic twins, where concordance rates are approximately 25%.

Comparison of concordance rates between half-siblings reared together and those reared apart showed no significant difference, suggesting that environment does not account for the slightly higher rate of MS in half-siblings of affected persons. Furthermore, it did not matter whether the shared biologic parent was the mother or the father, arguing against a mitochondrial inheritance pattern. Hence, it is unlikely that any single gene is responsible for conferring susceptibility; a polygenic mode of transmission is assumed.

Pathology

Because the disease process has such protean manifestations and a variable course, demyelinating disorders have a broad clinical spectrum, ranging from a single benign episode to one that is potentially fatal. With classic MS, the primary process is one of **demyelination** leading to loss of myelin from CNS axons. **Myelin loss** (a nonspecific term) occurs concurrently with other pathologic processes that also affect the vasculature, glial elements, or axons.

CNS oligodendrocytes are responsible for the elaboration of brain myelin. Myelin is predominantly lipid based (70%), and the remainder is protein based. One part, myelin basic protein, is

MULTIPLE SCLEROSIS AND ACUTE DISSEMINATED ENCEPHALOMYELITIS

particularly immunologically susceptible and experimentally encephalitogenic.

Inspection of the gross brain does not suggest any sign of abnormalities that indicate the myriad microscopic histologic changes. However the optic nerves, optic chiasm, and spinal cord may be atrophic. Sometimes, areas of patchy demyelination are seen on the basis pontis surface, the cerebellar peduncles, and the surface of the medulla and floor of the fourth ventricle.

Coronal brain sections reveal changes similar to those noted on MRI, where variously sized MS plaques are apparent. Recently acquired lesions are pink and soft, whereas chronic MS lesions are gray, translucent, and firm (Figure 62-1). It is often difficult to correlate the multiple lesions found at autopsy or by MRI throughout the neuraxis with a patient's history. Sometimes classic MS plaques exist in patients who were never clinically suspected of harboring it.

Figure 62-1 **Multiple Sclerosis: Central Nervous System Pathology**

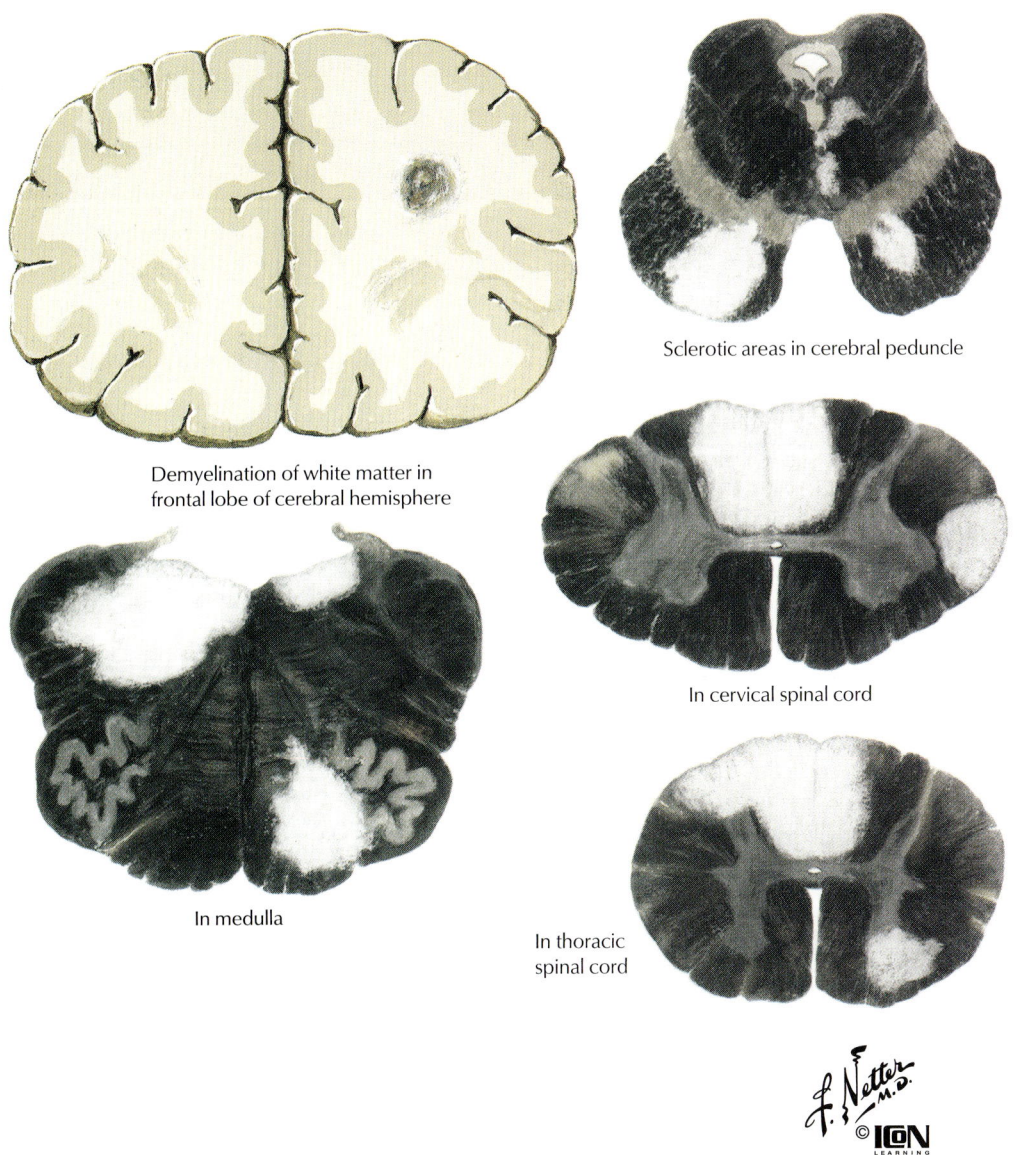

Demyelination of white matter in frontal lobe of cerebral hemisphere

Sclerotic areas in cerebral peduncle

In cervical spinal cord

In medulla

In thoracic spinal cord

MULTIPLE SCLEROSIS AND OTHER DEMYELINATING DISORDERS

Microscopic analysis demonstrates that many plaques have no relation to specific nerve tracts. Often, the plaques have a perivenular and paraventricular distribution frequently seen in the optic nerves, optic tracts, and spinal cord. Myelin loss from a nerve fiber is distinct and best defined by toluidine blue stains. Macrophage accumulation is a frequent accompaniment. Active plaques contain myelin debris. Severe loss of oligodendrocytes within MS plaques is associated with the concomitant nonspecific finding of hypertrophic astrocytes. Signs of leptomeningeal inflammation not unlike that found in acute disseminated MS may be evident.

Subtypes

The natural history of MS varies with the subtype of disease. Functional consequences may relate to some degree of axonal loss occurring after demyelination.

Benign

Clinical Vignette

A 62-year-old woman experienced a generalized tonic-clonic seizure immediately after a closed head injury. Her neurologic examination results were normal, with the exception of optic pallor confined to the temporal margin of the right optic disk.

She was otherwise healthy but recalled 2 bouts of optic neuritis at 21 and 32 years of age. On both occasions, she had complete recovery of visual acuity and no other transient or permanent sequelae until this seizure. She was neurologically asymptomatic for the next 30 years. The results of intermittent neurologic examinations had always been normal.

Because of the recent head injury and subsequent seizure, brain MRI was obtained, demonstrating 15 bilateral periventricular and subcortical white matter T2 and flair hyperintensities, none of which enhanced with contrast. Additionally, there was a large lesion in the posterior corpus callosum. She was treated with anticonvulsants for 2 years, during which no changes were seen in her MRI. Drug therapy was then discontinued, and she had no further neurologic symptoms until she died of a pulmonary embolism at the age of 76 years.

The patient described in the preceding vignette experienced 2 temporally distinct episodes of optic neuritis as a young adult, usually a common harbinger of later-onset, more generalized MS. However, clinical signs of more diffuse disease never developed. Approximately 30 years later, when the patient required an MRI subsequent to a mild head injury with a seizure, clinically inactive more widespread MS that never caused further symptoms became evident. Knowing what was present within her immune system that prevented eventual development of more widespread signs of MS might be the key for specific therapeutic intervention of this disorder.

Relapsing-Remitting

Clinical Vignette

A 26-year-old woman was seen in the ED for several days of right arm numbness. When bending forward and flexing her neck to dry her hair, she had noticed an odd "shiver" radiating from the base of her neck into both arms. She had experienced transient numbness in either foot on a number of occasions in the previous 5 years, with symptoms never persisting more than 24 hours. Neurologic examination results had always been normal.

The majority of patients with MS (85%) start with a relapsing-remitting (**RRMS**) course that may initially be benign. A minority of these patients never have any major disability despite fulfilling the criteria for an MS diagnosis. Most MS cases are characterized by 1 or more exacerbations over each year or two, although this average has decreased considerably with the advent of immunomodulatory therapy.

Secondary Progressive

Clinical Vignette

A 50-year-old woman had many bouts of optic neuritis, transient dizziness, and short-lived problems with her balance. She was diagnosed with RRMS in the 1970s and had a few steroid infusions over the years, but no specific therapy since 1984. She briefly received treatment with interferon beta-1b in the mid-1990s but stopped that therapy after a year because of insurance problems. Subsequently, a few minor episodes occurred; she had become dependent on a cane 2 years previously. Since then, she had insidious progression of lower extremity weakness and urinary incontinence that interfered with her work as a kindergarten teacher.

Examination revealed an internuclear ophthalmoplegia (INO), optic pallor, and spastic hemiparesis. Ultimately, the patient required an electric wheelchair to maintain her activities of daily living.

Typically, RRMS continues over many years, gradually leading to incremental decline in various neurologic functions. However, most enter this secondary progressive phase developing varying degrees of neurologic disability. Eventually, the severity and discreteness of relapsing symptoms tends to wane, but dysfunction concomitantly becomes more insidious, resulting in secondary progressive MS. Rarely, MS begins with a fulminant course followed by poor recovery, rapid progression, or both, ending in significant disability or death in a relatively short period after disease onset.

Primary Progressive

Clinical Vignette

A 43-year-old man encountered increasing difficulty with ambulation when walking any distance. He had always been an avid skier and attributed his lack of interest in sports in recent years to aging and lack of motivation. His wife noticed that he had a left foot drop. During the previous 6 months, he had occasionally tripped when going up stairs.

Neurologic examination demonstrated a spastic gait with circumduction of the right leg, mild weakness of the iliopsoas, brisk muscle stretch reflexes in the legs greater on the right, bilateral Babinski signs, and loss of vibration perception at the ankles and knees.

In approximately 15% of patients with MS, the clinical course is more chronically progressive from the outset, without the classic remissions and exacerbations of relapsing-remitting disease, thereby defining another group of patients, those with primary progressive MS. Most of these individuals have clinical evidence of significant spinal cord disease but a paucity of intracranial findings. Typically, progressive gait dysfunction and spasticity characterize their clinical course. Unlike RRMS, this subtype exhibits a male predominance, older age of onset, and poor response to disease-modifying strategies.

Therefore, the MS clinical spectrum can range from a relatively asymptomatic disorder, after an initial few benign episodes of CNS or optic nerve disorder, to an acute life-threatening illness that may mimic a brain tumor.

Differential Diagnosis

Because MS can affect any CNS area from the optic nerves to the distal spinal cord, patients present during the late second into the early sixth decade of life with extremely varied manifestations. Therefore, a broad differential diagnosis must be considered depending on the patient's initial symptomatology. When confronted with neurologic processes primarily affecting the CNS in a previously healthy young person, the physician must consider whether the clinical set could be the initial presentation of MS.

Ocular

Blurred vision, likely a manifestation of acute optic neuritis, is often one of the initial symptoms of MS patients. When temporally associated with a myelopathy, the combination is known as **Devic syndrome** or **neuromyelitis optica**. Vision changes may also be related to a poorly expressed diplopia secondary to an INO, one of the most common neuro-ophthalmologic manifestations of MS (Figure 62-2). In the first instance, the differential diagnosis includes any process affecting the retina or cornea, and in the second, the diplopia may be related to a pseudo-INO, mimicking MS. This is typical of myasthenia gravis. Sometimes a true INO secondary to a stroke may occur in older hypertensive patients.

Inner Ear or Cerebellum

A vague feeling of unsteadiness, dizziness, and sometimes a whirling vertigo with nausea are frequent symptoms of MS. The most common cause of true vertigo is a vestibular neuronitis or Ménière syndrome, both benign processes originating within the inner ear. Patients with a primary CNS lesion causing vertigo are often found to have vertical nystagmus, an important clue sometimes identified in the neurologic examination. This finding alone requires MRI to look for primary CNS disease. Downbeat nystagmus, often the hallmark requiring consid-

MULTIPLE SCLEROSIS AND ACUTE DISSEMINATED ENCEPHALOMYELITIS

Figure 62-2

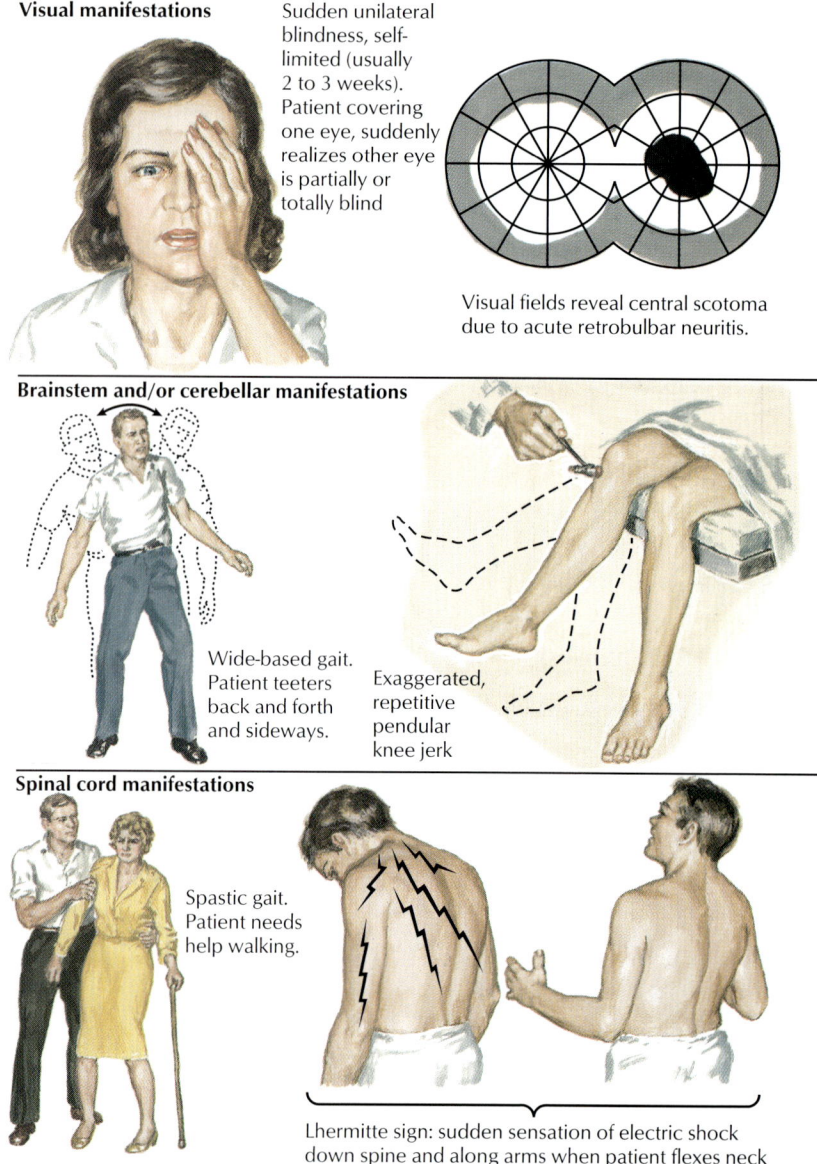

eration of an Arnold-Chiari malformation, may also occur in MS patients with feelings of dizziness.

Precise definition of exactly what patients mean by "*dizzy*" is essential. Frequently, patients are actually reporting a sense of dysequilibrium likely representing cerebellar dysfunction and less commonly reflecting corticospinal involvement. In these instances, patients demonstrate a broad-based gait, various signs of dysmetria, a tremor not seen in patients with a primary vestibular lesion, and often vertical nystagmus.

MULTIPLE SCLEROSIS AND ACUTE DISSEMINATED ENCEPHALOMYELITIS

Figure 62-2

Multiple Sclerosis: Clinical Manifestations (continued)

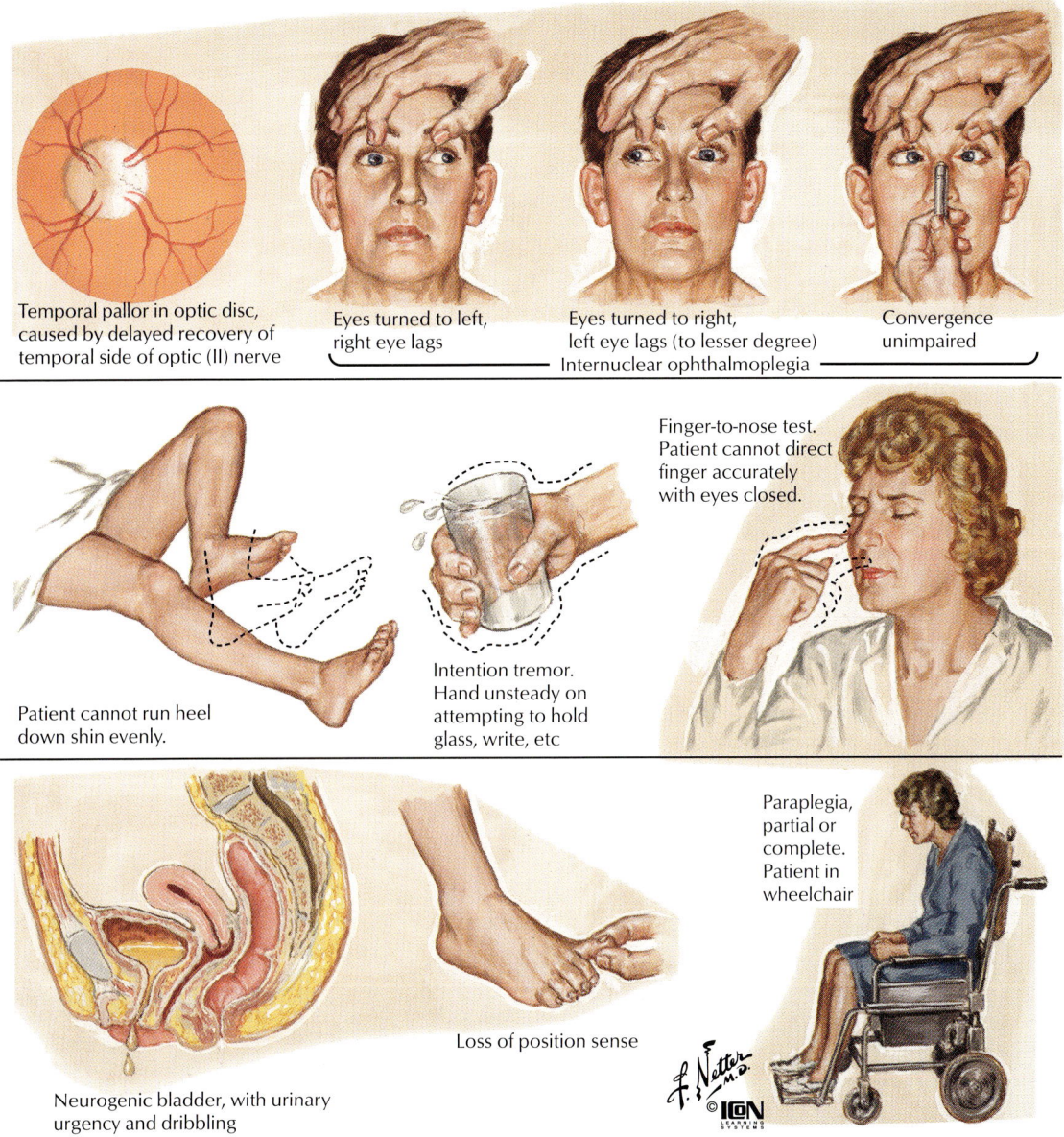

Myelopathies

Sensations of tingling, pins and needles, tightness, and electric shocks are other common symptoms. Relatively early in the disease course, some MS patients report an electric shock–like sensation when they bend their neck that usually radiates down the back or arms. Although the Lhermitte sign is nearly pathognomonic of MS, it can be reported with almost any form of spinal cord disease, including spondylosis with cervical spinal stenosis, a space-occupying lesion, or vitamin B_{12} (cobalamin) deficiency.

MULTIPLE SCLEROSIS AND OTHER DEMYELINATING DISORDERS

MULTIPLE SCLEROSIS AND ACUTE DISSEMINATED ENCEPHALOMYELITIS

Other patients with MS frequently report a tight bandlike distribution of numbness. When circumferential or hemicircumferential, particularly in the midtrunk, the immediate concern is a possible transverse myelitis or primary spinal cord mass lesion. Sometimes patients describe a distribution suggestive of a polyneuropathy with bilateral symmetric numbness. On other occasions, numbness may occur acutely in the hand, compatible with mononeuropathy or stroke. Other myelopathies deserving consideration relate to tropical spastic paraparesis or AIDS.

Strokes and TIAs

Although MS is one of the most common neurologic disorders in young to middle-aged adults, stroke must always be considered. Carotid or vertebrobasilar dissection or both, paradoxical emboli, and CNS vasculitis require differential consideration in potential MS patients.

Cerebral Mass Lesions

Gliomas, meningiomas, and even primary CNS lymphoma should always be considered in young patients with recent onset of functional neurologic dysfunction. Lymphomas particularly may mimic MS because of their periventricular distribution on MRI. Additionally, the relatively promising response of lymphoma to corticosteroids mimics that witnessed in some patients with MS.

When patients present with cerebellar ataxia, cerebellar astrocytomas, hemangioblastomas, or other mass lesions must be excluded. Similarly, patients with evolving paraparesis may have a mass lesion anywhere in the spinal axis, particularly meningiomas at the cervical medullary junction.

Clinical Vignette

A 48-year-old right-handed woman presented with a 2-day history of right leg weakness. She had no history of neurologic symptoms but was previously treated for hypertension, psoriasis, and stress incontinence. There was a strong family history of stroke. One sister had "had an MS attack."

Neurologic examination demonstrated severe right leg weakness with hyperreflexia, ankle clonus, and a questionable plantar response. Brain MRI demonstrated a focal enhancing mass lesion in the high left frontal region. A glioblastoma multiforme was suspected. However, stereotactic biopsy showed demyelination with axonal sparing, sparse perivascular lymphocytic infiltration, and numerous periodic acid-Schiff–positive macrophages.

The patient received a short course of methylprednisolone, and administration of phenytoin was begun. She recovered normal right leg function within 1 month. MRI 6 months later revealed near-complete resolution of the masslike area.

It was initially suspected that this patient had the most malignant type of brain tumor, but biopsy revealed a rare monofocal form of MS, monofocal acute inflammatory demyelination (MAID). This can mimic a primary brain tumor or abscess, is a rare and unique demyelinating disorder that may be superimposed on more typical MS, may herald the development of MS, or may be seemingly unassociated with MS.

Acute myelitis or optic neuritis are more common examples of a monofocal demyelinating process. In contrast, MAID usually affects the cerebral hemispheres, and its clinical and radiologic features suggest a brain tumor. Patients with the "cerebral form" of demyelinating disease have symptoms atypical for MS, including an acute hemiplegia, hemisensory complaints, and visual field deficits. Less common symptoms include headaches, seizures, aphasia, an alteration in level of consciousness and cognitive or psychiatric manifestations.

Rarely, patients with a similar acute clinical presentation have multifocal CNS lesions, diagnosed as acute disseminated encephalomyelitis (ADEM). This process may develop with or without preceding vaccination, viral syndrome, or previous neurologic abnormalities compatible with otherwise occult MS. ADEM usually has widespread or multifocal MRI abnormalities.

Arteriovenous Malformations

Patients with MS typically experience evanescent or waxing and waning symptomatology. However, 2 different forms of vascular anomalies sometimes present with a similar temporal profile.

Clinical Vignette

A vigorous 45-year-old woman presented with a 7-month history of intermittent paresthesias character-

ized by a swollen sensation from her buttocks to her feet, associated gait difficulties, and nocturnal leg cramps. She had one particularly severe event wherein her walking was impaired, but it resolved within hours. Low back pain, difficulty voiding, and diminished sexual responsiveness developed a few months later. On one occasion, after a routine 50-mile drive, she was unable to walk for 1 hour.

Neurologic examination demonstrated diminished vibration perception in the legs. A tethered cord was noted on MRI. CSF protein level was 65 mg/L (mildly increased). Neurologic examination 1 month later demonstrated a slightly broad-based gait, mild tandem ataxia, bilateral proximal leg weakness, and diminished perception of pain and temperature from L5 to S2. MS was one possible diagnosis.

Another spinal MRI demonstrated serpiginous epidural blood vessels at T10-11. Laminectomy revealed a T10-11 dural AVM; the large feeding vessels to this dural AVM were coagulated and ligated. Postoperatively, the patient's course was markedly improved. She had no significant recurrent symptoms for 9 years.

Intermittent myelopathic symptoms should always suggest a spinal dural arteriovenous fistula or MS. Careful inspection of the MRI is essential to not miss the epidural lesion. Surgical treatment or an embolization procedure should be performed to obliterate the abnormal cord vasculature.

Similarly with intermittent brainstem symptoms such as diplopia, hemiparesthesias, and bilateral Babinski signs, **pontine cavernous hemangiomas** also deserve consideration in the differential.

Peripheral Neuropathy

Numbness is another common but variable MS symptom. When both legs are involved in a relatively symmetric fashion, a polyneuropathy should be considered. If the onset is relatively acute, Guillain-Barré syndrome is a possibility. More chronic presentations should include vitamin B_{12} deficiency, particularly when associated with a myelopathy manifested by Babinski signs, Lyme disease, or even the relatively unusual migrant sensory neuritis of Wartenberg in the differential diagnosis.

Neuromuscular Transmission Defects

Like MS, myasthenia gravis tends to occur in young women. It is characterized by combinations of intermittent visual difficulties, particularly diplopia, dysarthria, and fatigue, symptoms that also occur in MS. Lambert-Eaton myasthenic syndrome, a presynaptic autoimmune, often paraneoplastic disorder also may cause intermittent weakness, bulbar signs, and fatigue (chapter 101).

Myopathies

Limited extraocular muscle function and an increased tendency to muscular fatigue occur with mitochondrial myopathies and some dystrophies. Individuals with periodic paralysis have intermittent symptomatology; however, these events usually start in childhood and adolescence, are symmetric, are relatively short-lived, and rarely affect bulbar musculature.

Conversion Hysteria

Conversion hysteria is absolutely only a diagnosis of exclusion but should always be considered with variable symptomatology in a young adult, particularly a woman. These individuals invariably have normal examination results, although their subconscious attempts to demonstrate neurologic abnormalities often result in findings of "*give-way*" weakness or gait problems known as "*astasia-abasia.*" Judgment in this setting is not appropriate. Repeated neurologic examinations, MRI, evoked potentials, and CSF examinations are all warranted to search for organic disease. When tests are repeatedly normal, certain psychiatric disorders should be carefully considered. Incest has occasionally been revealed as an inciting factor.

Diagnostic Approach

No diagnostic criteria exist for MS based solely on laboratory testing. Neuroimaging is the most helpful adjunct to the clinical history and physical findings and has replaced CSF analysis, the oldest methodology, as the primary diagnostic method. However, similar to spinal fluid evaluation, MRI is not entirely sensitive or specific for MS.

Magnetic Resonance Imaging

The diagnosis of MS has become more certain with advanced MRI technology. Classic MRI findings are multiple well-demarcated ovoid lesions whose long axes are situated perpendicularly within the corpus callosum (Dawson fingers), in the periventricular and subcortical white matter, middle cerebellar peduncle, pons, or medulla (Figure 62-3).

FLAIR and T2-weighted images with contrast-enhanced T1 images are the most revealing when looking for areas of active demyelination. Increasingly powerful magnets and techniques, able to resolve variations from the norm that sometimes mimic MS but may not be pathologic, complicate interpretation of abnormalities. "Unidentified bright objects" are the classic imitators seen in those who smoke, have hypertension, or have migraine headaches or are present for unknown reasons. Similarly, Virchow-Robin spaces, dilated CSF-filled vascular areas, may give high T2 signal intensity. However, these can be distinguished from demyelinated plaques of MS by their absence on proton density images.

MRI of the spinal cord may be particularly useful in substantiating a diagnosis. In clinically suspicious cases with normal or equivocal brain MRI, spinal cord lesions can be compelling, even without symptoms referable to the spinal cord. Spinal cord lesions, however, are frequently less easily identified because of the constraints of motion artifact and the necessity of a high-field magnet for adequate resolution.

Patients with MS sometimes present with symptoms that seem appropriate to other intercurrent conditions. They undergo MRI scanning to assuage patient fears of an unlikely structural abnormality only to uncover unexpected white matter lesions that do not necessarily explain the presenting symptoms.

Clinical Vignette

A previously healthy 27-year-old man saw his primary care physician for persistent neck pain after a concussion sustained in a motor vehicle accident in which he lost consciousness for less than 1 minute. Afterward, he had a normal head CT and plain C-spine images. Subsequently, he reported pain in the left cervical paraspinal muscles associated with transient left hand numbness. Cervical spine MRI demonstrated normal vertebrae and intervertebral discs. However, T2-weighted images showed an area of hyperintensity in the left lateral spinal cord at C6 that enhanced with contrast. Brain MRI revealed 3 small areas of T2 hyperintensity in both cerebellar hemispheres and a single linear focus adjacent to the right lateral ventricle.

Clinical Vignette

An 18-year-old man began to have recurrent frontal headaches during his freshman year in college. Both parents had a history of migraine. A paternal aunt had a diagnosis of migraines in childhood and died of a ruptured intracranial aneurysm at the age of 25 years. The primary care physician obtained brain MRI and MRA to rule out a familial aneurysm. No aneurysm was identified, but multiple bilateral linear periventricular T2 hyperintensities and gadolinium-enhanced lesions compatible with active CNS demyelination were present.

These 2 vignettes emphasize how MRI can serendipitously demonstrate findings of MS in the absence of active clinical symptoms, raising the question, "How early is too early to offer immunomodulatory therapy?" There is no consensus on the approach to such patients. How to identify patients with a potentially benign course versus those at risk for significant future disease with later disability remains unknown. MRI will be a keystone as this algorithm is developed.

Cerebrospinal Fluid

Lumbar puncture for CSF is becoming superfluous when the diagnosis is established by history, examination, and supportive MRI images. It is useful in excluding other diagnoses, particularly Lyme disease, sarcoidosis, lymphoma, or multi-infarcts secondary to a primary CNS vasculitis. When indicated, this procedure is typically performed by neurologists.

The typical CSF profile of a patient with MS (Figure 62-4) demonstrates a normal cell count of less than 6 mononuclear cells/mm^3. Occasionally, and in up to 33% of acute instances, a mild pleocytosis is seen, but it usually does not exceed 25 cells/mm^3. Lymphocyte counts greater than 100/mm^3 arouse suspicion of other processes, particularly inflammatory or neoplastic in character. Given the expectation of subtle, if any, pleocytosis, it is paramount to strive for an atraumatic tap. The number of cells present may correlate with enhancing MRI lesions and thus with disease activity. However, there is no apparent correlation between cell count and T2 lesion burden. CSF glucose level is expected to be

Multiple Sclerosis

Figure 62-3

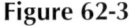

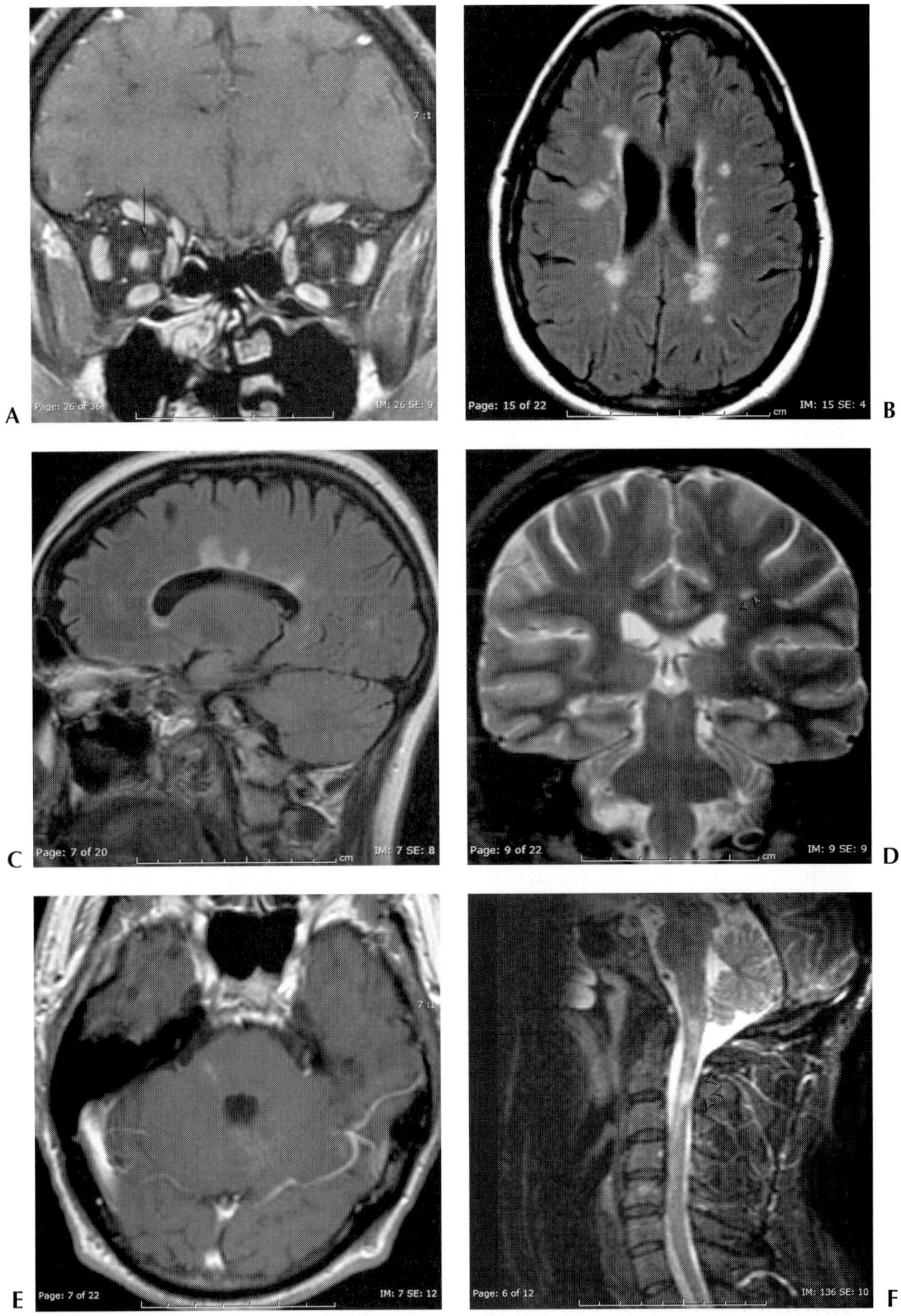

(A) Coronal T1-weighted, fat-saturated, post–gadolinium-enhanced image shows enhancement and enlargement of the right optic nerve (arrow). (B and C) Axial and sagittal FLAIR images with increased T2 signal within the corpus callosum and paraventricular white matter with extension into central white matter along vascular pathways, also illustrated in D, coronal T2, where the typical oval lesions are oriented along vascular pathways, typical of "Dawson fingers" (arrowheads). (E) Axial T1-weighted post–gadolinium-enhanced image shows enhancement of T2 bright lesion shown in other sequences in the right cerebellar penduncle. The enhancement suggest disease activity. (F) Sagittal T2-weighted image shows T2 bright lesion in posterior cord at C2-3.

MULTIPLE SCLEROSIS AND ACUTE DISSEMINATED ENCEPHALOMYELITIS

Figure 62-4   Multiple Sclerosis: Diagnostic Tests—Spinal Fluid

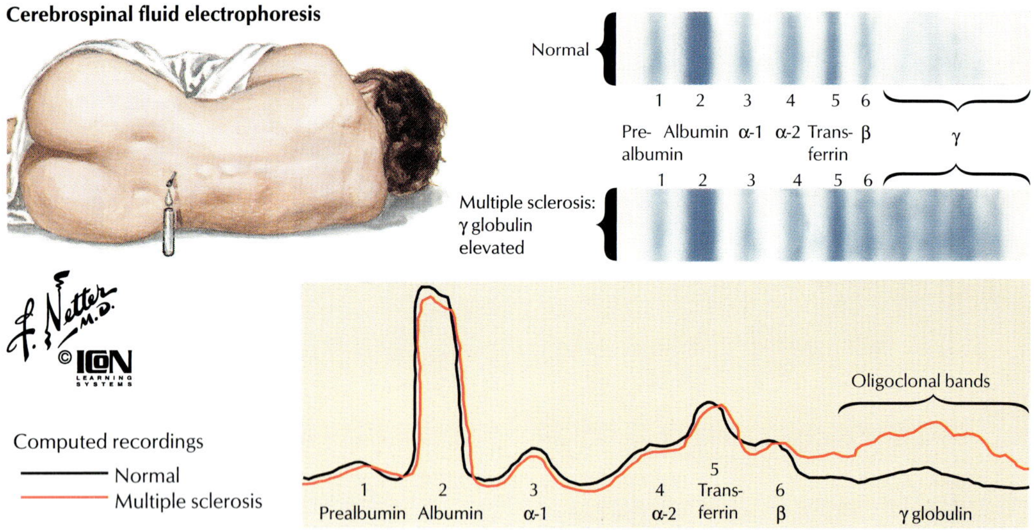

normal, appropriate to the generally benign cell counts.

Normal total protein is present in 60% of MS cases; rarely is it greater than 70 mg/dL. CSF IgG is relatively increased compared with albumin and with that found in serum of the same subject because of changes in the permeability of the blood-brain barrier and IgG synthesis by plasma cells within the abnormal CNS. Abnormal IgG synthesis is associated with CSF oligoclonal bands, the bandlike staining pattern of CSF immunoglobulins when subjected to electrophoresis. In normal CSF, there is no discrete banding; instead, a diffuse single band represents a mixture of polyclonal immunoglobulins that do not segregate into distinct groups. When a few well-defined B-cell clones migrate to the CNS, they begin to produce distinct populations of immunoglobulins that separate into the bands seen on electrophoresis. Even in healthy individuals, there may be a banding pattern seen in serum immunoglobulin electrophoresis, but if CSF bands outnumber serum bands, this suggests an abnormal CNS immune response. Associated oligoclonal bands that are not specific for MS may occur with any in situ CNS hyperimmune response, such as in other CNS inflammatory or infectious diseases.

Myelin basic protein is a large component of myelin that can be detected in a degraded form by CSF immunoassay. Its presence is thought to correlate with active demyelination. When detected, the level seems to be related to the amount and rate of myelin destruction. As such, smoldering MS is not typically associated with the presence of myelin basic protein. Other pathologic processes that destroy large amounts of myelin rapidly (eg, stroke) also produce high levels of CSF myelin basic protein.

Evoked Potentials

Neurophysiologic studies offer objective analysis of the integrity of neuronal pathways in the central and peripheral nervous systems that sometimes help to identify subclinical CNS disease. Testing is relatively easy to perform and requires little patient cooperation, particularly when testing the auditory and visual pathways.

A peripheral stimulus, typically a reversing high-contrast checkerboard pattern for visual evoked responses (VERs) and a series of clicks for brainstem auditory evoked responses (BAERs), evokes an electric potential that can be tracked through the white matter tracts to the cerebral cortex (Figure 62-5). The response latencies can yield objective data regarding the

MULTIPLE SCLEROSIS AND ACUTE DISSEMINATED ENCEPHALOMYELITIS

Figure 62-5 **Multiple Sclerosis: Diagnostic Tests—Evoked Responses I**

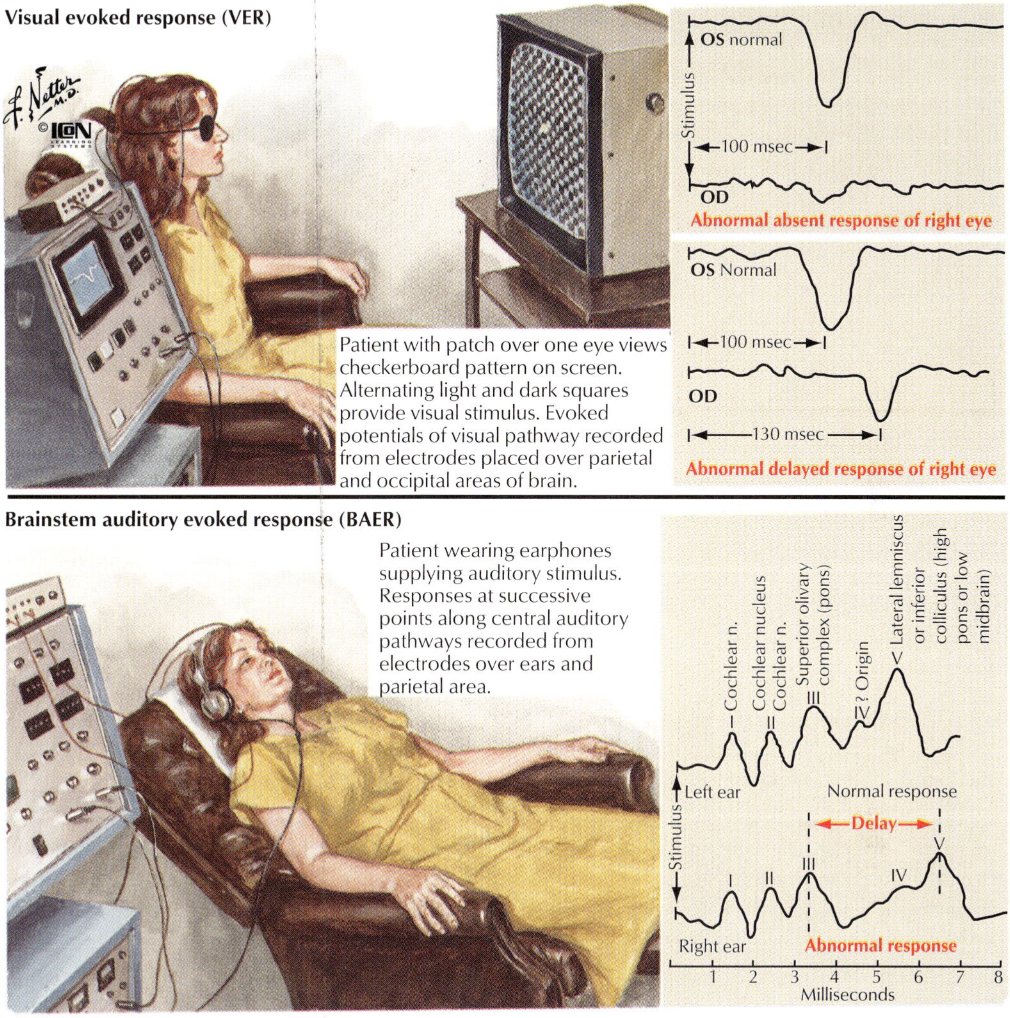

Visual evoked response (VER)

Patient with patch over one eye views checkerboard pattern on screen. Alternating light and dark squares provide visual stimulus. Evoked potentials of visual pathway recorded from electrodes placed over parietal and occipital areas of brain.

OS normal
←100 msec→
OD
Abnormal absent response of right eye

OS Normal
←100 msec→
OD
←130 msec→
Abnormal delayed response of right eye

Brainstem auditory evoked response (BAER)

Patient wearing earphones supplying auditory stimulus. Responses at successive points along central auditory pathways recorded from electrodes over ears and parietal area.

Cochlear n.
Cochlear nucleus
Cochlear n.
Superior olivary complex (pons)
?? Origin
Lateral lemniscus or inferior colliculus (high pons or low midbrain)

Left ear — Normal response
←Delay→
Right ear — Abnormal response
Milliseconds

---

ability of the nervous system to transmit impulses efficiently. These potentials become delayed, attenuated, or blocked when passing through a demyelinated pathway.

Visual evoked responses are recorded at the occipital scalp and depend on the integrity of the optic nerves and radiations. Poor visual acuity may prolong latency and simulate an abnormal study, particularly if there is a pronounced discrepancy of acuity in the 2 eyes. **Somatosensory evoked potentials**, obtained by tracking median and tibial nerve responses through the CNS, can elucidate abnormal conduction through white matter tracts within the spinal cord and brain that may not have an obvious or easily resolved associated MRI abnormality (Figure 62-6). **Brainstem auditory evoked potentials** are recorded by placing a set of headphones over the ears and having the patient listen to clicks. Generated responses are recorded as the evolving waveform is sent to the brain.

Diagnostic Criteria

Most clinicians define evidence of clinically definite RRMS as at least 2 episodes of neurologic dysfunction, abnormal neurologic exami-

MULTIPLE SCLEROSIS AND ACUTE DISSEMINATED ENCEPHALOMYELITIS

Figure 62-6 Multiple Sclerosis: Diagnostic Tests—Evoked Responses II

Somatosensory evoked responses (SER)

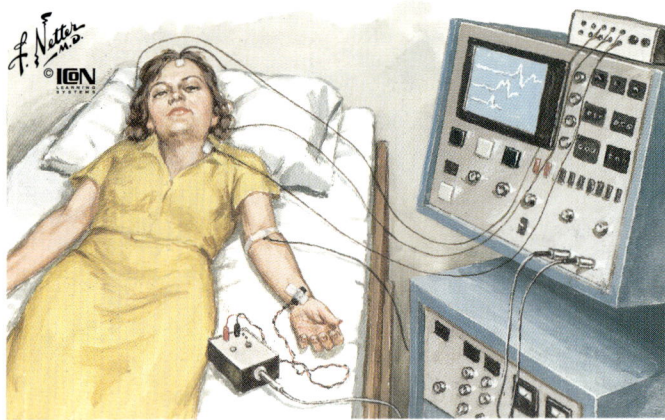
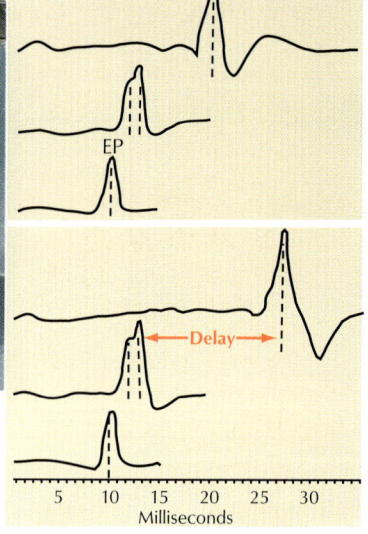
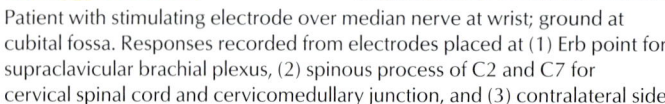

Patient with stimulating electrode over median nerve at wrist; ground at cubital fossa. Responses recorded from electrodes placed at (1) Erb point for supraclavicular brachial plexus, (2) spinous process of C2 and C7 for cervical spinal cord and cervicomedullary junction, and (3) contralateral side

nation results consistent with MS, or both, before a diagnosis is given and treatment is offered. An abnormal brain or spinal cord MRI or both are insufficient to make this diagnosis. However, classic CNS demyelination on MRI is the primary diagnostic adjunct to confirm a diagnosis of MS. When lacking, an abnormal evoked potential finding, a visual evoked response or a somatosensory evoked potential with oligoclonal bands, and increased myelin basic protein findings are useful to confirm clinical suspicion of CNS demyelination compatible with an MS diagnosis. When this is confirmed, the issue of when to initiate therapy becomes paramount.

Management and Therapy

"The Prevention of Relapses and Disability by Interferon Beta-1a Subcutaneously in MS study" suggested that delaying treatment until disability or deficit becomes evident may have significant consequences. It was initially designed to determine whether a higher dose of subcutaneous interferon beta-1a was superior to a lower dose in reducing the relapse rate in RRMS. An extension of the 2-year study allowed patients in all groups to adopt or continue therapy. Those originally assigned to placebo were assigned to 1 of 2 groups: one was given a higher dose of interferon, and the other was given a lower dose. The two groups originally randomized to the higher and lower dosages of interferon beta-1a were permitted to continue their therapy after already receiving 2 years of treatment. Thus, a comparison of different dose levels and of treatment delay was derived. The group that received the higher dose of interferon for the full 4 years fared the best with progressive reduction in relapse rate for each year of therapy and longer intervals of stability before advancement of sustained disability.

The dilemma of whether to treat patients with incidental but suspicious demyelinating lesions remains. The diagnosis of MS remains a clinical one that requires multiple symptoms and signs characteristic of the disease to be documented in time and space, but questionable areas abound. With the advent of disease altering drugs, abnormalities defined with MRI technology carry more weight. Findings on physical examination or extended MS workup may corroborate the impression of probable MS. Whether immunomodulatory therapy is more appropriate for symptom-free patients with hyperreflexia, Babinski responses, abnormal visual evoked potentials, and evolving radiographic evidence of demyelination than for patients with 1 episode of optic neuritis, periodic complaints of transient hand numbness, and a normal physical examination and normal serial brain and C-spine MRI may be answered by future clinical studies.

Immunomodulatory Therapy

Patients newly diagnosed with MS are relieved to know that it has a broadly based prognostic spectrum; some have a benign course, and others encounter a debilitating disease. Most patients have an experience between these extremes. Only 10% of patients have "benign" MS. Of MS patients, 85% begin with a relapsing/remitting course, and 90% of these eventually enter a secondary progressive phase; in the preponderance of patients with a diagnosis of MS, a long-term life-altering morbidity eventually develops. Overall mortality is only a few years less than that of the general population. However, there are exceptions wherein MS follows a relentlessly progressive course over relatively few years, leading to death much earlier than anticipated. If untreated, 20% of patients with MS are unable to walk without assistance 5 years after diagnosis. At 15 and 30 years after diagnosis, this increases to 50% and 80%, respectively.

Medical management of MS was once limited to palliative care. Although symptom treatment remains integral to MS care, immunomodulatory therapies are changing treatment. Pharmacologic interventions modify the course of MS through the reduction of relapse rate and MRI lesion burden, both of which are likely to affect disease progression.

Four drugs are approved by the US FDA for treatment of RRMS: interferon beta-1b, intramuscular interferon beta-1a, glatiramer acetate, and subcutaneous interferon beta-1a. Subcutaneous interferon beta-1b (8 million U every other day) became available early in the 1990s, followed by intramuscular interferon beta-1a (30 µg once weekly) later in that same decade. Flu-like symptoms, the most prominent adverse effect, occur in approximately 60% of those who use interferons, but these effects are mitigated over time and can be treated effectively with NSAIDs. An alternative subcutaneous form of interferon beta-1a used in Europe became available in the United States in 2002 and is injected 3 times per week (22-44 µg), delivering a greater weekly dose of interferon beta-1a.

Glatiramer acetate (20 mg subcutaneously daily) is an unrelated compound of polypeptides that may have fewer potential adverse effects and perhaps more than 1 mechanism of action on the aberrant immune response. Some of its benefit may be realized later in the course of treatment than with the interferons.

Each of these agents reduces relapse rates and decreases CNS MRI burden, but differences in trial design make effective drug-to-drug comparisons difficult. Preexisting factors may influence the choice of therapy in treatment-naive patients. For example, a history of depression, suicidal ideation, or both, which may be adverse effects of the interferon drugs, may make glatiramer acetate the drug of choice in certain individuals.

Mechanisms of Immunomodulatory Therapies. Interferons and glatiramer acetate alter the mechanism of antigen presentation in MS. A host of immune mechanisms are stimulated by the presentation of a candidate antigen, perhaps an intrinsic myelin protein or a viral antigen cross-reacting with a native myelin protein. Myelin reactive T cells become activated and cross the blood-brain barrier, where they can initiate inflammation of myelin-rich white matter. Interferons do not actually enter the CNS and hence exert their effects external to it. Although, like interferons, glatiramer acetate does not itself cross the BBB, it does affect activity within the CNS.

Neutralizing Antibodies. Although the long-term safety of available first-line immunomodulating therapies is unclear, each type seems to be relatively well tolerated. However, neither the interferons nor glatiramer acetate are naturally occurring human proteins and, as such, are prone to inducing antibodies in human recipients. The propensity for antibody production depends on the agent, dose, and route of administration. Substantial controversy exists as to the impact of these antibodies on long-term effectiveness of immunomodulatory medications.

Drug induced antibodies simply bind to the molecules of the active agent and may have no significant function. Neutralizing antibodies are a subset of these binding antibodies that might interfere with drug activity by a steric hindrance of drug binding to its receptor or via remote effects on drug activity through binding at distant sites.

Some agents are more "foreign" than others and have a higher likelihood of inducing antibodies. Glycosylation renders substances more soluble in suspension; without it, aggregates that may be immunogenic are likely to form. This may account for the higher incidence of neutralizing antibodies with the use of interferon beta-1b (30-35%) compared with interferon beta-1a (15%), which is glycosylated, has no amino acid substitutions, and looks almost exactly like naturally occurring IFN-β. Higher doses of the drug, more frequent exposures, and delivery via subcutaneous injection may affect antibody induction.

Treatment of More Severe Multiple Sclerosis

The protocol for treating recalcitrant MS is not formulaic. Only 2 agents are approved by the US FDA for rapidly progressive MS: mitoxantrone and interferon beta-1b. Mitoxantrone (12 mg/m^2 IV given every 3 months to a cumulative maximum dose of 144 mg) is a chemotherapeutic agent used to treat other immune-mediated disorders. Usually considered a treatment of last resort after multiple treatment failures, its categorization is due to its potential toxicities, the most worrisome of which is cardiac toxicity.

Two trials offered some evidence that interferon beta-1b favorably impacts secondary progressive disease with respect to various outcome measures (progression of disability scores, relapse rate reduction, MRI activity), not all of which were significant in both studies. High-dose interferon beta-1a has also been investigated in secondary progressive disease; 2 studies demonstrated efficacy compared with placebo. Although heterogeneity of study populations and outcome measures make these studies difficult to compare, they offer some rationale for choosing a new therapy in patients who have advanced from relapsing-remitting disease to a more aggressive RRMS or secondary progressive disease, regardless of previous treatments. Multi-interferon therapy and interferon plus glatiramer acetate are being investigated. Despite multiple investigations focused on other treatment strategies, their efficacies have remained largely anecdotal.

Azathioprine, Cyclosporine, and Cyclophosphamide. The equivocal benefits of **azathioprine** (2-3 mg/kg daily) in MS are realized in decreasing relapse rates and MRI lesion burden. **Cyclosporine** inhibits the production of lymphokines and seems to foster the expansion of certain populations of suppressor T cells. One cyclosporine and azathioprine comparison showed no differences between the 2 agents with respect to relapse frequency or expanded disability status scale, but therapy complications were more than twice as likely in the cyclosporine group as in the azathioprine group. Other studies of cyclosporine have been marred by high attrition in the treatment groups due to toxicities (renal failure, hypertension) that likely occur before any benefit is achieved. These observations have taken cyclosporine out of the usual arsenal of immunosuppressive therapy for the treatment of MS in many centers.

Cyclophosphamide is another immunosuppressive agent widely used to treat various neoplastic and autoimmune disorders. One study suggested some response based on expanded disability status scale scores to induction with booster infusions in patients younger than 40 years. Toxicities include hemorrhagic cystitis, leukopenia, myocarditis, pulmonary interstitial fibrosis, malignancy, interstitial pulmonary fibrosis, and infertility. **Mitoxantrone** tends to be better tolerated, with fewer adverse effects, and has better evidence of efficacy in secondary progressive MS.

Methotrexate. Low-dose weekly oral methotrexate is not approved for use in MS but is used as an adjunct therapy in off-label use based on a limited number of studies in patients with MS and its efficacy in rheumatoid arthritis, another autoimmune disease. Methotrexate is a competitive inhibitor of dihydrofolate reductase and interferes with the production of reduced cofactors required for the synthesis of DNA and RNA. It seems to have both immunosuppressive and antiinflammatory effects and immunoregulatory action. Toxicities include pulmonary and liver fibrosis, cirrhosis, and bone marrow suppression.

Monthly Intravenous Methylprednisolone. In addition to its efficacy as acute therapy in relapses, cyclical infusions of 500 to 1000 mg IV glucocorticoids can be useful as a scheduled monthly or bimonthly treatment in patients whose frequent relapses signal a transition from RRMS to secondary progressive MS. This is generally a safe, well-tolerated approach for patients who have waning response to other conventional immunomodulators but are unwilling to undertake chemotherapeutic options.

Plasma Exchange. Plasmapheresis intervenes primarily at the level of humoral responses, thought to be less important in MS than cellular responses. There is no data supporting a significant treatment effect.

Intravenous Immunoglobulin. Limited data exist regarding IV immunoglobulin for MS. There are few long-term adverse effects but no evidence that it is more effective than other approved therapies for MS. Because MS is not a US FDA–approved indication for IV immunoglobulin, the expense of treatment is usually prohibitive.

Adjuvant Medical Problems and Treatments

Despite new therapies, for most people, MS eventually involves some adaptation in lifestyle. It may mean adopting a less frenetic pace with curtailed work hours, help with household management, less travel, napping, or avoidance of excessive heat. The demand for lifestyle modification can be one of the more frustrating aspects of MS.

Clinical Vignette

A 32-year-old woman who generally enjoyed good health presented with a subacute history of advancing fatigue. In high school, she was active in track and field hockey. She attended college on a partial athletic scholarship and had no difficulty maintaining her academic responsibilities and social life during her undergraduate years. Subsequently, she went to law school and married, enjoying hiking vacations with her husband and regularly exercising at the gym.

Six months postpartum from her first child, she began to note a precipitous decline in her energy level. Although her child was sleeping easily through the night and she had not returned to work, she found herself struggling to get through the simplest routine household activities. She had no overt weakness, numbness, pain, or other constitutional symptoms, but 3 weeks previously, she had had a few days of blurred vision and transient diplopia that had fully resolved.

Neurologic examination confirmed the presence of optic pallor, a slight INO, and minimal spastic ataxia, with diminished vibratory perception in the feet. MRI revealed multifocal areas of demyelination.

The patient in this vignette was unaware of having a significant neurologic disorder; she sought medical attention for fatigue, one of the most common symptoms that will affect her activities of daily living as MS increasingly influences her life.

Fatigue. Fatigue is often the most debilitating symptom, particularly early in MS. The primary "lassitude" of MS is an overwhelming sense of physical and mental exhaustion that has no identifiable cause but significantly interferes with normal activity. The majority of patients with MS rank it as their most disabling symptom, eclipsing bowel and bladder dysfunction, weakness, and balance problems in affecting daily living. Although fatigue can be secondary to deconditioning, the advanced symptoms of MS that limit physical activity are not a prerequisite for fatigue. It has been associated with every stage of the disease, regardless of clinical subtype, and is often present in an apparently well-compensated individual who otherwise has little objective disability.

Persistent but ineffective neuronal firing of short-circuited neural pathways that do not effect movement in weak limbs, transmit cohesive visual impulses, or recruit the reflexes necessary to maintain balance may be a pathophysiologic correlate of primary MS fatigue. No link is evident to objective measures of disease activity such as commonly used functional scales or MRI findings.

Additionally, some evidence exists of an association among MS-related fatigue, depression, and cognitive dysfunction. That this is true in patients without significant deficits and in patients who have not received a diagnosis suggests that the mental fatigue is not simply an epiphenomenon of a reactive depression. The fatigue of MS is likely a direct consequence of demyelination, inflammation, and axonal injury along shared neuronal networks that affect attention, depression, and cognitive dysfunction. Hypometabolism in the frontal cortex and basal ganglia resulting from this type of damage has been implicated in primary MS fatigue.

Sufficient rest is critical to managing fatigue in MS, but pharmacologic therapy is a useful adjunct to behavioral and lifestyle strategies. Despite the incomplete understanding of the pathophysiology of MS-related fatigue, clearly valuable pharmacotherapies mitigate a profoundly low energy level through modification of altered neurochemistry that results from damage to the CNS.

Wakefulness involves various arousal systems with complex circuits that project between the reticular activating system, limbic system, and frontal cortex. From the brainstem, monoamine-mediated pathways (dopamine, norepinephrine, serotonin, acetylcholine) ascend through the reticular activating system. Several useful agents operate along this pathway. The stimulant medications (methylphenidate, amphetamine salts, dextroamphetamine [Dexedrine], pemoline) affect this mesocorticolimbic system by enhancing global CNS activation but may produce undesirable side effects such as dependence through stimulation of central "reward mechanisms" (governed by the nucleus accumbens in the striatum), insomnia, appetite suppression, and peripheral autonomic effects including tachycardia, dysrhythmia, and hypertension. Amantadine enhances dopamine release and seems to have some benefit in improving central attention and processing speed. Modafinil, used to treat narcolepsy, is also helpful in treating MS fatigue by increasing activity in the frontal cortex via activation of histaminergic neurons arising from the hypothalamus.

Pain. Multiple sclerosis is usually regarded as a disease of progressive neurologic dysfunction without significant pain. However, pain is a common problem deserving appropriate attention. Years of gait disturbance, abnormal forces on joints, repetitive motion injuries, wheelchair confinement, disuse, and painful muscle spasms are all typical sources of pain in MS. A regular exercise program is essential to prevent additional disability from deconditioning.

NSAIDs, gabapentin, and tricyclic antidepressants are often useful. For pain, narcotic medications are probably best avoided because they are likely to exacerbate fatigue and cognitive dysfunction. Aqua therapy is an excellent form of exercise that does not put undue stress on joints and provides buoyant support for weak limbs, allowing patients to maximize range of motion. Yoga is helpful for relaxation and flexibility maintenance. Shiatsu massage therapy may help to prevent contractures, but deep muscle massage may be overzealous and increase rather than mitigate pain. Acupuncture may disrupt aberrant pain pathways.

Bladder Dysfunction. Bladder symptoms, one of the most vexing problems commonly experienced, significantly influence quality of life in 50% to 80% of patients with MS. The degree of impairment usually parallels the degree of other neurologic deficits. Bladder hygiene is compromised by increased spasticity, loss of strength, and diminished mobility. Although bladder dysfunction rarely leads to life-threatening infection or secondary renal failure, the resultant recurrent or chronic urinary tract infections can potentiate other MS symptoms and are a common trigger for significant exacerbations.

Control of urination depends on the complex coordination of reflexive and volitional activities that rely on the integrity of complex pathways that traverse the subcortical white matter, spinal cord tracts, and reflex spinal cord centers. Lateral and posterior cervical spinal tracts are among the most common sites of demyelination in MS and are critical for all aspects of coordinating voluntary voiding.

Bladder dysfunction in MS is managed both pharmacologically and with adaptations in toileting. The most common pharmacologic agents diminish bladder contraction, eg, an antispasmodic anticholinergic, oxybutynin chloride, beginning at 5 mg to a maximum 20 mg daily. These are generally more effective than attempts to improve bladder emptying with cholinergic agents. α-Adrenergic agents increase bladder outlet resistance and sometimes help to treat urinary incontinence. Emptying the hyporeflexic or areflexic bladder is best accomplished by clean, intermittent self-catheterization.

Pregnancy. Pregnancy in women with MS seems to have no long-term effects on MS progression. It may have some **protective value**, because the incidence of exacerbations is actually lower during pregnancy. In the 6 to 12 months after pregnancy, the exacerbation rate is higher than expected. The decision to bear children should probably take into account the prepregnancy tempo of disease and whether a woman with MS feels physically capable of keeping up with the rigorous demands of raising children. Family support and financial resources are also factors.

Heat. High ambient temperatures and high levels of humidity are often associated with MS worsening and possibly even exacerbations. During summer months, especially within temperate countries, patients are advised to avoid the stress of overexposure to high ambient temperatures, especially during heat waves. Where possible, air conditioning, ceiling fans, or avoidance of strenuous activities may lessen the chances for causing deterioration in the overall status of patients with MS.

ACUTE DISSEMINATED ENCEPHALOMYELITIS

Acute disseminated encephalomyelitis is an acute monophasic demyelinating CNS disorder characterized by multifocal white matter involvement. ADEM usually occurs without any recognized antecedent cause or within 6 weeks of an antigenic challenge after exanthems (measles, rubella, variola, varicella), vaccination (rabies, smallpox and pertussis), or respiratory infections (*Mycoplasma* pneumoniae, Epstein-Barr virus, and cytomegalovirus). An uncommon disease, it affects children more than adults. Its pathogenesis is postulated to be a T-cell–mediated autoimmune response against myelin basic protein triggered by infection or vaccination. The entire clinical spectrum, epidemiology, imaging characteristics, and pathology are often initially indistinguishable from severe MS.

Clinical Presentation

The clinical manifestations of ADEM reflect the CNS disseminated involvement and include encephalopathy associated with pyramidal, cerebellar and brainstem signs. Seizures can be seen at onset in approximately 25% of patients. Bilateral optic neuritis and transverse myelitis are particularly suggestive of a demyelinating disease such as ADEM.

Diagnosis and Treatment

The most useful diagnostic tool for this condition is MRI, which commonly shows multifocal asymmetric lesions throughout the brain and spinal cord (Figure 62-7). The lesions may enhance with gadolinium. Enhancing lesions can show different patterns, including nodular, gyral, amorphous, spotty, and ringlike shapes. The CSF is abnormal in 70% of patients, showing a modest lymphocytosis, increased protein, and normal glucose. Immunoglobulins can be increased in some patients with 60% having oligoclonal bands. EEG often shows diffuse slowing compatible with an encephalopathic process. Epileptiform spike discharges are unusual in ADEM.

The differential diagnosis of ADEM includes acute MS, metabolic leukoencephalopathies, various acute aseptic meningoencephalitides, and vasculitides. Cerebral biopsy is often necessary to confirm the diagnosis, especially in adults and atypical cases. Perivenous mononuclear cell infiltration associated with demyelination within the cellular cuff is the typical finding in patients with ADEM. In contrast to MS (where the periventricular white matter is most commonly involved), these abnormalities most often occur at cortical gray and subcortical white matter interface.

Most patients with ADEM improve with methylprednisolone. However, if that fails, immunoglobulins, plasmapheresis, or cytotoxic drugs are given.

MULTIPLE SCLEROSIS AND ACUTE DISSEMINATED ENCEPHALOMYELITIS

Figure 62-7

Acute Disseminated Encephalomyelitis

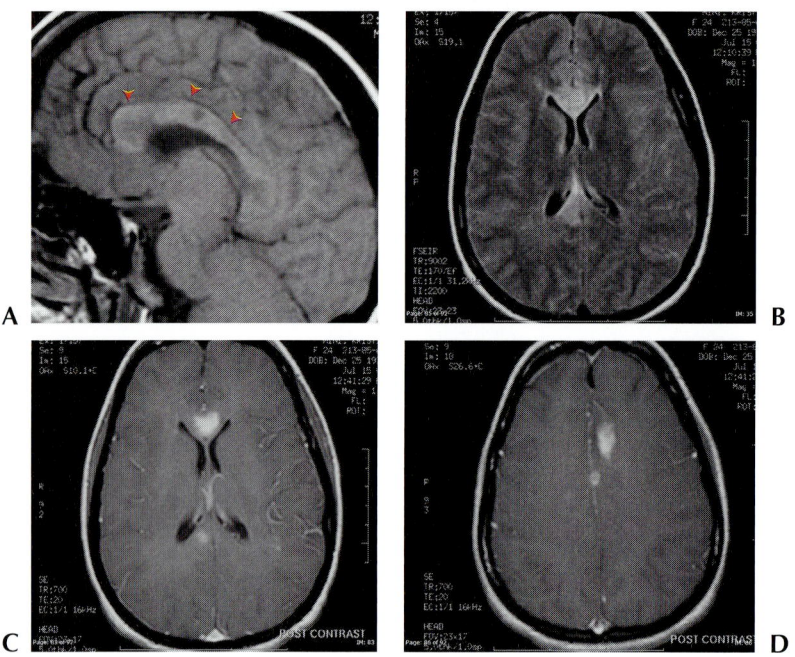

(**A**) Sagittal T1-weighted image shows expanded corpus callosum with mixed signal characteristics (arrowheads). (**B**) Axial FLAIR image demonstrates enlargement and increased T2 signal in corpus callosum. (**C and D**) Axial T1-weighted, gadolinium-enhanced scans with multiple enhancing lesions within corpus callosum and beyond.

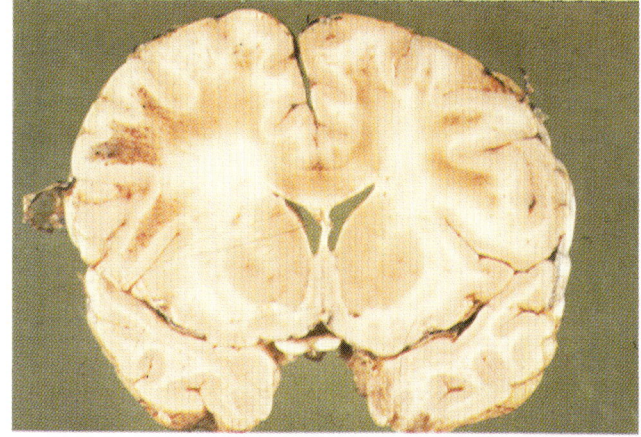

Coronal section of cerebral hemispheres at level of corpus striatum showing punctate hemorrhagic lesions in subcortical white matter

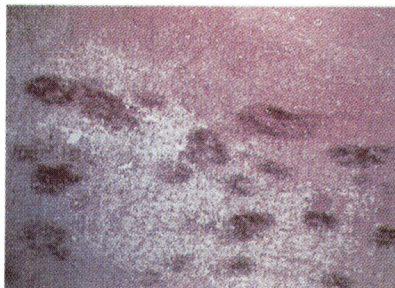

Cerebral white matter with scattered deep hemorrhages in pale, edematous areas (H and E stain, ×10)

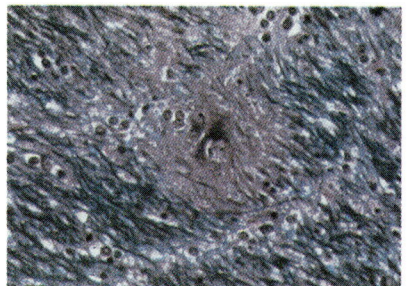

Cingulate gyrus white matter showing area of perivenous demyelination (Luxol-fast blue-Holmes, ×100)

MULTIPLE SCLEROSIS AND OTHER DEMYELINATING DISORDERS

Acute disseminated encephalomyelitis is usually associated with a very good prognosis. Most patients achieve complete recovery or are left with mild deficits.

ACUTE HEMORRHAGIC LEUKOENCEPHALOPATHY

Acute hemorrhagic leukoencephalopathy (AHL) is considered a hyperacute form of ADEM. As in ADEM, AHL is a monophasic disease. It is usually postinfectious, secondary to an autoimmune process directed against the CNS myelin. However, the clinical course of AHL is much more fulminant than that of ADEM and more frequently fatal.

Clinical Presentation

Early symptoms of AHL include fever, headaches, and malaise. These rapidly progress to confusion, decreased level of consciousness (obtundation) and coma. Aphasia, hemiparesis, brainstem signs, and seizures are common focal signs.

Diagnosis and Treatment

Peripheral leukocytosis is often present in AHL, with WBC counts as high as $40,000/mL^3$. The lesions on MRI are usually larger and have more edema than in ADEM. Hemorrhages are frequently seen. CSF usually shows polymorphonuclear pleocytosis, increased protein, and normal glucose. Although AHL is associated with petechiae, the number of RBCs can vary from none to thousands. Increased levels of CSF γ globulins may be present.

The pathologic findings in AHL are unique and show widespread edema in the white matter, ball and ring hemorrhages, perivascular exudates, and perivenous foci of microglial proliferation. Areas of demyelination are seen around the vessels.

Early and aggressive treatment with high-dose steroids is indicated and may occasionally lead to an improved clinical outcome.

REFERENCES

Case records of the Massachusetts General Hospital (case 1-1999). *N Engl J Med.* 1999;340:127-135.

Dale RC. Acute disseminated encephalomyelitis. *Semin Pediatr Infect Dis.* 2003;14:90-95.

IFNB Multiple Sclerosis Study Group. Interferon beta-1b in relapsing-remitting multiple sclerosis: clinical results of a multicenter, randomized, double-blind, placebo-controlled study. *Neurology.* 1993;43:651-661.

Interferon beta-1b is effective in relapsing remitting multiple sclerosis: II. MRI analysis results of a multicenter, randomized, double-blind trial. *Neurology.* 1993;43:662-667.

Jacobs LD, Cookfair DL, Rudick RA, et al. Intramuscular interferon beta-1a for disease progression in relapsing multiple sclerosis. *Ann Neurol.* 1996;39:285-294.

Keegan BM, Noseworthy JH. Multiple sclerosis. In: Johnson RT, Griffin JW, Mc Arthur JC. *Current Therapy of Neurologic Disease.* 6th ed. St Louis, MO: Mosby; 2002:181-187.

Placebo-controlled multicentre randomized trial of interferon beta-1b in treatment of secondary progressive multiple sclerosis. *Lancet.* 1998;352:1491-1497.

Rust RS. Multiple sclerosis, acute disseminated encephalomyelitis, and related conditions. *Semin Pediatr Neurol.* 2000;7:66-90.

Samuels M, Fiske S. *Office Neurology.* 2nd ed. Philadelphia, PA: Churchill-Livingstone; 2003:408-425.

Sustained clinical benefits of glatiramer acetate in relapsing multiple sclerosis patients observed for 6 years. *Multiple Sclerosis.* 2000;6:255-266.

Section XV
INFECTIOUS DISEASE

Chapter 63
Bacterial Meningitis 560

Chapter 64
Parameningeal Infections 566

Chapter 65
Neurosyphilis 570

Chapter 66
Viral Infections of the Nervous System 574

Chapter 67
Brain and Spine Tuberculosis 583

Chapter 68
Infections in Immunocompromised Hosts 586

Chapter 69
Tetanus 594

Chapter 70
Poliomyelitis 597

Chapter 63
Bacterial Meningitis

Donald E. Craven, Francesco G. De Rosa, Daniel P. McQuillen, and Robert A. Duncan

Clinical Vignette

An 18-year-old woman presented to the ED with mild sore throat, arthralgia, myalgia, and low-grade fever of 3 days' duration. One day previously, she had experienced a severe headache with neck stiffness, nausea, and vomiting. She had no other symptoms. Her college dorm mates were well.

On physical examination, although alert and oriented, she had an inappropriate affect. Her temperature was 98.6°F, her pulse was 100 beats/min, respirations were 20/min, and her blood pressure was 110/70 mm Hg. Although her neck was stiff, Kernig and Brudzinski signs were absent. The pharynx was slightly injected without exudate. Heart and lung examination results were normal. No rash was present.

Neurologic examination revealed intact cranial nerves, normal reflexes, and no motor or sensory deficits. The patient's WBC count was 21,800/mm^3 with 26% bands and 67% PMNs. Her platelet count was 200,000/mm^3. Her electrolytes were normal, and here glucose level was 131 mg/dL. A chest radiograph was normal. A lumbar puncture revealed normal CSF.

The patient was admitted for IV hydration and observation. Twelve hours later, she became acutely lethargic. Repeat lumbar puncture revealed cloudy CSF with 871 WBCs (90% PMNs), a glucose level of 1 mg/dL, and a protein level of 350 mg/dL. Gram stain revealed rare gram-negative diplococci that on culture grew Neisseria meningitidis. The patient was treated with 24 million U/d IV penicillin G and recovered completely. Before discharge, she was given rifampin to eliminate nasopharyngeal carriage of N meningitidis.

One of the most serious neurologic emergencies involves the evaluation and care of patients with bacterial meningitis. Patients are often vigorous and previously healthy when they suddenly develop a severe headache, fever, and stiff neck. Despite more than 50 years of experience with antibiotic therapies, meningitis is a potentially lethal disease. Expedient diagnosis is essential. In the preceding vignette, typical for meningococcal meningitis, despite the history and findings suggestive of a meningeal infection, the initial CSF examination results were normal. Emergency physicians wisely admitted the patient for observation. When she experienced sudden deterioration, repeated CSF examination led to diagnosis and appropriate therapy. With this illness, any delay in therapy can be irretrievable because death may occur soon after a clinical change unless antibiotic therapy is begun immediately.

PATHOPHYSIOLOGY

Classically, any bacterial infection involving the leptomeninges within the subarachnoid space is called *meningitis* (Figure 63-1). Typically, microbial seeding of the leptomeninges occurs via the bloodstream or from a contiguous site of infection, such as otitis media, sinusitis, or mastoiditis. Rare causes include a defect in the anatomical barriers, as with a perforating cranial or spinal injury or congenital dural defect.

The responsible microorganisms may differ between children and adult patients. Those commonly responsible for meningitis in adults include *Streptococcus pneumoniae*, *N meningitidis*, and *Listeria monocytogenes*. *Haemophilus influenzae* still causes 20% to 50% of meningitis in developing countries, but in the United States, this rate has been reduced 90% with the *H influenzae* type b vaccine. In neonates, *Escherichia coli* and group B β-hemolytic streptococci comprise most cases. *L monocytogenes* can cause meningitis in immunocompromised patients and rarely in the newborn. *N meningitidis* infection often occurs with a primary sepsis, petechial and/or purpuric skin lesions, or disseminated intravascular dissemination. Conditions predisposing to pneumococcal meningitis in adults in-

BACTERIAL MENINGITIS

Bacterial Meningitis—I

Figure 63-1

Most common causative organisms

H influenzae still causes ~25-50% of meningitis in developing countries (90% reduction in US with Hib vaccine)

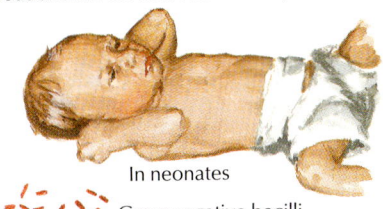

In neonates

Gram-negative bacilli
(*E coli*, *Klebsiella pneumoniae*, etc)
Streptococci
Other (*S aureus*, *Listeria monocytogenes*, *H influenzae*, etc)

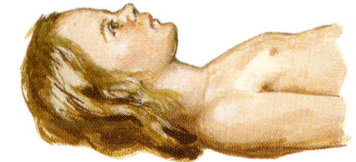

In children

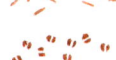
N meningitidis, *S pneumoniae*, *H influenzae*
Other (*Listeria* etc)

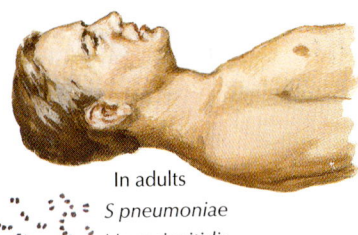

In adults

S pneumoniae
N meningitidis
Gram-negative bacilli
Other (*Listeria* etc)

Sources of infection

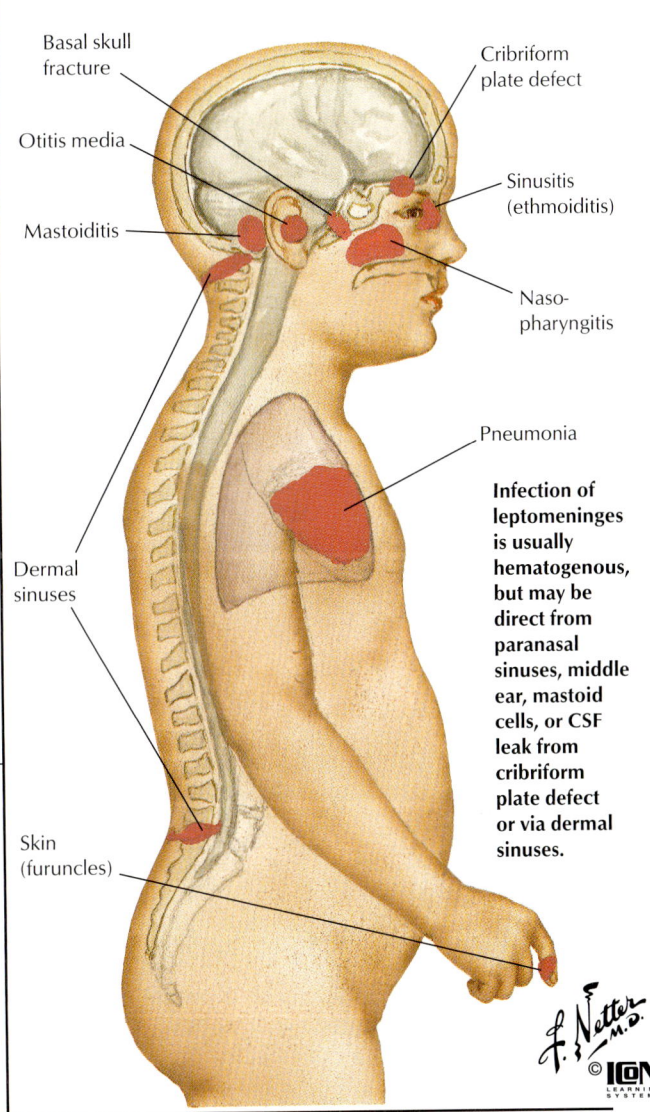

- Basal skull fracture
- Cribriform plate defect
- Otitis media
- Sinusitis (ethmoiditis)
- Mastoiditis
- Nasopharyngitis
- Dermal sinuses
- Pneumonia
- Skin (furuncles)

Infection of leptomeninges is usually hematogenous, but may be direct from paranasal sinuses, middle ear, mastoid cells, or CSF leak from cribriform plate defect or via dermal sinuses.

Diagnosis

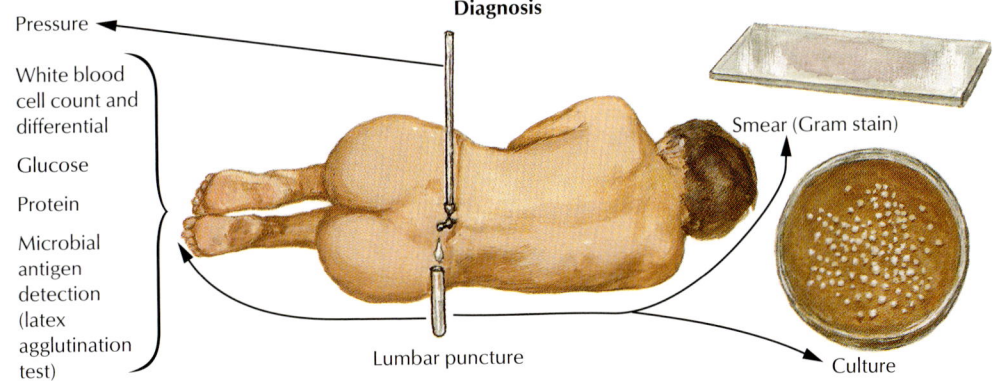

- Pressure
- White blood cell count and differential
- Glucose
- Protein
- Microbial antigen detection (latex agglutination test)
- Lumbar puncture
- Smear (Gram stain)
- Culture

INFECTIOUS DISEASE

561

clude sickle cell disease and immune deficiencies including alcoholism, cirrhosis, splenectomy, and HIV/AIDS.

Gram-negative bacilli (*E coli, Proteus, Pseudomonas, Serratia, Klebsiella,* and *Citrobacter*) are rarely found in community-acquired meningitis but may be found in association with head or spinal trauma or after neurosurgery and should always be considered in immunocompromised hosts. Meningitis due to *Staphylococcus aureus* may follow penetrating trauma, neurosurgery, or bacteremia. Coagulase-negative staphylococci (*Staphylococcus epidermidis*) or *S aureus* and other organisms are associated with infected ventricular shunts.

CLINICAL PRESENTATION AND DIAGNOSIS

The onset of acute bacterial meningitis is rapid: hours to a day or so. Clinical findings that are almost always present include signs of a CNS disorder, with fever and specific signs of meningeal involvement manifested by severe neck stiffness, called *meningismus*. The patient rapidly becomes sleepy and confused, obtunded, and often comatose. Clinically significant nuchal rigidity is typified by the examiner's inability to move the neck regardless of which maneuver is used. Two clinical maneuvers reflect inflamed meningeal coverings involving the lumbosacral nerve roots: Kernig and Brudzinski signs (Figure 63-2). The **Kernig sign** is elicited by flexing the patient's hip to a 90° angle and then attempting to passively straighten the leg at the knee; pain and tightness in the hamstring muscles prevent maneuver completion. This sign should be present bilaterally to support the meningitis diagnosis. The **Brudzinski sign** is positive if the patient's hips and knees flex automatically when the examiner flexes the patient's neck while the patient is supine. The relative sensitivity of these meningeal irritation signs must be correlated with the etiologic agent and the host responsiveness to the infection. These findings are not invariably present, especially in debilitated and elderly patients and infants. When signs of meningitis are elicited, further history and examination to elicit a parameningeal source is vital (Figure 64-1).

Dermatologic findings often provide clues suggesting an early clinically specific diagnosis; however, these are not a substitute for CSF examination, the only means to establish a specific bacteriologic etiology. A maculopapular or petechial/purpuric rash usually indicates infection with *N meningitidis*. Usually secondary to vasculitis, it is rarely related to concomitant coagulation defects or a combination of the two. A similar, less severe rash rarely accompanies aseptic meningitis caused by echovirus (wherein CSF findings are totally different). The rash of meningococcal infection more commonly affects the trunk and extremities in contrast to the echo viral exanthem that usually involves the face and neck early in the infection. Purpuric lesions may be rarely found in fulminant pneumococcal bacteremia with meningitis and staphylococcal endocarditis, the latter primarily involving the finger pads.

DIAGNOSTIC APPROACH

CSF examination is essential to the diagnosis of bacterial and other microbial forms of meningitis. Generally, CT should precede CSF examination to rule out primary brain abscess or parameningeal focus with significant mass effect lesion, potentially causing cerebral herniation with a sudden change in CSF dynamics. Lumbar puncture is contraindicated in patients with suspected meningitis and concomitant signs of increased intracranial pressure including papilledema, coma, and focal neurologic findings of dilated pupils, hemiparesis, aphasia, and rarely bradycardia, Cheyne-Stoke respirations, and projectile vomiting. When CT is needed before lumbar puncture, administration of empiric antibiotics is essential before the scan. CSF examination can be safely performed if none of the above contraindications or clinical signs of increased intracranial pressure exist.

CSF analysis provides the only conclusive proof of bacterial infection of the subarachnoid space. It must include a Gram-stained smear to define the offending organism morphology. The Gram stain correlates with the etiology results of the more specific bacteriologic culture in approximately 80% of patients. The Gram stain is a simple technique that may allow better selection

BACTERIAL MENINGITIS

Bacterial Meningitis—II

Figure 63-2

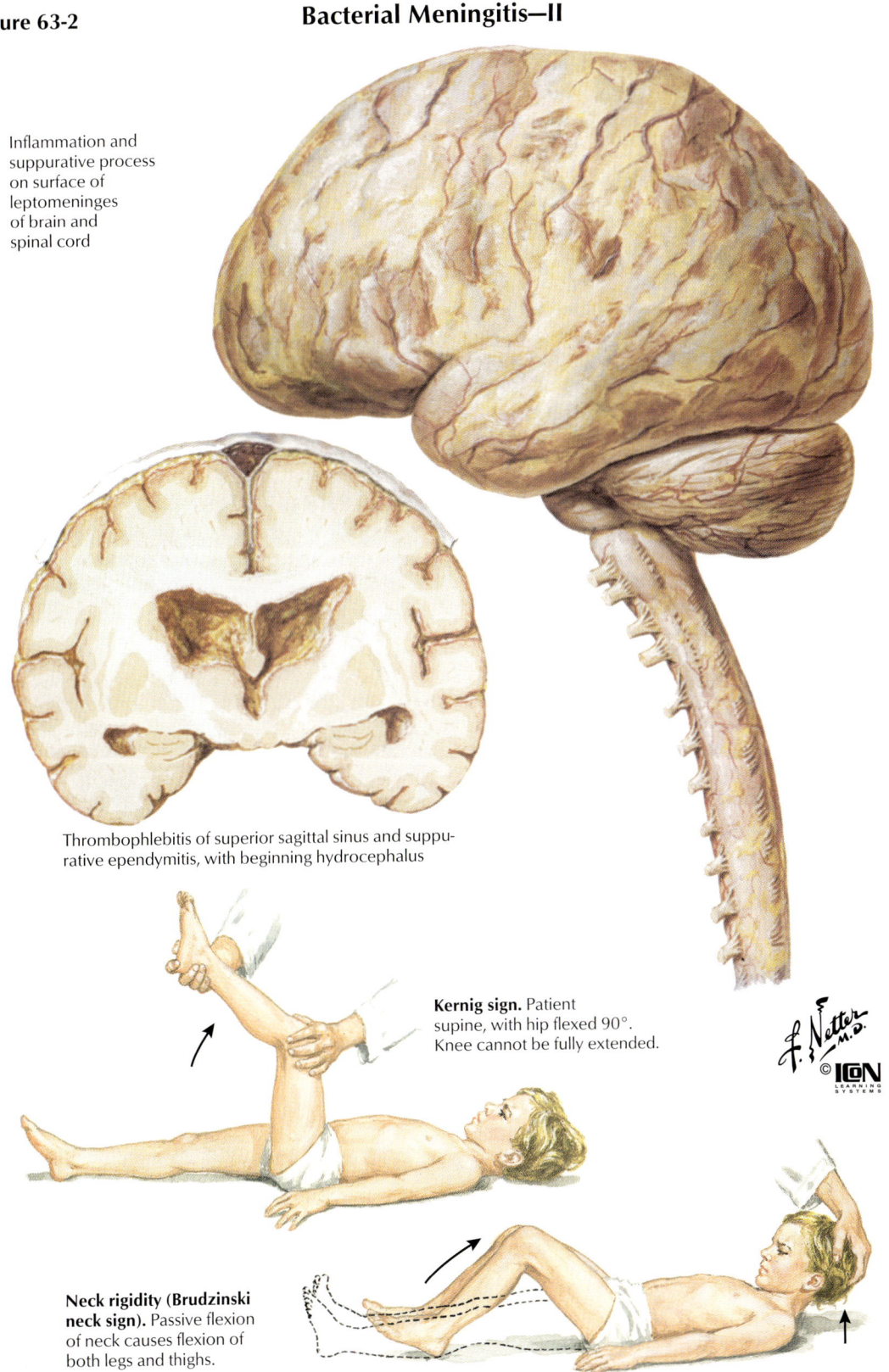

Inflammation and suppurative process on surface of leptomeninges of brain and spinal cord

Thrombophlebitis of superior sagittal sinus and suppurative ependymitis, with beginning hydrocephalus

Kernig sign. Patient supine, with hip flexed 90°. Knee cannot be fully extended.

Neck rigidity (Brudzinski neck sign). Passive flexion of neck causes flexion of both legs and thighs.

INFECTIOUS DISEASE

BACTERIAL MENINGITIS

of appropriate antibiotic therapy before definitive culture and sensitivity data are available, but it should not delay initiation of appropriate antibiotic therapy. Rapid detection of microbial antigens by counterimmunoelectrophoresis or latex agglutination tests can aid diagnosis when CSF Gram stain and cultures are not diagnostic. Newer molecular diagnostic techniques are anticipated.

The initial CSF analysis should also include measurement of the opening pressure, color, WBC count and differential, and the levels of glucose and protein. Typically in bacterial meningitis, CSF opening pressure is increased (>200 mm of CSF lying down and >35 mm Hg upright). The fluid is usually turbid or frankly purulent and contains predominantly (>90%) polymorphonuclear leukocytes. The CSF glucose level is very low, usually less than 50% that found in concomitant serum glucose. Low glucose levels (<40 mg/100 mL) are found in some cases of meningitis with clear CSF, such as cases from *Listeria monocytogenes*, *M tuberculosis*, and *Cryptococcus neoformans*. Normal glucose levels are common in viral meningitis. Usually, CSF protein levels are increased, often greater than 100 mg/dL (reference range, <45 mg/dL). In patients with parameningeal foci, such as a brain or epidural spinal abscess, or with multiple septic emboli, CSF glucose may not be as low as with typical bacterial meningitis, even though its protein level is significantly increased.

TREATMENT

Bacterial meningitis is life threatening. Any delay in its diagnosis by not assessing the patient initially or not beginning therapy at the first consideration of this critical diagnosis can increase morbidity and mortality. Antibiotic treatment must be initiated as soon as possible, guided by CSF examination results. When CSF examination cannot be performed promptly, empiric therapy must be instituted immediately. Patients must receive at least 10 days of high-dose IV antibiotics that easily cross the blood-brain barrier. Empiric IV therapy with a third-generation cephalosporin, such as ceftriaxone or cefotaxime plus vancomycin, must commence pending results of the bacterial cultures. High-dose corticosteroids, administered before antibiotic therapy, are recommended for all children and should be seriously considered for adults with community-acquired meningitis. When culture and sensitivity data are available, a specific antimicrobial therapy can be defined. Penicillin G is recommended for documented meningococcal meningitis.

Antimicrobial therapy for meningitis caused by *S pneumoniae* should be based on antibiotic sensitivity test results. If the strain is susceptible to penicillin, penicillin or ceftriaxone is recommended. Ceftriaxone or cefotaxime are recommended when the strain is not susceptible to penicillin and is susceptible to cephalosporins. If the strain is susceptible to neither cephalosporins nor penicillin, vancomycin should be added to a third-generation cephalosporin (cefotaxime or ceftriaxone). In patients older than 50 years, empiric therapy with ampicillin should be added to vancomycin and a third-generation cephalosporin to provide coverage for *Listeria monocytogenes*.

COMPLICATIONS

Of patients with bacterial meningitis, approximately 15% experience acute and chronic complications, including cranial nerve dysfunctions, particularly those affecting extraocular function (CN-III, -IV, and -VI), CN-VII, and sometimes CN-VIII, although this is less common today with the antibiotics lacking in specific ototoxicity or vestibular toxicity. However, permanent sensorineural hearing loss occurs occasionally, most likely with pediatric meningococcal infections. Assorted cranial neuropathies are generally secondary to the exudate common with the more purulent forms of bacterial and tuberculosis meningitis.

Focal or generalized seizures, various focal cerebral signs, coma, and acute cerebral edema also sometimes occur. Findings mimicking a stroke, such as a hemiparesis, dysphasia, and hemianopsia, are seen relatively infrequently; persistence of such findings suggests secondary cerebral arteritis, cerebral venous thrombosis, or rarely a mass lesion, particularly an abscess. Even with astute and early diagnosis, mortality rates are still at least 10% for meningococcal and 30% for pneumococcal meningitis. Without immediate diagnosis and treatment, mortality and morbidity are significantly higher.

Chemoprophylaxis

Chemoprophylaxis is particularly recommended for persons in close contact with patients who acquired meningococcal meningitis, especially in confined settings such as college dormitories and army barracks. Rifampin is preferred; ciprofloxacin is also effective.

Vaccines

Vaccines are available for 3 common organisms. *H influenzae*, type b protein-polysaccharide vaccine, is highly effective in preventing meningitis in newborns and young infants. *N meningitidis* (meningococcus) serogroups A, C, Y, and W135 polysaccharide vaccine is recommended for high-risk adults and contacts of persons with meningococcal disease. *S pneumoniae* (pneumococcus), pneumococcal protein-polysaccharide heptavalent vaccine, is recommended for children and is under study in adults. Currently, 23-valent pneumococcal polysaccharide vaccine is recommended for adults. Several new vaccines are in development.

REFERENCES

deGans J, vande Beek D. Dexamethasone in adults with bacterial meningitis. *N Engl J Med*. 2002;347:1549-1556.

Durand ML, Calderwood SB, Weber DJ, et al. Acute bacterial meningitis in adults. *N Engl J Med*. 1993;328:21-28.

Fiore AE, Moroney JF, Farley MM, et al. Clinical outcomes of meningitis caused by Streptococcus pneumoniae in the era of antibiotic resistance. *Clin Infect Dis*. 2000;30:71-77.

Friedland IR, Paris MM, Ehrett S, et al. Evaluation of antimicrobial regimens for treatment of experimental penicillin and cephalosporin-resistant pneumococcal meningitis. *Antimicrob Agents Chemother*. 1993;37:1630-1636.

McMillan DA, Lin CY Aronin SI, Quagliarello VJ. Community-acquired bacterial meningitis in adults: categorization of causes and timing of death. *Clin Infect Dis*. 2001;33:969-975.

Odio CM, Faingezicht I, Paris M, et al. The beneficial effects of early dexamethasone administration in infants and children with bacterial meningitis. *N Engl J Med*. 1991;324:1525-1531.

Schuchat A, Robinson K, Wenger J, et al. Bacterial meningitis in the United States. *N Engl J Med*. 1997;337:970-976.

Syrogiannopoulos GA, Olsen KD, Reisch JS, McCracken GH Jr. Dexamethasone in the treatment of experimental Haemophilus influenzae type b meningitis. *J Infect Dis*. 1987;155:213-219.

Chapter 64
Parameningeal Infections

Donald E. Craven, Francesco G. De Rosa, and H. Royden Jones, Jr

Clinical Vignette

A diabetic 46-year-old man experienced typical flu symptoms. Two days later, right hip and leg pain developed, followed by vomiting, dehydration, and upper thoracic spine pain. These difficulties rapidly worsened over 6 to 8 hours, when the patient lost some sensation in his legs and then became unable to walk or urinate. His spouse called 911 for transportation to the ED.

Neurologic examination demonstrated a spastic paraparesis with a T8 sensory level. The patient required urinary catheterization. Physicians were concerned about possible bacteremia or a rapidly evolving spinal cord lesion.

Spinal MRI demonstrated a paraspinal abscess extending from T6 to T10. Emergency neurosurgical decompression was performed. The patient had an incomplete recovery.

Relatively uncommon disorders, parameningeal infections are always important in the differential diagnosis of acute cerebral or spinal lesions. These processes can easily go unrecognized until it is too late to prevent permanent neurologic deficits. Although these abscesses are easily considered within the setting of an overt infection, a precise microbial source is not always clear in the clinical presentation. Consideration of whether any acute spinal or cerebral lesion could have an infectious basis is essential, particularly in patients with chronic illnesses such as diabetes mellitus. These clinical settings, particularly a spinal epidural abscess, require the highest diagnostic and therapeutic priority. They are among the most urgent neurologic emergencies and demand immediate attention. Even when appropriate diagnostic and therapeutic focus occurs, outcome may still be guarded, as in the vignette in this chapter.

SPINAL EPIDURAL ABSCESS

Patients usually present with fever and back pain, sometimes with varying degrees of leg weakness. There are 4 clinical stages: focal vertebral pain, pain radiation along the course of involved nerve roots, spinal cord compression, and paralysis below the lesion level.

A purulent or granulomatous collection within the spinal epidural space may overlie or encircle the spinal cord, nerve roots, and nerves (Figure 64-1). Although the infection is usually localized within 3 to 4 vertebral segments, it rarely extends the length of the spinal canal.

Staphylococcus aureus is the most common organism leading to a spinal epidural abscess, but aerobic or anaerobic streptococci and gram-negative organisms also may be isolated. Mixed anaerobic and aerobic organisms are sometimes responsible. When no organism is isolated or if granulomas are identified, *Mycobacterium tuberculosis* of the spine, or Pott disease, should be considered. The most common focus for hematogenous spread to the epidural space is a skin infection, especially a furuncle. Antecedent hematogenous vertebral osteomyelitis comprises approximately 40% of spinal epidural abscess. Dental and upper respiratory infections are also frequent sources.

Any patient presenting with back pain, fever, and localized tenderness or signs of cord compression requires immediate MRI. Surgical or CT-guided needle aspiration is needed for accurate diagnosis and possible decompression. Blood cultures are recommended. Lumbar puncture should not be performed. Appropriate parenteral antibiotics are necessary for 3 to 4 weeks in uncomplicated cases and for up to 8 weeks or more if osteomyelitis is present.

PARAMENINGEAL INFECTIONS

Figure 64-1
Parameningeal Infections

Brain abscess

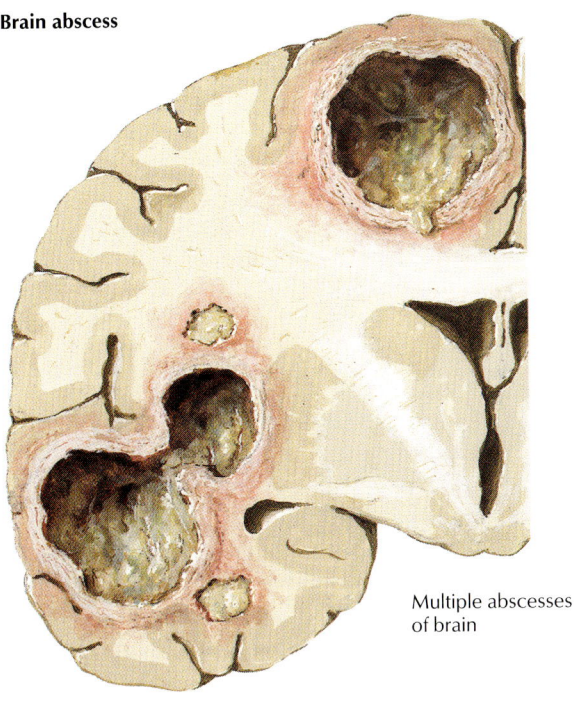

Multiple abscesses of brain

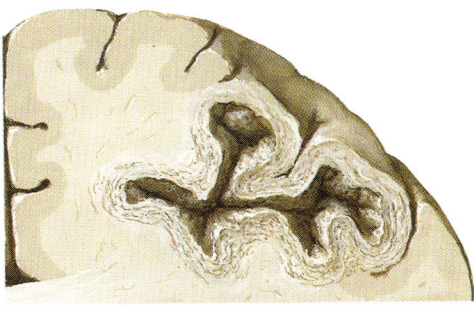

Scar of healed brain abscess, with collapse of brain tissue into cavity

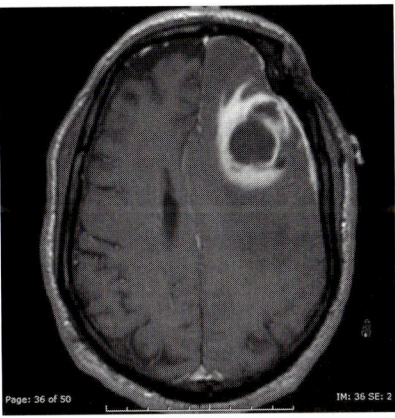

Axial T1-weighted, gadolinium-enhancing left frontal mass with central hypointensity

Subdural abscess

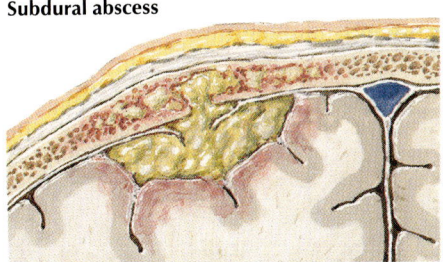

Osteomyelitis of skull, with penetration of dura to form subdural "collar button" abscess

Epidural abscess

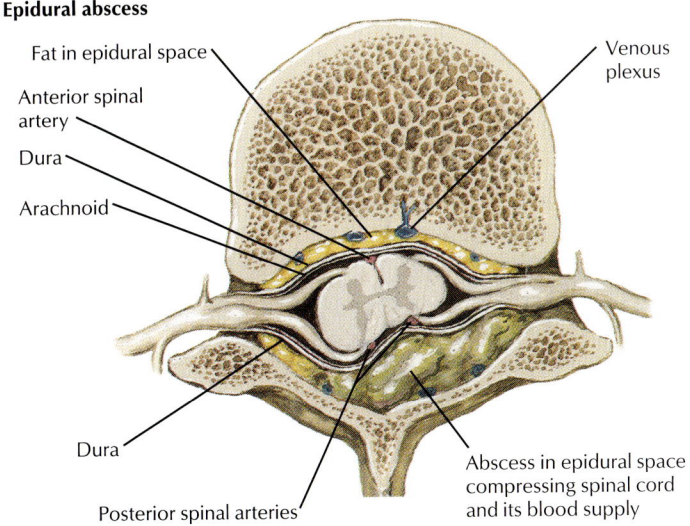

- Fat in epidural space
- Anterior spinal artery
- Dura
- Arachnoid
- Venous plexus
- Abscess in epidural space compressing spinal cord and its blood supply
- Dura
- Posterior spinal arteries

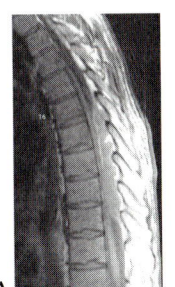
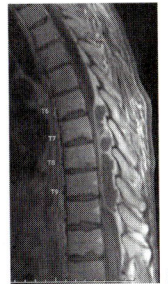

Epidural abscess. Sagittal T1-weighted images without (**A**) and with (**B**) gadolinium enhancement demonstrate an extensive posterior epidural process from T6 to T11. Enhancement of the granulation tissue allows appreciation of nonenhancing focal pus collections.

INFECTIOUS DISEASE

PARAMENINGEAL INFECTIONS

BRAIN ABSCESS

Brain abscess, which may be indolent or fulminant, results from direct extension from a contiguous focus, such as middle ear or sinus infections; congenital heart disease, with a right-to-left shunt or pulmonary AVMs with similar shunt mechanisms; hematogenous spread from distant infection sites in the head and neck, heart (infectious endocarditis), lung, or abdomen; or direct introduction of bacteria after penetrating head injuries. The cardinal symptom of brain abscess is relentless and progressive headache, usually followed by focal neurologic manifestations. Only two thirds of patients have fever. Papilledema and other signs of increased intracranial pressure may develop.

Most brain abscess cases are polymicrobial. Etiologic agents often include aerobic bacteria, such as streptococci, Enterobacteriaceae, and staphylococci. *Streptococcus milleri* normally resides in the oral cavity, appendix, and female genital tract and has a proclivity for abscess formation. Anaerobic microorganisms, such as *Bacteroides* and *Prevotella* species, are present in up to 40% of cases. Fungi are uncommon but increasingly recognized among immunosuppressed patients.

CT enables an early diagnosis (Figure 64-1). The characteristic appearance is a focal cerebral lesion with a hypodense center and a peripheral uniform ring enhancement after contrast material injection. Sometimes there is a concomitant area of surrounding edema. Lumbar puncture should be avoided to prevent abscess herniation or rupture into the ventricular system.

Therapeutically, the abscess may be directly aspirated. Empiric medical therapy is started with a third- or fourth-generation cephalosporin or penicillin plus metronidazole, depending on the setting. Surgery may not be necessary if follow-up CT demonstrates decreased abscess size. Brain edema associated with acute brain abscess necessitates use of steroids and mannitol, as well as phenytoin to prevent convulsions.

SUBDURAL EMPYEMA

Another form of life-threatening neurologic infection, subdural empyema, is typically characterized by a purulent collection within the potential space between the dura mater and arachnoid membrane (Figure 64-1). An active paranasal sinusitis, particularly originating within the frontal sinuses or mastoid air cells, usually precedes extension of the infection into the subdural space. Occasionally, it is directly introduced through operative or traumatic wound sites.

Streptococci usually comprise 50% of cases; *S aureus*, gram-negative bacteria, and anaerobic bacteria such as microaerophilic streptococci, *Bacteroides* species, and *Clostridium perfringens* are sometimes identified. Occasionally, polymicrobial infections occur.

Localized swelling, erythema, headache, or tenderness of the site overlying the primary infection may occur. As the illness progresses, the headache becomes generalized and severe, with a high fever, vomiting and nuchal rigidity developing. Seizures, hemiparesis, visual field defects, and papilledema sometimes occur.

CSF contains 1 to 1000 WBCs; protein level is increased, and glucose level is normal. CT or MRI demonstrates a low-absorption extracerebral mass. A thin, moderately dense margin may be visualized with contrast medium.

Treatment includes a combination of prompt surgical drainage and intensive antimicrobial therapy. The initial antibiotic choice requires intravenous third- or fourth-generation cephalosporin for aerobic bacteria and metronidazole for anaerobic bacteria. Prophylactic use of anticonvulsants and corticosteroids may also be required.

REFERENCES

Brook I. Aerobic and anaerobic bacteriology of intracranial abscesses. *Pediatr Neurol*. 1992;8:210-214.

Chun CH, Johnson JD, Hofstetter M, Raff MJ. Brain abscess: a study of 45 consecutive cases. *Medicine (Baltimore)*. 1986;65:415-431.

Giannoni CM, Stewart MG, Alford EL. Intracranial complications of sinusitis. *Laryngoscope*. 1997;107:863-867.

Heilpern KL, Lorber B. Focal intracranial infections. *Infect Dis Clin North Am*. 1996;10:879-898.

Ng PY, Seow WT, Ong PL. Brain abscesses: review of 30 cases treated with surgery. *Aust N Z J Surg*. 1995;65:664-666.

Nussbaum ES, Rigamonti D, Standiford H, Numaguchi Y, Wolf AL, Robinson WL. Spinal epidural abscess: a report of 40 cases and review. *Surg Neurol*. 1992;38:225-231.

Schliamser SE, Backman K, Norrby SR. Intracranial abscesses in adults: an analysis of 54 consecutive cases. *Scand J Infect Dis*. 1988;20:1-9.

Seydoux C, Francioli P. Bacterial brain abscesses: factors influencing mortality and sequelae. *Clin Infect Dis.* 1992;15:394-401.

Wheeler D, Keiser P, Rigamonti D, Keay S. Medical management of spinal epidural abscesses: case report and review. *Clin Infect Dis.* 1992;15:22-27.

Yamamoto M, Fukushima T, Ohshiro S, et al. Brain abscess caused by Streptococcus intermedius: two case reports. *Surg Neurol.* 1999;51:219-222.

Yang SY, Zhao CS. Review of 140 patients with brain abscess. *Surg Neurol.* 1993;39:290-296.

Chapter 65
Neurosyphilis

Daniel P. McQuillen

Clinical Vignette

A 73-year-old man experienced acute-onset dizziness with nausea and diaphoresis. He reported unsteadiness and decreased hearing in his right ear, which had developed over several months. His medical history included hypertension and hyperlipidemia.

The patient was afebrile, with a BP of 170/88 mm Hg and a pulse of 88 beats/min. His pupils were small and irregular, accommodating to near vision but not reactive to light or painful stimuli; cranial nerves were otherwise intact. He had a mildly ataxic gait and a positive Romberg sign, but his muscle stretch reflexes and vibratory sense were normal.

Head CT, CBC, chemistry, and liver function test results were normal. RPR (1:2) and fluorescent treponemal antibody absorption (2+) test results were positive. CSF examination revealed a WBC count of 23/mm³ (78% lymphocytes), protein of 59 mg/dL, glucose of 68 mg/dL, and positive VDRL test results.

Intravenous penicillin G was initiated for 10 days. The patient's symptoms gradually resolved.

Syphilis, or lues, is an uncommon disorder occurring primarily within the immune-compromised population, particularly in those with AIDS. *Treponema pallidum*, a spiral bacterium that is difficult to culture in the laboratory, causes syphilis. The diagnosis is made by spirochete identification in material from primary lesions using dark-field microscopy or serologic methods. CNS syphilis occurs in less than 20% of patients with primary infection. Typical of many patients with CNS lues, diagnosis is made only by clinical signs, particularly the disparate pupillary responses to light and accommodation, along with often subtle findings of posterior spinal cord column and dorsal root ganglion involvement.

Untreated, *T pallidum* causes chronic inflammation of CNS cellular and interstitial tissues, culminating in a granulomatous process, producing endarteritis and gummatous lesions. In the United States, syphilis occurs primarily in persons aged 20 to 39 years. Reported rates in men are 1.5 times those of women. The incidence is highest in women aged 20 to 29 years and men aged 30 to 39 years.

Cases of primary and secondary syphilis in the United States increased 2.1% between 2000 and 2001 and 12.4% between 2001 and 2002. Increases were observed only in men; several outbreaks, associated with high rates of HIV coinfection and high-risk sexual behavior, were seen among men who had sex with men. From 2000 to 2002, the number of primary and secondary syphilis cases decreased 19.0% among women and 10.3% among African-Americans. Poverty, inadequate health care access, and lack of education are associated with disproportionately high syphilis incidence in certain populations.

CLINICAL PRESENTATION

There are 5 classic neurologic presentations: meningitis, meningovascular syphilis, tabes dorsalis, general paresis, and gumma.

Syphilitic meningitis develops early after primary infection, usually coinciding with the secondary-stage syphilis rash. Common symptoms are nocturnal headache, malaise, stiff neck, fever, and cranial nerve palsies. CSF shows increased lymphocyte count and total protein; serum RPR test results are usually positive.

Meningovascular syphilis, as described in the vignette at the beginning of this chapter, is a more chronic disorder. Usually evident 20 or more years after initial exposure, it rarely occurs as early as 2 years after the primary untreated infection. Chronic inflammation produces brain or spinal cord infarction leading to cranial nerve palsies, cerebrovascular accidents, seizures, or paraplegia. Argyll Robertson pupils, which are

NEUROSYPHILIS

small and irregular and accommodate to near vision but do not react to light or painful stimuli, are present.

Tabes dorsalis develops 10 to 20 years after primary infection, usually in persons aged 25 to 45 years. Both direct invasion by the spirochete and an immunologic reaction may occur, producing degenerative and sclerotic changes in the posterior nerve root fibers of the spinal cord, spinal ganglia cells, long fibers of the posterior columns of the spinal cord, optic nerves, and oculomotor nuclei. Symptoms may include lightning nerve root pains, gastric crisis, spastic gait, failing vision, and urinary and sexual function disturbances. Optic nerves show progressive primary atrophy; Argyll Robertson pupils are small and irregular. Impaired vibration sense, ataxia, and a positive Romberg sign are present. Knee and ankle jerks are absent. RPR test results in blood and VDRL test results in CSF are positive in only 59% of patients.

General paresis (dementia paralytica) occurs most commonly in patients older than 40 years, from direct spirochete invasion of neural tissue causing neuronal degeneration, astrocytic proliferation, and meningitis (Figure 65-1). Resultant degenerative and sclerotic changes produce a thickened dura mater, chronic subdural hematoma, cortical cell atrophy, and astrocyte proliferation. The frontal lobes are disproportionately affected. Progressive dementia occurs in 60% of patients, but headaches, insomnia, personality change, impaired judgment, disturbed emotional responses, slurred speech, and tremors can also develop. Argyll Robertson pupils are characteristic. RPR test results in blood and VDRL test results in CSF are positive in more than 90% of patients.

Gumma of the brain and spinal cord are rare. Symptoms are consistent with expanding CNS lesions.

DIAGNOSIS AND TREATMENT

Clinical Vignette

Treatment for neurosyphilis in a 49-year-old man resolved his headaches. However, 6 months later, he began exhibiting changes in personality, behavior, and memory, which continued during the next 8 months. He began losing money without recollection of where he left it and driving recklessly, leading, at his wife's request, to forfeiture of his driver's license. He became increasingly distractible and restless and began doing things repetitively. Delusional behaviors were witnessed, including what seemed to be conversations with angels and a declaration that Jehovah was talking through him. He stuffed toilet paper in his mouth, apparently because of a bad taste. Although normally of even temperament, he became increasingly irritable and verbally abusive. Neurologic examination showed orientation to person but not date. He could not perform serial sevens and had difficulty with categorizing words, relying on descriptions. He had Argyll Robertson pupils but normal cranial nerves, sensory and motor examination results, muscle stretch reflexes, and flexor plantar responses.

CT and MRI findings were normal. Results of EEG were abnormal because of 5-Hz generalized slow activity. CSF examination demonstrated a WBC count of 6/mm^3, protein of 72 mg/dL, and a positive VDRL test result of 1:16. The serum RPR ratio was 1:256. The patient was treated again with 2 weeks of IV penicillin G followed by 3 weeks of IM benzathine penicillin.

This vignette illustrates the importance of early diagnosis and appropriate therapy of primary syphilis. When the pathologic condition evolves to general paresis, treatment is usually unsuccessful in resolving personality changes.

Diagnosis is based on serologic tests with blood RPR and CSF VDRL tests for screening and fluorescent treponemal antibody absorption test or microhemagglutination–*T pallidum* test for specific confirmation. CSF usually demonstrates a modest increase in primarily lymphocytic cells, with a moderate protein increase and normal glucose level.

The treatment for all forms of syphilis is penicillin. Repeated therapeutic blood and CSF levels are necessary to effect a cure if the syphilis stage is treatable.

Future Directions

Although no large-scale randomized trial has compared azithromycin directly to benzathine penicillin, preliminary studies support the efficacy of azithromycin (a single oral dose of 1 or 2 g) in treatment of early-stage syphilis. Evidence does not yet support its use in late- or tertiary-stage disease. Additional data support the use of ceftriaxone in early-stage disease. Ceftriaxone (2 g IM once daily for 10 days) produced similar CSF responses for treatment of neurosyphilis in HIV-infected individuals. In aggregate, the data

NEUROSYPHILIS

Figure 65-1

Neurosyphilis

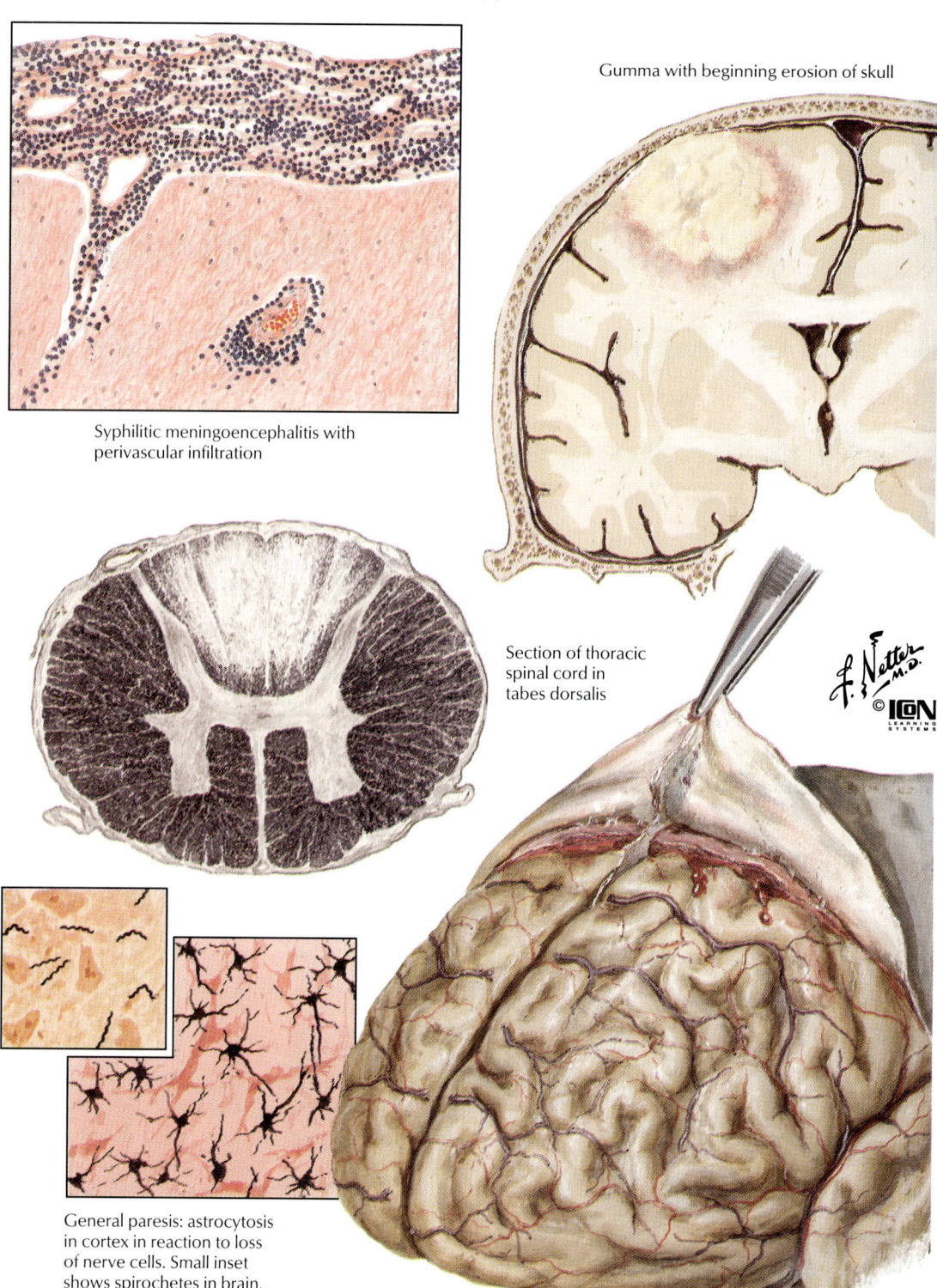

Syphilitic meningoencephalitis with perivascular infiltration

Gumma with beginning erosion of skull

Section of thoracic spinal cord in tabes dorsalis

General paresis: astrocytosis in cortex in reaction to loss of nerve cells. Small inset shows spirochetes in brain.

General paresis: atrophy of brain and chronic subdural hematoma

INFECTIOUS DISEASE

do not establish the equivalence or superiority of these agents to standard penicillin regimens but support their use as alternatives when penicillin is not a therapeutic option. Concurrent HIV infection may modify the natural history of syphilis, but the overall response to standard therapy has been no different than in HIV-seronegative individuals.

REFERENCES

Augenbraun MH. Treatment of syphilis 2001: nonpregnant adults. *Clin Infect Dis*. 2002;35:S187-S190.

Chesney AM, Kemp JE. Incidence of *Spirocheta pallida* in cerebrospinal fluid during early stage of syphilis. *JAMA*. 1924;83:1725-1728.

Golden MR, Marra CM, Holmes KK. Update on syphilis: resurgence of an old problem. *JAMA*. 2003;290:1510-1514.

Johns DR, Tierney M, Felsenstein D. Alteration in the natural history of neurosyphilis by concurrent infection with the human immunodeficiency virus. *N Engl J Med*. 1987;316:1569-1572.

Merritt HH, Adams RD, Solomon HC. *Neurosyphilis*. New York, NY: Oxford University Press; 1946.

Merritt HH, Moore M. Acute neurosyphilitic meningitis. *Medicine (Baltimore)*. 1935;7:161-167.

Primary and secondary syphilis: United States, 2002. *MMWR*. 2003;52;1117-1120..

Scheck DN, Hook EW III. Neurosyphilis. *Infect Dis Clin North Am*. 1994;8:769-795.

Chapter 66
Viral Infections of the Nervous System

Francesco G. De Rosa, Daniel P. McQuillen, Donald E. Craven, John Markman, and H. Royden Jones, Jr

ENCEPHALITIDES

A wide spectrum of etiologic agents may cause viral encephalitis, and diagnosis and management are dependent on identifying specific causative agents. Only a few are amenable to specific antiviral therapy, so prevention strategies are particularly important, especially for arthropod-borne viruses such as West Nile virus (WNV).

Herpes Simplex Encephalitis

Herpes simplex encephalitis (HSE) is the most common acute encephalitis in the United States, with an annual incidence of 1 in 250,000 to 1 in 500,000. It affects all ages and both sexes equally, without significant seasonal variation. Early antiviral treatment significantly reduces mortality, but morbidity remains unacceptably high.

Etiology

Most cases of HSE are caused by oral herpes (herpes simplex virus [HSV] type 1), but genital herpes (HSV-2) is more common in neonates with disseminated disease. HSE may occur during primary infection or, more commonly, recurrent infection. Animal data support a retrograde virus transport via olfactory or trigeminal nerves, but in human disease pathogenic pathways are not fully clarified. The disease most often involves the medial temporal and frontal lobes. The histologic picture includes hemorrhagic necrosis, inflammatory infiltrates, and cells containing intranuclear inclusions.

Clinical Vignette

An active 84-year-old woman with chronic obstructive pulmonary disease and type 2 diabetes presented with fever. No source was identified. She was sent home without treatment. Two days later, a neighbor found her acutely confused and brought her back to the hospital. This former smoker was dyspneic and wheezing. She was started empirically on clarithromycin and admitted to the hospital. She remained febrile, with a temperature up to 38.4°C, and hyponatremic (123 mEq/L). Ceftriaxone was started empirically. Her confusion and fever persisted. On the fourth day, a neurologist was consulted.

The patient was not responsive to verbal stimuli and had left eye deviation, neck stiffness, and bilateral palmar grasps. She withdrew to noxious stimuli; plantar responses were flexor. Findings of a head CT were unremarkable. CSF examination demonstrated a WBC count of 30/mm³, predominantly lymphocytes, protein of 110 mg/dL, and a normal glucose level. Acyclovir was begun.

Head MRI showed increased signal in the left insular cortex region extending inferiorly into the subthalamic nucleus region and the inferior temporal region into the parahippocampal gyrus and hippocampus, suggestive of HSV encephalitis. EEG demonstrated periodic lateralizing epileptiform discharges. This diagnosis was confirmed by HSV PCR 11 days after symptom onset. The patient had no neurologic improvement. She was discharged to hospice.

Clinical Presentation and Differential Diagnosis

Subacute or acute focal encephalitis causes signs and symptoms without characteristic diagnostic findings. Fever, headache, and altered consciousness are common, followed by seizures and hemiparesis (Figure 66-1). Dysphasia, ataxia, personality changes, cranial nerve de-

Figure 66-1

HSV Encephalitis

Possible Route of Transmission in Herpes Simplex Encephalitis

HSV
Ophthalmic branch
Meningeal branches
Trigeminal ganglion
Maxillary branch
Mandibular branch
CN-V
Temporal lobe

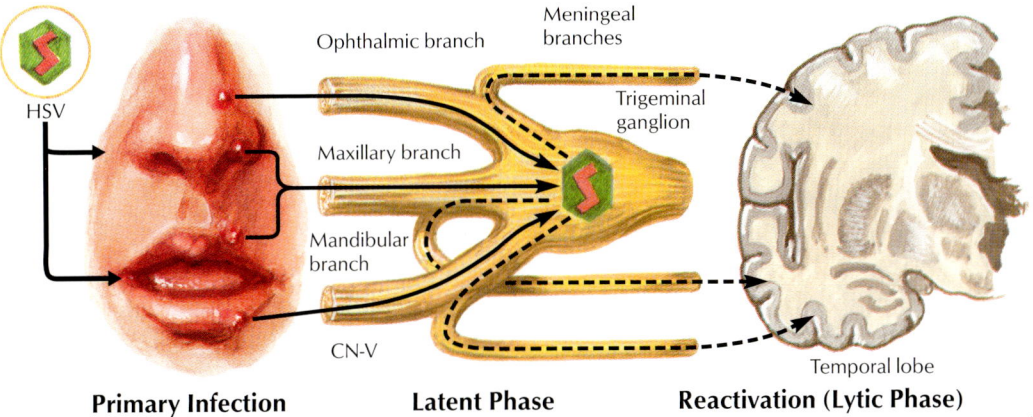

Primary Infection

Virus enters via cutaneous or mucosal surfaces to infect sensory or autonomic nerve endings with transport to cell bodies in ganglia.

Latent Phase

Virus replicates in ganglia before establishing latent phase.

Reactivation (Lytic Phase)

Reactivation of HSV in trigeminal ganglion can result in spread to brain (temporal lobe) via meningeal branches of CN-V.

Clinical Features of HSV Encephalitis

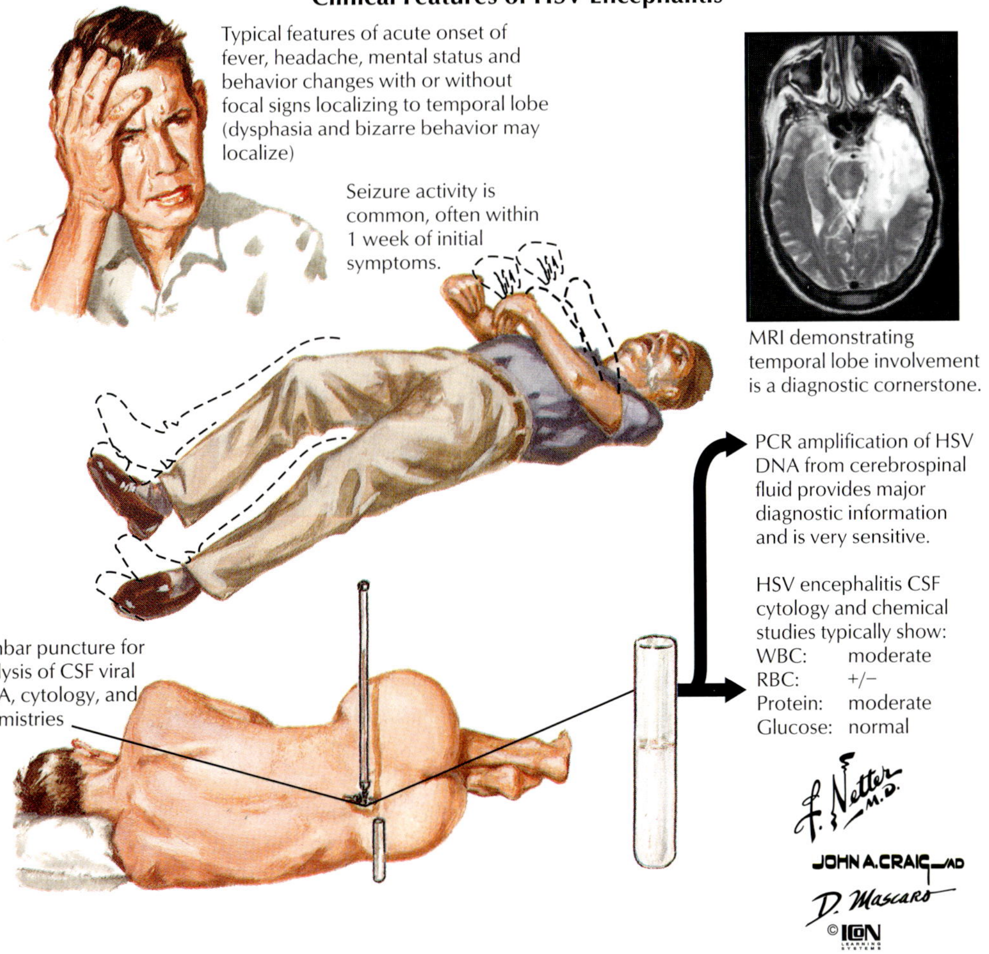

Typical features of acute onset of fever, headache, mental status and behavior changes with or without focal signs localizing to temporal lobe (dysphasia and bizarre behavior may localize)
Seizure activity is common, often within 1 week of initial symptoms.
MRI demonstrating temporal lobe involvement is a diagnostic cornerstone.
PCR amplification of HSV DNA from cerebrospinal fluid provides major diagnostic information and is very sensitive.
HSV encephalitis CSF cytology and chemical studies typically show:
WBC: moderate
RBC: +/−
Protein: moderate
Glucose: normal
Lumbar puncture for analysis of CSF viral DNA, cytology, and chemistries
F. Netter M.D.
JOHN A.CRAIG AD
D. Mascaro
© ICON

VIRAL INFECTIONS OF THE NERVOUS SYSTEM

fects, and papilledema are also found. The differential diagnosis includes vascular diseases, tuberculosis, tumors, other forms of viral encephalitis, bacterial abscesses, cryptococcal infections, and toxoplasmosis.

Diagnostic Approach and Treatment

For patients with suspected encephalitis, the diagnosis should include a CT scan (rule out a mass effect) and CSF examination. MRI and EEG may be used for further investigation (Figure 66-2).

CT scan results are abnormal in 50% of cases and usually demonstrate localized edema, low-density lesions, mass effects, contrast enhancements, or hemorrhage. If results are negative, the more sensitive MRI should be performed. Some recommend MRI as the method of choice.

CSF findings are nonspecific, often including a lymphocytic pleocytosis with a slight protein increase. Abnormal CSF findings are found in 96% of biopsy-proven HSE cases. EEG may show spike and slow waves localized to the involved area often as periodic lateralized epileptiform discharges (PLEDs).

Brain biopsy is the gold standard for specificity, but it is rarely used because of the availability of PCR. Biopsy specimens should be examined for histopathologic changes and for HSV antigens by immunofluorescence testing and appropriate culture techniques.

PCR for HSV-DNA detects HSV-1 and -2 in CSF, compares favorably with brain biopsy-proven cases, and has good sensitivity and specificity (90-98% for both). The viral sequence for HSV may be detected months after the acute episode and may be negative in early disease phases. PCR should not be used to monitor therapy success. No standardized commercial assay is available.

The course of the patient in the first vignette in this chapter emphasizes the need for primary care physicians always to consider HSE in individuals of any age who experience relatively acute changes in mental status. Immediate initiation of acyclovir is indicated the moment HSV is suspected; this relatively benign medication has the greatest chance of efficacy when initiated early. Otherwise, the outcome is usually poor, with minimal chance of return to independent living.

Prognosis

Before the availability of IV acyclovir, mortality from HSE was approximately 70%. Early antiviral therapy for 10 to 21 days has reduced mortality and morbidity substantially. Although morbidity remains high, mortality is 10% to 20%.

Rabies

Rabies is an acute viral CNS disease caused by an RNA virus of the rhabdovirus family. Although usually transmitted to humans through wounds contaminated by the saliva of a rabid animal, rare airborne transmission has occurred in bat-infested caves. Transmission by corneal transplant has also been rarely reported.

Animals predominantly infected and involved in rabies transmission vary by geographic area. In the United States in 1995, of the 7887 cases of animal rabies, 50% were raccoons, 23% were skunks, and 10% were bats (Figure 66-3). Dogs and cats are unusual sources of animal rabies in the United States because of rabies vaccinations; nevertheless, dog and cat bites account for 90% of human rabies cases worldwide.

Etiology

After a rabid dog bite, the rabies virus may travel through the nerves to the spinal cord and into the brain, where it disseminates widely, traveling centrifugally along nerves to retina, cornea, salivary glands, skin, and other organs. The incubation period ranges from 15 days to more than 1 year. If the virus involves the salivary glands, it usually manifests in 10 to 14 days. Quarantined animals always manifest the disease within 2 weeks if infected.

Clinical Presentation and Diagnosis

Two main syndromes have been described: encephalitic (furious) and paralytic (dumb) rabies. The prodrome includes anxiety, fever, and headache, often with paresthesias at the bite site. Two to 10 days after the prodrome, the **encephalitic form** presents with agitation, autonomic instability, delirium, seizures, nuchal rigidity, severe pharynx spasms, stridor, and possible

VIRAL INFECTIONS OF THE NERVOUS SYSTEM

Herpes Simplex Encephalitis

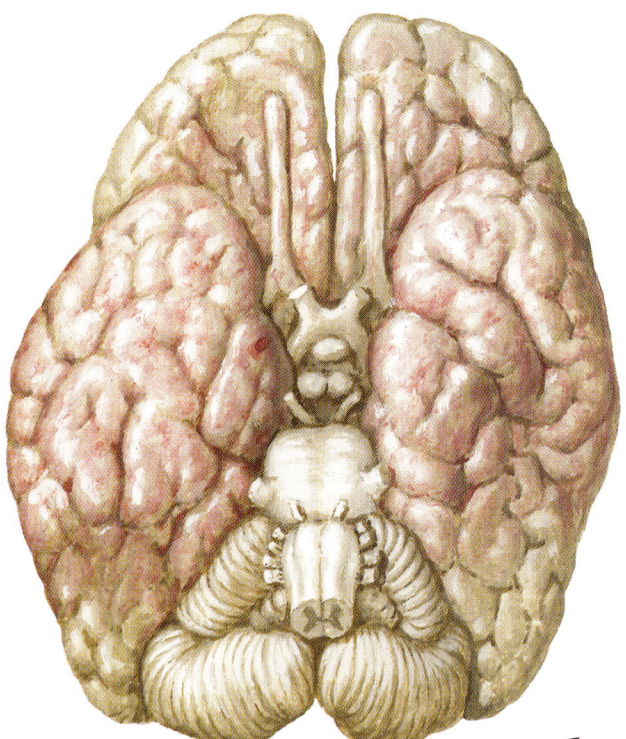

Swelling and patchy hemorrhagic areas, most marked in right temporal lobe

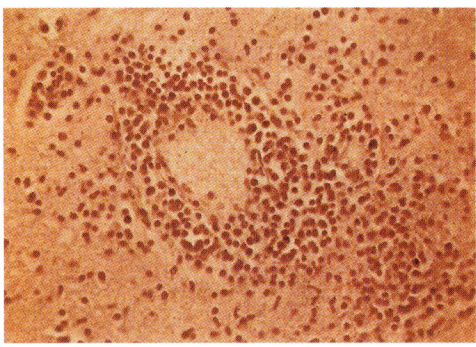

Perivascular infiltration with mononuclear cells in disrupted brain tissue

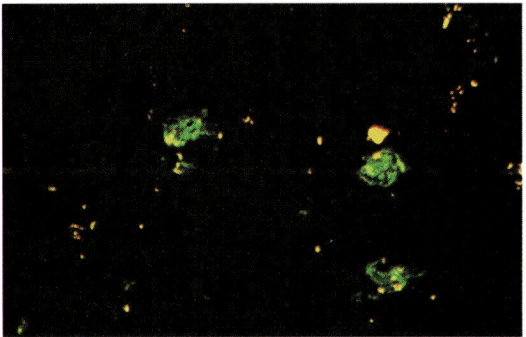

Immunofluorescent staining shows presence of herpesvirus antigen in neurons

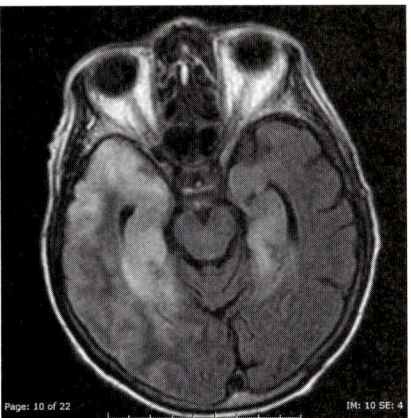

Axial FLAIR image with extensive intracranial signal in right temporal lobe and medial left temporal lobe

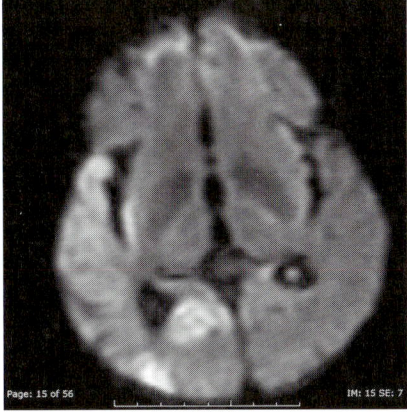

Diffusion with right temporal and insular changes

INFECTIOUS DISEASE

VIRAL INFECTIONS OF THE NERVOUS SYSTEM

Figure 66-3

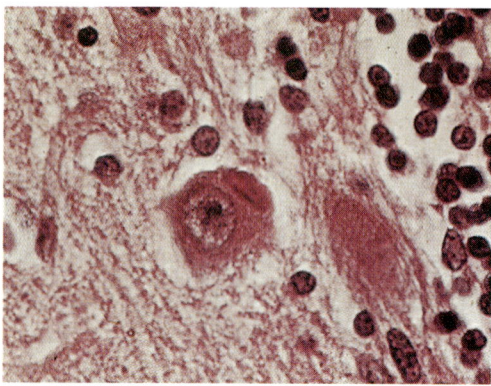

Negri inclusion body in Purkinje cell of brain

Rabies

Common animal disseminators

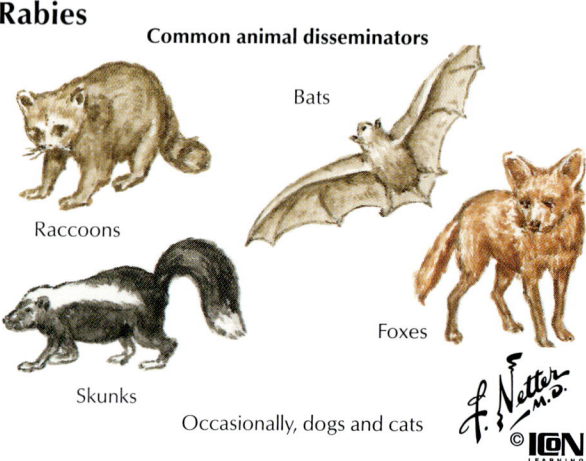

Raccoons

Bats

Skunks

Foxes

Occasionally, dogs and cats

---

hydrophobia or aerophobia. The **paralytic form** (20% of cases) presents with progressive paralysis until death. The clinical course is more indolent, with a clear sensorium sometimes preserved until late in the course.

Diagnosis is made through demonstration of anti-rabies glycoprotein antibodies in serum or CSF or through immunofluorescence for glycoprotein antigens in the nuchal skin or brain biopsy. Molecular techniques detect the virus nucleoprotein in CSF, saliva, or biopsy samples.

Clinical manifestations contrast strikingly with neuropathologic findings. Only mild congestion and perivascular inflammation are noted. The Negri body, a neuronal cytoplasmic inclusion with a dark central inner body, is pathognomonic (Figure 66-3).

Prognosis

Improvements in vaccine grown in human cells and human anti-rabies globulin have made early postexposure prophylaxis safe and effective. The Centers for Disease Control's postexposure prophylaxis for rabies includes immediate and thorough wound cleansing with soap and water, administration of human rabies immune globulin around the wound, and rabies vaccine IM on days 0, 3, 7, 14, and 28. No effective treatment is available after clinical illness develops.

West Nile Virus

West nile virus is a flavivirus usually found in Africa, West Asia, and the Middle East. The Middle Eastern strains are most closely related genetically to the St Louis encephalitis virus found in the United States. The virus can infect humans, birds, mosquitoes, horses, and some other mammals. It was not documented in the Western Hemisphere until 1999.

In the temperate zones of the world, West Nile encephalitis cases occur primarily in the late summer or early fall. In southern climates, where temperatures are milder, WNV can be transmitted year-round.

Clinical Vignette

A 54-year-old man with no significant medical history presented with malaise, weakness, anorexia, watery diarrhea, and mild headache of 2 days' duration. He was treated conservatively for presumed viral gastroenteritis. He was admitted to the ED 2 days later with increasingly severe frontal headache and fever.

Physical examination was remarkable for a temperature of 39.6°C and nuchal rigidity without focal neurologic signs or impaired sensorium. The peripheral WBC count was 7900/mm³, the CSF WBC count was 140/mm³ (11% polymorphonuclear leukocytes, 88% lymphocytes, 1% monocytes), protein was 105 mg/dL, and glucose was 45 mg/dL. CSF gram stain results were negative. Head CT findings were unremarkable.

INFECTIOUS DISEASE

The patient was treated empirically with ampicillin and ceftriaxone. Blood cultures remained negative. He slowly defervesced; his headache improved, and he was discharged to home.

After discharge, results of IgM and IgG antibody and enzyme-linked immunosorbent assays returned positive for WNV. One week after discharge, a transient morbilliform rash developed on the patient's chest, back, and arms.

Clinical Presentation

West Nile fever is a mild disease characterized by flulike symptoms that develop 3 to 15 days after the bite of an infected mosquito. West Nile fever typically lasts only a few days and does not seem to cause any long-term health effects. Mild fever, headache, body aches, occasional skin rash, and swollen glands are the most common symptoms.

More severe disease can manifest as encephalitis, meningitis, or meningoencephalitis. Cases of acute proximal and asymmetric flaccid paralysis have occurred in recent outbreaks in the United States. Neurophysiologic, radiologic, and pathologic studies suggest WNV causes acute flaccid paralysis by damaging anterior horn cells in the spinal cord. The clinical presentation is similar to poliomyelitis.

Diagnosis is made by serologic assays of blood and CSF. Treatment is supportive; there is no specific drug treatment or vaccine available.

HERPES ZOSTER, SHINGLES

Shingles is the most common neurologic disease. In America, it is estimated that 15% of the population will experience shingles during their lifetime. An aging population, increasing prevalence of immunosuppressed hosts from myriad causes, and widespread adoption of varicella vaccination in children are causing these rates to rise. Advancing age is the most significant risk factor for acute herpes zoster reactivation and development of the chronic neuropathic pain of postherpetic neuralgia (PHN).

The growing use of varicella vaccine reduces the rates of chickenpox in children. As a consequence, fewer adults have experienced viral exposure. Waning varicella-specific immunity in older adults leads to higher rates of shingles. The precise breach of immune surveillance that allows for varicella reactivation remains unknown.

Although most cases affect healthy adults, 10% of all patients with lymphoma will develop shingles. In addition to treatment of acute symptoms, further diagnostic evaluation for underlying carcinoma or lymphoma needs to be considered. Other patients at high risk for herpes zoster include organ-transplant recipients and those receiving corticosteroid therapy. Immunocompromised persons can experience recurrent, multifocal, protracted bouts of acute neuralgia.

Pathophysiology and Diagnosis

Focal reactivation of latent varicella-zoster virus (VZV) in sensory ganglia causes the distinctive rash known as ***shingles*** (Figure 66-4). This viral peripheral nervous system disease occurs in 2 discrete stages. Initially, human herpes virus causes varicella (chickenpox), primarily during childhood. After chickenpox, VZV becomes latent in the peripheral nervous system ganglia, where it persists. Later in the life of the host, the dormant virus regains virulence and produces new disease, most commonly shingles. In immunocompetent hosts, reactivation of the herpes virus is typically an isolated event. Reactivation is associated with declining, virus-specific, cell-mediated immune response.

The dorsal root ganglion is the primary site of infection. The virus spreads transaxonally to the skin. Cellular level examination reveals hemorrhagic inflammation extending from the sensory ganglion to its projections in the nerve, skin, and adjacent soft tissue. Virions also spread centrally into the spinal cord, causing an occult focal poliomyelitis in the anterior horn cells. VZV can spread to the large cerebral arteries to cause a spectrum of large-vessel vascular injury, ranging from vasculopathy to vasculitis with resultant stroke. The damage may ascend into the CNS at the level of the dorsal columns and brainstem. Cellular scrapings from the base of fresh skin lesions are the most efficient way to confirm the diagnosis of VZV infection. Immunofluorescence assays reveal infected epithelial cells.

Clinical Manifestations

A vesicular skin rash in a dermatomal distribution forms the clinical signature of VZV reactivation in the dorsal root ganglion. Although any spinal segment or cranial nerve may be in-

VIRAL INFECTIONS OF THE NERVOUS SYSTEM

Figure 66-4

Herpes Zoster

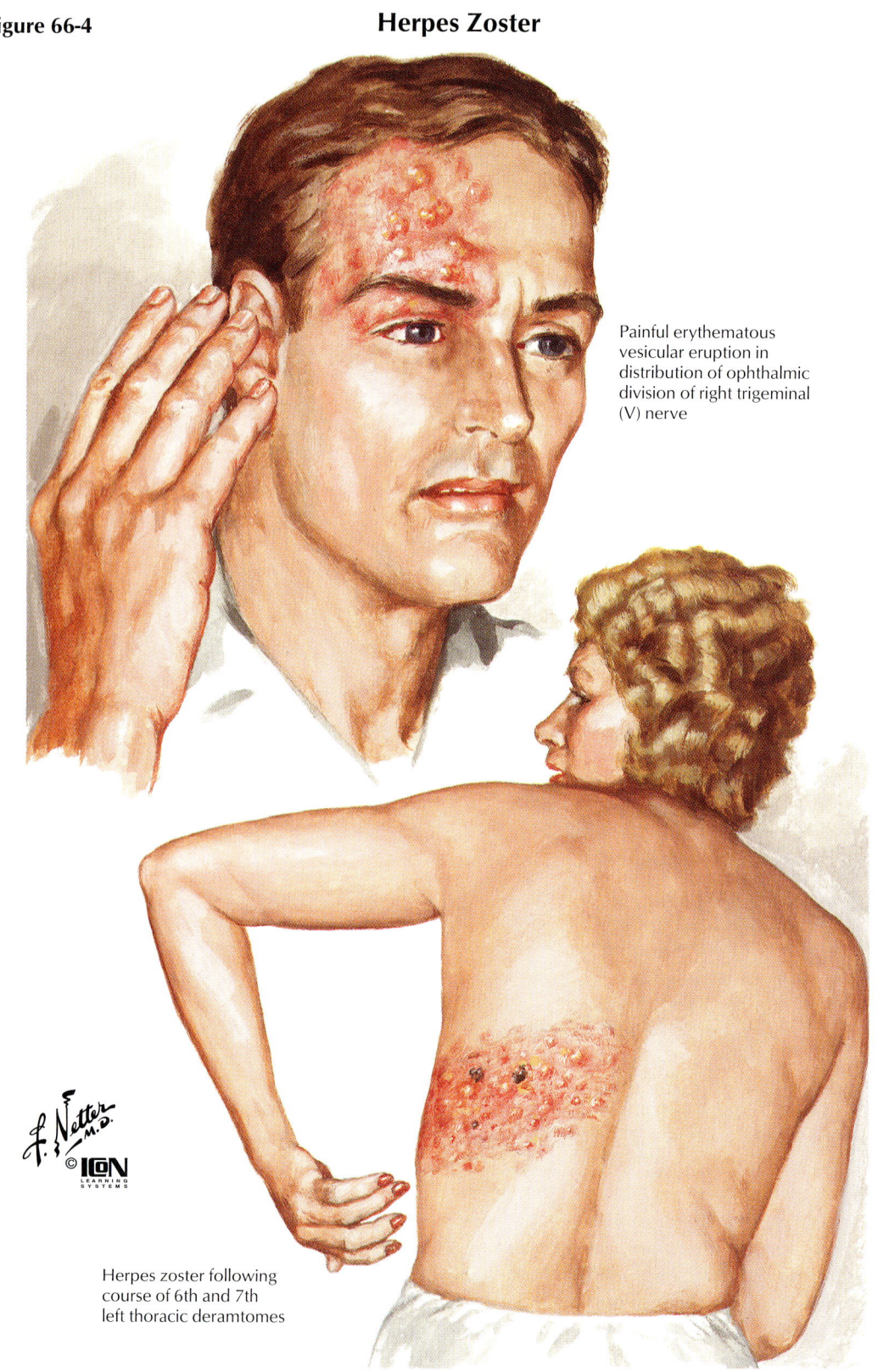

Painful erythematous vesicular eruption in distribution of ophthalmic division of right trigeminal (V) nerve

Herpes zoster following course of 6th and 7th left thoracic deramtomes

INFECTIOUS DISEASE

volved, the lower thoracic roots and the ophthalmic sensory ganglia are most commonly affected. Onset is often heralded by a few days of severe localized pain or nonspecific discomfort in the affected area. The eruption is unilateral and does not cross the midline. Vesicles follow 72 to 96 hours later (Figure 66-4). The lesions have an erythematous base with a tight, clear bubble that becomes opaque and crusts after 5 to 10 days. The localized cutaneous eruption is typically confined to the distribution of a specific spinal nerve root or cranial nerve but overlaps adjacent dermatomes in 20% of cases. Rarely, VZV produces pain without a rash (**zoster sin herpete**).

The acute pain of shingles is characterized by burning discomfort associated with volleys of a severe lancinating sensation. Nociceptive pain from soft tissue inflammation and itching may also be associated. Persistence of neuropathic symptoms beyond 3 months fulfills diagnostic criteria for PHN. The chronic, devastating neuropathic pain of PHN, rather than the nociceptive pain, is the most common significant consequence of shingles. Patients experiencing neuropathic pain report the paradox of numbness and pain in the same region. Affected regions also commonly manifest motor and autonomic deficits. Age, rash severity, a prodrome, intensity of acute pain, and associated neurologic abnormalities are all risk factors for PHN. In most instances, PHN resolves within 6 months after the initial rash.

Ophthalmic herpes zoster with involvement of the first division of the trigeminal nerve is the second most common dermatome affected. If the rash involves the tip of the nose, it is likely that ophthalmic herpes zoster is present (Figure 10-5). All patients with ophthalmic shingles require formal evaluation with a slit lamp and fluorescein study to assess any zoster dendrites and subsequent risk of corneal scarring. Surveillance is warranted because iritis and retinal necrosis may have delayed onset.

Ramsay Hunt syndrome is secondary to herpes zoster of the facial nerve, which affects the geniculate ganglion. Usually associated with vesicles in the external ear, it sometimes causes tinnitus, vertigo, and deafness.

Patients with radicular involvement of the arm or leg uncommonly may have concomitant loss of motor function. Rarely, severe spinal cord involvement may produce generalized meningoencephalitis with a variable prognosis. Even more unusual, an acute meningoencephalitis, mimicking a bacterial process with many polymorphonuclear leucocytes, may be followed a few days later by the appearance of the classic zoster rash.

Treatment

Acute patient care combines treatment of the underlying viral infection, host inflammatory response, and accompanying neuropathic pain. Once the diagnosis of shingles has been made, PHN risk is assessed. Early treatment of infection and associated pain has important ramifications for the risk of chronic symptoms. Formal assessment of pain quality and intensity is critical to analgesic decision-making, especially in elderly patients who tend to minimize pain symptoms. Multiple validated verbal, numeric, and visual scales may be used to gauge pain intensity throughout the illness course.

Antiviral medications are the mainstay of acute herpes zoster treatment and need to be administered within 72 hours after rash onset. Acyclovir (800 mg, 5 times daily for 1-1.5 weeks) is the treatment of choice for immunocompetent hosts. When treating an immunocompromised host, acyclovir should be given intravenously to prevent a generalized zoster rash dissemination. These agents accelerate cutaneous healing, shorten the duration of viral shedding, and reduce the risk of ophthalmic complications.

The effect of medications such as acyclovir on chronic pain is less clear. The potential benefit of combined treatment with corticosteroids is controversial with regard to cutaneous healing and alleviation of acute pain. To reduce the risk of bacterial superinfection, cutaneous lesions need to be kept clean and dry.

Oral opioids are first-line therapy and have clearly proven efficacy in reducing neuropathic pain intensity in acute and chronic stages. Opioids are used in combination with a tricyclic drug (eg, ortriptyline or gabapentin). Early use of low-dose tricyclic antidepressants (eg, amitriptyline), for 90 days within the initial months after shingles, reduces the likelihood of developing PHN. The most severe cases require IV opioids and regional anesthetic approaches, such as epidural catheter placement.

Because of the clearly defined cause and onset of PHN, the efficacy of analgesics has been studied extensively. Research supports the use of 4 medication categories: tricyclic antidepressants, anticonvulsants, opioids, and topical agents. Tricyclic antidepressants were the first category with demonstrated efficacy, and they remain first-line agents. However, the limitations of anticholinergic side effects and tolerability often prompt trials with other medications if moderate-to-severe pain persists. The anticonvulsant agent gabapentin and topical sodium channel blockers (lidocaine patches) are standards of care. Adverse effects (most commonly somnolence and dizziness) are minimized, and patient adherence to treatment is improved when gabapentin is initiated at low doses. The opioid analgesics oxycodone and morphine significantly relieve neuropathic pain. In one study, patients with PHN preferred controlled-release morphine to tricyclic antidepressants because of improved outcomes in pain relief and sleep improvement.

REFERENCES

Galer BS, Rowbotham MC, Perander J, Friedman E. Topical lidocaine patch relieves postherpetic neuralgia more effectively than a vehicle topical patch: results of an enriched enrollment study. *Pain.* 1999;80:533-538.

Jeha LE, Sila CA, Lederman RJ, Prayson RA, Isada CM, Gordon SM. West Nile virus infection: a new acute paralytic illness. *Neurology* 2003;61:55-59.

Kleinschmidt-DeMasters BK, Gilden DH. Varicella-zoster virus infections of the nervous system: clinical and pathologic correlates. *Arch Pathol Lab Med* 2001;125:770-780.

Laothamatas J, Hemachudha T, Mitrabhakdi E, Wannakrairot P, Tulayadaechanont S. MR imaging in human rabies. *Am J Neuroradiol.* 2003;24:1102-1109.

Noah DL, Drenzek CL, Smith JS, et al. Epidemiology of human rabies in the United States, 1980 to 1996. *Ann Intern Med.* 1998;128:922-930.

Raja SN, Haythornwaite JA, Pappagallo M, et al. Opioids versus antidepressants in postherpetic neuralgia: a randomized, placebo-controlled trial. *Neurology.* 2002;59:1015-1021.

Rowbatham MC, Harden N, Stacey B, Bernstein P, Magnus-Miller L, Gabapentin Postherpetic Neuralgia Study Group. Gabapentin for the treatment of postherpetic neuralgia: a randomized controlled trial. *JAMA.* 1998;280:1837-1842.

Rupprecht CE, Hanlon CA, Hemachudha T. Rabies re-examined. *Lancet Infect Dis.* 2002;2:327-343.

Sampathkumar P. West Nile virus: epidemiology, clinical presentation, diagnosis, and prevention. *Mayo Clin Proc.* 2003;78:1137-1143.

Shi PY, Wong SJ. Serologic diagnosis of West Nile virus infection. *Expert Rev Mol Diagn.* 2003;3:733-741.

Whitley RJ, Gnann JW. Viral encephalitis: familiar infections and emerging pathogens. *Lancet.* 2002 9;359:507-513.

Chapter 67
Brain and Spine Tuberculosis

Daniel P. McQuillen

Clinical Vignette

A 51-year-old Vietnamese woman presented with 7 days of headache, vomiting, and episodic left facial and arm tingling numbness while visiting the United States. She reported diplopia, having fallen twice and fractured her nose. Some seizurelike activity was witnessed.

The patient's temperature was equivocably febrile. On neurologic examination, she was confused and only intermittently fluent. She had bilateral CN-VI palsies and early papilledema. Her neck was stiff, and her lungs were clear.

A lumbar puncture revealed a CSF opening pressure of 500 mm CSF, protein of 218 mg/dL, glucose of 22 mg/dL (serum glucose level 137 mg/dL), an RBC count of 190/mm^3, and a WBC count of 1390/mm^3 (4% polymorphonuclear leukocytes, 94% lymphocytes). The patient's serum sodium level decreased to 117 mEq/dL. CSF acid-fast bacilli smear and PCR results were negative. Cranial CT and MRI results were normal.

The patient was treated with isoniazid, rifampin, ethambutol, pyrazinamide, and solumedrol. The CSF ultimately grew Mycobacterium tuberculosis.

The incidence of CNS tuberculosis in the United States has markedly decreased; it most commonly occurs in foreign-born adults and those infected with HIV. Neurologically, it presents as a meningitis, mass lesion, or vertebral lesion. Because tuberculosis is still endemic in Southeast Asia, it must be considered in the differential diagnosis of patients from this area who have a meningoencephalopathy with cranial neuropathies; the vignette in this chapter is classic. It is important to make a clinical diagnosis and begin treatment while awaiting CSF culture results.

TUBERCULOUS MENINGITIS

Tuberculous meningitis usually results from hematogenous meningeal seeding or contiguous spread from a tuberculoma or parameningeal granuloma, with subsequent rupture into the subarachnoid space (Figure 67-1). Local foci of infection along the meninges, brain, or spinal cord, thought to be present from hematogenous seeding of the primary infection, also release bacilli directly into the subarachnoid space. Infection then spreads along the perivascular spaces into the brain. An intense inflammatory reaction at the brain base causes an occlusive arteritis, with small vessel thrombosis and resultant brain infarction. Direct cranial nerve compression and obstruction of CSF flow at the foramina of the fourth ventricle or at the basal cisterns may result in subarachnoid block and cerebral edema.

Clinical Presentation and Diagnosis

Tuberculous meningitis progresses rapidly, with headache, fever, meningismus, and cranial nerve deficits, especially CN-VI palsy. Focal cerebral or cerebellar deficits are followed by altered sensorium and coma.

CSF examination is critical in establishing the diagnosis. Classically, the CSF glucose level is less than two thirds that of the serum glucose level; the CSF protein level is greater than 50 mg/dL; and the WBC count is increased, with a lymphocyte predominance. Acid-fast (Ziehl-Neelsen) smears are positive only 25% of the time, more commonly with concentrated CSF specimens. PCR analysis and culture are the most sensitive diagnostic tools. PCR can detect fewer than 10 organisms in clinical specimens compared with the 10,000 necessary for smear positivity. False-negative PCR results have been reported (sensitivity in acid-fast smear negative cases varies from 40% to 77%).

BRAIN AND SPINE TUBERCULOSIS

Figure 67-1   Tuberculosis of Brain and Spine

TB with involvement of basal cisterns with vasculitis and ischemia

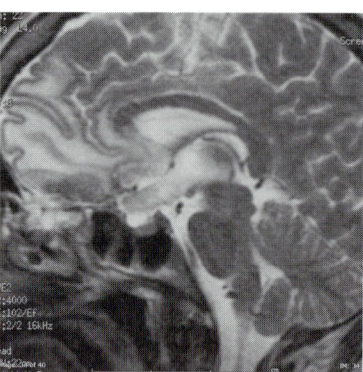

Midsagittal T2-weighted image shows increased T2 signal within ischemic frontal lobe.

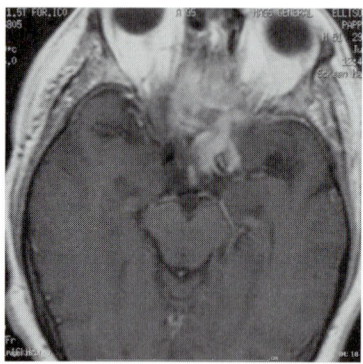

Axial T1-weighted, gadolinium-enhanced image with enhancing mass at left basal cisterns and subfrontal region.

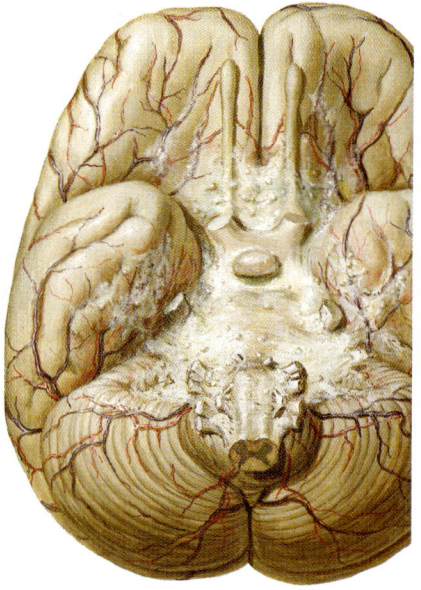

Tuberculous basilar meningitis

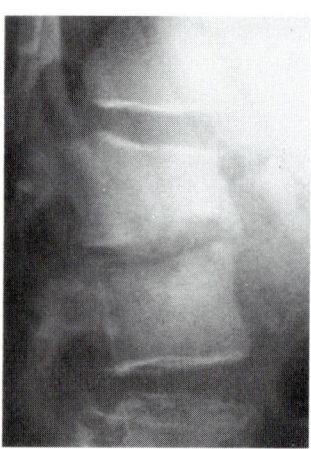

X-ray film: destruction of disc space and adjacent end plates of vertebrae

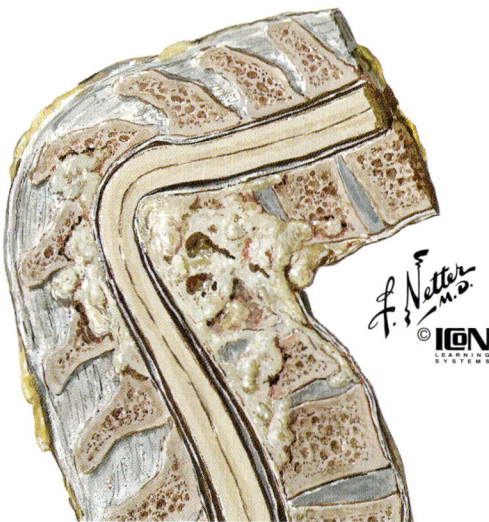

Tuberculosis of spine (Pott disease) with marked kyphosis

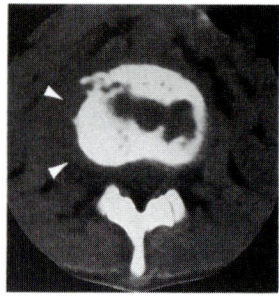

CT scan: paraspinous abscess in addition to bony destruction

INFECTIOUS DISEASE

Treatment

Death follows within weeks in untreated CNS tuberculosis. Because of worldwide increases in drug resistance, therapy for presumptive tuberculous meningitis must be instituted immediately on clinical suspicion with isoniazid, rifampin, ethambutol, and pyrazinamide until diagnostic identification and sensitivity testing are available. Typical medications include isoniazid, pyrazinamide (both of which achieve CSF concentrations equaling those in blood), rifampin (which crosses the blood-brain barrier adequately), and ethambutol. Corticosteroids are added when cerebral edema, subarachnoid block, or both occur. Mortality is greatest at the extremes of age (20% at <5 years and 60% at >50 years) or if illness has been present more than 2 months (80%). HIV infection does not seem to alter the clinical course or prognosis of tuberculous meningitis, although CNS mass lesions are more likely.

CEREBRAL TUBERCULOMAS

Cerebral tuberculomas are less common than tuberculous meningitis, often calcified, and usually located in the posterior fossa (cerebellum). Although most frequently multiple, they can be single. Antituberculous therapy should be attempted before surgery is contemplated unless there are signs of impending herniation because standard medical therapy is usually successful without multidrug resistance. Contrast-enhanced MRI is generally considered the modality of choice in detecting and assessing CNS tuberculosis (Figure 67-1). PCR and CSF culture or culture of biopsied lesional material confirms the diagnosis.

VERTEBRAL TUBERCULOSIS (POTT DISEASE)

Skeletal joints most subject to trauma are primarily affected. The spine—typically the disc space and adjacent vertebral bodies, the epidural space, or both—is involved in approximately 50% of tuberculosis cases. Back pain and fever are often followed by progressive spinal cord compression from unrecognized epidural infection or fracture, collapse, or angulation of vertebral segments.

Standard spinal radiographs reveal disc space infection with spread to adjacent vertebrae (Figure 67-1). MRI and/or CT myelography are the diagnostic procedures of choice. Bone biopsy or disc space aspiration is required for culture diagnosis before therapy.

A 9- to 12-month regimen of isoniazid and rifampin is appropriate. Prolongation of therapy is indicated for tuberculosis in sites that are slow to respond.

FUTURE DIRECTIONS

Reliable methods for rapid determination of *M tuberculosis* drug susceptibility are needed. Multiple investigators have identified chromosomal mutations associated with drug resistance. Genotypic assays are highly specific but of variable sensitivity. Phenotypic susceptibility assays under development use mycobacteriophages to detect metabolically active mycobacteria grown in the presence of antituberculous drugs. Although these assays are not widely clinically available, they reduce turnaround time for results from 3 weeks to as little as 54 to 94 hours.

REFERENCES

Bernaerts A, Vanhoenacker FM, Parizel PM, et al. Tuberculosis of the central nervous system: overview of neuroradiological findings. *Eur Radiol.* 2003;13:1876-1890.

Centers for Disease Control and Prevention. Nucleic acid amplification tests for tuberculosis. *MMWR.* 1996;45:951.

Dube MP, Holtorn PD, Larsen RA. Tuberculous meningitis in patients with and without human immunodeficiency virus infection. *Am J Med.* 1992;93:520-524.

Garcia-Monco JC. Central nervous system tuberculosis. *Neurol Clin.* 1999;17:737-759.

Haas DW. Current and future applications of polymerase chain reaction for *Mycobacterium tuberculosis. Mayo Clin Proc.* 1996;71:311-313.

Hazbon MH, Guarin N, Ferro BE, et al. Photographic and luminometric detection of luciferase reporter phages for drug susceptibility testing of clinical *Mycobacterium tuberculosis* isolates. *J Clin Microbiol.* 2003;41:4865-4869.

Kennedy DH, Fallon RJ. Tuberculous meningitis. *JAMA.* 1979;241:264-268.

Taylor GR, Dannecker, GE, Hoppe JE, et al. Negative polymerase chain reaction in a child with tuberculous meningoencephalitis. *Infection.* 1997;25:256-257.

Chapter 68
Infections in Immunocompromised Hosts

Donald E. Craven, Francesco G. De Rosa, Daniel P. McQuillen, and H. Royden Jones, Jr

Clinical Vignette

A 65-year-old woman with recent successful immunosuppressive treatment of Wegener granulomatosis presented with a 3-week history of rapidly progressive difficulty in walking and slurring of speech. In the previous few days, she had became unable to walk on her own, even with a walker. She had no other neurologic symptoms. On examination, her speech was dysarthric, there was a breakdown in her eye movement saccades with bilateral nystagmus, she had a broad-based ataxic gait, and she was unable to walk unassisted. Finger-to-nose testing demonstrated past pointing on the left side greater than the right. Her mental status, cranial nerves, muscle strength, all reflexes, and sensation were normal.

Findings of brain CT scan and CSF examinations were normal; MRI could not be performed because of an implanted pacemaker. Paraneoplastic antibody and chest CT results were normal. When the patient continued to progress, her pacemaker was removed. MRI demonstrated prominent white matter lesions in the cerebellum, pons, and midbrain. A biopsy of one of these cerebellar white matter lesions demonstrated abnormal oligodendrocytes containing in situ hybridization of JC virus. This was diagnostic of progressive multifocal leukoencephalopathy (PML), a rare opportunistic viral brain infection occurring most commonly among immunocompromised patients. Ara-C therapy was unsuccessful. This patient died 2.5 months after the onset of symptoms.

Immunocompromised hosts are particularly susceptible to infections from a wide spectrum of bacterial pathogens (including those endemic to specific geographic areas), mycobacterial diseases, opportunistic viruses or fungi and, less commonly, parasites. In addition, certain infections are more likely to occur in relation to the onset of immune suppression, the duration of immune compromise, or the type of immune suppression. Some pathogens, such as neurocysticercosis, also occur in nonimmunocompromised hosts.

ENCEPHALITIS
Progressive Multifocal Leukoencephalopathy
JC Virus

JC virus is a human polyomavirus (a small nonenveloped virus with a circular, double-stranded DNA genome). Infection is acquired during childhood and persists in the kidney. JC virus is the cause of PML, a rare demyelinating disease of immunosuppressed patients.

Patients with PML present with rapidly progressive focal neurologic deficits, without signs of increased intracranial pressure. At presentation, the most common neurologic deficits include hemiparesis, visual field deficits, and cognitive impairment. Aphasia, ataxia, or cranial nerve deficits may also be noted. Patients can have severe neurologic deficits late in the course of PML, including cortical blindness, quadriparesis, profound dementia, and coma.

Lesions are generally located in the cerebral white matter or sometimes in the cerebellum and brainstem (Figure 68-1). Spinal cord involvement is rare. PML is an AIDS-defining illness, but the clinical presentation in HIV patients is no different than in those with other immunodeficiencies.

A definitive diagnosis of PML requires identification of the characteristic pathologic changes on brain biopsy: multiple asymmetric foci of demyelination at various stages of evolution in the cerebral white matter. The oligodendrocytes demonstrate characteristic cytopathic effects, including nuclear enlargement, loss of normal chromatin pattern, and intranuclear accumulation of deeply basophilic homogenous staining

INFECTIONS IN IMMUNOCOMPROMISED HOSTS

Slow Virus Infections

Figure 68-1
Progressive multifocal leukoencephalopathy

Coronal section of brain showing many minute demyelinating lesions in white matter, which have coalesced in some areas to form irregular cavitations

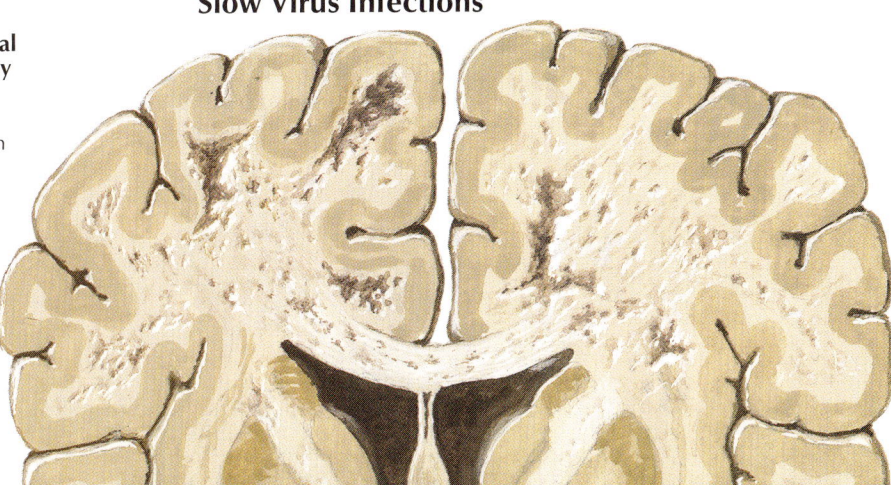

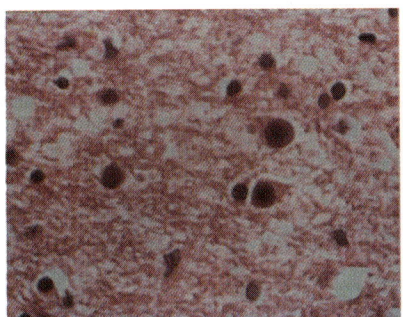

Section from edge of demyelinated focus showing abnormal oligodendrocytes with large hyperchromatic nuclei (H and E stain)

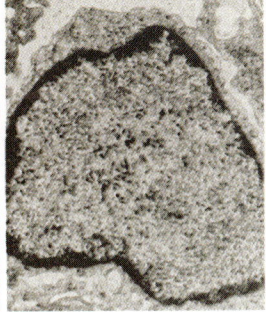

Electron micrograph showing giant glial nucleus with inclusion bodies

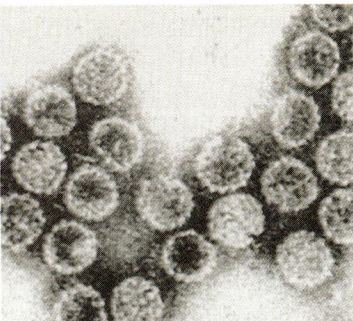

Electron micrograph showing papovavirus virions isolated from brain

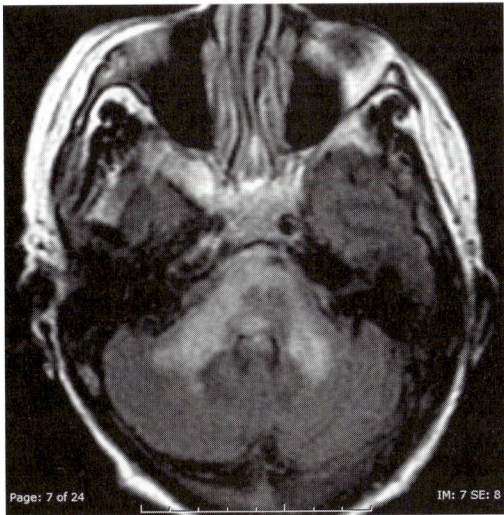

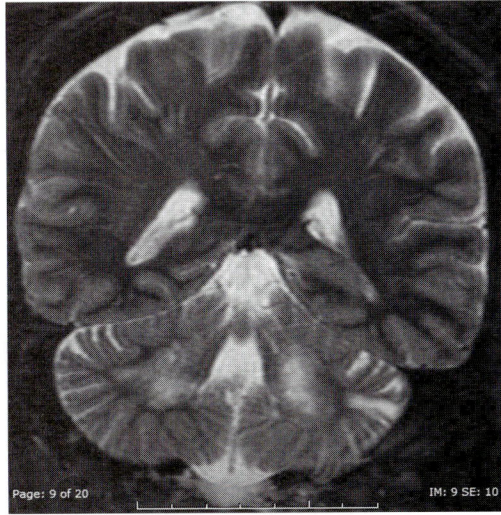

(**A**) Axial FLAIR image demonstrates increased signal in pons and bilateral cerebellar peduncles. (**B**) Coronal T2-weighted image with increased signal in central cerebellar white matter.

INFECTIOUS DISEASE

587

material. Electron microscopy reveals polyomavirus particles in enlarged oligodendrocyte nuclei.

CT scans reveal hypodense, nonenhancing lesions of the cerebral white matter. The severity of clinical findings is often greater than is suggested by the extent of involvement on CT scan. PCR has been used to amplify JC virus DNA in CSF samples (sensitivities range from 60 to 100%). CSF cell count and chemistry results are usually normal. EEG may reveal focal slowing or may be normal early in the course of PML.

Differential Diagnosis

MRI typically helps to differentiate brain tumors, especially lymphoma, or abscesses in the immunocompromised. A spongiform encephalopathy caused by a prion, *Creutzfeldt-Jakob disease* is a fatal infectious disease that sometimes presents with a progressive cerebellar syndrome or various focal cerebral lesions (chapter 36).

Treatment

No specific antiviral therapy has been reported effective in PML, although positive results have been reported with cidofovir, a nucleoside analog active against polyomaviruses. This is being studied in a larger trial. Marked clinical and radiographic improvement in HIV-infected patients with PML has been seen after treatment with combination antiretroviral regimens that include a protease inhibitor. Aggressive antiretroviral treatment of underlying HIV infection seems to be the most reasonable therapeutic approach to management in HIV-infected patients.

CHRONIC SEIZURE DISORDERS
Cysticercosis

Cysticercosis is a relatively common cause of seizure disorders, particularly in individuals from Central and South America, including those who have immigrated to the United States. It may occur in both immunocompromised and nonimmunocompromised individuals. It results from infection with the larval form of the porcine tapeworm *Taenia solium*. Humans acquire the adult tapeworm by eating undercooked pork and become infected with the larval stage (cysticercus) by ingesting tapeworm eggs. Eggs hatch within the small intestine, burrow into venules, and are carried to distant sites, including the CNS and muscle. Because the larvae are relatively large, they may lodge in the subarachnoid space, ventricles, or brain tissue (Figure 68-2). Cysts in the subarachnoid space may result in chronic meningitis and arachnoiditis; cysts in the ventricular system may lead to obstruction hydrocephalus, and cysts in the cerebrum may mimic brain tumors. Symptoms may not occur for 4 to 5 years, when larvae die and provoke an inflammatory response. Old nonviable cysts eventually calcify, simplifying detection.

MRI or contrast-enhanced CT may reveal signs of CNS infection. Serum or CSF serologic study and biopsy of subcutaneous cysts or skeletal muscle calcifications support the diagnosis.

Albendazole or praziquantel are the therapies of choice for cysticercosis. Steroids are used to decrease inflammation. Traditional anticonvulsants are indicated to control seizures.

MENINGITIS AND MASS LESIONS

The same pathogens commonly found in healthy hosts may cause meningitis in immunocompromised patients. *Listeria monocytogenes* (Figure 68-2) or *Cryptococcus neoformans* should always be considered potential causes of meningitis in such patients. Similarly, immunocompromised patients who develop space-occupying lesions should be evaluated for opportunistic bacteria, fungi, or parasitic infections, including *Nocardia* species, *Toxoplasma gondii*, *Aspergillus fumigatus*, *Mucormycosis*, or *C neoformans*.

Nocardiosis

Nocardia are present in the soil and decaying vegetable matter. When *Nocardia asteroides* causes a brain abscess, it enters through the respiratory tract, even though the pulmonary focus may not be prominent. The initial pulmonary focus is suppurative and not well localized, allowing infection to spread to the brain. Meningitis is infrequent in the absence of a contiguous abscess.

Brain biopsy is the most reliable diagnostic technique if the diagnosis cannot be made by evaluation of pulmonary or skin lesions (Figure

INFECTIONS IN IMMUNOCOMPROMISED HOSTS

Figure 68-2

Cysticercosis

Ovum of *Taenia solium* (pork tapeworm); indistinguishable from that of *T saginata* (beef tapeworm)

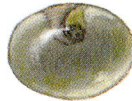
Cysticercus (larval stage) of pork tapeworm; fluid-filled sac (bladder) containing scolex (head) of worm

T solium ova hatch after ingestion by hogs; embryos migrate to hog tissues and form cysticerci. When humans eat infested pork, intestinal tapeworms develop. However, if humans ingest ova instead of larvae, or if ova reach stomach by reverse peristalsis from intestinal worm, human cysticercosis may occur.

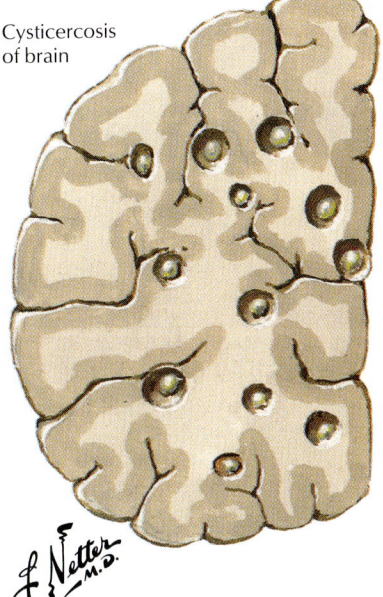
Cysticercosis of brain

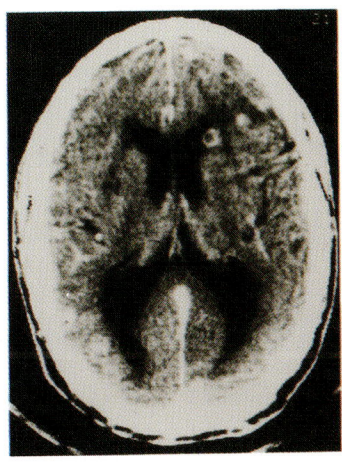
CT scan: punctate calcifications, cystic lesions (some with ring enhancement) and noncystic areas, which enhance

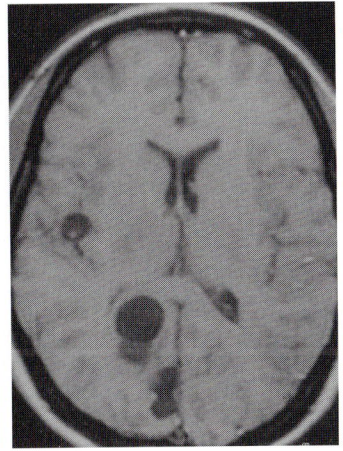
T1-weighted image with multiple cystic masses, one with eccentric intradural signal region (seen as calcification on CT—calcification of dead larvae)

68-3). *Nocardia* are weakly acid-fast and can be stained with the modified Ziehl-Neelsen method. They may be isolated on Sabouraud's medium or brain-heart infusion agar, but growth may not be visible for 2 to 4 weeks.

Sulfonamides are the drugs of choice for nocardiosis. Therapy should continue for at least 3 months or several weeks after clinical resolution of the lesion.

Toxoplasmosis

Toxoplasma gondii is a parasite that infects most mammalian species (Figure 68-4). Humans may acquire *T gondii* infections by ingestion, transplacental transmission, blood transfusion, or organ transplantation. Oral route infection results from ingestion of *T gondii* cysts in undercooked food (pork, lamb) or *T gondii* oocysts found in the feces of 1% of cats. Human intestinal tract enzymes liberate *T gondii* trophozoites, which cause clinical toxoplasmosis. Serologic evidence of *Toxoplasma* infection is present in 50% of the US population. Most cases are subclinical infections primarily manifested by cervical lymphadenopathy.

Four major *T gondii* clinical syndromes occur: congenital, ocular, lymphadenopathic, and severe neurologic or disseminated disease. The last occurs in at least 50% of immunocompromised patients. Diffuse encephalitis, meningoencephalitis, or cerebral mass lesions may result in predominant neurologic abnormalities.

INFECTIOUS DISEASE

INFECTIONS IN IMMUNOCOMPROMISED HOSTS

Figure 68-3   Nocardiosis

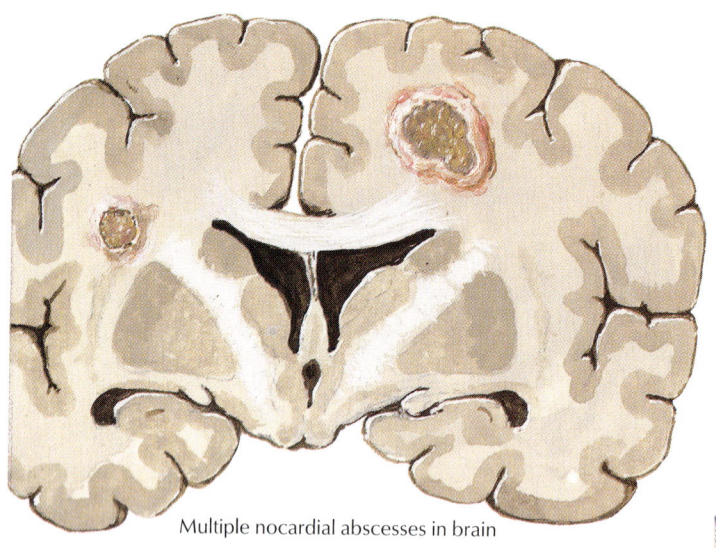

Multiple nocardial abscesses in brain

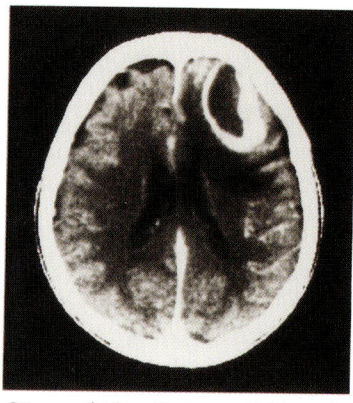

CT scan: thick-walled nocardial frontal lobe abscess in immunocompromised patient

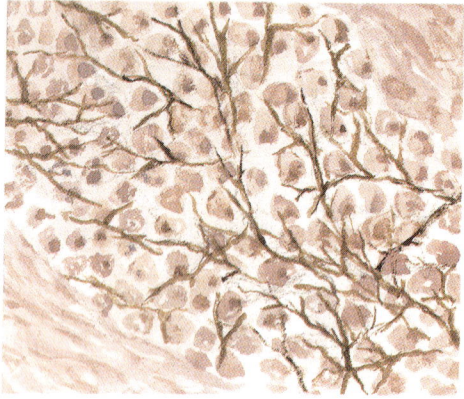

Branching hyphae of *Nocardia asteroides* in brain abscess (methenamine-silver strain)

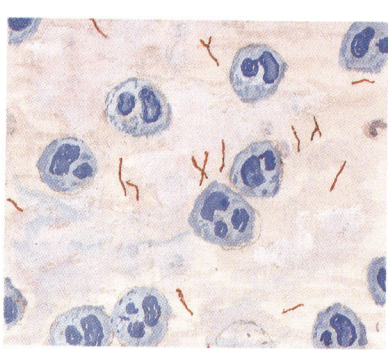

Modified acid-fast organisms as they may appear in pus, sputum, or tissues. They may be mistaken for tubercle bacilli, but are actually fragmented nocardial hyphae.

Focal masses (which may be multiple) and encephalitis are common presentations in patients with advanced AIDS or HIV with toxoplasmosis. Invariably, the CD4-helper lymphocyte count in patients with AIDS is less than $100/mm^3$ (normal is $>800/mm^3$). CSF shows mild lymphocytic pleocytosis and increased protein; the glucose level remains normal.

The indirect fluorescent antibody test measuring IgG antibodies is the most widely used diagnostic procedure. Results become positive 1 to 3 weeks after infection, and positive titers persist for many years. Definitive diagnosis requires a fourfold increase in IgG titer or a single high IgM titer. CSF examination is not required. Brain MRI with gadolinium is the most sensitive diagnostic technique for patients with HIV or AIDS. The multiple mass lesions present in patients with HIV usually show dramatic improvement after 2 weeks of therapy.

Chemotherapy is recommended for CNS toxoplasmosis. Pyrimethamine and sulfadiazine are the most active agents. Treatment is continued for 4 to 6 weeks. In patients with AIDS, maintenance therapy is often needed until immune reconstitution occurs with combination antiretroviral therapy.

Cryptococcus

This chronic, subacute or, rarely, acute CNS infection is caused by *C neoformans*, a yeastlike fungus. Distributed worldwide in soil, fruits, and

INFECTIONS IN IMMUNOCOMPROMISED HOSTS

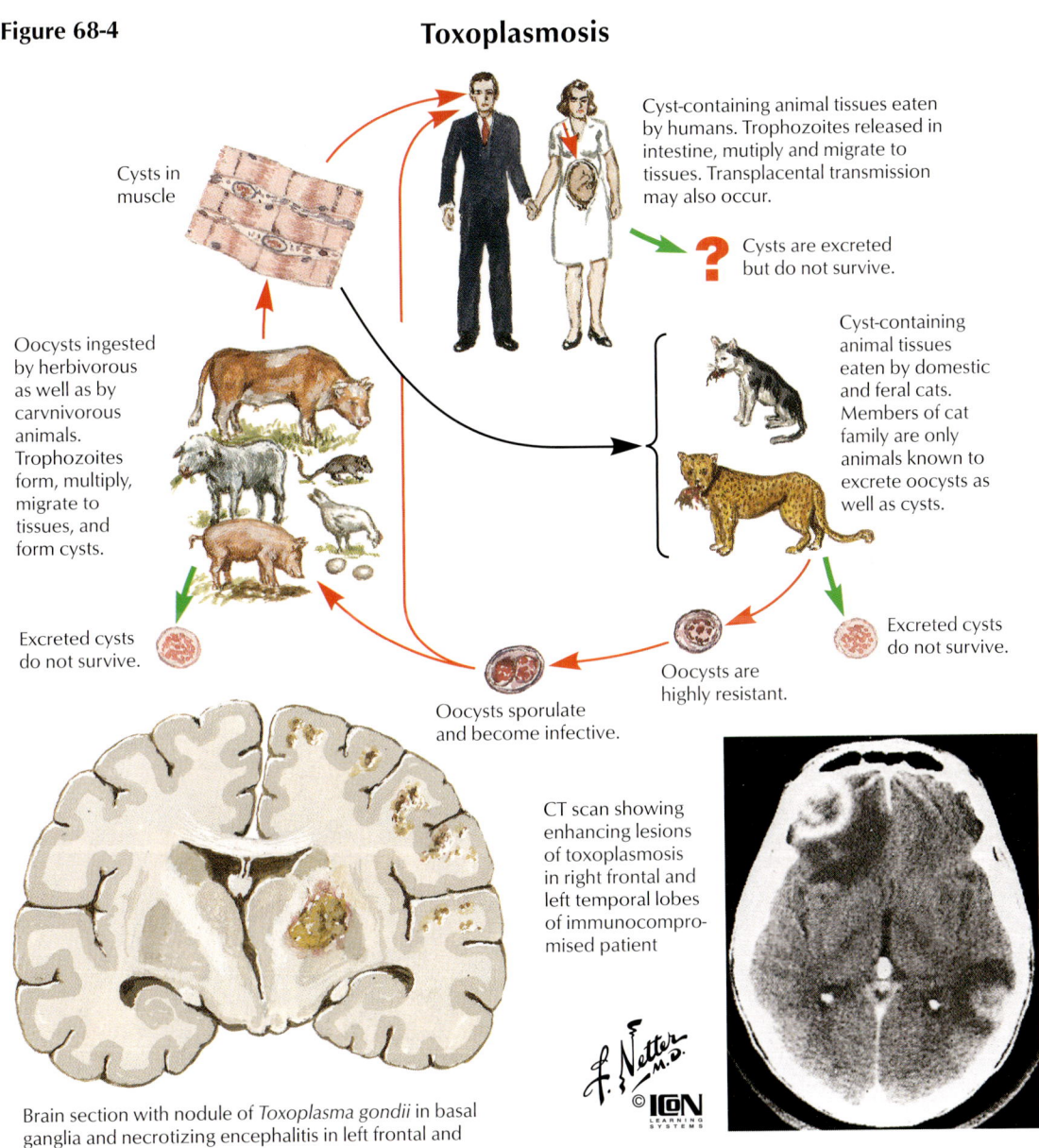

Figure 68-4

Toxoplasmosis

Cyst-containing animal tissues eaten by humans. Trophozoites released in intestine, mutiply and migrate to tissues. Transplacental transmission may also occur.

Cysts are excreted but do not survive.

Cysts in muscle

Oocysts ingested by herbivorous as well as by carvnivorous animals. Trophozoites form, multiply, migrate to tissues, and form cysts.

Cyst-containing animal tissues eaten by domestic and feral cats. Members of cat family are only animals known to excrete oocysts as well as cysts.

Excreted cysts do not survive.

Excreted cysts do not survive.

Oocysts are highly resistant.

Oocysts sporulate and become infective.

CT scan showing enhancing lesions of toxoplasmosis in right frontal and left temporal lobes of immunocompromised patient

Brain section with nodule of *Toxoplasma gondii* in basal ganglia and necrotizing encephalitis in left frontal and temporal corticomedullary zones

matter contaminated by pigeon excreta, this organism probably enters the body through the lungs and then disseminates to all organs (Figure 68-5). Mild, self-limited infections are common. Clinical disease develops in healthy and immunocompromised patients.

Meningeal involvement is the most common form of cryptococcosis. The onset is usually insidious, with symptoms often present for months. Patients typically have nonspecific complaints, ie, headache, nausea, irritability, somnolence, and clumsiness. Cranial nerve involvement occurs in 20% of patients and may cause decreased visual acuity, diplopia, and facial numbness. Patients are often afebrile, with minimal nuchal rigidity. Papilledema is noted in some

INFECTIOUS DISEASE

INFECTIONS IN IMMUNOCOMPROMISED HOSTS

Figure 68-5
Cryptococcosis

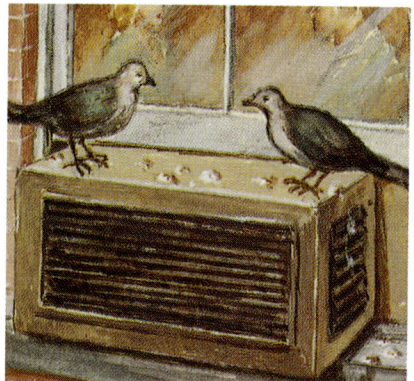
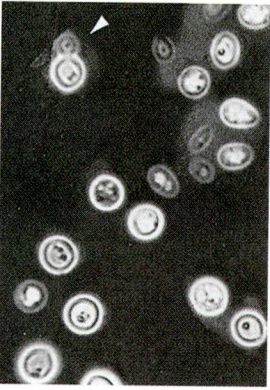
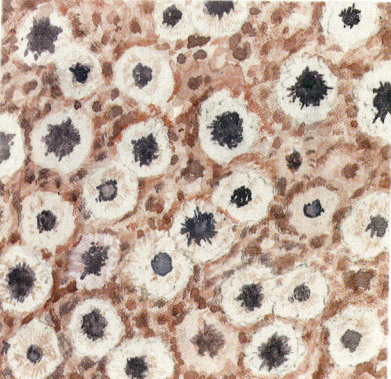

Infection is by respiratory route. Pigeon dung and air conditioners may be factors in dissemination.

India ink preparation showing budding and capsule

Accumulation of encapsulated cryptococci in subarachnoid space (PAS or methenamine-silver strain)

Listeriosis

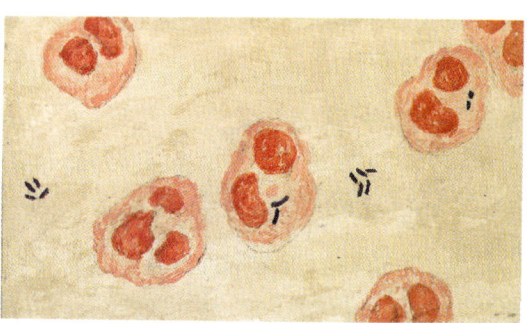

Smear of CSF showing white blood cells and *Listeria* organisms, which appear as gram-positive rods. They may be very short, to resemble cocci, and they often orient in palisades suggestive of Chinese characters. They cause severe purulent meningitis, most commonly in immunocompromised patients or newborns.

patients. Direct cerebral involvement may cause dementia.

CSF examination reveals elevated opening pressure, lymphocytic leukocytosis with a WBC count of 40 to 400/mm^3 (lymphocytes predominating), increased protein concentration, and decreased glucose level in 50% of patients. India ink preparations can define the organism, but isolation of *C neoformans* by culture is the single best diagnostic test. Less commonly, diagnosis is made by culturing or identifying the organism with periodic acid-Schiff or methenamine-silver stain in a CNS specimen. PCR is not used yet.

Latex agglutination for detection of cryptococcal capsular antigen (in serum and CSF) is also available and is helpful in monitoring therapy response. Urine cultures are positive in approximately 33% of patients.

Treatment depends on disease severity. It usually consists of IV amphotericin B with or without flucytosine for at least 2 weeks. Thereafter, oral fluconazole should be given for at least 6 weeks. Maintenance therapy is recommended for patients with HIV or AIDS until immune reconstitution occurs with combination antiretroviral therapy.

Listeriosis

Listeria monocytogenes is a gram-positive rod that occurs pathologically in neonates and immunocompromised adults. The bacteria is widespread and has been isolated from soil, water, animal feed, and sewage. This organism should always be suspected in patients with AIDS and those receiving prednisone or azathioprine. Neurologic presentation is similar to that of acute bacterial meningitis. Headache, fever, meningismus, and, occasionally, seizures and focal symptomatology predominate.

Diagnosis is based on CSF identification of gram-positive rods in association with polymorphonuclear leucocytosis and a low CSF sugar-level (<50% of serum glucose) (Figure 67-2). The treatment of choice is IV ampicillin and gentamicin.

REFERENCES

Baker AS. Infections in immunocompromised host. In: Netter FH, Jones HR Jr, Dingle RV, eds. *The Netter Collection of Medical Illustrations*. Vol 1, Part 2. Teterboro, NJ: Icon Learning Systems; 2000:161-162.

Chang KH, Han MH. MRI of CNS parasitic diseases. *J Magn Reson Imaging*. 1998;8:297-307.

Cinque P, Koralnik IJ, Clifford DB. The evolving face of human immunodeficiency virus-related progressive multifocal leukoencephalopathy: defining a consensus terminology. *J Neurovirol*. 2003;9(suppl 1):88-92.

Clifford DB. Challenges for clinical trials to treat progressive multifocal leukoencephalopathy. *J Neurovirol*. 2003;(9 suppl 1):68-72.

Cohen BA. Neurologic manifestations of toxoplasmosis in AIDS. *Semin Neurol*. 1999;19:201-211.

Cunha BA. Central nervous system infections in the compromised host: a diagnostic approach. *Infect Dis Clin North Am*. 2001;15:567-590.

Garcia HH, Evans CA, Nash TE, et al. Current consensus guidelines for treatment of neurocysticercosis. *Clin Microbiol Rev*. 2002;15:747-756.

Mylonakis E, Hohmann EL, Calderwood SB. Central nervous system infection with *Listeria monocytogenes*: 33 years' experience at a general hospital and review of 776 episodes from the literature. *Medicine (Baltimore)*. 1998;77:313-336.

Powderly WG. Recent advances in the management of cryptococcal meningitis in patients with AIDS. *Clin Infect Dis*. 1996;22:S119-S223.

Threlkeld SC, Hooper DC. Update on management of patients with Nocardia infection. *Curr Clin Top Infect Dis*. 1997;17:1-23.

Chapter 69
Tetanus

H. Royden Jones, Jr

Tetanus is caused by a potent neurotoxin, tetanospasmin, released by a gram-positive spore-forming obligate anaerobe, *Clostridium tetani*, from a wound infection. This bacterial infection can be introduced at any site; contaminated wounds or retained foreign bodies are particularly dangerous. Although common in developing countries, tetanus occurs in North America mostly after the age of 60 years. Rarely, patients contract tetanus despite adequate immunization.

Tetanus results from the release of tetanospasmin into the bloodstream from a focus of infection by *C tetani*; subsequently, it binds to the neuromuscular junction and then attaches to peripheral motor neuron nerve endings. It travels **centrally** up the nerve, in retrograde fashion (**antidromically**), to the anterior horn cells, where it enters adjacent spinal inhibitory interneurons, exerting its primary pathophysiologic effect by blocking inhibitory neurotransmitter release to the anterior horn cell. This leads to the classic muscular hypertonia and muscle spasms (Figure 69-1).

CLINICAL PRESENTATION
Generalized Tetanus

Generalized tetanus varies from mild to severe, depending on the incubation period, usually 2 to 14 days. It is occasionally delayed by weeks to months after the injury. A more severe clinical picture occurs when the incubation period is less than 8 days and the onset period is less than 48 hours.

In patients with partial or complete immunization, tetanus sometimes occurs as a mild form. It is often more severe in nonimmunized patients. Muscles close to the infection site are more severely affected initially. Typically trismus (lockjaw) and risus sardonicus (a spasmodic tetanic involuntary smile) are early and constant signs.

Subsequently shocklike painful spasms of all muscles are provoked by the slightest disturbance, including sight, sound, or touch, or occur spontaneously. Between the intermittent severe spasms, continuous muscle rigidity is often characterized by the clenched jaw, **risus sardonicus**, and a stiff back, neck, abdominal wall, and limbs, sometimes associated with laryngeal and respiratory muscle spasms that may cause airway obstruction.

Tetanus patients are fully conscious because this toxin does not affect cortical function or sensory nerves. They experience severe pain with every muscle contraction. The spasms become progressively severe in the first week after onset, gradually improving over 1 to 4 weeks. Sympathetic overactivity may occur with tachycardia, labile hypertension, and arrhythmias.

Focal Tetanus

Focal tetanus, an unusual manifestation, is limited to muscles at the wound site. It is thought to occur when circulating antitoxin neutralizes the toxin. However, this does not prevent the spread of the tetanus toxin regionally. Painful muscle spasms adjacent to the wound site last a few weeks. Sometimes, focal tetanus proceeds to generalized tetanus. If generalization does not occur, there is eventually good recovery.

DIAGNOSIS

Abdominal rigidity, generalized spasms, trismus, and risus sardonicus are highly characteristic of tetanus. They may be mistaken for encephalitis, encephalomyelitis, meningitis, intracranial haemorrhage, or even stiff man syndrome. Normal CSF and absence of an altered level of consciousness differentiate tetanus from primary CNS infections. Certain local conditions, including dental and peritonsillar abscesses, may also

TETANUS

Figure 69-1

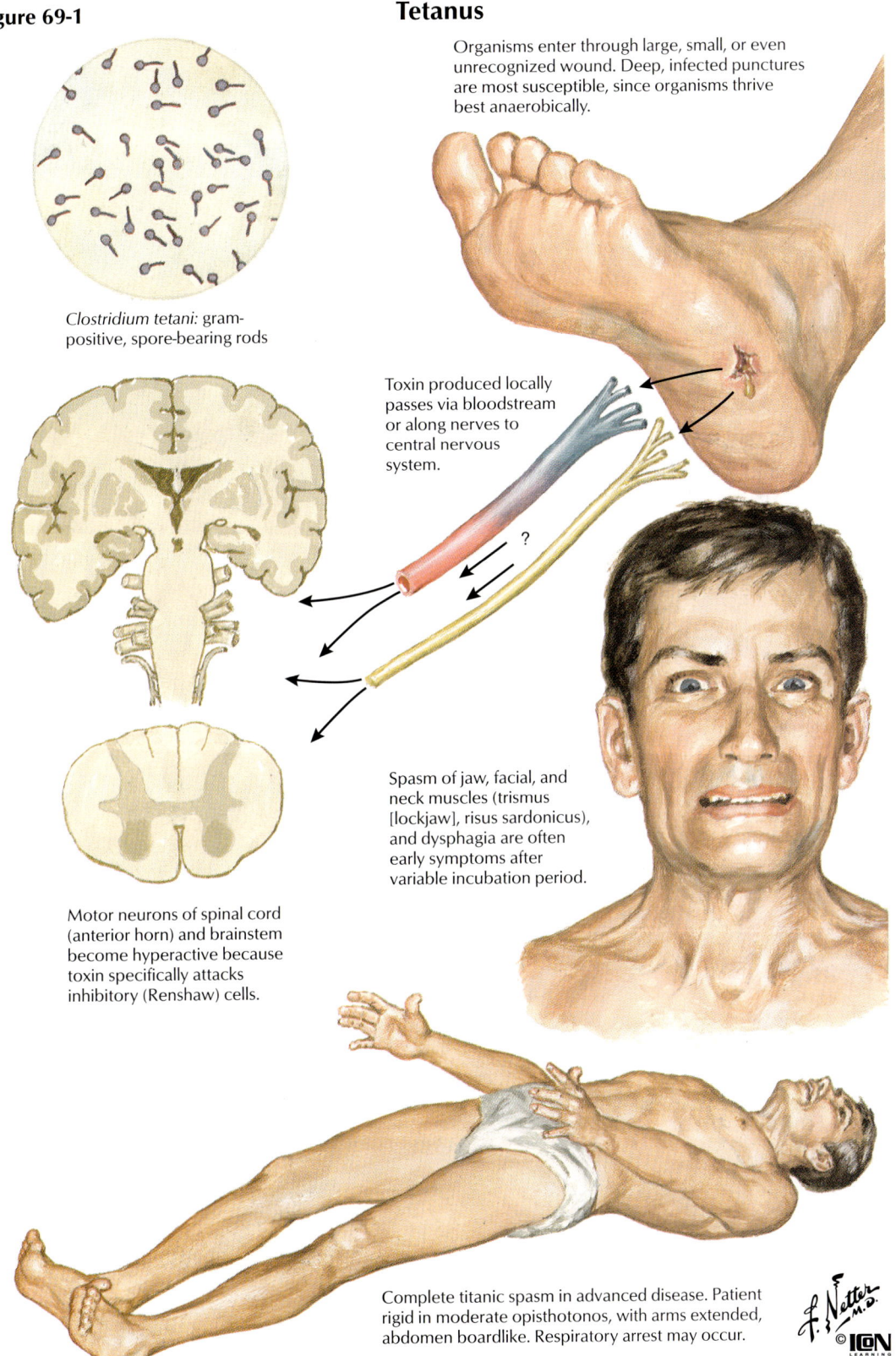

Tetanus

Clostridium tetani: gram-positive, spore-bearing rods

Organisms enter through large, small, or even unrecognized wound. Deep, infected punctures are most susceptible, since organisms thrive best anaerobically.

Toxin produced locally passes via bloodstream or along nerves to central nervous system.

Motor neurons of spinal cord (anterior horn) and brainstem become hyperactive because toxin specifically attacks inhibitory (Renshaw) cells.

Spasm of jaw, facial, and neck muscles (trismus [lockjaw], risus sardonicus), and dysphagia are often early symptoms after variable incubation period.

Complete titanic spasm in advanced disease. Patient rigid in moderate opisthotonos, with arms extended, abdomen boardlike. Respiratory arrest may occur.

INFECTIOUS DISEASE

mimic tetanus. Hypocalcemic tetany is usually distinguished by carpopedal spasms and a positive Chovstek sign. Phenothiazine toxicity sometimes results in dystonia and opisthotonus mimicking tetanus; prompt response to IV diphenhydramine helps to distinguish this situation. Epileptic seizures and drug withdrawal reactions also deserve consideration in the differential diagnosis.

Fortunately, tetanus has a characteristic clinical picture, because *C tetani* organisms are isolated from the wound in only one third of affected patients. There are no specific confirmatory blood studies or CSF analyses for tetanus. Sometimes electromyography supports the diagnosis.

TREATMENT AND PROGNOSIS

Tetanus is entirely preventable with immunizations. Treatment modalities include appropriate antibiotics and tetanus immunoglobulin, local wound care, control of spasms with muscle relaxants and or anticonvulsants, ventilatory support, meticulous nursing care, and maintenance of adequate nutrition and hydration.

The incubation period and time to onset are important predictors of prognosis. If the incubation period is less than 8 days, the onset period is less than 48 hours, and reflex spasms have been present during more than 12 of 24 hours, the prognosis is generally poor. With treatment, mortality from tetanus is substantially reduced throughout the world.

REFERENCES

Bardenheimer B, Prevots DR, Khetsurani N, Wharton M. Tetanus surveillance: United States 1995-1997. *MMWR CDC Surveill Summ.* 1998;47:1-13.

Case records of the Massachusetts General Hospital. Weekly clinicopathological exercises. Case 12-2001: A 16-year-old boy with an altered mental status and muscle rigidity. *N Engl J Med.* 2001;344:1232-1239.

Engrand N, Guerot E, Rouamba A, Vilain G. The efficacy of intrathecal baclofen in severe tetanus. *Anaesthesiology.* 1999;90:1773-1776.

Steinegger T, Wiederker M, Ludin H, Roth F. Electromyography as a diagnostic aid in tetanus. *Schweiz Med Wochenschr.* 1996;126:379-385.

Warren JD, Kimber TE, Thompson PD. The silent period after magnetic brain stimulation in generalized tetanus. *Muscle Nerve.* 1999;22:1590-1592.

Chapter 70
Poliomyelitis

Daniel P. McQuillen and Michael P. McQuillen

Clinical Vignette

An 18-year-old man, raised by parents who sought their medical care in faith and not from physicians and particularly refused immunizations, reported headache, fever, nausea and general malaise 1 week after camping. Two days later, he felt better, but 48 hours after that, the general symptoms returned, with more headache, generalized muscle aching and pain, and some drowsiness. When weakness supervened a week after illness onset, he was brought to the ED.

The patient's temperature was 39.5°C, his pulse was pulse 100 beats/min, and his BP was 130/70 mm Hg. He had a stiff neck, generalized muscle tenderness, asymmetric weakness (right arm and left leg more than elsewhere) preserved though hypoactive muscle stretch reflexes, flexor plantar responses, normal sensation, and intact cranial nerves.

His cough was weak, with a vital capacity of barely 1 L. His WBC count was 15,000/mm^3 (40% lymphocytes). Lumbar puncture revealed somewhat cloudy fluid under increased pressure (220 mm Hg), 170/mm^3 nucleated cells (60% polymorphonuclear leukocytes), 150 mg/dL protein, and 80 mg/dL glucose. Spinal MRI showed enhancement of the cord anteriorly, especially the right cervical region.

The word *poliomyelitis* is derived from the Greek polio (gray) and myelon (marrow, indicating the spinal cord). Spinal cord infection with poliomyelitis virus leads to the classic paralysis. The incidence of polio peaked in the United States in 1952 with more than 21,000 cases but rapidly decreased after introduction of effective vaccines in 1954. The last case of wild-virus polio acquired in the United States was in 1979, and the Global Polio Eradication Program dramatically reduced transmission elsewhere.

Poliovirus transmission now occurs primarily in the Indian subcontinent, the Eastern Mediterranean, and Africa. Humans are the only known reservoir. Transmission occurs most frequently with inapparent infection. An asymptomatic carrier state occurs only in those with immunodeficiency. Person-to-person spread occurs predominantly via the fecal-oral route. Infection typically peaks in summer in temperate climates, with no seasonality in the tropics. Poliovirus is highly infectious and may be present in stool up to 6 weeks; seroconversion in susceptible household contacts of children is nearly 100%, and that of adults is greater than 90%. Persons are most infectious from 7 to 10 days before and after symptom onset.

Inactivated poliovirus vaccine (IPV) was licensed in 1955 and used until the early 1960s, when trivalent oral poliovirus vaccine (OPV), containing attenuated strains of all 3 serotypes of poliovirus in 10:1:3 ratios, largely replaced it. Enhanced potency trivalent poliovirus vaccine (IPV) was introduced in 1988. The viruses are grown in monkey kidney (Vero) cells and are inactivated with formaldehyde.

An occasional live vaccine-associated case of paralytic polio continued to occur in infants after their first immunization at approximately 3 months of age until the Centers for Disease Control mandated in the late 1990s that initial vaccinations must be with the Salk IPV. Since then, no such incidents have been reported. Between 1980 and 1999, 152 confirmed cases of paralytic polio occurred in the United States. Of these, 145 (95%) were vaccine-associated. For this reason, in 2000, the recommendation was made to use IPV exclusively in the United States. Vaccine-associated paralytic polio is thought to occur from a reversion or mutation of the vaccine virus to a more neurotropic form.

Live attenuated polioviruses replicate in the intestinal mucosa and lymphoid cells and draining lymph nodes. Vaccine viruses are excreted in

INFECTIOUS DISEASE

POLIOMYELITIS

stool for up to 6 weeks, with maximal shedding in the first 1 to 2 weeks after vaccination. IPV is highly effective in producing immunity (99% after 3 doses) and protection from paralytic poliomyelitis. IPV seems to produce less local gastrointestinal immunity than OPV. Thus, persons immunized with IPV could still become infected with wild-type poliovirus and shed it on return to the United States, with subsequent potential spread. Although most individuals in economically privileged countries are immunized, occasionally, an instance such as described in the vignette in this chapter is seen. Asymmetric weakness distribution and CSF findings help to differentiate it from Guillain-Barre syndrome.

ETIOLOGY AND PATHOGENESIS

Poliovirus is a member of the family Picornaviridae, enterovirus subgroup. Enteroviruses are transient inhabitants of the gastrointestinal tract and are stable at acid pH. Picornaviruses have an RNA genome; the 3 poliovirus serotypes (P1, P2, and P3) have minimal heterotypic immunity among them. The virus enters through the mouth and multiplies primarily at the implantation site in the pharynx and gastrointestinal tract; usually, it is present in the throat and stool before clinical onset (Figure 70-1). Within 1 week of clinical onset, little virus exists in the throat, but it continues to be excreted in the stool for several weeks. The virus invades local lymphoid tissue, enters the bloodstream, and then may infect CNS cells. Viral replication in anterior horn and brainstem motor neuron cells results in cell destruction and paralysis.

CLINICAL PRESENTATION

The incubation period for poliomyelitis is usually 6 to 20 days, with a range of 3 to 35 days. Conical response to poliovirus infection varies. Up to 95% of all polio infections are asymptomatic even though infected persons shed virus in stool and are contagious.

Abortive poliomyelitis occurs in 4% to 8% of infections. It causes a minor illness, without evidence of CNS infection. Complete recovery characteristically occurs within 1 week. Upper respiratory infection (sore throat and fever), gastrointestinal disturbances (nausea, vomiting, abdominal pain, constipation, or rarely diarrhea), and influenzalike illness can all occur and are indistinguishable from other enteric viral illnesses.

Nonparalytic aseptic meningitis, usually occurring several days after a prodrome similar to the minor illness, occurs in a few percent of infections. Increased or abnormal sensations may occur with stiffness in the neck, back, leg, or a combination of those areas, typically last 2 to 10 days, and are then followed by complete recovery.

Flaccid paralysis occurs in less than 1% of polio infections. Paralytic symptoms typically begin 1 to 10 days after the prodromal symptoms and evolve for 2 to 3 days. Paralysis does not usually progress after defervescence. In children, the prodrome may be biphasic, with initial minor symptoms separated by 1 to 7 days from major symptoms. Initially, severe muscle aches and spasms are typically seen with significant meningismus and a Kernig sign. The illness evolves into asymmetric flaccid paralysis with diminished muscle stretch reflexes, typically reaching a plateau within days or weeks. Some strength gradually returns. No sensory or cognitive loss occurs. Most patients recover some function, and many recover completely; however, weakness or paralysis present 12 months after onset is usually permanent.

Three types of paralytic polio are described. Most common is spinal polio (approximately 79% of cases in the 1970s), characterized by asymmetric paralysis usually involving the legs (Figure 70-2). Bulbar polio (2%) causes weakness of muscles innervated by cranial nerves. Bulbospinal polio (19%) is a combination of the two. Mortality in paralytic polio cases is lower in children (2-5%) than in adults (15-30%) and highest (25-75%) with bulbar involvement.

Postpolio Syndrome

Postpolio syndrome occurs 30 to 40 years after paralytic poliomyelitis in childhood, when 25% to 40% of patients note seeming increased weakness. It does not constitute recurrence of a dormant infectious process. Rather, it is thought to involve failure of oversized motor units created during the recovery process from the initial paralytic syndrome.

POLIOMYELITIS

Figure 70-1   Poliomyelitis—I

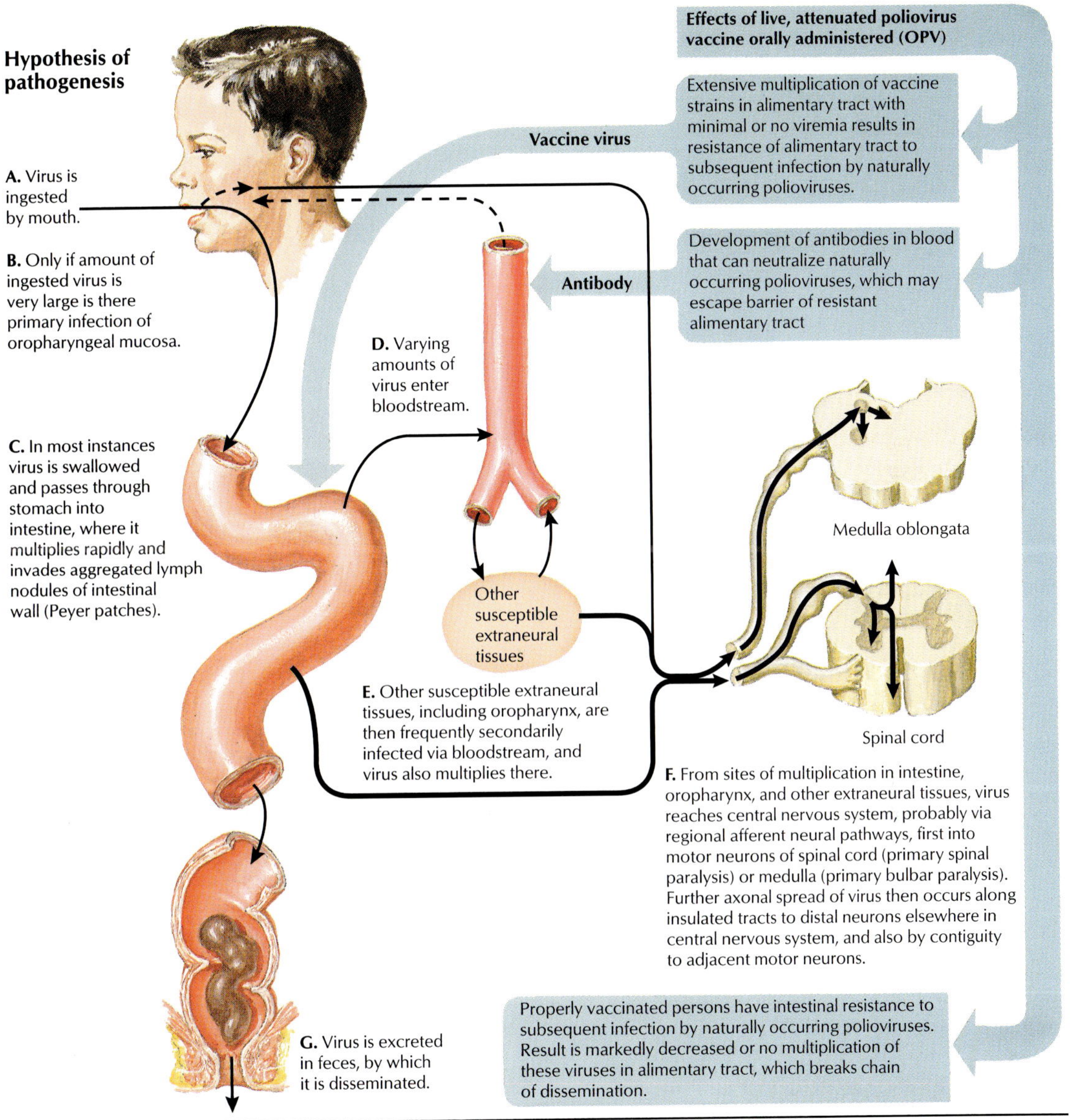

Hypothesis of pathogenesis

A. Virus is ingested by mouth.

B. Only if amount of ingested virus is very large is there primary infection of oropharyngeal mucosa.

C. In most instances virus is swallowed and passes through stomach into intestine, where it multiplies rapidly and invades aggregated lymph nodules of intestinal wall (Peyer patches).

D. Varying amounts of virus enter bloodstream.

E. Other susceptible extraneural tissues, including oropharynx, are then frequently secondarily infected via bloodstream, and virus also multiplies there.

F. From sites of multiplication in intestine, oropharynx, and other extraneural tissues, virus reaches central nervous system, probably via regional afferent neural pathways, first into motor neurons of spinal cord (primary spinal paralysis) or medulla (primary bulbar paralysis). Further axonal spread of virus then occurs along insulated tracts to distal neurons elsewhere in central nervous system, and also by contiguity to adjacent motor neurons.

G. Virus is excreted in feces, by which it is disseminated.

Effects of live, attenuated poliovirus vaccine orally administered (OPV)

Extensive multiplication of vaccine strains in alimentary tract with minimal or no viremia results in resistance of alimentary tract to subsequent infection by naturally occurring polioviruses.

Development of antibodies in blood that can neutralize naturally occurring polioviruses, which may escape barrier of resistant alimentary tract

Properly vaccinated persons have intestinal resistance to subsequent infection by naturally occurring polioviruses. Result is markedly decreased or no multiplication of these viruses in alimentary tract, which breaks chain of dissemination.

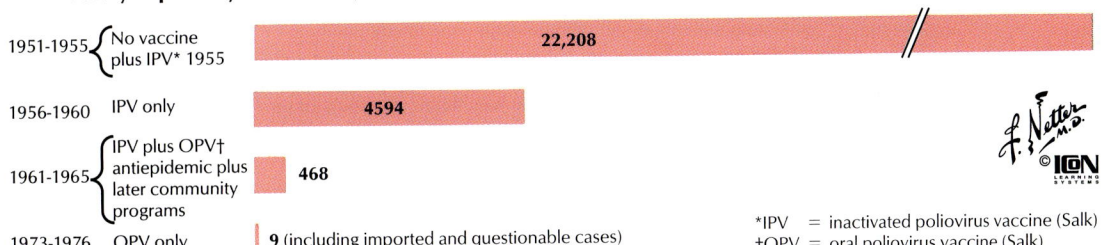

Paralytic poliomyelitis in USA, 1951 to 1976 (average number of cases per year) and effect of vaccine

Years	Vaccine	Cases
1951-1955	No vaccine plus IPV* 1955	22,208
1956-1960	IPV only	4594
1961-1965	IPV plus OPV† antiepidemic plus later community programs	468
1973-1976	OPV only	9 (including imported and questionable cases)

*IPV = inactivated poliovirus vaccine (Salk)
†OPV = oral poliovirus vaccine (Salk)

INFECTIOUS DISEASE

POLIOMYELITIS

Figure 70-2 Poliomyelitis—II

Stages in destruction of a motor neuron by poliovirus

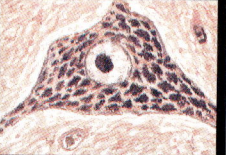 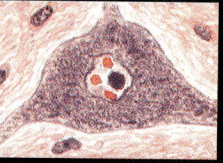 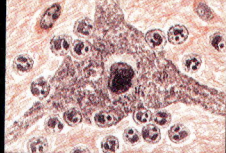 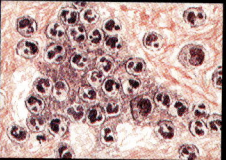

A. Normal motor neuron   B. Diffuse chromatolysis; 3 acidophilic nuclear inclusions around nucleolus   C. Polymorphonuclear cells invading necrotic neuron   D. Complete neuronophagia

Relative distribution of neuronal lesions in spinal and bulbar poliomyelitis

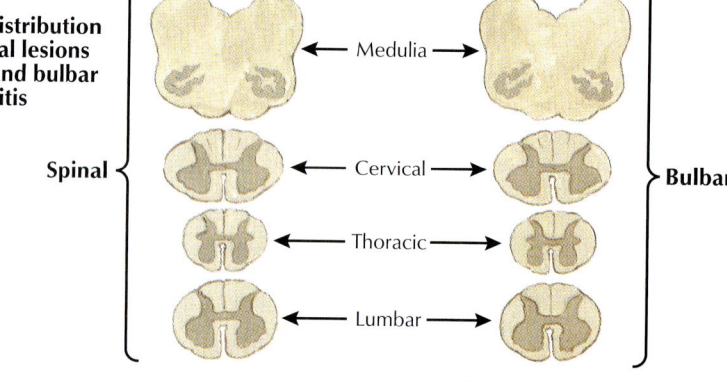

Spinal { Medulla, Cervical, Thoracic, Lumbar } Bulbar

Paralytic residua of spinal poliomyelitis

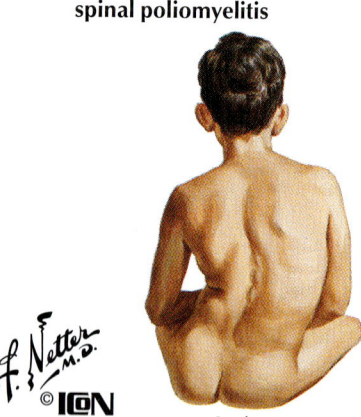

Scoliosis

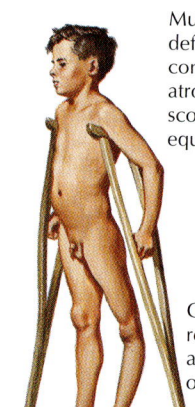

Multiple crippling deformities: contractures, atrophy, severe scoliosis and equinovarus

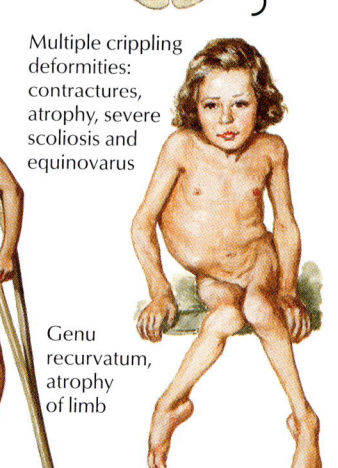

Genu recurvatum, atrophy of limb

DIAGNOSTIC APPROACH

Poliovirus can be isolated from the pharynx or stool but is rarely isolated from CSF. Sequencing can distinguish wild-type from vaccine-type virus in acute flaccid paralysis. Neutralizing antibodies are often present early and at high levels. CSF usually shows an increased WBC count (10-200 cells/mm^3, primarily lymphocytes) and a mildly increased protein level (generally 40-50 mg/dL).

REFERENCES

Baker AB. Bulbar poliomyelitis: its mechanism and treatment. *Am J Med.* 1949;6:614-619.

Dalakis MC, Sever JL, Madden DL, et al. Late postpoliomyelitis muscular atrophy: clinical, virologic, and immunologic studies. *Rev Infect Dis.* 1984;6:S562-S567.

Enders JF, Weller TH, Robbins FC. Cultivation of the Lansing strain of poliomyelitis virus in cultures of various human embryonic tissue. *Science.* 1949;109:85-87.

Horstmann DM. Clinical aspects of acute poliomyelitis. *Am J Med.* 1949;6:592-605.

Live Poliovirus Vaccines. First and Second International Conferences on Live Poliovirus Vaccines. Washington, DC: World Health Organization; 1959 and 1960.

Salk JE. Studies in human subjects on active immunization against poliomyelitis: I. A preliminary report of experiments in progress. *JAMA*. 1953;151:1081-1098.

Strebel PM, Sutter RW, Cochi SL, et al. Epidemiology of poliomyelitis in the United States: one decade after the last reported case of indigenous wild virus-associated disease. *Clin Infect Dis*. 1992;14:568-579.

Vermont State Department of Public Health. Infantile paralysis in Vermont. Brattleboro, Vt: Vermont Printing Co; 1924.

Weinstein L, Shelokov A, Seltser R, Winchell GD. A comparison of the clinical features of poliomyelitis in adults and children. *N Engl J Med*. 1952;246:297-302.

Wright PF, Kim-Farley RJ, de Quadros CA, et al. Strategies for the global eradication of poliomyelitis by the year 2000. *N Engl J Med*. 1991;325:1774-1779.

Section XVI
NEURO-ONCOLOGY

Chapter 71
Neuro-oncology Differential Diagnosis 604

Chapter 72
Malignant Brain Tumors 611

Chapter 73
Benign Brain Tumors 622

Chapter 74
Spinal Cord Tumors 635

Chapter 71
Neuro-oncology Differential Diagnosis

H. Royden Jones, Jr, Peter K. Dempsey, and Lloyd M. Alderson

The time course of a patient's illness is an important indicator of the disease process. Unlike stroke, which presents suddenly, brain tumor symptoms often progress over weeks or months. The exceptions are seizures, which can be focal or generalized, and are the presenting symptom of a cerebral tumor in one third of patients. Seizures represent cortical dysfunction, and focal seizures suggest involvement of the contralateral cerebral cortex. Occasionally, a patient thought to have a stroke is found to have a brain tumor.

Numerous conditions require consideration in patients presenting with new seizures versus gradual or rarely abrupt change in focal or generalized neurologic function. Also seen are patients without focal changes who present with papilledema and sixth nerve palsies strongly suggestive of a brain neoplasm or increased intracranial pressure but who may have basically unremarkable imaging study results.

IDIOPATHIC INTRACRANIAL HYPERTENSION

Clinical Vignette

A 38-year-old overweight woman presented with a recent onset of headaches and blurred vision. The headaches were increasingly severe and more bothersome to her when she bent forward. She noted intermittent double vision on lateral gaze.

Neurologic examination demonstrated bilateral limitation of lateral eye movements compatible with CN-VI paresis and modest papilledema. Brain imaging demonstrated diminished size of her lateral ventricles. Spinal fluid pressure was 350 mm CSF; its hematologic, cytologic, and chemical components were normal.

Idiopathic intracranial hypertension, also called *pseudotumor cerebri* (Figure 71-1), is a unique syndrome of relatively severe and often progressive headaches with diplopia, primarily presenting in healthy young women who are usually significantly overweight. Frequently poorly defined and nonspecific in character, the headaches are often severe, with a progressive intensity. Pseudotumor cerebri is associated with increased intracranial CSF pressure (>250 mm CSF).

Clinical Presentation and Diagnostic Studies

In addition to headaches and frequent horizontal diplopia, transient visual obscurations and pulsatile tinnitus are often significant in the clinical picture. Neurologic examination demonstrates papilledema, with a concomitant visual field defect, and sometimes a lateral rectus muscle weakness (pseudo–sixth nerve palsy). Patients are awake, alert, and have no focal neurologic deficits.

Hypervitaminosis A or various antibiotics such as tetracycline, minocycline, nitrofurantoin, ampicillin, or nalidixic acid may induce this syndrome. Other possible offending medications include oral contraceptives, corticosteroids, estrogens and progestational therapies, NSAIDs, amiodarone, perhexiline, and the anesthetic agents ketamine and nitrous oxide.

Neuroimaging studies are mandatory to exclude other causes of increased intracranial pressure (Figure 71-2). With a normal MRI, brain tumor is eliminated from the differential diagnosis.

When the CSF has an increased (>250 mm Hg) intracranial pressure but a normal cell count and chemical profile, the possibility of a medication-induced pseudotumor cerebri must be ex-

NEURO-ONCOLOGY DIFFERENTIAL DIAGNOSIS

Pseudotumor Cerebri

Figure 71-1

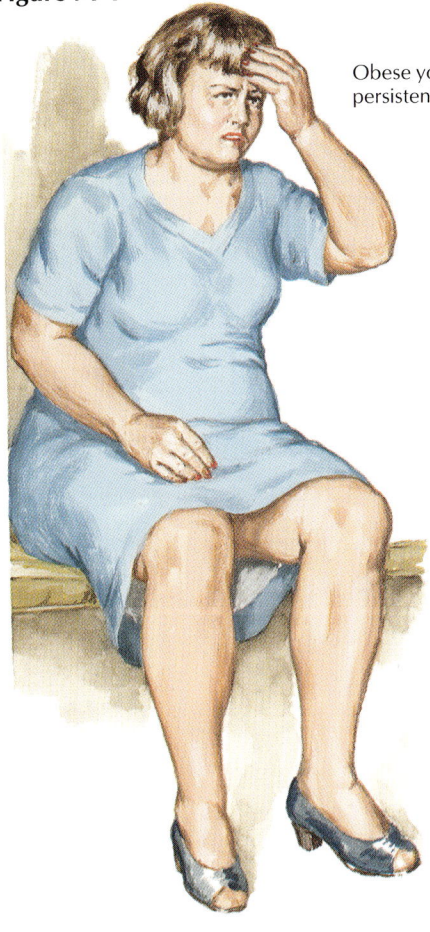

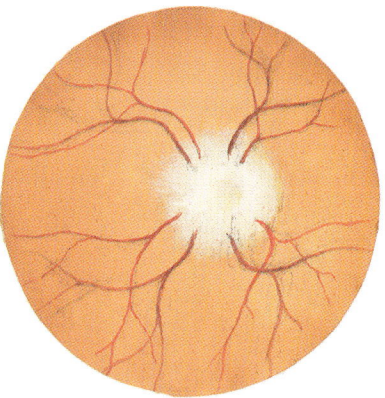

Obese young woman: persistent headache

Papilledema: nasal blurring of optic disc vessels

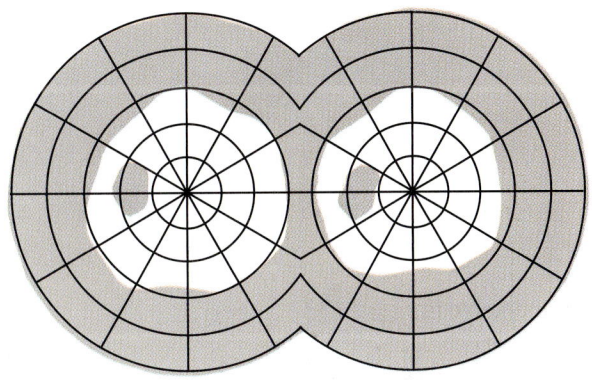

Concentrically contracted visual fields, large blind spots

Often related to pregnancy; menstrual disturbances; hypervitaminosis A; use of steroids, tetracycline, or nalidixic acid; chronic otitis media with dural sinus occlusion; endocrinopathy (Addison or Cushing disease, hypoparathyrodism)

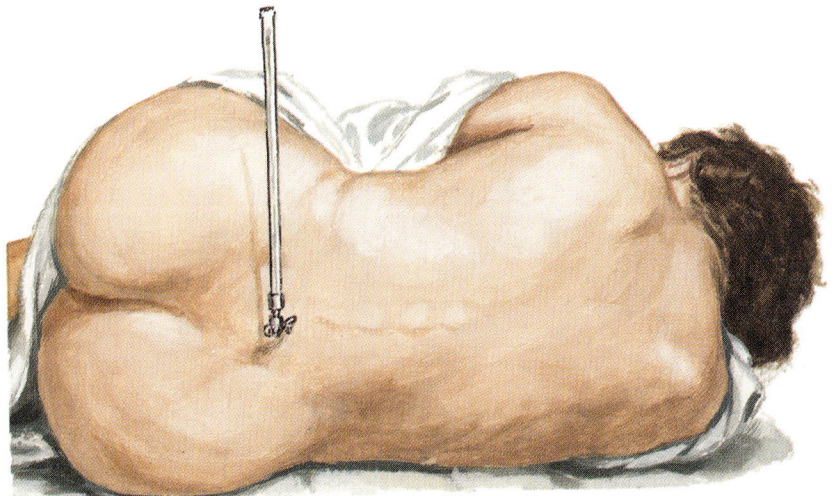

Cerebrospinal fluid pressure elevated

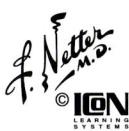

NEURO-ONCOLOGY

605

NEURO-ONCOLOGY DIFFERENTIAL DIAGNOSIS

Figure 71-2 **Some Common Manifestations of Brain Tumors**

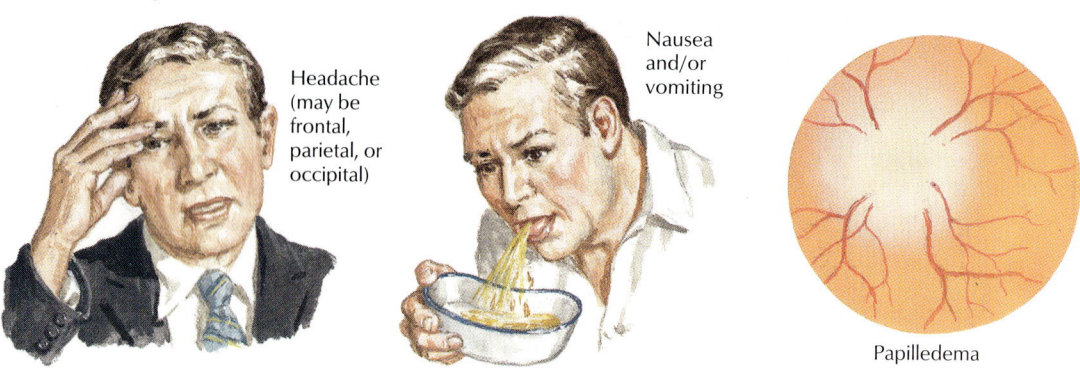

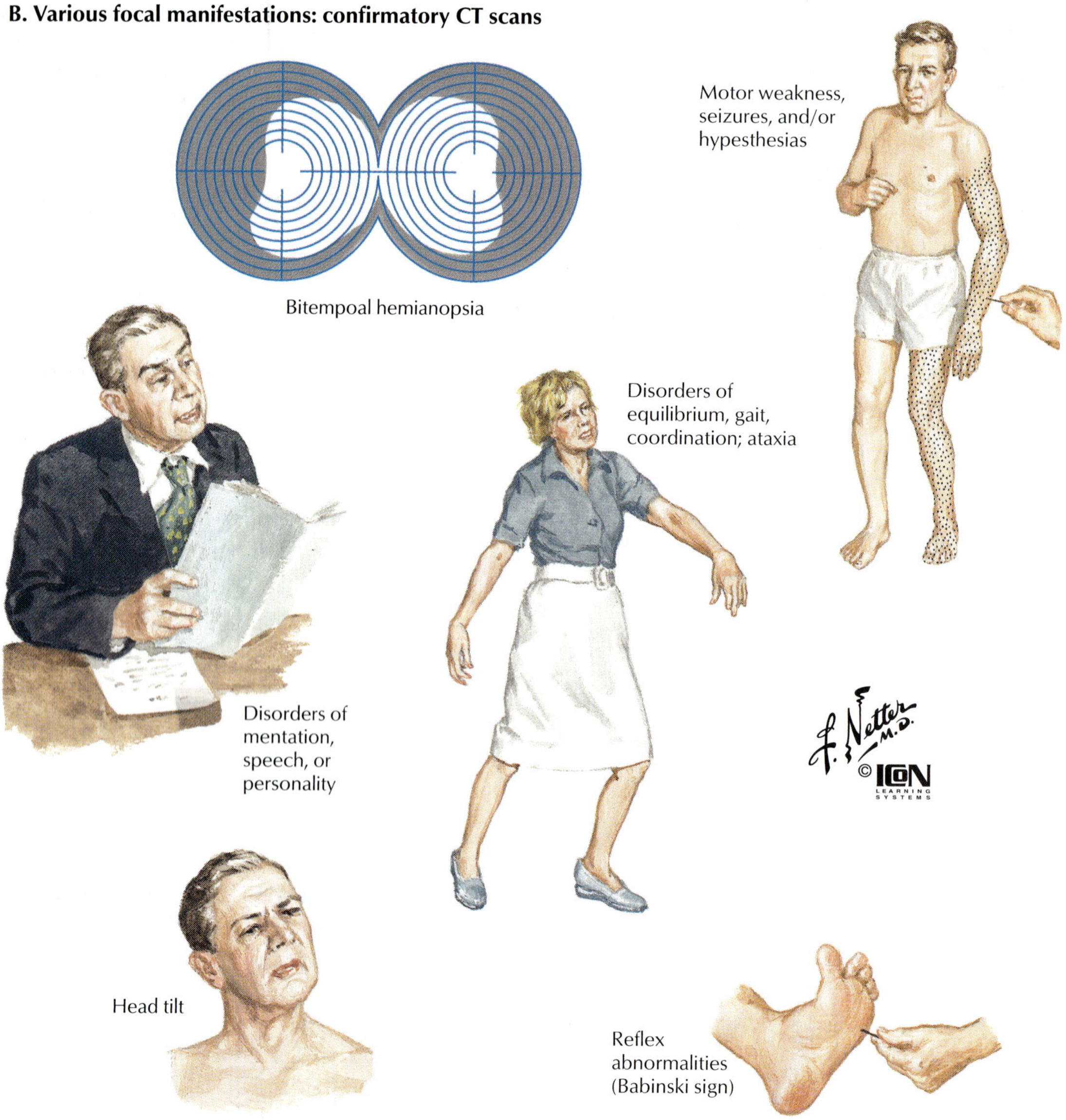

NEURO-ONCOLOGY DIFFERENTIAL DIAGNOSIS

Figure 71-2   Some Common Manifestations of Brain Tumors (continued)

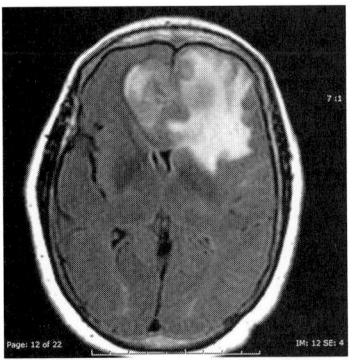

Glioblastoma. Axial FLAIR image demonstrates edema involving both frontal lobes, left more so than right, and the intervening expanded corpus callosum (arrowheads).

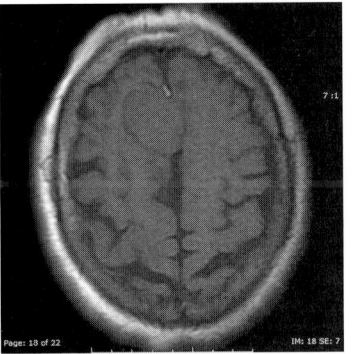
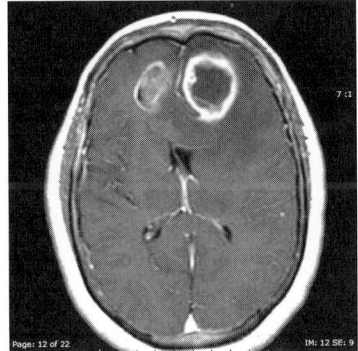
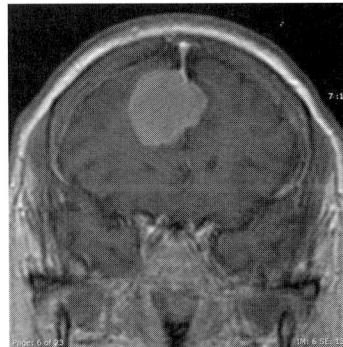

Meningioma of falx. Axial T1-weighted FLAIR and coronal post-gadolinium-enhanced T1-weighted images with fat saturation demonstrate an extraaxial, right falx-based mass, which extends through the falx to the left. The lesion is isointense to brain on T1- and T2-weighted sequences and enhances homogeneously.

---

cluded before assigning the diagnosis of pseudotumor cerebri.

Treatment

Discontinuation of an offending medication often reverses the entire clinical picture. With idiopathic pseudotumor cerebri, treatment generally consists of weight loss, low salt diet, diuretics, and symptomatic headache control.

Frequent visual monitoring with formal visual field testing is essential. Chronic increased intracranial pressure causes loss of visual acuity, secondary to the optic nerve head swelling, ie, papilledema, measured by increasing size of the blind spots on formal visual field testing.

Although diuretics occasionally help to control the increased CSF pressure, with any sign of visual compromise, more aggressive therapy is indicated. However, in individuals refractory to these benign measures, corticosteroids, optic nerve sheath fenestration (if progressive visual loss is present), and one of the CSF shunting procedures is indicated.

LOW-CSF-PRESSURE HEADACHE SYNDROME

Classic low-CSF-pressure headaches are severe, exacerbated by postural factors, and often mimic the ball valve effect seen in some intraventricular brain tumors. They commonly arise after a lumbar puncture for spinal anesthesia, CSF analysis, or a seemingly benign closed head injury. MRI with gadolinium is essential to the diagnosis (Figures 71-3 A and B). The headaches must be differentiated from leptomeningeal neoplastic or inflammatory processes. Sometimes a lumbar blood patch can provide relief and a therapeutic diagnosis (chapter 18).

NEURO-ONCOLOGY DIFFERENTIAL DIAGNOSIS

Figure 71-3

Low-Pressure Headache

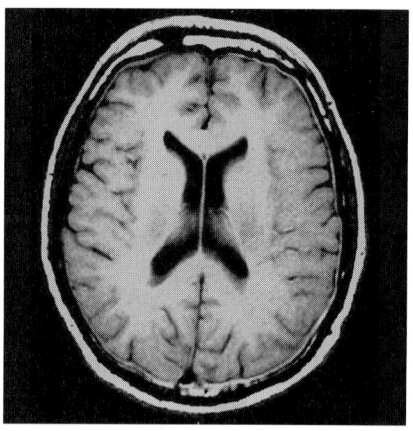
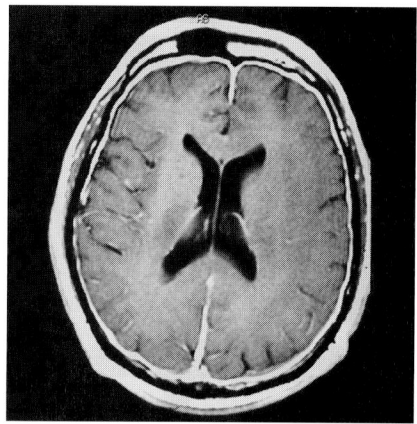

(**A**) Axial T1-weighted image with dural thickening. (**B**) Axial T1-weighted, gadolinium-enhanced image with striking enhancement of the thickened dura.

Brain Abscess

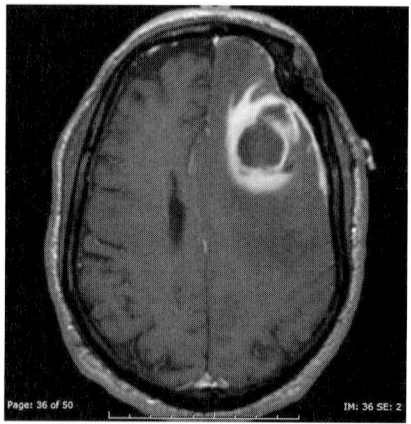
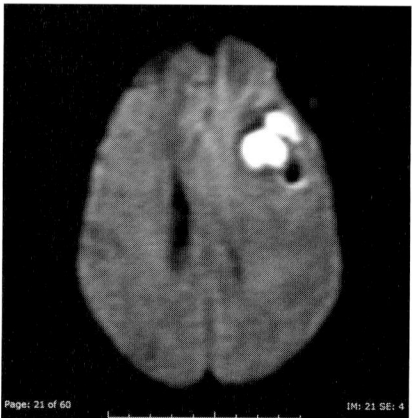

(**C**) Axial T1-weighted, gadolinium-enhancing left frontal mass with central hypointensity. (**D**) Diffusion image shows restricted diffusion within the pus as very bright signal.

Herpes Encephalitis

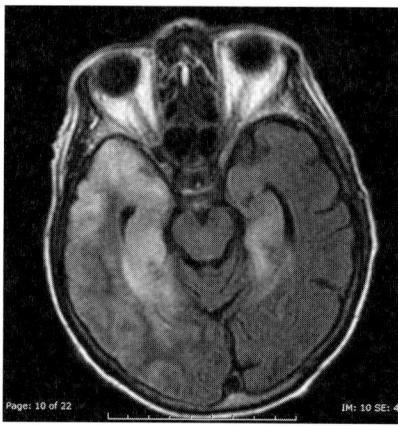
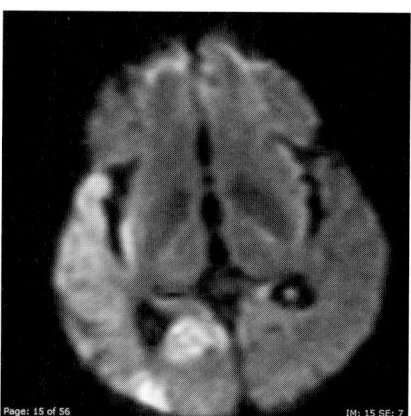

(**E**) Axial FLAIR image with extensive intracranial signal in right temporal lobe and medial left temporal lobe. (**F**) Diffusion with right temporal and insular changes.

NEURO-ONCOLOGY DIFFERENTIAL DIAGNOSIS

BRAIN TUMOR

Either malignant or benign brain tumors are the usual mechanism in patients presenting with headaches, seizures, focal deficits, or changes in level of consciousness. These entities are discussed in chapters 72 and 73.

BRAIN ABSCESS

A solitary intraparenchymal brain abscess is always within the differential diagnosis of individuals presenting with evolving focal brain lesions. A contiguous or systemic source, including sinus, ear, dental, or pulmonary infections, are some of the most common infectious sources for a cerebral abscess (Figures 71-3 C and D). Recent open head injury should also alert the examiner to possible infection. Similarly but less commonly, certain systemic illnesses, such as bacterial endocarditis in patients with fever and heart murmur, may lead to focal or even multifocal cerebritis. Patients with sarcoidosis or tuberculosis may produce focal intracerebral noncaseating or caseating granulomas that may also present with focal brain lesions suggestive of a primary tumor (chapter 64).

HERPES ZOSTER ENCEPHALITIS

Herpes zoster encephalitis is the most common focal viral encephalitis (Figures 71-3 E and F). Although it has a relatively acute onset, it can mimic fulminating glioblastoma multiforme. Often, these patients present with complex partial seizures or personality changes not unlike those associated with a brain tumor. They occasionally have a more subacute onset over 4 to 8 weeks, more reflective of a primary CNS malignancy than of focal viral encephalitis.

While this differential diagnosis is being settled, it is wise to "cover the patient" with appropriate therapy for the viral infection, namely acyclovir, 800 mg 3 times daily, until a specific lesion is confirmed. CSF polymerase chain reactivity may offer a relatively immediate means to confirm herpes zoster infection. When not diagnostic, a stereotactic or open brain biopsy may be needed to confirm a specific diagnosis.

ARTERIOVENOUS MALFORMATIONS

Congenital vascular malformations usually present in a young adult as a focal seizure appropriate to the site of the lesion, headaches, or an acute intracerebral parenchymal hemorrhage. With focal seizures, patients may initially be suspected of harboring a focal malignancy, likely a glioma. However, imaging studies usually differentiate distinctly from an intrinsic cerebral neoplasm (chapter 24).

SUBDURAL HEMATOMA

Although subdural hematomas usually present after recognized head trauma, they may be relatively subtle and unsuspected, especially in the elderly. Caution is advised with findings on CT that may progress from acute blood that is hyperdense to isodense to hypodense. During the subacute clinical phase, this lesion may not be appreciated without careful evaluation of the imaging study in the patient presenting with headaches, focal neurologic symptoms, or both, perhaps mimicking a brain neoplasm.

DEMYELINATING DISORDERS

Occasionally, patients with ingravescent focal neurologic histories seemingly compatible with a cerebral malignancy have specific localized lesions on imaging studies. At surgery, the neuropathologist finds evidence of a primary demyelinating process otherwise known as *monofocal acute inflammatory demyelination*. These lesions usually are self-limited and may be seen in multiple sclerosis and are treatable with corticosteroids. On occasion, new lesions appear over time in different portions of the cerebral cortex.

In contrast, **immunocompromised hosts** receiving long-term immunosuppressive therapy such as corticosteroids or azathioprine and patients with HIV are at risk for development of progressive multifocal leukoencephalopathy. Usually, these individuals have an evolving focal neurologic lesion. Primary CNS lymphoma and certain parasites, such as toxoplasmosis or cytomegalovirus, also require consideration in this differential.

Diagnostic Modalities and Treatment

Brain MRI is the most specific means to differentiate these lesions (Figures 71-3 A-F). EEG may sometimes be helpful because of the relatively specific pseudoperiodic discharges seen in herpes simplex encephalitis. CSF analysis, direct brain biopsy, or both may be indicated to finalize the diagnosis. Treatment depends on results of clinical diagnostic modalities and their respective findings.

REFERENCES

Binder DK, Horton JC, Lawton MT, McDermott MW. Idiopathic intracranial hypertension. *Neurosurgery*. 2004;54:538-551.

Gutrecht JA, Berger JR, Jones HR, Mancall AC. Monofocal acute inflammatory demyelination (MAID): a unique disorder simulating brain neoplasm. *South Med J*. 2002;95:1180-1186.

Kennedy PG. Viral encephalitis: causes, differential diagnosis, and management. *J Neurol Neurosurg Psychiatry*. 2004;75(suppl 1):i10-i15.

Koss SA, Ulmer JL, Hacein-Bey L. Angiographic features of spontaneous intracranial hypotension. *AJNR Am J Neuroradiol*. 2003;24:704-706.

Maarouf M, Kuchta J, Miletic H, et al. Acute demyelination: diagnostic difficulties and the need for brain biopsy. *Acta Neurochir (Wien)*. 2003;145:961-969.

Mokri B. Headaches caused by decreased intracranial pressure: diagnosis and management. *Curr Opin Neurol*. 2003;16:319-326.

Rapport RL, Hillier D, Scearce T, Ferguson C. Spontaneous intracranial hypotension from intradural thoracic disthoracic disc herniation: case report. *J Neurosurg*. 2003;98(suppl):282-284.

Raschilas F, Wolff M, Delatour F, et al. Outcome of and prognostic factors for herpes simplex encephalitis in adult patients: results of a multicenter study. *Clin Infect Dis*. 2002;35:254-260.

Chapter 72
Malignant Brain Tumors

Peter K. Dempsey and Lloyd M. Alderson

EPIDEMIOLOGY

The chance of development of a malignant brain tumor in the United States is small (5.8 per 100,000 person-years). However, most primary care physicians encounter such a patient every few years. Most have a **glioma**; unfortunately, **glioblastoma** is the most common type. The incidence of brain tumors in several US regions as collected by the Central Brain Tumor Registry of the United States and the Surveillance, Epidemiology, and End Results consortia demonstrates 5.1 gliomas per 100,000 person-years in adults; approximately 2.5 cases for glioblastoma alone. Brain cancer incidence increases with age, peaking at 65 to 70 years. For glioblastoma alone, the highest incidence occurs at 60 years of age. Although Central Brain Tumor Registry of the United States data demonstrate that glioma incidence decreases in people older than 75 years, other investigators report an increasing incidence in this population. The male:female ratio for malignant glioma is 1.5 to 2.0:1. Brain cancer incidence also varies regionally; the incidence in Hawaii is roughly half that in New England.

PRIMARY INTRAAXIAL BRAIN TUMORS

Gliomas, the most common primary brain tumor in adults, can show features of **astrocytes**, **oligodendrocytes**, or both (mixed glioma) (Figure 72-1). The World Health Organization uses a 3-tiered classification system in which tumor grade reflects the extent to which tumor cells are morphologically abnormal (anaplasia), their apparent growth rate, and the presence of necrosis. Low-grade tumors may contain a high density of almost normal-appearing cells with less than 2% growth rate. **Anaplastic gliomas** have more atypical cells with pleomorphic nuclei with growth rates in the 5% to 10% range but no evidence of necrosis. Gliomas with high growth rates (>20%) and necrosis are classified as **glioblastoma multiforme** (GBM). Similar criteria are used to classify tumors into 1 of 4 grades. Grade I is reserved for **pilocytic astrocytoma**. Grades II, III, and IV correspond to **low-grade glioma**, **anaplastic glioma**, and **glioblastoma**, respectively (Table 72-1). Tumor grade is the most reliable predictor of prognosis. Even if the lesion cannot be safely excised, a needle biopsy is often indicated. A classification system is being developed that relies more on genetics than on cellular morphology. Whether it will more accurately predict therapy response and prognosis is unknown.

Low-Grade Glioma

Clinical Vignette

A 26-year-old, right-handed man with an unremarkable medical history had 2 generalized tonic-clonic seizures and was brought to the ED. He noted a progressive headache for several weeks. Evaluation revealed some postictal confusion. His gait was initially unsteady but improved within a few hours. The remainder of his examination results were normal.

Brain MRI showed a right frontal lobe lesion, bright on T2 and FLAIR imaging but hypointense on T1, with no evidence of enhancement after gadolinium. The patient was treated with phenytoin and admitted to the hospital. Stereotactic biopsy revealed a mixed low-grade glioma with a Ki-67 index of less than 2%.

Low-grade gliomas are slow growing and, although seen on MRI, often do not enhance with gadolinium. Even though these tumors carry better initial prognoses than glioblastomas, most patients with low-grade gliomas eventually progress to glioblastoma and succumb to their disease.

MALIGNANT BRAIN TUMORS

Figure 72-1

Gliomas

Glioblastoma

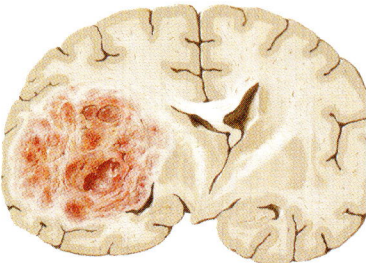

Large, hemispheric glioblastoma multifome with central areas of necrosis; brain distorted to opposite side

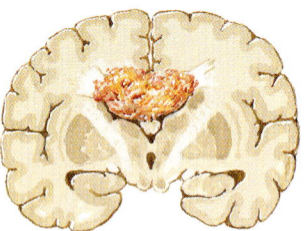

Coronal section of corpus callosum glioma

Stereotactic brain biopsy using modified Gouda frame

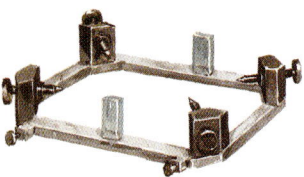

Basic frame for interfacing with CT scanner fastens to patient's head by steel pins.

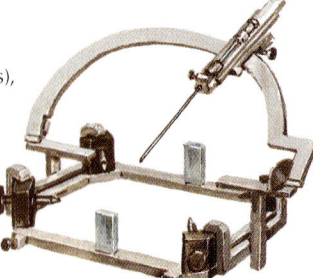

Side arms (for Y axis), vertical bars (for Z axis, which relates to level of CT cut), and horizontal bars (for X axis), plus arc with biopsy needle affixed to frame

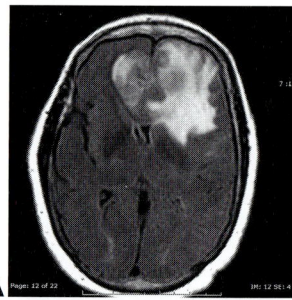
A

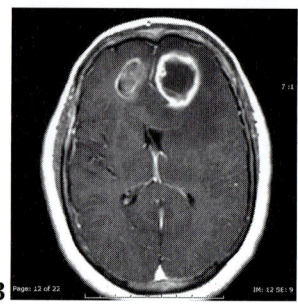
B

(**A**) Axial FLAIR image demonstrates edema involving both frontal lobes, left more so than right, and the intervening expanded corpus callosum (arrowheads). (**B**) T1-weighted, post–gadolinium-enhanced image shows rim-enhancing lesions with irregular margins and central hypointensity. This central hypointensity represents necrosis, and the enhancing region represents the more active regions within this butterfly glioma.

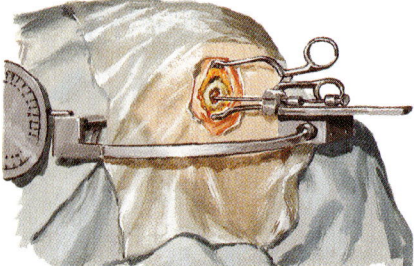

Patient, head draped, on operating table; biopsy specimen taken via blurrhole under local anesthesia

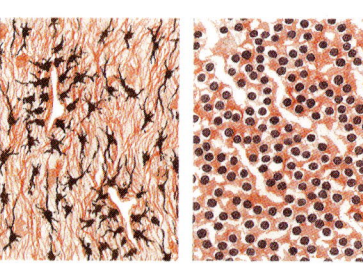
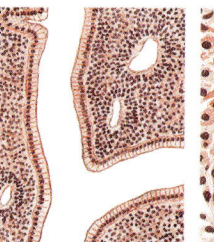
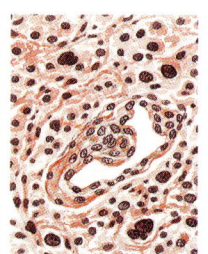

Astrocytoma — Oligodendroglioma — Ependymoma — Glioblastoma multiforme

Neuro-oncology

612

MALIGNANT BRAIN TUMORS

Table 72-1
Grades of Gliomas

	Low-Grade Glioma	*Anaplastic Glioma*	*Glioblastoma*
Grade	Grade II	Grade III	Grade IV
Symptom duration	Years	Months	Weeks
Patient age at diagnosis, y	5-30	30-50	>50
MRI enhancement	−	+/−	+/+
Pathology	Hypercellular	Anaplastic	Necrosis, endothelial cell, proliferation
Mitotic index (Ki-67)	<2%	5-10%	>10%
Treatment	Observe	Radiation therapy and chemotherapy	Radiation therapy and chemotherapy
Survival	5-10 years	3-4 years	12 months

Histologically, low-grade gliomas are classified as **astrocytomas**, **oligodendrogliomas**, or **oligoastrocytomas** (mixed glioma). Symptom history can extend from months to years. These tumors may be relatively stable for several years before progressing. A low mitotic index (as measured by Ki-67 or mib-1 immunostaining), younger patient age, and a supratentorial lesion that is amenable to resection predict a longer progression-free survival.

Treatment and Prognosis
The choice of therapeutic modalities is always an issue. Retrospective studies suggest that gross total resection for tumors that can be safely removed provide longer progression-free survival. However, the surgeon can never remove all tumor tissue when dealing with infiltrative gliomas, which eventually progress even after gross total resection. Therefore, disabling resections in patients with astrocytomas or oligodendrogliomas are neither wise nor helpful.

Subtotal resection is indicated in most gliomas remediable to decompression without leaving a significant disability (such as aphasia) and where the mass effect of the tumor is causing disability. In patients with pilocytic astrocytoma, surgical indications differ slightly; a complete resection may provide a cure, and a more aggressive surgical approach is often indicated.

The next therapeutic decision is whether to recommend external beam radiation therapy (RT). Preliminary data suggest that RT does not prolong overall survival in patients with low-grade glioma. There was an increase in progression-free survival for treated patients; however, this benefit may be offset by a higher incidence of cognitive impairment in the treated group. Survival is not the only factor when considering RT. Patients with large symptomatic tumors often benefit functionally from RT, which may also reduce seizure frequency in some patients who are refractory to anticonvulsant drugs.

Radiation therapy is recommended for patients with large symptomatic residual disease. Otherwise, therapy can be withheld until radiographic or clinical evidence of tumor progression exists. Focal radiation (radiosurgery or gamma knife) is used in some patients with low-grade glioma, but long-term follow-up data does not show a clear benefit.

Chemotherapy is usually not part of the initial management of low-grade glioma, except for patients with oligodendroglial tumors who are older or whose tumors have a relatively high mitotic index. These patients may benefit from PCV (procarbazine, CCNU, and vincristine) chemotherapy, which delays the use of RT with its primary risk of long-term cognitive impairment, particularly in elderly patients. However, chemotherapy

NEURO-ONCOLOGY

MALIGNANT BRAIN TUMORS

is not without risk, and chemotherapy-induced leukemia occurs in approximately 1% to 2% of patients treated with PCV who survive for 5 years.

Although patients with low-grade tumors have a much better prognosis than those with anaplastic glioma and GBM, low-grade gliomas are usually fatal. The median survival is 5 to 7 years for patients with astrocytoma and 7 to 10 years for patients with oligodendroglioma.

Anaplastic Glioma

Clinical Vignette

A 39-year-old, right-handed man presented with 3 weeks of progressive clumsiness in the left hand and a right frontal headache that was worse in the morning and improved during the day.

Examination revealed papilledema and decreased rapid movements in the left hand. Brain MRI revealed a 3 × 4-cm cystic mass centered in the medial aspect of the right frontal lobe, significant adjacent edema with right-to-left shift of the brain, and heterogeneous enhancement with gadolinium.

After oral dexamethasone was initiated, the patient's headache and clumsiness improved. Lesion resection revealed an anaplastic oligodendroglioma. Postoperatively, he was treated with a combination of chemotherapy (PCV × 6 cycles) followed by external beam RT.

Anaplastic gliomas are intermediate-grade tumors with a higher mitotic index than low-grade gliomas but lacking the necrosis of glioblastomas. They commonly affect patients in the 35- to 50-year age range, who often present with a relatively recent, few weeks' history of symptoms.

Treatment and Prognosis

Theoretically, complete surgical resection is the best initial intervention; however, a heroic but neurologically disabling procedure is not truly beneficial and therefore is not indicated. It is not acceptable to attempt a major resection of a glioma when confronted by a tumor originating within **elegant** cerebral tissue, the loss of which would leave the patient significantly incapacitated by the loss of ability to speak, form memory, or use extremities, particularly motor structures within the dominant hemisphere, where preservation of functional mobility is particularly important.

Most patients with anaplastic tumors are treated with combined radiation and chemotherapy. Most patients with anaplastic astrocytomas are offered RT soon after surgery. There is controversy about the value, if any, of adjuvant PCV chemotherapy; studies have not confirmed a survival advantage.

Temozolomide is an oral, well-tolerated chemotherapeutic drug approved for the treatment of recurrent anaplastic gliomas. Unlike any other form of glioma treatment, there is a relatively high chance of response (40-50%) resulting in complete or partial improvement or stable disease. Temozolomide is being evaluated as an adjuvant to radiation and concomitant with RT in patients with anaplastic astrocytoma.

The postsurgical approach is somewhat different in patients with anaplastic oligodendrogliomas and mixed anaplastic gliomas. There is approximately a 70% chance that patients will respond to PCV chemotherapy. Therefore, PCV (6 cycles, if tolerated) can be recommended before RT in most patients. A chromosomal marker (loss of heterozygosity at 1p and 19q) can predict with 95% sensitivity whether a patient will respond to PCV chemotherapy. Patients who lack this marker have only a 30% chance of responding, and their prognosis is much worse. This and other genetic markers may soon affect decisions about which therapies to use.

Anaplastic astrocytoma is associated with a median survival of approximately 3 years. Unlike astrocytomas, anaplastic oligodendrogliomas respond better, particularly if the tumor has the chromosomal abnormalities described in this chapter. Aggressive chemotherapy (with bone marrow transplantation) has not significantly prolonged survival.

Glioblastoma Multiforme

Clinical Vignette

A 62-year-old, left-handed woman presented to the ED with headache and confusion after a motor vehicle accident. She struck a parked car with the left side of her vehicle, her third accident within 3 weeks. Her medical history was remarkable for type 2 diabetes and mild hypertension. Evaluation in the ED revealed that

MALIGNANT BRAIN TUMORS

she was disoriented, had a left homonymous hemianopsia, and was unsteady on her feet, falling to the right.

Brain MRI revealed multifocal right occipital lobe and right cerebellar hemisphere lesions. There was ring enhancement with gadolinium and some fourth ventricle compression.

The patient was treated with IV dexamethasone and admitted to the hospital. Resection of the cerebellar lesion revealed GBM. Postoperative treatment with external beam RT was complicated by symptomatic swelling of the residual lesion, necessitating surgical decompression. After completion of RT 4 months later, tumor progression was noted. The patient was enrolled in an experimental chemotherapy trial but later succumbed to her illness.

Glioblastoma multiforme is the most common and most aggressive of the gliomas and the least likely to respond to therapy. The average age at presentation is 62 years, and the male:female ratio is 1.5 to 2:1. *Multiforme* refers to the gross appearance of the tumor. Often, areas of necrosis, hemorrhage, and fleshy tumor exist within the same tumor focus.

When clinical and molecular behavior of GBM tumors is reviewed, a developmental dichotomy emerges. Younger patients with GBM sometimes have a long history of seizures, suggesting that the tumor developed from a lower-grade precursor, whereas older patients with GBM tend to have relatively sudden symptom onset, suggesting that the malignancy did not evolve from a less aggressive tumor.

Genetic studies confirm this dichotomy. Tumors from older patients with GBM frequently have amplification of the gene encoding the epidermal growth factor receptor, whereas GBM in younger patients often exhibits mutation of p53 and loss of portions of chromosome 19, changes that are also seen in low-grade and anaplastic tumors.

Treatment and Prognosis

The first treatment step is to perform as wide a surgical resection as is functionally tolerable. Younger patients with normal examination results who have had a gross total resection have the best prognosis. Postoperative RT clearly benefits many patients and continues as the standard of care. In a large randomized study in the 1970s, patients with GBM who received RT had a median survival roughly twice that of those who did not. Additionally, when a small volume of residual disease (<3 cm in diameter) remains, a focal radiation boost has also prolonged survival.

Chemotherapy is more controversial. Bis-2-chloroethylnitrosourea (BCNU) is an IV chemotherapy that penetrates the brain, but most studies suggest that only 20% to 25% of patients benefit. BCNU can also be delivered directly to the brain in a biodegradable wafer (polifeprosan/carmustine) during surgery, which has resulted in a modest improvement in survival when used at the initial surgery or at tumor recurrence.

Temozolomide is now the most commonly used US FDA–approved drug for patients with recurrent GBM. Its response rates are higher than those attained with BCNU (30-40%), and it is better tolerated. Clinical trials of new agents for patients with recurrent or recently diagnosed GBM are ongoing.

The median survival for patients with GBM who have received RT is slightly less than 1 year. The chance of survival at 2 years is 5% to 10%, and that at 5 years is less than 5%. Long-term survivors are often those relatively younger patients who have had complete resection and received RT and some form of chemotherapy. That survival rates for patients with GBM have not significantly changed in 30 years is discouraging and emphasizes the need for more basic science and clinical research to find a reasonable treatment.

METASTATIC BRAIN TUMORS

Clinical Vignette

A 49-year-old, right-handed woman with a 2-year history of locally metastatic breast cancer, for which she received surgery, radiation, and chemotherapy, experienced progressive headache, confusion, and left-sided weakness. Neurologic evaluation revealed anomia, a moderate left hemiparesis, and a homonymous left upper quadrantanopsia.

Gadolinium-enhanced brain MRI demonstrated multiple, round ring-enhancing lesions consistent with metastases, abdominal CT revealed hepatic lesions, and bone scan results revealed a femoral tumor. The patient was treated with whole brain RT followed by systemic chemotherapy with paclitaxel (Taxol).

MALIGNANT BRAIN TUMORS

For the medical oncologist and internist, metastatic brain tumors are the most common neuro-oncologic challenge. Of all patients with cancer, CNS metastases develop in 25%, usually after the primary tumor has been diagnosed but occasionally as the initial sign. Typically, CNS metastasis is a solid tumor compressing the brain and spinal cord, or cancer cells infiltrating the CSF and nerve roots.

Lung cancer is the most common primary tumor that metastasizes to the CNS (50%), followed by breast (33%), colon (9%), and melanoma (7%) (Figure 72-2). The interval between the primary diagnosis and presentation of a CNS metastasis depends on the tumor type. For lung cancer, the median interval is 4 months; for breast cancer, the median interval is 3 years. CNS metastasis is an indicator of poor prognosis and portends a survival of less than 6 months for most patients.

Clinical Presentation and Diagnosis

As with primary CNS malignancies, clinical presentation depends entirely on the tumor site. The onset can be almost precipitous, mimicking a stroke, or can be indolent, with gradual development of focal neurologic deficit: motor, sensory, language, visual, gait, or coordination. In other instances, patients may have focal or generalized seizures or present with nonspecific symptoms possibly suggesting increased intracranial pressure, such as positional headaches, cranial neuropathies, and rarely nausea, vomiting, or both.

Gadolinium-enhanced MRI typically defines these focal metastases. Patients may present with a single focal symptom complex, or evidence of multiple other lesions may indicate the likelihood of metastatic disease. A hemorrhagic component of a tumor may signal an underlying melanoma, often a lesion that the patient had forgotten or thought irrelevant. When there is carcinomatous leptomeningeal invasion, the gadolinium enhancement of the meninges on the brain surface may suggest the need for CSF analysis, where cytologic evaluation of the increased number of CSF cells can lead to diagnosis.

Treatment

Although treatment is clearly palliative, most patients benefit from CNS-directed therapy. Whole brain RT is indicated for most patients with parenchymal brain lesions. The rare patient with an isolated, single brain lesion, who has no evidence of systemic recurrence, is a candidate for surgical resection. In fact, some resected solitary lesions have an entirely different pathology, including benign tumors such as meningioma. Focal radiation is helpful only in patients with 1 to 2 lesions who are otherwise stable. In the rare patient with a solitary brain metastasis who has received surgery or focal RT, it is reasonable to consider withholding whole brain RT until there is evidence of tumor progression in the brain.

The treatment of carcinomatous meningitis involves direct infusion of chemotherapy (methotrexate or cytarabine) into the spinal fluid via lumbar puncture or preferably a ventricular reservoir. Prognosis is typically very poor.

OTHER PRIMARY BRAIN TUMORS
Ependymoma

Ependymomas are unusual tumors of glial origin that can arise anywhere along the neuraxis. When they occur intracranially, it is usually within the floor of the fourth ventricle. Histologically, ependymomas often have a cellular appearance characterized by a pseudorosette perivascular pattern. There is also a more malignant version with an anaplastic appearance. Another variant of ependymoma, the **myxopapillary ependymoma**, occurs only in the filum terminale at the end of the spinal cord.

Treatment of ependymomas usually involves surgical resection. Like other primary brain tumors, tumor location determines whether a complete resection is achievable.

Medulloblastoma

Medulloblastomas belong to a class of uncommon tumors called ***primitive neuroectodermal tumors***. More prominent in children, they comprise 3% of all primary brain tumors in some series (Figure 72-4). They usually occur in the posterior fossa, often in the midline, and can cause hydrocephalus, nausea, vomiting, and

MALIGNANT BRAIN TUMORS

Figure 72-2
Tumors Metastatic to Brain

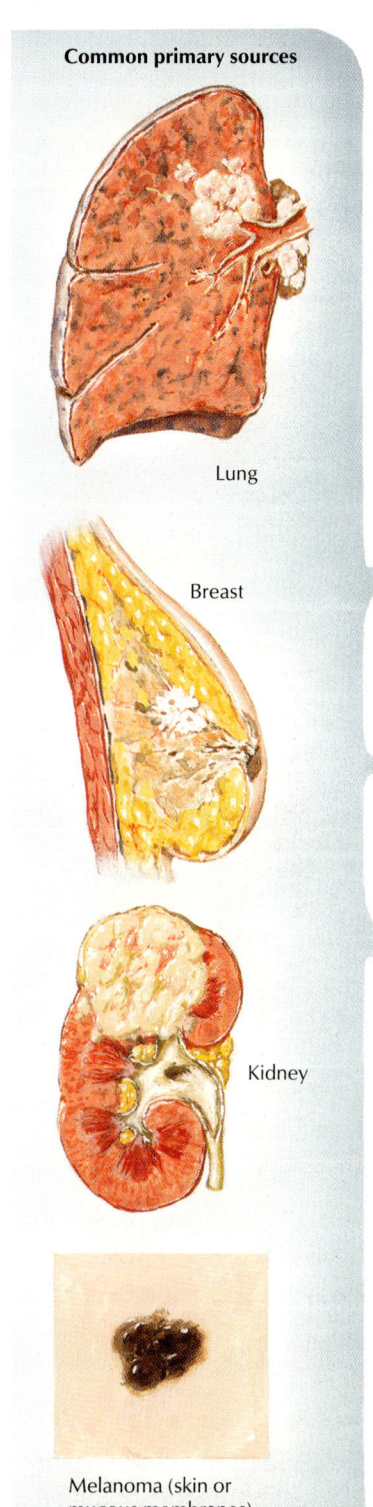

Common primary sources: Lung, Breast, Kidney, Melanoma (skin or mucous membranes)

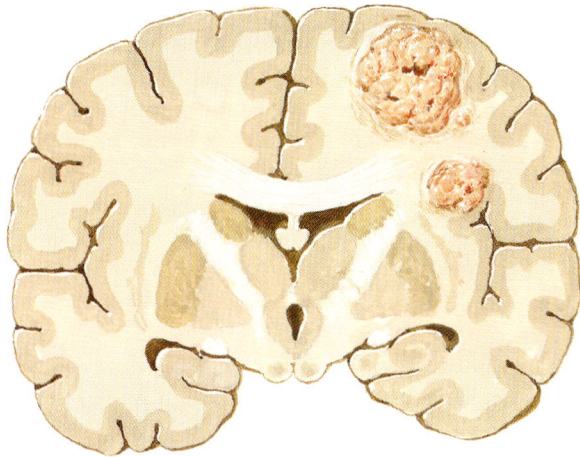

Metastatic metastases of small cell anaplastic (oat cell) carcinoma of lung to brain

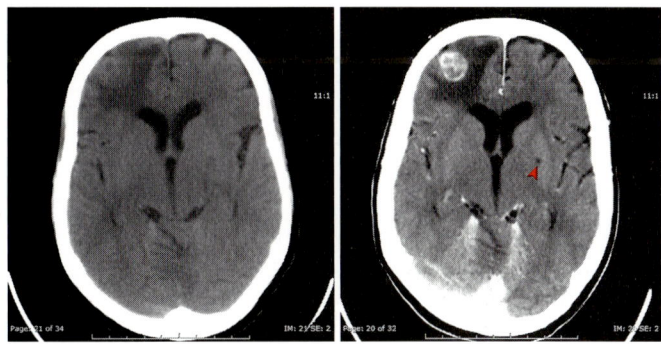

Axial CT demonstrates edema within the right frontal pole. An ill-defined heterogeneous region is seen peripherally, which enhances after iodinated contrast administration. Incidental small remote lacunar infarct is seen within the left putamen (arrowhead).

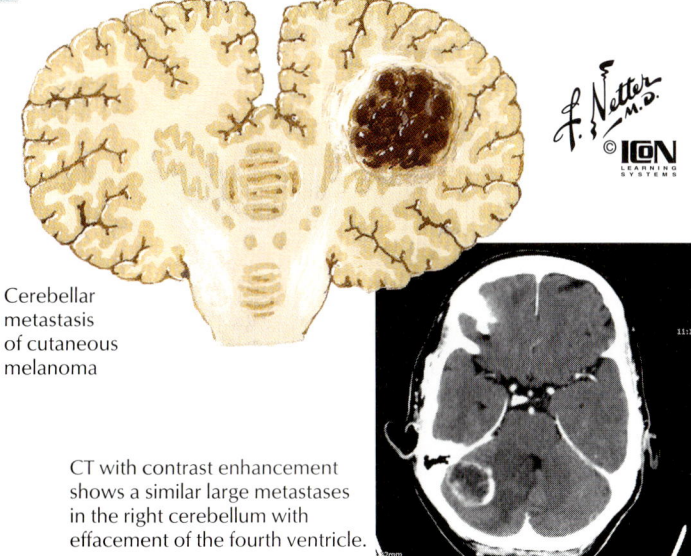

Cerebellar metastasis of cutaneous melanoma

CT with contrast enhancement shows a similar large metastases in the right cerebellum with effacement of the fourth ventricle.

NEURO-ONCOLOGY

MALIGNANT BRAIN TUMORS

ataxia. In adults, medulloblastomas also can arise within the cerebellar hemisphere. Surgical resection is the first treatment step; however, incomplete removal usually occurs. Because of the propensity to spread along the leptomeninges and through the CSF, additional treatment is required. Patients with medulloblastomas should undergo evaluation of the entire craniospinal axis to establish the extent of disease. Irradiation to the entire brain and spine is usually recommended. Chemotherapy after external beam RT improves survival.

Primary CNS Lymphoma

Previously a rare tumor, **primary CNS lymphoma** has increased dramatically in incidence, possibly consequent to the AIDS epidemic or the increasing use of immunosupression. Lymphoma can arise anywhere within the brain but is often located in the periventricular region. Radiographically, it is often hyperdense on noncontrast CT with enhancement. MRI reveals an irregular shape with enhancement. Although often solitary, it can occur in multiple locations (Figure 72-3B).

Given the nonspecific radiographic appearance of lymphoma, a biopsy is mandated. Surgical resection is usually not helpful; needle biopsy establishes the diagnosis. A systemic workup is also advised to evaluate for other lymphoma locations.

CNS lymphoma is markedly radiosensitive, and most patients show a positive response to external beam radiation. The addition of chemotherapy may also prolong survival. The usual regimen involves intrathecal methotrexate delivery through an indwelling ventricular catheter. Despite aggressive treatment and a positive initial response, most lymphomas recur.

Cerebellar Astrocytoma

Most childhood primary brain tumors are in the glioma family, and many of these occur in the cerebellum (Figure 72-5). **Pilocytic astrocytomas** are the most common variant in the posterior fossa and tend to arise within the cerebellar hemisphere. A second form of cerebellar astrocytoma, the **diffuse** or **fibrillary form**, often arises in the midline and produces obstruction of the fourth ventricle and hydrocephalus. **Cerebellar astrocytomas** are often cystic in appearance, with an enhancing mural nodule.

Surgical resection can sometimes be curative, particularly with pilocytic astrocytomas. Incompletely resected tumors often require postsurgical irradiation. The survival rate of patients with cerebellar astrocytomas is often much greater than those with supratentorial glial tumors.

Figure 72-3   **Primary CNS Lymphoma**

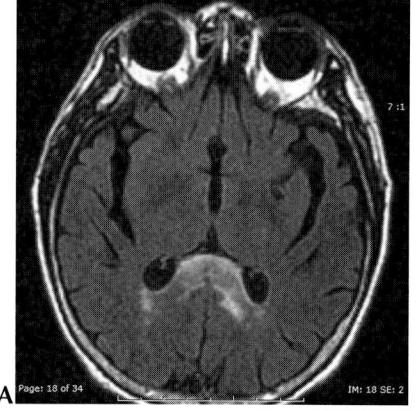 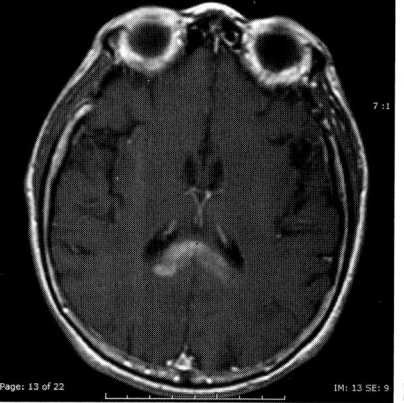

(**A**) Axial FLAIR image demonstrates increased signal within a diffusely expanded splenium of the corpus callosum. (**B**) Axial T1-weighted, post–gadolinium-enhanced image shows enhancement within the same region.

MALIGNANT BRAIN TUMORS

Brain Tumors in Children

Figure 72-4

Medulloblastoma

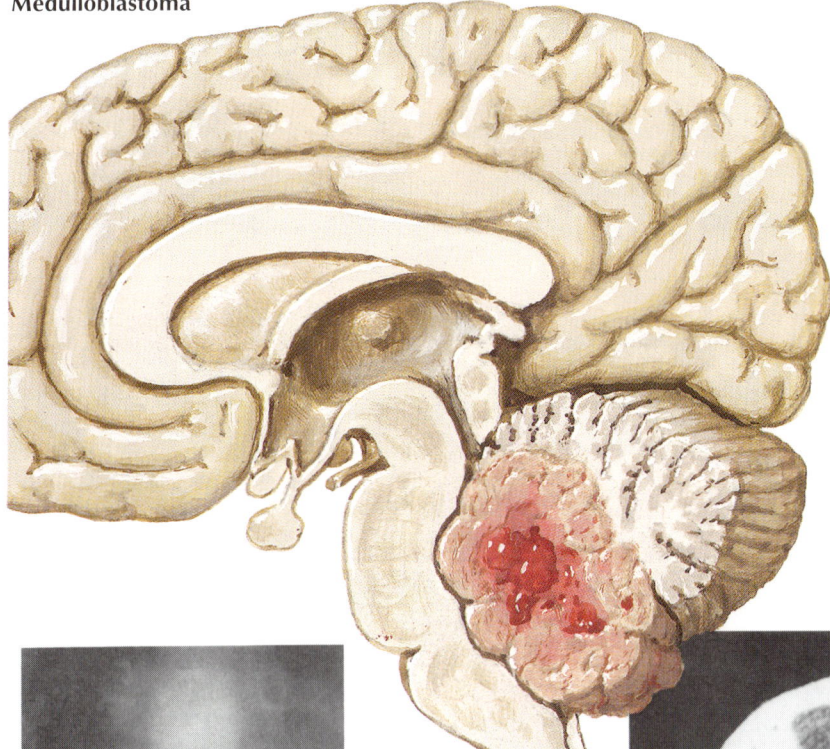

Medulloblastoma arising from vermis of cerebellum, filling 4th ventricle and protruding into cisterna magna

CT scan showing enhancing medulloblastoma in region of 4th ventricle; obstructive hydrocephalus indicated by dilated temporal horn

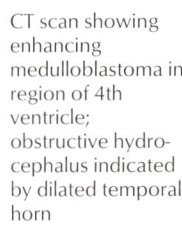

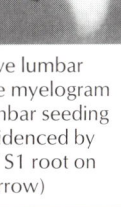

Postoperative lumbar metrizamide myelogram showing lumbar seeding of tumor evidenced by nonfilling of S1 root on right side (arrow)

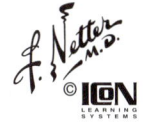

Positive CSF cytologic findings in patient with medulloblastoma; malignant tumor cells clumped on Millipore filter

NEURO-ONCOLOGY

MALIGNANT BRAIN TUMORS

Figure 72-5

Cystic Astrocytoma of Cerebellum

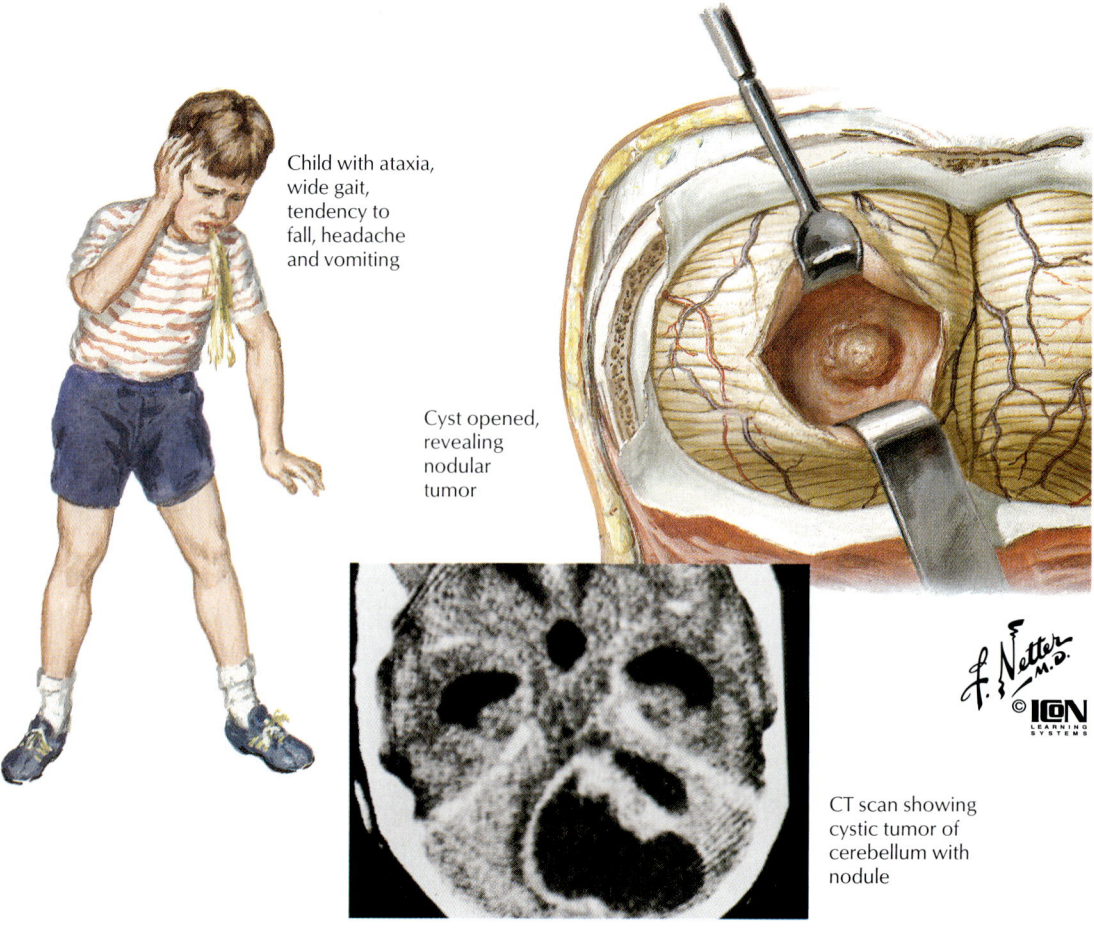

Child with ataxia, wide gait, tendency to fall, headache and vomiting

Cyst opened, revealing nodular tumor

CT scan showing cystic tumor of cerebellum with nodule

Pontine Glioma

Pontine gliomas occur primarily in childhood. They tend to be higher-grade tumors that expand the pons and infiltrate into the surrounding tissue (Figure 72-6). Presenting symptoms are consistent with their location, namely hydrocephalus from fourth ventricle obstruction or long tract signs from impairment of axonal pathways. Isolated cranial neuropathies may also arise from compression of brainstem nuclei. The infiltrative nature of these tumors often precludes surgical resection, and RT is usually ineffective at achieving long-term growth control.

FUTURE DIRECTIONS

Treatment of malignant brain tumors remains challenging and often unsuccessful. Advances in treatment are being made in the field of imaging, where PET and MR spectroscopy are often able to distinguish recurrent tumors from necrotic, posttreatment change. Image guidance in the operating room allows for smaller, more precisely located incisions and provides real-time information on the extent of tumor resection.

Radiation therapy remains the mainstay for treating malignant brain neoplasm, and stereotactic radiosurgery is being used more fre-

Brain Glioma

Figure 72-6

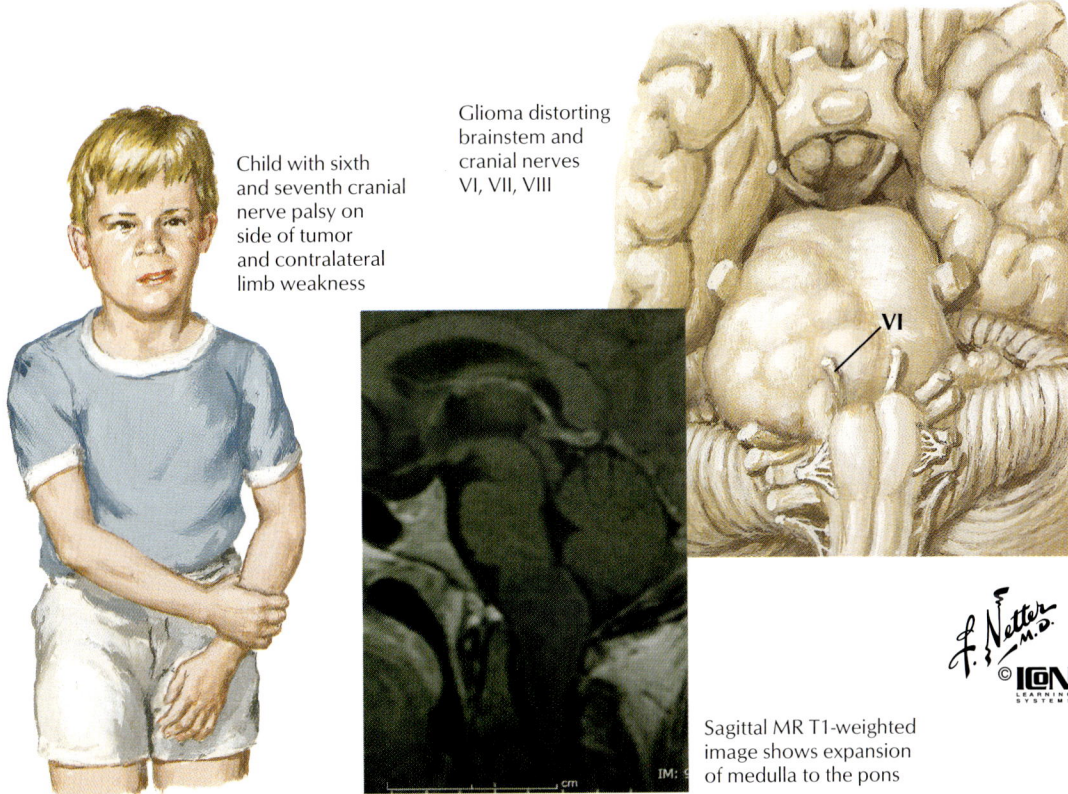

Child with sixth and seventh cranial nerve palsy on side of tumor and contralateral limb weakness

Glioma distorting brainstem and cranial nerves VI, VII, VIII

Sagittal MR T1-weighted image shows expansion of medulla to the pons

---

quently to provide additional doses to previously irradiated tissue, improving the control of tumor growth.

Perhaps the greatest improvements in treating gliomas are the novel chemotherapy treatments, such as temozolamide, that are showing promise in controlling tumor growth. Gene therapy and other targeted, biochemically based treatments are also showing promise.

REFERENCES

Ahsan H, Neugut AI, Bruce JN. Trends in incidence of primary malignant brain tumors in USA, 1981-1990. *Int J Epidemiol.* 1995;24:1078-1085.

Daumas-Duport C, Scheithauer BW, O'Fallon J, Kelly P. Grading of astrocytomas: a simple and reproducible method. *Cancer.* 1988;62:2152-2165.

Karim AB, Afra D, Cornu P, et al. Randomized trial on the efficacy of radiotherapy for cerebral low-grade glioma in the adult: European Organization for Research and Treatment of Cancer Study 22845 with the Medical Research Council study BRO4: an interim analysis. *Int J Radiat Oncol Biol Phys.* 2002;52:316-324.

Prados MD, Scott C, Curran WJ Jr, Nelson DF, Leibel S, Kramer S. Procarbazine, lomustine, and vincristine (PCV) chemotherapy for anaplastic astrocytoma: a retrospective review of radiation therapy oncology group protocols comparing survival with carmustine or PCV adjuvant chemotherapy. *J Clin Oncol.* 1999;17:3389-3395.

Walker MD, Green SB, Byar DP, et al. Randomized comparisons of radiotherapy and nitrosoureas for the treatment of malignant glioma after surgery. *N Engl J Med.* 1980;303:1323-1329.

Chapter 73
Benign Brain Tumors

Peter K. Dempsey and Lloyd M. Alderson

MENINGIOMAS

Clinical Vignette

A 56-year-old healthy woman experienced the onset of intermittent episodes of tingling in her left leg. She was unaware of any precipitating factors. Within a few weeks, the symptoms spread in a "marchlike" fashion into the left arm and eventually into the left side of her face. Each episode lasted approximately 3 minutes, resolving with no residual deficit. Neurologic history was otherwise unremarkable. Her only abnormal finding on neurologic examination was sensory; she had diminished graphesthesia, ie, diminished ability to identify numbers drawn in her left palm.

Contrast-enhanced CT results demonstrated a homogeneously enhancing lesion overlying the cortical surface of the right hemisphere. Brain MRI confirmed this mass was superficially located and showed concomitant dura mater enhancement within the area immediately adjacent to the tumor.

EEG demonstrated abnormal focal epileptiform activity within the right parietal region, which correlated with her report of focal sensory seizures secondary to this mass lesion. Phenytoin was initiated, and a complete surgical resection of the tumor was performed. A meningioma was identified. Focal seizures ceased; subsequently, the patient has been asymptomatic.

Meningiomas typically occur in middle-aged and older individuals, especially women, but can occur at any age. They arise from arachnoid meningeal cells, and although usually they are benign, rare malignant varieties occur. Found at any level of the neuraxis, they are primarily located intracranially; approximately 1 of 7 intracranial tumors is a meningioma. Several typical locations are the falx cerebri separating the 2 hemispheres, the meninges covering the hemispheres, along the sphenoid bone at the skull base, and the olfactory groove along the anterior skull base.

Because meningiomas are classic slow-growing tumors, they typically attain large size before becoming symptomatic, particularly within the frontal regions where they may not produce definitive symptoms until they gradually compress the brain surface (Figure 73-1). Meningiomas also provide the classic example of an intradural, extramedullary spinal tumor. Most commonly, they have a thoracic predilection although they occur at every level including the cervical medullary junction.

Clinical Presentation

Meningiomas present with a variety of symptoms, especially seizures, gait difficulties, progressive, sometimes long-standing headache, cranial nerve palsies, or other progressive neurologic impairment. Many meningiomas are identified incidentally on CT and MRI during evaluation of unrelated causes. Usually, no further radiographic studies are necessary. However, meningiomas located at the base of the skull near blood vessels are often evaluated with angiography if their setting demands surgical resection.

Treatment

The decision to treat meningiomas rests on several factors. First, because many are asymptomatic, it is important to determine that neurologic symptoms arise from the lesion. In the absence of neurologic symptoms, continued radiographic follow-up is often recommended. No treatment is necessary in patients who remain asymptomatic when follow-up CT and MRI demonstrate no change in tumor size or config-

BENIGN BRAIN TUMORS

Meningiomas

Figure 73-1

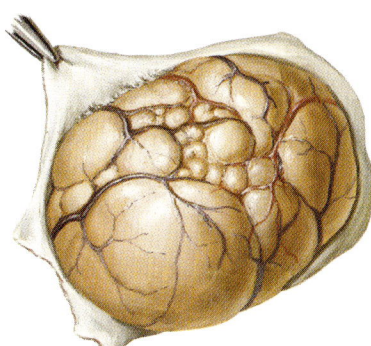

Meningioma with attached dura mater removed from brain, leaving depressed bed

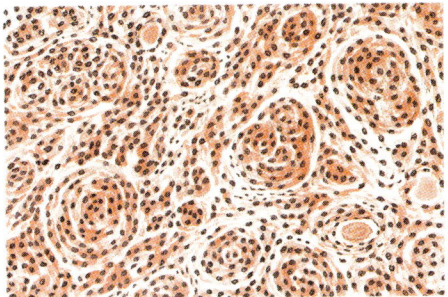

Histologic section showing whorl formation

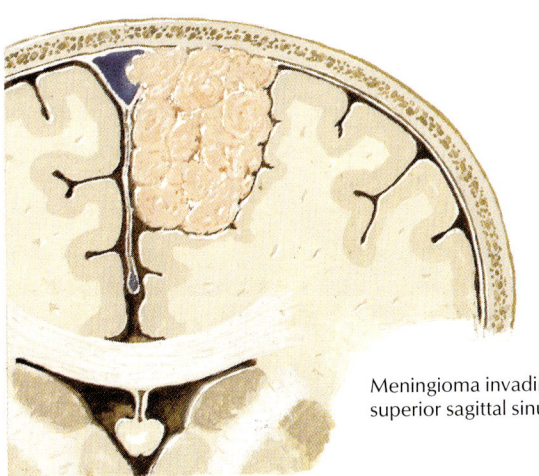

Meningioma invading superior sagittal sinus

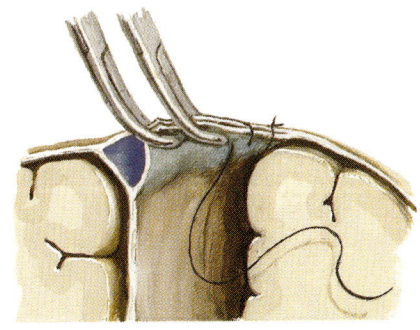

Repair of sinus following removal of tumor

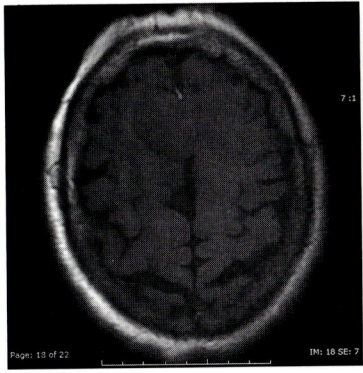
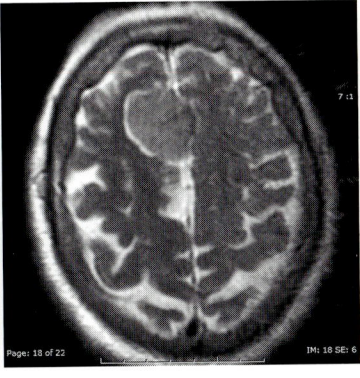
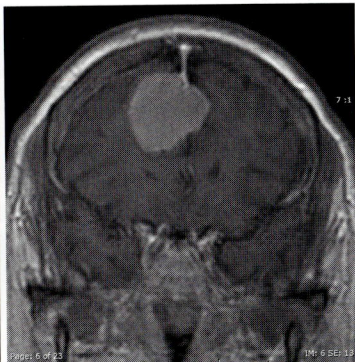

Meningioma of falx. Axial T1-weighted FLAIR and coronal post–gadolinium-enhanced T1-weighted images with fat saturation demonstrate an extraaxial, right falx-based mass, which extends through the falx to the left. The lesion is isointense to brain on T1-weighted sequences and enhances homogeneously.

Neuro-oncology

623

BENIGN BRAIN TUMORS

uration. Given the typical slow growth of these benign tumors, scans are usually scheduled at 6- to 12-month intervals. If progressive symptoms develop or follow-up imaging indicates lesion growth, treatment is mandated.

Surgical resection is the primary treatment for meningiomas. The surgical complexity is directly related to tumor location; those on the brain convexity or along the falx cerebri are often easily resected. Skull base tumors located near blood vessels and cranial nerves often pose a surgical challenge when the meningioma becomes entwined with these structures.

Radiation therapy, chemotherapy, or both are rarely used to treat typical benign meningiomas. Antiprogesterone agents to slow the growth of the meningiomas are being investigated.

ACOUSTIC NEUROMAS

Clinical Vignette

A previously healthy 58-year-old woman noted left-sided hearing loss and mild tinnitus that had gradually worsened over several years. In recent months, she noticed that she could not use her left ear for the telephone. She believed that her right-sided hearing was normal. She did not report any other neurologic symptoms. Her medical history was unremarkable.

On examination, the patient was bright and alert with mild nystagmus on left lateral gaze. Facial sensation was intact and there was no facial asymmetry. Her hearing was grossly diminished only in the left ear. The remainder of her examination results were normal.

Audiometric examination demonstrated a markedly decreased pure tone average and diminished speech discrimination in the left ear. Brainstem auditory evoked response testing showed prolonged I-II latency on the left. Gadolinium MRI revealed a homogeneously enhancing 2 × 1.5-cm mass in the left cerebellar pontine angle emanating from the internal auditory canal, leading to mild pontine distortion.

The history of slowly progressive, unilateral hearing loss associated with tinnitus is consistent with the slow growth of a benign **acoustic neuroma** (also called ***vestibular schwannoma***). These benign tumors arise from the Schwann cells of the vestibular nerve within the eighth cranial nerve complex.

Acoustic neuromas comprise approximately 6% to 8% of primary intracranial tumors. The incidence is 2% within the general population and peaks between the ages of 40 and 60 years. Unless patients have neurofibromatosis type II, it is unusual to see acoustic neuromas before the age of 20 years. They are predominantly unilateral lesions, although those associated with type II neurofibromatosis often are bilateral (Figure 73-2).

Clinical Presentation and Diagnostic Studies

Although acoustic neuromas arise from the vestibular portion of CN-VIII, hearing loss is usually the most prominent symptom (Figure 73-2). Anatomically, CN-VII (facial nerve) is closely related to CN-VIII; however, it is unusual to see CN-VII involvement as a presenting symptom. Because of CN-VIII's relation to the vestibular nerve and its proximity to the brainstem and cerebellum, patients with larger acoustic neuromas often have gait instability or ataxia initially, sometimes as presenting signs. With large tumors, hydrocephalus can occur if CSF flow is impaired near the fourth ventricle. This also can contribute to gait problems and cause headaches.

Cranial nerve evaluation is of the utmost importance. Hearing loss from CN-VIII involvement is the hallmark of these tumors. Lateral gaze nystagmus is notable on extraocular movement testing. Acoustic neuromas often cause pressure on the brainstem, affecting CN-V with resultant ipsilateral facial sensory loss and diminished corneal reflex. Larger tumors may cause CN-VII impairment with ipsilateral facial weakness. Lower cranial nerve involvement and brainstem compression that produce hemiparesis or sensory loss are unusual.

MRI is the best means of evaluation. Its clarity, resolution, and ability to scan in multiple planes allow for 3-dimensional assessment. Because lesion size and its relation to adjacent neurologic structures, such as the pons and various cranial nerves, often determine treatment, MRI is crucial. However, CT is often the first study obtained. Typically, these well-demarcated, homogeneously enhancing tumors arise within the cerebellar pontine angle and extend into the internal auditory canal.

BENIGN BRAIN TUMORS

Figure 73-2

Acoustic Neurinomas

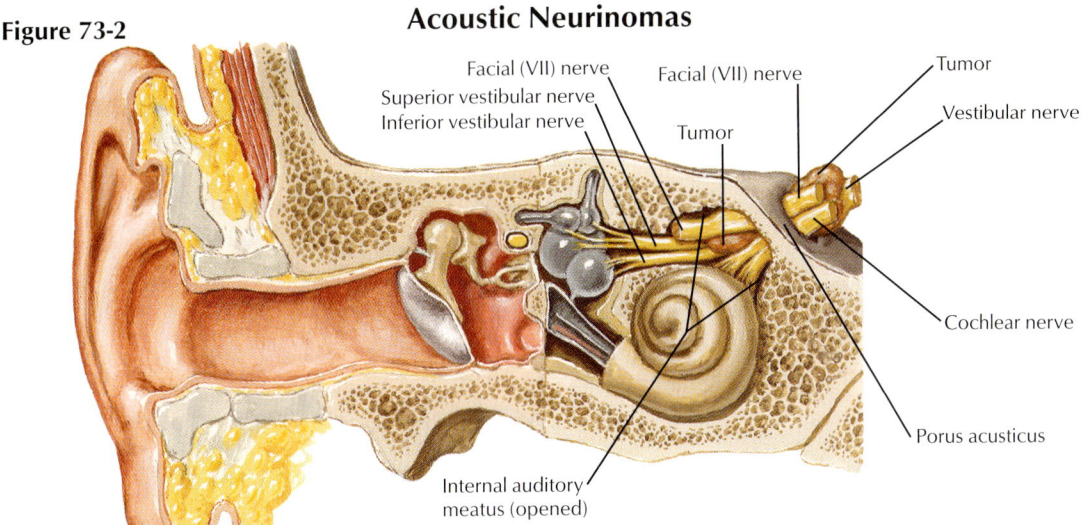

Neurofibromatosis, Type II

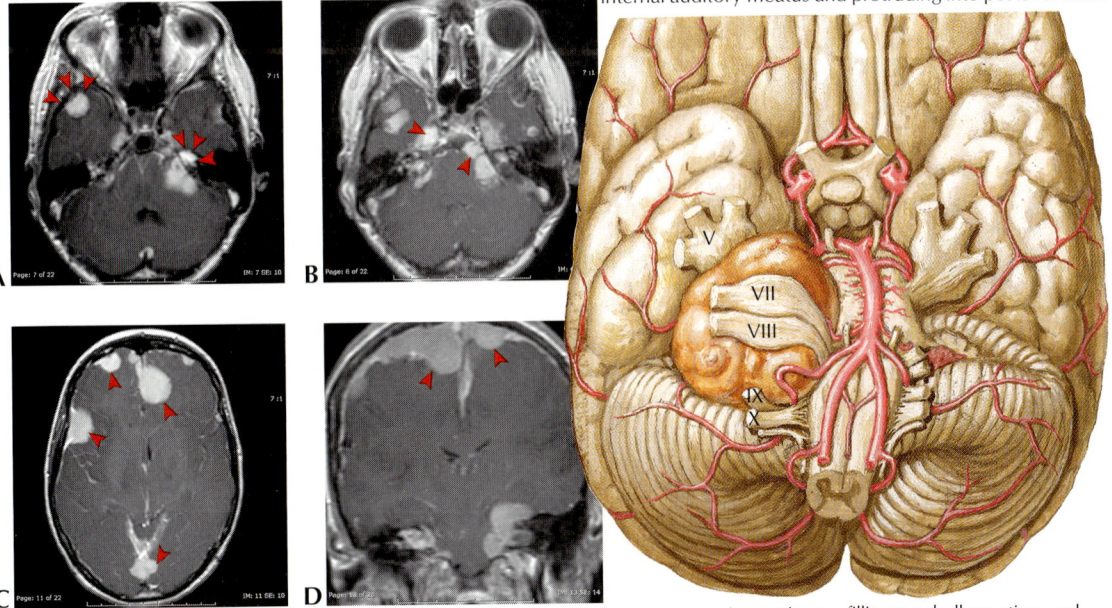

(**A-C**) Axial and coronal (**D**) T1-weighted post–gadolinium-enhanced images demonstrating bilateral vestibular schwannomas (arrowheads) and multiple dural-based meningiomas (arrowheads). Both types of tumors enhance avidly.

Small neurinoma arising from superior vestibular nerve in internal auditory meatus and protruding into posterior fossa

Large acoustic neurinoma filling cerebellopontine angle, distorting brainstem and cranial nerves V, VII, VIII, IX, X

Brainstem auditory evoked response (BAER) in patient with acoustic neurinoma on right side. There is delay in action potentials of cochlear nerve (wave I) and cochlear nuclei (wave II) on affected side.

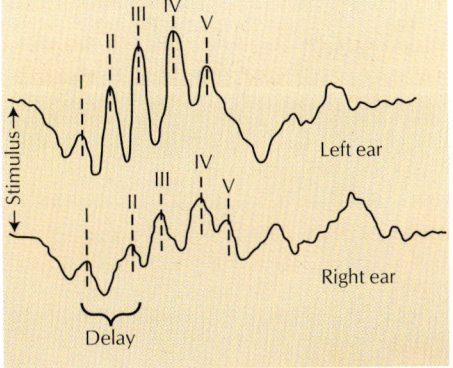

NEURO-ONCOLOGY

625

BENIGN BRAIN TUMORS

Treatment

Surgery is the traditional and primary therapeutic modality; stereotactic radiosurgery is occasionally used. Acoustic neuromas often grow slowly. It is reasonable to observe some tumors temporally, if clinically warranted. Elderly patients with unilateral hearing loss, particularly with other medical issues, are often best treated with serial imaging. When MRI evidence of tumor growth occurs, or patients have progressively worsening symptoms, especially in addition to hearing loss, specific treatment is indicated.

Surgical resection of acoustic neuromas is often performed with neurosurgery and otorhinolaryngology specialists. The surgical goal is tumor resection and preservation of CN-VII and CN-VIII when possible, particularly important with large volume tumors exhibiting brainstem compression. Hearing preservation in patients with these large lesions is often impossible because the cochlear nerve becomes indistinguishable from the tumor. Success rates for hearing preservation vary directly with tumor volume. When CN-VII is densely adherent to the tumor capsule, a subtotal resection is often indicated, because facial nerve preservation is more important than complete surgical removal.

Stereotactic radiosurgery involves a single nonsurgical treatment using high-dose radiation to a precisely localized 3-dimensional volume. Radiosurgical treatment can control approximately 80% to 85% of acoustic tumors. It retains many of the same risks as conventional surgery but is an excellent option for patients with small tumors (<2-3 cm) who have no useful hearing. Control of tumor growth is achieved and operative risks are avoided. With improved imaging, acoustic neuromas are being detected earlier; therefore, greater potential exists to achieve a complete cure with this modality.

PITUITARY ADENOMA

Clinical Vignette

A 26-year-old woman noticed milk drainage from her breasts. She had stopped having menstrual periods during the past few months. She had no other symptoms. Her medical history was unremarkable. She had previously given birth to a healthy child but was not pregnant. Her cranial nerves and visual fields were intact, and she showed no neurologic deficits.

Endocrinologic workup revealed an increased prolactin level and decreased follicle-stimulating and luteinizing hormone levels in the blood. Brain MRI showed a mass lesion within the sella turcica consistent with a pituitary adenoma.

The presentation in this vignette with gonadal dysfunction is typical of **prolactinomas**, one of the most common endocrinologically active pituitary tumors. Although histologically benign, **pituitary adenomas** may have serious consequences when undiagnosed early because their proximity to the optic nerves, the optic tracts, the cavernous sinus, and the temporal lobe tip may lead to significant neurologic consequences. These intrinsic pituitary lesions represent approximately 10% of all intracranial tumors. These tumors are classified according to whether they are endocrinologically active.

The majority of pituitary adenomas arise from the anterior portion of the pituitary gland (**adenohypophysis**). Endocrinologically active tumors secrete hormones, often resulting in symptoms appropriate to the target glands to which the specific active cell type is directed. For example, in the preceding vignette, abnormal galactorrhea was directly related to the production of increased amounts of prolactin-secreting tumor cells. **Cushing disease** occurs when these tumors primarily secrete adrenocorticotropic hormone with subsequent increases in serum cortisol. Pituitary adenomas that primarily secrete growth hormone lead to the clinical syndrome of **acromegaly**.

Nonsecreting tumors frequently reach a large size before symptoms develop. Typically, their diagnosis depends on the presentation of mass effect symptoms. Bitemporal visual field cuts result when pituitary macroadenomas extend above the sella and compress the overlying optic chiasm.

Pituitary apoplexy is a relatively rare clinical presentation of pituitary adenomas. Classically, an acute-onset severe headache sometimes mimics a ruptured intracranial aneurysm, associated with significant visual impairment and decreased mental status. The cause is often hemorrhage into a preexisting pituitary adenoma.

BENIGN BRAIN TUMORS

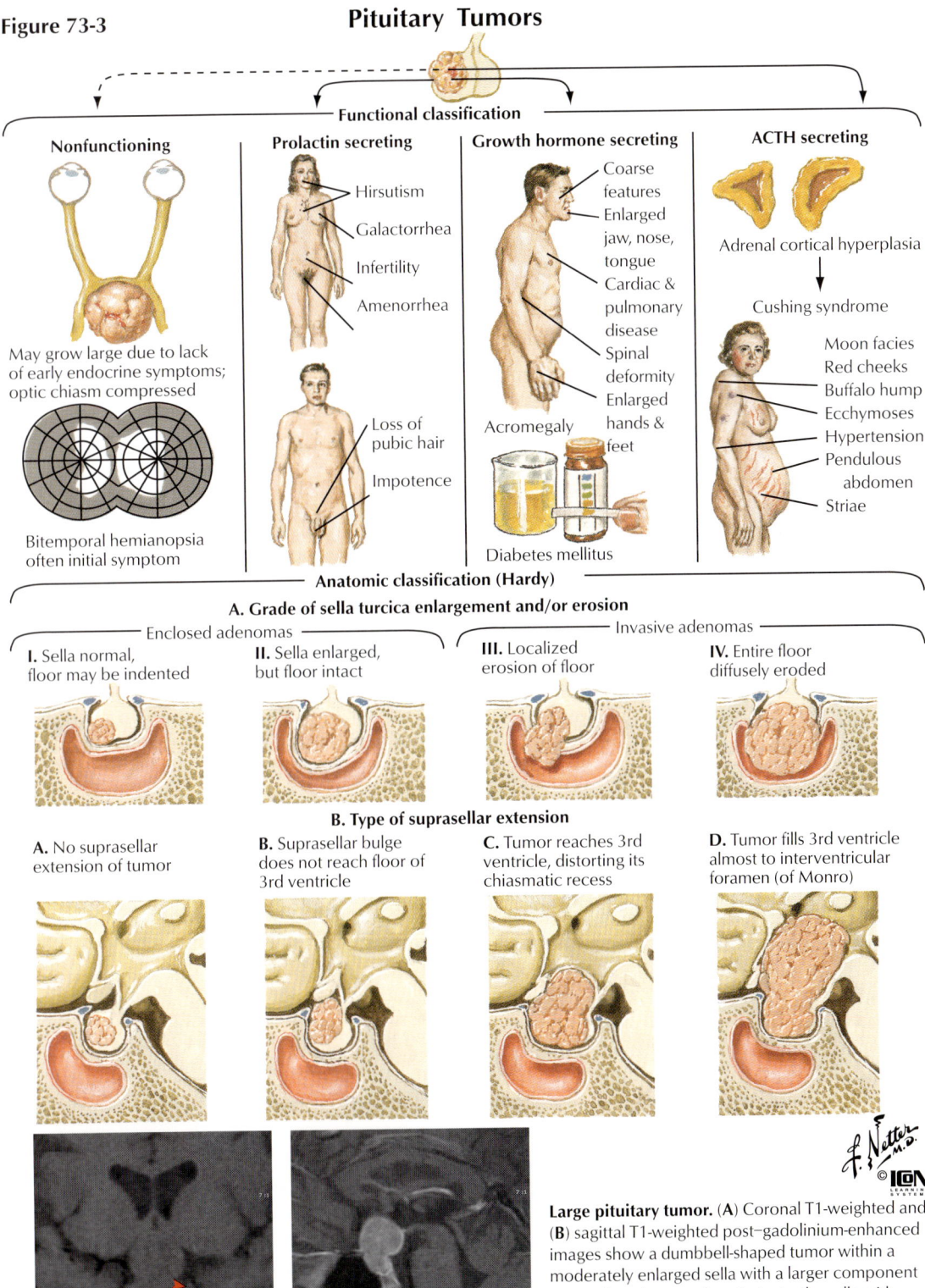

Figure 73-3 Pituitary Tumors

Large pituitary tumor. (**A**) Coronal T1-weighted and (**B**) sagittal T1-weighted post–gadolinium-enhanced images show a dumbbell-shaped tumor within a moderately enlarged sella with a larger component protruding above and posterior to the sella with elevation and distortion of the optic chiasm. There is more compression of the cavernous sinus on the left.

NEURO-ONCOLOGY

Diagnostic Approach

Patients with suspected pituitary adenomas are evaluated with a combination of endocrinologic and imaging studies. A thorough endocrine evaluation includes serum levels of prolactin, follicle stimulating hormone and luteinizing hormone, cortisol, and growth hormone and thyroid function parameters.

Brain MRI is the best means to identify pituitary tumors. Sellar expansion, diminished enhancement within the sella, and shifting of the pituitary stalk to one side are all clues for a possible **pituitary microadenoma**. In contrast, **macroadenomas** (measuring >25 mm) extend above the sella or into the cavernous sinus on either side of the sella and are easily identified with MRI (Figure 73-3).

Treatment

Primary medical therapy is the initial treatment for many patients with pituitary adenomas. Prolactin secreting tumors may be successfully controlled with bromocriptine, a dopamine agonist that suppresses prolactin production and concomitantly decreases tumor volume. Growth hormone–secreting tumors are often controlled with octreotide, a somatostatin analog. Small, nonsecreting pituitary tumors may often be observed with combined clinical and MRI modalities. Treatment is not necessary unless they enlarge.

Surgical treatment is indicated for macroadenomas causing mass effect and for endocrinologically active tumors that cannot be controlled with medication. Surgical treatment of macroadenomas usually involves a transsphenoidal approach wherein the sella turcica is entered through the nasal cavity and the sphenoid sinus. Using an operating microscope, the contents of the sella can be visualized and the tumor can be removed, often sparing the pituitary gland.

Postoperatively, patients require follow-up for signs of hypopituitarism, particularly patients who initially present with Cushing disease and, subsequently, have diminished adrenocorticotropic hormone secretion. These patients usually require postoperative and sometimes lifelong steroid replacement. Although pituitary adenomas occur in the anterior hypophysis, antidiuretic hormone secretion is occasionally impaired from the posterior pituitary subsequent to surgery. In these individuals, diabetes insipidus develops with concomitant problems in sodium balance and fluid intake, necessitating careful follow-up and sometimes treatment with DDAVP to replace the antidiuretic hormone.

OTHER BENIGN INTRACRANIAL TUMORS

Craniopharyngioma

Craniopharyngiomas are uncommon tumors thought to arise from the Rathke pouch as a remnant of the brain's embryologic development. Comprising 2% to 3% of intracranial tumors, with greater incidence in children, they are cystic lesions often occurring in the region of the sella, hypothalamus, or third ventricle (Figure 73-4). Because of their location, they often present with visual impairment, pituitary dysfunction, and hydrocephalus. The radiographic features of craniopharyngiomas distinguish them from other tumors of the suprasellar region. Cystic changes, variable contrast enhancement, and calcification seen on CT occur frequently.

The treatment of choice for symptomatic craniopharyngiomas is usually surgery. Resection is difficult because of the intense glial reaction of the surrounding brain, causing adherence to critical brain structures and nearby blood vessels. The suprasellar location also limits tumor access, making incomplete resections common. Although radiation therapy and possibly radiosurgery can decrease recurrence rates, craniopharyngiomas have a high rate of local recurrence.

Chordoma

Chordomas are very rare tumors that arise from the same embryologic elements from which intervertebral disks arise. Usually benign, they typically occur in the clivus or sacrum (Figure 73-5). Chordomas often cause significant bony destruction and can recur locally at a high rate, making a surgical cure difficult to achieve.

Intracranial chordomas arise from within the skull bone and cause local destruction, while also entering the intradural space and affecting structures such as the brainstem and cranial nerves.

BENIGN BRAIN TUMORS

Figure 73-4 Craniopharyngiomas

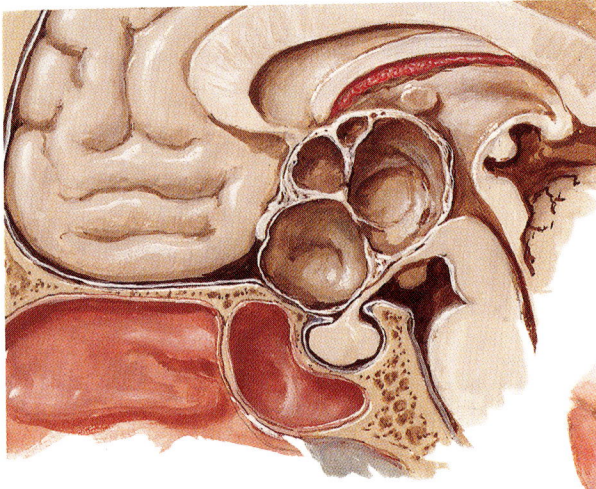

Large cystic suprasellar craniopharyngioma compressing optic chiasm and hypothalamus, filling 3rd ventricle up to interventricular foramen (of Monro), thus causing visual impairment, diabetes insipidus, and hydrocephalus

Tumor gently teased forward from under optic chiasm after evacuation of cystic contents via frontotemporal flap

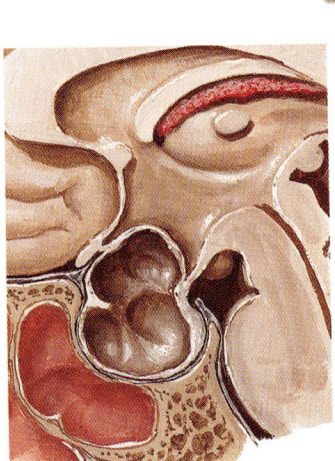

Intasellar cystic craniopharyngioma compressing pituitary gland to cause hypopituitarism

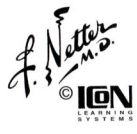

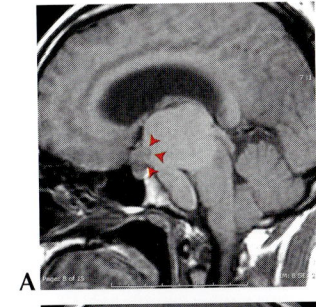

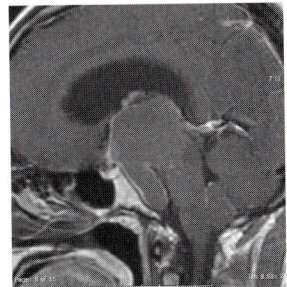

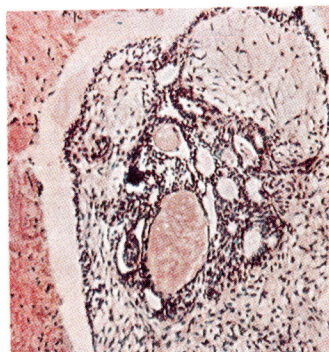

Histologic section: craniopharyngioma (H and E stain, ×125)

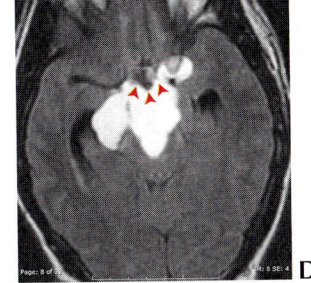

(A-D) Sagittal T1-weighted images without (A) and after (B) gadolinium enhancement and coronal T1-weighted gadolinium-enhanced images demonstrate a multilobulated mass above the sella and normal pituitary extending into the interpeduncular cistern and into the prepontine cistern. The posterior portion above the sella is solid (arrowheads), whereas the remainder is cystic with faint rim enhancement. The T2-weighted axial image shows the darker solid component (arrowheads) and the T2-bright cystic portions.

NEURO-ONCOLOGY

BENIGN BRAIN TUMORS

Figure 73-5 — Chordomas

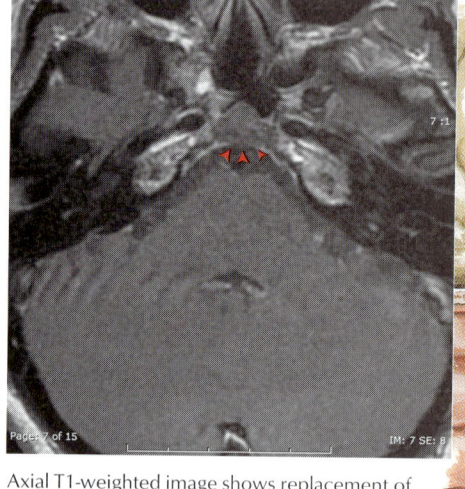

Axial T1-weighted image shows replacement of normal marrow fat (arrowheads).

Chordomas of clivus compressing pons and encroaching on sella turcica and sphenoid sinus

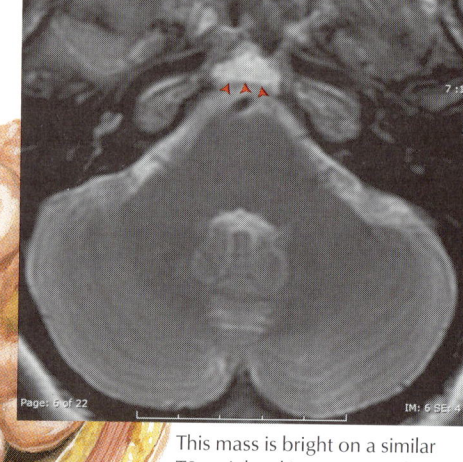

This mass is bright on a similar T2-weighted image (arrowheads).

Chordoma of sacrum bulging into pelvis, compressing rectum and other pelvic organs, as well as vessels and nerves

NEURO-ONCOLOGY

BENIGN BRAIN TUMORS

Figure 73-6

Tumors of Pineal Region

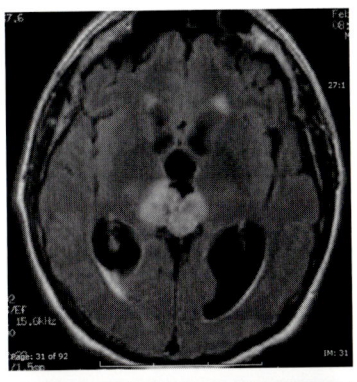

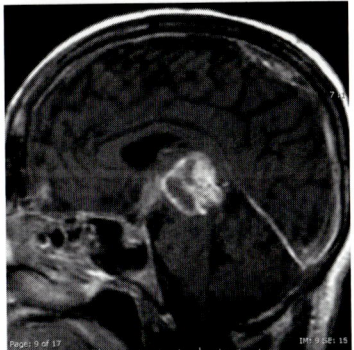

Pineoblastoma. Axial, FLAIR, and sagittal T2-weighted gadolinium-enhanced images show a large mass in the pineal region, bright on T2 imaging, heterogeneous after gadolinium enhancement, compressing the aqueduct with enlargement of the third and lateral ventricles.

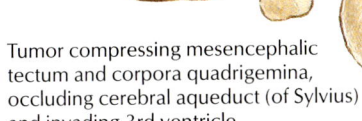

Tumor compressing mesencephalic tectum and corpora quadrigemina, occluding cerebral aqueduct (of Sylvius) and invading 3rd ventricle

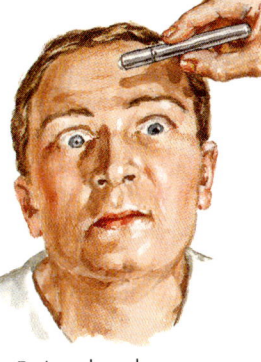

Parinaud syndrome: paresis of upward gaze, unequal pupils, loss of convergence

Diabetes insipidus in some patients

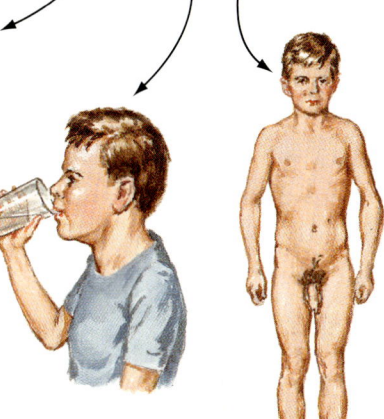

Sexual precocity in boys may occur

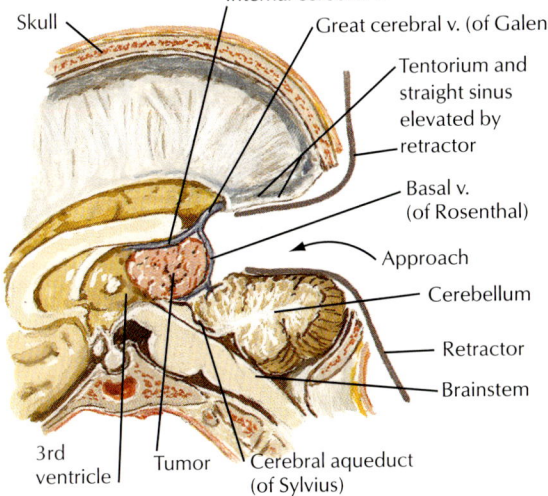

Anatomic aspects of exposure

- Skull
- Internal cerebral v.
- Great cerebral v. (of Galen)
- Tentorium and straight sinus elevated by retractor
- Basal v. (of Rosenthal)
- Approach
- Cerebellum
- Retractor
- Brainstem
- 3rd ventricle
- Tumor
- Cerebral aqueduct (of Sylvius)

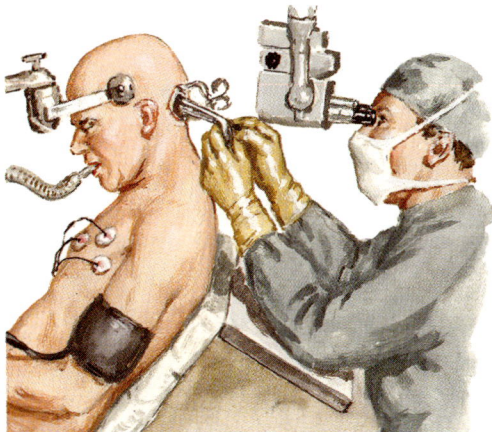

Position of patient (undraped to show detail), surgeon, and microscope for resection of pineal region tumors

NEURO-ONCOLOGY

BENIGN BRAIN TUMORS

Figure 73-7   Intraventricular Tumors

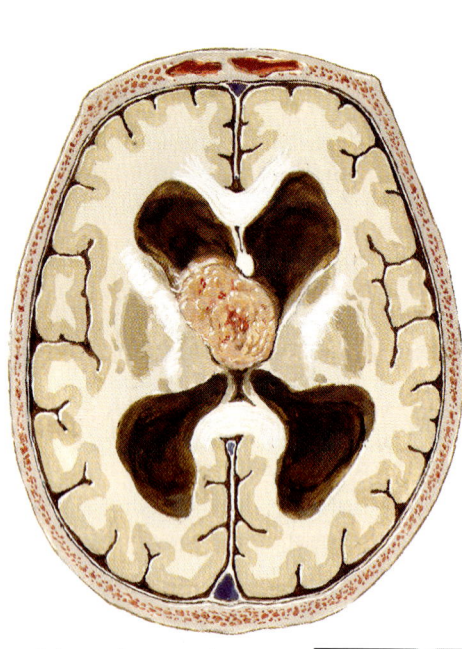

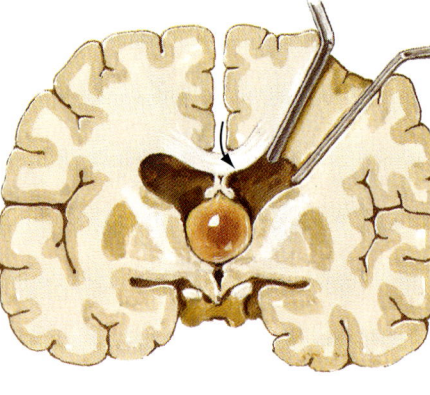

Colloid cyst of 3rd ventricle and surgical approach via right prefrontal (silent) cerebral cortex. May also be approached through corpus callosum (arrow). Note enlarged lateral ventricles (posterior view).

Subependymoma of anterior horn of left lateral ventricle obstructing interventricular foramen (of Monro), thus producing marked hydrocephalus

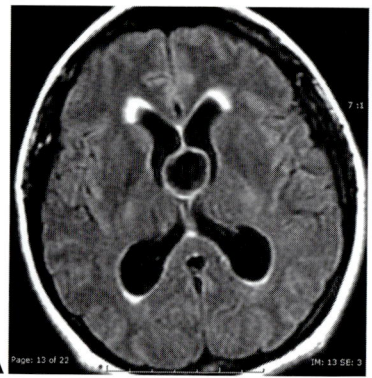
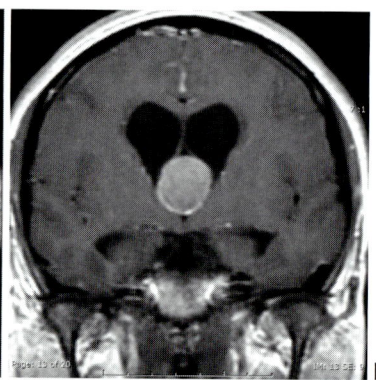

Colloid cyst. (**A**) Axial, FLAIR and (**B**) coronal, T1-weighted gadolinium enhanced images demonstrate a round cystic mass in the region of the foramina of Monro, with dilatation of the lateral ventricles. The signal characteristics are variable. This cyst is hypointense on T2-weighted images and bright on T1-weighted imaging, with minimal peripheral enhancement.

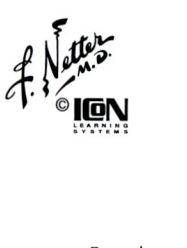
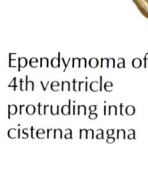
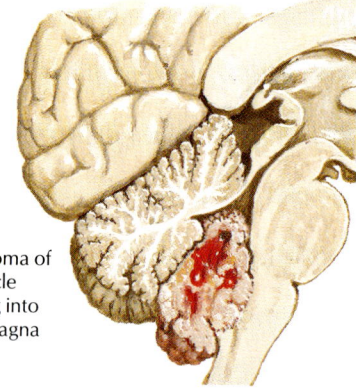

Ependymoma of 4th ventricle protruding into cisterna magna

NEURO-ONCOLOGY

Histologically, chordomas are notable for large, mucous-filled cells called **physaliferous cells**. Few chordomas show features of frank malignancy, but their aggressive local invasion of the surrounding bone confers malignant potential.

Surgical resection is often used initially, but complete resection is often impossible because of anatomical constraints. Although generally used, the role of radiation therapy in treatment of residual tumor is unclear. Radiosurgery and proton beam irradiation have been proposed, but the benefit is uncertain. Chemotherapy has no role in chordoma treatment.

Pineal Region Tumors

Tumors occurring in the region of the pineal gland are uncommon, comprising approximately 1% of intracranial tumors. Tumors in this group include **germ cell tumors**, **tumors of glial origin**, and **tumors of the pineal parenchyma** (Figure 73-6). In the pineal region, tumors of germ cell origin are the most common and usually occur in younger patients. **Gliomas** can arise from within the pineal gland itself or from the glial cells in the surrounding tissue. In this region, glial tumors tend to be of lower grade. Tumors arising from the pineal parenchyma comprise approximately 20% of pineal region tumors.

These neoplasms are further classified into **pineoblastomas** and **pineocytomas**. *Pineoblastomas* are poorly differentiated tumors that can spread throughout the spinal fluid pathways or into adjacent brain tissue. *Pineocytomas* are usually well-encapsulated cellular tumors that do not invade surrounding tissue. A mixed form of pineal parenchymal tumor contains features of both pineocytoma and pineoblastoma. **Teratomas**, **embryonal carcinomas**, **endodermal sinus tumors**, and **choriocarcinomas** are also found in the pineal region.

With the increasing use of MRI, asymptomatic pineal region cysts are being described more commonly. These cysts are usually incidental findings and rarely require any treatment. Serial MRI scans are used to track any growth over time.

Colloid Cysts

Colloid cysts are tumors that usually occur in the third ventricle and are thought to arise from remnants during embryologic development. They often become symptomatic during adulthood but can be seen in children. They are histologically benign tumors. and the cells lining the walls of the cyst are ciliated. Colloid cysts typically present with signs and symptoms of hydrocephalus. Because of their location, they often obstruct CSF pathways at the foramina of Monro (Figure 73-7). Cases of sudden death from colloid cysts have been reported, presumably from acute hydrocephalus; however, most patients present with a more gradual course. Diagnosis can often be made on the basis of imaging, which reveals a cystic-appearing mass.

Treatment of symptomatic colloid cysts is usually surgical, and complete resection is often possible. Care must be exercised during surgical resection because the fornix, adjacent to the tumor, can be injured, resulting in severe memory impairment. If surgery for resection is not possible, CSF diversion through shunting can often relieve the symptoms of hydrocephalus.

With the increased use of MRI, many more cystic tumors within the third ventricle are being described. These asymptomatic lesions are followed with serial scans; treatment is reserved for those patients whose cysts increase in size.

FUTURE DIRECTIONS

Treatment of benign intracranial tumors has improved with better MRI imaging and the development of new surgical techniques that exploit bone removal rather than brain manipulation. These skull base techniques allow for exposure and resection of tumors in previously inaccessible locations within the skull. Intraoperative monitoring of cranial nerve function is being used more frequently to limit the morbidity of these operations.

Improvements in stereotactic radiosurgery continue to allow for tumor growth control while causing fewer radiation adverse effects. Further research into the relation of hormonal receptors in meningiomas may someday allow for a medical means of controlling these tumors.

REFERENCES

MacFarlane R, King TT. Acoustic neuronoma: vestibular schwannoma. In: Kaye AH, Larz ER Jr, eds. *Brain Tumors*. Philadelphia, Pa: Churchill Livingstone; 1995:577-622.

Larijani B, Bastanhagh MH, Pajouhi M, Kargar Shadab F, Vasigh A, Aghakhani S. Presentation and outcome of 93 cases of craniopharyngioma. *Eur J Cancer Care (Engl)*. 2004;13:11-15.

Black PM. Meningiomas. *Neurosurgery*. 1993;32:643-657.

Ciric I. Long-term management and outcome for pituitary tumors. *Neurosurg Clin N Am*. 2003;14:167-171.

Menezes AH, Gantz BJ, Traynelis VC, McCulloch TM. Cranial base chordomas. *Clin Neurosurg*. 1997;44:491-509.

Mathiesen T, Grane P, Lindgren L, Lindquist C. Third ventricle colloid cysts: a consecutive 12-year series. *J Neurosurg*. 1997;86:5-12.

Chapter 74
Spinal Cord Tumors

Peter K. Dempsey, Lloyd M. Alderson, and H. Royden Jones, Jr

Primary **spinal cord tumors** occur infrequently. Their clinical presentation can be relatively subtle, particularly with intradural tumors. In contrast, extradural metastatic tumors are relatively common in patients with malignancies. These individuals with metastatic cancer often have a relatively precipitous onset. Typically, spinal cord and spinal column tumors are classified into 2 categories: **extradural**, occurring outside of the dura, and **intradural**, contained within the dura mater (Table 74-1).

Extradural tumors generally are derived from metastatic lesions to vertebral bodies with extension into the epidural space causing external compression of the thecal sac and its contents. Primary bony vertebral tumors—both malignant, such as myeloma, and benign, including hemangiomas and osteoid osteomas—also occur (Figure 74-1).

Intradural tumors are further categorized as **extramedullary** or **intramedullary**, depending on their relation to the spinal cord. **Intradural extramedullary tumors**, usually **meningiomas** or **schwannomas**, generally arise outside of the spinal cord parenchyma. However, they often grow so large that they eventually cause spinal cord compression. In contrast, **intradural intramedullary tumors**, such as **gliomas** and **ependymomas**, originate within the spinal cord parenchyma. Because these malignancies primarily expand within the spinal cord, important neurologic pathways and cell populations are subsequently destroyed (Figure 74-2).

EXTRADURAL SPINAL TUMORS

Clinical Vignette

A 70-year-old man presented with lumbar pain and bilateral leg weakness with sensory change. For 24 hours, he had been unable to stand and support his weight. His lower back discomfort was centered in the spine and extended into the buttocks and posterior thighs, particularly when he attempted to stand. The right leg was affected more than the left. For the past 12 hours, he was unable to void urine. He had a history of prostate cancer.

Neurologic examination demonstrated intact cranial nerves and upper extremity function. Lower extremity motor examination showed markedly diminished dorsiflexion and plantar flexion, diminished knee extension, and somewhat limited hip flexor strength. Sensory examination showed loss of response to pinprick and light touch throughout the lumbar and sacral dermatomes. The patient had mild tenderness to palpation in the upper lumbar spine. Rectal examination showed diminished sphincter tone, and the patient was incontinent of urine. Knee and ankle muscle stretch reflexes were absent. Plantar stimulation was flexor.

Plain lumbar radiographs revealed destruction of the L2 pedicle. MRI showed a soft tissue mass involving most of the L2 body, extending into the pedicle, and epidural extension of the tumor into the spinal canal with marked compression of the thecal sac and cauda equina. CT was confirmatory.

Metastatic cancer is the most common neoplasm affecting the spine; 5% to 35% of patients with cancer have spinal metastases. Lung, breast, prostate, and hematopoietic system tumors are the most common cancers causing spinal cord compression (Figure 74-1). The metastatic mass in the preceding vignette caused a **cauda equina syndrome** consistent with an L2 vertebral body tumor extending into the spinal canal. The tumor location at the cauda equina level was thus below the inferior aspect of the spinal cord.

Clinical Presentation

Progressive pain confined to the spine is one of the most common presenting symptoms. Distinguishing pain secondary to tumor involvement from the pain of mechanical lower back

SPINAL CORD TUMORS

Figure 74-1
Extradural Spinal Tumors

Metastatic tumors

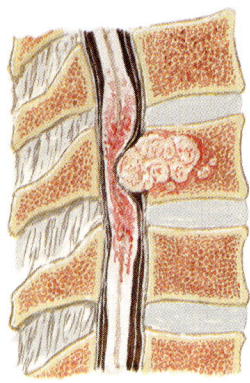

Common primary sites, noted on history examination

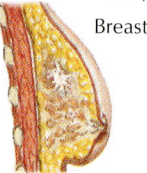
Breast

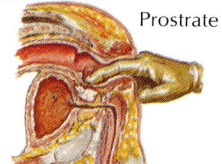
Prostrate

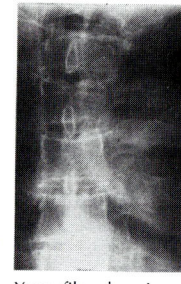
Lung

Melanoma (skin or mucous membrane)

Lymphoma (may be primary)

X-ray film showing destruction of pedicle and vertebral body by metastatic carcinoma

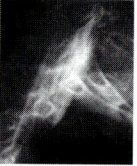
Myelogram showing extradural block caused by metastatic tumor

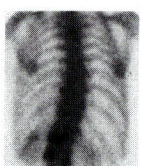
Bone scan showing multiple metastases

Benign tumors

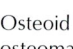
Osteoid osteoma

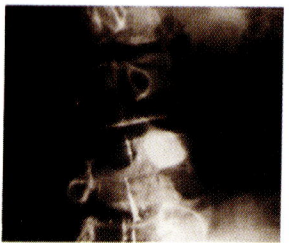
Hemangioma

Primary, malignant tumors

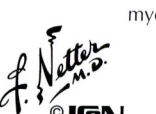
Multiple myeloma

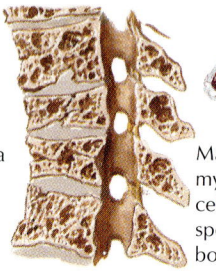
Malignant myeloma cells in biopsy specimen of bone marrow

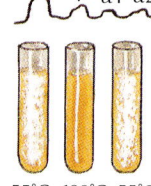
γ spike on serum electrophoresis

Bence Jones protein in urine in 60% of cases (precipitates at 45° to 60°C, redissolves on boiling, and reprecipitates on cooling to 60° to 45°C)

55°C   100°C   55°C

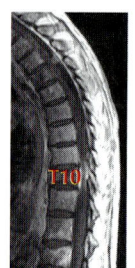

A   B

Metastatic tumor. (**A**) Sagittal T1-weighted image demonstrates loss of normal marrow fat at multiple levels. (**B**) Sagittal T1-weighted, gadolinium-enhanced image shows enhancement within the vertebral lesions and epidural extension with spinal cord compression at T10.

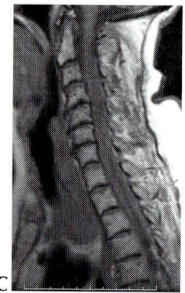

C   D

Epidural hematoma. (**C**) T1-weighted sagittal image shows a vague posterior epidural mass better seen on D. (**D**) T2-weighted image extending from C2 into the thoracic region.

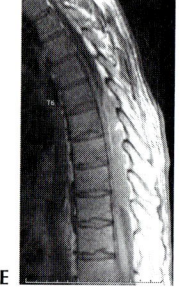

E   F

Epidural abscess. Sagittal T1-weighted images without (**E**) and with (**F**) gadolinium enhancement demonstrate an extensive posterior epidural process from T6 to T11. Enhancement of the granulation tissue allows appreciation of nonenhancing focal pus collections.

SPINAL CORD TUMORS

Table 74-1
Classification of MRI Abnormalities*

Extradural	Intradural Extramedullary	Intramedullary
Disc disease	Tumor	Syringomyelia

Tumor
    Metastatic
    Lymphoma
    Sarcoma
    Plasmacytoma
    Primary bone
	Neurinoma
	Meningioma
	Intracranial tumor seeding
	    Ependymoma
	    Medulloblastoma
	    Glioma
		Tumor
		    Ependymoma
		    Glioma
		    Hemangioblastoma

Abscess	Eypertrophic neuropathy	Edema
Scar	Cauda equina lesions Scarring	Myelitis
Hemangioma	—	Lipoma

Rare lesions
    Hemorrhage
    Neurilemmoma
    Meningioma
    Chordoma
	Rare lesions
	    Lymphoma
	    Metastasis
	    Hemangioblastoma
	    Lipoma
	    Dermoid
	    Epidermoid
	    Cyst
	    Clot
		Rare lesions
		    Abscess
		    Hematoma
		    Varix with AVM
		    Lymphoma
		    Neuroblastoma
		    Metastasis

*Dermoid or epidermoid teratoma, lipoma, and cysts are often associated with spinal dysraphism. In this setting, many tumors are intradural, although they may involve all 3 areas.

disorders, such as degenerative osteoarthritis, is often challenging. However, unlike mechanical back pain, pain having a tumor origin is frequently unrelated to position and tends to increase at night.

Progressive neurologic symptoms often vary and are related to the precise level of spinal column involvement (Figure 74-3). **Tumors in the cervical and thoracic spinal cord** areas often present with progressive weakness, numbness, or both at levels below the tumor. Examination usually reveals hyperreflexia and other long tract signs at levels below the tumor involvement. **Conus medullaris tumors** at the distal tip of the spinal cord frequently lead to bladder and bowel dysfunction and poor motor function.

Diagnosis

Although the clinical presentation can be similar to that of neurogenic claudication secondary to spinal stenosis, the course of metastatic spinal tumors is more rapid, sometimes producing significant neurologic compromise within hours or days.

In many instances, a history of cancer provides the information to define the nature of the lesion. However, occasionally a metastatic spinal tumor is the initial presentation of the malignancy, so a histologic diagnosis is needed. This can be accomplished as part of an open surgical procedure or by percutaneous CT-guided needle biopsy.

Clinical differentiation between compressive lesions arising at the level of the conus medullaris or the spinal cord tip and those within the cauda equina may be difficult. However, symmetric lesions involving both lower extremities tend to arise from lesions of the conus medullaris, whereas cauda equina lesions often cause a more patchy or asymmetric distribution of signs and symptoms.

MRI is the standard for evaluating metastatic spine lesions, especially those with cord compression. When MRI is contraindicated because of a pacemaker, CT myelogram is a useful and valid study. CSF evaluation is usually unnecessary with MRI.

Neuro-oncology

SPINAL CORD TUMORS

Figure 74-2

Intradural Spinal Tumors

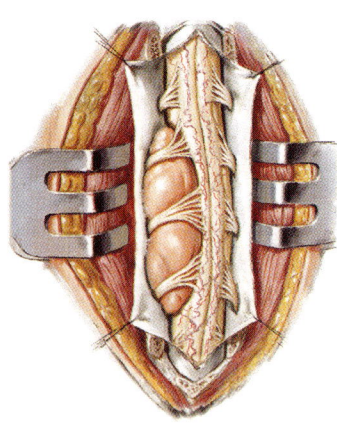

Intradural extramedullary tumor (meningioma) compressing spinal cord and deforming nerve roots

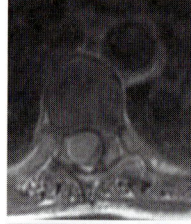
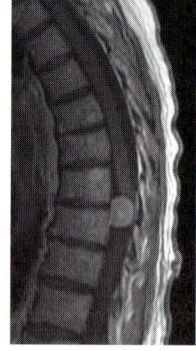

Thoracic meningioma: axial and sagittal T1-weighted, gadolinium images show that the enhancing mass occupies the right anterior 70% of the spinal canal.

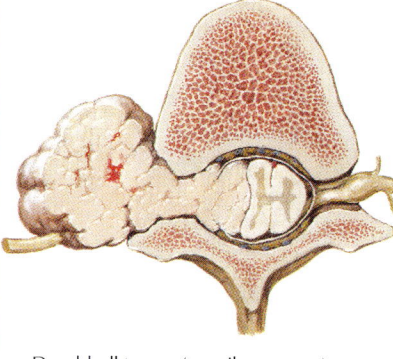

Dumbbell tumor (neurilemmoma) growing out along spinal nerve through intervertebral foramen (neurofibromas of von Recklinghausen disease may act similarly)

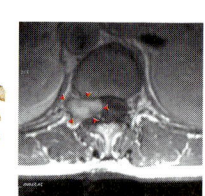

Foraminal neurolemmoma seen on axial T1-weighted, gadolinium-enhanced image (arrowheads)

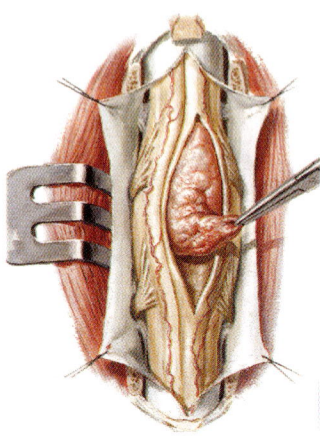

Intramedullary tumor and myelogram showing widening of spinal cord

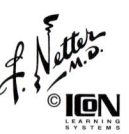

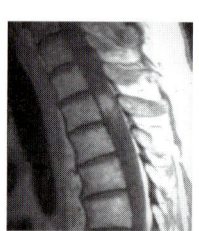

Astrocytoma on gadolinium-enhanced T1-weighted image with diffuse cord enlargement and focal enhancement

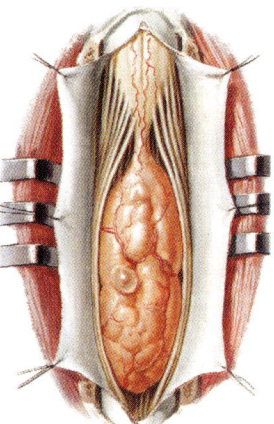

Tumor of filum terminale compressing cauda equina: enlarged vessels feed tumor

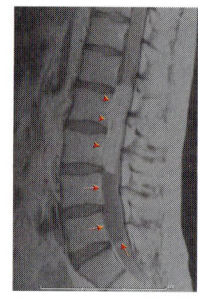

Ependymoma of filum with cyst: sagittal T1-weighted, gadolinium-enhanced image with large, moderately enhancing mass (arrowheads) and cyst distal to it (thin arrows)

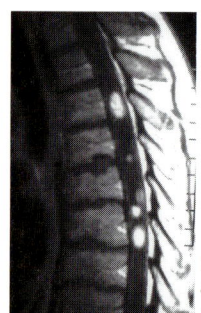

Intramedullary metastases: multiple enhancing masses within the spinal cord

NEURO-ONCOLOGY

SPINAL CORD TUMORS

Figure 74-3 Evolution of Symptoms

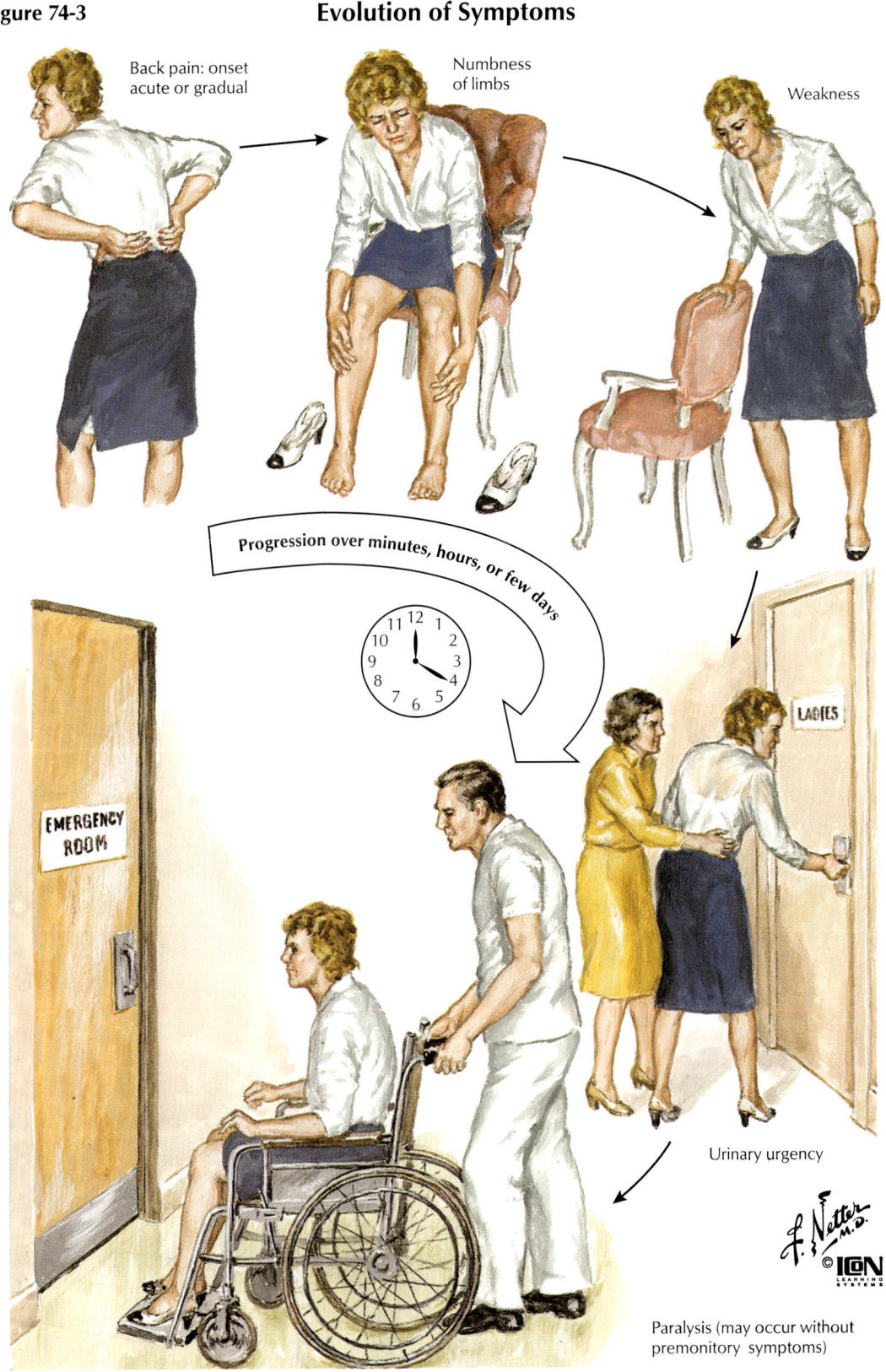

Neuro-oncology

SPINAL CORD TUMORS

Treatment and Prognosis

In most cases, treatment for spinal column metastatic disease is indicated to prevent further destruction, to attempt to prevent progression of the neurologic deficits, and to control pain. Typically, large-dose corticosteroids, ie, 10 to 20 mg dexamethasone, followed by 4 to 6 mg every 4 to 6 hours, are administered at diagnosis and continued throughout the initial treatment stages for their protective effect on the neural elements.

Surgical decompression and radiation therapy are the primary treatment modalities. When patients present with neurologic symptoms and signs, surgery is often indicated. It allows rapid decompression of the neural elements and preserves previously unaffected neurologic function. Surgical intervention generally requires removal of as much tumor as possible. In many instances, when spinal column destruction has caused significant spinal instability, fusion is also required. Subsequent radiation treatment to the area is also indicated.

If there is no serious neurologic involvement, radiation is often the treatment of choice. Administered in multiple fractions, radiation is delivered precisely to the involved vertebrae. In many instances, pain relief is apparent within a few days after radiation treatment commences. However, with radioresistant tumors, such as renal cell cancer, in which symptoms can evolve progressively despite radiation therapy, surgery is often indicated after completion of radiation treatment.

Prognosis for patients with metastatic disease to the spine depends on their clinical status on presentation. Individuals who have presented with a severe neurologic deficit, existing at least 24 to 36 hours, often do not regain significant neurologic function. However, many patients who present with acute deterioration and undergo rapid evaluation and treatment often experience improvement.

INTRADURAL EXTRAMEDULLARY TUMORS

Intradural extraaxial (extramedullary) tumors originate within the dural sleeve of the spinal column but outside of the spinal cord. They primarily arise within the leptomeninges or the nerve roots.

Clinical Vignette

A 36-year-old man noticed progressive numbness on the lateral aspect of his left foot, worsening over several months. He had no associated back or leg pain, leg weakness, contralateral leg symptoms, or sphincter dysfunction.

Neurologic examination demonstrated sensory loss to light touch and pinprick in the left S1 dermatome. The patient had full strength in both lower extremities. Muscle stretch reflexes were notable for an absent left Achilles reflex.

Lumbar spine MRI demonstrated an intradural mass lesion at the left S1 level, well demarcated from the surrounding structures with homogeneous enhancement after gadolinium administration. There was no bony destruction, but the nerve root foramen was widened compared with the contralateral side. Given the progressive nature of his neurologic symptoms, the patient underwent surgical resection. Histologic analysis revealed a nerve sheath tumor.

Tumors that arise from nerve sheaths are generally benign, slow-growing lesions that often have an indolent course. Eventually, they can lead to significant clinical symptomatology particularly when they are at the level of the spinal cord. They are more commonly found in middle-aged women. The painless numbness in the preceding vignette, with isolated evidence of focal nerve root damage, was more representative of a benign tumor than a disc lesion, which usually is associated with significant back pain.

Intradural extramedullary tumors are classified into 2 main groups, **schwannomas** and **neurofibromas**. Both often have a similar gross appearance and require microscopic analysis for differentiation. Neurofibromas have less dense cellular structure (Antoni B pattern) and often contain nerve elements. Usually benign, they occur as a solitary finding or as multiple nodules throughout the body. **Type I neurofibromatosis** (**von Recklinghausen disease**) is a familial condition with associated neurocutaneous findings such as café au lait spots, axillary freckling, optic gliomas, and Lisch nodules of the iris. Schwannomas have a dense pattern on microscopic analysis.

SPINAL CORD TUMORS

Clinical Presentation

If a single nerve root is involved without invasion of the spinal cord or cauda equina, symptoms mimic a more distal lesion such as a mononeuropathy or a radiculopathy but often without the typical pain (first Clinical Vignette). When tumors occur at the spinal cord level, they initially often have intermittent symptomatology not leading to significant neurologic signs at the first clinical evaluation. The clinician may therefore consider the possibility of primary CNS demyelinating syndrome. Eventually, patients often develop neurologic signs of involvement of the posterior columns and spinothalamic and corticospinal tracts (second Clinical Vignette).

Clinical Vignette

A 41-year-old woman presented with intermittent numbness in her left leg that was particularly prominent when she played tennis. The results of a detailed neurologic examination were normal, as was MRI of the lumbosacral spine. A follow-up appointment was scheduled for 2 months later. However, within 6 weeks, she noted more persistent numbness and, for the first time, difficulty walking.

Repeat neurologic examination demonstrated a slightly spastic gait, subtle weakness of the left iliopsoas, more brisk muscle stretch reflexes on the left, a left Babinski sign, and a subtle cord level to pinprick and temperature sensation at T6 on the right.

MRI confirmed the presence of a large intradural extramedullary tumor compressing the spinal cord. An encapsulated benign meningioma was surgically removed. The patient had an excellent recovery with no clinical residua.

Despite the significant size of and gradual spinal cord compression by the tumor in this vignette, the presentation was benign with intermittent leg numbness precipitated by exercise and body heat. When the initial lumbar MRI was normal, the possibility of early multiple sclerosis needed consideration.

Continued observation was therefore important, as were patient instructions to call with any new symptomatology and return for follow-up within a few months. On this occasion, another thorough neurologic examination demonstrated a subtle sensory cord level and contralateral corticospinal dysfunction, typical of a classic **Brown-Séquard syndrome** indicating a specific level of spinal cord dysfunction. Focused spinal MRI at a higher level led to the diagnosis of this treatable lesion.

Treatment

The management of **intradural extramedullary nerve sheath tumors** is dictated by the clinical scenario. Patients presenting with neurologic deficits are best treated by surgical resection. The slow-growing nature of these tumors allows for displacement of surrounding structures without compromising the basic anatomy. Often, intradural extramedullary nerve sheath tumors can be completely resected without a resultant neurologic deficit. The nerve fascicle on which the tumor arises can usually be separated from other fascicles, avoiding nerve root injury. Although the fascicle is amputated when the tumor is resected, the patient often has no deficit. Radiation and chemotherapy are not needed for these benign tumors. If an intradural extramedullary tumor is incidentally discovered, having no associated symptoms, observation is often appropriate because many of these lesions have benign courses.

INTRADURAL INTRAMEDULLARY TUMORS

Tumors that originate and grow within the substance of the spinal cord are designated as **intradural**, **intraaxial tumors**, ie, **intramedullary**. They account for approximately 15% of all primary intradural tumors and occur in children and adults.

Clinical Vignette

A 29-year-old woman noted clumsiness and loss of sensation in her right leg over a 4-month period. Previously an avid athlete, she began having difficulty walking, often catching her foot and losing her balance. Symptoms worsened slowly. She noted milder symptoms starting in the left leg but had no upper extremity symptoms and no back or neck pain.

Neurologic examination demonstrated mild right leg weakness with increased muscle stretch reflexes and a right Babinski sign. She had loss of position and vibratory sensation on the right side and diminished pinprick and temperature sensation on the left, a Brown-Séquard syndrome.

Spinal MRI revealed a T6 intraaxial spinal cord mass to the right of midline, which showed heterogeneous enhancement after gadolinium administration. There was extensive T2 signal change within the cord, extending rostral and caudal to the lesion, but no cystic component. Scans of the remainder of the spine and brain were unrevealing. Lumbar puncture, performed to exclude primary CNS demyelinating disease, showed an increased protein level but no oligoclonal bands. Cell counts were normal.

Surgery revealed an anaplastic astrocytoma of the spinal cord. Given its infiltrative nature, complete resection was not attempted. After surgery, symptoms worsened.

Although relatively rare, primary CNS spinal cord tumors always deserve consideration in the differential diagnosis of possible demyelinating disease. **Ependymomas** and **astrocytomas** comprise the majority of intramedullary spinal cord malignancies. Both are tumors of glial origin that also occur within the brain. **Spinal cord astrocytomas** are more infiltrative and non-encapsulated. Other less common intraaxillary tumors include **hemangioblastomas**, **lipomas**, and **dermoid**, **epidermoid**, and **metastatic tumors**.

Clinical Presentation

Intramedullary tumors often present with progressive, painless neurologic decline over several weeks. In the previous vignette, the patient had a **Brown-Séquard syndrome** with loss of motor function and diminished position and vibratory sensation ipsilateral to the lesion and loss of pain and temperature in the contralateral lower extremity. The fibers that supply pain and temperature cross to the opposite side of the spinal cord below the lesion level, resulting in this classic syndrome. Typically seen in tumors that occupy only half of the spinal cord, "pure" Brown-Séquard syndrome is rare; most patients have a mixed picture with spinal cord impingement.

Treatment

Total resection of ependymomas may be possible because a detectable plane often exists between the tumor and the normal spinal cord. Surgical resection of astrocytomas is difficult. The highly organized architecture of the spinal cord makes manipulation and resection of the malignant tissue difficult. Therefore, surgery in astrocytomas is usually restricted to biopsy and limited resection. Recent technological developments in the operating room, including ultrasonography, intraoperative MRI, and ultrasonic aspirators, have somewhat improved surgical outcomes.

Both chemotherapy and radiation therapy are advocated for treatment of spinal cord astrocytomas; however, results are equivocal. In contrast, observation with MRI follow-up is often the best course for ependymomas that are thought to have been completely resected.

FUTURE DIRECTIONS

Advances in the treatment of spinal cord tumors are being made in several areas. Imaging, such as MRI, is being used earlier as a screening tool in many patients with spine-related symptoms. Minimally invasive techniques and advances in instrumentation are improving surgical treatment. Intraoperative monitoring techniques provide improved outcomes for patients undergoing surgical resection of intramedullary and extramedullary tumors. Stereotactic radiosurgery, usually confined to treating intracranial pathology, is now being developed to administer high-dose radiation with surgical precision to lesions within the spine.

REFERENCES

Albanese V, Platania N. Spinal intradural extramedullary tumors: personal experience. *J Neurosurg Sci.* 2002;46:18-24.

Bowers DC, Weprin BE. Intramedullary spinal cord tumors. *Curr Treat Options Neurol.* 2003;5:207-212.

Chang UK, Choe WJ, Chung SK, Chung CK, Kim HJ. Surgical outcome and prognostic factors of spinal intramedullary ependymomas in adults. *J Neurooncol.* 2002;57:133-139.

Conti P, Pansini G, Mouchaty H, Capuano C, Conti R. Spinal neurinomas: retrospective analysis and long-term outcome of 179 consecutively operated cases and review of the literature. *Surg Neurol.* 2004;61:34-43.

Cooper P. Management of intramedullary spinal cord tumors. In: Tindall, Cooper, Barrow, eds. *The Practice of Neurosurgery.* Baltimore, Md: Williams & Wilkins; 1996:1335-1346.

Newton HB, Newton CL, Gatens C, Hebert R, Pack R. Spinal cord tumors: review of etiology, diagnosis, and multidisciplinary approach to treatment. *Cancer Pract.* 1995;3:207-218.

Ratliff JK, Cooper PR. Metastatic spine tumors. *South Med J.* 2004;97:246-253.

Section XVII
TRAUMA TO THE BRAIN AND SPINAL CORD

Chapter 75
Brain Trauma 644

Chapter 76
Trauma of the Spine and Spinal Cord 658

Chapter 75
Brain Trauma

Carlos A. David

Clinical Vignette

A vigorous 75-year-old newspaper editor, who had been able to downhill ski 3 weeks previously, experienced increasingly severe headaches that began awakening him from sleep. He also noted "spinning vertigo," particularly precipitated by standing or neck extension, decreased coordination of his hands, weakness of his legs, cloudiness of vision, problems reading, and inability to concentrate.

Although the patient did not initially report such, history revealed that he had slipped on the ice, striking his occiput, 7 weeks previously. Neurologic examination results were normal, with the exception of moderately severe inability to perform tandem gait (something most healthy 70-year-olds often cannot perform, but this was probably abnormal in this athletic man).

Despite the relatively normal examination results, head CT demonstrated large bilateral subdural hematomas (SDHs). Biparietal craniotomies provided drainage of both hematomas. He had an uneventful recovery.

This patient's history is classic for **subdural hematoma**. He had sustained a moderately significant closed head injury, something he had disregarded because of its lack of significant immediate sequelae; other than the immediate scalp contusion, he was symptom free for 5 weeks. In individuals of this age group, the bridging subdural veins are stretched as the diminished volume of the brain allows it to retract from the dura. Relatively minor to modest injury causes small venous tears and bleeding that gradually accumulates. This patient's symptoms were impressive. However, his brain compensated well, and the only abnormality on examination was tandem ataxia, which could easily be dismissed as appropriate for age. The entire clinical picture suggested subdural hematoma until proven otherwise. He had an uneventful recovery except for a few focal motor sensory seizures that responded to phenytoin therapy.

Traumatic head and spinal injuries are among the leading causes of morbidity and mortality in the United States. There is approximately 1 such injury every 15 seconds. Of the 2 million annual cases of traumatic head injury, 100,000 die within hours, 500,000 require hospital stays, and up to 100,000 have permanent disability. **Traumatic brain injuries** (TBIs) cost at least $25 billion per year. Major causes include motor vehicle accidents, falls, violent assaults, and sports and recreation accidents.

Head injuries can be classified by mechanism (closed vs penetrating), severity (mild, moderate, severe), presence of skull fractures (depressed versus nondepressed), and the presence of intracranial lesions (focal versus diffuse).

GENERAL PRINCIPLES OF HEAD INJURY CARE

The initial management of severe head injuries, as for any serious trauma victim, includes the "ABC" evaluation for airway, breathing, and circulation and a careful general and neurologic examination (Figure 75-1). Concomitantly, the patient's general level of responsiveness must be assessed using the **Glasgow coma scale**. The lowest possible score of 3 means that individuals have no ability to open the eyes, no motor response to verbal command or direct stimuli, and no verbal response to the physician's questions, giving a score of 1 or nil for each of the 3 components. The highest possible score is 15.

SCALP AND SOFT TISSUE INJURIES

Soft tissue injuries are commonly associated with more severe head injuries. A complete examination of the exterior surface of the face and head is vital. Blood loss can be extensive given

BRAIN TRAUMA

Figure 75-1 — **Initial Management of Severe Head Injuries**

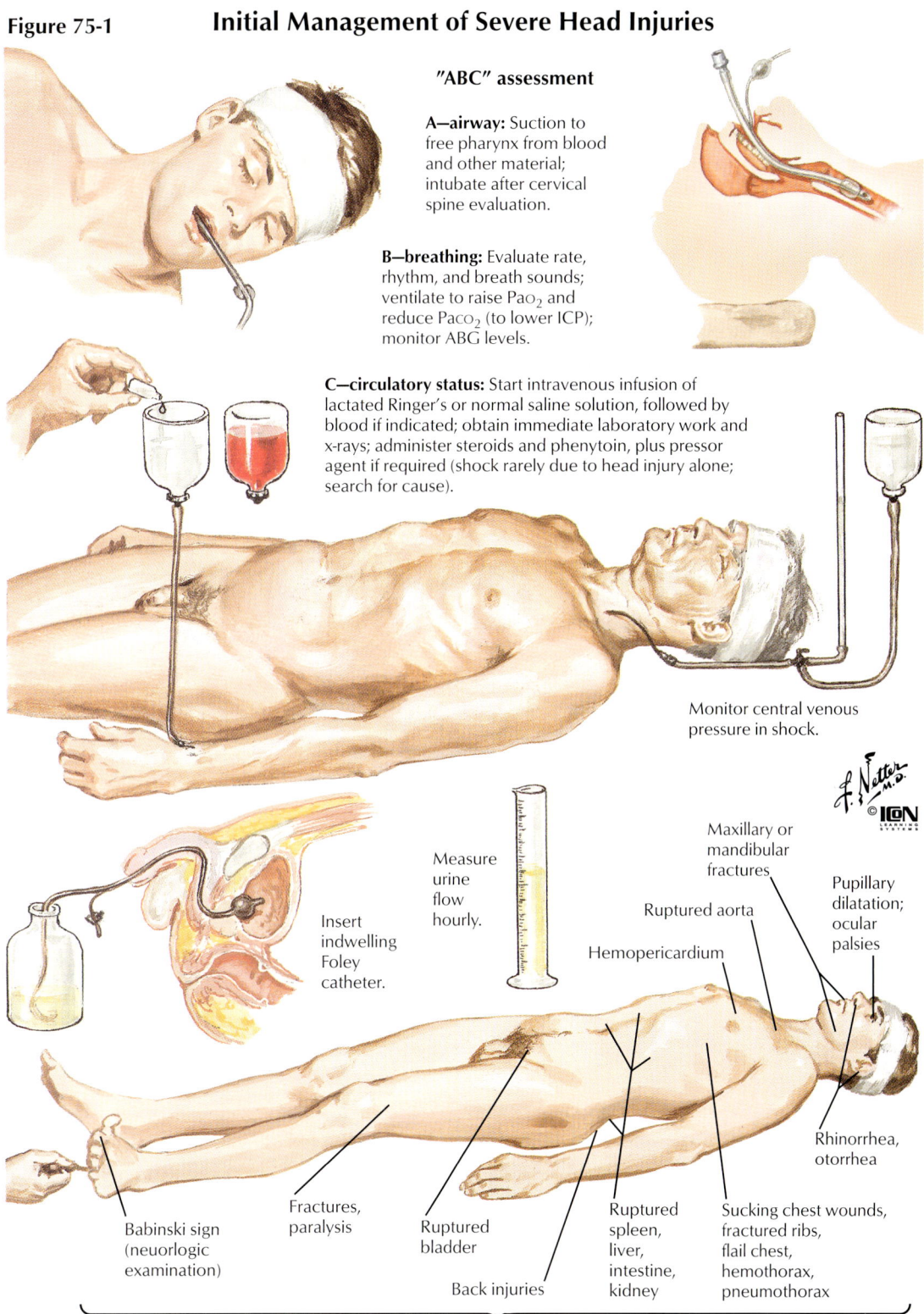

TRAUMA TO THE BRAIN AND SPINAL CORD

BRAIN TRAUMA

the location of blood vessels within the dense connective tissue of the scalp, which decreases retraction of cut vessels and promotes bleeding.

After more serious lesions are excluded, scalp injuries should be shaved, explored, and debrided. If lacerations extend to the skull, the galea must be included in primary closure sutures.

SKULL FRACTURES

Bone fractures can be located in the calvaria (vault) or in the basal skull. Fractures of the cranial vault carry a 20-times-greater incidence of intracranial hematoma in comatose patients and a 400-times-greater incidence in conscious patients. Therefore, considerable concern is appropriate for TBI even in neurologically intact patients with skull fractures. **Basal skull fractures** are often difficult to identify on head CT, even with thin-cut sections. They can present with certain signs, including **raccoon** or **Panda bear eyes**, **Battle signs** (ecchymoses over the mastoid), and CSF leakage from the nose, throat, or ears (Figure 75-2). There are approximately 150,000 cases of basal skull fracture–related CSF leaks per year. Many of these leaks resolve spontaneously. Persistent leaks necessitate operative treatment. There is no need for prophylactic antibiotic therapy with basal skull fractures.

Fractures are classified as **linear** or **stellate**, depressed or nondepressed, open or closed, and by location. Linear skull fractures not associated with an underlying brain injury do not necessitate surgery. However, depressed (outer skull table forced beneath normal level of inner table) and stellate (comminuted) skull fractures often necessitate operative elevation and possible evacuation of underlying hematomas (Figure 75-3; see also Figure 28-1).

Depressed fractures and those along the temporal bone are more commonly associated with injury to the brain or blood vessels. A fracture line across the middle meningeal artery indicates a possibility for **epidural hematoma**. A depressed skull fracture that injures an underlying dural sinus can precipitate massive blood loss. Open fractures involve communication between the intracranial vault and the external environment and are associated with higher risks of spinal fluid leaks and infection.

EXTRAAXIAL TRAUMATIC BRAIN INJURIES

Traumatic Subarachnoid Hemorrhage

Subarachnoid hemorrhage (SAH) is the most common sequela of TBI. Depending on the severity of the initial injury and the types of injured vessels, the SAH can range from clinically insignificant to fatal. SAH is typically associated with other types of intracranial lesions.

The most concerning effect of posttraumatic SAH is the risk of hydrocephalus. The blood products in the SAH can obstruct the reabsorption of CSF and lead to increased **intracranial pressure** (ICP).

Treatment of SAH often involves placement of ventricular drains and shunting systems for secondary hydrocephalus.

Epidural Hematomas

Most **epidural hematomas**, acute blood collections contained between the dura and inner table of the skull, result from traumatic injury, although they occur in only 2% of TBIs (Figure 75-4). Common in the temporal and parietal regions, 90% are associated with a skull fracture. Nearby intraparenchymal lesions such as contusions, lacerations, and bone fragments occur infrequently. Epidural hematomas are less common in those older than 60 years because the dura becomes more adherent to the inner skull surface.

Arterial lacerations, particularly of the middle meningeal, or, less commonly, venous injuries initiate the formation of hematomas. Contiguous lacerations of the dura mater allow this blood into the epidural space.

Clinical Presentation and Diagnosis

The classic picture for patients with epidural hematomas includes a **lucid interval**. Typically, it is an initial loss of consciousness secondary to a primary concussive injury, then a return of wakefulness, and finally a lapse into coma as the epidural hematoma enlarges in size. However, this presentation occurs in less than one third of affected patients. The rate of symptom progression depends on associated brain injuries, the etiology of the injury, and the rate of blood accumulation.

BRAIN TRAUMA

Figure 75-2 Basilar Skull Fractures

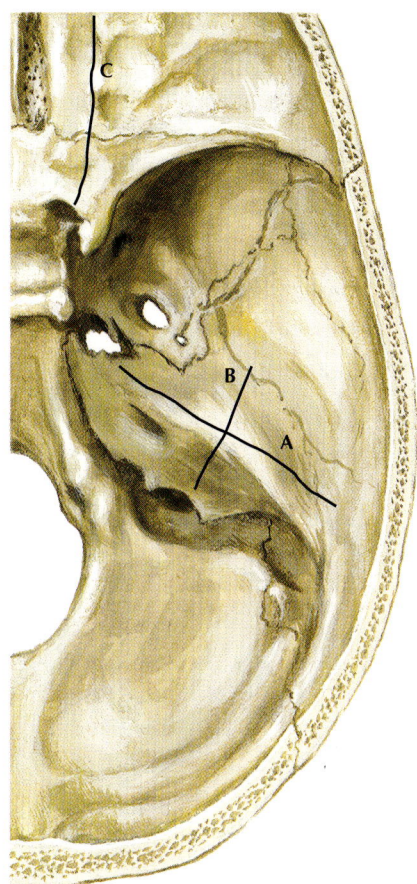

Longitudinal (**A**) and transverse (**B**) fractures of petrous pyramid of temporal bone, and anterior basal skull fracture (**C**)

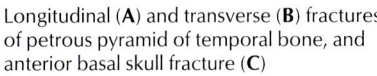

Rhinorrhea

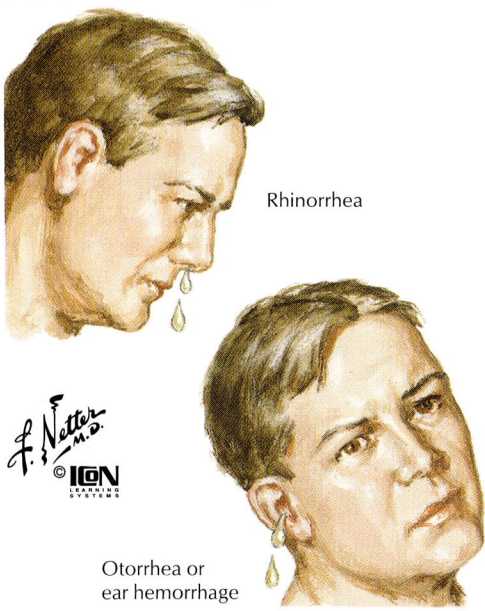

Otorrhea or ear hemorrhage

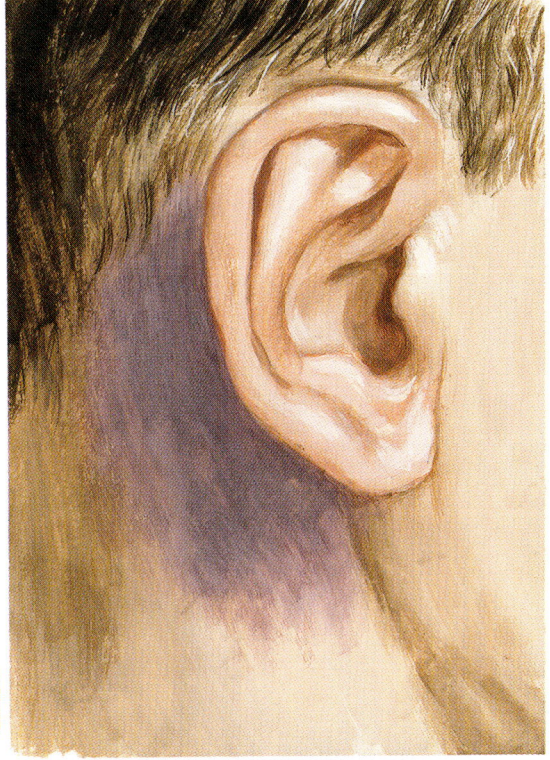

"Panda bear" or "raccoon" sign due to leakage of blood from anterior fossa into periorbital tissues. Absence of conjunctival injection differentiates fracture from direct eye trauma.

Battle sign: postauricular hematoma

TRAUMA TO THE BRAIN AND SPINAL CORD

BRAIN TRAUMA

Figure 75-3 — Signs Suggesting Need for Operation

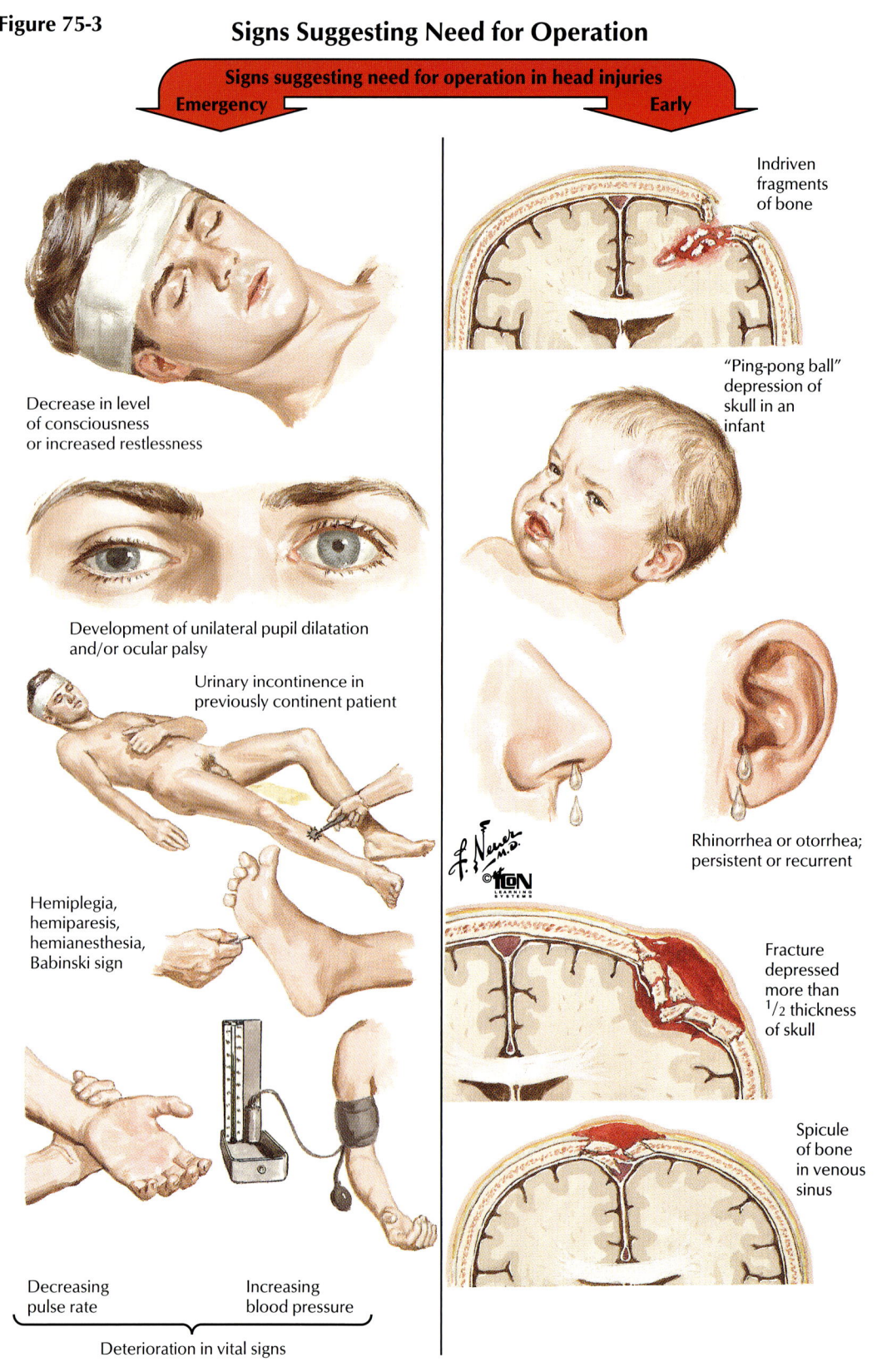

TRAUMA TO THE BRAIN AND SPINAL CORD

BRAIN TRAUMA

Figure 75-4

Epidural Hematoma

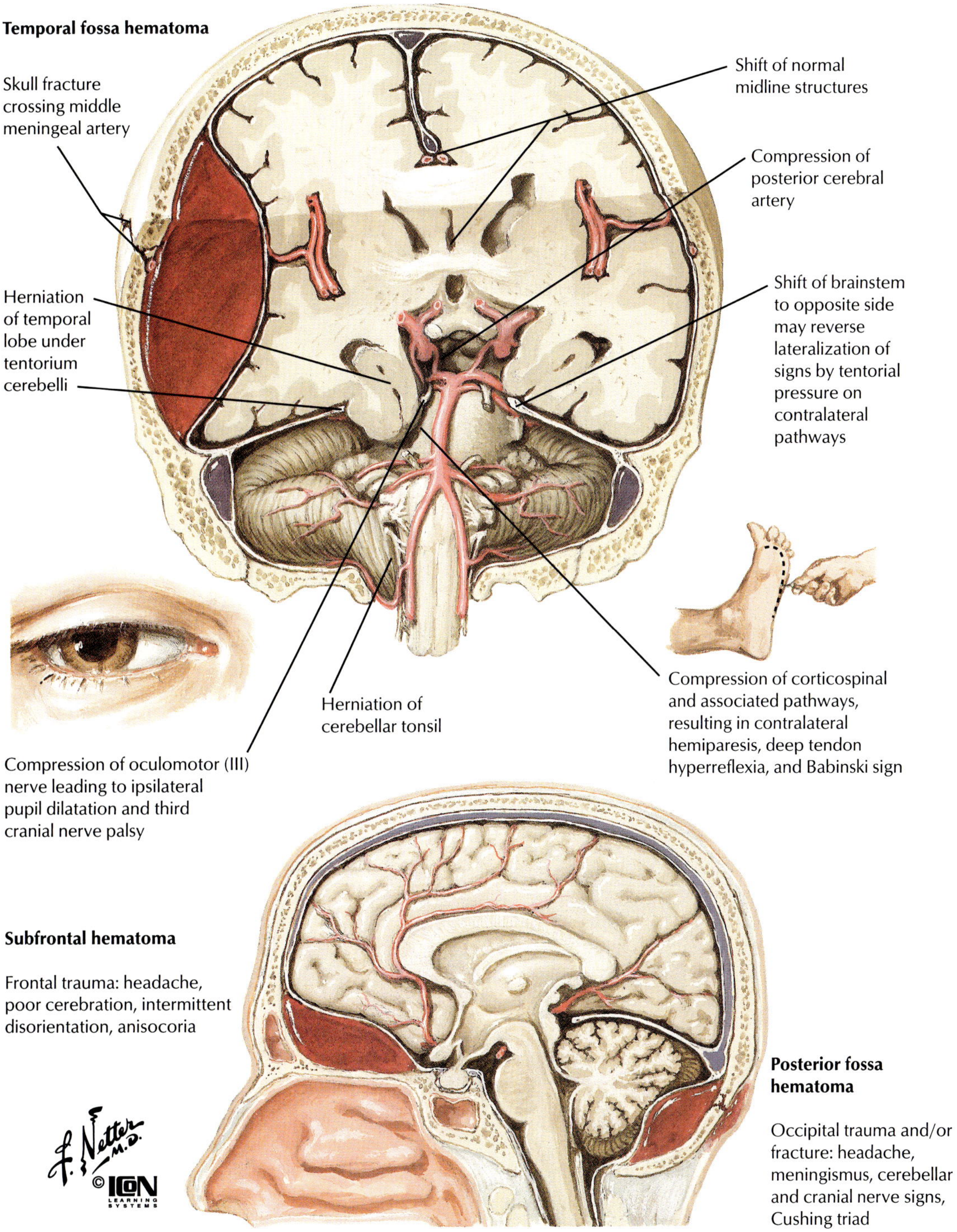

Temporal fossa hematoma

Skull fracture crossing middle meningeal artery

Herniation of temporal lobe under tentorium cerebelli

Shift of normal midline structures

Compression of posterior cerebral artery

Shift of brainstem to opposite side may reverse lateralization of signs by tentorial pressure on contralateral pathways

Herniation of cerebellar tonsil

Compression of corticospinal and associated pathways, resulting in contralateral hemiparesis, deep tendon hyperreflexia, and Babinski sign

Compression of oculomotor (III) nerve leading to ipsilateral pupil dilatation and third cranial nerve palsy

Subfrontal hematoma

Frontal trauma: headache, poor cerebration, intermittent disorientation, anisocoria

Posterior fossa hematoma

Occipital trauma and/or fracture: headache, meningismus, cerebellar and cranial nerve signs, Cushing triad

TRAUMA TO THE BRAIN AND SPINAL CORD

BRAIN TRAUMA

Usually, a hyperdense, biconvex collection between the skull and brain is seen (Figure 75-5). The typical CT appearance of epidural hematomas in certain at-risk patients, even with an initial negative head CT, is a delayed epidural formation in as many as 30% of individuals. Therefore, it is essential to be prepared to repeat the CT scan for the slightest indication.

Treatment and Prognosis

Treatment for epidural hematomas is surgical removal in most cases. There is significant concern for acute deterioration in patients who may otherwise look well, and therefore patients are taken promptly to surgery. Occasionally, small hematomas in select patients may be watched closely with clinical exams and serial CT.

Delay in diagnosis and failure to recognize a hematoma have the strongest association with morbidity and mortality. Overall mortality is 5% to 40% depending on patient age, time of treatment, hematoma size, and associated injuries.

Acute Subdural Hematoma

Subdural hematomas are blood collections located between the brain parenchyma and the dural membranes. Major distinctions between acute and chronic SDH are the therapeutic approaches they call for and the clinical outcomes they produce.

Acute SDHs occur in 5% to 22% of patients with TBI. Older individuals are at greater risk because they commonly have increasing space in the subdural compartment secondary to brain atrophy. During traumatic impact, the brain accelerates and decelerates in relation to fixed dural structures. Tearing of bridging veins and injury to cortical arteries can cause bleeding into the subdural space. Patients with TBI commonly present with other injuries, including parenchymal contusions, hemorrhages, skull fractures, and diffuse brain swelling.

Clinical Presentation and Diagnosis

The initial severity of the injury determines the patient's initial presentation, which can range from neurologically intact to altered mental states to comatose with signs of decorticate or decerebrate posturing. Common clinical findings of expanding hematomas include altered mental states, pupil inequality, and motor weakness. The lucid interval, a classical finding with epidural hematoma, is also commonly seen with acute SDH. Specific clinical signs often help to localize the lesion.

Brain CT is the initial test of choice for detecting SDH and concomitant brain injuries (Figure 75-5). An acute SDH is recognized by its hyperdense crescent shaped image between the brain and skull. Unlike epidural hematomas, SDH typically cross skull suture lines, and sometimes extend along the falx cerebri. Head CT sometimes underestimates the size of the SDH given the similar imaging density of the nearby bone.

Treatment and Prognosis

If the patient has mental status changes or other signs of focal cerebral compromise, treatment of acute SDH begins with medical management for increased ICP. Treating the patient with 1 g/kg IV mannitol as rapidly as possible and then 25 g every 4 to 6 hours if the serum osmolarity remains less than 320 mOsm/L is very useful. Surgical intervention is appropriate for individuals whose SDHs have mass effect causing various neurologic deficits; when this strategy is determined, the procedure must be performed as quickly as possible. Extensive craniotomy, with wide dural opening, and clot resection is required (Figure 75-6). A burr hole trephine evacuation is inadequate because the clot is solid. Outcomes do not improve after a simple decompressive craniectomy wherein the bone flap is not replaced.

Cerebral edema is common with acute SDH, resulting in increased postoperative ICP in almost 50% of patients. Intensive medical management is required (Figure 75-7). Residual and recurrent hematomas are also postoperative concerns.

An acute SDH is often associated with a poor outcome. The combination of the hematoma and other injuries, particularly those affecting the brain parenchyma, is associated with a 50% mortality rate. Unfortunately, a significant number of surviving patients have permanent mental and physical disabilities. Outcomes are strongly predicted by patient age and initial presentation. Mortalities of 20% are recorded for individuals younger than 40 years, but this number in-

BRAIN TRAUMA

Figure 75-5   **CT Scans and Angiograms of Intracranial Hematomas**

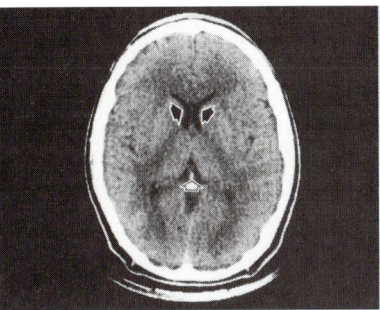

A. Normal brain. CT scan demonstrating normal anatomy at level of frontal horns of lateral ventricles (black arrows). Pineal gland (white arrow) is in normal midline location.

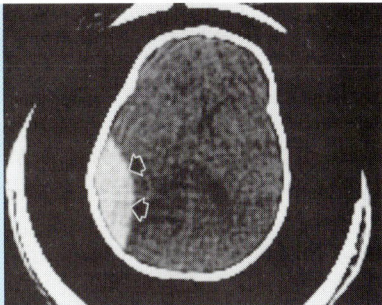

B. Epidural hematoma. CT scan demonstrating hyperdense right parietal epidural hematoma (black arrows), which has assumed classic lenticular configuration secondary to adherence of dura to inner table of skull. Other structures are compressed and shifted.

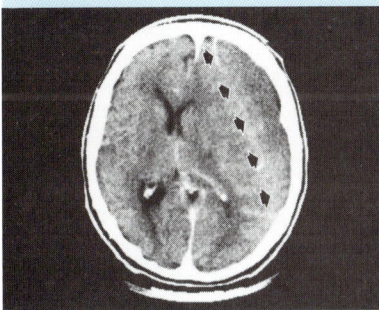

C. Subacute subdural hematoma. CT scan demonstrating large isodense mass over left cerebral convexity. Compressed cerebral cortex (black arrows) shows enhanced density delineating inner border of subacute subdural hematoma. Normal structure are shifted across midline.

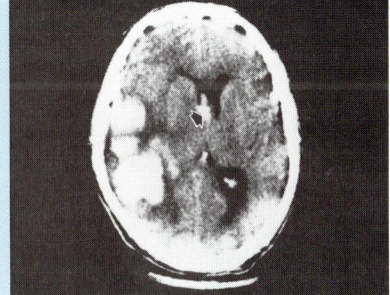

D. Acute intracerebral hematoma. CT scan demonstrating hyperdense mass in right parietotemporal area. Large acute intracerebral hematoma has shifted lateral ventricle toward midline. Blood is visualized within ventricular system (black arrow).

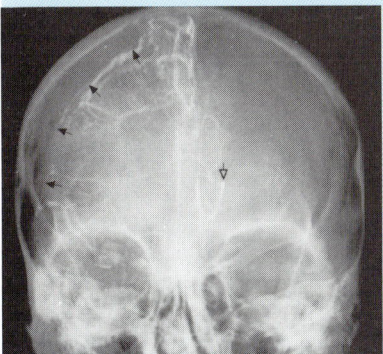

E. Acute subdural hematoma. Cerebral angiogram, venous phase, demonstrating displacement of cortical veins (solid arrows) away from skull by acute subdural hematoma. Typical shape is due to relatively free spread of blood within subdural space. Internal cerebral vein (open arrow) is shifted across midline.

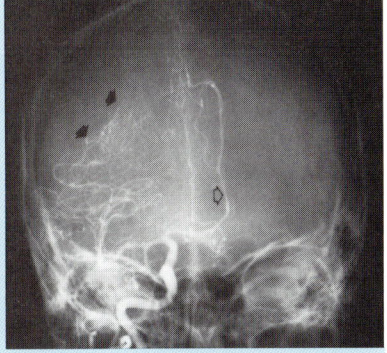

F. Chronic subdural hematoma. Cerebral angiogram, arterial phase, demonstrating displacement of cortical vessel (solid arrows) away from inner table of skull by chronic subdural hematoma. Lenticular shape is secondary to subdural membrane formation. Anterior cerebral artery (open arrow) is shifted across midline.

TRAUMA TO THE BRAIN AND SPINAL CORD

BRAIN TRAUMA

Figure 75-6
Acute Subdural Hematoma

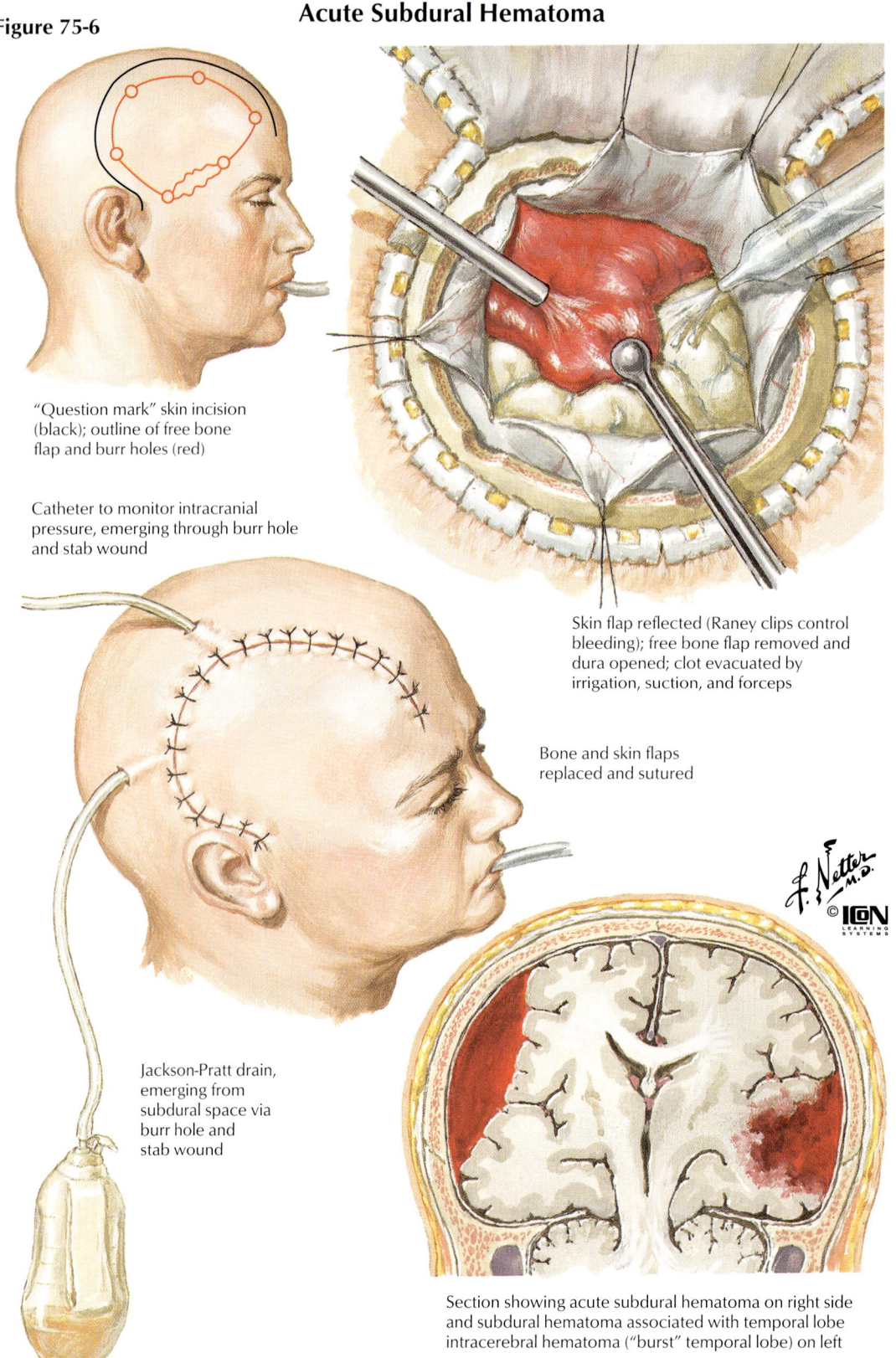

"Question mark" skin incision (black); outline of free bone flap and burr holes (red)

Catheter to monitor intracranial pressure, emerging through burr hole and stab wound

Skin flap reflected (Raney clips control bleeding); free bone flap removed and dura opened; clot evacuated by irrigation, suction, and forceps

Bone and skin flaps replaced and sutured

Jackson-Pratt drain, emerging from subdural space via burr hole and stab wound

Section showing acute subdural hematoma on right side and subdural hematoma associated with temporal lobe intracerebral hematoma ("burst" temporal lobe) on left

TRAUMA TO THE BRAIN AND SPINAL CORD

BRAIN TRAUMA

Figure 75-7   Intensive Medical Management of Severe Head Injury

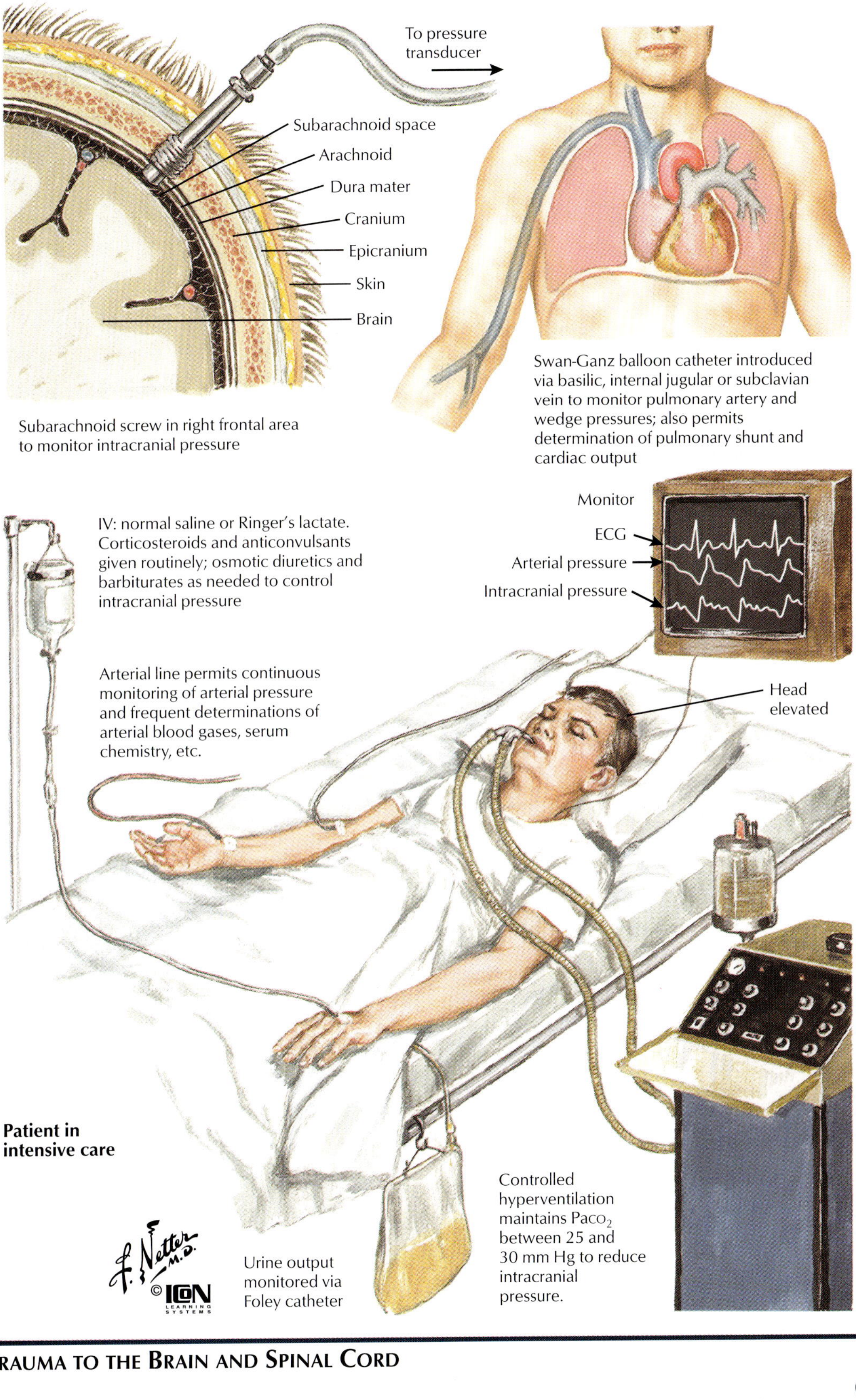

- Subarachnoid space
- Arachnoid
- Dura mater
- Cranium
- Epicranium
- Skin
- Brain

To pressure transducer

Subarachnoid screw in right frontal area to monitor intracranial pressure

Swan-Ganz balloon catheter introduced via basilic, internal jugular or subclavian vein to monitor pulmonary artery and wedge pressures; also permits determination of pulmonary shunt and cardiac output

IV: normal saline or Ringer's lactate. Corticosteroids and anticonvulsants given routinely; osmotic diuretics and barbiturates as needed to control intracranial pressure

Arterial line permits continuous monitoring of arterial pressure and frequent determinations of arterial blood gases, serum chemistry, etc.

Monitor
- ECG
- Arterial pressure
- Intracranial pressure

Head elevated

Patient in intensive care

Urine output monitored via Foley catheter

Controlled hyperventilation maintains $Paco_2$ between 25 and 30 mm Hg to reduce intracranial pressure.

TRAUMA TO THE BRAIN AND SPINAL CORD

creases to 65% for individuals older than 40 years, reaching 88% for octogenarians. The initial consciousness level provides a guide to prognosis. Conscious patients have a mortality rate of less than 10%, whereas unconscious patients have 45% to 60% mortality. The timing of surgical intervention also affects the outcome.

Chronic Subdural Hematoma

Chronic SDHs are blood collections within the subdural space, commonly appearing 2 to 3 weeks after an injury, which may initially seem trivial, as in the clinical vignette. Their incidence is 1 to 2 per 100,000 persons in the population each year. Most of these patients are older than 50 years and often are chronic alcoholics or have coagulopathies, particularly from iatrogenic sources such as anticoagulants. A history of trauma can be defined, with careful querying in 50% to 75% of cases. Often, the inciting injury is relatively mild and has been disregarded by tenacious individuals.

Initially, blood collections enter the subdural space after trauma or spontaneous hemorrhages. Membranes begin to form at the inner and outer aspects of the hematoma. One theory postulates that these membranes are prone to low-grade bleeding, leading to slow enlargement of the SDH. Another theory suggests that higher osmotic pressure within the subdural hematoma draws in CSF, causing SDH accumulation. In some patients, the SDH continues to enlarge, whereas in others it slowly reabsorbs. It is difficult to predict which course will result.

Clinical Presentation and Diagnosis

Often variable, presentation may range from subtle focal signs of cerebral compromise to those symptoms of the various **herniation syndromes**. A high clinical suspicion of SDH must be held for at-risk individuals whenever a remote history of head trauma exists.

CT is the study of choice (Figure 75-5). During the initial weeks after the head injury, pathologic evolution leads to blood clot liquification, consequently changing its CT appearance. Unlike the hyperdense character of acute SDH, chronic SDH evolves from an initial brainlike isodense image to a hypodense picture of extraaxial fluid collections. Sometimes, variable amounts of retained hyperdense fluid represent ongoing subdural hemorrhage from the vascular membranes. Occasionally, a brain MRI serendipitously leads to a diagnosis of SDH in patients presenting with strokelike or seizure symptoms.

Treatment and Prognosis

A patient's presentation and comorbidities determine the treatment of chronic SDH. Medical management and observation is recommended for individuals with subtle clinical symptoms and signs: discontinuation of anticoagulant medications, close observation in a hospital or by a reliable adult, and serial CT.

Surgical therapy is advisable for chronic SDH that is causing significant mass effect or is associated with other serious clinical signs or symptoms. Approaches include bedside twist drill drainage, operative burr holes, and craniotomy. Twist drill drainage can be performed in an ICU or ED setting, where a small hole is drilled into the skull over the SDH and a small catheter is passed into the fluid and allowed to drain slowly over a few days. Slow drainage avoids rapid brain shifts associated with operative drainage. The risk of twist-drill drainage is causing new bleeding and converting a chronic SDH to an acute SDH.

Other patients with SDH, especially those with significant membranes, should undergo surgery. Often, 1 or 2 burr holes adequately drain the subdural fluid. Formal craniotomy is indicated when burr holes have led to inadequate fluid drainage, in patients with excessive subdural membranes, and for those with a large acute SDH component.

Usually, removal of just 10% of the SDH fluid leads to clinical improvement. Although the ideal therapeutic goal is complete evacuation, up to 45% of chronic SDHs reaccumulate. Complications of chronic SDHs include seizures (10%) and infections (1%).

Postsurgical mortality is approximately 10%. Outcomes are closely related to patient status at treatment. Unlike acute SDH, most chronic subdural patients are able to return to their previous levels of functioning.

INTRAAXIAL TRAUMATIC INJURIES
Cerebral Contusions

Contusions, the second most common post-traumatic lesions, are bruises of the brain comprising hemorrhage, infarcted tissue, and necrosis, usually of the frontal and temporal lobes. *Coup lesions* are those found under the sites of direct injury; *contrecoup lesions* are located at sides opposite to impact sites, **where the brain decelerates against the skull (often the frontal and temporal poles). Cortical** contusions are most common, but they can also occur in the deep white matter.

Clinical presentation of contusions varies widely and is predicated on their location and size. Patients with small frontal lobe contusions primarily present with headache. Many contusions enlarge during 2 to 3 days after injury, secondary to necrosis and edema, which can become significant in higher impact cases. Contusions that develop over a few days may not have been identifiable on initial CT scans.

Surgical intervention is usually not required for intracerebral contusions, especially for small, deep subcortical contusions; they can be managed medically. However, larger lobar contusions with significant signs of mass effect sometimes require craniotomy and evacuation. It is difficult to predict which patients will deteriorate from their specific contusions. Temporal lobe contusions are potentially the most dangerous given their location near the brainstem. Repeat CT scanning is essential to follow these lesions.

Depending on the number and sizes of the contusions, their anatomical locus, and the severity and mechanism of the injury, mortality rates for cerebral contusions range from 25% to 60%.

Intraparenchymal Hematomas

Up to 25% of patients who sustain head trauma develop **intraparenchymal hematomas**: localized, well-defined regions of acute hemorrhage. The basic pathophysiology is similar to contusions. Most (90%) occur within the frontal and temporal lobes. Shear injury leads to deep cerebral white matter hematomas. Two thirds of intraparenchymal hematomas are associated with extraaxial hematomas. An **intraventricular hemorrhage** is a common association and is often complicated by hydrocephalus.

Depending on the severity of the injury, almost half of these patients present with a loss of consciousness. Other signs and symptoms relate to the size and location of the hemorrhage.

Medical management is the treatment of choice for deep or small hemorrhages and for unstable patients. Surgical resection is indicated for large superficial lobar hematomas associated with clinical signs of mass effect. ICP monitors can be placed to follow patients with poor neurologic examination results. The best ICP monitor is a ventricular drain that drains CSF and monitors pressure.

Mortality rates vary from 25% to 75%, depending on level of consciousness at presentation, size and location of hematoma, severity of trauma, patient age, and associated injuries.

Diffuse Axonal Injury

Diffuse axonal injury or **shear injury** results from rotational acceleration and deceleration of the brain during traumatic impact. Damage is sustained through the shearing of diffuse axonal pathways and small capillaries. This contrasts with focal mass lesions that may occur concomitantly. Shear injury is commonly associated with other intraaxial and extraaxial traumatic injuries. Motor vehicle accidents are the most common causes of diffuse axonal injury.

CT often does not show mass lesions specifically associated with shear injury. However, obvious cerebral edema may become more significant during the first 48 to 72 hours after the injury. Small areas of punctate contusions can also be found in areas of diffuse axonal injury. Often, other associated cerebral injuries are defined with brain CT.

The brains of patients with diffuse axonal injury can become edematous, with resulting increased ICP. Pressure monitors are required in patients whose clinical examination results are not reliable. Intraparenchymal monitors are usually used because the ventricles are often so compressed that ventricular catheter placement is difficult.

Patients with severe forms of diffuse axonal injury may remain comatose for extended periods, a clinical picture classified as a **persistent vege-**

BRAIN TRAUMA

Figure 75-8
Exploratory Burr Holes and Removal of Posterior Fossa Hematoma

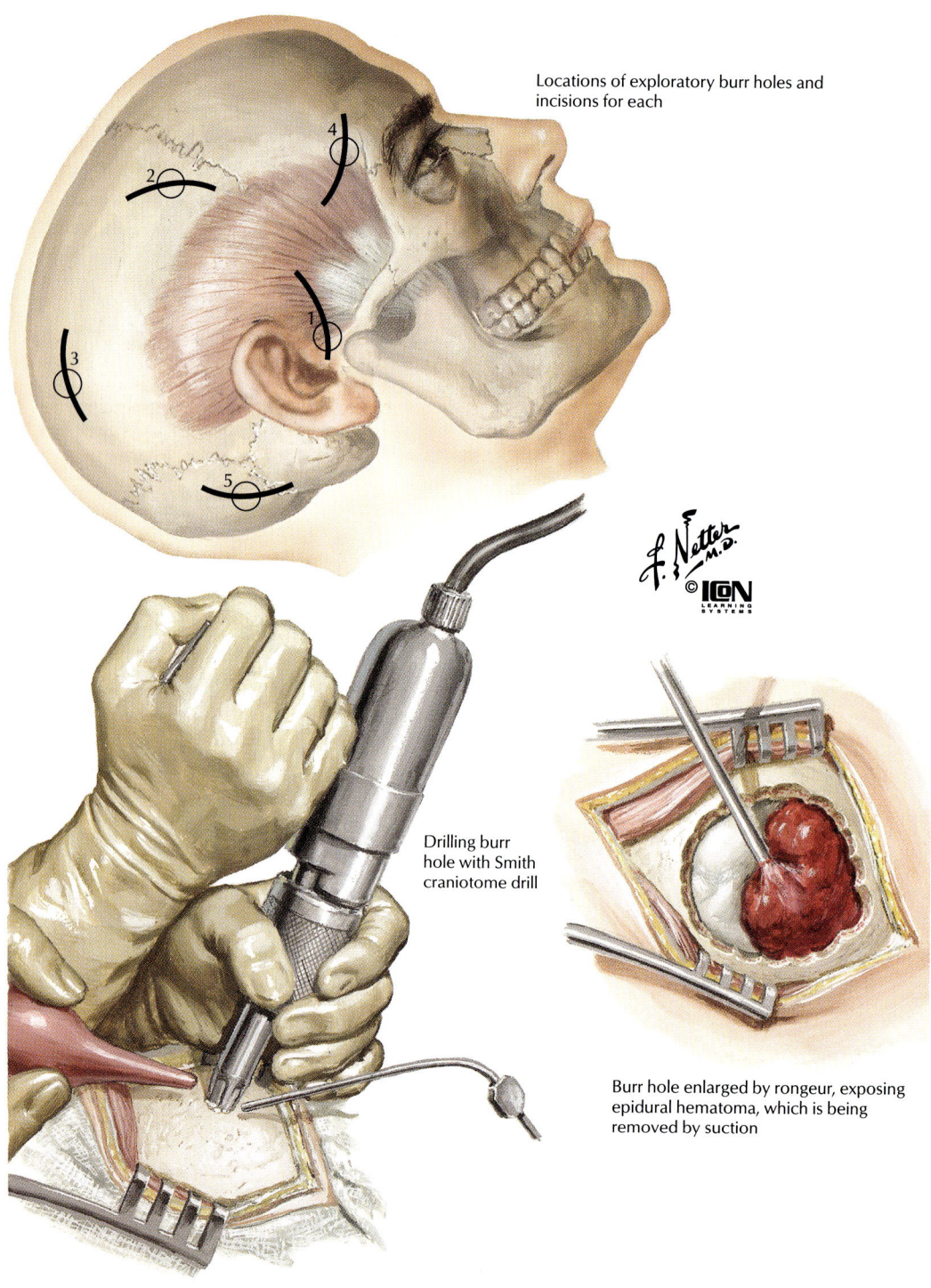

Locations of exploratory burr holes and incisions for each

Drilling burr hole with Smith craniotome drill

Burr hole enlarged by rongeur, exposing epidural hematoma, which is being removed by suction

tative state that carries an extremely poor prognosis (Figure 28-5). Outcomes are significantly worse for patients with evidence of moderate to severe shear injury.

POSTERIOR FOSSA LESIONS

Lesions of the cerebellum and posterior fossa are less common than supratentorial traumatic injuries, comprising only 5% of post-TBI sequelae. The most common lesions are **epidural hematomas**, **SDH**, and **intracerebellar hematomas**. These lesions can cause rapid neurologic decline given the small amount of space in the posterior fossa, with possible early brainstem compression and hydrocephalus. Because of bony artifacts, routine brain CT frequently does not identify posterior fossa TBI. Therefore, MRI is more commonly used in this setting. Careful assessment of patients for these injuries is critical, especially in high-risk individuals, particularly those with basal skull fractures.

Most **posterior fossa lesions** are treated with **posterior fossa craniectomy** with evacuation of the hematoma (Figure 75-8). In contrast, a ventricular drain is adequate for intraventricular bleeds.

OUTCOMES FROM TRAUMATIC BRAIN INJURY

Patient prognosis is always first on a family's mind. Unfortunately, it is often difficult to determine a patient's chance for recovery accurately. It is relatively easy to identify individuals at the ends of the trauma severity spectrum but more difficult in the middle gray area. Useful factors include injury severity, the Glasgow coma scale score at presentation, initial response to therapy, global versus focal injuries, associated injuries, age, medical comorbidities, and timing of medical and surgical interventions (Figure 75-8).

Reliable outcome scales, including the Glasgow outcome scale and the disability rating scale, show that neurologic recovery often stabilizes 6 months to 1 year after TBI.

REFERENCES

Chesnut RM. Management of brain and spine injuries. *Crit Care Clin*. 2004;20:25-55.

Brain Trauma Foundation, American Association of Neurological Surgeons, Joint Section on Neurotrauma and Critical Care. Guidelines for the management of severe head injury. *J Neurotrauma*. 1996;13:641-734.

Fakhry SM, Trask AL, Waller MA, et al. Management of brain-injured patients by an evidence-based medicine protocol improves outcomes and decreases hospital charges. *J Trauma*. 2004;56:492-500.

Henderson WR, Dhingra VK, Chittock DR, et al. Hypothermia in the management of traumatic brain injury: a systematic review and meta-analysis. *Intensive Care Med*. 2003;29:1637-1644.

Liao CC, Lee ST, Hsu WC, et al. Experience in the surgical management of spontaneous spinal epidural hematoma. *J Neurosurg*. 2004;100(suppl):38-45.

Tokutomi T, Morimoto K, Miyagi T, et al. Optimal temperature for the management of severe traumatic brain injury: effect of hypothermia on intracranial pressure, systemic and intracranial hemodynamics, and metabolism. *Neurosurgery*. 2003;52:102-112.

Chapter 76
Trauma of the Spine and Spinal Cord

Stephen R. Freidberg and Subu N. Magge

Trauma to the spine and spinal cord is one of the most devastating injuries in terms of morbidity, life change, and costs to patients, families, and society. Caring for the acute and long-term needs of patients with spinal cord injury (SCI) is estimated to cost $4 billion per year. The costs to patients and families are incalculable. Of more than 22,000 citations in a review of the National Library of Medicine database for *spinal cord injury*, many titles dealt with the problems of acute surgical management, but most were related to physiology, biochemistry, and drug trials. Many were related to rehabilitation problems and long-term urologic, skin, medical, social, and psychological issues of those with SCI.

Spinal cord injury is associated with a mortality rate of 50%, mostly at the scene of the accident. Of patients brought to major trauma centers, 1 in 40 has SCI. Patients who come to the hospital have a 16% mortality rate. Young males predominate (85%). There is a high correlation with alcohol, motor vehicle accidents, and certain sport-related injuries (Figures 76-1 and 76-2). In older individuals, there is a higher incidence of SCI from falls associated with concomitant spinal deformities including spondylosis and stenosis, ankylosing spondylitis, and congenital fusion (Figure 76-3).

Spinal cord injury problems last a lifetime. Patients with SCI must adjust to limited mobility, psychiatric issues, urologic problems, pulmonary difficulty, skin deterioration, sexual dysfunction, and frequently the inability to perform their jobs. The higher the level of neurologic injury, the more difficult are patients' adjustments to it (see Figure 60-2). Nonetheless, most SCI patients live active, productive lives. The Americans With Disabilities Act removed many physical barriers to wheelchair accessibility and has prevented discrimination in the workplace. Patients with SCIs race in marathons, play basketball, and compete in international tournaments.

Clearly, SCI presents a condition where prevention is preferred over treatment. The American Association of Neurological Surgeons sponsors an effective and aggressive program, "Think First," bringing the message of safety to more than 8 million high school and elementary school pupils in the United States and 7 foreign countries.

PATHOPHYSIOLOGY

It is usually not possible to focus on the problems of spine and spinal cord trauma as isolated phenomena. There are frequently multisystem injuries with problems of hypotension, hypoxia, infection, and the need for surgery on other organ systems complicating the treatment of the spine injury.

Advanced Trauma Life Support's ABCs—airway, breathing, and circulation—are the first priority. Hypotension and hypoxia worsen the SCI, so minimizing secondary injury to the contused spinal cord caused by inadequate blood supply and oxygen is essential. Pathologic microvascular injury with thrombosis within the cord leads to hemorrhage and necrosis secondary to infarction. The hemorrhage is probably venous in origin. Toxic excitatory amines produced by the trauma worsen the secondary injury.

DIAGNOSTIC APROACH
Cervical Spine

If the trauma victim is alert, with no evidence of alcohol or drugs, and has no neck pain or tenderness, with full painless range of neck motion and

TRAUMA OF THE SPINE AND SPINAL CORD

Figure 76-1   **Cervical Spine Injury: Flexion and Flexion-Rotation**

Mechanism

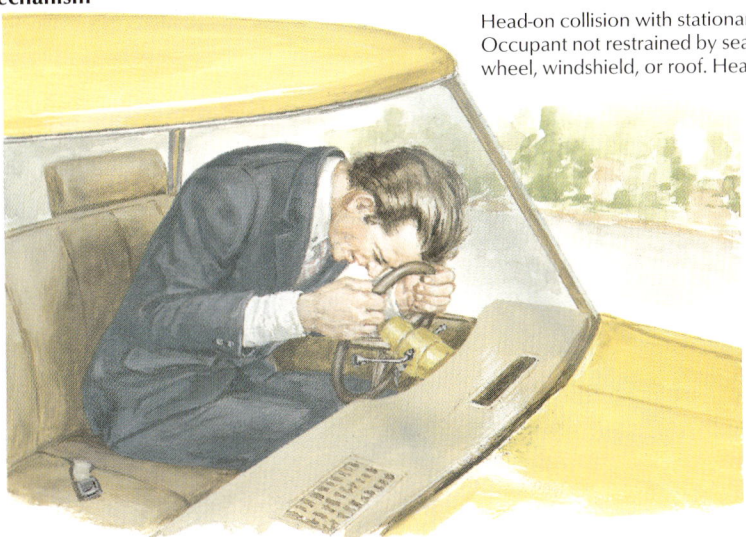

Head-on collision with stationary or moving object. Occupant not restrained by seat belt: head strikes steering wheel, windshield, or roof. Head hyperflexed on trunk.

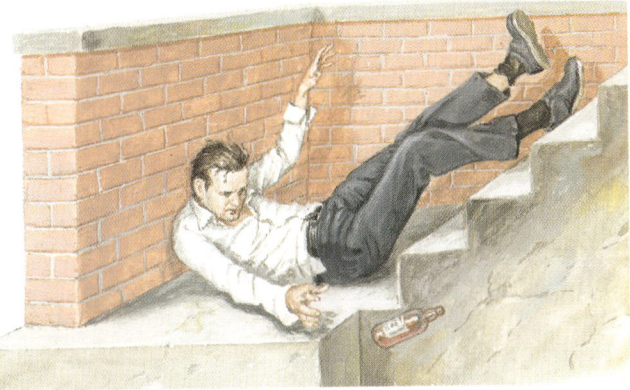

Blow to back of head from falling against hard surface when balance is compromised

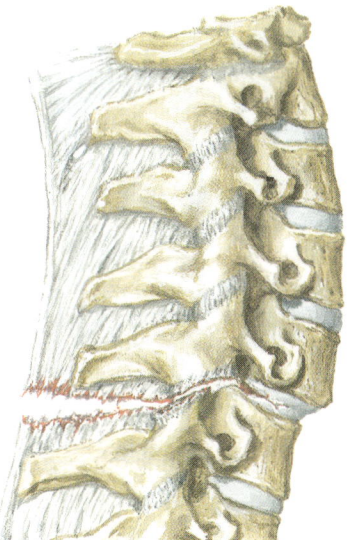

Anterior dislocation of C5-6 with tear of interspinal ligament, facet capsules, and posterior fibers of intervertbral disc

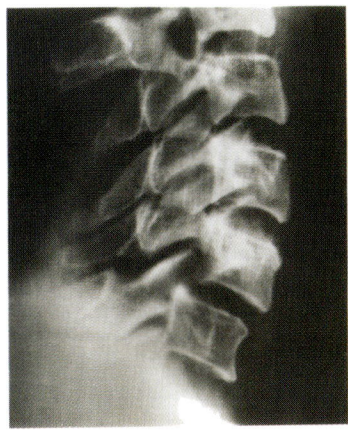

X-ray film (lateral view) showing bilateral interfacet dislocation at C5-6

TRAUMA TO THE BRAIN AND SPINAL CORD

TRAUMA OF THE SPINE AND SPINAL CORD

Figure 76-2   Cervical Spine Injury: Compression

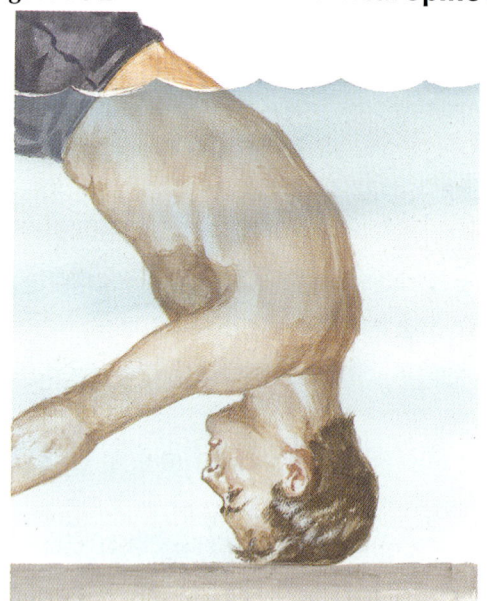
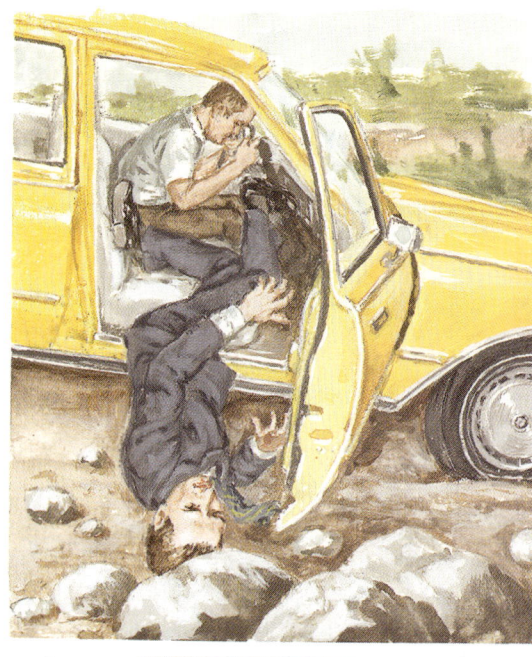

Mechanism. Vertical blow on head as in diving or surfing accident, being thrown from car, or football injury

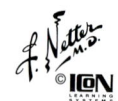

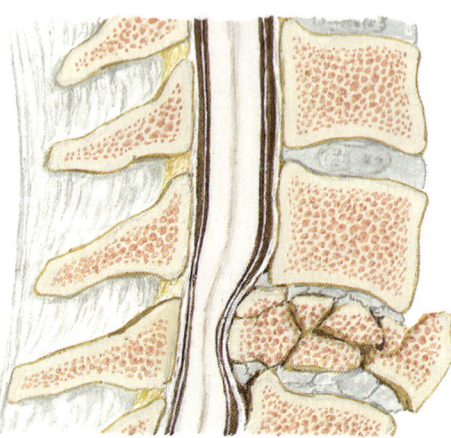

Burst fracture with characteristic vertical fracture through vertebral body

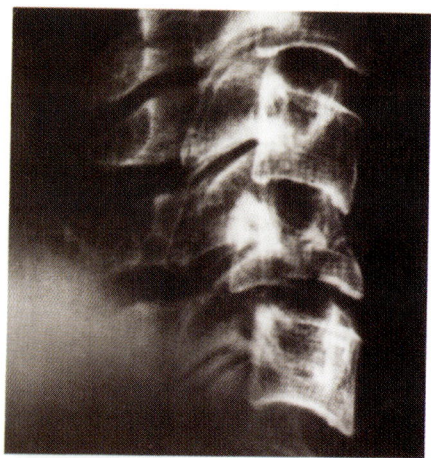

X-ray film showing fracture of C5

More severe trauma explodes vertbral body. Posteriorly displaceed bone fragments frequently produce spinal cord injury.

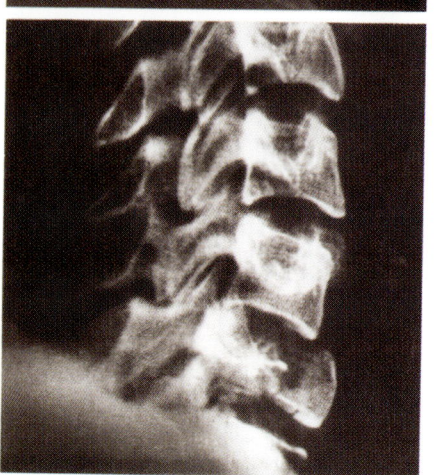

X-ray film showing fracture of C6

TRAUMA TO THE BRAIN AND SPINAL CORD

TRAUMA OF THE SPINE AND SPINAL CORD

Figure 76-3   Cervical Spine Injury: Hyperextension

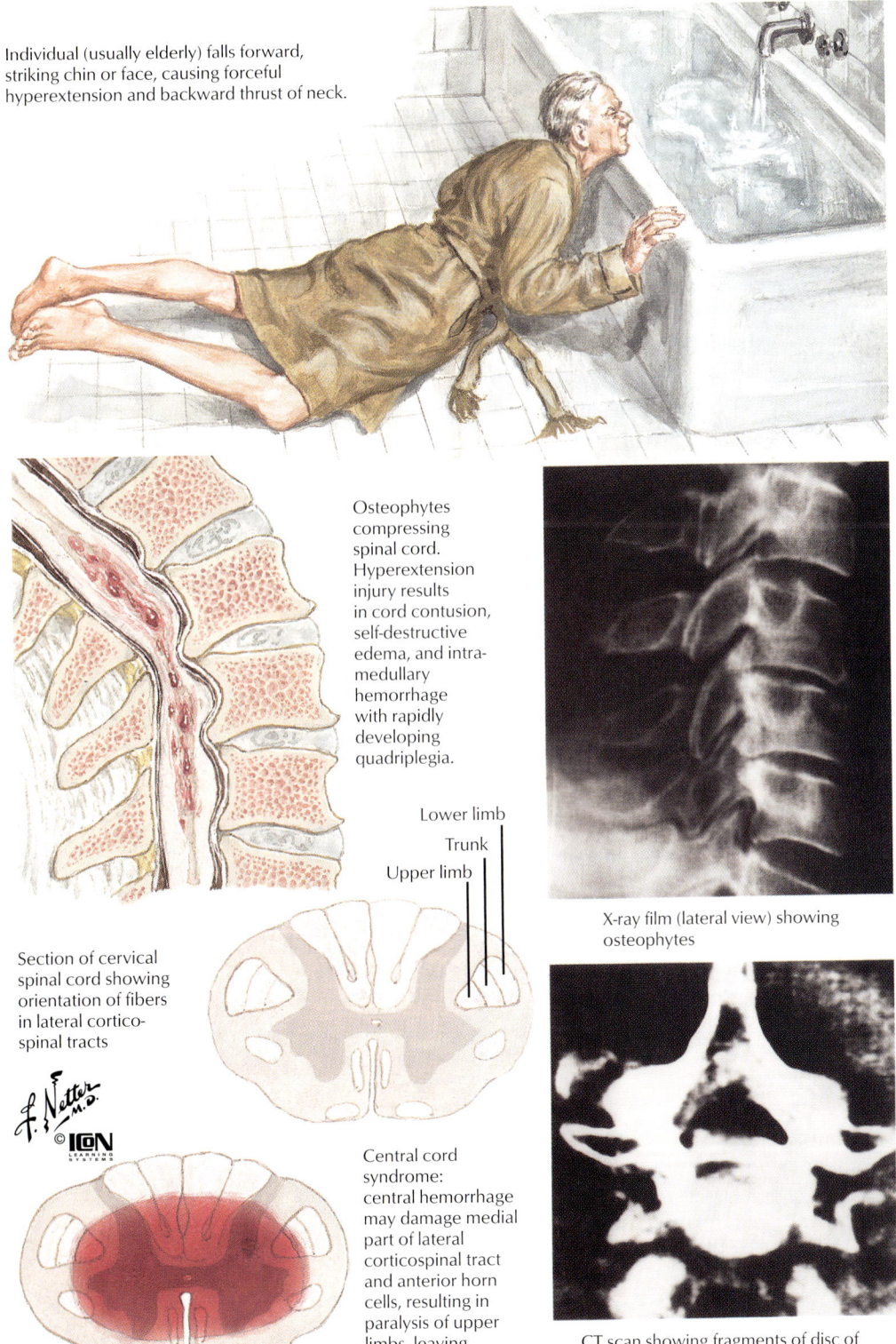

TRAUMA TO THE BRAIN AND SPINAL CORD

normal neurologic examination results, no imaging is necessary. If the patient is alert, with neck pain, tenderness or both and without neurologic deficit, while the neck is immobilized, 3-view radiographs of the cervical spine should be performed: lateral, anteroposterior, and open mouth of the odontoid. It is essential that the spine be visualized from the skull base to the cervicalthoracic junction. Should the imaging not be adequate, thin-cut CT with reconstruction through the questionable areas must be performed. If the head is being scanned, CT must be carried to the upper cervical spine. Most trauma patients require some CT examination. With CT scanning, the spinal examination is rapid, and the reconstruction of the CT data in sagittal, coronal, or any angled plane is so elegant as to be more useful than plain radiographs, especially if the plain spine films are performed using a portable technique in the ED. If portable x-ray examination is not adequate the first time, CT examination is preferable to repeating the plain films.

For patients with neck pain and normal spinal radiographs or CT, it is essential to use dynamic, lateral flexion/extension films or fluoroscopy. Excursion can be performed by patients, if they are cooperative. If patients are not cooperative or are obtunded, they should be kept in a rigid collar until the flexion/extension films can be done passively, by a neurosurgeon, orthopedic spine physician, neuroradiologist, or other experienced trauma physician.

With any neurologic injury, MRI is usually performed before removing the collar or instituting therapy. MRI can demonstrate SCI, pressure on the nerve roots, disc herniation, and ligamentous soft tissue injury. MRI of the obtunded patient will demonstrate ligamentous injury. A negative examination allows removal of the collar support and early mobilization.

Thoracolumbar Spine

For injuries to the thoracic, thoracolumbar, and lumbar spines, plain radiography, CT, and MRI are also used. Plain radiographs may demonstrate bony injuries. However, to see the extent of the fracture and compromise of the spinal canal, CT with reconstruction is the imaging method of choice. With any question of neurologic injury or disc rupture, MRI is mandatory.

TREATMENT

Problems to be addressed are alignment and stability of the spine and compression of neural structures including the spinal cord and individual nerve roots. Treatment begins at the accident scene. EMT personnel are trained to extract injured patients from the accident location, whether it is a motor vehicle, a football helmet, or an awkward position in the bathroom of an elderly person. The spine must be immobilized on a backboard with the neck in a collar, taped to the board (Figure 76-4). This position must be maintained until the entire spine is cleared by appropriate physicians. To prevent secondary SCI, the bony spine must be stabilized. Because of spinal instability, 4% of patients with SCI deteriorate after treatment. Nonoperative stabilizing techniques include a collar, craniocervical traction, a halo, a rotating frame, or a rocking bed (Figure 76-5).

Early mobilization is in patients' best interest and is a primary treatment goal. Deconditioning and morbidity associated with immobility are major drawbacks of bed rest treatment that make patients more susceptible to deep venous thrombosis, pneumonia, and skin deterioration.

When these techniques are not successful, surgery must be considered for spinal misalignment or neural compression. Generally, earlier surgical decompression and stabilization is suggested because, even with complete lesions, it allows for early mobilization and rehabilitation and reduces the morbidity of prolonged bed rest. Early surgery is also suggested for facet fractures to improve nerve root function. Some wait until patients' neurologic recovery has plateaued before surgery. It is generally thought that, regardless of the timing, surgical decompression and fusion provide better neurologic results than nonoperative treatment even after a long delay and whether spinal cord, root function, or both are concerns. However, controversy exists as to whether early surgery improves neurologic function compared with delayed surgery.

Others recommend decompression for those with a central cord syndrome and persistent spinal cord compression. The central cord injury is usually associated with the initial injury, and the persistent compression may not be contributing to the myelopathy.

Corticosteroids

In 1990, the National Acute Spinal Cord Injury Study recommended that patients with acute SCI be treated with a 24-hour course of high-dose methylprednisolone. This protocol became the accepted treatment in the United States. However, those data has been reanalyzed, and the conclusions have been questioned. Several studies demonstrate increased risk of complications with steroid use. In 2002, a consensus concluded that there is insufficient evidence to support steroid treatment as either a standard or a guideline. Corticosteroids are currently recommended as an option "that should be undertaken only with the knowledge that the evidence suggesting harmful side effects is more consistent than any suggestion of clinical benefit."

Surgery

The goals of surgery are 2-fold: to decompress the neural elements and to stabilize the spine. This allows early mobilization. The degree of neural compression may be assessed by CT and MRI. Significant spinal cord or nerve root compression necessitates surgical decompression. The issue of stability can be more difficult to evaluate.

Axial Cervical Spine

In the cervical spine, open mouth odontoid films should show the relation of the lateral masses of C1 with the articular pillars of C2. With C1-2 instability and in the setting of a Jefferson fracture, an axial load injury causes a 4-point fracture of the C1 ring. Treatment, typically involves halo vest immobilization or occipital-cervical fusion (Figure 76-6).

Dens fractures can be type 1 through the dens tip above the transverse ligament, which are rare and may be associated with atlantoaxial instability, necessitating arthrodesis, or type 2, the most common, which occur through the dens base and are usually unstable. Considerable controversy exists regarding treatment of dens fractures. Generally, displacement of more than 6 mm, instability in a halo, and painful nonunion are indications for surgery. Options include anterior odontoid screw placement and posterior C1-2 fusion. Otherwise, treatment consists of immobilization in a halo or hard cervical collar.

Type 3 fractures occur through the body of C2 and are usually stable, healing with immobilization in a hard collar or a halo vest. Surgery is generally reserved for patients with nonunion with immobilization.

Traumatic spondylolisthesis of the axis caused by bilateral fractures of the C2 pars interarticularis, called *hangman's fracture*, is caused by hyperextension and axial loading (Figure 76-7). Type 1 fractures have minimal angulation, less than 3 mm of subluxation, and are considered stable. Treatment involves reduction of the fracture and stabilization in a hard collar or a halo. Type 2 fractures have 4 mm or more of subluxation, are usually unstable, and necessitate reduction and stabilization in a halo. Type 3 fractures involve marked disruption of C2-3 posterior elements and wide subluxation; they are often fatal. They necessitate open reduction and stabilization via C2-3 anterior discectomy and fusion or posterior C1-3 fusion.

Subaxial Cervical Spine

An injury to the anterior elements tends to cause instability in extension, whereas posterior spine injury causes more instability in flexion, particularly when subluxation exceeds 3.5 mm or angulation is greater than 11°. Flexion-extension films showing sagittal plane translation greater than 3.5 mm or rotation greater than 20° also suggest instability. Injuries resulting in stable fractures usually heal well with immobilization in a hard collar. Grossly unstable injuries necessitate surgical stabilization via anterior decompression and fusion, posterior decompression and fusion, or both.

Thoracolumbar Spine

The thoracolumbar spine accounts for most noncervical spinal injuries; 64% of the noncervical spinal fractures occur at the thoracolumbar junction.

PROGNOSIS

Prognosis for improvement is poor with a complete spinal cord lesion. However, partial lesions, with even residual autonomic function, have greater potential for neurologic improvement. SCI is a devastating injury; functional improvement in cases of complete neurologic loss

TRAUMA OF THE SPINE AND SPINAL CORD

Figure 76-4

Suspected Cervical Spine Injury: Treatment at Site of Accident

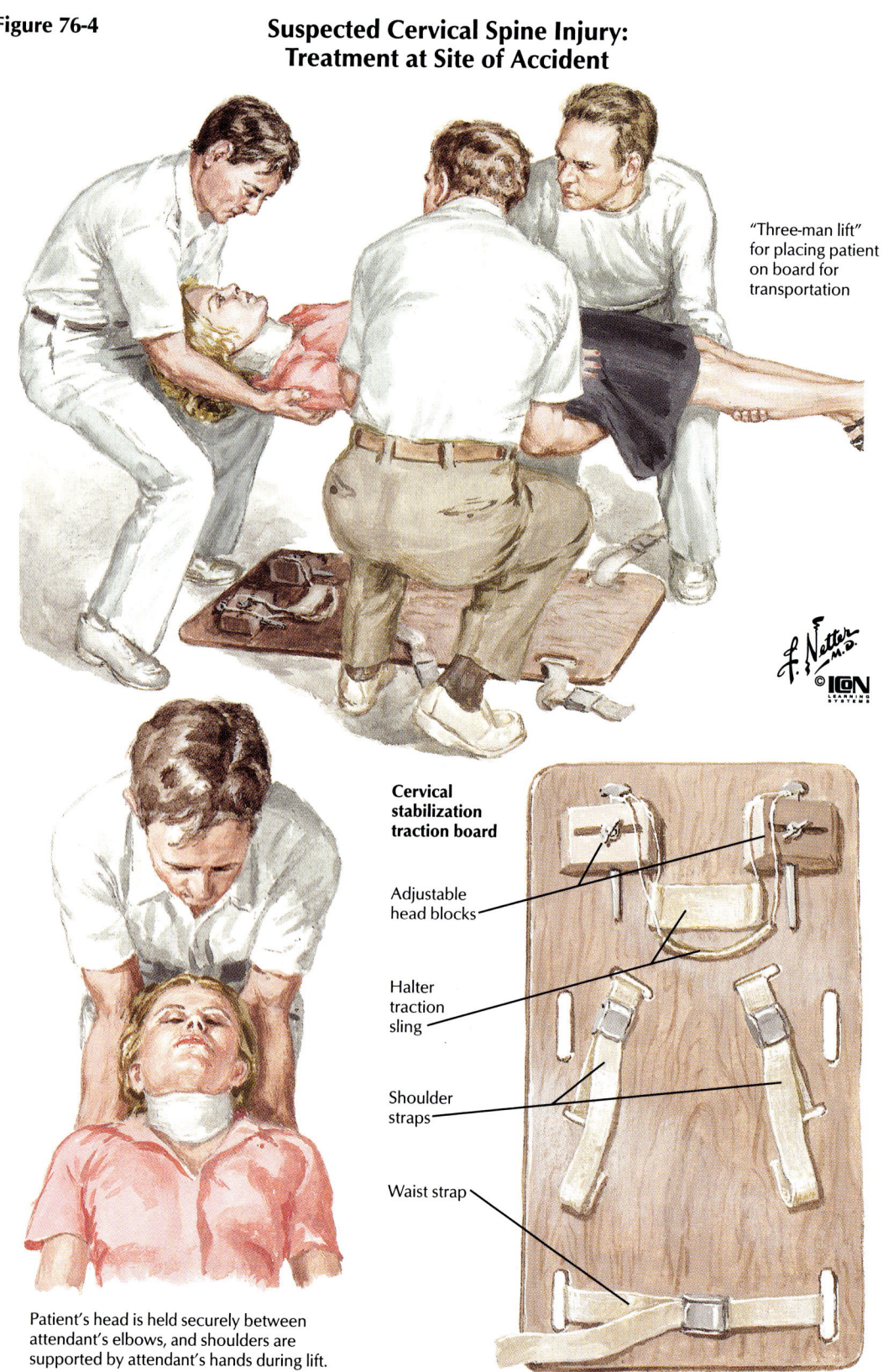

"Three-man lift" for placing patient on board for transportation

Cervical stabilization traction board

Adjustable head blocks

Halter traction sling

Shoulder straps

Waist strap

Patient's head is held securely between attendant's elbows, and shoulders are supported by attendant's hands during lift.

TRAUMA TO THE BRAIN AND SPINAL CORD

TRAUMA OF THE SPINE AND SPINAL CORD

Figure 76-4

Surgical Spine Injury: Treatment at Site of Accident (continued)

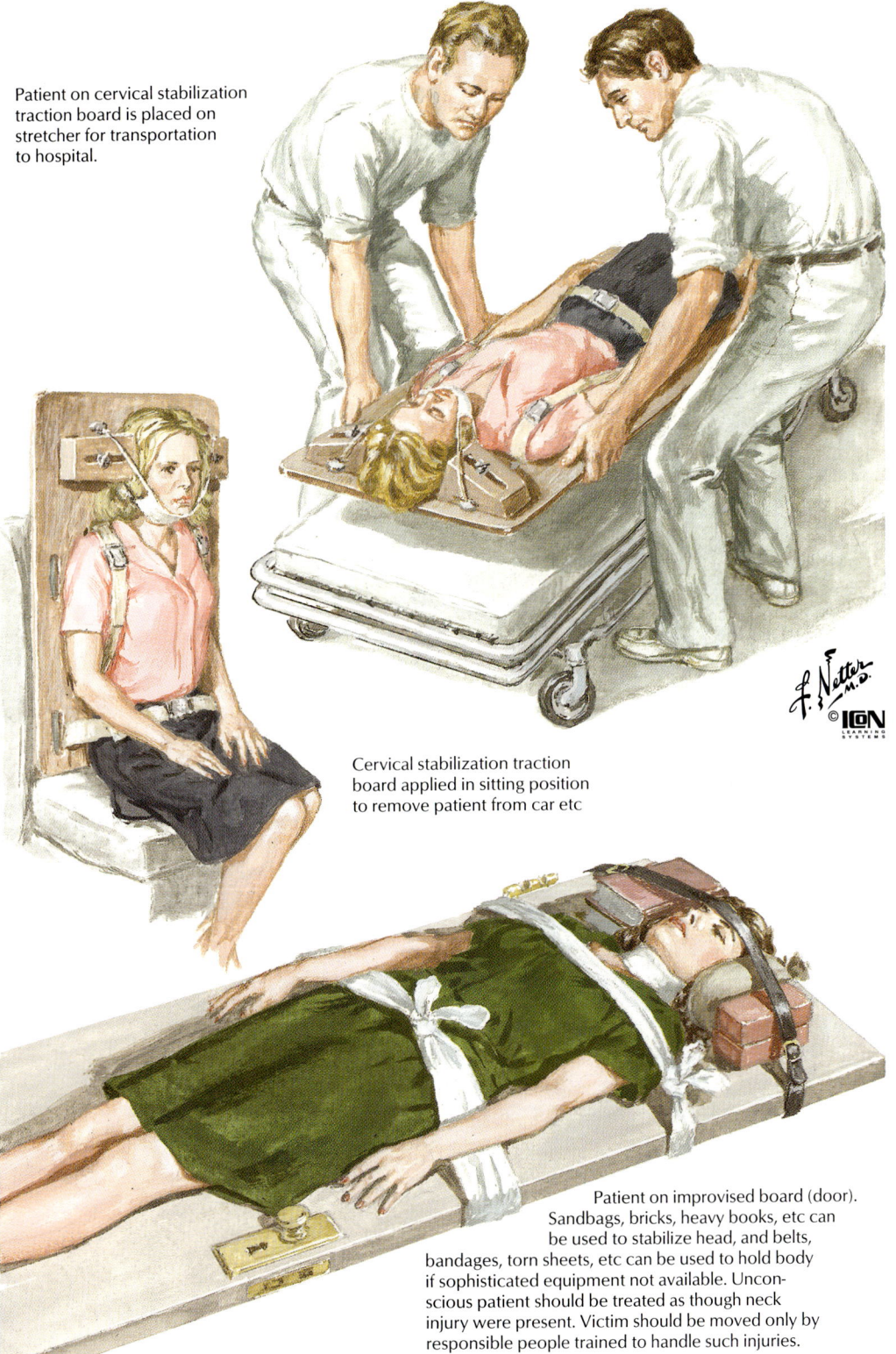

Patient on cervical stabilization traction board is placed on stretcher for transportation to hospital.

Cervical stabilization traction board applied in sitting position to remove patient from car etc

Patient on improvised board (door). Sandbags, bricks, heavy books, etc can be used to stabilize head, and belts, bandages, torn sheets, etc can be used to hold body if sophisticated equipment not available. Unconscious patient should be treated as though neck injury were present. Victim should be moved only by responsible people trained to handle such injuries.

TRAUMA TO THE BRAIN AND SPINAL CORD

TRAUMA OF THE SPINE AND SPINAL CORD

Figure 76-5

Cervical Spine Injury: Traction and Bracing

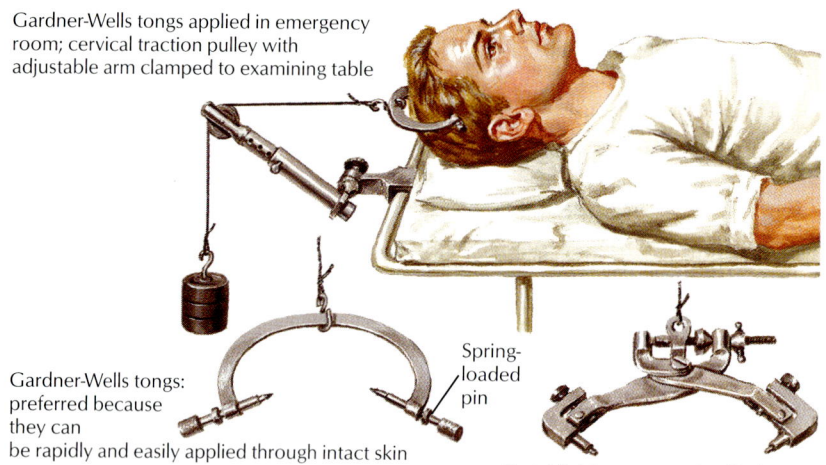

Gardner-Wells tongs applied in emergency room; cervical traction pulley with adjustable arm clamped to examining table

Gardner-Wells tongs: preferred because they can be rapidly and easily applied through intact skin

Spring-loaded pin

Crutchfield tongs: require skin incision and drill holes in skull for application

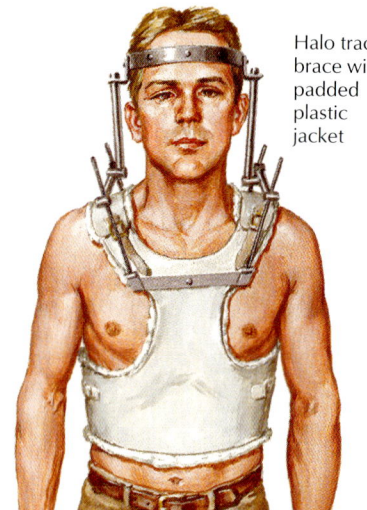

Halo traction brace with padded plastic jacket

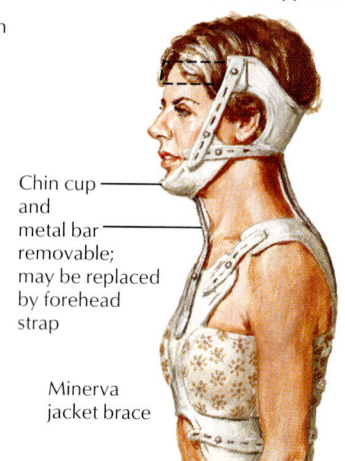

Chin cup and metal bar removable; may be replaced by forehead strap

Minerva jacket brace

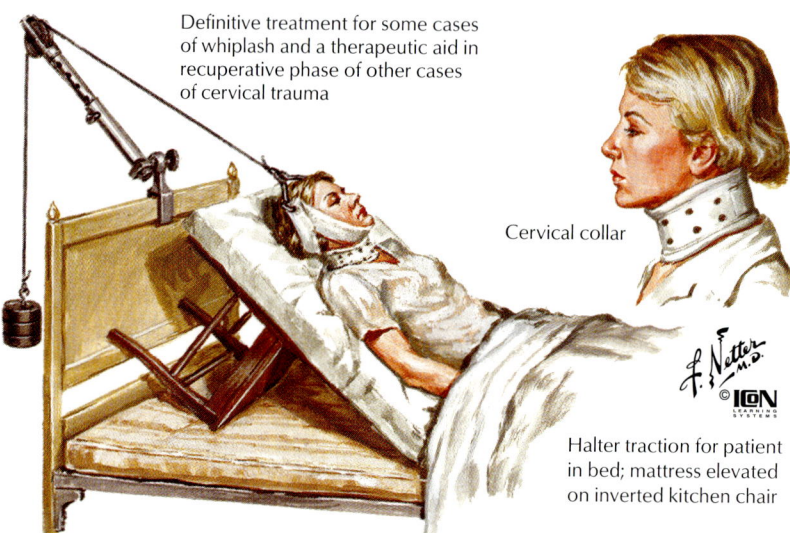

Definitive treatment for some cases of whiplash and a therapeutic aid in recuperative phase of other cases of cervical trauma

Cervical collar

Halter traction for patient in bed; mattress elevated on inverted kitchen chair

TRAUMA OF THE SPINE AND SPINAL CORD

Figure 76-6 ## Wiring of Cervical Spinous Processes

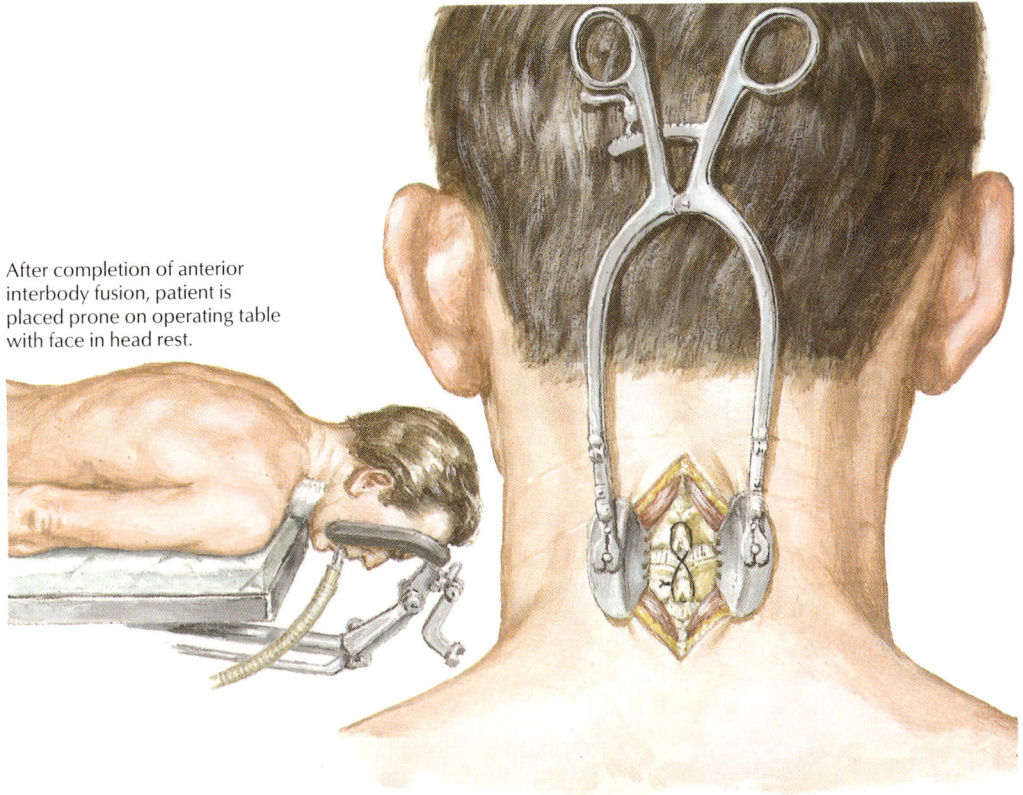

After completion of anterior interbody fusion, patient is placed prone on operating table with face in head rest.

Two spinous processes exposed through small incision using self-retaining retractor, and secured with figure-8 wire

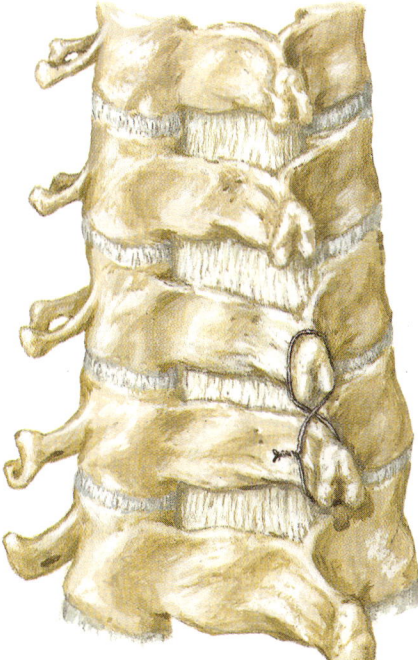

Enlarged view showing wire passed around spinous processes and twisted securely for additional stabilization of anterior interbody fusion

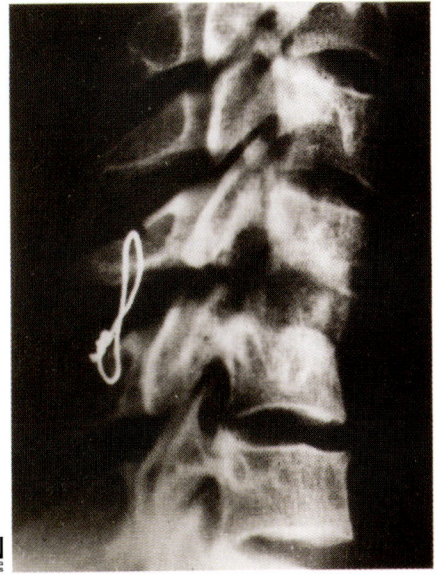

Postoperative x-ray film after dowel fusion and wiring of spinous processes for 3rd-degree dislocation of C5. Here, the wire was passed through the 6th spinous process instead of around it.

TRAUMA TO THE BRAIN AND SPINAL CORD

TRAUMA OF THE SPINE AND SPINAL CORD

Figure 76-7 **Fracture and Dislocation of Cervical Vertebrae**

Fracture of odontoid process
- Type I. Fracture of tip
- Type II. Fracture of base or neck
- Type III. Fracture extends into body of axis

Superior articular facet
Inferior articular facet

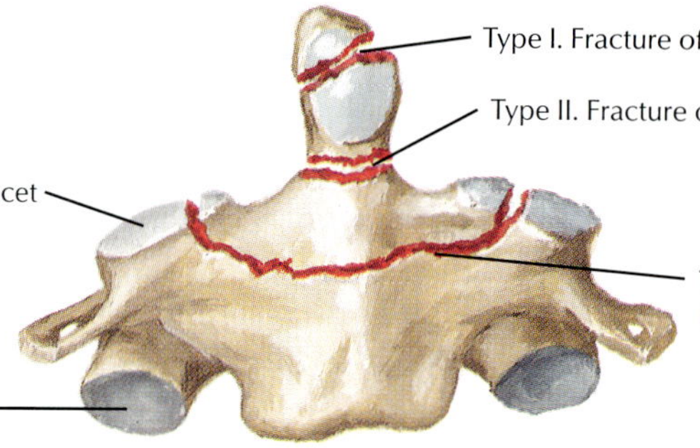

Jefferson fracture of atlas (C1)
Each arch may be broken in 1 or more places

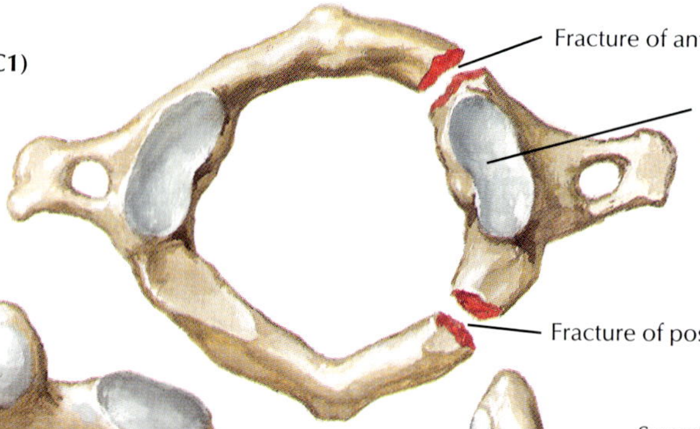

- Fracture of anterior arch
- Superior articular facet
- Fracture of posterior arch

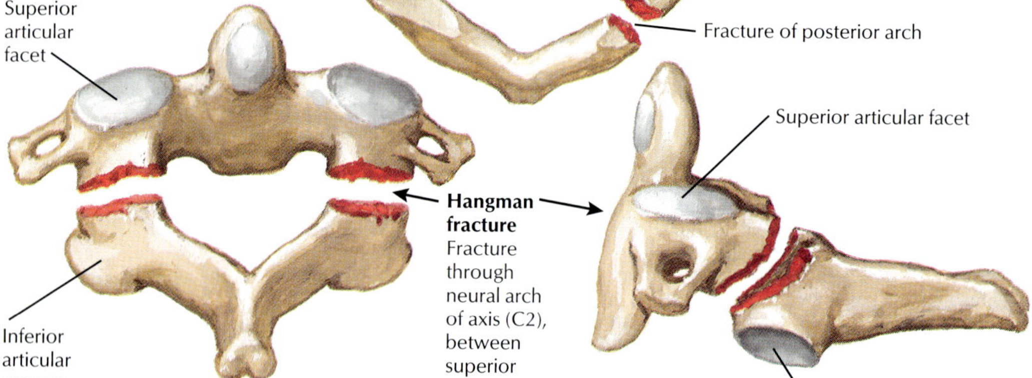

Superior articular facet
Inferior articular process

Hangman fracture
Fracture through neural arch of axis (C2), between superior and inferior articular facets

Superior articular facet
Inferior articular facet

Superior view

C6
C5

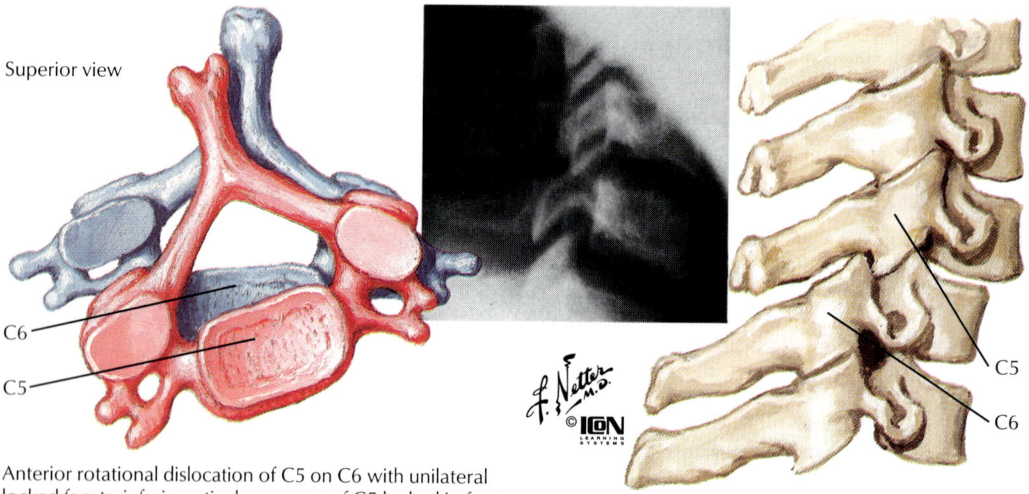

Anterior rotational dislocation of C5 on C6 with unilateral locked facets; inferior articular process of C5 locked in front of superior articular process of C6

C5
C6

Lateral view

TRAUMA TO THE BRAIN AND SPINAL CORD

TRAUMA OF THE SPINE AND SPINAL CORD

Cervical Spine Injury: Rehabilitation of Patient

Figure 76-8

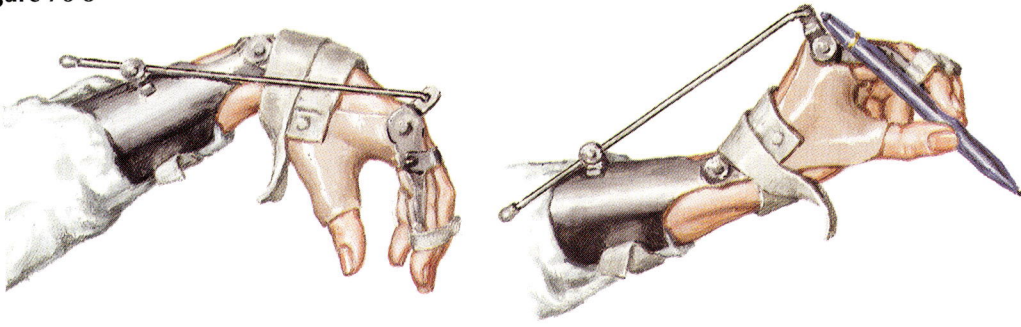

Functional wrist orthotic device aids in prehension and in maintaining metacarpophalangeal alignment. Extension of wrist opposes fingers to thumb, providing grasping action.

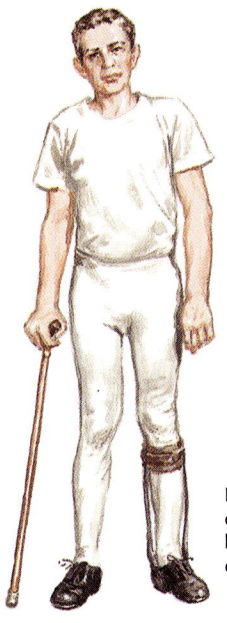

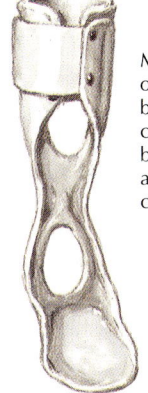

Molded polypropylene orthotic device preferred by many patients to conventional braces because of lighter weight and more pleasing cosmetic appearance

Paraplegic girl wearing full-length lower limb braces, facilitating ambulation by "swing-through" gait

Patient wearing conventional double-metal upright below-knee brace for weakness of foot dorsiflexors and evertors

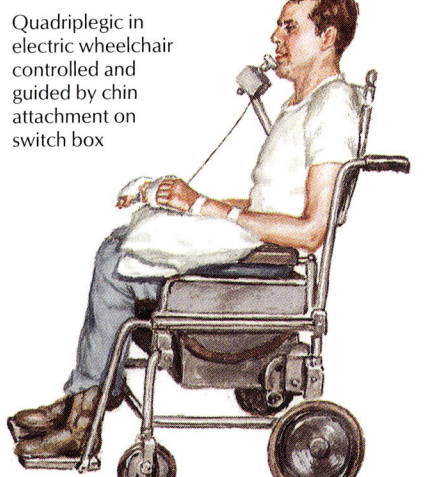

Quadriplegic in electric wheelchair controlled and guided by chin attachment on switch box

Pegs on hand rim of wheelchair allow patient with paralyzed lower limbs and weak upper limbs to grasp rim and push more easily.

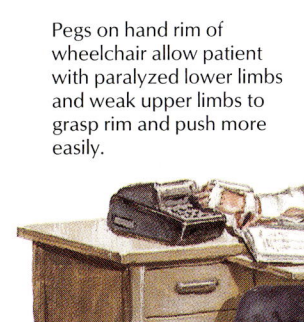

TRAUMA TO THE BRAIN AND SPINAL CORD

relates to rehabilitation rather than anatomical regeneration (Figure 76-8).

One case of neurologic improvement 5 years after a clinically complete C2 SCI has been attributed to patterned neural activity. Perhaps stem cell research will discover a means to bypass the injured spinal segment and reestablish communication between the brain and peripheral structures.

REFERENCES

D'Alise MD, Benzel EC, Hart BL. Magnetic resonance imaging evaluation of the cervical spine in the comatose or obtunded trauma patient. *J Neurosurg (Spine)*. 1999;91:54-59.

Guidelines for the management of acute cervical spine and spinal cord injuries. *Neurosurgery* (suppl) 50 (No 3), Section on Disorders of the Spine and Peripheral Nerves of the American Association of Neurological Surgeons and the Congress of Neurological Surgeons.

Hadley MN, Fitzpatrick BC, Sonntag VKH, Browner CM. Facet fracture-dislocation injuries of the cervical spine. *Neurosurgery*. 1992;30:661-666.

Hugenholtz H. Methylprednisolone for acute spinal cord injury: not a standard of care. *Can Med Assoc J*. 2003;168:1145.

Kilburn MPB, Hadley MN. Contemporary treatment paradigms in spinal injury. *Clin Neurosurg*. 2000;46:153-169.

Maiman DJ, Barolat G, Larson SJ. Management of bilateral locked facets of the cervical spine. *Neurosurgery*. 1986;18:542-547.

Marshall LF, Knowlton S, Garfin SR, et al. Deterioration following spinal cord injury. *J Neurosurg*. 1987;66:400-404.

McDonald JW, Becker D, Sadowsky CL, Jane JA, Conturo TE, Schultz LM. Late recovery following spinal cord injury. *J Neurosurg (Spine)*. 2002;97:252-265.

Pasqual M, Fabian TC. Practice management guidelines for trauma from the Eastern Association for the Surgery of Trauma. *J Trauma*. 1998;44:945-946.

Sonntag VKH, Francis PM. Patient selection and timing of surgery: contemporary management of spinal cord injury. *American Association of Neurological Surgeons*. 1995:97-107.

Section XVIII
RADICULOPATHIES

Chapter 77
Cervical Radiculopathy 672

Chapter 78
Lumbar Radiculopathy 679

Chapter 79
Lumbar Spinal Stenosis 691

Chapter 80
Rheumatologic, Functional, and Psychosomatic Back Pain 694

Chapter 77
Cervical Radiculopathy

Subu N. Magge and Stephen R. Freidberg

Clinical Vignette

A 57-year-old man presented with a 3-week history of increasingly severe neck pain with radiation to the right scapula and posterior arm. He had mild numbness with tingling in the index and middle fingers while noting difficulty fully extending his arm. There were no myelopathic symptoms. During the previous 3 years, he had experienced similar intermittent pain and numbness. Neurologic examination demonstrated significant right triceps muscle weakness and an absent right triceps muscle stretch reflex.

MRI demonstrated a herniated disc at C6-7. An anterior cervical discectomy and fusion at C6-7 provided immediate relief of his radicular pain. The weakness improved to almost normal within 4 months.

This vignette presents the classic history of recurrent C7 nerve root irritation. Often, this resolves with conservative therapy. However, as in with this case, increasingly severe pain and unresolved weakness are the 2 major indications for operative intervention.

Cervical radiculopathy, related to pressure on a cervical nerve root, is a common clinical problem. It affects most adult age groups but is uncommon in adolescents and children. Symptoms may be relatively minor and chronic, or acute pain can be associated with weakness and sensory disturbance. Although cervical root symptoms often begin spontaneously, clinical presentation less frequently begins with a specific incident such as a mild twist, carrying a heavy briefcase, or significant acute trauma.

CLINICAL PRESENTATION

Symptoms of a cervical radiculopathy depend on the specific root involved (Figure 77-1). Simultaneous multiple nerve root compression is unusual. Neck or interscapular pain commonly accompanies cervical root compression; occasionally, shoulder or arm pain is present. Evidence of arm weakness and sensory disturbances are typical clinical findings. Frequently, neck movement exacerbates the pain radiating into the arm, often with an electriclike sensation. With pressure on the spinal cord as well as the nerve root, evidence of myelopathy may be present. In any patient with cervical radiculopathy, clinical examination requires evaluation for evidence of myelopathy.

C5 is the least frequent cervical radiculopathy level. Because it exits the spine between C4 and C5, its compression of this nerve root produces pain radiating into the medial scapula and the upper arm, which rarely goes beyond the elbow. Muscle weakness manifests as difficulty performing tasks with the arm elevated. Sensory loss is either mild, primarily affecting the shoulder, or unnoticed by the patient. Therefore, some individuals present only with limited arm abduction.

One of the most common cervical nerve roots affected is C6, which exits the spine between C5 and C6. Typical pain with C6 compression occurs at the medial scapula, frequently radiating into the arm and the lateral hand. Motor loss overlaps that occurring from C5 root irritation with weakness in the proximal arm muscles, particularly with difficulty flexing the arm and sometimes abducting the arm at the shoulder. Classic paresthesias are experienced in the thumb and index finger.

The most common cervical radiculopathy affects the C7 nerve root, which exits the spine between C6 and C7. Typically, its compression leads to pain in the posterior arm. Unlike in C5 and C6 lesions, C7 usually has little functional overlap with other roots. C7 innervates the triceps muscle, which extends the elbow. Unless patients perform activities such as rowing or

CERVICAL RADICULOPATHY

Figure 77-1   Dermatomes and Myotomes of Upper Limb

Note: Schematic demarcation of dermatomes (according to Keegan and Garrett) shown as distinct segments. There is actually considerable overlap between adjacent dermatomes. An alternative dermatome map is that provided by Foerster.

A. C2 to T1 Sensory Representation

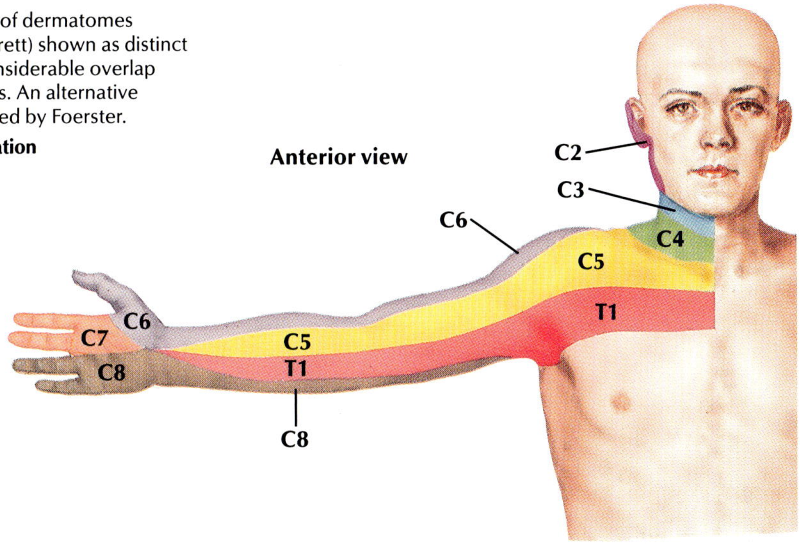

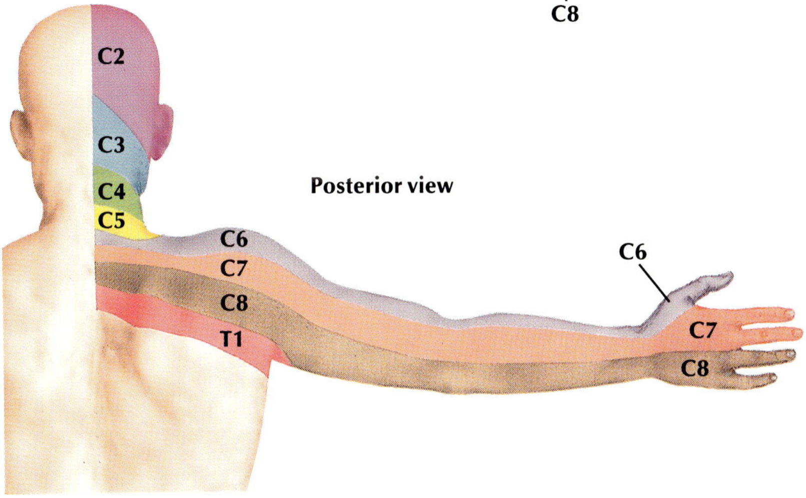

B. Motor Impairment Related to Level of Cervical Root Lesion

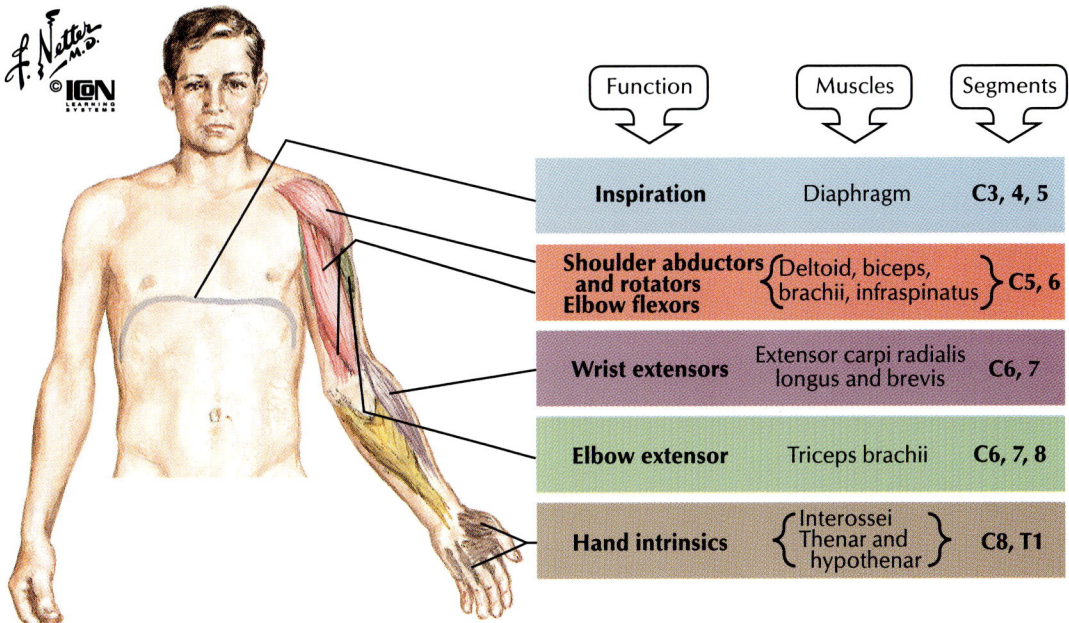

Function	Muscles	Segments
Inspiration	Diaphragm	C3, 4, 5
Shoulder abductors and rotators / Elbow flexors	Deltoid, biceps, brachii, infraspinatus	C5, 6
Wrist extensors	Extensor carpi radialis longus and brevis	C6, 7
Elbow extensor	Triceps brachii	C6, 7, 8
Hand intrinsics	Interossei, Thenar and hypothenar	C8, T1

RADICULOPATHIES

CERVICAL RADICULOPATHY

push-ups, many individuals are not aware of their significant triceps weakness. Gravity extends the elbow in most cases. Paresthesias and sensory loss are typically experienced in the index and middle fingers.

The lowest of the cervical roots, C8, exits between the C7 and T1 vertebrae. When it is affected, pain radiates from the neck into the medial arm and forearm. Paresthesiae affect the fourth and fifth fingers. Patients may have significant weakness of intrinsic hand function with sensory loss appropriate to the paresthesias.

The temporal profile is crucial to obtain during the history because it helps in diagnostic and therapeutic decisions. Has there been slow progression or rapid worsening? Has there been a plateau or improvement in the condition? How long have the symptoms persisted? Pain quality and provocative factors are also important. Does the arm pain worsen with neck movement? Is the pain of an electric quality? These symptoms are characteristic of root compression. A Tinel phenomenon with palpation of the axilla or supraclavicular fossa could be associated with extraspinal or brachial plexus tumors.

Concomitant with cervical radiculopathy symptoms, neurologic signs provide confirmation of the specific nerve root involved (Figure 77-1 and Table 77-1). Because of the overlap between C5 and C6, weakness of the supraspinatus and infraspinatus are seen with lesions of either root. However, the deltoid is more specific for C5, and the biceps brachii is more specific for C6. In contrast, the C7 and C8 roots have little overlap, with the C7 primarily affecting the triceps muscle and the C8 primarily affecting the intrinsic hand muscles. A careful physical examination must include a search for causes of pain other than cervical root compression.

DIFFERENTIAL DIAGNOSIS

Many pathologic conditions affect the cervical spine and require consideration. Radiculopathies secondary to herniated cervical discs are the most common cause (Figure 77-2). Degenerative encroachment of the neural foramina by spondylosis is also common. Although an experienced physician may assume that the patient with neck and arm pain and neurologic symptoms has a disc herniation, a tumor or vertebral infection can present similarly.

A metastatic extradural tumor is the most common neoplasm of the cervical spine. The typical sites of origin are lung, breast, prostate, and plasmacytoma. Although statistically less common, intradural extramedullary tumors, schwannomas and meningiomas, fall within the differential diagnosis. Intramedullary lesions originating within the spinal cord substance, including primary tumors or syringomyelia, do not usually present with symptoms mimicking a radiculopathy but rather a myelopathy (chapters 59-61). MRI greatly aids in the diagnosis.

Spinal infection, particularly epidural abscesses, has increased in frequency. They are related to sepsis associated with infection in the skin, other wounds, or urinary tract and dental manipulation. Drug abusers have a particularly high incidence. Typical presentation includes significant spinal discomfort and nerve root pain. Myelopathic signs signal a condition more severe than cervical radiculopathy.

Brachial plexus neoplasms, invading or less commonly arising within the medial brachial plexus, occasionally mimic a C8 radiculopathy. These occur with occult superior sulcus apical lung tumors, either cancer or lymphoma. Schwannomas are the most common primary nerve tumors arising within the brachial plexus.

Table 77-1
Cervical Roots

Root	Motor Weakness	Sensory Loss	Reflex Loss
C5	Deltoid	Small patch lateral shoulder	None
C6	Biceps	Thumb, index finger	Biceps and brachioradialis
C7	Triceps	Index and middle fingers	Triceps
C8	Intrinsic muscles of hand	Fourth and fifth fingers	None

CERVICAL RADICULOPATHY

Figure 77-2   Cervical Disc Herniation: Clinical Manifestations

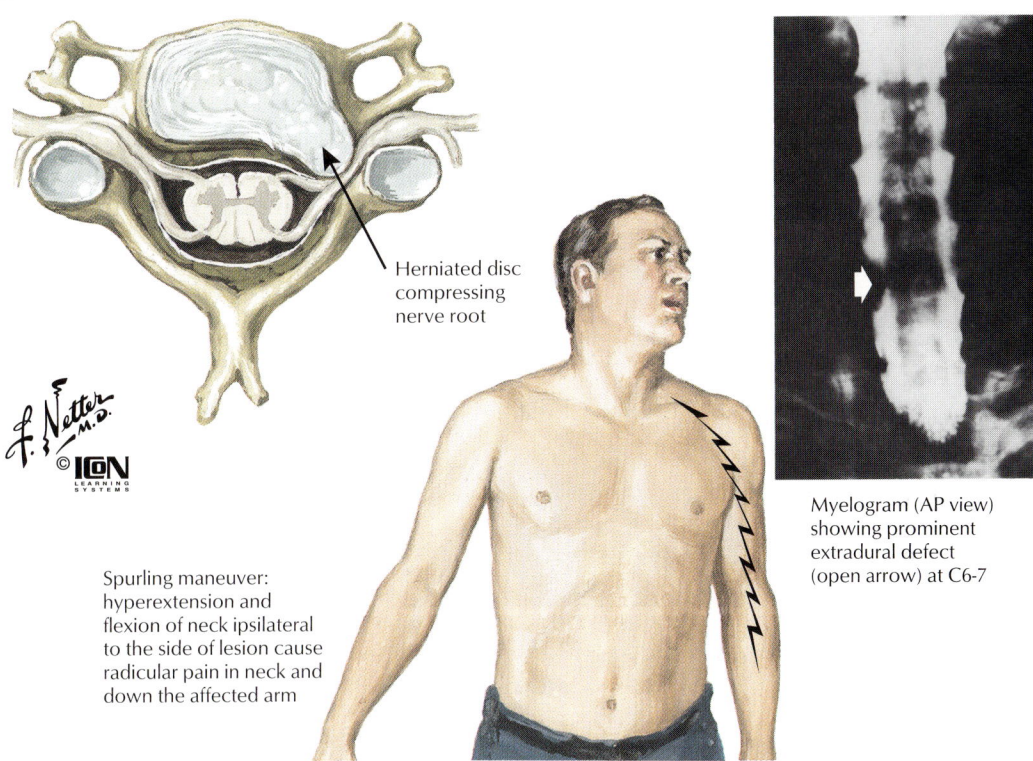

Spurling maneuver: hyperextension and flexion of neck ipsilateral to the side of lesion cause radicular pain in neck and down the affected arm

Myelogram (AP view) showing prominent extradural defect (open arrow) at C6-7

Level	Motor signs (weakness)	Reflex signs	Sensory loss
C5	Deltoid	0	
C6	Biceps brachii	Biceps brachii — Weak or absent reflex	
C7	Triceps brachii	Triceps brachii — Weak or absent reflex	
C8	Interossei	0	

RADICULOPATHIES

CERVICAL RADICULOPATHY

Primary brachial plexitis may mimic a C5 radiculopathy (chapter 81). The differential diagnosis also includes ulnar neuropathy or the rare thoracic outlet syndrome.

DIAGNOSTIC APPROACH

Because 80% of patients with cervical radiculopathy improve spontaneously, imaging is frequently deferred. However, MRI is initially important for patients with unusual presentations and those who are not improving. The use of imaging depends on the clinical setting. All available modalities are required for various situations. The evaluation of the patient referred with symptoms of a potential cervical radiculopathy whose previous accompanying abnormal images do not correlate with the clinical picture necessitates caution. It is common for asymptomatic or minimally symptomatic persons to have significant MRI or CT myelogram findings that are of no clinical consequence. The images and clinical findings must correlate if surgical treatment is to be considered.

Although frequently omitted, **plain spinal radiographs** often have significant diagnostic value. In particular, "**spine films**" provide excellent visualization of the degree of spondylosis, disc degeneration, or, of even greater importance, increased kyphosis. Flexion and extension lateral views are particularly valuable for demonstrating abnormal movement between the vertebrae.

MRI is the imaging modality of choice for most conditions affecting the cervical spine and spinal cord (Figure 77-3). Nerve root compression caused by spondylosis or disc herniation is usually clearly defined, as are intrinsic spinal cord pathologies. MRI is particularly useful in the setting of acute spinal cord compression. Tumors within the bone or epidural space and intradural tumors with their relation to the nerve root and spinal cord are clearly demonstrated. Extramedullary tumors usually readily enhance with gadolinium. Intramedullary tumors are often difficult to differentiate from primary demyelinating myelopathies. A bright signal in the spinal cord noted on the T2-weighted image indicates an injury to the cord.

As a primary imaging modality, **spinal CT** has limited value. However, it is useful for patients unable to have MRI because of cardiac pacemakers or claustrophobia. Additionally, a "reconstructed" CT is invaluable in understanding complex bony deformities of the spine.

Myelography, in conjunction with CT scanning, remains a valuable diagnostic modality when MRI is not possible. Also, MRI is occasionally not technically adequate. A myelogram with postmyelogram CT can adequately demonstrate nonfilling of nerve root sleeves or direct nerve root compression. It may also reveal pressure on or deformity of the spinal cord. CT can also demonstrate ossification of the posterior longitudinal ligament, another potentially pathologic condition. Although some institutions rarely use myelography, it can add valuable data.

TREATMENT AND PROGNOSIS

Treatment of cervical radiculopathy depends on the patient's initial clinical status. The usual temporal profile of cervical radiculopathy caused by disc herniation or foraminal narrowing is of spontaneous improvement in up to 80% of patients within 1 to 3 months. Because most cases improve spontaneously, early imaging and active treatment are rarely needed unless there is history of recent trauma or initial signs of a concomitant myelopathy. Acute cases can be treated with restriction of heavy activity, particularly anything that exerts tension on the cervical nerve roots and worsens the pain secondary to muscular spasms, eg, carrying a heavy briefcase, reaching into closed spaces, or even driving a vehicle with frequent neck movement and straining; patients can be scheduled for reexamination in a few weeks. Occasionally, a benzodiazepine muscle relaxant, an NSAID, or both are also used. Usually, these modalities are successful. This conservative management compares favorably with a host of other treatments including traction, acupuncture, chiropractic, and massage. The good results of these conservative modalities probably owe their success to the overall benign natural history of cervical radiculopathies in many individuals.

For patients whose pain is severe and does not improve and for those with significant neurologic deficit including a myelopathy, imaging is requested. Where appropriate, surgery is performed.

CERVICAL RADICULOPATHY

Figure 77-3   **Cervical Disc Herniation**

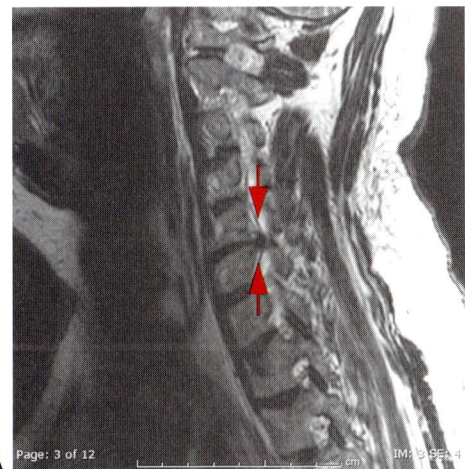
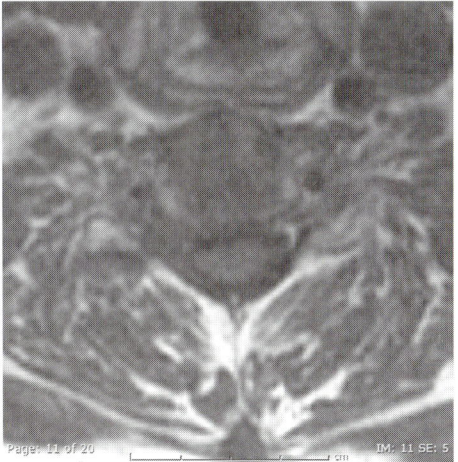
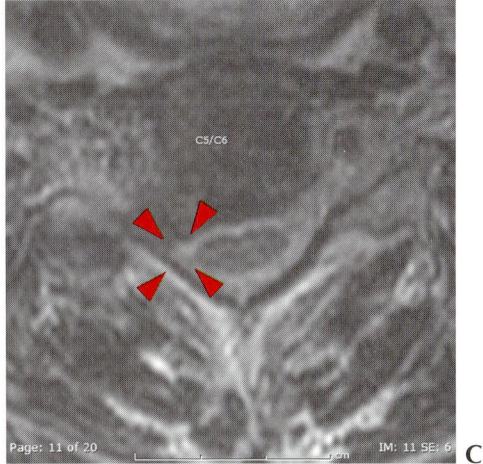

(**A**) Right sagittal T2-weighted image shows small disc herniation at C5-6 (thin arrows). Axial T1-weighted (**B**) and T2-weighted (**C**) images show a small mass in the right lateral recess (arrowheads).

Spine surgeons differ on the best approach—anterior or posterior—to the ruptured cervical disc because treatment can be satisfactory from either. Although more uncomfortable for the patient, a posterior medial facetectomy is preferred for a lateral disc herniation, with nerve root elevation and disc removal. Exposure of the nerve root by facetectomy does not require fusion and, therefore, prevents the late problems of fusion that may occur with anterior discectomy. The less common midline disc herniations causing cord or root symptoms, or both, are more safely decompressed via an anterior approach. Because significant risk exists for development of a postoperative kyphotic deformity, disc space height and overall cervical lordosis should be preserved by combining anterior decompressive surgery with fusion.

When imaging demonstrates diagnoses other than either a ruptured cervical disc or degenerative disorders, eg, a tumor or infection, the treatment can be tailored appropriately. In the near future, replacement of the degenerative disc with an artificial disc may become an important therapeutic option.

REFERENCES

Boutsen Y, De Coene B, Hanson P, Deltombe T, Gilliard C, Esselinckx W. Axillary schwannoma masquerading as cervical radiculopathy. *Clin Rheumatol.* 1999;18:174-176.

Celli P. Treatment of relevant nerve roots involved in nerve sheath tumors: removal or preservation? *Neurosurgery.* 2002;51:684-692.

Ellenberg MR, Honet JC, Treanor WJ. Cervical radiculopathy. *Arch Phys Med Rehabil*. 1994;75:342-352.

Freidberg SR, Pfeifer BA, Dempsey PK, et al. Intraoperative computerized tomography scanning to assess the adequacy of decompression in anterior cervical spine surgery. *J Neurosurg (Spine 1)*. 2001;94:8-11.

Misamore GW, Lehman DE. Parsonage-Turner syndrome (acute brachial neuritis). *J Bone Joint Surg Am*. 1996;78:1405-1408.

Shafaie FF, Wippold FJ II, Gado M, Pilgram TK, Riew KD. Comparison of computed tomography myelography and magnetic resonance imaging in the evaluation of cervical spondylotic myelopathy and radiculopathy. *Spine*. 1999;24:1781-1785.

Sundaresan N, Rothman A, Manhart K, Kelliher K. Surgery for solitary metastases of the spine: rationale and results of treatment. *Spine*. 2002;27:1802-1806.

Tay BK, Deckey J, Hu SS. Spinal infections. *J Am Acad Orthop Surg*. 2002;10:188-197.

Wainner RS, Gill H. Diagnosis and nonoperative management of cervical radiculopathy. *J Orthop Sports Phys Ther*. 2000;30:728-744.

Wilson DW, Pezzuti RT, Place JN. Magnetic resonance imaging in the preoperative evaluation of cervical radiculopathy. *Neurosurgery*. 1991;28:175-179.

Wirth FP, Dowd GC, Sanders HF, Wirth C. Cervical discectomy: a prospective analysis of three operative techniques. *Surg Neurol*. 2000;53:340-346.

Chapter 78
Lumbar Radiculopathy

Stephen R. Freidberg and Subu N. Magge

Clinical Vignette

A 47-year-old man had a long history of occasional, severe episodes of low back pain. They usually occurred 1 to 2 times per year after activities such as shoveling snow or playing basketball with his teenagers. Treatment included muscle relaxants, simple analgesics, and instruction to "take it easy." He had never lost work because of these episodes.

Three weeks previously, he was awakened with severe left sciatic pain radiating from his lumbar spine to his buttock, down the back of his left leg to his ankle. The pain was improved by lying down. Sitting or bending forward in attempt to put his socks on was the most uncomfortable position. He limped when he walked, and a scoliosis leaning toward the right had developed. He had no subjective weakness but reported a burning sensation on the foot's lateral aspect, sole, and heel. Coughing or straining produced an electric sensation along the sciatic nerve. He had not slept or been able to work since the onset. He was not improving.

Physical examination demonstrated a positive straight leg sign on the left, normal muscle strength, an absent left ankle reflex, and altered sensation on the lateral aspect of the foot. MRI of the lumbar spine revealed a large extruded disc fragment on the left at L5-S1 with pressure on the S1 nerve root. Because of the severe unremitting pain and MRI findings, surgical decompression was recommended. A microhemilaminectomy was performed, the disc was removed, and the nerve root was decompressed. The patient left the hospital with no sciatic pain the next morning. He returned to work at home in 2 days and to his office pain free in 1 week.

This vignette describes a typical course for a healthy individual with an extruded disc. Although the patient had previously improved with conservative therapy, the persistence and severity of his pain, documented by MRI, necessitated surgical repair.

Lumbar radiculopathy, frequently called *sciatica*, is one of the most common afflictions, typically affecting 1% of the population per year. Most individuals with sciatica experience some degree of low back pain. These symptoms are a major cause of disability and the primary cause of workers' compensation disability in the United States.

CLINICAL PRESENTATION

Sciatic pain may occur acutely or evolve more gradually, sometimes exacerbated from a long-standing problem. When the onset is sudden, it may be spontaneous or related to a specific incident, sometimes seemingly a relatively trivial event, such as bending over to make a bed, or even sleeping. The symptoms may be minor and clinically inconsequential or significant, necessitating urgent evaluation and treatment.

Depending on the specific nerve root involved, the pain may be classic sciatica with radiation down the posterior aspect of the leg into the foot, as noted with compression of the L5 or S1 roots (Figure 78-1). At higher levels, L3 or L4, the pain may radiate to the anterior thigh.

There may or may not be associated neurologic signs. Like symptoms, the signs of lumbar radiculopathy are related to the specific level of involvement (Table 78-1). The most common levels involved are L5 and S1 roots; L4 and L3 radiculopathies are less common. It is rare to have involvement of the higher roots (L1 and L2).

Because the spinal cord ends between L1 and L2, the nerve root compressed depends on whether the lesion is medial in the spinal canal or lateral in the neural foramen. The exiting root passes around the pedicle with the same designated number, cephalad to the disc space. A lesion occurring at the disc space in the spinal canal compresses the passing root, the root with the next lower number. For example, a medial disc rupture in the spinal canal at L4-5 will compress the L5 root, whereas the disc rupturing lat-

LUMBAR RADICULOPATHY

Figure 78-1A   Lumbar Disc Herniation: Clinical Manifestations

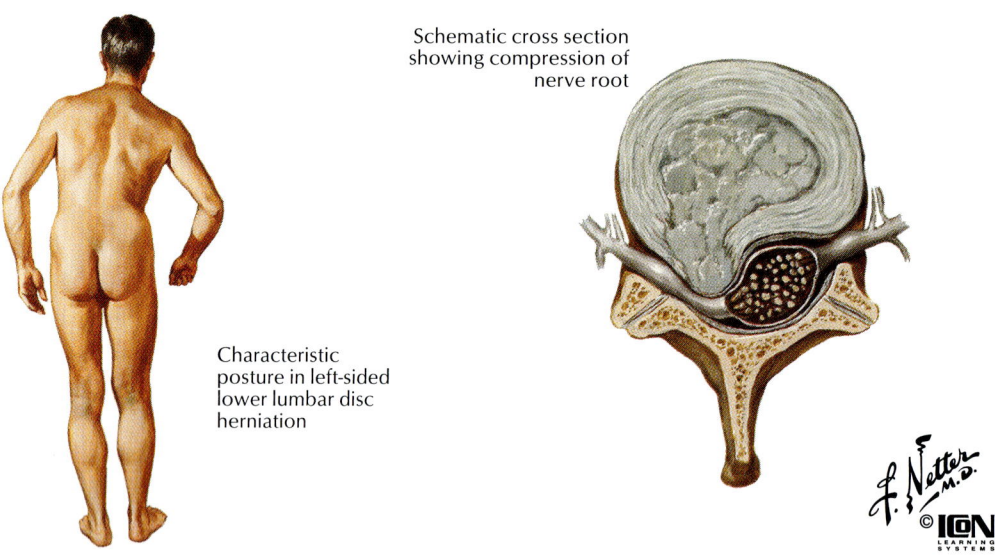

LUMBAR RADICULOPATHY

Figure 78-1B Examination of Patient With Low Back Pain

A. Standing

Body build
Posture
Deformities
Pelvic obliquity
Spine alignment
Palpate for:
   muscle spasm
   trigger zones
   myofascial nodes
   sciatic nerve tenderness
Compress iliac crests
for sacroiliac
tenderness

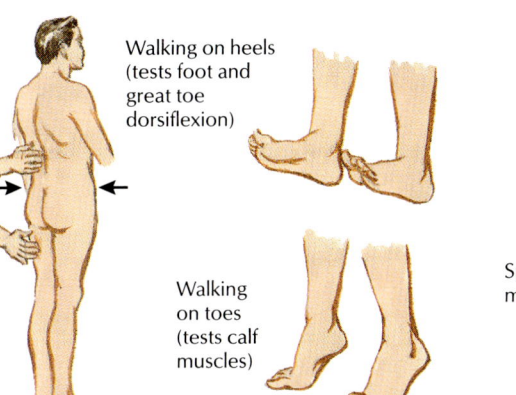

Walking on heels (tests foot and great toe dorsiflexion)

Walking on toes (tests calf muscles)

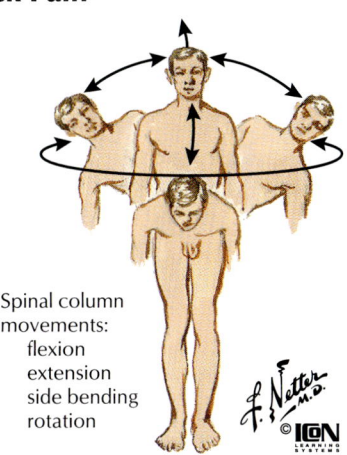

Spinal column movements:
   flexion
   extension
   side bending
   rotation

B. Kneeling on chair

Ankle jerk

Sensation on calf and sole

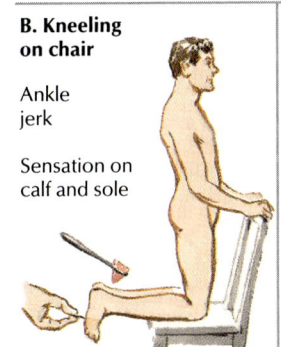

C. Seated on table

Straight leg raising

Knee jerk

Measure calf circumference

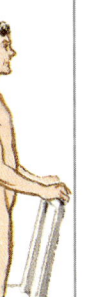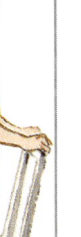

D. Supine

Straight leg raising: flex thigh on pelvis and then extend knee with foot dorsiflexed (sciatic nerve stretch)

Palpate abdomen; listen for bruit (abdominal and inguinal)

Palpate for peripheral pulses and skin temperature

Palpate for flattening of lumbar lordosis during leg raising

Measure leg lengths (anterior superior iliac spine to medial malleolus) and thigh circumferences

Test sensation and motor power

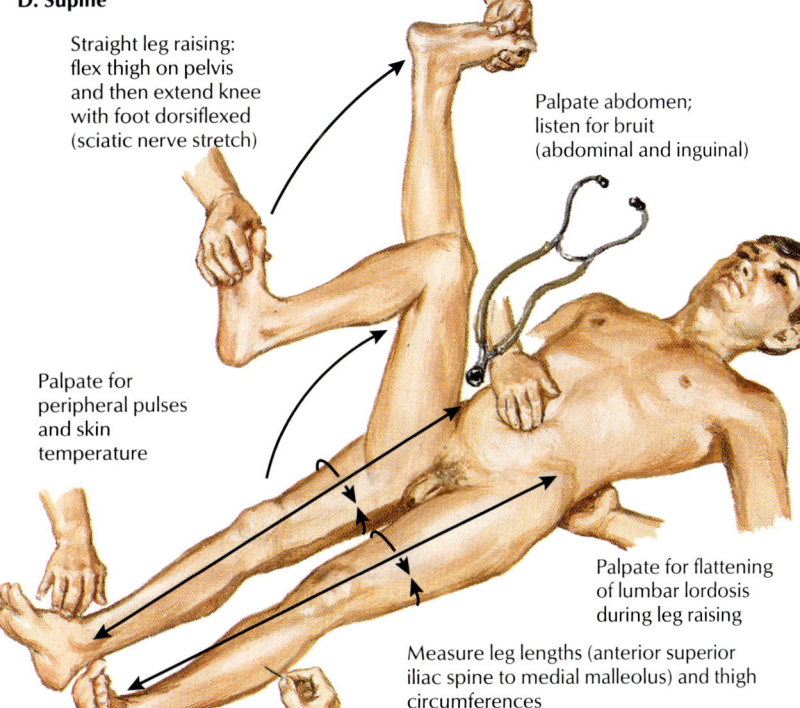

E. Prone

Spine extension

Test for renal tenderness

Palpate for local tenderness or spasm

Femur extension

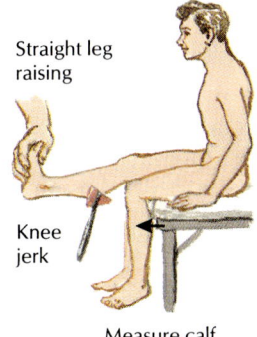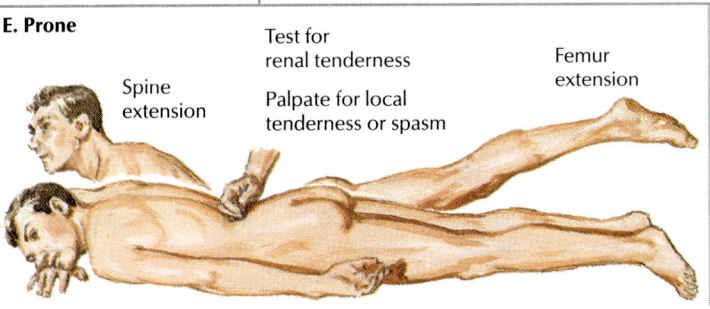

F. Rectal and/or pelvic examination

G. MRI and/or CT and/or myelogram of
1. lumbosacral spine
2. abdomen/pelvis

H. Laboratory studies
Serum Ca^{2+} and PO_4^{-}, alkaline phosphatase, acid phosphatase (males over 40), CBC, ESR, and urinalysis

RADICULOPATHIES

LUMBAR RADICULOPATHY

Table 78-1
Nerve Root Signs of Lumbar Radiculopathy

Root	Motor Weakness	Sensory Loss	Muscle Stretch Reflexes
L3	Iliopsoas/quadriceps	Anterior thigh	KJ diminished but still present
L4	Quadriceps	Anterior thigh to below knee	KJ absent
L5	Tibialis anterior	Dorsum and medial foot	Internal hamstring
S1	Gastrocnemius	Lateral aspect of foot, sole, and heel	AJ absent

eral in the neural foramen will compress the L4 root.

DIFFERENTIAL DIAGNOSIS
Herniated Lumbar Disc

The most frequent cause of lumbar radiculopathy is a herniated lumbar disc, usually occurring with an equal frequency at the lowest 2 levels, L4-5 and L5-S1 (Figures 78-2 and 78-3). Only approximately 5% of lumbosacral herniations occur at higher levels. Herniation is the last manifestation of disc degeneration that is an ongoing process in all humans. Hence, disc herniation is uncommon in youth, although occasionally teenagers and rarely toddlers have symptomatic herniations. It is less common in the very elderly but does occur. Herniation is occasionally seen with spinal stenosis and may be the cause of rapid deterioration in those cases.

Most lumbar radiculopathies are unilateral and related to the mechanical issues germane to a single herniated nucleus pulposus. Thus bilateral sciatica has more ominous significance, suggesting compression of the cauda equina and not just a single nerve root. These patients are at serious risk for loss of sphincter functions as well as potency in males. Early recognition is essential, as even after expeditious decompression, sphincter control and potency may not always return. Although most cases of lumbar radiculopathy are caused by disc rupture, an extensive differential diagnosis cannot be overlooked. For example, spondylosis with foraminal encroachment resulting from disc degeneration is a common cause of radiculopathy.

Spinal Stenosis

Spinal stenosis is becoming more prevalent with the increasingly aged population (Figure 78-4). It may occur at one or frequently multiple spinal levels. Unlike the classic lumbosacral radiculopathies, it rarely affects L5-S1 unless one vertebral body is subluxated on the next.

Patients typically report an exercise-precipitated neurogenic claudication–type anterior thigh or sciatic pain. Neurologic examination is usually normal. MRI is the diagnostic modality of choice. Surgical decompression is usually successful (see chapter 79).

Spondylolisthesis

Spondylolisthesis, the anterior slippage of the superior vertebral body with respect to the inferior, is another common cause of lumbar root and low back pain. The misalignment entraps roots in the neural foramen. It may cause significant stenosis at the affected level, leading to a combination of cauda equina compression with exiting nerve root symptoms and findings. The 2 common causes of spondylolisthesis involve spinal degenerative (spondylotic) changes and congenital defects of the vertebral pars interarticularis. Patients with degenerative spondylolisthesis tend to be older. Those with a pars defect usually present in their third or fourth decade of life with significant lumbar and root pain, usually related to postural change. Neurologic deficits are rarely associated with spondylolisthesis.

Synovial Cysts

Relatively uncommon, synovial cysts may produce symptoms identical to disc herniation. The cysts develop from hypertrophy of synovial tissue in the facet joint. Neurosurgeons sometimes encounter these cysts pushing into the paraspinal muscles when reflecting them for exposure of the spine. In this location, they indicate degenerative joint disease, but by themselves,

LUMBAR RADICULOPATHY

Figure 78-2 — Pain Patterns in Lumbar Disease

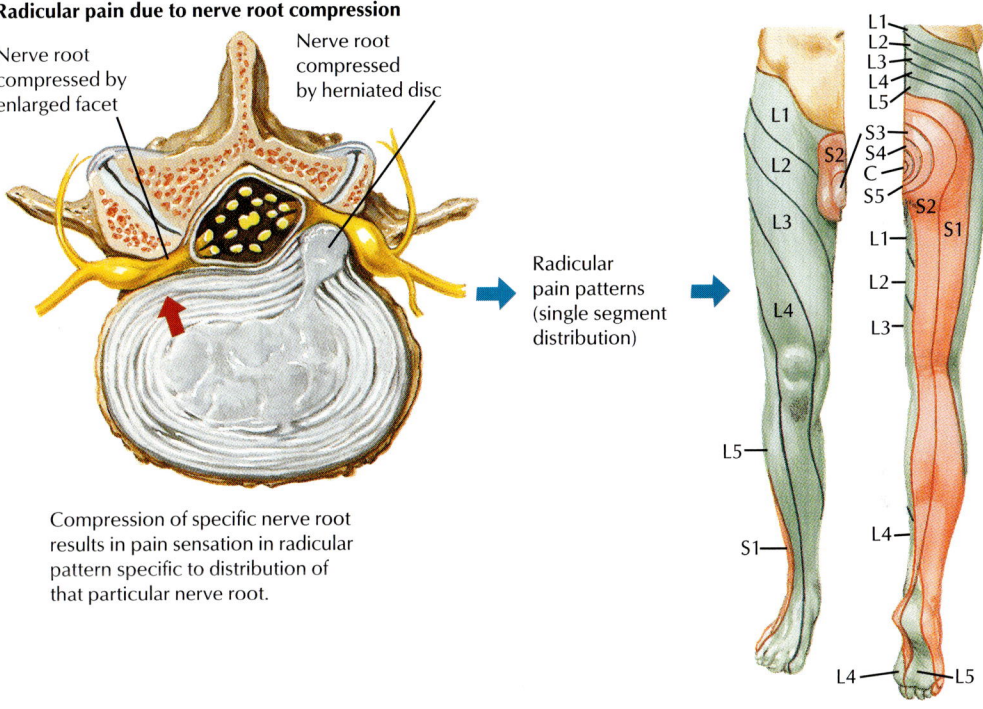

Radicular pain due to nerve root compression

Compression of specific nerve root results in pain sensation in radicular pattern specific to distribution of that particular nerve root.

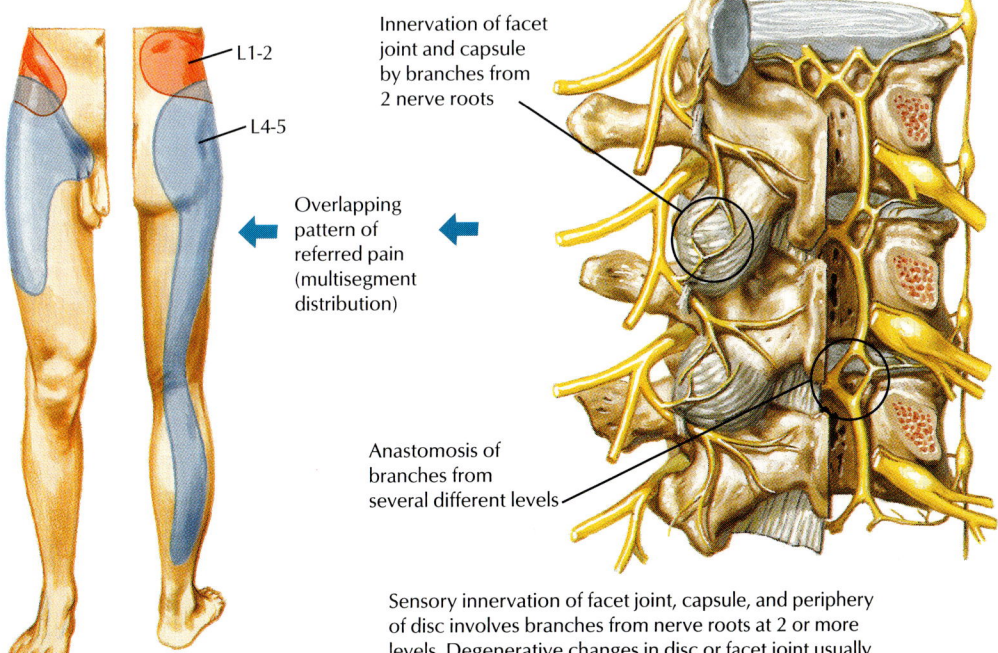

Nonradicular, referred pain due to facet or disc disease

Sensory innervation of facet joint, capsule, and periphery of disc involves branches from nerve roots at 2 or more levels. Degenerative changes in disc or facet joint usually cause overlapping pattern of referred pain.

RADICULOPATHIES

LUMBAR RADICULOPATHY

Figure 78-3 Role of Inflammation in Lumbar Pain

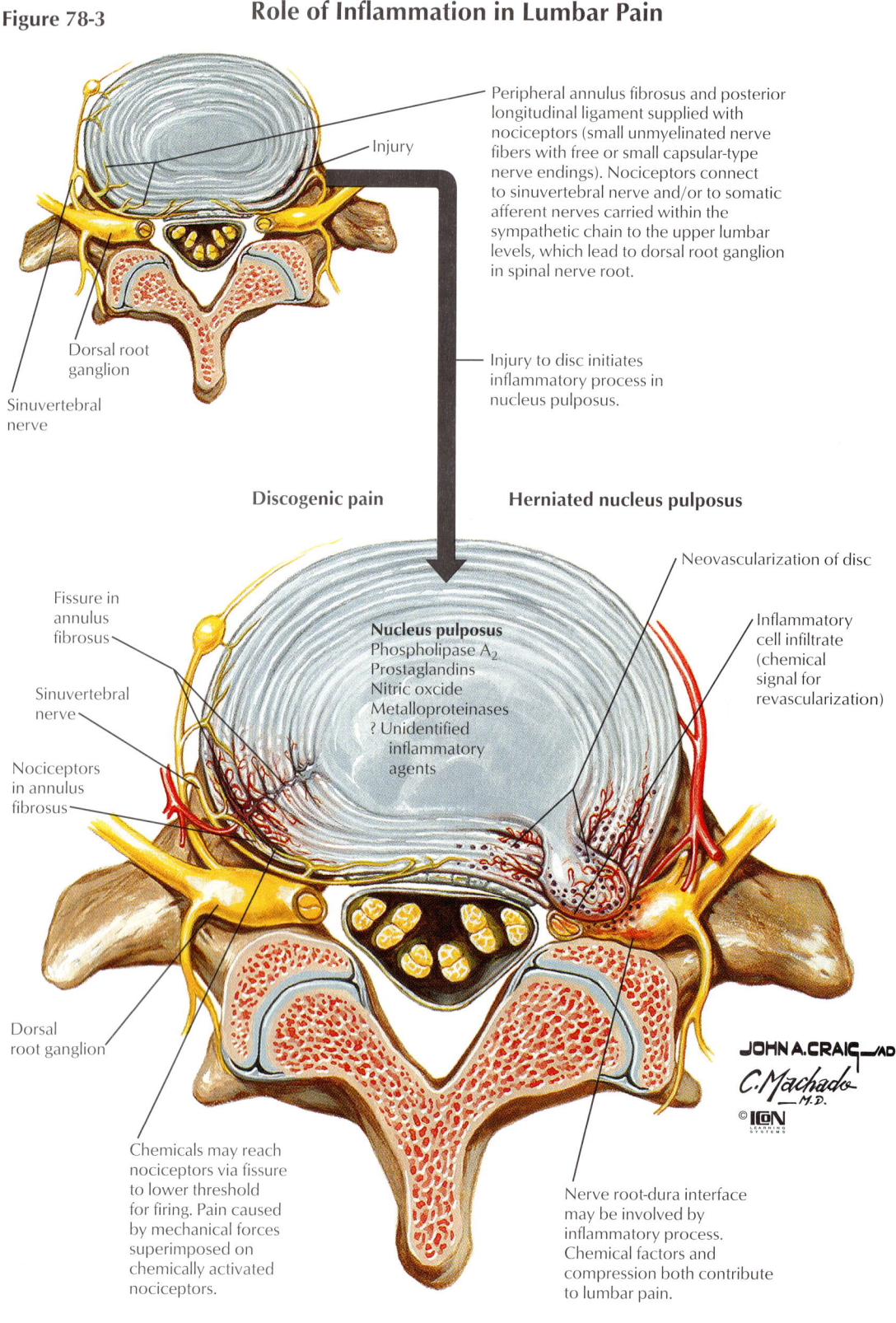

LUMBAR RADICULOPATHY

Figure 78-4

L4-5 Disc Extrusion

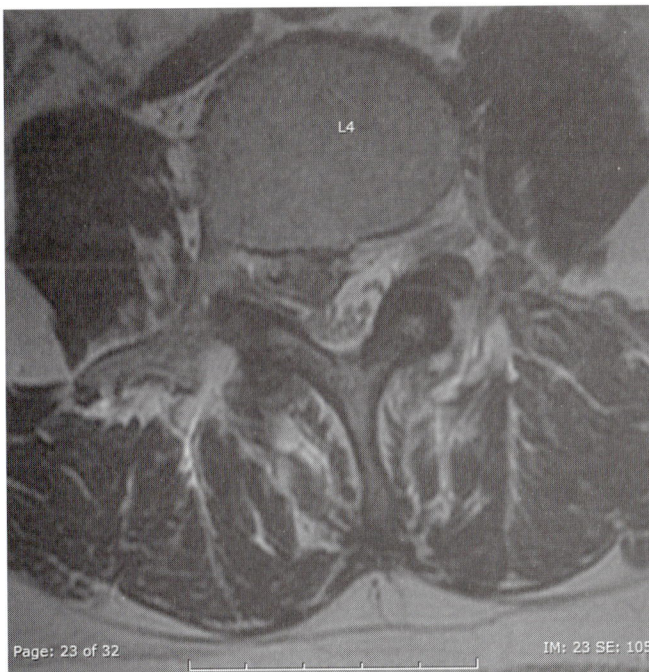
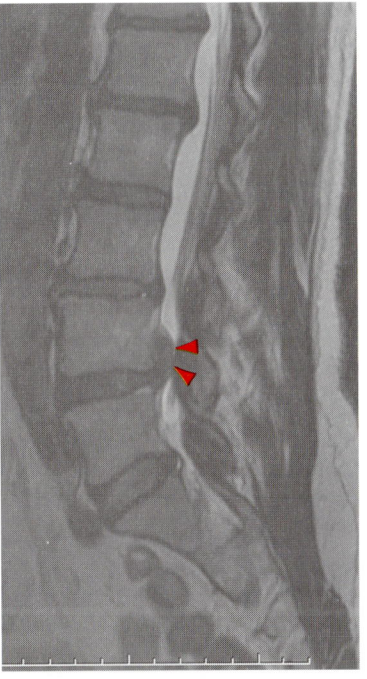
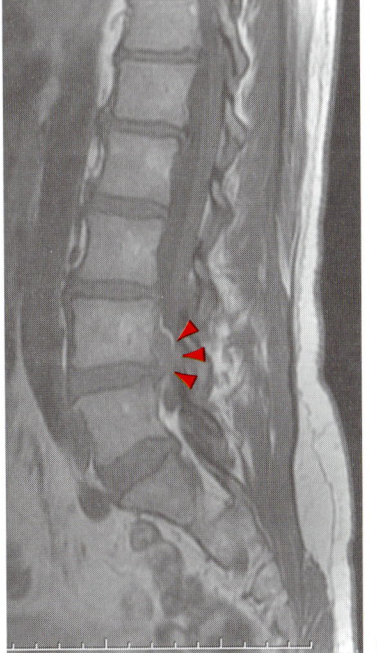

(**A**) Axial T2-weighted image at L4 shows large hypointense mass in the right lateral recess and foramen. (**B** and **C**) Right center T2 and sagittal images show mass extending cephalad from the L4-5 disc (arrowheads).

RADICULOPATHIES

LUMBAR RADICULOPATHY

they are not symptomatic. When cysts become intraspinal, they compress the nerve root. Unlike herniated discs, synovial cysts create an inflammatory reaction and must be carefully dissected free from the dura of the nerve roots. Resection of lumbar epidural synovial cysts usually relieves patients' pain.

Epidural Infection

Epidural infections can occur secondary to disc surgery or via hematogenous spread. Unlike metastatic tumors that primarily involve the vertebral bodies, abscess involves the disc space with secondary spread to the adjacent vertebral bodies. Both spinal and secondary nerve root pain are usually severe. Common causative organisms in the United States are *Staphylococcus*, coagulase positive and negative, from surgical or hematogenous spread. Gram-negative organisms are seen from urinary sepsis. Intravenous drug users and people who are immunocompromised have higher incidences of epidural abscess. Worldwide, the most common spinal infection is tuberculosis. The incidence of spinal tuberculosis seems to be increasing with widespread HIV in susceptible populations.

Tumors

Although degenerative spondylotic disease is listed first in the lumbosacral pain differential, the serious potential of neoplasia or infection must always be considered. Metastatic extradural cancers to the spine are the most common tumors, although primary bone and intradural tumors also mimic discogenic disorders. The common primary sites include prostate, breast, lung, melanoma, and myeloma. Usually symptoms begin with spine pain that worsens gradually. Root pain starts as the neural elements become involved, which may be gradual or acute with significant and sometimes sudden neurologic deterioration. Evaluation and treatment in this situation is urgent, and recovery after treatment may not be complete.

Schwannoma, meningioma, myxopapillary ependymoma, and lipoma are the common lumbar spinal intradural tumors. The symptoms of schwannoma, meningioma, and ependymoma are gradually progressive. Patients with a lipoma, a congenital tumor, usually have a history of baseline neurologic deficit and a later progression.

DIAGNOSTIC APPROACH

The evaluation of patients having their initial bout of acute sciatica or low back pain does not routinely necessitate any diagnostic testing. Most individuals recover spontaneously. However, for those who do not fit the classic pattern of nerve root compression or acute low back strain and for patients with a typical clinical picture who do not improve, neurodiagnostic testing is necessary.

Lumbar spine plain radiographs, including lateral flexion and extension views, serve 2 purposes. The anatomy of the spine, with its degenerative changes, is demonstrated, as are subluxations and instability. Destructive lesions in the vertebral bodies and disc space can be seen.

MRI is the primary spinal imaging modality (Figure 78-5). Good-quality MRI demonstrates disc herniation or spinal stenosis and differentiates an uncommon tumor or infection. However, on occasion, for technical reasons, MRI does not clearly demonstrate the pathology. The patient may have moved, been too obese, or been claustrophobic. The appropriate nerve roots may not be visualized.

Myelogram with CT continues to be a valuable adjunct to the diagnostic repertoire. Myelography with water-soluble contrast, followed by axial CT scanning, can demonstrate nerve root filling or lack thereof with more clarity than MRI. Sagittal and coronal reconstructions of CT data add excellent information.

TREATMENT

Treatment of lumbar radiculopathy is usually successful if the history, physical examination, and imaging components all correlate. Most acute episodes of lumbar or root pain, without significant neurologic deficit, necessitate only judicious rest. Strict bed rest should be avoided because it leads to rapid deconditioning and more serious problems, including deep venous thrombosis, pulmonary embolism, and very rarely fatal paradoxical cerebral emboli. Patients must be encouraged to get up as much as possible but to avoid activities that exacerbate their symptoms.

LUMBAR RADICULOPATHY

Figure 78-5   **Spondylotic Subluxation With High-Grade Stenosis**

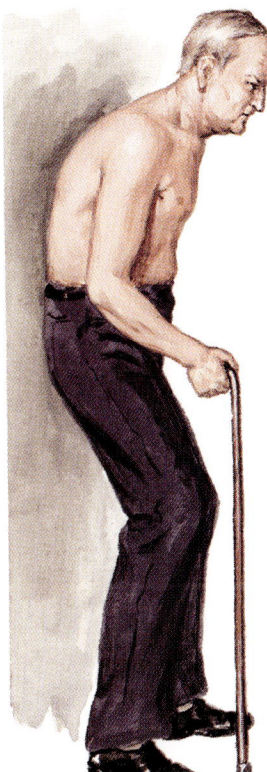

Patient assumes characteristic bent-over posture, with neck, spine, hips, and knees flexed; back is flat or convex, with absence of normal lordotic curvature. Pressure on cauda equina and resultant pain thus relieved.

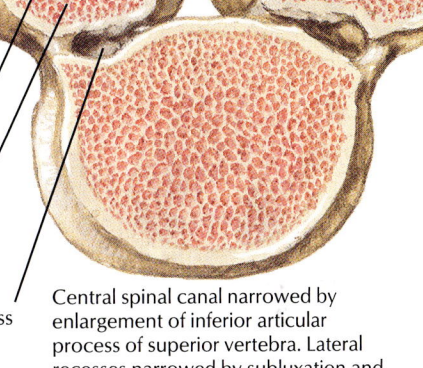

- Inferior articular process of superior vertebra
- Superior articular process of inferior vertebra
- Lateral recess

Central spinal canal narrowed by enlargement of inferior articular process of superior vertebra. Lateral recesses narrowed by subluxation and osteophytic enlargement of superior articular processes of inferior vertebra.

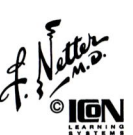

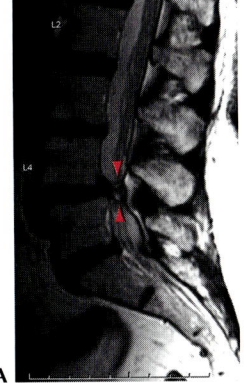

(**A** and **B**) Center and left sagittal T2-weighted images demonstrate grade 1 forward subluxation of L4 on L5 showing high-grade stenosis with thickening of ligamentum flavum and with cystic changes (arrowheads). (**C**) Axial T2-weighted image shows severe facet arthropathy with cystic changes from the left facet.

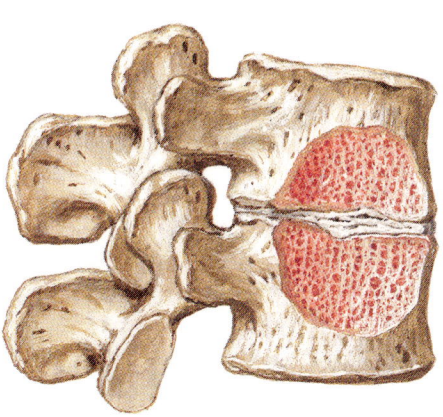

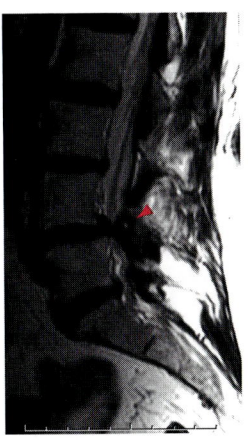

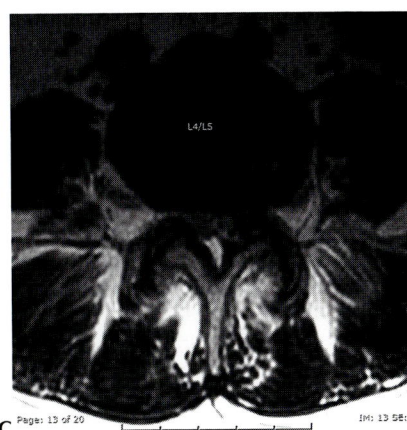

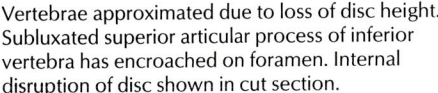

Vertebrae approximated due to loss of disc height. Subluxated superior articular process of inferior vertebra has encroached on foramen. Internal disruption of disc shown in cut section.

RADICULOPATHIES

LUMBAR RADICULOPATHY

Figure 78-6 — Laminectomy and Discectomy

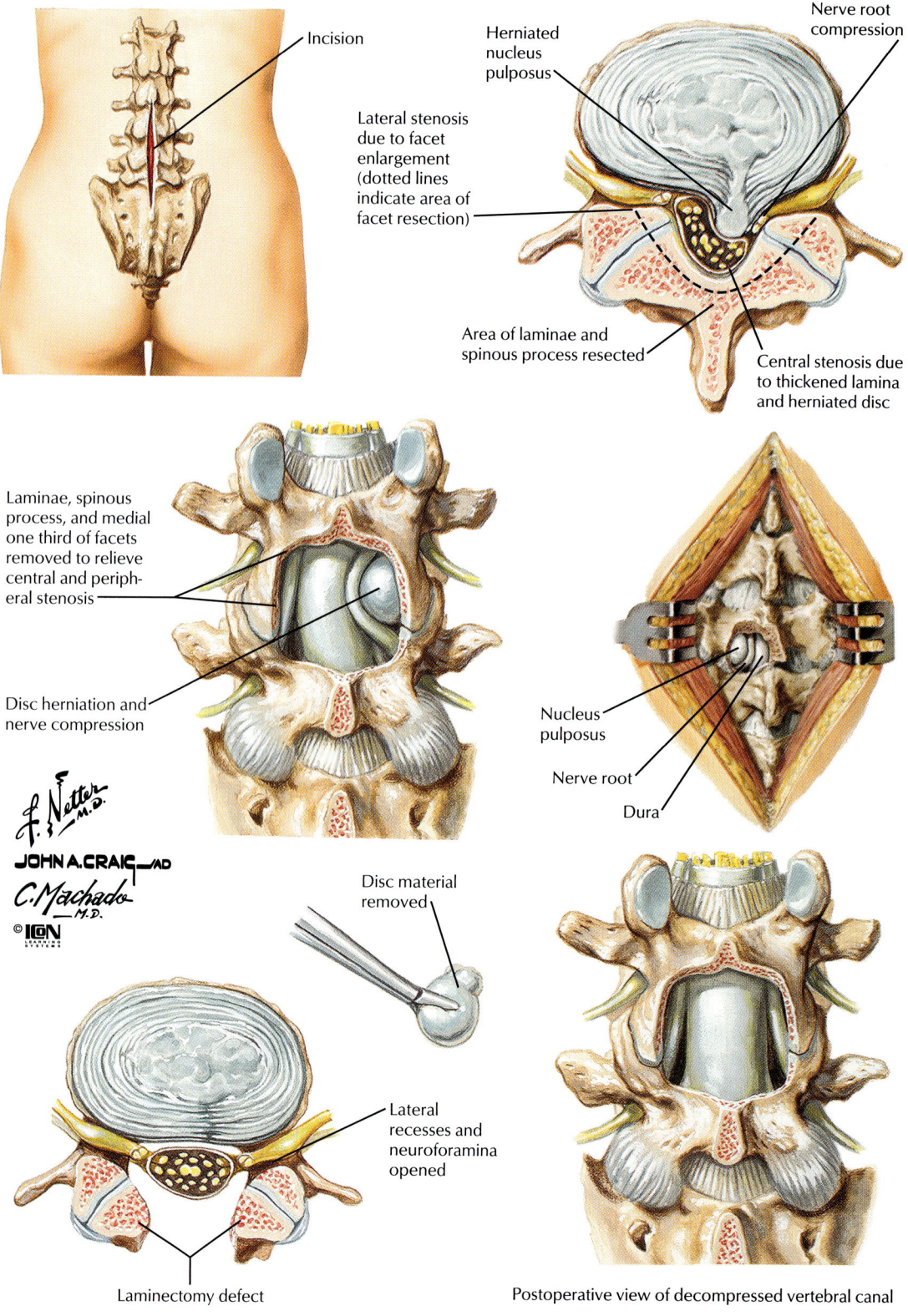

RADICULOPATHIES

When patients have recovered from their acute symptoms, they can begin a judicious exercise program, graduating to heavy exercise. Analgesics, antiinflammatory medication, and occasional steroids help patients to function until this usually self-limited problem improves. With this approach, 80% of patients improve within 1 to 3 months, the normal natural history of discogenic nerve root compression. Therefore, care is advised when evaluating therapeutic claims for chiropractic, acupuncture, and other purported treatment modalities. Supportive care results in an 80% cure of most cases of acute low back pain and sciatica.

For patients with more chronic, nondisabling pain, lifestyle changes with weight loss and health club membership are the best approach. Unfortunately, few patients change their behavior patterns.

When acute symptoms do not improve or the chronic degenerative disc related pain persists and when the diagnosis is clear, specific indications exist for surgery. The first and most important is the presence of a significant persistent neurologic deficit such as foot drop. However, severe unrelenting nerve root pain that disrupts a patient's life is the common reason to proceed with nerve root decompression. When advising patients who are making decisions about surgery, they must be informed that postponing surgery will not place them in neurologic jeopardy, but the discomfort will likely persist.

Surgical goals for patients with degenerative disease or disc rupture relate to the origin of the pain (Figure 78-6). If the patient has root pain with corresponding root compression on imaging, the root or roots should be decompressed, and the herniated disc or synovial cyst must be removed. This approach results in total or significant relief of root pain in a high percentage of cases. If posture-related lumbar pain is the primary symptom, root decompression alone will not resolve the symptoms. Spinal segmental instability, with abnormal spinal motion, can also cause significant pain secondary to intermittent compression of nerve roots, causing radicular pain. It can also increase degeneration around the facet joints and disc annulus, causing primary back pain. In these uncommon situations, spinal fusion is a reasonable consideration.

Surgery for an extruded disc requires removal of the extruded fragment with freeing of the compressed nerve root. The disc space should be entered, and the loose fragments should be removed. With this technique, more than 90% of patients obtain symptomatic relief. However, large series have experienced a greater than 5% reherniation at the same site.

The treatment of a patient with a tumor depends on the tumor histology and the extent of neurologic involvement. If the initial presentation of a potentially metastatic tumor is in the spine, needle biopsy of the spinal tumor or biopsy of an obvious tumor demonstrated in the lung, breast, prostate, or skin can provide the diagnosis. Radiotherapy is appropriate when the tumor is radiosensitive, the spine is stable, and there is relatively minimal neural compression. However, if those considerations are not met, surgery must be considered. A major destructive lesion involving most of the vertebral body and both pedicles usually requires a 360° decompression and fusion. Neurologic deterioration can be rapid, and after paresis has occurred, the patient may not recover, even after emergency surgery.

Appropriate therapy of an epidural infection is controversial (chapter 64). Some reports demonstrate good results with antibiotic treatment. However, because of the potential rapid loss of neurologic function, surgical drainage of frank pus is advised to reduce pain rapidly and prevent paraplegia. Rapid deterioration can occur in patients treated nonoperatively with antibiotics. Subsequently, these patients still require long-term specific IV antibiotic treatment.

REFERENCES

Anderson RE, Drayer BP, Braffman B, et al. Acute low back pain—radiculopathy. American College of Radiology. ACR appropriateness criteria. Radiology. 2000;215(suppl):479-485.

Bartynski WS, Lin L. Lumbar root compression in the lateral recess: MR imaging, conventional myelography, and CT myelography comparison with surgical confirmation. AJNR Am J Neuroradiol. 2003;24:348-360.

Fager CA. Identification and management of radiculopathy. Neurosurg Clin North Am. 1993;4:1-12.

Freidberg SR, Fellows T, Thomas CB, Mancall AC. Experience with spinal epidural cysts. Neurosurgery. 1994;34:989-993.

LUMBAR RADICULOPATHY

Gerszten PC, Welch WC. Current surgical management of metastatic spinal disease. *Oncology (Huntingt).* 2000;14:1013-1024.

Herzog RJ, Guyer RD, Graham-Smith A, Simmons ED Jr. Magnetic resonance imaging: use in patients with low back or radicular pain. *Spine.* 1995;20:1834-1838.

Javedan S, Sonntag VK. Lumbar disc herniation: microsurgical approach. *Neurosurgery.* 2003;52:160-162.

Lauerman WC, Cain JE. Isthmic spondylolisthesis in the adult. *J Am Acad Orthop Surg.* 1996;4:201-208.

Reihsaus E, Waldbaur H, Seeling W. Spinal epidural abscess: a meta-analysis of 915 patients. *Neurosurg Rev.* 2000;23:175204.

Webster BS, Snook SH. The cost of 1989 workers' compensation low back pain claims. *Spine.* 1994;19:1111-1115.

Chapter 79
Lumbar Spinal Stenosis

H. Royden Jones, Jr, and Stephen R. Freidberg

Clinical Vignette

A previously vigorous 85-year-old man developed intermittent painful paresthesiae in his anterior thighs. Typically, walking initially precipitated these; they were distance related and occurred after a distance of approximately 1 block. If the man stopped and rested for a minute or so, he could continue walking; gradually, his reserve lessened to the point that he often became symptomatic after only a hundred yards. Although this symptom constellation had the characteristics of vascular claudication, his internist found no evidence of vascular insufficiency. Therefore, this patient had a "pseudoclaudication syndrome." The pain became more incapacitating over several months and was even present particularly when the patient was at rest or even when he attempted to sit in a chair.

On neurologic examination, the patient had mild diminished strength in his iliopsoas, with hypoactive muscle stretch reflexes at both knees, and subjective hypesthesias over his anterior thighs. He was claustrophobic, and MRI could not be performed. A CT myelogram demonstrated severe lumbosacral spinal stenosis. A lumbar spinal decompression was performed. The patient had a dramatic improvement in the claudication symptoms and, by 6 months, regained his mobility.

The patient in this vignette had a relatively long clinical course with symptoms of progressive bilateral lumbar nerve root compression. Initially, he had normal neurologic examination results, emphasizing the importance of performing appropriate imaging studies after the first symptoms develop. As in the vignette, decompressive laminectomies can result in significant improvement. Often, relief occurs relatively rapidly when surgery is performed early in the clinical course.

Spinal stenosis is becoming more prevalent with the increasingly aging population. It rarely occurs before the age of 60 years, although individuals with achondroplasia or other congenital processes predisposed to spinal stenosis have a particularly early onset (Figure 79-1). Patients typically have multilevel spinal canal compression of the lumbosacral nerve roots primarily at L3-4 or L4-5. It rarely occurs at L5-S1. This is unlike a herniated nucleus pulposus, whose presentation reflects a single, specific nerve root irritation, particularly at L4-5 or L5-S1.

Spondylosis is the primary pathologic process, characterized by an overgrowth of the vertebral facets, bodies, and laminae. Lumbar spinal stenosis has a relatively distinct clinical picture of multilevel radiculopathy. Although a similar process occurs within the cervical spinal canal, its narrowing leads to spinal cord compression and a consequent myelopathy (chapters 59-61).

CLINICAL PRESENTATION

Characteristically, the patient has a neurogenic claudication pain pattern mimicking arteriosclerotic occlusive disease of the legs. Most individuals become symptomatic with standing or ambulating (Figure 78-5). They are able to walk a set distance and then feel the need to sit. Relief is usually rapid with sitting. Characteristically patients are more comfortable flexed at the waist. Therefore, walking uphill may be easier than walking downhill, wherein spinal hyperextension may precipitate symptomatology. Patients may be more comfortable leaning on a walker or a grocery cart. In the most severe instances, patients are unhappy even seated.

Often, patients have normal neurologic examination results. Occasionally, with long-standing symptomatic spinal stenosis, there may be significant associated neurologic deficits.

DIAGNOSIS

The primary issue is often the differentiation of spinal stenosis from vascular claudication. The

LUMBAR SPINAL STENOSIS

Figure 79-1   Lumbar Spinal Stenosis

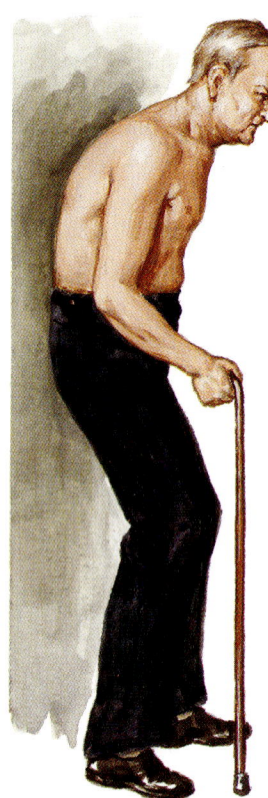

Patient assumes characteristic bent-over posture, with neck, spine, hips, and knees flexed; back is flat or convex, with absence of normal lordotic curvature. Pressure on cauda equina and resultant pain thus relieved.

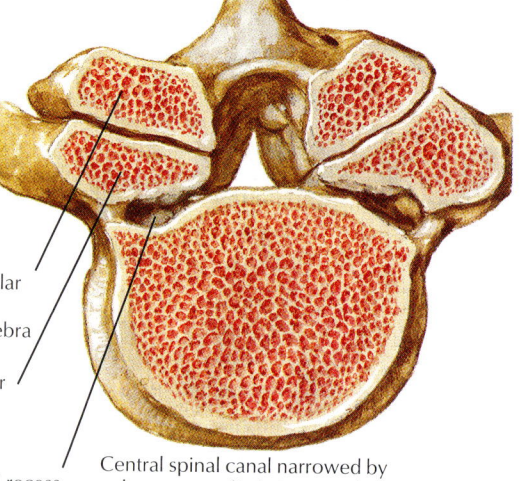

Inferior articular process of superior vertebra

Superior articular process of inferior vertebra

Lateral recess

Central spinal canal narrowed by enlargement of inferior articular process of superior vertebra. Lateral recesses narrowed by subluxation and osteophytic enlargement of superior articular processes of inferior vertebra.

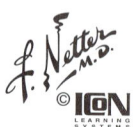

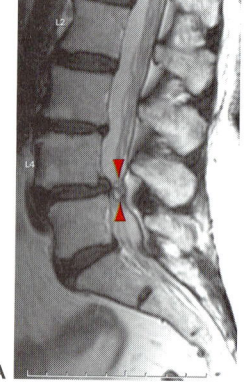

(**A** and **B**) Center and left sagittal T2-weighted images demonstrate grade 1 forward subluxation of L4 on L5 showing high-grade stenosis with thickening of ligamentum flavum and with cystic changes (arrowheads). (**C**) Axial T2-weighted image shows severe facet arthropathy with cystic changes from the left facet.

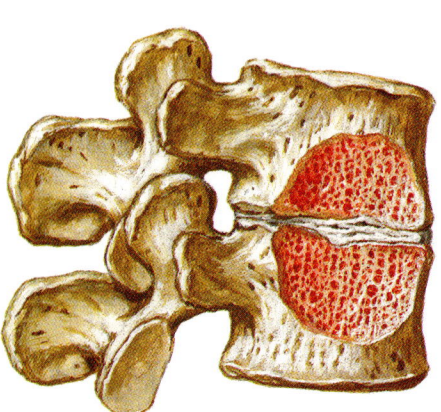

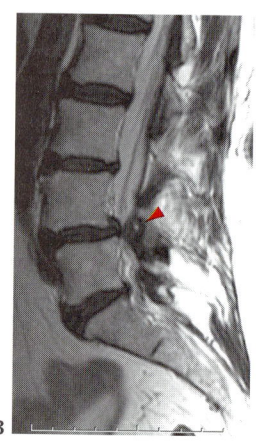

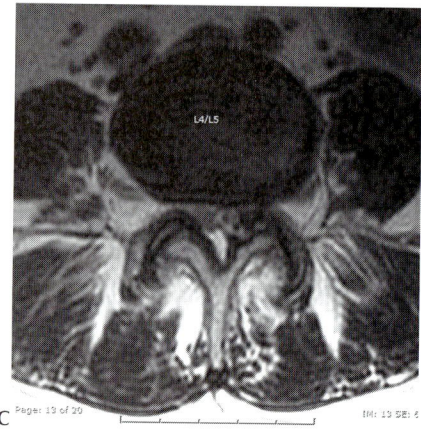

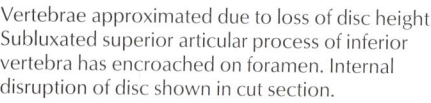

Vertebrae approximated due to loss of disc height. Subluxated superior articular process of inferior vertebra has encroached on foramen. Internal disruption of disc shown in cut section.

Figure 79-1   Lumbar Spinal Stenosis (continued)

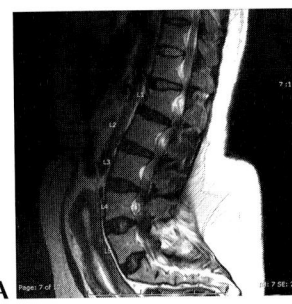 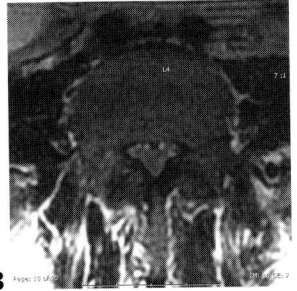 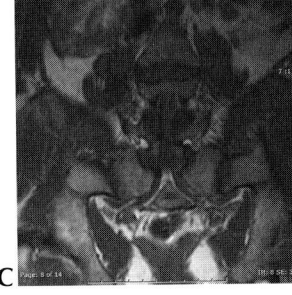

(**A**) Sagittal T2-weighted image shows multilevel stenosis. Narrow AP dimension of the canal and prominent concavity of the lumbar vertebrae are typical of achondroplasia. (**B**) Axial T1-weighted images show small lumbar canal with trefoil configuration. (**C**) Coronal T1-weighted image showing coronal narrowing of the canal, which increases inferiorly, and typical champagne-glass configuration of the pelvic cavity.

demographic population for both conditions is similar. Individuals with spinal stenosis tend to have pain of a more dysesthetic burning character in contrast to the squeezing tight discomfort typical for arteriosclerotic occlusive disorders. Another physical differentiating point is that those with spinal stenosis can ride a bicycle long distances while in the flexed spinal posture, whereas the exercise per se still predictably limits arteriosclerotic patients just as if they are walking.

Patients with spinal stenosis often have normal arterial pulsations, although occasionally, some have poor pulses. In contrast, those with vascular claudication may have some component of spinal stenosis; therefore, these clinical tools sometimes overlap and are not always helpful.

Unlike nerve root disorders, patients with spinal stenosis are typically comfortable at rest, showing no signs of paraspinal spasm, difficulty with straight leg raising testing, or problems bending forward to put on their socks.

Plain radiographs provide a good means to recognize severe spondylotic changes, although MRI is the diagnostic modality of choice. Myelography or CT is used if the patient cannot tolerate MRI. MRI often demonstrates high-grade obstruction or even suggests a complete spinal block, particularly from L3 to L5.

TREATMENT

For individuals who have relatively modest symptomatology, when the diagnosis is confirmed and other more serious conditions are excluded, there is no urgency to proceed with surgery. However, when the patient is physically limited by inability to walk or is increasingly uncomfortable particularly even when seated, a wide decompressive laminectomy and foraminotomy at appropriate spinal levels brings significant relief of pseudoclaudication for a high percentage of patients. For patients whose stenosis may be associated with spondylolisthesis, fusion may be indicated.

REFERENCES

Berven S, Tay BB, Colman W, Hu SS. The lumbar zygapophyseal (facet) joints: a role in the pathogenesis of spinal pain syndromes and degenerative spondylolisthesis. *Semin Neurol*. 2002;22:187-196.

Binder DK, Schmidt MH, Weinstein PR. Lumbar spinal stenosis. *Semin Neurol*. 2002;22:157-166.

Katz JN, Dalgas M, Stucki G, et al. Degenerative lumbar spinal stenosis: diagnostic value of the history and physical examination. *Arthritis Rheum*. 1995;38:1236-1241.

Schultz IZ, Crook JM, Berkowitz J, et al. Biopsychosocial multivariate predictive model of occupational low back disability. *Spine*. 2002;27:2720-2725.

Storm PB, Chou D, Tamargo RJ. Lumbar spinal stenosis, cauda equina syndrome, and multiple lumbosacral radiculopathies. *Phys Med Rehabil Clin North Am*. 2002;13:713-733, ix.

Chapter 80
Rheumatologic, Functional, and Psychosomatic Back Pain

H. Royden Jones, Jr

Clinical Vignette

A 28-year-old man had increasingly incapacitating back pain during the previous year. He delivered milk, lifting heavy cases daily, and dated the inception of his difficulties to lifting an extra-large load approximately 1 year previously, wherein he recalled "wrenching" his back. The discomfort was primarily limited to his low back and was rarely associated with a brief twinge of right-sided sciatica. When arising from bed to go to work, he had an extreme feeling of stiffness, particularly in his back and hips. Paradoxically, he noted that his body would loosen up so that after 45 to 90 minutes of exercise or work, he felt much less limited.

These symptoms had progressed significantly in the previous 2 months, increasingly limiting the patient's work capacity so that he felt unable to complete his job responsibilities in a reasonable time frame. Therefore, believing that his physically demanding occupation must be responsible for his difficulties, and particularly so subsequent to the event 1 year previously, he had applied to his company for workers' compensation.

Neurologic examination revealed loss of lumbar lordosis, diminished chest excursion, and mildly positive straight leg testing on the right. The patient's leg strength, muscle stretch reflexes, and sensation were normal. General examination revealed a mild aortic diastolic murmur.

Spinal and hip radiographs demonstrated findings typical for ankylosing spondylitis, including sclerosis of the sacroiliac joints. A serum HLA-B27 test was positive. The patient was referred to a rheumatologist, who concurred with the diagnosis and began appropriate therapy.

The patient in this vignette sought care for a job-related injury. Instead, he was found to have ankylosing spondylitis, a serious rheumatologic disorder that, if not appreciated early on, could eventually lead to total spinal ankylosis. Nevertheless, despite this early diagnosis of a treatable condition, and paradoxically so, he was disappointed with his care. Before the evaluation, he thought that he was entitled to long-term disability benefits and therefore wished that the appropriate but non–occupationally-related diagnosis had not been made.

HISTORY

Issues of work- and accident-related back pain are common. Frequently, the clinician is confronted with many potential causes of the patient's back pain, not only the classic well-defined organic mechanisms, but often occupation-related symptoms in which overt or covert psychologic factors combine to provide a confusing milieu. Secondary gain issues are commonly confounding factors. It is vital not to impugn patients' veracity by applying pejorative labels such as *"hysteric," "a crock," "functional,"* or even *"having psychological overlay."* Too often, these labels have led to inadequate evaluations, and serious illness is occasionally overlooked, as in this vignette.

It is understandable that sincere physicians have some difficulties dealing with disingenuous patients seeking a "free ride" or a "green poultice" (Figure 80-1). Although secondary gain is often a factor, particularly through workers' compensation, it is often not the primary cause of pain and disability. Therefore, the examining neurologist must carefully evaluate each patient, whether a straightforward, easily defined neurologic illness, such as carpal tunnel syndrome, or one that is embellished by ill-defined relations to a "work-related injury" exists. Unfortunately, sometimes patients focus on their backs, seeking to prove the presence of a posttraumatic mechanically related disorder. Often, they have not considered that they have a specific neurologic disorder.

RHEUMATOLOGIC, FUNCTIONAL, AND PSYCHOSOMATIC BACK PAIN

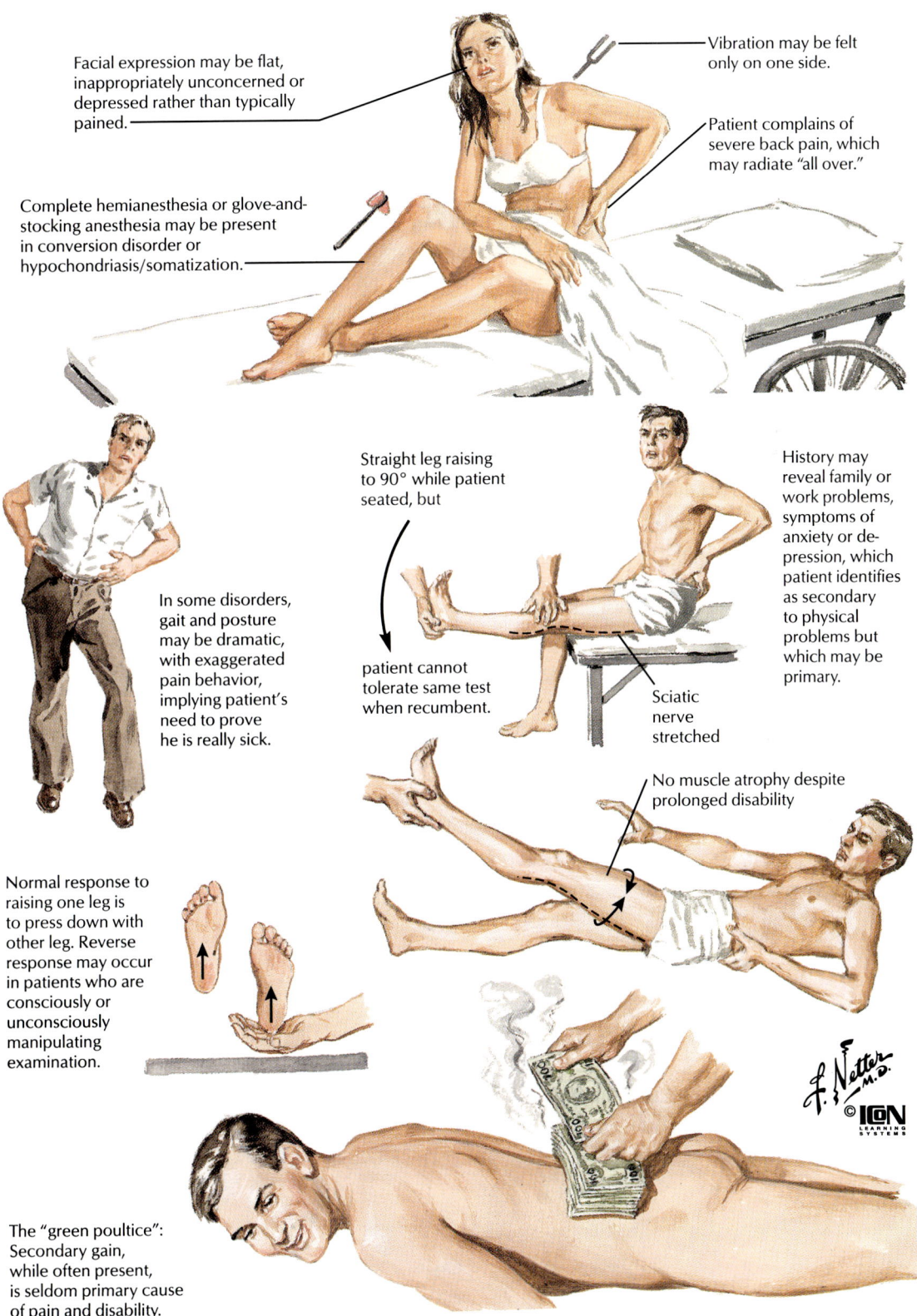

Figure 80-1 Psychosomatic Back Complaints

RADICULOPATHIES

RHEUMATOLOGIC, FUNCTIONAL, AND PSYCHOSOMATIC BACK PAIN

Like many organic physical disorders, several primary psychiatric illnesses have psychosomatic features including back pain. Diagnoses to consider include depression, conversion disorder, psychophysiologic disorder, chronic pain syndrome, hypochondriasis, factitious disorder, and even schizophrenia.

As the physician gains the patient's confidence during the interview and examination, certain life stressors may become apparent, including family, job, personal issues, and inappropriate use of medications or even street drugs.

DIAGNOSIS
Neurologic Examination

Each patient requires a comprehensive general neurologic examination, not only to evaluate the affected extremity and back, but also to confirm that other neurologic systems and anatomical structures are healthy. Certain specific means can distinguish an organic lesion from one that is embellished or inconsistent. The straight leg raise is an excellent example. A patient with organic nerve root compression becomes uncomfortable when lying supine while the physician attempts to bring the patient's leg to the perpendicular and is similarly affected when seated for a similar maneuver. Stretch on the sciatic nerve and its already compromised origins within the L5-S1 nerve roots cause the discomfort. In contrast, an inconsistent response is often noted wherein individuals seeking secondary gain report pain with movement in the supine but not the seated posture.

Another example is the well-known observation that when denervation occurs with significant peripheral nerve injury, it is followed by significant muscular atrophy. Such is generally lacking in the nonorganic setting. However, the quadriceps femoris is an exception; it may undergo significant disuse atrophy without a true peripheral nerve injury. Other useful clues and testing modalities can help to verify psychosomatic back pain (Figure 80-1).

Evaluation

It is essential to carefully investigate patients' concerns even when confident of a psychosomatic or compensation disorder diagnosis. Patients need physicians to take their complaints with an appropriate degree of seriousness, which may mean ordering imaging studies such as MRI or, when MRI is contraindicated, CT/myelography, neurophysiologic investigations including electromyography, and, on occasion, evoked potentials. Finding a symptom-specific organic lesion that can be readily treated occasionally rewards the conscientious physician.

However, if the results of these investigations are all normal, the physician can appropriately reassure patients that no organic mechanism is present. When a true organic neurologic, musculoskeletal, or primary psychiatric disorder is excluded, only then should the physician consider psychologic mechanisms or secondary gain. A number of clues help in these diagnoses; perhaps the most important observation is the patient's tendency to be "consistently inconsistent" in some features of the history or neurologic examination.

TREATMENT

Whether a conversion disorder is diagnosed or no specific surgically remediable disc disease is defined, various behavioral and rehabilitative interventions are supportive and often helpful to patients. A flexible approach combining patient reassurance, rehabilitative medicine techniques, group therapy, and, in more refractive instances, individual psychiatric intervention often improves outcomes. Unfortunately, some individuals with chronic low back pain have multiple surgeries for less than standard reasons and do not improve. The surgeries then provide justification for continuing disability. Another subset of individuals continues to complain until a legal settlement is reached; then they discontinue care, implying that a component of the "green poultice syndrome" was present.

REFERENCES

Hayes J. Psychosomatic back complaints. In: Vol I: *Nervous System*. Part II: Neurologic and Neuromuscular Disorders. Prepared by Frank Netter. West Caldwell, NJ: Ciba; 1986;198. Jones HR. *The Ciba Collection of Medical Illustrations*.

Murphy PL, Volinn E. Is occupational low back pain on the rise? *Spine*. 1999;24:691-697.

Schultz IZ, Crook JM, Berkowitz J, et al. Biopsychosocial multivariate predictive model of occupational low back disability. *Spine.* 2002;27:2720-2725.

Storm PB, Chou D, Tamargo RJ. Lumbar spinal stenosis, cauda equina syndrome, and multiple lumbosacral radiculopathies. *Phys Med Rehabil Clin North Am.* 2002;13:713-733, ix.

Webster BS, Snook SH. The cost of 1989 workers' compensation low back pain claims. *Spine.* 1994;19:1111-1115.

Section XIX
PLEXOPATHIES

Chapter 81
Brachial Plexus and Brachial Plexopathies 700

Chapter 82
Lumbosacral Plexopathies 708

Chapter 81
Brachial Plexus and Brachial Plexopathies

Ted M. Burns and H. Royden Jones, Jr

Clinical Vignette

Four hours postpartum, a 28-year-old previously healthy woman had sudden onset of severe left shoulder girdle and forearm pain and tingling. This was her first pregnancy. Her medical history was unremarkable. She was taking no medications. Her family history was striking in that 9 of 11 women experienced episodic postpartum brachial plexus neuropathies.

Pertinent findings on the initial neurologic examination included weakness of the left deltoid, infraspinatus, and flexor pollicis longus with a diminished left biceps muscle stretch reflex.

EMG confirmed an acute left brachial plexopathy, principally involving the upper plexus. Hereditary brachial plexus neuropathy (HBPN) was diagnosed. Treatment with IV methylprednisolone, 500 mg/d for 4 days, was associated with near-complete resolution of pain and gradual improvement in weakness.

The brachial plexus is susceptible to many pathologic processes, including traumatic (usually stretch) injuries, contusion, compression, inflammation, invasive tumors, ischemia, and genetic disorders (Table 81-1). Often the primary pathophysiologic cause is deduced from the history. In the preceding vignette, the family history of postpartum brachial plexopathies was well documented, and there was no history of other mechanisms of plexus injury. Therefore, HBPN was the most likely etiology.

Knowledge of the processes most likely to injure the plexus provides important information. For example, if an infant was injured during delivery, a neonatal plexopathy is suspect, although other mechanisms should be considered. Infants typically have a predominantly upper and middle plexus lesion because of shoulder traction during delivery (Duchenne-Erb palsy). Recent trauma, such as a fall from a bicycle or motorcycle, suggests a closed traction injury; how the patient landed becomes important. Usually, injury results from sudden, forceful depression of the shoulder, so upper plexus injury is likely. The presentation of a medial plexopathy is always suspect for neoplastic invasion, with a few exceptions. If localization by examination and EMG testing does not match the working hypothesis, the differential diagnosis may require expansion. Anatomical definition also guides therapy, particularly if surgical exploration, repair, or both are being considered.

CLINICAL PRESENTATION

Patients with brachial plexopathies experience upper extremity or shoulder girdle weakness or both, often associated with sensory symptoms including pain, numbness, and, less commonly, vague paresthesias (Figure 81-1). Pain is often severe, especially in HBPN, neoplastic infiltration, or the early stage of neuralgic amyotrophy and sometimes after severe traction injury.

When evaluating a patient with shoulder or arm pain and weakness, one initially determines whether the symptoms have a neuropathic mechanism, eg, plexopathy, mononeuropathy, or radiculopathy, or whether they reflect a non-neuropathic origin. For example, rotator cuff tendonitis, adhesive capsulitis, or shoulder bursitis are common and may initially mimic a brachial plexopathy. In such instances, the patient's pain sometimes limits muscle strength testing and can suggest that the patient is weak. However, true weakness can usually be differentiated from that resulting from splinting (inactivation because of pain), unless secondary gain is the mo-

Table 81-1
Brachial Plexus Etiologies*

Mechanism	Examples	Comments
Trauma, traction	Motorcycle injury, cardiothoracic surgery	Often severe degree, poor prognosis
Stinger	Football etc	Good prognosis
Perinatal	Mixed mechanisms	Generally good prognosis
Idiopathic	Autoimmune?	Self-limited
Hereditary	Genetically determined	Recurrent, benign
Malignancy	Infiltration of tumor cells	Poor prognosis
Radiation	RoRx-induced ischemia	Prognosis guarded but not suggestive of recurrent tumor
Knapsack, rucksack, etc	Compression	Usually self-limited
Thoracic outlet	Entrapment	Rare, confused with CTS
Heroin induced	Indeterminate	

*CTS indicates carpal tunnel syndrome; RoRx, radiation therapy.

tivator, by encouraging the patient to momentarily ignore the pain and "give just one good effort." Most individuals with a primary orthopedic problem will cooperate enough to allow testing of their abilities and strength preservation. Furthermore, with a primary joint problem, the muscle stretch reflexes are normal, and sensory symptoms such as numbness are not involved.

In contrast, with a brachial plexus lesion, weakness typically exists within the distribution of the principally affected nerves, primarily including the shoulder girdle when the upper, lateral plexus is involved and predominantly the hand with lower, medial plexus lesions. Sensory loss is usually present but variable. It is often best defined with a medial plexus lesion causing numbness of the fourth and fifth fingers. Usually, at least 1 muscle stretch reflex is affected, with the occasional exception of medial plexus lesions. Autonomic disturbances, caused by disruption of the sympathetic fibers traversing the lower trunk to the superior cervical ganglia, are variable: trophic skin changes, edema, reflex sympathetic dystrophy (complex regional pain syndrome), and Horner syndrome (miosis, ptosis, ipsilateral facial anhidrosis).

ANATOMICAL CORRELATIONS

Next, one must localize the nerve injury. This requires a detailed appreciation of brachial plexus anatomy. The brachial plexus is formed from the ventral rami of cervical roots 5 to 8 and thoracic root 1 (Figure 81-2). The ventral rami of the fifth and sixth cervical roots together form the upper trunk; the seventh cervical root ventral ramus becomes the middle trunk; and the eighth cervical and first thoracic root ventral rami join to become the lower trunk. The trunks of the brachial plexus are located above the clavicle between the scalenus anterior and scalenus medius muscles, in the posterior triangle of the neck, posterior and lateral to the sternocleidomastoid muscle. The dorsal scapular, long thoracic, and suprascapular nerves originate from the brachial plexus above the clavicle.

Behind the clavicle and in front of the first rib, each trunk separates into anterior and posterior divisions. The anterior divisions of the upper and middle trunks unite to become the lateral cord, whereas the anterior division of the lower trunk forms the medial cord. The posterior divisions of all 3 trunks unite to become the posterior cord. The 3 cords are named for their positions relative

BRACHIAL PLEXUS AND BRACHIAL PLEXOPATHIES

Figure 81-1

Brachial Plexopathy

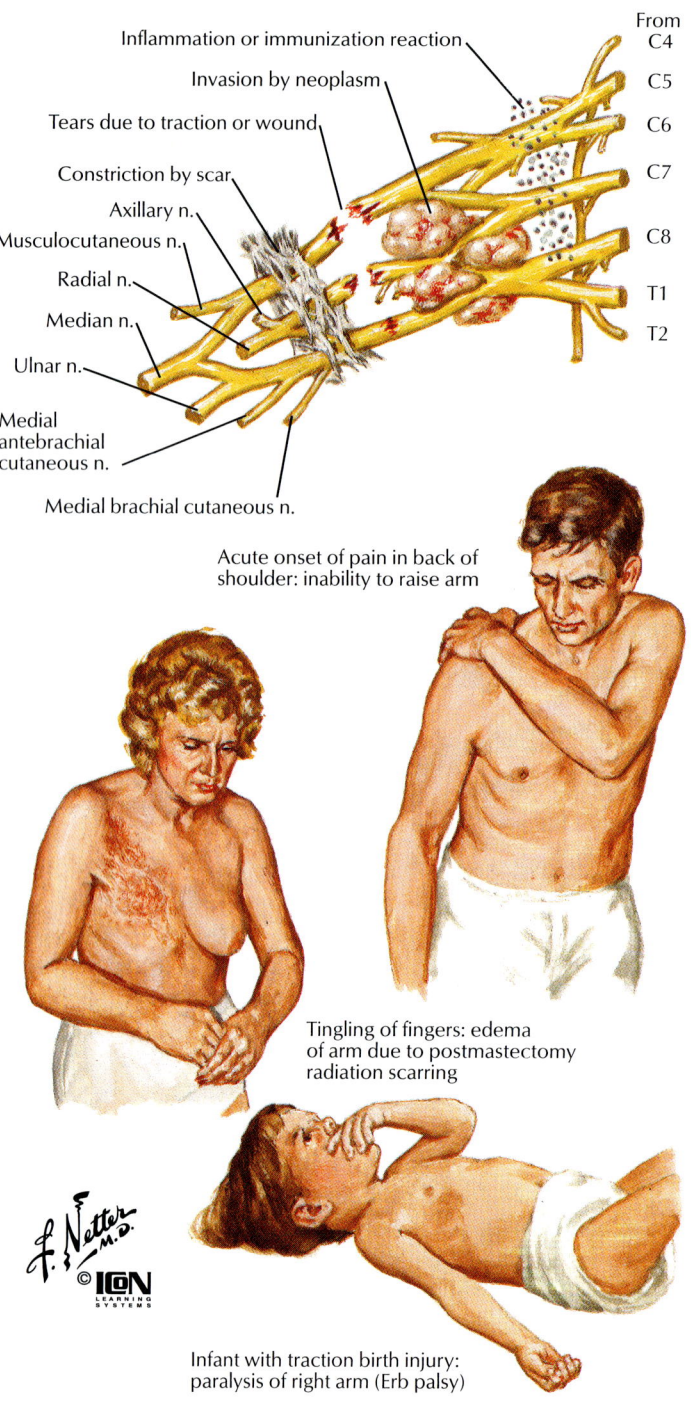

BRACHIAL PLEXUS AND BRACHIAL PLEXOPATHIES

Figure 81-2A

Comparison of Embryonic Limb Organization to the Plan of the Brachial Plexus

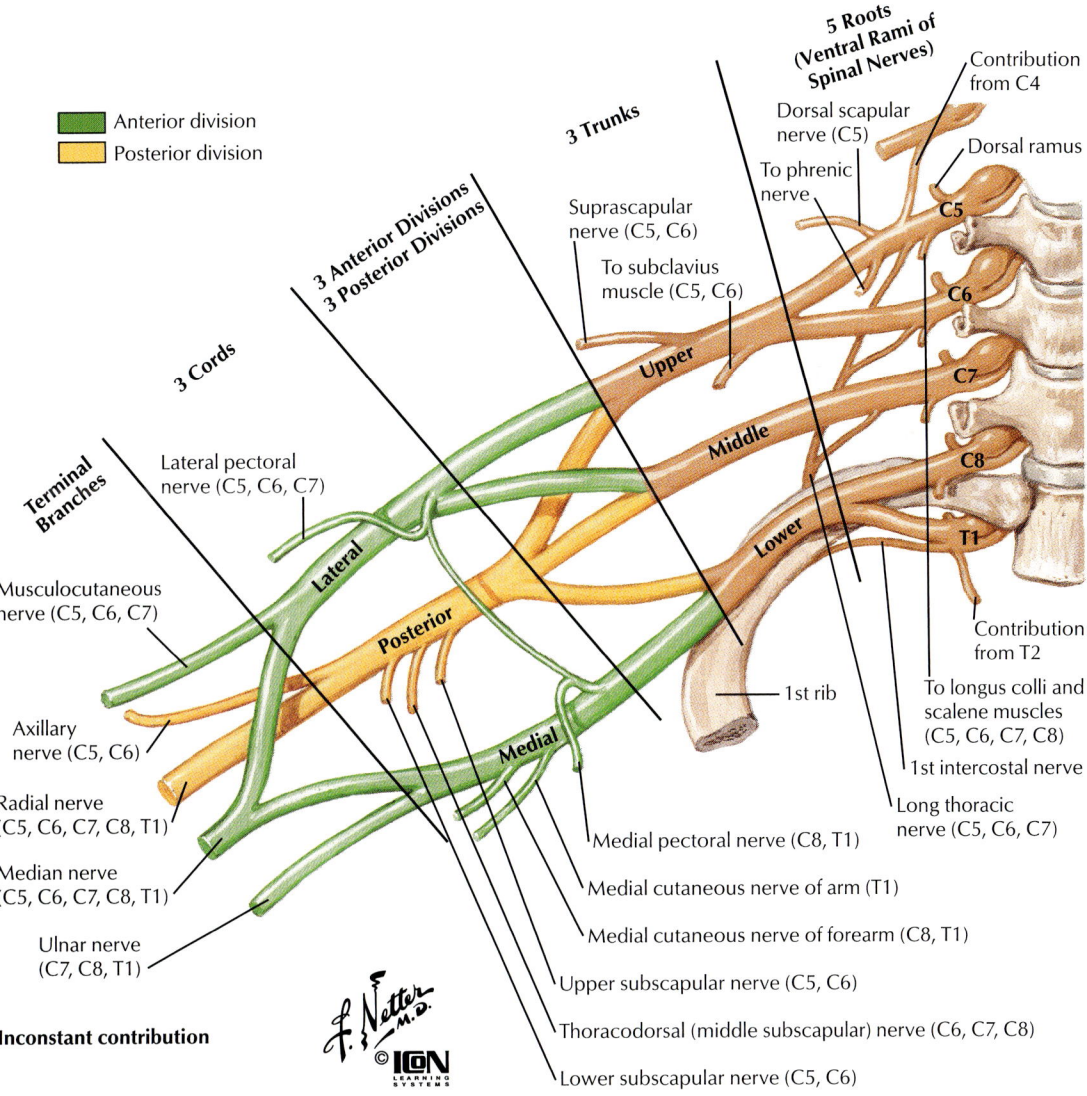

PLEXOPATHIES

703

BRACHIAL PLEXUS AND BRACHIAL PLEXOPATHIES

Figure 81-2B   Axilla (Dissection): Anterior View

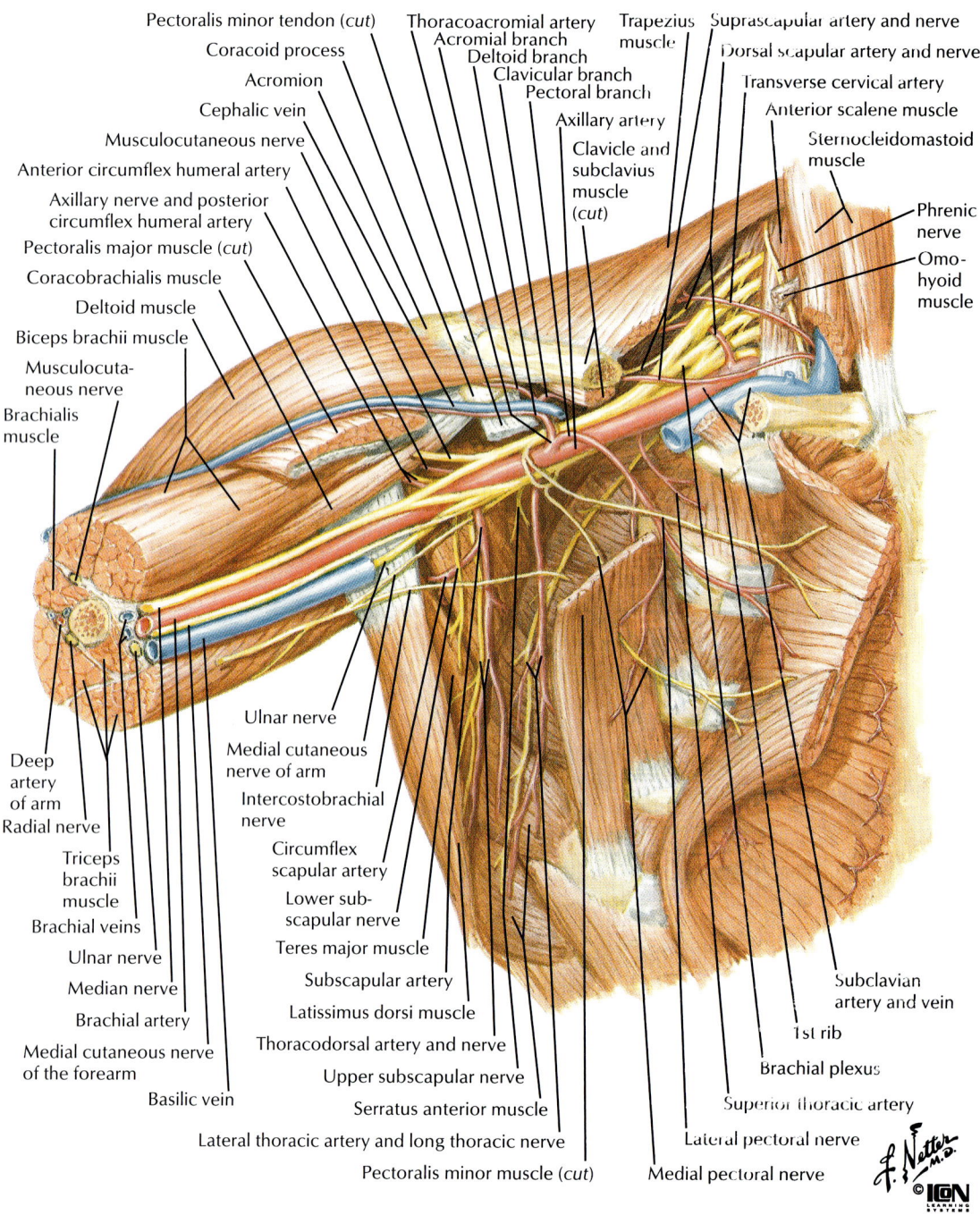

704

PLEXOPATHIES

to the axillary artery. Below the clavicle, the upper extremity nerves arise from the cords. From the lateral cord arises the musculocutaneous, the lateral head of the median, and the lateral pectoral nerves. From the medial cord comes the ulnar, the medial head of the median, the medial pectoral, and the medial brachial and antebrachial nerves. From the posterior cord arise the radial, axillary, subscapular, and thoracodorsal nerves.

DIAGNOSTIC APPROACH

EMG with nerve conduction studies is useful in the evaluation of potential plexopathies. Nonneuropathic causes produce normal results, unlike the abnormal findings of brachial plexus lesions. EMG defines the precise anatomical distribution of the lesion differentiating a mononeuropathy or a radiculopathy from a plexopathy.

CT and MRI help to assess brachial plexus lesions. Occasionally, a patient has a combined plexopathy and radiculopathy with either trauma or some tumors. Sometimes, pain is not present as in most cervical radiculopathies, suggesting an upper, lateral plexus lesion until the disc is seen compromising a cervical root. Chest imaging may show evidence of a Pancoast tumor originating in the pulmonary apex that compresses the lower trunk, medial cord plexus, producing a pseudo-"C8" weakness and numbness.

DIFFERENTIAL DIAGNOSIS

Trauma, particularly secondary to high-speed cycling accidents, is the most common pathophysiologic mechanism for a brachial plexopathy. The superficial anatomical location of the brachial plexus with close proximity to bony and vascular structures within the shoulder and neck predisposes it to this risk. Traumatic mechanisms include compression, traction, ischemia, laceration, or a combination. Motor vehicle accidents, gunshot or knife wounds, and, rarely, falls can be causative. Some events may be iatrogenic, eg, cardiothoracic surgery maximally abducts the arm, stretching the most lateral brachial plexus.

Sporting activities causing **"burners"** or **"stingers"** are common mechanisms. Despite their relative frequency, their pathophysiology is unclear. Proposed etiologies include (1) compression, traction or both of the C5-6 cervical nerve roots and (2) mild stretch injury to the upper trunk of the brachial plexus. Because the clinical presentation is consistent with lesions at either of these anatomical sites and because no apparent long-term sequelae exist, the primary etiology remains undefined. Child abuse is another cause for neurologic trauma that should be considered when the primary lesion is presumed to be idiopathic.

No etiologic or pathophysiologic implications are inherent in the designation, ***idiopathic brachial plexus neuropathy*** (IBPN), (also called **neuralgic amyotrophy or Parsonage-Turner syndrome),** although an autoimmune basis is presumed. Most common in adults, IBPN typically occurs after a viral illness, vaccination, or mild trauma or during the immediate postpartum period. Usually, patients present with relatively acute shoulder pain and partial loss of brachial plexus function. Typically, IBPN predominantly affects nerves of the shoulder girdle muscles, although other portions of the plexus and its terminal branches are occasionally involved, especially the anterior interosseous segment of the median nerve. Approximately one third of patients with IBPN have bilateral, asymmetric involvement.

Hereditary brachial plexus neuropathy is an autosomal dominant disorder characterized by periodic, often recurrent, episodes of unilateral or asymmetric pain, weakness, atrophy, and sensory alterations in the shoulder girdle and upper extremity. Genetically, HBPN localizes to chromosome 17q25. HBPN is presumably an immune-mediated disorder.

In the vignette at the beginning of this chapter, the description of acute onset of shoulder girdle pain within the immediate postpartum period, affecting a previously healthy woman who had a strong family history of similar events, is typical for individuals having the genetic predisposition to recurrent brachial plexopathies.

Malignant tumors, particularly apical lung or postradiation breast cancer, are common causes of brachial plexus lesions. With apical lung tumors, the lesion may insidiously advance, causing lost sensation in the fourth and fifth fingers, weakness in the ulnar and median hand intrinsic

BRACHIAL PLEXUS AND BRACHIAL PLEXOPATHIES

musculature, and Horner syndrome (**Pancoast tumor**). Often, pain is significant, secondary to the infiltration of the tumor into the plexus. This clinical constellation sometimes precedes recognition of the lung tumor. Every patient who smokes and presents in this fashion requires a chest CT or MRI.

Clinical Vignette

A 62-year-old woman was in an automobile accident 8 months previously. The left front end of the car was struck. The woman was wearing a 3-point seat belt. Subsequently, she noted numbness in all of her left fingers except her thumb. In the recent 3 months, she had experienced progressive loss of fine motor control of her left hand. Thirteen years previously, she had had breast cancer treated by lumpectomy and radiation therapy. Her lymph nodes were normal. Litigation was pending regarding the findings of a brachial plexopathy on a recent EMG thought to be related to her automobile trauma.

Neurologic examination demonstrated weakness of all forearm and intrinsic hand musculature. No muscle stretch reflexes were elicited in the left arm, and sensation was diminished in digits 2 through 5.

EMG demonstrated significant myokymia as well as active and chronic denervation of median, radial, and ulnar muscles on needle examination. Motor and sensory nerve conduction findings were surprisingly normal.

A brachial plexopathy in a woman with previous **breast cancer** suggests possible radiation-induced injury, recurrent tumor, or metastatic disease. Usually, plexopathies related to radiation for breast cancer are painless and associated with lymphedema. Typically, this occurs years later as a delayed consequence of radiation, and EMG is particularly helpful. Myokymia, the repetitive semirhythmic firing of simple or complex motor unit potentials at rates of 0.1 to 10 Hz, is almost specific for radiation damage in this setting. The findings in the preceding vignette are specific for a radiation-induced plexopathy and not related to the automobile trauma.

In **heroin-induced brachial plexopathy**, typical onset of plexitis occurs within a few hours to 1 day after the most recent heroin injection. Its pathogenesis is not defined. A recurrent plexopathy can develop, and some affected individuals also have primary lumbosacral plexus lesions. Heroin should be considered in the differential diagnosis of unexplained plexopathies.

Neurogenic thoracic outlet syndrome is another rare disorder. Most patients present with hand weakness, atrophy, or both. Pain is usually mild but is not usually the primary symptom. Classic nerve conduction study findings are usually documented. A cervical rib or increased length of the C7 transverse process is the typical mechanism.

Cervical radiculopathies often present with symptoms of shoulder pain, arm or hand weakness, and paresthesias. Because these are similar to a brachial plexopathy, clinical differentiation can be important. EMG testing may reveal abnormalities of sensory nerve action potentials with plexopathies, whereas with radiculopathies, they are usually normal. The sensory dorsal root ganglia are unaffected in radiculopathies because they are located distal to pathologies that cause nerve root injury (eg, herniated discs, spondylotic bony changes, nerve root inflammation, etc).

Mononeuropathies should also be considered in patients with shoulder girdle weakness: **axillary** nerve for the deltoid and teres major muscles, and **suprascapular** nerve for the infraspinatus and supraspinatus muscles, unlike a lateral cord lesion. When evaluating a patient with a presumed **radial** neuropathy, lesions affecting the posterior cord of the brachial plexus require exclusion. Certain mononeuropathies, eg, radial neuropathies, are sometimes misdiagnosed as brachial plexopathies because radial nerve weakness impairs the ability to stabilize the wrist and thumb. Consequently, examination may spuriously suggest weakness of the ulnar and median hand muscles in addition to actual radial nerve weakness. Careful examination after wrist stabilization helps to distinguish the nerve involvement. Also, **ulnar** nerve lesions may mimic plexopathies.

Patients with **primary intraspinal lesions**, including syringomyelia and motor neuron disease, may present with an atrophic hand. Occasionally, painless progressive upper extremity weakness with atrophy is the presenting symptom. Patients with segmental cervical spinal muscular atrophy, Hirayama disease, usually present in the late teens with primarily unilateral weakness of 1 distal forearm and hand. Self-limited, initially progressive, Hirayama disease stabilizes by the age of 20 to 25 years.

Less commonly, **strokes** presenting as upper extremity weakness may mimic brachial plexopathies.

TREATMENT AND PROGNOSIS

The severity, extent, and etiology of injury dictate treatment and prognosis. Options often include symptomatic therapies with analgesics and supportive care, such as physical therapy. With severe traction lesions, common with motorcycle accidents, root avulsion characteristically causes disabling, unrelenting pain necessitating medical and sometimes surgical intervention. With milder traction or compression lesions, such as neonatal palsy or postoperative brachial plexopathy, physical therapy including range-of-motion exercises is beneficial. Rarely with severe cases, surgical intervention may be necessary. Infrequently, treatment may include surgical exploration or specific therapy for the underlying mechanism.

Idiopathic brachial plexus neuropathy or HBPN treatment frequently includes steroids, which seem to relieve symptoms, but whether they alter the natural history is unknown. No effective treatment for radiation plexopathy exists other than symptomatic support. Although often unsuccessful, primary oncologic intervention is needed for neoplastic brachial plexopathy. Surgical exploration is frequently necessary for open injuries to the plexus, eg, gunshot injuries. Recovery is usually complete in mild cases of neonatal palsy and incomplete in severe cases with Horner syndrome and intrinsic hand muscle weakness.

FUTURE DIRECTIONS

Any progress in brachial plexopathies must include efforts in minimizing the risk of brachial plexopathy, especially those of trauma. Public education, safety campaigns, and tougher laws could decrease the number of traumatic brachial plexopathies. Scientific advances in neuroimmunology and oncology will affect brachial plexopathies of autoimmune and oncologic etiology. Likewise, identification of the gene or genes involved in HBPN will greatly improve understanding and may lead to targeted treatments.

REFERENCES

Harper CM, Thomas JE, Cascino TL, Litchy WJ. Distinction between neoplastic and radiation-induced brachial plexopathy, with emphasis on the role of EMG. *Neurology.* 1989;39:502-506.

Jones HR, Miller TA, Wilbourn A. Brachial and lumbosacral plexus lesions. In: Jones HR, De Vivo D, Darras BT. *Neuromuscular Disorders of Infancy, Childhood, and Adolescence.* Philadelphia, Pa: Butterworth-Heinemann, Elsevier; 2003:245-277.

Klein CJ, Dyck PJB, Friedenberg SM, Burns TM, Windebank AJ, Dyck PJ. Inflammation and neuropathic attacks in hereditary brachial plexus neuropathy. *J Neurol Neurosurg Psych.* 2002;73:45-50.

Kori SH, Foley KM, Posner JB. Brachial plexus lesions in patients with cancer: 100 cases. *Neurology.* 1981;31:45-50.

Lederman RJ, Wilbourn AJ. Postpartum neuralgic amyotrophy. *Neurology.* 1996;47:1213-1219.

Parsonage MJ, Turner JWA. Neuralgic amyotrophy: the shoulder-girdle syndrome. *Lancet.* 1948;1:973-978.

Pellegrino JE. Rebbeck TR, Brown MJ, Bird TD, Chance PF. Mapping of hereditary neuralgic amyotrophy (familial brachial plexus neuropathy) to chromosome 17q. *Neurology.* 1996;46:1128-1132.

Suarez GA, Giannini C, Bosch EP, et al. Immune brachial plexus neuropathy: suggestive evidence for an inflammatory-immune pathogenesis. *Neurology.* 1996;46:559-561.

Tsairis P, Dyck PJ, Mulder DW. Natural history of brachial plexus neuropathy. *Arch Neurol.* 1972;27:109-117.

Wilbourn AJ. Brachial plexus disorders. In: Dyck PJ, Thomas PK, Griffin JW, Low PA, Poduslo JF, eds. *Peripheral Neuropathy.* 3rd ed. Philadelphia, Pa; WB Saunders; 1993:911-950.

Chapter 82
Lumbosacral Plexopathies

Ted M. Burns and Monique M. Ryan

Clinical Vignette

A 14-year-old boy reported gradually evolving right buttock and posterior thigh pain that eventually caused him to limp. Dysesthesias developed over the outer right foot and were exacerbated by walking and direct pressure on the sciatic nerve. Weakness was limited to the superficial peroneal innervated muscle group.

EMG demonstrated borderline peroneal motor and tibial compound motor action potentials. The sural sensory nerve action potential was absent. Active denervation was confined to the sciatic and gluteal innervated musculature, with no changes in the distribution of the femoral or paraspinal nerves.

Subsequently, the patient experienced fatigue, abdominal pain, nausea and vomiting, and 3-kg weight loss. A serum uric acid level of 17.2 mg/dL (reference range, 4.0-8.5 mg/dL) was the only abnormality on screening blood studies. Ultrasonography demonstrated hepatosplenomegaly and retroperitoneal masses. Bone marrow evaluation revealed an undifferentiated lymphoma. CT demonstrated a pelvic malignancy invading the sacral plexus.

At autopsy, 3.5 months after the onset of symptoms, the sacral plexus was compressed and infiltrated by lymphomatous masses at the pelvic brim.

The lumbosacral plexus is susceptible to many pathologic processes, including acute compression from hematomas (especially iatrogenic), inflammation, invasive tumors, ischemia, genetic disorders, and trauma—particularly stretch injuries, with or without contusions. Although rare, the possibility of a localized or metastatic tumor should be considered when any patient reports persistent leg pain with an evolving femoral or sciatic neuropathy. EMG abnormalities in this vignette demonstrated sciatic and gluteal nerve involvement compatible with a sacral plexus lesion. The cause of a lumbosacral plexopathy often can be surmised through the medical history of the patient.

CLINICAL PRESENTATION

Nerve lesions of the lumbar and sacral plexuses are relatively uncommon. Most cases of lumbosacral plexopathy are idiopathic or arise as complications of systemic diseases, such as diabetes mellitus, tumors, or radiation-induced injury.

Plexus lesions commonly result in unilateral lower extremity muscle weakness and sensory loss that does not conform to the distributions of single roots or nerves. Upper plexus lesions cause weakness of thigh flexion, adduction, and leg extension. Lower plexus lesions result in weakness of thigh extension, knee flexion, and ankle flexion and extension and in sensory changes over the lower leg and foot. Complete lumbosacral plexus involvement produces weakness and muscle atrophy throughout the lower extremity, with total areflexia and anesthesia. Concurrent autonomic loss results in warm, dry skin and peripheral edema.

Back pain may interfere with the examination of the patient; however, its most common cause is an L5 or S1 radiculopathy. Usually, these individuals have severe paraspinal muscle spasm and significant limitation of straight leg raising. Primary orthopedic problems, including trochanteric bursitis, hip joint arthritis, or ankylosing spondylitis, should be considered because patients may seem weak because they are splinting to avoid joint discomfort. Significant limitation of joint movement is common; attempts to rotate the leg externally or internally are uncomfortable.

ANATOMICAL CORRELATIONS

Although the term *lumbosacral plexus* is used for organization, a clinical lesion may occasionally predominate in either the lumbar or the sacral component.

The femoral nerve, innervating the iliopsoas and the quadriceps femoris muscles, is the predominant derivative of the lumbar portion of the lumbosacral plexus (Figure 82-1). Its sensory supply includes the anterior and lateral thigh, and the medial foreleg as the saphenous nerve. The obturator nerve innervating the adductor magnus also originates from the lumbar plexus.

The sacral portion of the lumbosacral plexus innervates the remainder of the lower extremity muscles, including posterior thigh and buttocks muscles and all leg musculature below the knee. The superior and inferior gluteal nerves, the most proximal nerves originating from the sacral derivative of the lumbosacral plexus, innervate the gluteal muscles (medius, minimus, and maximus).

The sciatic nerve innervates the hamstring group and bifurcates into the peroneal and tibial nerves, providing all motor innervation below the knee. The sciatic nerve provides sensory innervation to the posterior thigh and the entire leg below the knee, with the exception of the medial foreleg, which is supplied only by the saphenous nerve.

The peroneal nerve is derived from the lateral portion of the sciatic nerve within the thigh; it supplies only 1 muscle above the knee, the short head of the biceps femoris. This site provides a means to differentiate atypical proximal peroneal or sciatic nerve lesions from common peroneal nerve compression or entrapment syndromes at the fibular head, where the peroneal nerve bifurcates into the superficial and deep peroneal nerves, the latter innervating all anterior compartment muscles. The superficial peroneal motor nerve supplies the lateral compartment.

The tibial nerve, the other primary sciatic nerve derivative, supplies the calf. The superficial peroneal sensory, the sural, and the medial and lateral plantar nerves are the primary superficial sensory nerves below the knee, in addition to the saphenous. The L5 lumbosacral trunk and S1 portion of the plexus are injured more often because of the proximity of the sacrum and the sacroiliac joint.

DIAGNOSTIC APPROACH

EMG testing helps to localize the anatomical distribution of a lesion, differentiating a plexopathy from a mononeuropathy or a radiculopathy. Needle examination demonstrates denervation in involved muscles, defining the affected nerves and often demarcating a plexus lesion, particularly when sensory potentials are absent. The results are normal for primary orthopedic-related mechanisms.

Routine radiographs, CT, and MRI of the lumbosacral spine and pelvis are often required to exclude inflammatory or mass lesions within the spine or pelvis. CSF examination may be indicated to exclude infection. CSF protein is increased in approximately 50% of patients with idiopathic lumbosacral plexopathy, suggesting that the nerve roots are also involved by the process. In diabetic, vasculitic, and idiopathic lumbosacral plexopathy, nerve biopsy may reveal ischemic nerve injury caused by microvasculitis or vasculitis. When no cause is evident, the diagnostic workup should include a search for systemic vasculitis and undiagnosed diabetes.

DIFFERENTIAL DIAGNOSIS

Diagnosis includes differentiation of radiculopathies from plexopathies and then determination of the cause of the plexopathy. Weakness, sensory loss, and loss of muscle stretch reflexes can arise from any lesion of the lower motor neuron. Cord lesions usually cause sphincter involvement and long tract signs; lumbar radiculopathies are more common than lumbar plexopathies. Radiculopathies may be associated with significant back pain and evidence of paraspinal muscle denervation on EMG testing. Distinguishing between a lumbar plexopathy and a radiculopathy can be challenging because these conditions present similarly and involve the same levels. However, they have different causes and disparate treatment strategies.

For example, lumbar radiculopathies are usually caused by structural lesions, such as disc herniation or spondylosis, and are therefore amenable to surgical treatment, whereas spinal surgery is of no value in plexopathies. The clinical setting, the risk factors, and the temporal course often provide information to differentiate plexopathies from radiculopathies. For example, a radiculopathy is more likely if pain onset occurred related to heavy lifting that caused a her-

LUMBOSACRAL PLEXOPATHIES

Figure 82-1A

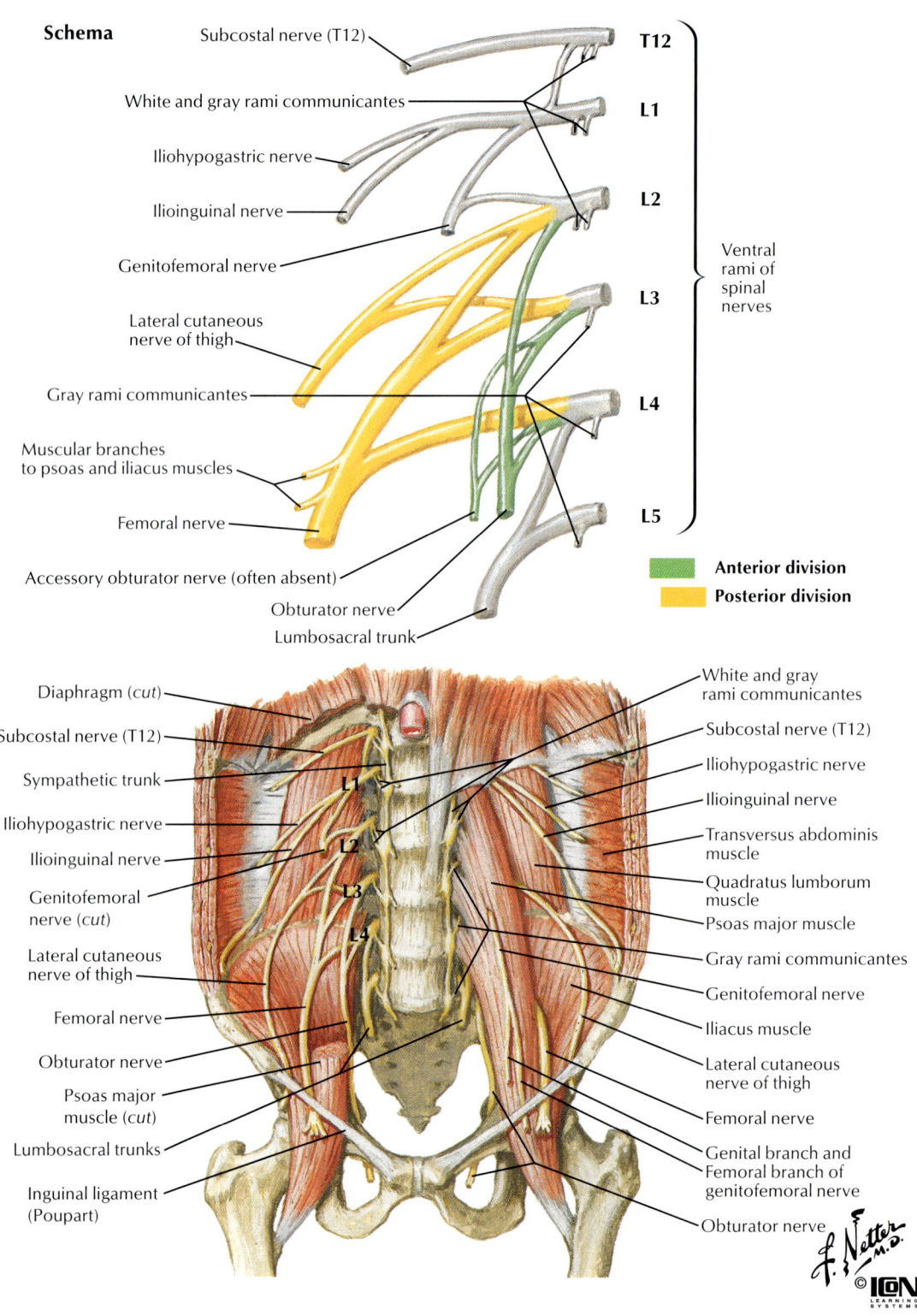

Lumbar Plexus

PLEXOPATHIES

LUMBOSACRAL PLEXOPATHIES

Figure 82-1B   Sacral and Coccygeal Plexuses

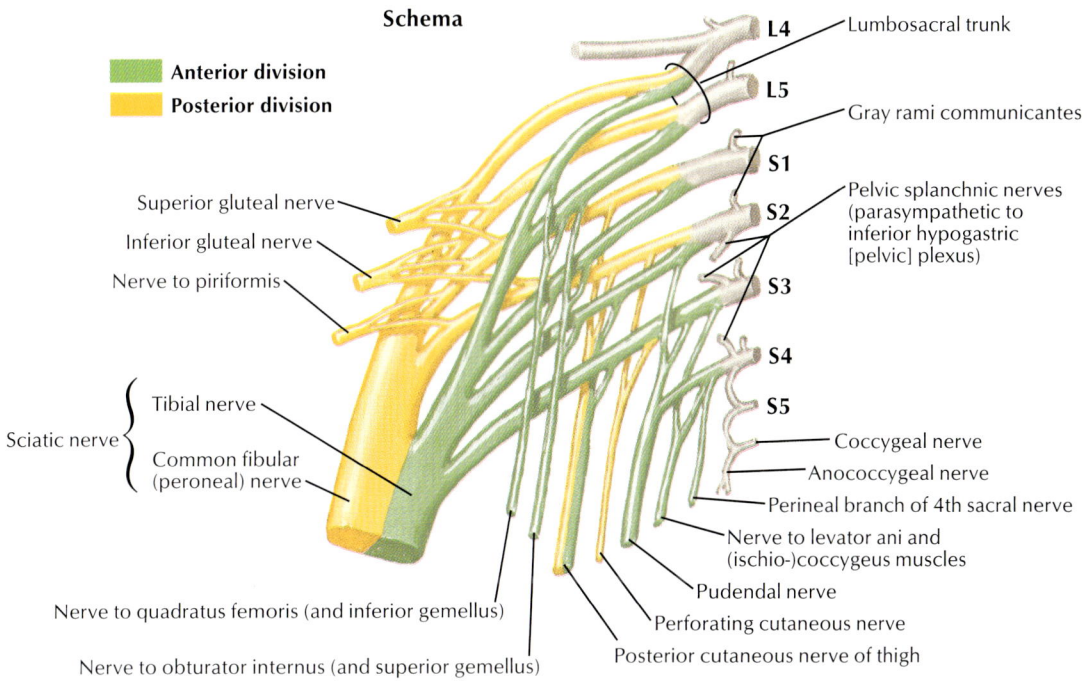

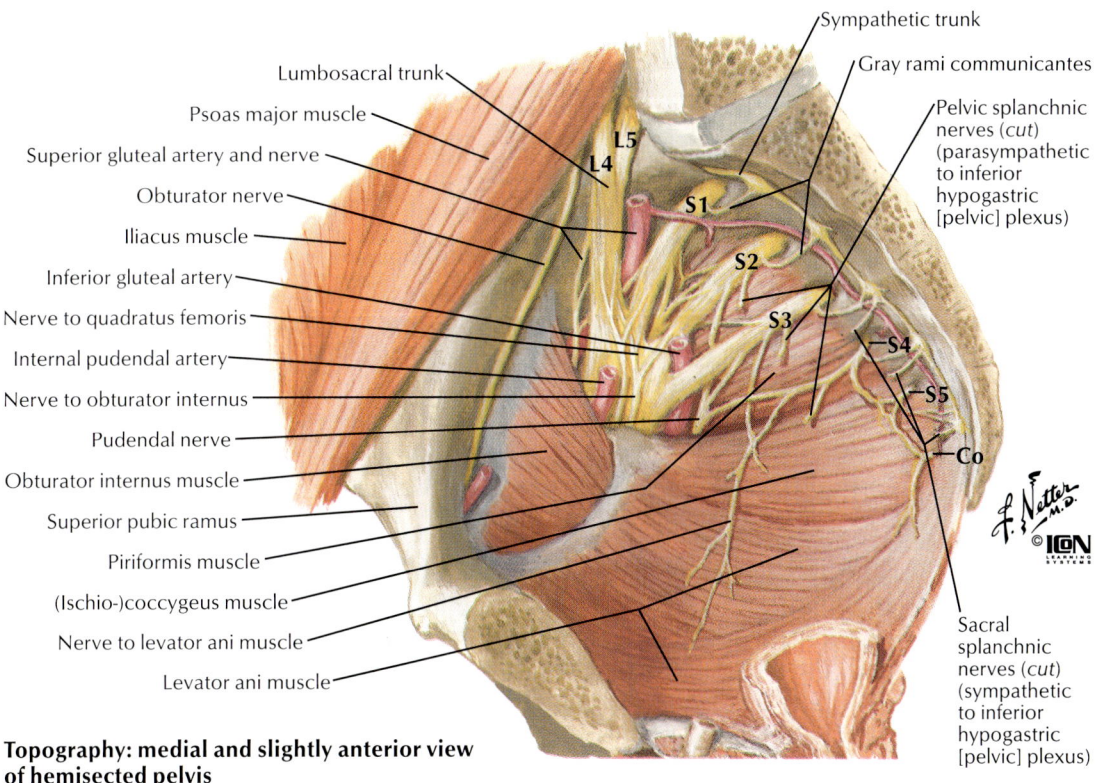

PLEXOPATHIES

711

LUMBOSACRAL PLEXOPATHIES

niated disk. With an insidiously evolving process such as that described in the vignette at the beginning of this chapter, a plexopathy caused by neoplasm is more likely in patients with a history of a malignancy or with systemic symptoms of cancer, such as unexplained weight loss.

Lumbar and sacral plexopathies are distinguished from femoral and sciatic neuropathies by involvement of muscles that do not conform to a single nerve (Figure 82-2). Femoral and sciatic mononeuropathies are uncommon.

Clinical Vignette

A previously healthy 48-year-old woman presented with a 3-week history of lancinating right thigh pain and recent right calf pain. She had difficulty sleeping and obtained minimal relief from analgesics. Neurologic examination revealed weakness of knee extension and ankle dorsiflexion. Right knee jerk was absent. Sensory examination was normal, except for severe allodynia (hyperpathia) over the right calf.

Results of ESR testing, CSF examination, and MRI of the lumbosacral spine were unremarkable. An EMG revealed denervation in the distribution of the right femoral, obturator, and peroneal nerves. The right peroneal compound motor action potential amplitude was decreased, and the superficial peroneal sensory nerve action potential was absent. All other lower extremity motor and sensory action potentials were normal.

During the following weeks, the patient's pain decreased, but atrophy of the right thigh and calf developed, and she experienced increased weakness, with development of a right drop foot. Twelve months after the onset of symptoms, her weakness had improved markedly, and her pain had resolved completely.

This vignette is a typical example of an idiopathic, possibly autoimmune lumbosacral plexitis perhaps related to a microvasculitis or vasculitis. Systemic vasculitides, particularly polyarteritis nodosa, occasionally present in this fashion. This diagnosis should be suspected in patients with other manifestations of systemic vasculitis, including abdominal pain, arthritis, rash, kidney disease, unexplained fever, and weight loss.

Diabetic amyotrophy (DA) is the most common cause of lumbosacral plexopathy. Although DA is classified as a plexopathy, it often concomitantly affects the nerve roots and peripheral nerves, resulting in its alternate terms, **diabetic lumbosacral radiculoplexus neuropathy** or **proximal diabetic neuropathy**. Typically, DA presents in older patients who have type 2 diabetes mellitus, with abrupt or subacute onset of hip and thigh pain. Weakness and muscle atrophy occur 1 to 2 weeks later, when pain may improve. Muscle stretch reflexes may be lost, especially at the knee. DA often begins unilaterally but frequently progresses to bilateral involvement. Commonly associated with unexplained weight loss, this monophasic disorder is usually disabling. DA is thought to originate from peripheral nerve microvasculitis.

Tumors occasionally invade the lumbosacral plexus by primary extension from pelvic, abdominal, or retroperitoneal malignancies. Pain in the distribution of the affected nerves is the cardinal symptom. Late symptoms and signs may include numbness and paresthesias, weakness and gait abnormalities, and lower extremity edema.

Trauma to the lumbosacral plexus is uncommon, because the nerves are relatively immobile and protected by the vertebrae, psoas muscle, and pelvis. Most traumatic injuries are associated with pelvic or acetabular fractures, frequently with soft-tissue injuries to other pelvic organs.

Retroperitoneal hematomas can compress the lumbar or sacral plexuses or both. Patients present with unilateral pelvic or groin pain, with the hip flexed to minimize pressure on the plexus. This condition is typically a complication of anticoagulation therapy, or less commonly bleeding diatheses, and immediate surgical decompression can be beneficial.

Idiopathic lumbosacral plexus neuropathy is a rare primary plexopathy, similar to idiopathic brachial plexus neuropathy (Parsonage-Turner syndrome). It is also manifested by rapid onset of pain, leg weakness, and atrophy. Patients often experience a viral illness 3 to 10 days before symptoms begin. Lumbar plexus involvement often affects the most proximal musculature, decreasing strength in the iliopsoas, quadriceps, and adductor muscles. Often, significant recovery occurs within 3 months.

Compressive lumbosacral plexopathies may also occur from a number of other mechanisms, including late pregnancy or childbirth and abdominal aortic aneurysms. A retroperitoneal in-

LUMBOSACRAL PLEXOPATHIES

Figure 82-2 Radiculoplexopathies

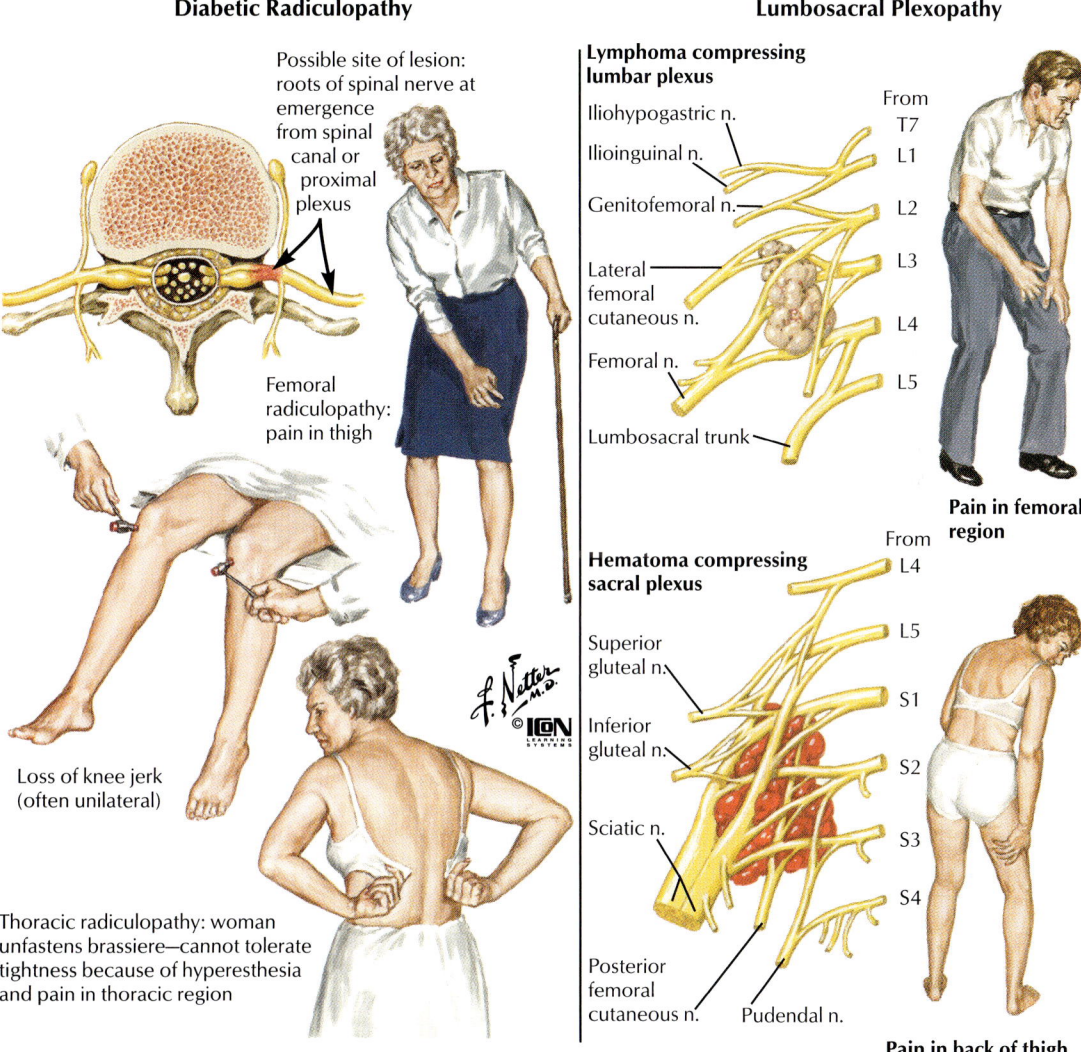

fection such as a psoas abscess rarely affects the lumbosacral plexus. Radiation-induced lumbosacral plexopathies develop months to years after radiotherapy to pelvic malignancies. The lumbar plexus is more commonly affected in radiation-induced lesions, whereas the sacral plexus is more frequently affected by neoplastic plexopathies. Painless weakness develops at a variable rate, ultimately causing asymmetric but significant weakness of both lower extremities. Paresthesias and pain are common but usually mild. Sphincter involvement is rare.

TREATMENT AND PROGNOSIS

Treatment of lumbosacral plexus lesions comprises management of the primary condition. Careful glucose control probably hastens DA recovery and may improve outcome. The efficacy of steroids or IV immunoglobulin in the acute or subacute phase of DA is not proven, but anecdotal reports suggest clinical benefit. One of these treatments is commonly used, although both have potentially significant adverse effects. Corticosteroid treatment of systemic vasculitis is required because systemic vasculitis is often fatal if untreated. Most traumatic lesions are treated conservatively, although pelvic fractures and gunshot wounds may necessitate surgery. No effective treatment for radiation-induced lumbosacral plexopathy exists. Oncologic intervention is necessary for neoplastic lumbosacral plexopathy.

Symptomatic pain management is usually necessary. Pain control can be difficult in the acute phase of DA, idiopathic plexopathy, vasculitic plexopathy, and in neoplastic plexopathies.

Prognosis is predicated on the severity, extent, and cause of nerve injury. Most patients with diabetic or idiopathic lumbosacral plexopathies experience a monophasic course, with a slow (commonly incomplete) recovery during 1 to 2 years. Prognosis of plexopathies caused by vasculitis or neoplasm depends on the underlying condition. In traumatic plexopathies, recovery is usually complete in mild cases and incomplete in severe cases.

FUTURE DIRECTIONS

A better understanding of the basic pathomechanisms of the underlying causes of lumbosacral plexopathies will lead to better treatments. For example, it has been only during the past few years that investigators have reached a consensus that DA is a systemic microvasculitis, which is just now leading to detailed investigation of the mechanism involved and to treatment trials. It is also thought that nondiabetic lumbosacral plexus neuropathies share similar mechanisms of disease, but work remains to be done. As for plexopathies associated with malignancies, improved treatments will depend on advances in the field of oncology.

REFERENCES

Bradley WG, Chad D, Verghese JP, et al. Painful lumbosacral plexopathy with elevated erythrocyte sedimentation rate: a treatable inflammatory syndrome. *Ann Neurol.* 1984;15:457-464.

Dyck PJ, Norell JE, Dyck PJ. Microvasculitis and ischemia in diabetic lumbosacral radiculoplexus neuropathy. *Neurology.* 1999;53:2113-2121.

Dyck PJ, Norell JE, Dyck PJ. Non-diabetic lumbosacral radiculoplexus neuropathy: natural history, outcome and comparison with the diabetic variety. *Brain.* 2001;124:1197-207.

Evans BA, Stevens JC, Dyck PJ. Lumbosacral plexus neuropathy. *Neurology.* 1981;31:1327-1330.

Sander JE, Sharp FR. Lumbosacral plexus neuritis. *Neurology.* 1981;31:470-473.

Thomas JE, Cascino TL, Earle JD. Differential diagnosis between radiation and tumor plexopathy of the pelvis. *Neurology.* 1985;35:1-7.

Triggs W, Young MS, Eskin T, Valenstein E. Treatment of idiopathic lumbosacral plexopathy with intravenous immunoglobulin. *Muscle Nerve.* 1997;20:244-246.

Verma A, Bradley WB. High dose intravenous immunoglobulin therapy in chronic progressive lumbosacral plexopathy. *Neurology.* 1994;44:248-250.

Section XX
MONONEUROPATHIES

Chapter 83
Overview of Mononeuropathies 716

Chapter 84
Mononeuropathies Presenting With Upper Extremity Symptoms 726

Chapter 85
Mononeuropathies Presenting With Shoulder Pain and Weakness 741

Chapter 86
Mononeuropathies Presenting With Lower Extremity Weakness 746

Chapter 87
Primary Sensory Neuropathies of the Lower Extremity 757

Chapter 83
Overview of Mononeuropathies

N. George Kasparyan and James A. Russell

Mononeuropathies are one of the most frequently encountered problems in clinical neurology and clinical medicine. Most occur from prolonged or excessive external compression or entrapment at anatomically vulnerable sites, such as the carpal tunnel. Compression explains their prevalence in postoperative or ICU patients after prolonged immobilization in potentially compromising postures. Patients with diabetes have increased susceptibility to nerve compression and entrapment injuries.

EPIDEMIOLOGY

Epidemiology, socioeconomic effects, and public perception of mononeuropathies have changed significantly during the past 50 years. Thoracic outlet syndrome, now recognized as an extremely rare disorder, was previously thought to account for most cases of what is now diagnosed as carpal tunnel syndrome (CTS). The prevalence of CTS was appreciated only after EMG became clinically available. Public perception holds that excessive computer use is a common cause of CTS. A large population-based study, using clinical and EMG parameters, does not support this speculation. Primary risk factors are female sex, pregnancy, diabetes, and rheumatoid arthritis.

Predisposition for specific mononeuropathies also relates to the micro and gross anatomy of peripheral nerves as interrelated to their specific anatomical sites (Figures 83-1 and 83-2). Examples include superficial locations within extremities, such as the peroneal nerve at the fibular head or the ulnar nerve at the elbow. Similarly, proximity to areas frequently used for medical interventions may predispose to nerve injury; the superficial radial sensory branch of the forearm may be injured by IV access lines, as may the accessory nerve at the posterior cervical triangle by lymph node biopsy.

MECHANISMS AND PATHOPHYSIOLOGY OF INJURY

Clinical Vignette

A 43-year-old woman with type 2 diabetes and a history of obesity reported tingling and numbness of the thumb and index fingers bilaterally. Although not painful, these paresthesias kept her awake at night. They responded to massaging of the hands, and she usually slept with her hands elevated on pillows. Her physical examination revealed normal thenar musculature strength. No objective sensory deficits could be identified.

The paresthesias were reproduced by tapping over the carpal tunnel (Tinel sign). Nerve conduction studies showed prolongation of the median sensory latencies bilaterally, with slowed sensory nerve conduction over the distal segment, suggesting focal demyelination. The patient underwent bilateral surgical releases, with subsequent complete resolution of her symptoms.

Entrapment and **compression** cause many peripheral nerve lesions. Although these terms are sometimes used interchangeably, they differ conceptually and pragmatically. *Entrapment* defines a nerve injury within a pathologically compromised anatomical structure, often by seemingly innocuous processes, such as ligamentous thickening. Symptoms are often of insidious onset but are frequently progressive. CTS, a median nerve lesion at the wrist, is the most notable example. *Compression* neuropathy describes the effect of prolonged or excessive pressure inadvertently applied to a peripheral nerve, usually at a site of anatomical vulnerability (Figures 83-3 and 83-4). Classic examples are the radial nerve within the spiral groove of the humerus and the peroneal nerve at the fibula head. Clinical presentation is usually acute or subacute. The inherent pathophysiologic mechanism common to both entrapment and compression mononeuropathies is primary demyelination with or without evidence of associated axon loss (Figure

OVERVIEW OF MONONEUROPATHIES

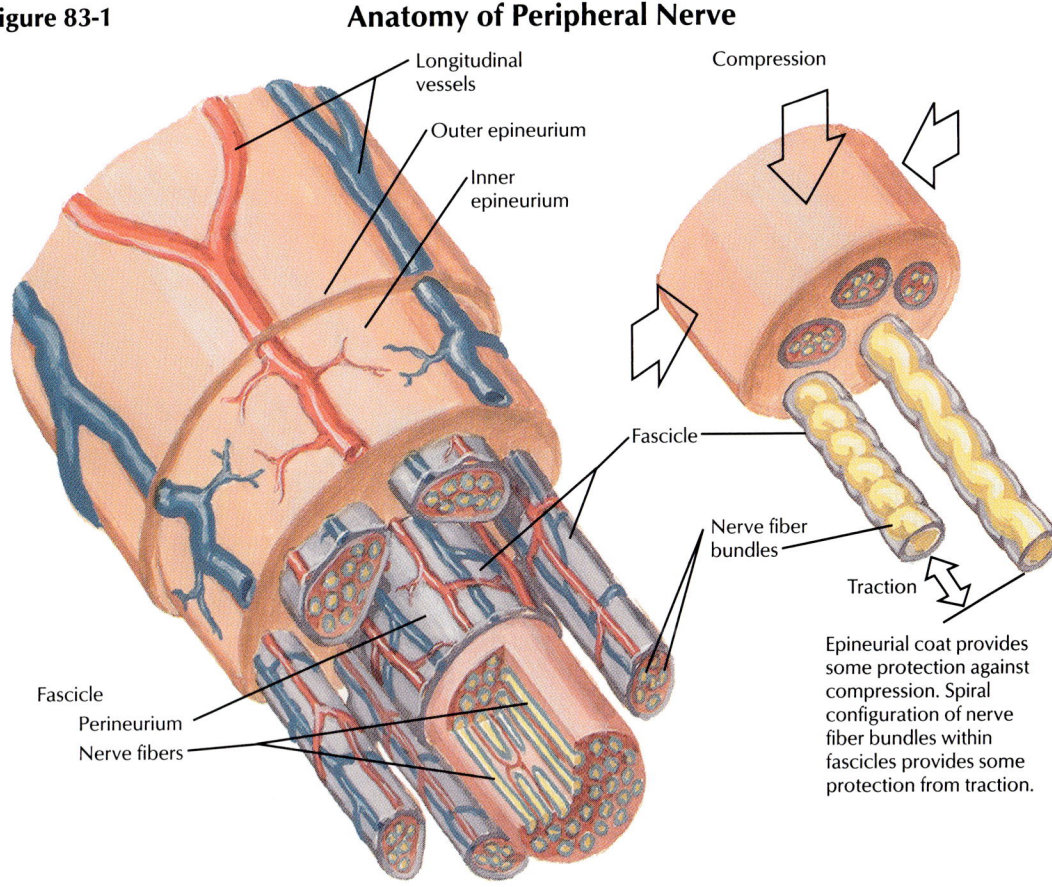

Figure 83-1

MONONEUROPATHIES

OVERVIEW OF MONONEUROPATHIES

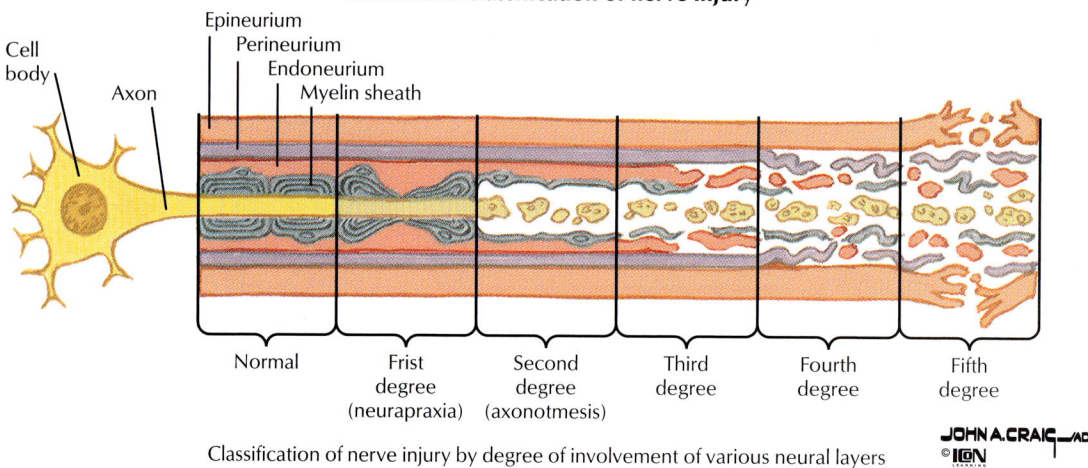

Figure 83-2 Nerve Injury in Compression Neuropathy

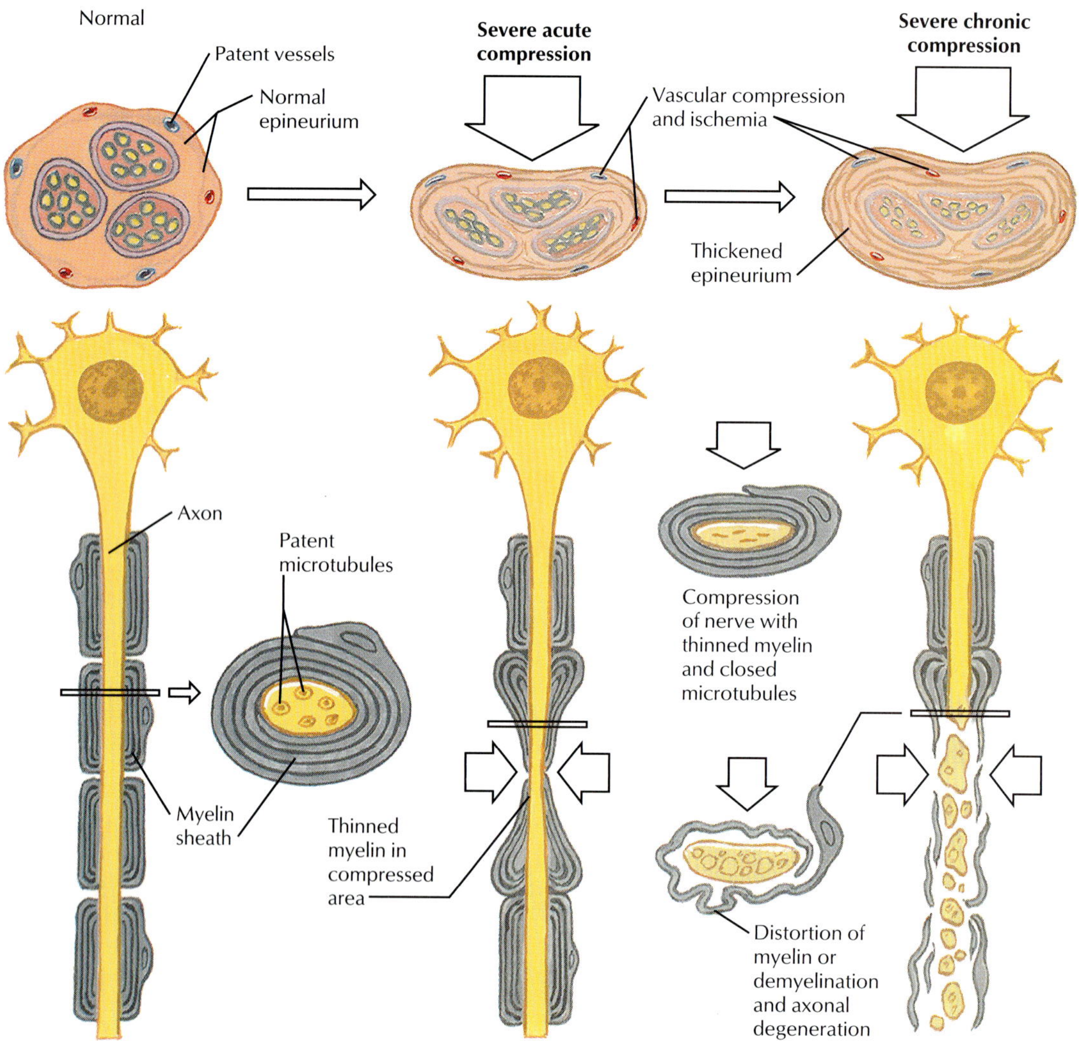

Sunderland classification of nerve injury

Classification of nerve injury by degree of involvement of various neural layers

OVERVIEW OF MONONEUROPATHIES

Figure 83-3

Compression Neuropathy in Workplace

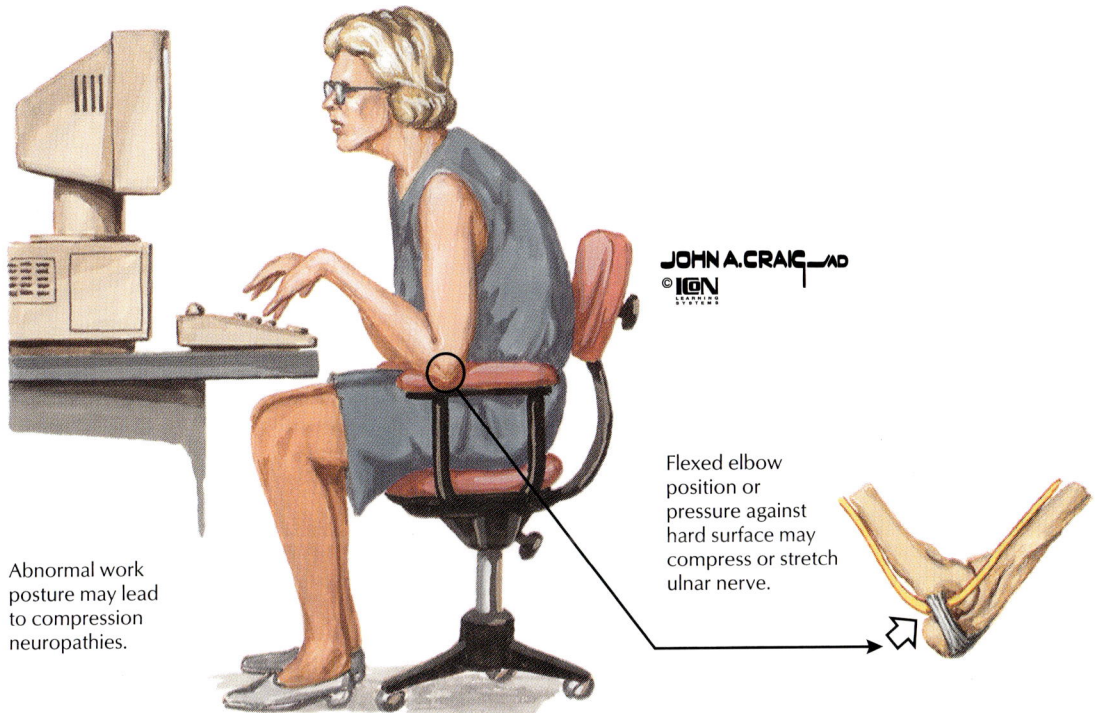

Abnormal work posture may lead to compression neuropathies.

Flexed elbow position or pressure against hard surface may compress or stretch ulnar nerve.

83-2). Less commonly, mononeuropathies occur secondary to acute trauma, especially stretch injuries and penetrating trauma, such as laceration of a peripheral nerve. Fractures sometimes cause acute entrapment.

Uncommon causes of peripheral nerve lesions include vasculitis or microemboli promoting occlusion of the vasa nervorum, leading to loss of blood supply, nerve infarction, and axon loss. Peripheral nerves are rarely infiltrated by tumors (eg, lymphoma), bacterial organisms (eg, leprosy), or products of abnormal metabolism (eg, amyloid). When peripheral nerve infarction or infiltration occurs, although a mononeuropathy may be the presenting feature, it is rarely the sole clinical finding. Concomitant involvement of other peripheral nerves and organ systems, such as the kidneys, lungs, and skin, typically provides diagnostic clues.

Nerve ischemia is important not only in the pathogenesis of vasculitic neuropathies, but also in syndromes of nerve entrapment and compression. Compression-induced venous ischemia may explain the phenomenon of intermittent nocturnal symptoms in CTS, with subsequent relief by position change and "shaking out" of the hands. Symptomatic relief is often provided by resolution of microscopic ischemia, promoted by nerve decompression. The earliest findings of low-grade peripheral nerve compression occur when epineural blood flow is reduced to 20 to 30 mm Hg.

Some systemic disorders (of which diabetes is the best known and most widely accepted) increase nerve susceptibility to injury from external force. A more infrequent mechanism relates to mutations within the myelin PMP22 gene, leading to a hereditary liability for pressure palsy. Nerves of affected individuals are particularly susceptible to physical forces, such as compression. Other mechanisms that may enhance peripheral nerve injury susceptibility include radiation exposure, contact with industrial solvents, and normal aging.

OVERVIEW OF MONONEUROPATHIES

Figure 83-4 **Compression Neuropathy in Athletes and Musicians**

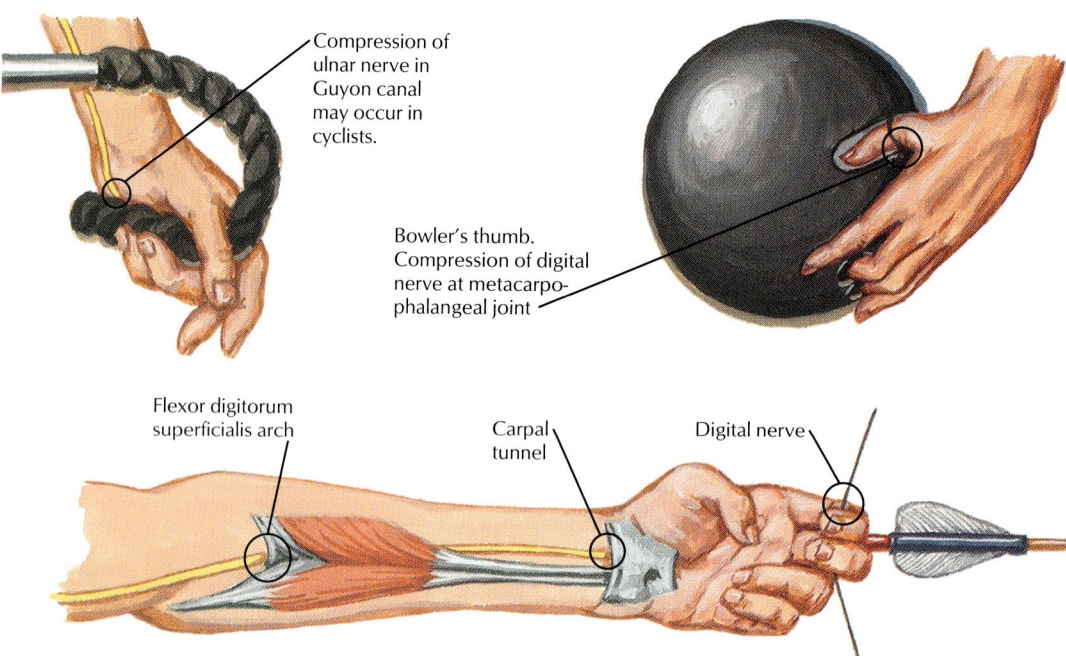

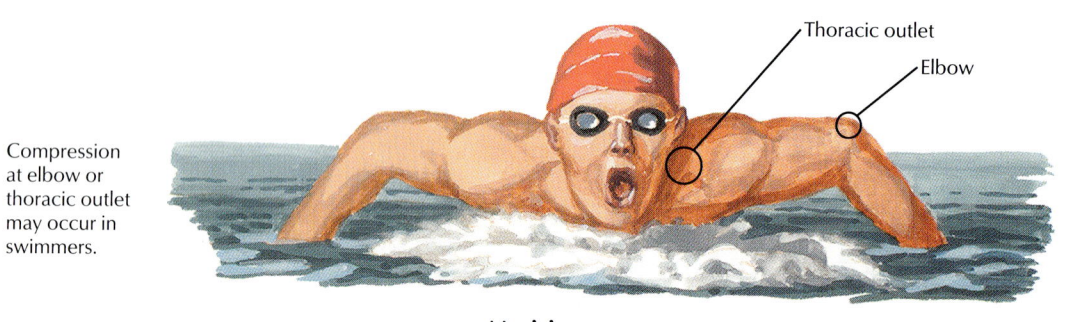

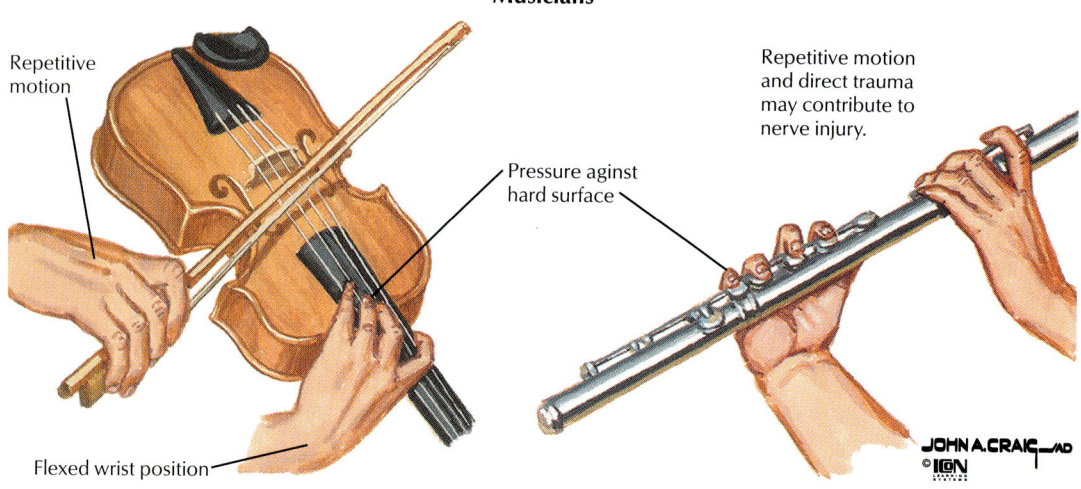

MONONEUROPATHIES

Reasonable correlation exists between the mechanism of mononeuropathies (eg, entrapment or compression), the pathophysiology (eg, axon loss or demyelination), and the resulting clinical symptomatology and prognosis. Myelin is more susceptible to external compression than are axons (Figure 83-2). Although variable axon loss occurs in many mononeuropathies, myelin loss provides the basis for precise electrodiagnostic localization and possibly a more optimistic prognosis than if there is concomitant axonal damage.

EMG Correlates

Myelin loss manifests electrodiagnostically in 3 ways: focal slowing, differential slowing (also known as temporal dispersion), and conduction block. **Focal slowing** occurs when all nerve fibers are affected, approximately to the same extent, in one precise anatomical area. Impulse transmission is slowed uniformly in all fibers at that location. Hence, the only clinical manifestations are pain and paresthesias; weakness, atrophy, and demonstrable sensory loss are absent, unless secondary axonal degeneration occurs, as is eventually seen in most chronic lesions. Focal nerve slowing is the hallmark of neurophysiologic abnormalities in CTS and other entrapment neuropathies.

When patients have evidence of differential slowing, ie, **temporal dispersion**, demyelination is typically multifocal, varying in severity in different fibers within the same nerve. Temporal dispersion is the EMG hallmark of acquired demyelinating polyneuropathies, particularly Guillain-Barré syndrome, but is atypical of focal mononeuropathies. When this occurs, clinical modalities requiring synchrony of impulse transmission, such as muscle stretch reflexes and vibratory perception, are typically lost. Because impulse transmission remains successful in all or most fibers, the strength, muscle bulk, and pain and thermal sensory modalities, mediated by nonmyelinated nerve fibers, are spared in these patients.

Primary **conduction block** is consistent with a demyelinating process in one or more locations that is sufficient to prohibit impulse transmission across involved sections of affected nerve fibers. This causes weakness. Because axonal integrity is not compromised, muscle wasting does not occur. Because unmyelinated fibers are also not affected, pain and thermal sensation are relatively spared. Conduction block commonly occurs with ulnar neuropathies at the elbow, radial neuropathies at the spiral groove, and peroneal neuropathies at the fibular head.

Prognosis is based on the nature of the primary nerve injury and the specific EMG findings that define the extent of **axonal damage.** With motor axonal disruption, the axon portion separated from the anterior horn cell degenerates. Myofibers are deprived of the trophic influence provided by that axon, with resultant atrophy far greater than that produced by disuse, leading to the classic findings of axonal damage as documented by needle EMG. The loss of trophic influences on muscle fiber leads to the appearance of abnormal spontaneous activity on needle examination, characterized by fibrillation potentials, positive waves, and a significant decrease in the number of activated motor unit potentials.

Similarly, the loss of unmyelinated axons mediating nociceptive, thermal, and autonomic functions usually produces clinical features different from primary demyelinating insults. These are characterized by loss of pain and thermal perception, hypersensitivity to touch, changes in sweat production, and sometimes vasomotor changes secondary to focal dysautonomia. Clinical features of axon loss are typically superimposed upon those associated with the demyelinating component of the nerve injury.

CLINICAL PRESENTATION

Mononeuropathies result in focal disruption of motor, sensory, or autonomic function and sometimes pain. The specific types of fibers damaged within the nerve and the precise pathophysiologic mechanism determine the clinical presentation of the neuropathy (Figure 83-5). Nerve injury symptoms are often intermittent if mechanically induced transient ischemia occurs, as in CTS. After axon damage occurs, patients experience continuous symptomatology.

It is generally thought that **sensory fibers** are more susceptible to injury than their contiguous motor components. Therefore, sensory symptoms are often the presenting manifestation of

OVERVIEW OF MONONEUROPATHIES

Figure 83-5 **Clinical Evaluation of Compression Neuropathy**

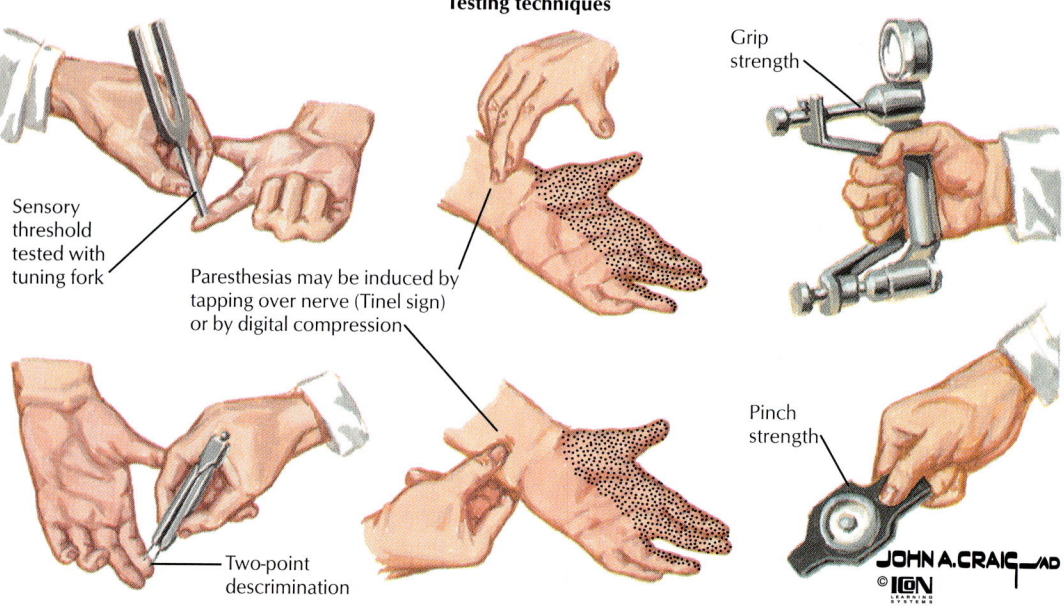

Motor and sensory functions of each nerve assessed individually throughout entire upper extremity to delineate level of compression or entrapment mononeuropathies. Patients may describe numbness or loss of sensation; "falling asleep," tingling, or swollen sensations; or abnormal sensations such as burning, hypersensitivity, or itching. Objective assessment of sensory function by bedside testing is less sensitive than patient perception. Often, asking patients to draw on their bodies the precise area of sensory change or loss improves the anatomical definition of sensory loss. The results are frequently the most credible diagnostic finding, even if not precisely confirmed by clinical examination.

Weakness, with or without atrophy, may occur relatively late in certain mononeuropathies (eg, CTS), as the presenting or major manifestation in others (eg, peroneal or radial neuropathies), or not at all in still others (eg, meralgia paresthetica). Clinical caveats include that not all muscles innervated by a nerve distal to the site of injury may be involved. For example, the ulnar-innervated forearm muscles are commonly spared in ulnar neuropathies at the elbow. This is thought to result from "selective fascicular injury," in which fascicles carrying the fibers innervating ulnar forearm muscles are theoretically deeper and therefore less susceptible to compressive injury.

Mononeuropathies may promote the falsely weak appearance of muscles not innervated by that nerve, especially with radial neuropathies. For example, the full expression of finger abduction strength (ulnar function) requires wrist extension. With a radial neuropathy and resultant wrist drop, finger abductors may seem weak unless the wrist and forearm are supported on a flat surface. Without this knowledge, diagnostic error may readily occur.

DIFFERENTIAL DIAGNOSIS

Intuitively, the diagnosis of mononeuropathy depends upon clinical demonstration of deficits confined to the distribution of a single nerve, with or without electrodiagnostic confirmation. The differential diagnosis between mononeuropathies and monoradiculopathies is sometimes difficult, because nerve and segmental distributions overlap considerably (eg, peroneal and L5) and because either process can cause pain, motor, and sensory deficits. A precise knowledge of peripheral neuroanatomy is crucial for accurate clinical and neurophysiologic diagnosis.

Plexopathies are recognized when motor and sensory deficits extend beyond a single nerve or segmental distribution. Early expression of a plexopathy may be readily confused with a mononeuropathy, eg, C8 radiculoplexopathy after sternotomy is often confused with ulnar neuropathy.

Several disorders may present with focal motor weakness and are in the differential diagnosis of mononeuropathies with predominantly motor symptoms and signs: motor neuron disease, multifocal motor neuropathy, myasthenia gravis, and brachial plexus neuritis. Rarely, CNS disorders present with sensory or motor deficits or both in a distribution so restrictive as to mimic a mononeuropathy. However, these CNS pathologies located above the foramen magnum are not associated with limb pain.

DIAGNOSTIC APPROACH

Electrodiagnosis can define the existence, location, pathophysiology and, to some extent, prognosis of mononeuropathies (Figure 83-6). Rarely does it define cause. Localization of a mononeuropathy is ascertained by one of two electrodiagnostic parameters: demonstration of focal demyelination and/or the pattern of axon loss. Focal demyelination is more accurate but is limited by anatomical and pathophysiologic considerations. Nerve conduction studies are the primary means by which demyelination is identified, based on the demonstration of conduction slowing or alteration in waveform morphology across a focal area of nerve. To demonstrate this, the electromyographer must be able to position the demyelinated nerve segment between the stimulating and recording electrodes. This can be technically difficult, even impossible, with proximal nerve segments that are deep and in close proximity to other nerve elements. Additionally, not all mononeuropathies have demyelinating components.

Localization can also be predicted by the pattern of muscles demonstrating changes of denervation on needle examination. However, the major limitation of this methodology is anatomical; nerve branching is erratic. For example, the ulnar nerve has no branches in the arm, two in

OVERVIEW OF MONONEUROPATHIES

Figure 83-6　Electrodiagnostic Studies in Compression Neuropathy

Electromyography (EMG)

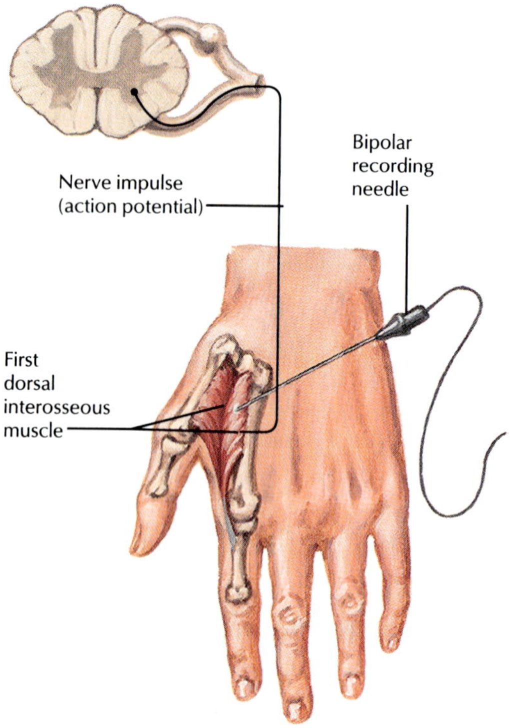

EMG detects and records electric activity or potentials within muscle in various phases of voluntary contraction.

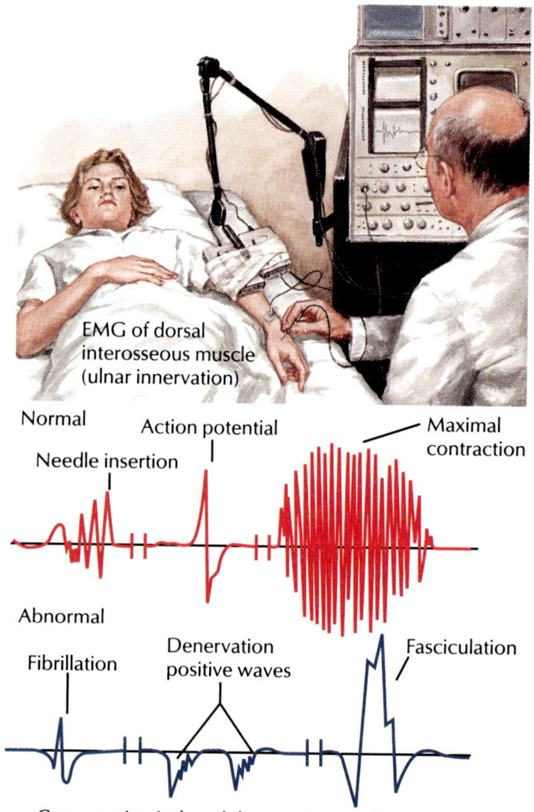

Compression-induced denervation produces abnormal spontaneous potentials.

Nerve conduction studies

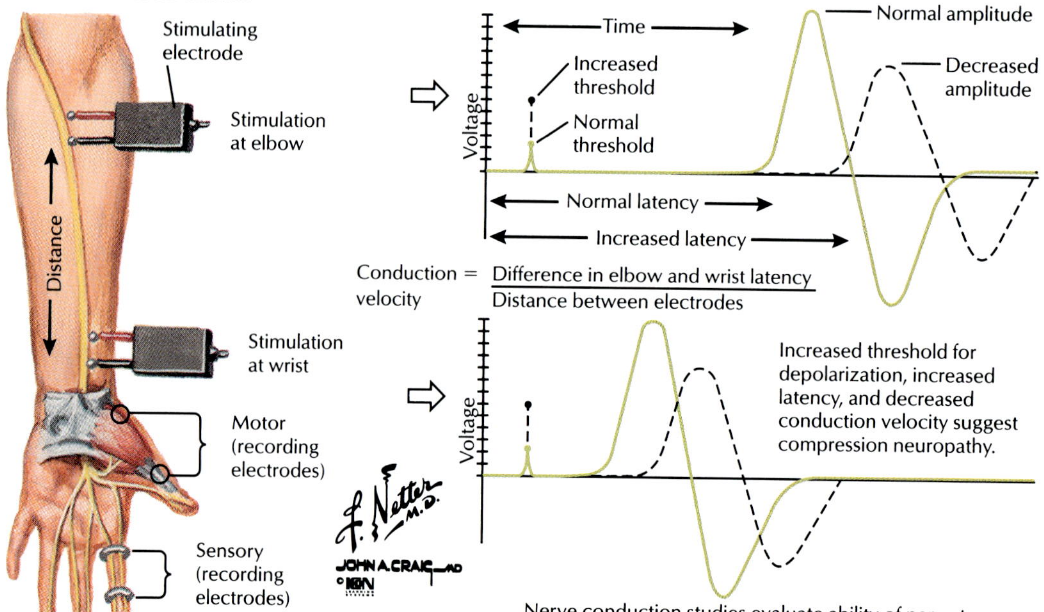

$$\text{Conduction velocity} = \frac{\text{Difference in elbow and wrist latency}}{\text{Distance between electrodes}}$$

Increased threshold for depolarization, increased latency, and decreased conduction velocity suggest compression neuropathy.

Nerve conduction studies evaluate ability of nerve to conduct electrically evoked action potentials. Sensory and motor conduction stimulated and recorded.

MONONEUROPATHIES

724

close proximity at the elbow, and then none until the hand. The other limitation is selective fascicular involvement, whereby a nerve injury at a given location may not result in denervation of all muscles innervated distal to that injury. Understandably, a false estimate of nerve injury location may result.

Imaging modalities, used primarily when a mononeuropathy develops without apparent cause, are of limited value in compression neuropathies. Plain x-rays in 2 planes may demonstrate bony deformities, cervical ribs, evidence of neoplasm, or posttraumatic deformity. CT and MRI are sometimes indicated. MRI can be particularly useful in identifying soft tissue compressive lesions or focal inflammatory conditions. MRI T2-weighted images can delineate nerve sheath tumors (schwannomas) from nerve axonal tumors (neurofibromas) and associated soft tissue cysts and masses. MR inversion recovery and gradient echo sequences also add diagnostic capacity in differentiating malignant and benign lesions.

THERAPY AND PROGNOSIS

In acute penetrating trauma with complete functional loss of a peripheral nerve, immediate exploration and primary reanastomosis is generally recommended. If a nerve transection is recognized subacutely, a delayed exploration may be attempted with cable grafting, which is performed in specialized centers and may enable limited functional recovery.

Acute nerve compression associated with a recognized cause of nerve injury is usually managed conservatively by removing the inciting mechanism. Padding or splinting the affected segment may minimize further pressure or stretch and expedite healing.

Mononeuropathies may develop insidiously without recognized cause. In such instances, imaging may identify an external source of compression, eg, a bony spur and fibrous band or an intrinsic nerve sheath tumor. Rarely, surgical exploration may be warranted depending on imaging results or when the lesion seems progressive.

With nerve entrapment, conservative management is usually advisable in mild cases, typically by avoidance of provocative positions or activities and by splints or padding. Nerve decompression or transposition is typically considered in cases with clinical or electrodiagnostic evidence of significant axon loss or if life-altering morbidity persists despite conservative treatment. Caution is necessary in patients with diabetes whose nerves may have a compromised blood supply. Manipulation, and particularly transposition of those nerves, may worsen rather than improve the problem.

Prognosis in mononeuropathies is determined by etiology, pathophysiology, location, degree of injury, patient age, and comorbidities. In general, predominantly demyelinating neuropathies caused by monophasic compressive insults in young, otherwise healthy individuals often improve considerably, particularly when injuries are not far from the innervated muscle or cutaneous region. Conversely, a significant axonal injury in the axilla of an elderly patient with diabetes to a nerve innervating a hand muscle rarely allows recovery of sensation or strength in the hand.

FUTURE DIRECTIONS

Development of high-resolution functional nerve scanning will enormously benefit neurologists and others caring for patients with mononeuropathies. This will augment electrodiagnosis in the localization of nerve injury and theoretically allow for more accurate assessment of conservative treatment efficacy. Better studies to guide the determination of optimal timing and treatment nature are also needed.

REFERENCES

Andersen JH, Thomsenn JF, Overgaard E, et al. Computer use and carpal tunnel syndrome: a 1-year follow-up study. *JAMA.* 2003;289:2963-2969.

Preston DC, Shapiro BE. *Electromyography and Neuromuscular Disorders.* Boston, Mass: Butterworth-Heinemann; 1998.

Stewart JD. *Focal Peripheral Neuropathies.* 3rd ed. Baltimore, Md: Lippincott Williams & Wilkins; 2000.

Sunderland S. *Nerves and Nerve Injuries.* Edinburgh, Scotland: Churchill Livingstone; 1978.

Chapter 84
Mononeuropathies Presenting With Upper Extremity Symptoms

Steven W. Margles and James A. Russell

MEDIAN MONONEUROPATHIES

The median nerve provides essential motor and sensory function to the lateral aspect of the hand (Figure 84-1). One of 2 primary nerves supplying the intrinsic hand muscles (primarily the thenar eminence) and innervating the muscles of the forearm, it also has a major sensory role, providing innervation for the thumb, index, and long fingers and the lateral half of the ring finger. The distal median nerve at the wrist is the primary site of clinical involvement. More proximal lesions at the elbow are far less common.

Distal Median Entrapment

Clinical Vignette

A 50-year-old woman, an avid gardener, presented with a 2-year history of her right hand "falling asleep." Initially, this occurred only in the morning on awakening. Three months before evaluation, these symptoms began to awaken her at night and were also noted while driving a car or blow-drying her hair. She reported that "all" her digits were affected and that her paresthesias were sometimes accompanied by aching of the wrist and forearm. She did not report problems with hand strength. More recently, she was experiencing similar but milder symptomatology in her left hand.

Neurologic examination disclosed minimal weakness of right thumb abduction, without loss of thenar eminence bulk. Results of reflex and sensory examinations were normal, including 2-point discrimination and graded monofilament touch. Her symptoms were reproduced by foraminal compression maneuvers, such as nerve percussion (Tinel sign) over the median nerve at the wrist.

Clinical Presentation and Testing

The presentation in the preceding vignette is typical for carpal tunnel syndrome (CTS). The tendency for symptoms to occur on awakening, or with activities such as sewing or painting, provides important diagnostic clues. The diagnosis can be confirmed by careful EMG. Median nerve entrapment at the wrist is the primary neuropathy presenting with intermittent symptoms, often at night or with provocative posturing (Figure 84-2). The perception that paresthesias (abnormal sensations) affect all digits (rather than just the $3\frac{1}{2}$ innervated by the median nerve) is common and likely related to the greater cortical representation of the thumb and first 2 fingers. As CTS progresses, persistent numbness ensues, alerting the patient that the precise sensory distribution involves the volar surface of the first $3\frac{1}{2}$ digits.

Neurologic examination, particularly in mild CTS cases, may offer few clues. It is helpful in severe cases, in which atrophy of the thenar eminence is common. Median hand functions, primarily thumb abduction and opposition, are weak. Having the patient supinate the forearm so the palm is flat, and then raise the thumb vertically against resistance, tests these functions. Other forearm muscles supplied by the median nerve, particularly the flexor pollicis longus, are spared.

Provocative tests offer supportive but not diagnostic evidence in suspected CTS (Figure 84-3). A positive Tinel sign consists of an electric, shooting sensation (not just local discomfort) radiating into the appropriate digits with wrist percussion. The Tinel and Phalen maneuvers (reproduction of paresthesias on forceful flexion of the wrist) should be performed with nonleading questions to improve response credibility. The

MONONEUROPATHIES PRESENTING WITH UPPER EXTREMITY SYMPTOMS

Figure 84-1

Arteries and Nerves of Hand: Palmar Views

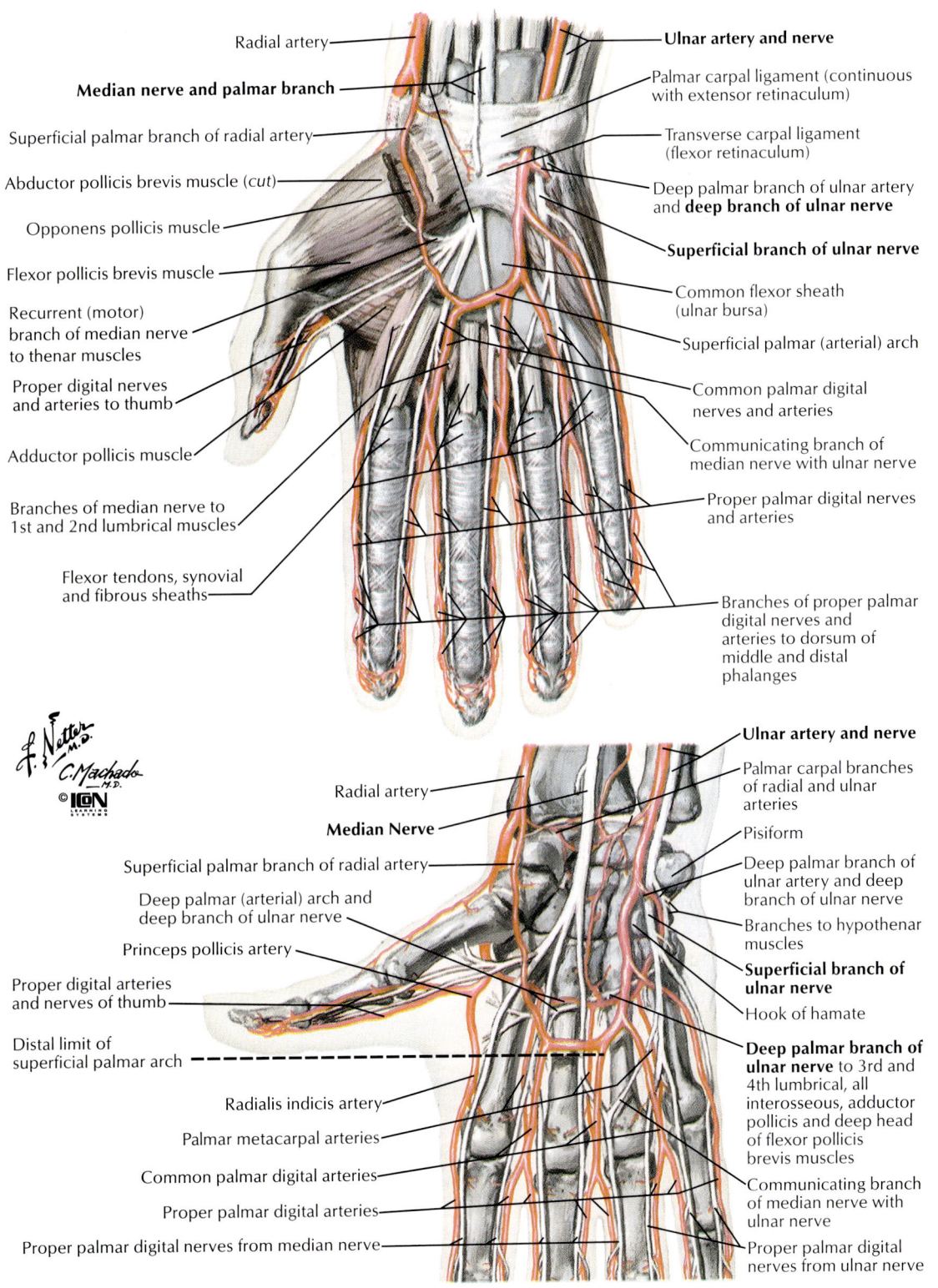

MONONEUROPATHIES

727

MONONEUROPATHIES PRESENTING WITH UPPER EXTREMITY SYMPTOMS

Figure 84-2

Carpal Tunnel Syndrome—I

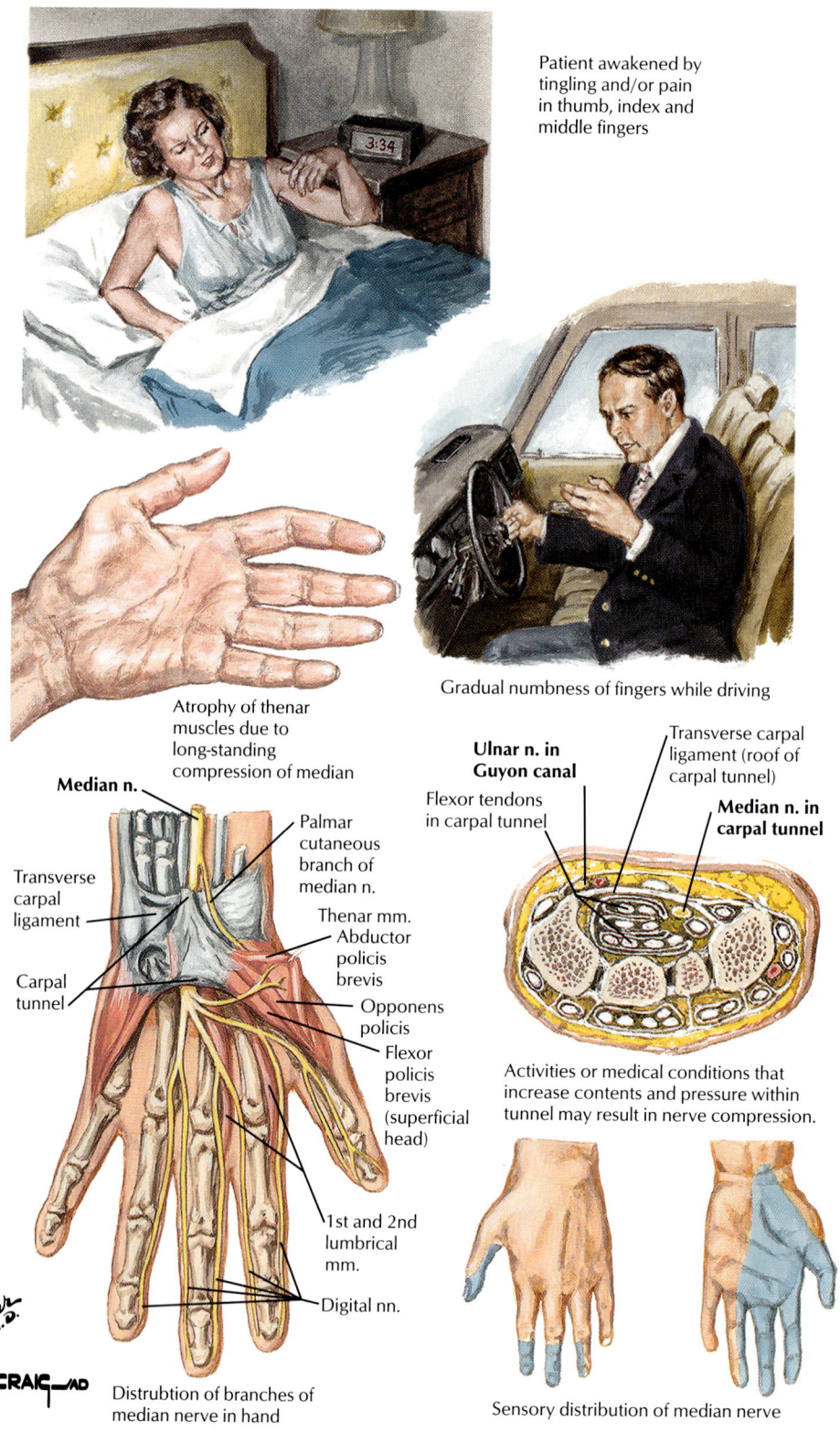

Mononeuropathies

MONONEUROPATHIES PRESENTING WITH UPPER EXTREMITY SYMPTOMS

Figure 84-3

Carpal Tunnel Syndrome—II
Provocative maneuvers

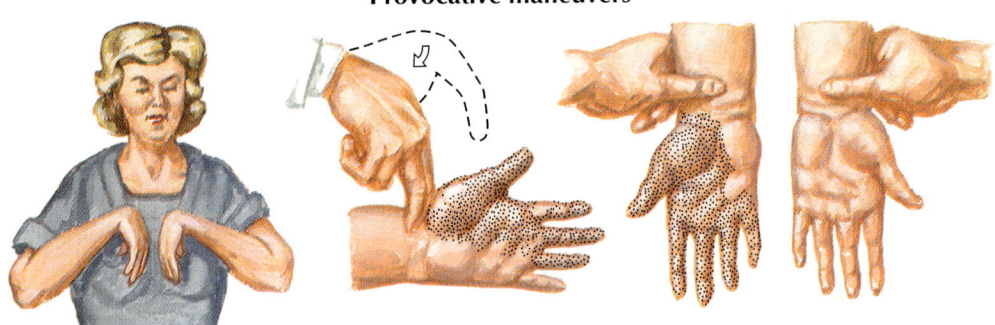

Phalen test (wrist flexion) — Tinel sign — Digital compression test
Provocative tests elicit paresthesia in hand.

Nonsurgical management

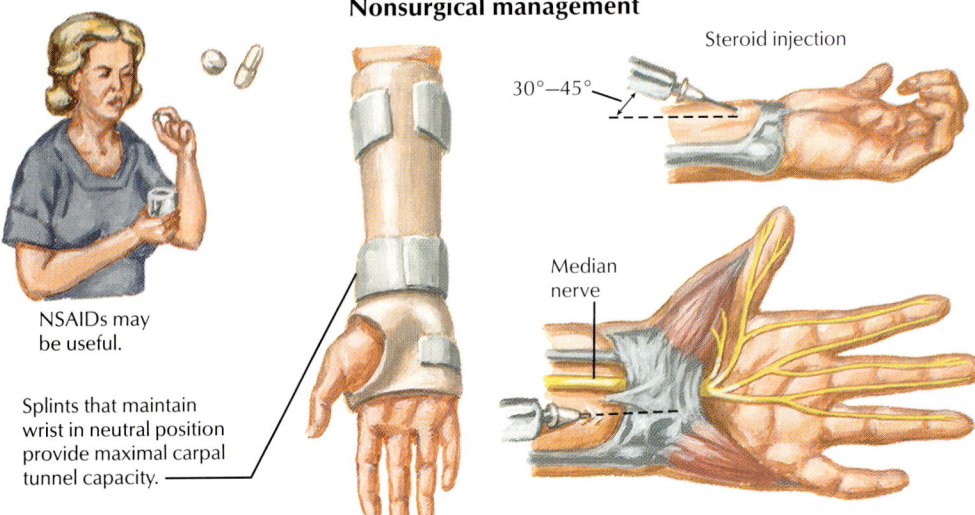

NSAIDs may be useful.

Splints that maintain wrist in neutral position provide maximal carpal tunnel capacity.

Steroid injection 30°–45°

Median nerve

Surgical decompression of carpal tunnel

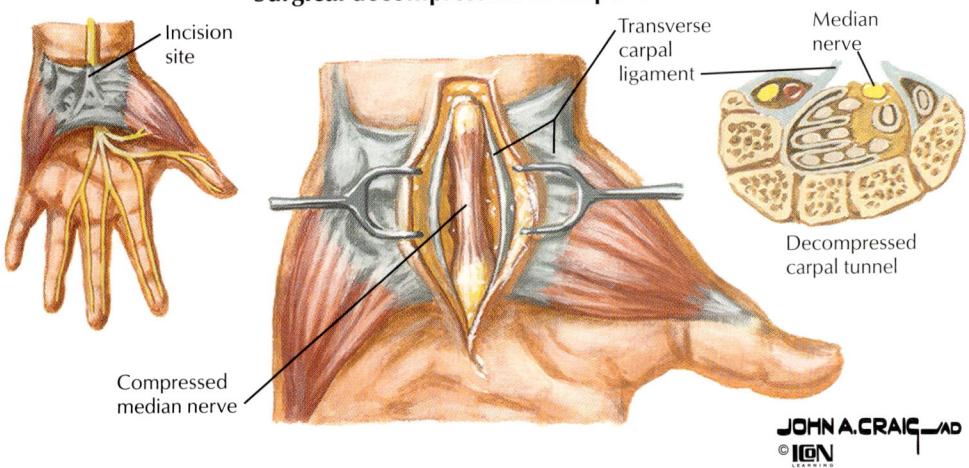

Incision site — Transverse carpal ligament — Median nerve

Compressed median nerve — Decompressed carpal tunnel

MONONEUROPATHIES

MONONEUROPATHIES PRESENTING WITH UPPER EXTREMITY SYMPTOMS

Phalen maneuver should be maintained for at least 1 minute before determining that the result is negative. The pressure test may be the most reliable of the 3 maneuvers; pressure is placed over the carpal tunnel (proximal palm, not wrist) for 20 to 30 seconds, attempting to reproduce paresthesias in a median nerve distribution.

Differential Diagnosis

Differentiation of CTS from other neurologic disorders is usually straightforward. The most common differential diagnosis is a C6-7 radiculopathy, in which numbness occurs in a similar distribution, ie, digits 1 through 3. Patients with a radiculopathy usually have neck or radicular pain.

Nerve conduction studies and needle EMG can differentiate these entities. Although the muscles of both thenar eminence and hypothenar eminence have a C8 innervation, the C8 root supplies digits 4 through 5. It also innervates the flexor pollicis longus (FPL) and the extensor indicis proprius muscles. Ulnar neuropathies have an entirely different pattern of motor and sensory loss.

Carpal tunnel syndrome virtually never presents with motor symptoms, except in pediatric storage disorders. If thumb abduction is weak, evidence of other motor involvement should be sought to confirm a different lesion. Weakness and atrophy confined to the median forearm muscles suggest a proximal median nerve lesion, particularly at the elbow (pronator syndrome). If more widespread weakness is demonstrated, with the absence of sensory signs or symptoms, motor neuron diseases or multifocal motor neuropathy require diagnostic consideration.

A more widespread polyneuropathy should be excluded, because CTS is often bilateral and patients frequently believe that all 5 digits are involved. This can occur particularly in patients with diabetes, who may not be as aware of sensory loss in their feet compared with their hands. Clinical examination and EMG usually clarify this issue.

Plexopathies typically produce motor and sensory dysfunction within multiple nerve and root distributions in a single extremity and pain in the shoulder region. They rarely enter the CTS differential diagnosis.

Although it is uncommon for CNS disorders to produce sensory signs and symptoms within the distribution of a single peripheral nerve, cervical spinal cord lesions occasionally and very rarely focal frontal parietal brain lesions mimic CTS. Vitamin B_{12} deficiency is a consideration in patients with bilateral hand numbness. Other cervical myelopathies, particularly spondylosis, cervical spinal stenosis, and rarely intrinsic cord tumors, require consideration in the differential diagnosis of CTS.

PROXIMAL MEDIAN NEUROPATHIES

Clinical Vignette

A 46-year-old man noted difficulty with putting keys into locks and increasing difficulty with handwriting. He had worked in a factory for 27 years, where he moved large barrels many times each day. He predominantly used his right arm to grasp the top of each cask and roll it across the floor, using a pronating motion.

Neurologic evaluation demonstrated weakness of the FPL and the median-innervated portion of the flexor digitorum profundus), manifested by inability to flex the distal phalanx of the thumb and the index and long fingers with weakness of the pronator teres (PT).

EMG confirmed active and chronic denervation in the FPL, PT, and pronator quadratus. Surgical exploration demonstrated median nerve entrapment by a ligament of Struthers arising from the distal humerus.

Median neuropathies arising rostral to the most proximal muscle innervated by the median nerve (the PT) occur at a frequency of less than 1% of that of CTS. The clinical and electrodiagnostic recognition of weakness in the distribution of the forearm muscles innervated by the median nerve is the diagnostic key (Figure 84-4). Median nerve compression by the ligament of Struthers, arising from a supracondylar spur on the medial distal humerus, is uncommon but well recognized.

The anterior interosseous nerve (AIN) may be primarily damaged or is sometimes affected as a component of acute brachial plexus neuritis. It may be more of a limited form of a multifocal neuropathy than a plexopathy. Individual nerves are sometimes affected as a forme fruste of brachial plexus neuritis. Proximal nerves, particularly the anterior interosseous, long thoracic, axillary, and suprascapular nerves, seem particularly vulnerable.

MONONEUROPATHIES PRESENTING WITH UPPER EXTREMITY SYMPTOMS

Figure 84-4: Proximal Compression of Median Nerve

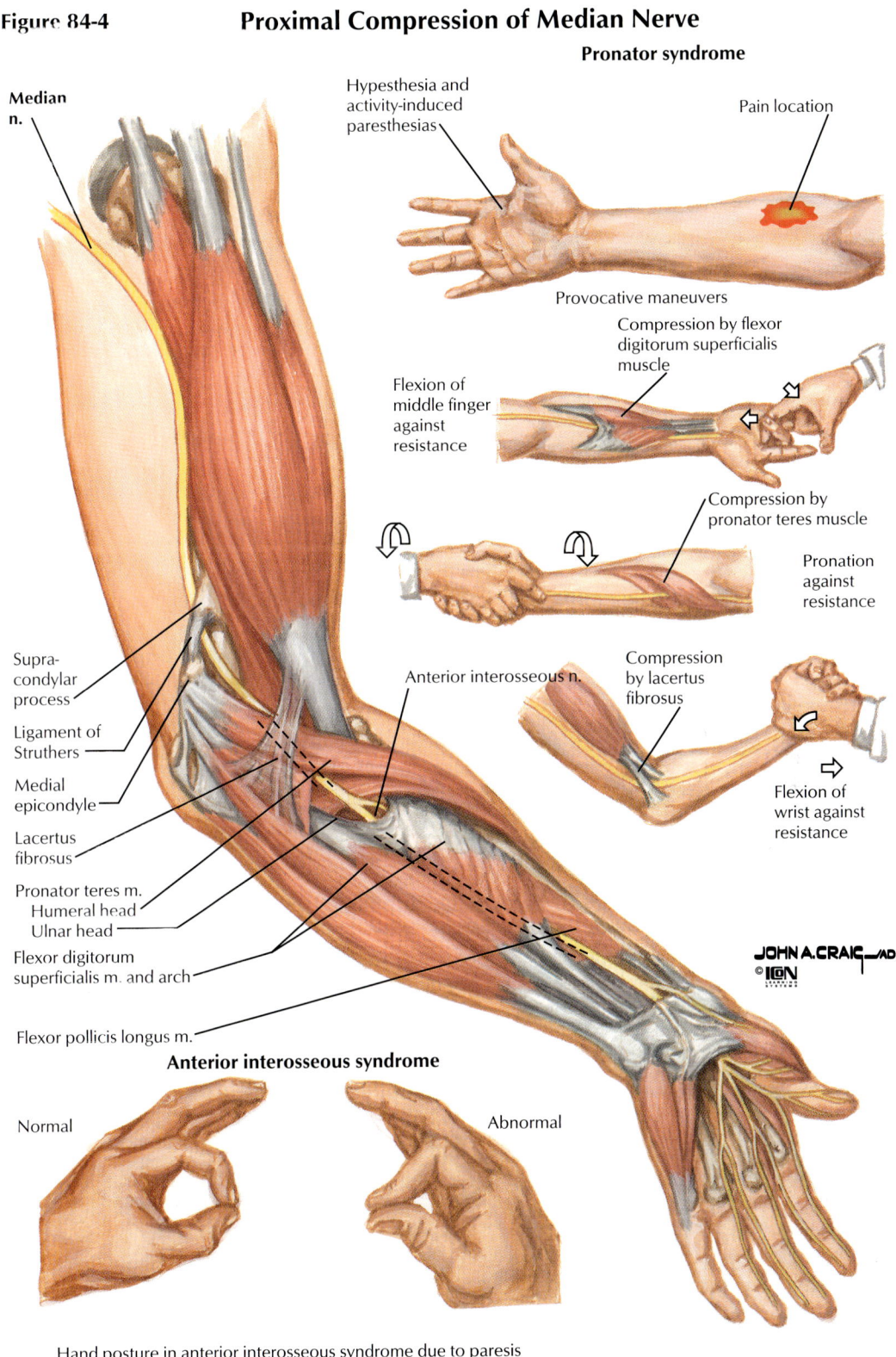

Mechanical lesions within the axilla, secondary to shoulder dislocation or penetrating injury, may also affect the proximal median nerve, although concomitant injury of other nerves often exists. More distal lesions of the proximal median nerve include humeral fractures, elbow dislocations, tourniquet compression, and forms of penetrating trauma, such as catheterization of the antecubital veins.

Anterior Interosseous Neuropathies

Typically, individuals with AIN present primarily with weakness of the distal flexors of the thumb, the FPL, the index and long fingers, and the median flexor digitorum profundus. This presentation is similar to proximal median neuropathies but without involvement of the PT. Patients report difficulty with pinching maneuvers, such as holding a pencil or key. There are no sensory symptoms or signs.

Pronator Teres Syndrome

When the median nerve lesion is most proximal, the PT is also affected. Clinical features include those of AIN and pain in the volar forearm worsened by physical use. In some individuals, the PT may be clinically weak and atrophied.

EMG is the crucial initial study in suspected AIN. Imaging studies, particularly MRI of the elbow region, are indicated when EMG results are positive. Focal lesions, such as the bony origin of a ligament of Struthers or a venous infarction secondary to tourniquet compression, may be defined on neuroimaging.

ULNAR MONONEUROPATHIES

The other major peripheral nerve supplying the hand, the ulnar nerve, primarily innervates all intrinsic hand muscles, with the exception of the thenar eminence, where it supplies just 2 muscles, the adductor pollicis and part of the flexor pollicis brevis (Figure 84-1). Only 2 forearm muscles have ulnar innervation, the flexor carpi ulnaris and the medial half of the flexor digitorum profundus. The ulnar nerve also supplies sensation to the medial $1\frac{1}{2}$ fingers (digits $4\frac{1}{2}$ and 5). Similarly to its median counterpart, the ulnar nerve typically is affected at 2 anatomical loci, the elbow and wrist; however, in reverse frequency; the majority of ulnar nerve lesions occur at the elbow (Figure 84-5).

Proximal Lesions

Proximal ulnar neuropathies are second only to CTS in frequency. Etiologies include external compression or entrapment at the elbow after remote elbow trauma (tardy ulnar palsy), from entrapment just distal to the elbow joint (cubital tunnel syndrome) or more rarely at the wrist or palm (Figure 84-6).

Manifestations of ulnar neuropathies vary with location and severity. Numbness and paresthesias of the fifth and sometimes half of the fourth digit are the rule and may be provoked by having the patient maintain a fully flexed elbow posture for 30 to 60 seconds. Sensory signs or symptoms should not extend proximal to the wrist. Weakness of the intrinsic muscles of the hand is more common in ulnar neuropathies than in CTS. The common ulnar lesion at the elbow is generally not associated with aching elbow or forearm pain. Clinically apparent involvement of ulnar forearm muscles is rarely detected.

Distal Lesions

Ulnar neuropathies within the palm are uncommon. They present with weakness confined to the ulnar muscles on the lateral aspect of the hand, particularly thumb adduction (Figure 84-7). This is secondary to weakness of the adductor pollicis, the only thenar muscle not primarily innervated by the median nerve. The first dorsal interosseous muscle is also affected, whereas abduction of the little finger may be preserved. Because the lesion is distal to the distribution of the last ulnar sensory fibers, these uncommon neuropathies have no associated sensory symptoms. The accompanying intrinsic muscle atrophy sometimes prompts consideration of motor neuron disease.

Ulnar neuropathies in the palm usually result from local trauma and repetitive injury, eg, from bicycling or from occupations that use tools requiring significant intermittent pressure over the distal ulnar motor fibers (ie, electricians, clam or oyster shuckers, and pizza cutters).

EMG is essential for diagnosis. When the pressure is discontinued, significant recovery of func-

MONONEUROPATHIES PRESENTING WITH UPPER EXTREMITY SYMPTOMS

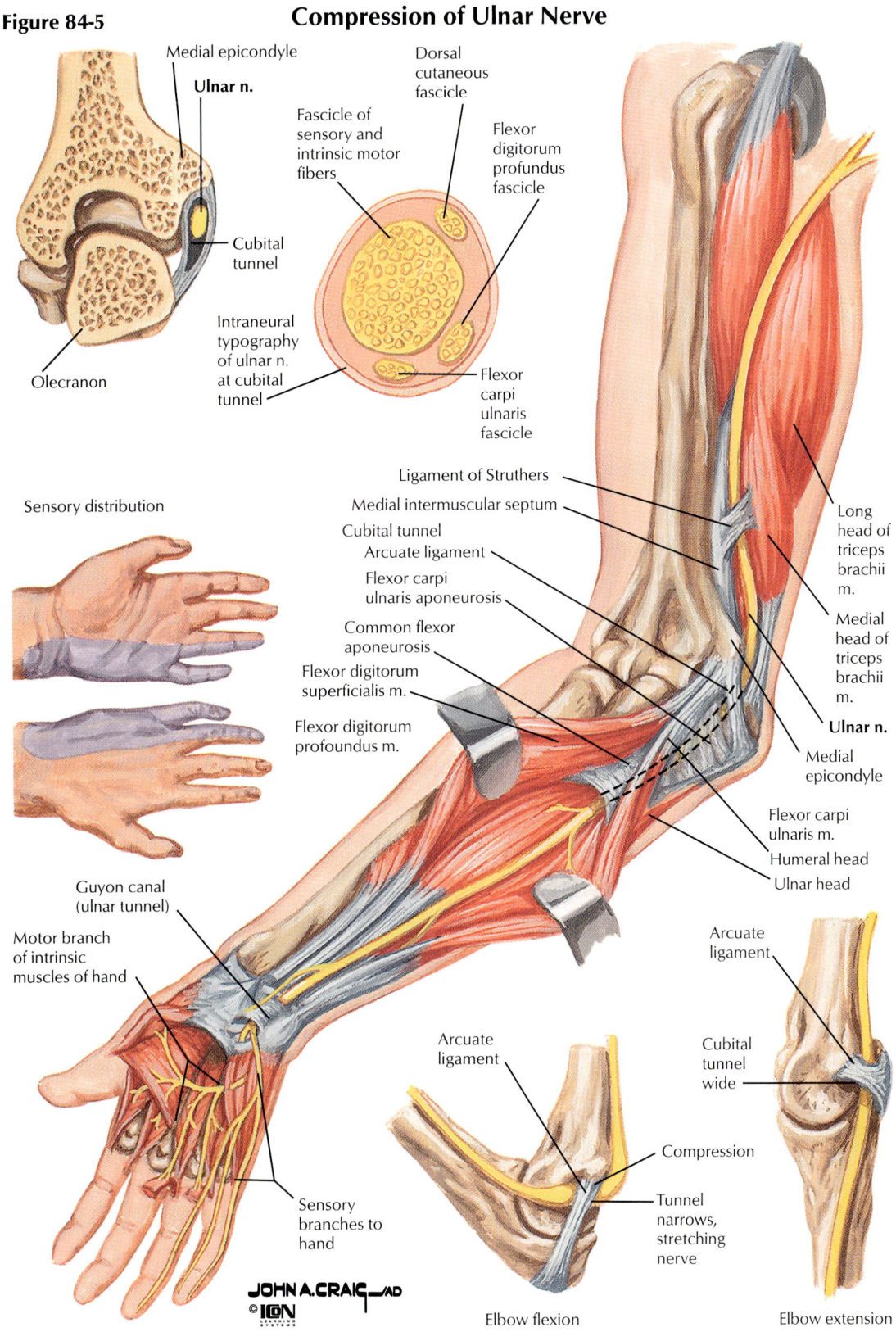

Figure 84-5. Compression of Ulnar Nerve

MONONEUROPATHIES PRESENTING WITH UPPER EXTREMITY SYMPTOMS

Figure 84-6

Cubital Tunnel Syndrome

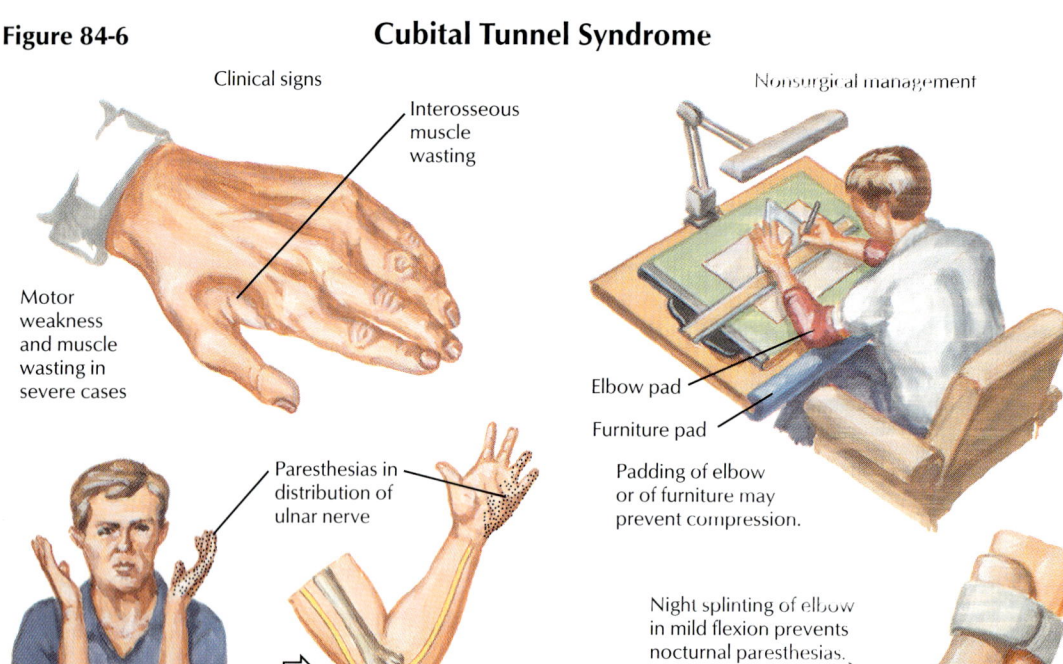

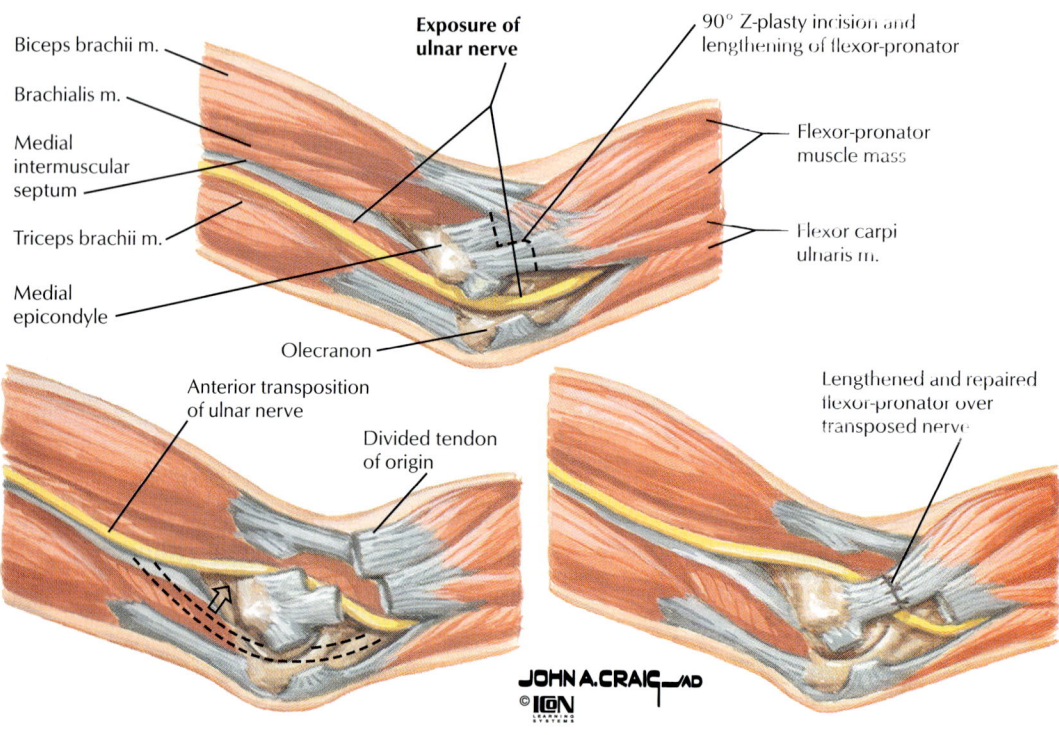

MONONEUROPATHIES

MONONEUROPATHIES PRESENTING WITH UPPER EXTREMITY SYMPTOMS

Figure 84-7 — Ulnar Tunnel Syndrome

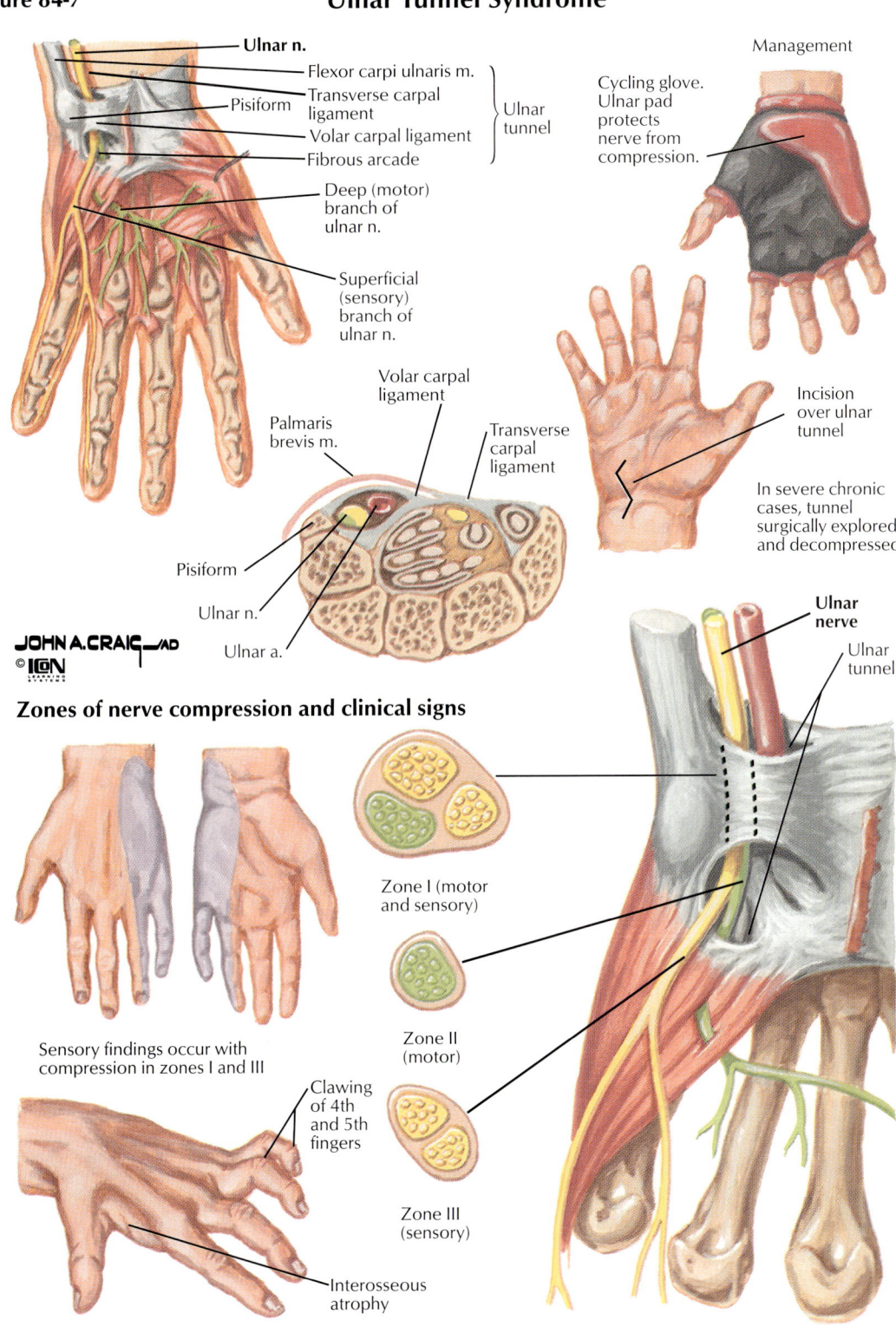

MONONEUROPATHIES PRESENTING WITH UPPER EXTREMITY SYMPTOMS

tion frequently occurs. Ulnar neuropathies at the wrist are rare and are most commonly seen in systemic diseases.

Differential Diagnosis

Brachial plexopathies typically produce pain in the shoulder region, accompanied by motor and sensory dysfunction in the distribution of multiple peripheral nerve and nerve root territories within a single extremity. Early in their course, some plexopathies may mimic mononeuropathy, particularly of the ulnar nerve.

Historically, **thoracic outlet syndrome**, a distal T1 radiculopathy or proximal lower trunk brachial plexopathy, was considered a common cause of upper extremity neurologic symptoms. Thoracic outlet syndrome is now recognized as a rare condition that is more likely to mimic an ulnar neuropathy than CTS. Perhaps many cases of CTS were erroneously diagnosed and treated as thoracic outlet syndrome before the recognition of the frequency of CTS in the late 1950s and early 1960s. EMG defined the relative frequency of these lesions.

C8 radiculopathy is less common than C7 or C6 radiculopathy but can easily be confused with an ulnar neuropathy because of its sensory distribution. Symptoms of medial forearm numbness and weak, non–ulnar innervated C8 muscles (ie, the thenar eminence, the FPL, and the extensor indicis proprius) provide the major diagnostic distinctions.

RADIAL NEUROPATHIES

The radial nerve primarily supplies the extensor muscles of the arm and forearm and 1 flexor of the arm, the brachioradialis. It also provides the sensory innervation to the lateral aspect of the hand and the dorsum of the first $3\frac{1}{2}$ fingers.

Predominant Motor Radial Neuropathies

Radial neuropathies most commonly occur at the **midhumeral level** near the spiral groove, secondary to external compression (Figure 84-8). These lesions primarily present with wrist and finger drop but little or no pain; sensory signs and symptoms are often elusive. Elbow extension is spared because the branches of the triceps originate proximal to the spiral groove. The brachioradialis reflex is typically diminished or lost, whereas the triceps and biceps reflexes are unaffected. A potentially confounding examination feature is a pseudoweakness of ulnar innervated finger abduction that appears concomitant with wrist drop. The full strength of these ulnar muscles requires at least partial wrist extension. Testing the strength of finger abduction while placing the hand and forearm flat on a hard and flat surface circumvents this problem and prevents false localization.

The **posterior interosseous nerve** (PIN) is analogous to the AIN because it is a distal, purely motor, branch of a major peripheral nerve trunk. Posterior interosseous neuropathies commonly occur with fractures of the proximal radius and sometimes have a delayed onset. The PIN may also be compromised by soft tissue masses. A syndrome of pain and weakness in the muscles innervated by the PIN may occur in patients who perform repetitious and strenuous pronation/supination movements, which in some instances leads to intermittent PIN compression by the fibrous edge of the arcade of Frohse. Entrapment may also develop secondary to an inordinately hypertrophied or anomalous supinator muscle. The extensor carpi radialis longus and brevis and the brachioradialis muscles are innervated by branches exiting the radial nerve before the origin of the PIN; therefore, finger drop, rather than wrist drop as with a more proximal radial nerve lesion, is the dominant manifestation. There are no sensory symptoms. Pain near the lateral epicondyle of the humerus, extending into the dorsal forearm without objective weakness, may or may not occur. Electrodiagnostic evidence of denervation is a proposed but unlikely manifestation of PIN neuropathy.

Predominant Sensory Radial Neuropathies

The **superficial radial nerve**, a primary distal sensory branch, may be injured in isolation with external pressure at the wrist, for example, with handcuff injuries. These injuries are readily recognized by the distribution of sensory symptoms on the dorsolateral portion of the hand. Weakness does not occur.

MONONEUROPATHIES PRESENTING WITH UPPER EXTREMITY SYMPTOMS

Figure 84-8

Radial Nerve Compression

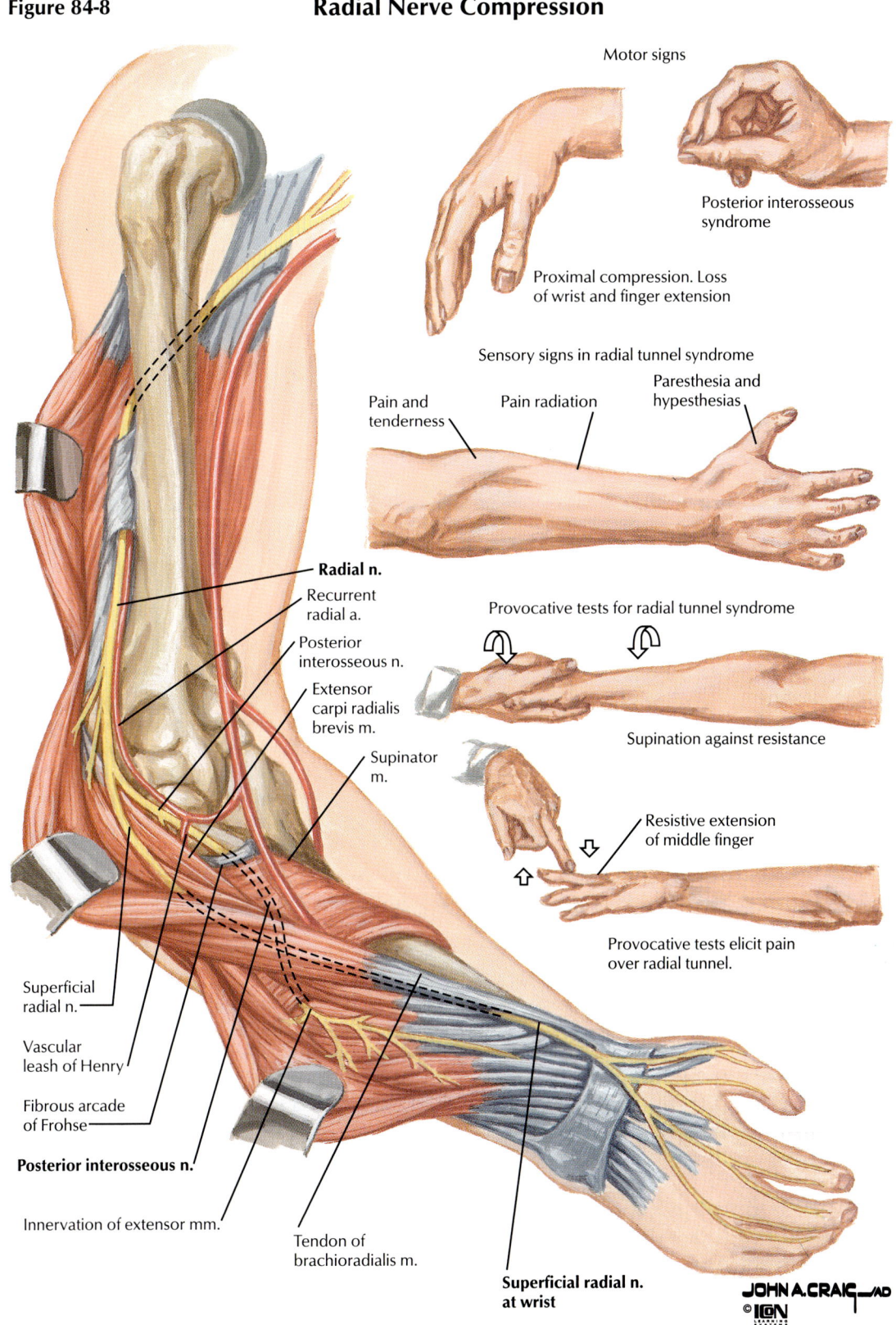

MONONEUROPATHIES PRESENTING WITH UPPER EXTREMITY SYMPTOMS

Figure 84-8   **Radial Nerve Compression (continued)**

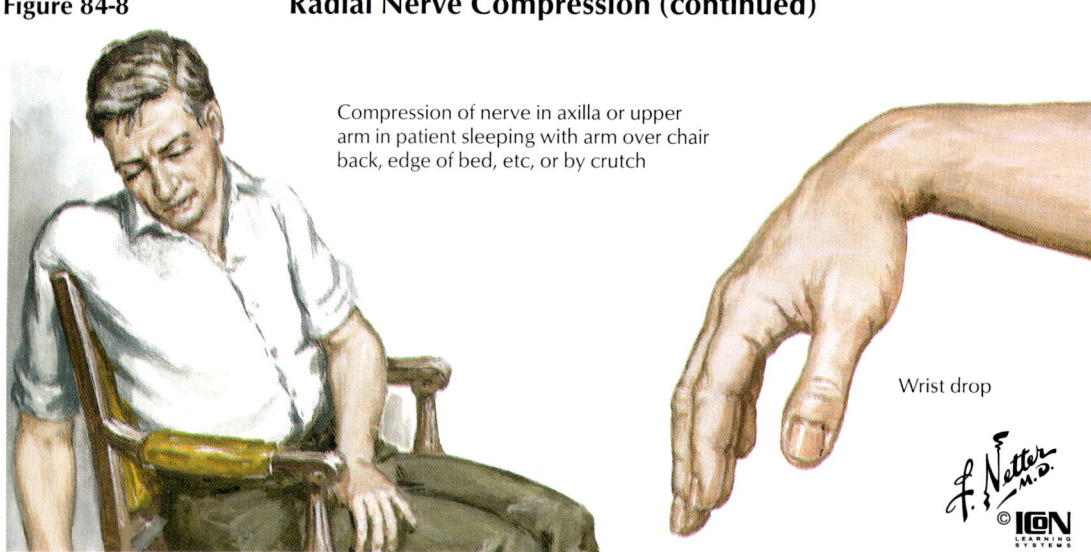

Compression of nerve in axilla or upper arm in patient sleeping with arm over chair back, edge of bed, etc, or by crutch

Wrist drop

UNUSUAL SENSORY NEUROPATHIES OF THE FOREARM

Reports of isolated, more proximal sensory symptoms on the lateral volar aspect of the forearm usually signify injury to the **lateral cutaneous nerve of the forearm**, a terminal sensory branch of the musculocutaneous nerve, therefore indicating a more proximal nerve injury. An associated weakness of elbow flexion and supination, with loss of the biceps reflex, also occurs. Injury to the lateral cutaneous nerve of the forearm is relatively uncommon but typically occurs with attempted cannulation of the cephalic or basilic vein in the antecubital fossa.

Similarly, isolated injuries of the **medial cutaneous nerve of the forearm** are rare. Sensory symptoms in the medial volar forearm are more commonly a result of more proximal injuries to the lower trunk or medial cord of the brachial plexus or to the C8 nerve root. Nerve injuries at these levels are associated with additional clinical findings, particularly hand weakness. Sensory symptoms on the posterior forearm from isolated injuries to the **posterior cutaneous nerve of the forearm** are equally rare.

DIAGNOSTIC APPROACH
EMG and Nerve Conduction Studies

EMG and nerve conduction studies provide the means to confirm the existence, location, pathophysiology, and severity of most mononeuropathies. Ideally, the injured nerve needs to be accessible to stimulation at multiple levels, including at least 1 site proximal to the site of injury. The various mononeuropathies do not have identical pathophysiologic signatures. Some, such as CTS, are initially characterized by focal slowing, whereas others may produce preferential demyelinating conduction block, such as an ulnar neuropathy at the elbow, axon loss as with a primary laceration, or a combination of the above.

Electrodiagnosis has important limitations. False-positive results can result from cold limb temperature, failure to recognize normal anatomic variants, or poor technique. Caution is required not to overcall on the basis of borderline data. Ideally, the presence of abnormalities in 2 concordant parameters enables conclusive diagnosis. False-negative results also occur. Ten percent of patients with histories that are strongly suggestive of CTS have normal electrodiagnostic evaluations.

Other Testing Modalities

Although most mononeuropathies occur secondary to recognizable compression, stretch, or entrapment mechanisms, some seem to be idiopathic. Additional testing, particularly MRI, may be diagnostic when mononeuropathies develop

MANAGEMENT
Median Neuropathies at the Wrist

Offending activities or positions need to be avoided. With CTS, neutral wrists splints, typically worn at night, provide conservative therapy by maximizing the carpal tunnel diameter and minimizing nerve pressure. Ergonomic workplace alterations should take place for patients with repetitive hand use occupations. If the patient acutely aggravates preexisting CTS, a local injection with corticosteroids may provide temporary pain relief, but this is rarely a permanent solution. Repeated injections increase the risk of flexor tendon rupture.

Surgical decompression is offered to patients with increasingly annoying sensory symptoms and is particularly indicated for those who have developed significant axon loss manifested by constant sensory symptoms and thenar atrophy (Figure 84-3).

Occasionally, elderly patients present with end-stage CTS and absent motor or sensory responses on nerve conduction studies. Resolution of pain, if still present, is the only realistic goal of surgical intervention for these patients. Meaningful return of sensation or thenar strength is unlikely this late in the course of the neuropathy. Endoscopic techniques are being used in carpal tunnel decompression but have no proven benefit compared with traditional decompressive surgery.

Ulnar Neuropathies at the Elbow

Conservative treatment consists of avoiding the stretch produced by a fully flexed elbow via a padded splint that prevents further direct nerve pressure. Surgical management of ulnar lesions is not as well defined as with CTS. It is less clear who is likely to benefit from surgery and which surgical procedure is appropriate. However, pain, progressive motor deficits, and to a lesser extent failure to improve after approximately 3 to 6 months of conservative management are reasons to consider surgery. With tardy ulnar palsy, surgeons typically transpose the nerve away from the offending epicondylar groove, often with concomitant epicondylectomy (Figure 84-6). This procedure is associated with some risk, particularly in patients with diabetes, because the microvasculature of the nerve can be easily compromised. For cubital tunnel lesions, it may be sufficient to decompress the nerve as it passes through the 2 heads of the flexor carpi ulnaris muscle.

Radial Neuropathies

Radial neuropathies usually result from monophasic external compression. They are almost always treated conservatively and successfully.

PROGNOSIS

Prognosis primarily depends on whether the injury has a demyelinating or axonal pathophysiologic mechanism or both. If axonal, recovery depends on the number of axons damaged, the persistence or resolution of the causative insult, the distance between the site of injury and the innervated muscle or cutaneous region, and the patient's age and comorbidities. Demyelinating lesions usually resolve spontaneously after removal of focal compression or entrapment.

REFERENCES

Arle JE, Zager EL. Surgical treatment of common entrapment neuropathies in the upper limbs. *Muscle Nerve*. 2000;23:1160-1174.

Beekman R, Van Der Plas JPL, Uitdehaag BMJ, Schellens RLLA, Visser LH. Clinical, electrodiagnostic, and sonographic studies in ulnar neuropathy at the elbow. *Muscle Nerve*. 2004;30:202-208.

Bozentka DJ. Cubital tunnel syndrome pathophysiology. *Clin Orthop*. 1998;351:90-94.

Brown RA, Gelberman RH, Seiler JG, et al. Carpal tunnel release: a prospective randomized assessment of open and endoscopic methods. *J Bone Joint Surg*. 1993;75A:1265-1275.

Dellon AL. Review of treatment for ulnar nerve entrapment at the elbow. *J Hand Surg*. 1989;14A:688-700.

Durkan JA. A new diagnostic test for carpal tunnel syndrome. *J Bone Joint Surg*. 1991;73A:535-538.

Gelberman RH, Aronson D, Weismann MH. Carpal tunnel syndrome: results of a prospective trial of steroid injection and splinting. *J Bone Joint Surg*. 1980;62:1181-1184.

Gross MS, Gelberman RH. The anatomy of the distal ulnar tunnel. *Clin Orthop RE Res*. 1985;196:238-247.

Grundberg AB. Carpal tunnel decompression in spite of normal electromyography. *J Hand Surg*. 1983;8:348-349.

Hartz CR, Linscheir RL, Gramse RR, et al. The pronator teres syndrome: compressive neuropathy of the median nerve. *J Bone Joint Surg.* 1981;63A:885-890.

Massy-Westropp N, Grimmer K, Bain G. A systematic review of the clinical diagnostic tests for carpal tunnel syndrome. *J Hand Surg.* 2000;25:120-127.

Merlevede K, Theys P, Van Hees J. Diagnosis of ulnar neuropathy: a new approach. *Muscle Nerve.* 2000;23:478-481.

Werner RA, Andary M. Carpal tunnel syndrome: pathophysiology and clinical neurophysiology. *Clin Neurophysiol.* 2002;113:1373-1381.

Chapter 85
Mononeuropathies Presenting With Shoulder Pain and Weakness

Alice A. Hunter and James A. Russell

Clinical Vignette

A 39-year-old right-handed avid tennis player was evaluated for a dull, aching pain in the posterior lateral aspect of his right shoulder. He described the pain worsening near the end of a tennis match, lingering, and then slowly improving. He was aware of weakness only when serving tennis balls. He had no recollection of injury or sensory symptoms.

Examination disclosed tenderness to palpation at the spinoglenoid notch. The patient's pain was reproduced only with cross-body adduction of the right arm. Shoulder position was normal; range of motion was full, and the glenohumeral and scapulothoracic dynamics were normal. Motor examination results were normal except for slight weakness of external rotation and mild atrophy of the infraspinatus muscle overlying the scapula. Reflex and sensory examination results were normal.

These findings of infraspinatus atrophy, weak external rotation of the shoulder, and point tenderness over the spinoglenoid notch were consistent with a focal suprascapular neuropathy. EMG demonstrated active denervation confined to the infraspinatus muscle consistent with the clinical diagnosis.

CLINICAL PRESENTATION

Mononeuropathies of the shoulder girdle are relatively uncommon and can be challenging. Unlike other mononeuropathies, pain is often the cardinal symptom, and the differential diagnosis involves orthopedic conditions with which the clinical neurologist may have little familiarity. Shoulder pain and weakness, real or perceived, can originate from disorders of the musculoskeletal system, cervical disc disease, mononeuropathies, or the aorta and other great vessels.

Shoulder girdle mononeuropathies are essentially caused by 1 of 5 mechanisms: brachial plexus neuritis, direct compression, transecting injury, stretch, or entrapment. Musculoskeletal mechanisms are the most prevalent. The history should focus on the precise location of the pain, positions and activities that provoke pain, defining the time of day of maximal discomfort, and any precipitating injury. True weakness can be difficult to separate from impaired effort due to pain and may be present in rotator cuff or other tendon tears in the absence of nerve injury.

Paresthesias or sensory loss, particularly if well defined within a recognized single nerve distribution, usually indicate peripheral nerve pathology. Atrophy can be related to axon loss or occasionally prolonged disuse; sometimes the clinical distinction is difficult. Shoulder motion is evaluated for abnormal dynamics of the glenohumeral, acromioclavicular, and scapulothoracic joints. Pain of shoulder joint origin may be relieved by local anesthetic injection into the joint.

Suprascapular Nerve

The suprascapular nerve may be injured at the suprascapular notch, before the innervation of the supraspinatus muscle, or distally at the spinoglenoid notch, affecting the infraspinatus alone (Figure 85-1). Acute-onset cases result from blunt shoulder trauma, with or without scapular fracture, or from forceful anterior rotation of the scapula. The suprascapular nerve may also be affected by brachial plexus neuritis in isolation or with other nerves. Suprascapular neuropathies

MONONEUROPATHIES PRESENTING WITH SHOULDER PAIN AND WEAKNESS

Figure 85-1

Neuropathy About Shoulder

Suprascapular Nerve

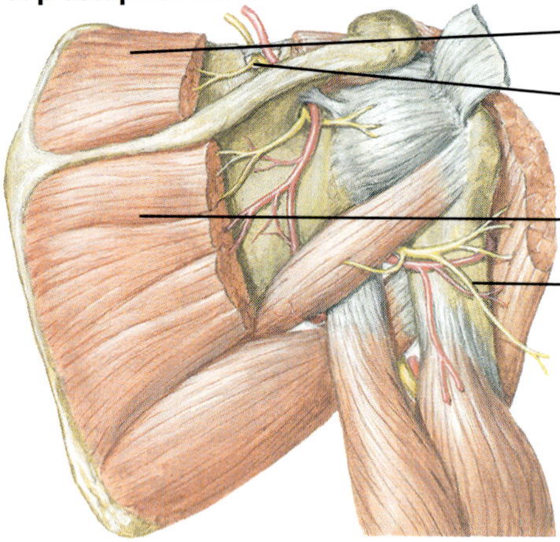

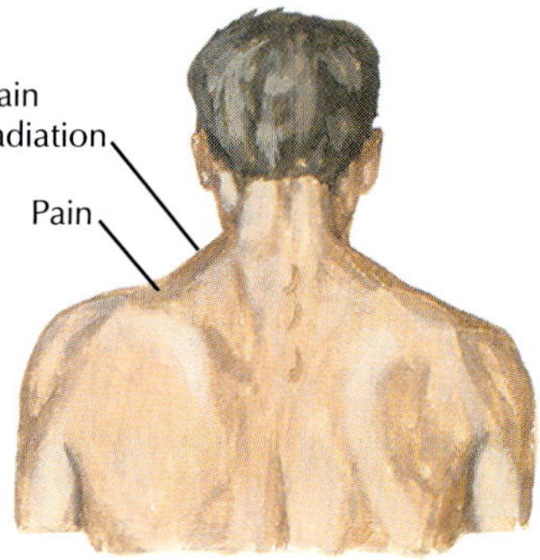

Compression of suprascapular nerve may cause lateral shoulder pain and atrophy of supraspinatus and infraspinatus muscles.

Musculocutaneous Nerve

Musculocutaneous nerve compression within coracobrachialis muscle causes hypesthesia in lateral forearm and weakness of elbow flexion.

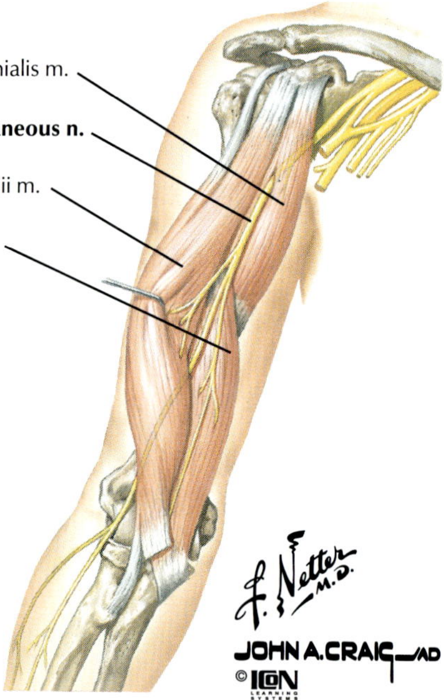

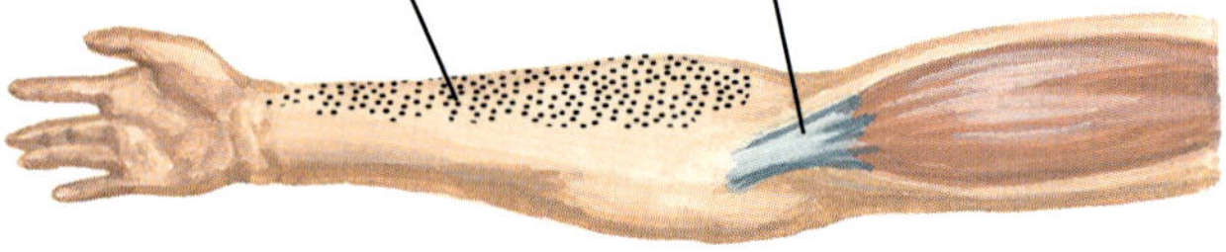

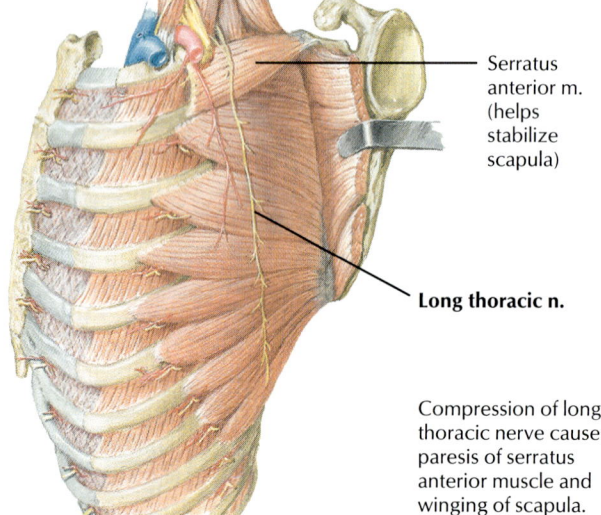

Long Thoracic Nerve

Compression of long thoracic nerve causes paresis of serratus anterior muscle and winging of scapula.

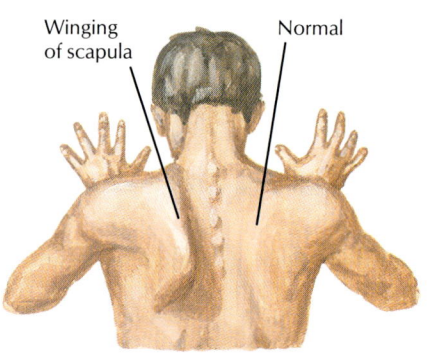

MONONEUROPATHIES

MONONEUROPATHIES PRESENTING WITH SHOULDER PAIN AND WEAKNESS

having an insidious onset often occur subsequent to fractures, from entrapment at the suprascapular or spinoglenoid notch, by compression from a ganglion or other soft tissue mass or by traction caused by repetitive overhead activity such as swimming or tennis.

DIFFERENTIAL DIAGNOSIS

The most common etiologies of shoulder pain are injuries to glenohumeral, subacromial, and acromioclavicular regions. Pain often may be reproduced by local pressure or provocative movements and positions. There should be no associated muscle weakness or sensory symptoms with musculoskeletal injury. Rotator cuff tears may mimic nerve injury because of apparent weakness of shoulder abduction (supraspinatus) and external rotation (teres minor and infraspinatus).

Motor neuron disease may begin in the shoulder region. It always must be considered in the differential diagnosis of weakness without associated sensory signs and symptoms.

C5 radiculopathy also enters the differential diagnosis in patients reporting shoulder pain sometimes extending into the upper arm with weakness and numbness. This pain often originates within the scapular region and not the neck. Having patients extend their neck laterally in the direction of the symptomatic limb may reproduce the pain. Patients with C5 weakness have problems with shoulder abduction (deltoid and supraspinatus muscles), external rotation (infraspinatus), and arm flexion (biceps brachii). The biceps stretch reflex is often diminished. Paresthesias or sensory loss occurs in a discrete triangular distribution on the lateral shoulder surface.

OTHER PROXIMAL MONONEUROPATHIES OF THE SHOULDER

Long Thoracic Nerve

The long thoracic nerve primarily innervates the serratus anterior muscle; it has no cutaneous sensory representation (Figure 85-1). Weakness of the **serratus anterior** is debilitating because it stabilizes the scapula for pushing movements and elevates the arm above 90°. This is the most common cause of scapular winging; it is best recognized by having the patient push against a wall. The inferior medial border is the most prominently projected away from the body wall. A dull shoulder ache may accompany this neuropathy. When severe acute pain occurs with the onset of scapular winging, brachial plexus neuritis should be considered.

The long thoracic nerve may be damaged by mechanical factors including repetitive or particularly forceful injuries to the shoulder or lateral thoracic wall and by surgical procedures including first rib resection, mastectomy, or thoracotomy. It is also one of the most common nerves to be affected by acute brachial neuritis, solely or in combination with others.

Scapular winging can also be related to scapular fracture and avulsion. Because they are surgically correctable, it is important to distinguish them from a primary long thoracic nerve injury. Winging is also a predominant feature in patients with facioscapulohumeral muscular dystrophy, where its strikingly asymmetric and bilateral representation immediately distinguishes it from long thoracic nerve palsy.

Spinal Accessory Nerve

Neuropathies affecting the spinal accessory nerve are easily missed because shoulder pain is the predominant presenting symptom. Sometimes weakness is not evident on standard manual muscle testing. The most common injury site is within the posterior triangle of the neck distal to sternocleidomastoid muscle innervation. Often, trapezius weakness is easier to detect by clinical observation than by manual muscle strength testing; patients have a characteristic "dropped shoulder" that hangs lower and has a steeper slope than its normal counterpart. There is no accompanying reflex or sensory loss.

The spinal accessory nerve is rarely injured intracranially, usually by meningiomas or schwannomas, which also affect the ipsilateral sternocleidomastoid. Injury at the jugular foramen by metastatic disease to the skull base also affects CN-IX and CN-X. Accessory neuropathies are most commonly iatrogenic, occurring during surgery to the posterior triangle of the neck, particularly with lymph node biopsy. These may also result from blunt trauma or slings or may occur idiopathically.

MONONEUROPATHIES PRESENTING WITH SHOULDER PAIN AND WEAKNESS

Axillary Nerve

The deltoid and the teres minor are weakened with axillary nerve lesions. Concomitantly, cutaneous sensibility of the lateral shoulder diminishes, overlapping the C5 dermatome. Because the teres minor is not the predominant external rotator of the shoulder, clinical isolation and testing are difficult. EMG may be necessary to define neurogenic injury to the teres minor.

Most axillary neuropathies are traumatic, related to anterior shoulder dislocations, fractures of the surgical humeral head, or both. Recognition of nerve injury may be delayed because of the shoulder injury. Acute axillary neuropathies can result from blunt trauma or as a component or sole manifestation of brachial plexus neuritis.

The idiopathic **quadrilateral tunnel syndrome** is hypothetically an axillary nerve entrapment syndrome. Characterized by an insidious onset of pain, it is often related to repetitive overhead activities. Pain in the area of the deltoid and down the arm is a common finding, as are paresthesias in an axillary nerve distribution. Compression of the posterior humeral circumflex artery within the quadrilateral tunnel is detectable by arteriography and Doppler ultrasonography. Evidence to support actual axillary nerve injury in this syndrome is circumspect.

Musculocutaneous Nerve

Damage to the musculocutaneous nerve results in weakness of forearm flexion and supination and sensory loss of the lateral volar forearm (Figure 85-1). The biceps reflex is diminished, but the brachioradialis reflex (same myotome, different nerve) is preserved.

Rupture of the biceps tendon is a significant differential diagnostic consideration. Pain varies, with the pain of nerve injury difficult to distinguish from that of the underlying injury.

Primary musculocutaneous neuropathies are unusual. They rarely occur from shoulder dislocation, sudden or severe forearm stretch, or as part of brachial plexus neuritis.

DIAGNOSTIC APPROACH

EMG is the primary diagnostic tool in the evaluation of suspected mononeuropathies. It is particularly helpful to identify mononeuropathies affecting the shoulder girdle for several reasons. Neurogenic injury may go unsuspected because pain is the predominant symptom. Weakness may be hidden by the observation of normal strength within unaffected muscles performing similar functions, eg, supraspinatus weakness obscured by normal deltoid function. Conversely, nerve injury may be suspected because of apparent weakness caused by tendon rupture, only to be refuted by the absence of denervation on needle EMG.

Although nerve conduction studies can be performed on the musculocutaneous, axillary, and accessory nerves, its value is limited by technical considerations. These nerves are typically accessible at only 1 stimulation site, precluding the determination of conduction velocities and accurate identification of conduction block. However, demyelination with conduction block may be suspected when a normal compound muscle action potential is obtained from a muscle with limited voluntary activation; often, this finding portends an excellent prognosis. This conclusion should be reached cautiously because the same pattern may result from axon loss when the study is performed within 5 days after injury.

Needle EMG is the primary electrodiagnostic tool in the evaluation of shoulder girdle mononeuropathies. Even subtle axon loss, which accompanies the majority of nerve injuries, can be identified by the detection of fibrillation potentials. The evaluating physician and the electromyographer should always examine the patient and consider every potential neuropathic cause of shoulder pain. Otherwise, uncommon neuropathies, eg, the accessory nerve, can easily be overlooked.

A common clinical dilemma occurs with patients who have nontraumatic shoulder girdle mononeuropathies. It is difficult to differentiate a primary idiopathic lesion from a limited form of brachial plexus neuritis and to determine whether entrapment or a related process necessitating surgical exploration is involved. A thorough clinical and electrodiagnostic examination is thus required. Subtle clinical or electrodiagnostic evidence of involvement of muscles innervated by a different nerve usually suggests that a conservative approach is indicated. This constellation of findings excludes the possibility that decompression of a single nerve could be the source.

Routine radiographs are useful to detect scapular fractures secondary to acute injuries, which sometimes predispose patients to suprascapular neuropathies or serratus anterior dehiscence from the scapula. MRI can define insidious-onset neuropathies that may be caused by expanding masses, eg, a ganglion cyst in the spinoglenoid notch.

MANAGEMENT AND PROGNOSIS

Unfortunately, shoulder bracing provides little benefit to patients with shoulder girdle weakness. Fixation of the scapula to the chest wall, a complex procedure that should be performed only by experienced surgeons, can improve strength in patients with chronic scapular winging but may decrease range of motion. With weakness of any shoulder girdle muscle, exercises to strengthen other shoulder girdle muscles may provide partial functional compensation.

If nerve transection from acute penetrating injury is suspected, surgical exploration and primary anastomosis should be considered, although results are mixed.

In acute nonpenetrating injury, exploration can be considered after 3 to 6 months provided no clinical or electrodiagnostic evidence exists of reinnervation. Nerve grafting is an option if unanticipated nerve transection is found.

For insidious-onset neuropathies without defined cause, imaging should be considered to exclude ganglion cysts or other masses. If no mass is demonstrable and the patient shows no evidence of improvement, exploration may be considered, particularly at potential sites of entrapment such as the suprascapular or spinoglenoid notches.

Despite apparent axonal injury in brachial plexus neuritis, there is a good prognosis for functional recovery, probably on the basis of the proximity of the injury to affected muscles, allowing for ease of reinnervation. Unfortunately, this recovery typically takes 6 months to 2 years. The prognosis for direct compressive injury is less predictable and probably depends on reinnervating distance, patient age, and attendant comorbidities. Stretch injuries and entrapment have the highest likelihood of a significant demyelinating component, with excellent outcome the rule, particularly if entrapment is recognized and removed before significant axon loss occurs.

FUTURE DIRECTIONS

Diagnosis and management of proximal neuropathies of the upper extremities will be improved by advances in nerve imaging and surgical management of nerve injuries. Improvement in methods of nerve anastomosis and grafting may offer new hope to patients with chronic morbidity from persisting nerve injury.

REFERENCES

Goslin KL, Krivickas LS. Proximal neuropathies of the upper extremity. *Neurol Clin.* 1999;17:525-548.

Leffert RD. Nerve lesions about the shoulder. *Orthop Clin North Am.* 2000;31:331-345.

Stewart JD. *Focal Peripheral Neuropathies.* 3rd ed. Baltimore, Md: Lippincott Williams & Wilkins; 2000.

Chapter 86
Mononeuropathies Presenting With Lower Extremity Weakness

Eric T. Tolo, James A. Russell, and H. Royden Jones, Jr

The principle nerves of the lower extremity are the femoral and obturator nerves and the sciatic nerve and its terminal branches, the tibial and common peroneal nerves. When any of these is injured, motor weakness is often the principal symptom.

PERONEAL NEUROPATHIES

Clinical Vignette

A 54-year-old football coach was evaluated for right foot drop first noted 6 weeks earlier when he tripped over his right foot. Tripping subsequently occurred with increasing frequency, especially when walking on uneven surfaces. He had no recent trauma or illness and no back, buttock, or radicular leg pain. Numbness developed over the dorsum of his foot. His medical history was unremarkable; there was no personal or family history of diabetes or nerve palsy.

Examination revealed a healthy man with normal-appearing lower extremities. However, he reported tenderness to palpation at the proximal lateral knee where there was an associated fullness without a discrete mass. Pain was not reproduced with various joint manipulations, all of which were normal. Motor examination disclosed weakness in right toe extension, foot dorsiflexion, and eversion. Plantar flexion and inversion of his right foot, knee flexion, and hip abduction were totally preserved. Sensation was diminished to pinprick and monofilament touch on the dorsum and first web space of the right foot. He had normal muscle stretch reflexes.

EMG defined a predominantly axonal, common peroneal neuropathy, with sparing of the short head of the biceps femoris. Because of the progressive course, lack of demyelinating features at the fibular head on EMG, and the local fullness and discomfort, MRI of the popliteal fossa was performed, demonstrating a large ganglion cyst emanating from the proximal tibiofibular joint. Surgical excision of the cyst with decompression of the common peroneal nerve at the proximal tibiofibular joint led to complete recovery of motor function within 3 months.

The anatomical pattern and clinical characteristics of this man's symptoms and signs reflect a common peroneal neuropathy. Isolated weakness of foot and toe dorsiflexion and foot eversion and the pattern of sensory loss are classic. In this example, there was no history implicating common predisposing mechanisms. Common peroneal neuropathy is the most common lower extremity mononeuropathy. Mainly supplied by L5 nerve root fibers, it is 1 of the 2 major divisions of the sciatic nerve and is most susceptible to external compression as it superficially crosses the fibular head (Figure 86-1).

Predisposing mechanisms include recent substantial weight loss, particularly in patients with habitual leg crossing or prolonged squatting. Similarly, external appliances such as casts, braces, and tight bandages can cause peroneal neuropathy. Occasionally diabetes mellitus, vasculitis, and rarely a hereditary tendency to pressure palsy are predisposing conditions. An acute posttraumatic **anterior** or **lateral compartment syndrome** below the knee sometimes leads to acute common, deep, or superficial peroneal neuropathies. Patients with insidious onset and progressive course, as described in the preceding vignette, require evaluation for mass lesions compromising this nerve, including a Baker cyst or ganglia, osteoma, or schwannoma.

The peroneal nerve is sometimes injured **iatrogenically**, eg, an inappropriate degree of traction after total hip arthroplasty, particularly if the ipsilateral leg is excessively lengthened. Knee positioning and padding to decrease pressure on this nerve in the operating room and ICU are important to prevent an acute compression neuropathy. Rarely, laceration of the peroneal nerve

MONONEUROPATHIES PRESENTING WITH LOWER EXTREMITY WEAKNESS

Figure 86-1

Peroneal Nerve

Compression of common peroneal nerve over fibular head by cast, in debilitated patient sitting with legs crossed, or in inebriate sleeping on side on hard surface

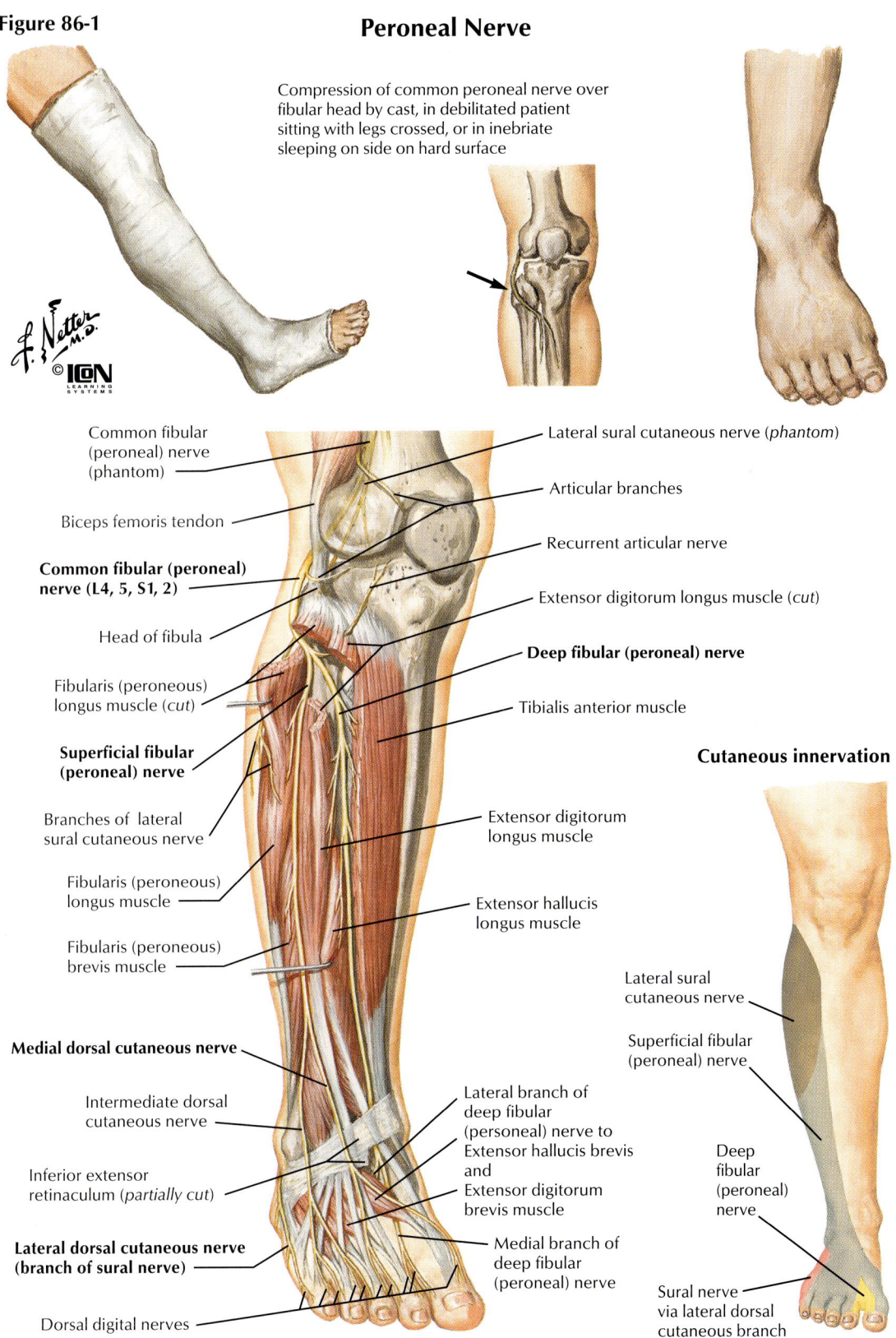

MONONEUROPATHIES

747

occurs with arthroscopic knee repair or direct penetrating trauma.

In the rare **anterior tarsal tunnel syndrome**, the deep peroneal nerve is injured at the ankle. Isolated superficial peroneal neuropathies are uncommon but usually result from lateral compartment syndrome, local trauma, or rarely an isolated schwannoma.

Clinical Presentation

Most peroneal neuropathies involve the common peroneal nerve at the fibular head causing weakness of foot dorsiflexion and eversion (Figure 86-1). With the less frequently occurring **deep peroneal** neuropathies, weakness is confined to the tibialis anterior, extensor hallucis, extensor digitorum longus, and brevis muscles. With primary **superficial peroneal** neuropathies, weakness is confined to the peroneus longus and brevis muscles, which are primarily responsible for foot eversion.

Sensory symptoms are limited to the web space between the first and second toes with deep peroneal neuropathies. Superficial peroneal neuropathies can diminish sensation on the dorsum of the foot and lateral distal half of the leg. Common peroneal sensory symptoms occur on the dorsal foot surface extending up the lateral half of the leg.

Differential Diagnosis
Sciatic Neuropathies

Because the peroneal division of the sciatic nerve is more superficial than its tibial portion, lesions as proximal as the hip can mimic a more common peroneal neuropathy. EMG involvement of the short head of the biceps femoris is the major distinguishing feature with proximal peroneal division sciatic neuropathies. Biceps femoris function cannot be isolated clinically; therefore, EMG is crucial to diagnosis. With most sciatic neuropathies, some tibial nerve functions are affected with weakness of knee flexion, foot plantar flexion, and foot inversion. Therefore, the subtle peroneal division lesion demands skillful investigation. Ankle jerk is characteristically depressed or lost if the tibial component of the sciatic nerve is affected, whereas it is typically preserved with primary peroneal neuropathies. Sensory loss is typical and affects the common peroneal territory described above and the plantar and lateral foot surfaces.

L5 Radiculopathy

An L5 lesion demands consideration in any patient who has foot drop. Back pain is expected with nerve root lesions and is uncommon in peroneal neuropathies. The pain is typically radicular with buttock, thigh, and leg components aggravated by positional change. The distribution of weakness is helpful. Isolated weakness of great toe extension is a common manifestation of L5 monoradiculopathies but rarely occurs with peroneal neuropathies. In more fully developed L5 radiculopathies, plantar foot inversion, dependent on posterior tibial muscle function, is an important L5-tibial innervated function. Careful evaluation of patients with an L5 root lesion should demonstrate this deficit in addition to those of the classic peroneal innervated musculature. Uncommonly, hip abduction weakness is discernible. The distribution of sensory symptoms in L5 radiculopathies overlaps significantly with common or superficial peroneal neuropathies. L5 nerve root lesions may extend more proximally onto the lateral leg than peroneal neuropathies.

Lumbosacral Plexopathy

Lumbosacral plexus lesions rarely enter the differential diagnosis of peroneal neuropathies but should be suspected in patients who have foot drop, proximal lower extremity pain, and motor and sensory findings extending beyond a single peripheral nerve or root distribution. Sometimes primary sciatic neuropathies are difficult to distinguish from sacral plexopathies. However, involvement of hip abduction and extension, clinically or with EMG or both, suggests plexus localization.

Other Peripheral Motor Unit Disorders

The possibility of motor neuron disease exists with insidious onset of foot drop with no associated pain or sensory findings. For example, in patients with myasthenia, unilateral foot drop can develop seemingly entirely from the neuromuscular transmission defect. Distal myopathies often produce foot drop but almost always do so bilaterally.

MONONEUROPATHIES PRESENTING WITH LOWER EXTREMITY WEAKNESS

Central Nervous System Lesions

Unilateral foot drop with or without sensory symptoms may occur with disorders of the spinal cord or parasagittal frontal lobe. MRI is important to these diagnoses.

SCIATIC NEUROPATHIES

Clinical Vignette

A 20-year-old college football player fell while running and trying to suddenly reverse direction, dislocating his hip. The lesion necessitated surgical repair. Postoperatively, the patient was placed in Buck traction with leg extension and prophylactic anticoagulation.

Two days later, he noted difficulty moving his toes and some discomfort in his right buttock. On examination, he was initially thought to have a foot drop secondary to peroneal nerve compression at the fibula head from a traction device strap. Within 24 hours, marked buttock pain and paralysis of all muscles below his right knee had developed. A large hematoma was identified over his right buttock. Despite drainage of more than 2 L of blood, there was little improvement in sciatic nerve function. Follow-up EMG 8 months later confirmed a primary sciatic nerve injury.

This vignette points to the importance of carefully considering the possibility of a proximal lesion affecting the peroneal division of the sciatic nerve in any patient in whom a foot drop develops. In this case, the possibility of traction strap–induced compression neuropathy at the fibula head slowed identification of the more proximal sciatic neuropathy.

The sciatic is the body's largest nerve, receiving contributions primarily from the L5 and S1/2 nerve roots (Figure 86-2). It has 2 primary divisions: the laterally situated peroneal, which is more superficial, and the more medially placed tibial nerves (Figure 86-3). These mixed nerves innervate the hamstrings, distal adductor magnus, anterior and posterior leg compartments, and intrinsic foot musculature. Through sensory branches of the tibial nerve (sural, medial, and lateral plantar and calcaneal) and the superficialis peroneal nerve, the sciatic nerve also supplies sensation to the skin of the entire foot and posterior lower leg.

Sciatic neuropathies can occur from hip arthroplasty, fracture, or posterior dislocation. Like femoral neuropathies, they can result from prolonged lithotomy position, presumably from stretching in individuals who are anatomically predisposed, perhaps by a persistent umbilical artery branch to this nerve. Occasionally, sciatic neuropathies result from external pressure in patients who are comatose or immobilized for protracted periods such as with drug overdose. They may result from traumatic mechanisms including misplaced injections into the inferior medial quadrant of the buttock. Mass lesions including nerve sheath tumors and external compression from hematoma, aneurysm, endometriosis, and other mechanisms have been described. Sciatic neuropathies commonly occur in patients with systemic vasculitis.

Clinical Presentation

As with peroneal neuropathies, patients with sciatic neuropathies also typically present with foot drop, weakness of other movements of the ankle and the toes, and concomitant knee flexion weakness. The ankle jerk and internal hamstring reflex are depressed or lost. Sensory loss occurs in the lateral foot (sural nerve), the plantar foot surface (medial plantar, lateral plantar, and calcaneal branches of the tibial nerve) and the dorsal foot surface extending up the lateral half of the leg (common peroneal nerve).

Clinical Vignette

A 12-year-old boy presented with a 3-year history of tingling and difficulty with running. Neurologic examination showed distal weakness in his right leg, with the EMG examination showing an absent right sural response. The right tibial and peritoneal F waves and right tibial H response could not be elicited. MRI of the thigh failed to demonstrate a mass lesion or congenital anomaly. However, because of his progressive course, surgical exploration of the sciatic nerve in the thigh was performed, demonstrating a myofascial band of the distal thigh entrapping the sciatic nerve. Sectioning of the band resulted in marked recovery of nerve function.*

Although the correct clinical diagnosis was made in this situation, MRI was unrevealing and surgical exploration was needed to specifically define the diagnosis. Good clinical judgment is an essential tool in the management of progressive and seemingly unexplained mononeuropathies.

---

*Venna et al, 1991.

MONONEUROPATHIES PRESENTING WITH LOWER EXTREMITY WEAKNESS

Figure 86-2

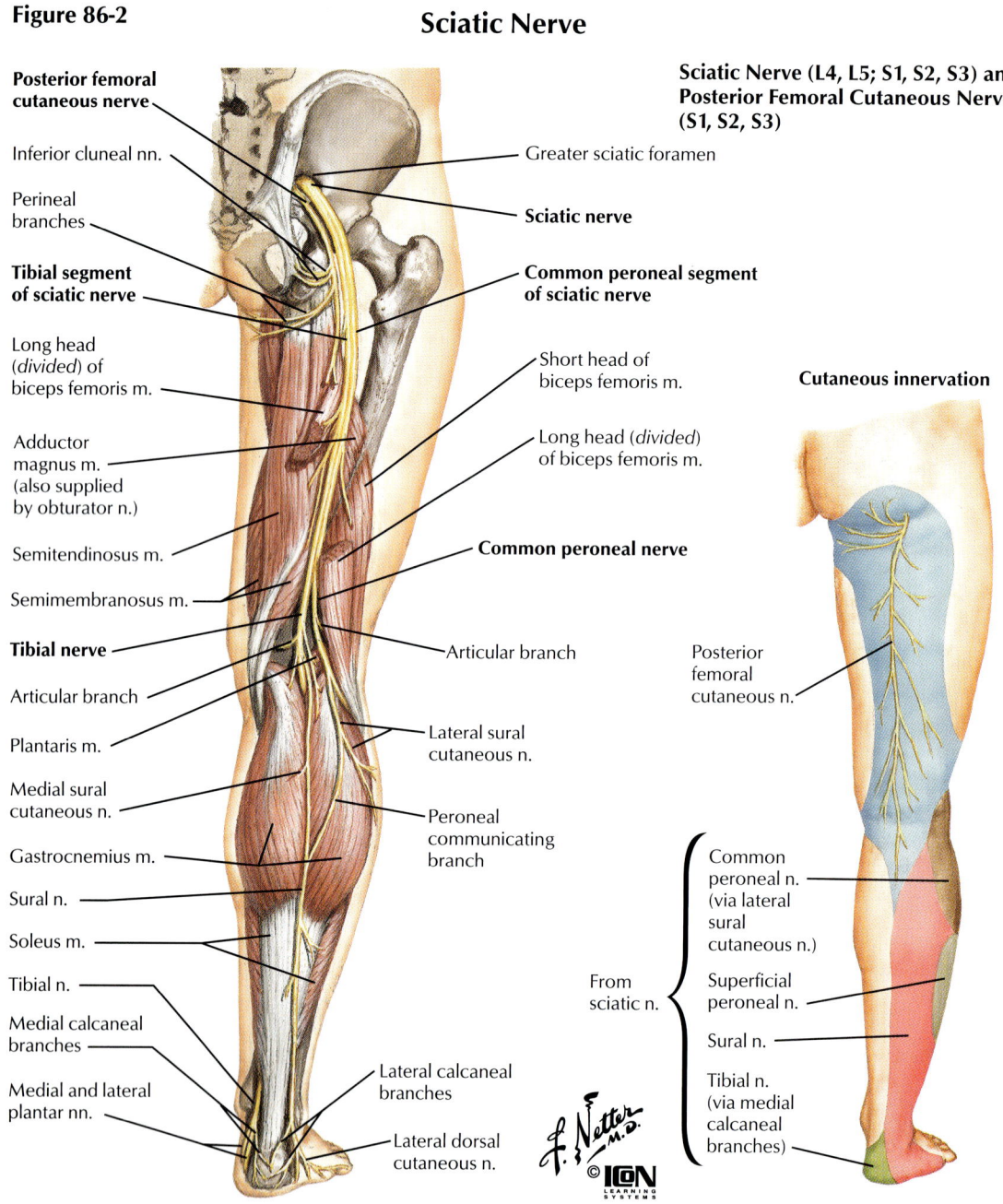

Differential Diagnosis

A **lumbosacral plexus** lesion is the primary consideration in most patients with sciatic neuropathies, when findings clearly encompass a territory outside the peroneal nerve. Hamstring weakness with sensory loss in the posterior thigh suggests a sciatic lesion. However, when clinical or EMG evidence suggests gluteal muscle involvement, primary lesions within the pelvis should be considered, especially benign tumors such as **schwannoma** or malignant processes, particularly **lymphoma**.

Piriformis syndrome is an unsubstantiated disorder that is phenomenologically similar to

MONONEUROPATHIES PRESENTING WITH LOWER EXTREMITY WEAKNESS

Figure 86-3 Tibial Nerve

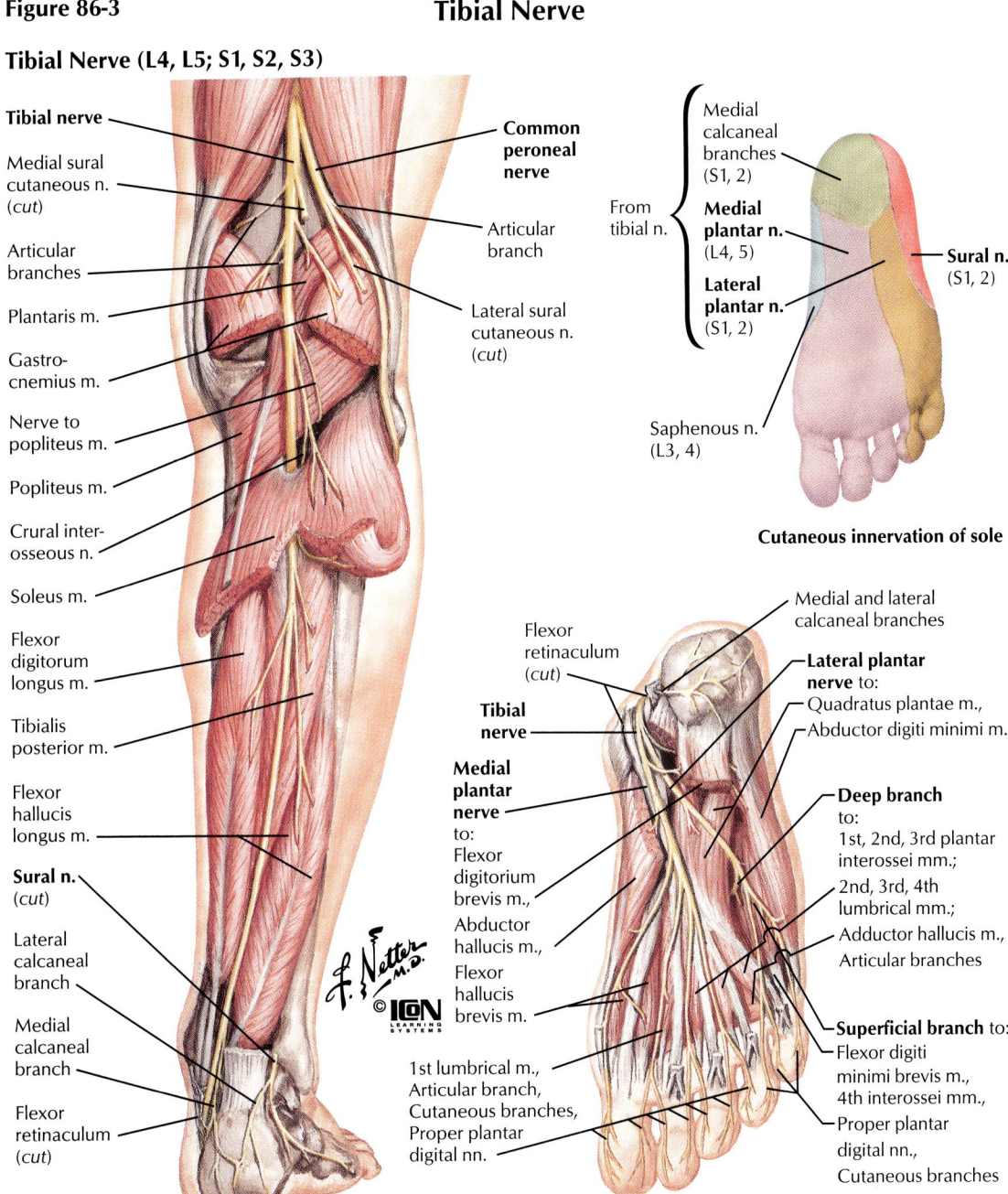

the thoracic outlet and tarsal tunnel syndromes. Descriptively, it is a syndrome of gluteal and posterior thigh pain theoretically resulting from sciatic nerve compression as it passes under or through the piriformis muscle. There are no objective clinical or electrodiagnostic signs of sciatic neuropathy in most patients in whom piriformis syndrome is suspected.

TIBIAL NEUROPATHIES

Tibial neuropathies rarely occur in isolation. They are characterized by weakness of foot plan-

MONONEUROPATHIES PRESENTING WITH LOWER EXTREMITY WEAKNESS

tar flexion and inversion, and flexion, abduction, and adduction of the toes, the latter functions being difficult to evaluate clinically. The ankle jerk is affected if the neuropathy occurs proximal to the branch points of the gastrocnemius-soleus complex. Sensory loss occurs on the heel and plantar foot surface (Figure 86-3).

Proximal tibial neuropathies may result from Baker cysts, ganglia, or rarely from severe ankle strains, the latter presumably resulting from stretch. **Tarsal tunnel syndrome**, a distal tibial neuropathy, primarily presents with sensory symptoms (chapter 87).

FEMORAL NEUROPATHIES

The femoral nerve is the other primary nerve of the lower extremity. As the major nerve of the lumbar plexus, it receives contributions primarily from the L2-4 nerve roots. Within the pelvis, it innervates the iliopsoas muscle, the primary thigh flexor, where it is prone to compression from tumors or from intraparenchymal hemorrhage into the iliopsoas. It exits the pelvis anteriorly at the femoral triangle where it lies just lateral to the femoral artery. Within the thigh, it innervates the quadriceps femoris muscle and provides sensory innervation to the anterior, lateral, and proximal medial thigh and the medial foreleg through the saphenous nerve (Figure 86-4).

Clinical Vignette

A 72-year-old man presented with increasing left groin and upper thigh pain that had begun 1 week previously. Deep venous phlebitis was diagnosed, and the patient was treated with anticoagulation. Partial thromboplastin time and prothrombin time were well maintained. Four days later, the patient experienced left flank pain radiating into his left thigh that in a few days became more severe and extended below his knee into the medial leg. He could not raise his left leg off the bed. There was no back pain or sphincter dysfunction.

Neurologic examination demonstrated moderately severe weakness of the left iliopsoas and quadriceps muscles, absent left quadriceps muscle stretch reflex, and diminished sensation to touch and pinprick over the anterior thigh and medial leg below the knee.

Pelvic CT demonstrated asymmetric enlargement of the left iliacus and psoas muscles in the pelvis, consistent with a hemorrhage. Surgery revealed a large hematoma that medially compressed the femoral nerve. This was successfully drained. Postoperatively, the patient gradually improved, regaining significant function within a week.

The hematoma in the preceding vignette created an acute entrapment of the femoral nerve. Treatment is immediate decompression when lesions are as severe and large as in this case. Sometimes when the hematoma is recognized early, before significant motor compromise occurs, for clinical or CT signs of an enlarging lesion is justified.

Femoral mononeuropathies are infrequent. Historically, **diabetic femoral neuropathies** were considered common, although most of these were actually **diabetic radiculoplexus neuropathies** wherein the femoral component dominated. These may represent an autoimmune process, perhaps with a vasculitic component. Rarely, **polyarteritis nodosa** presents as **mononeuritis multiplex**; the femoral may be one of the affected nerves, presenting with an acute lesion.

Femoral neuropathies occasionally follow prolonged surgeries in the lithotomy position, presumably from anatomical predisposition to kinking beneath the inguinal ligament. Iliacus hematoma or abscess, misplaced attempts at femoral artery or vein puncture, or iatrogenic injury after nephrectomy or hip arthroplasty are other recognized causes.

Clinical Presentation

Patients with severe quadriceps weakness are unable to extend the leg or lock the knee; when severe, this often interferes with or precludes walking. Initially, mild femoral neuropathies may present with difficulty going down stairs because the knee buckles from mild quadriceps weakness. When the more proximal femoral nerve is involved, weakness of the iliopsoas manifests as limited hip flexion.

Iliopsoas weakness is not invariable. Mild hip flexion weakness may also occur with more distal femoral nerve involvement from poor function of the rectus femoris, the only head of the quadriceps muscle originating within the pelvis and contributing to hip flexion.

The patellar muscle stretch reflex is almost always diminished or absent in femoral neuropathies. Groin and thigh pain are frequent presenting symptoms. When patients experience

MONONEUROPATHIES PRESENTING WITH LOWER EXTREMITY WEAKNESS

Figure 86-4   Femoral Nerve and Lateral Cutaneous Nerve of Thigh

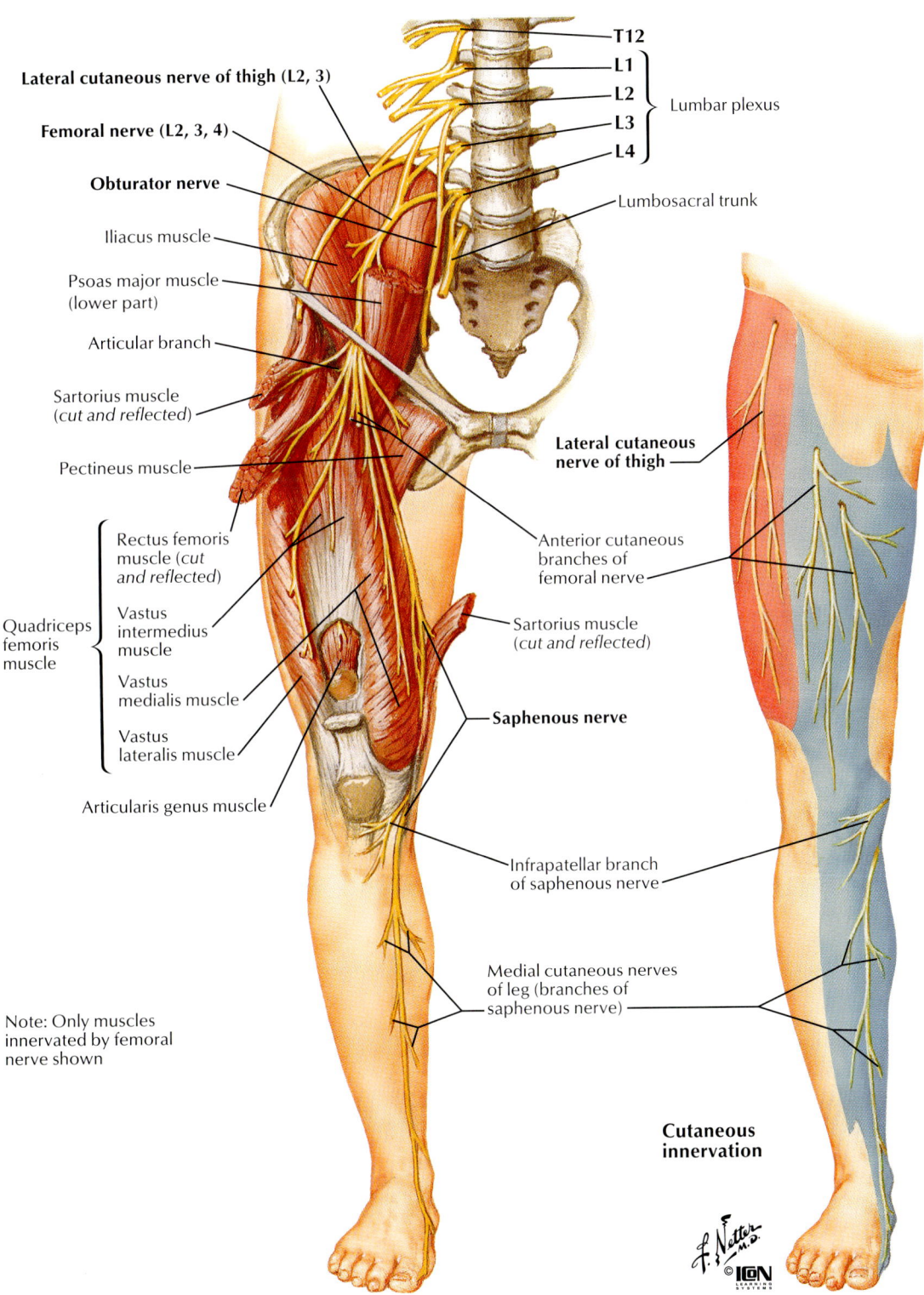

MONONEUROPATHIES

753

sensory symptoms, these typically involve the anterolateral thigh and anteromedial leg.

Differential Diagnosis

A nerve root lesion at L3-4 is the most common consideration. Unlike L5-S1 radiculopathies, a herniated nucleus pulposus infrequently involves L3-4.

OBTURATOR NEUROPATHIES

Obturator neuropathies are exceedingly uncommon focal nerve lesions that typically present with hip instability. Weakness and denervation are confined to the large hip adductors (Figure 86-5). Occasionally, they present with pain and sensory symptoms in the medial thigh without obvious weakness.

Obturator neuropathies may be caused by pelvic masses, difficult parturition, or obturator hernias or may be complications of hip arthroplasty.

Diagnostic Approach

Electrodiagnosis is one of 2 means of primary evaluation of suspected mononeuropathy. EMG helps to differentiate other lesions that mimic mononeuropathies, particularly at the respective plexus or nerve root level. Besides providing anatomical localization, EMG helps to assess prognosis. Etiology is rarely revealed, even with abnormal EMG. Demonstration of a predominantly demyelinating lesion provides the primary basis for localization; although it is useful in the evaluation of peroneal neuropathies, it is not particularly helpful in sciatic, femoral, and obturator neuropathies. An optimistic prognosis can be expected with a primary demyelinating lesion. However, when evidence of significant axonal damage exists, reinnervation, a process that progresses at a rate of 1 mm/day or approximately 1 inch/month, must occur.

Further testing is sometimes indicated, depending on the index of suspicion regarding causation. Plain radiographs can assess possible bone spurs or exostoses, arthritides, congenital deformities, fractures, or bony tumors that may contribute to nerve injury. MRI and occasionally ultrasonography are useful in assessing soft tissue lesions or sometimes localizing areas of entrapment and in providing a spatial image of the nerve and its surrounding structures. However, when EMG provides a defined localization without clinical evidence or imaging studies of a specific mechanism, surgical exploration is an important diagnostic tool that sometimes also provides a therapeutic option (see the second vignette under "Sciatic Neuropathies").

Occasionally, ESR provides a clue to an underlying vasculitis. Similarly serum glucose level may help to identify previously undiagnosed diabetes mellitus presenting with a possible femoral neuropathy. Rarely, CSF examination is indicated to distinguish a polyradiculopathy from a sciatic neuropathy.

Management and Prognosis

When a definable entrapment mechanism, a mass causing nerve compression, or a nerve laceration exists, surgery is indicated. If the neuropathy resulted from nerve traction from excessive squatting or compression from habitual leg crossing, the primary treatment is discontinuation of these activities. If a cast or brace is compressing the nerve, it must be modified to protect the nerve such as with the fibular head in peroneal compression.

An acute compartment syndrome is a surgical emergency and necessitates fasciotomy.

Foot drop can be effectively treated by an ankle-foot orthosis, its primary goal being prevention of falls. Patients also state that their walking endurance improves with this device. An ankle-foot orthosis should be prescribed cautiously in patients with significant quadriceps weakness. It may destabilize a patient's marginally compensated technique of "knee locking" and weight bearing, thus increasing the risk of falling.

Recovery depends on the nature, location, severity, and persistence of the injury and patients' underlying health and age. Primarily demyelinating lesions secondary to monophasic external compression or stretch typically recover within weeks to months. Persistent compression, if causing a predominantly demyelinating injury, improves when the compression is relieved. If recovery from axon loss is needed, a longer period (months to years) is required. The degree of axon loss and distance from the site of injury to the target site of reinnervation determine outcome.

MONONEUROPATHIES PRESENTING WITH LOWER EXTREMITY WEAKNESS

Figure 86-5

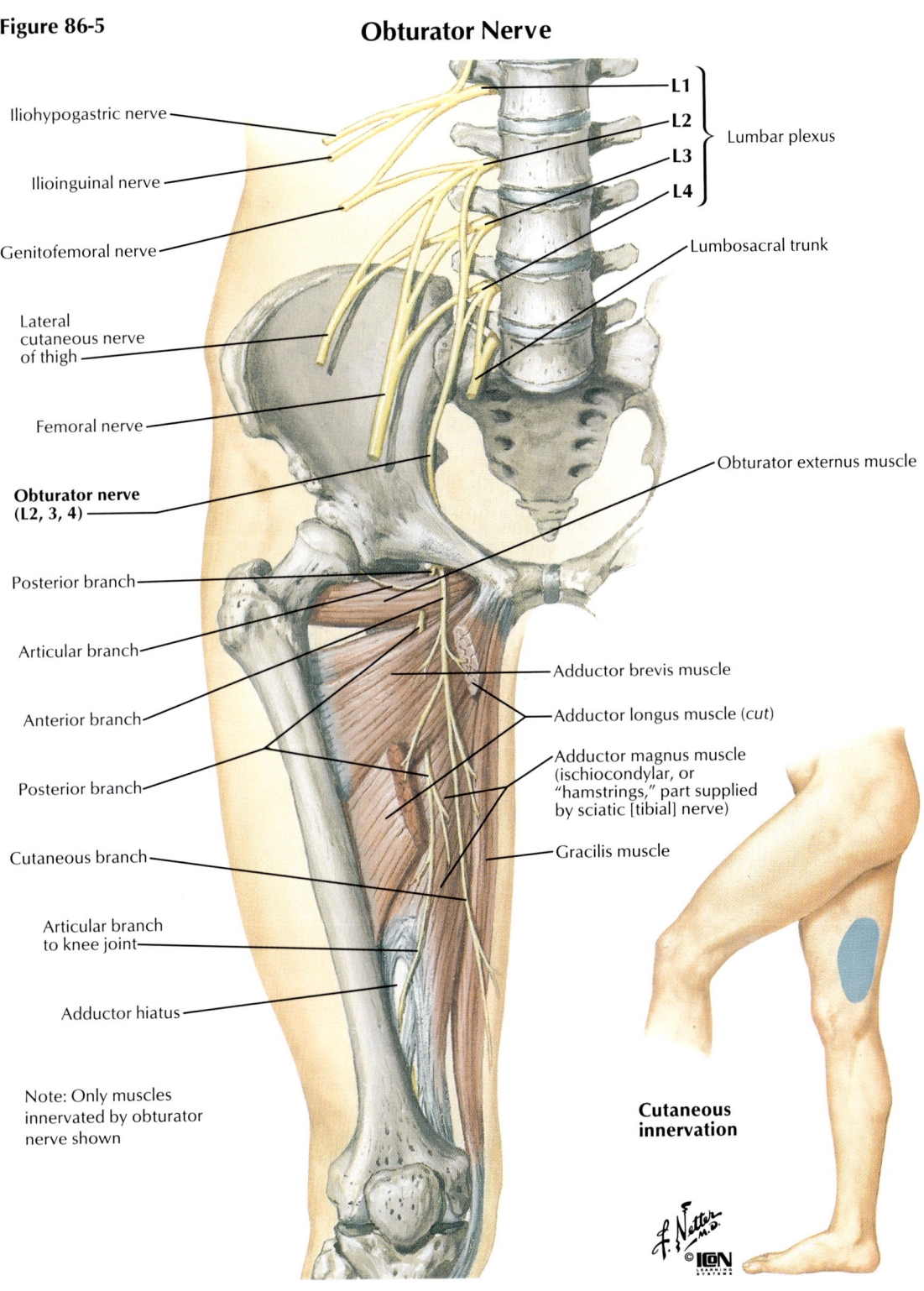

FUTURE DIRECTIONS

More sensitive neurophysiologic and neuroimaging techniques will lead to improved diagnosis of lower extremity mononeuropathies and more effective surgical treatment of nerve transection and traumatic injuries.

REFERENCES

Bradshaw C, McCrory P, Bell S, et al. Obturator nerve entrapment: a cause of groin pain in athletes. *Am J Sports Med.* 1997;25:402-408.

Busis NA. Femoral and obturator neuropathies. *Neurol Clin.* 1999;17:633-653.

Campbell WW. Diagnosis and management of common compression and entrapment neuropathies. *Neurol Clin.* 1997;15:549-567.

Katirji B. Peroneal neuropathy. *Neurol Clin.* 1999;17:567-591.

Kuntzer T, van Melle G, Regli F. Clinical and prognostic features in unilateral femoral neuropathies. *Muscle Nerve.* 1997;20:205-211.

Miller MD, Gomez BA. *Anatomy in Review of Orthopedics.* 3rd ed. Miller MD, Brinker MR, eds. Philadelphia, PA: WB Saunders; 2000:556-577.

Netter FH. *Atlas of Human Anatomy.* 3rd ed. Teterboro, NJ: Icon Learning Systems, LLC, 2003:502.

Seddon HJ. Three types of nerve injury. *Brain.* 1943;66:237-288.

Stewart JD. *Focal Peripheral Neuropathies.* 3rd ed. Baltimore, Md: Lippincott Williams & Wilkins; 2000.

Venna N, Bielawski M, Spatz EM. Sciatic nerve entrapment in a child: case report. *J Neurosurg.* 1991;75:652-654.

Chapter 87
Primary Sensory Neuropathies of the Lower Extremity

N. George Kasparyan and James A. Russell

Primary sensory neuropathies of the lower extremity generally result from iatrogenic injury or compression by mass lesions. Although neuropathy of the lateral femoral cutaneous nerve (LFCN) causing meralgia paresthetica (MP), medial and lateral plantar neuropathy causing tarsal tunnel syndrome (TTS), and rarely ilioinguinal neuropathy are sometimes thought to be entrapment syndromes, this thesis is difficult to prove.

LATERAL FEMORAL CUTANEOUS NERVE

Clinical Vignette

A 45-year-old overweight bartender was evaluated for sensory complaints of 4 months' duration of her left thigh. She described an aching discomfort extending from her buttock, across her hip, and down the lateral aspect of her thigh, intensified by standing or walking. She also described a burning numbness in the area where her hand would rest if put in her front pants pocket. There was associated cutaneous hypersensitivity with an aversion to having clothes or bed sheets rub against her. She was unaware of any other precipitating events.

Examination demonstrated an elliptically shaped area of sensory loss on the distal half of her anterolateral thigh. She had no atrophy, weakness, or reflex loss.

Patient history, detailing the distribution of sensory loss, provides the basis for the diagnosis of MP, an entrapment mononeuropathy of the LFCN. Often aggravated by standing or walking, symptoms include an uncomfortable positive component (burning, hypersensitivity) and negative features (numbness). Typically, the area of demonstrable sensory loss on examination is smaller than the LFCN territory in most anatomical diagrams (Figure 86-1). Because the LFCN contains only sensory fibers, no associated reflex or motor abnormalities exist, helping to distinguish MP from other disorders that deserve diagnostic consideration. MP often occurs in overweight individuals and is usually unilateral and idiopathic.

Cadaver studies suggest that MP is primarily an entrapment neuropathy due to "kinking" of the nerve as it passes through the inguinal ligament. Like many mononeuropathies, MP is more common in people with diabetes. Occasionally, the LFCN is injured within the thigh secondary to blunt or penetrating trauma, eg, a misplaced injection. Rarely, a soft tissue sarcoma within the thigh mimics MP.

Anatomy

The LFCN arises from the first and second lumbar roots and travels through the retroperitoneum, under the psoas muscle (Figure 87-1). It exits the pelvis under or through the inguinal ligament, the presumed usual site of entrapment. Subsequently, it supplies sensation to the lateral thigh.

Diagnosis

Although uncommon, L2 monoradiculopathy of any etiology, evidenced as weakness and denervation of L2 innervated hip flexors and adductors, is a major differential consideration. Sensory symptoms and signs extend over the anterior and medial aspects of the thigh. Lumbar spinal stenosis is also a consideration because it tends to be exacerbated by prolonged standing or walking, although it does not cause numbness in this specific distribution.

PRIMARY SENSORY NEUROPATHIES OF THE LOWER EXTREMITY

Figure 87-1

Lateral Femoral Cutaneous Nerve

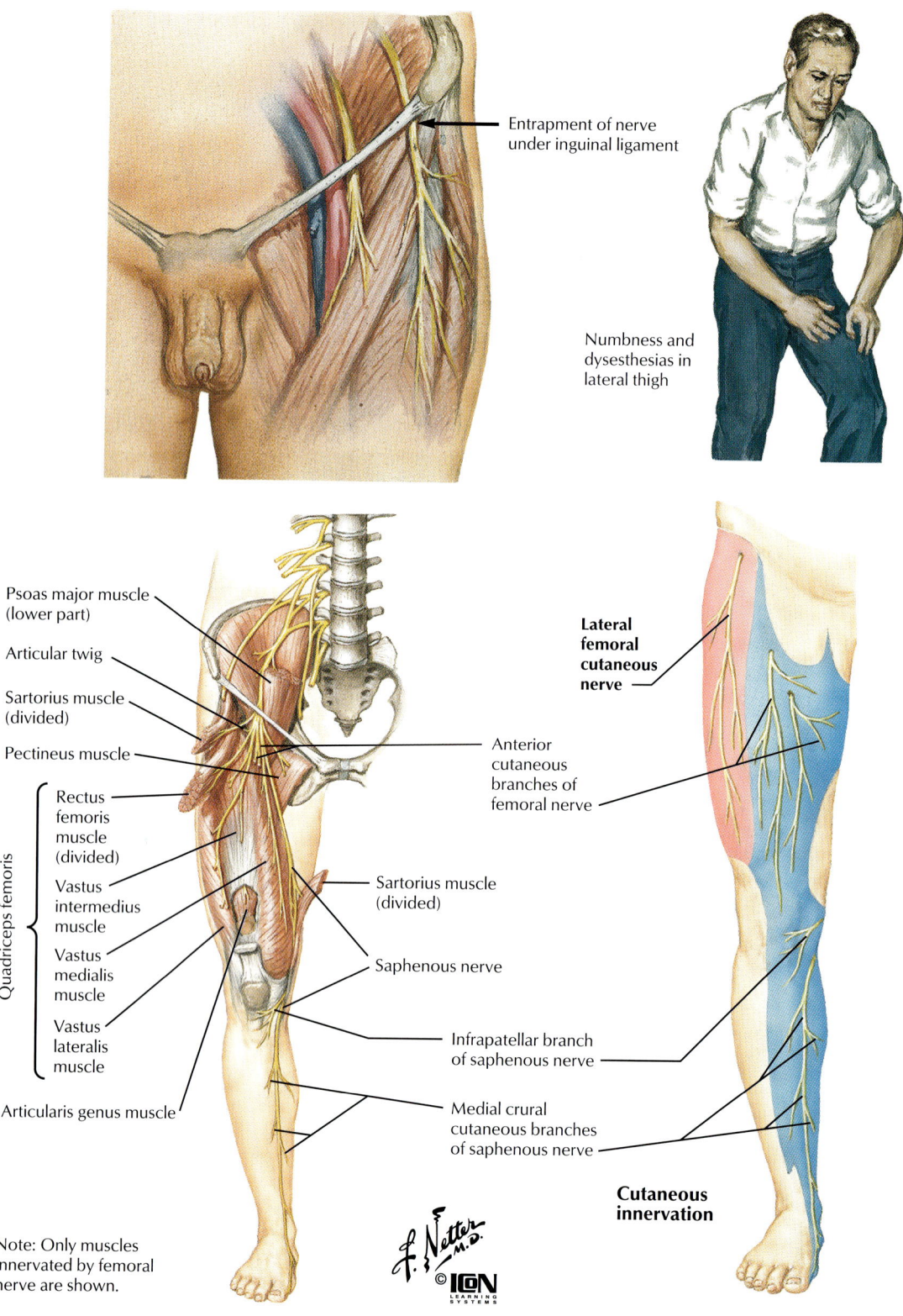

MONONEUROPATHIES

PRIMARY SENSORY NEUROPATHIES OF THE LOWER EXTREMITY

Disorders of the lumbosacral plexus may mimic MP, particularly in patients having insidious onset of invasive or compressive disorders in which pain and other sensory symptoms have no obvious motor component. Retroperitoneal neoplasms or hematomas and abdominal surgery are always considerations; however, they are unlikely to cause isolated MP. Instead, concomitant involvement of contiguous nerves eventually leads to motor, reflex, and more widespread anatomical sensory loss, indicating a plexus rather than a single nerve problem.

Isolated femoral neuropathies are uncommon and unlikely to be confused with MP because of the type and distribution of abnormalities. Sensory symptoms involve the anterior thigh and extend to the medial surface of the leg. Weakness of the quadriceps muscle and loss of its stretch reflex are other objective and distinguishing features.

Although the LFCN can be tested in the thigh distal to the inguinal ligament, technical difficulties interfere with detection of mild demyelinating injuries. A response cannot be reliably obtained from all, particularly in overweight individuals who are most susceptible to this syndrome. Nerve conduction studies of the LFCN are of greatest value when a normal response is readily obtained from the asymptomatic side and a low-amplitude or absent response is obtained from the symptomatic side. In patients with atypical symptoms, thigh MRI is indicated to exclude primary lesions such as soft tissue sarcoma. MRI and CT of the retroperitoneum and pelvis are also indicated in patients with unexplained LFCN neuropathy. Fasting blood sugar is appropriate in acute-onset, painful LFCN neuropathies without alternative explanation.

Management

The natural history of MP varies; approximately two thirds of affected individuals become asymptomatic within 2 years. Others have a more protracted and chronic course. MP is ideally managed by weight loss where applicable. Avoidance of tight garments may help.

Medications such as amitriptyline, carbamazepine, gabapentin, and venlafaxine may diminish pain intensity. Injections of local anesthetic and steroids near the anterior superior iliac spine may serve diagnostic and therapeutic roles and are sometimes "curative." Exploration at the presumed entrapment site is used in particularly intractable and lifestyle-altering cases, although few surgeons are experienced with the procedure.

UNCOMMON SENSORY NEUROPATHIES OF THE LOWER EXTREMITY

Four primary sensory mononeuropathies should be considered in the differential diagnosis of dysesthesias of the pelvis, groin, and feet with no clinically apparent motor deficits. Documentation of these syndromes is clinically difficult, and EMG is generally not helpful.

Iliohypogastric Nerve

Iliohypogastric neuropathies produce sensory symptoms in 2 distinct areas, the posterior aspect of the iliac crest and the suprapubic region just above the scrotum or labia. The anterior branch is most commonly injured by lower abdominal surgery, and the posterior branch is most commonly injured by major pelvic surgery. The prognosis for recovery is generally good in both.

Ilioinguinal Nerve

Loss of sensation along the inguinal ligament, with or without associated pain, characterizes ilioinguinal neuropathies. These most frequently result from herniorrhaphies, appendectomies, nephrectomies, suprapubic incisions, bone graft harvesting from the iliac crest, and parturition. Rarely, nerve entrapment occurs as it passes through the abdominal wall, causing groin pain relieved by hip flexion.

Genitofemoral Nerve

Genitofemoral neuropathy presents with pain and paresthesias of the suprapubic, upper thigh, and medial inguinal regions overlapping those of ilioinguinal and iliohypogastric neuropathies. Standing or hip extension may exaggerate symptoms. Retroperitoneal pathologies or abdominal wall surgery are common causes of genitofemoral neuropathy. Unlike the ilioinguinal and iliohypogastric nerves, the genitofemoral nerve has a motor branch innervating the cre-

PRIMARY SENSORY NEUROPATHIES OF THE LOWER EXTREMITY

master muscle. Unfortunately, the cremasteric reflex is not a reliable diagnostic clue.

Medial and Lateral Plantar Nerves

Tarsal tunnel syndrome is classified as an entrapment neuropathy of the posterior tibial nerve and of its 2 primary branches, the medial and lateral plantar nerves, at the ankle (Figure 87-2). This well-described neuropathy is infrequently documented, despite its being analogous to carpal tunnel syndrome. Whether this reflects its uncommon occurrence or the inadequate sensitivity of diagnostic procedures is unclear. Patients typically present with burning pain and numbness on the sole of 1 or both feet. Symptoms may occur while weight bearing but, consistent with nerve entrapment, are often exacerbated at night.

In well-established instances, examination may disclose intrinsic plantar surface muscle atrophy. However, weakness of these muscles is difficult to appreciate because the more proximal long toe flexors in the leg mask weakness from the involved short toe flexors within the foot. Toe abduction weakness occurs early but is difficult to assess even in healthy individuals. Sensory loss is confined to the sole of the foot, sparing the sural distribution of the lateral foot and the peroneal territory of the instep. Muscle stretch reflexes are unaffected. A Tinel sign elicited from the tibial nerve at the ankle is supportive, although not confirmatory.

Diagnosis

EMG is of limited value. The ilioinguinal, iliohypogastric, and genitofemoral nerves are inaccessible to nerve conduction techniques. Retroperitoneal and pelvic MRI and CT are indicated when a progressive ilioinguinal, iliohypogastric, or genitofemoral neuropathy develops without obvious cause. Ilioinguinal, iliohypogastric, and genitofemoral neuropathies may be addressed both diagnostically and therapeutically by a therapeutic trial of direct nerve injection.

If TTS results from nerve entrapment, simulating carpal tunnel syndrome, EMG should demonstrate demyelination via prolongation of the distal latencies. However, prolonged tibial motor and mixed nerve distal latencies from the medial and lateral plantar nerves are rarely demonstrated in patients with suspected TTS. Absent mixed nerve responses from the plantar nerves may be seen but have limited localizing value because they also occur in some seemingly healthy elderly individuals and in those with an underlying polyneuropathy. Fibrillation potentials in tibial innervated foot muscles must be interpreted with similar caution. Imaging in suspected TTS includes radiographs to detect osseous abnormalities involving the tarsal tunnel region and CT if severe ankle osteoarthritic changes and exostosis are considered.

Fasting blood sugar testing should be performed in cases of unexplained acute-onset, painful mononeuropathy.

Management

Most patients with postoperative neuropathies experience full recovery; persistent symptoms typically are seen only in those with unrepaired nerve transection or injury to the lumbosacral plexus.

Initial treatment of TTS is nonoperative, consisting of footwear modification, particularly avoidance of high-heeled and poorly fitting footwear. Antiinflammatory medications may help. Steroid injections, augmented with lidocaine, can be helpful if flexor tenosynovitis is suspected. Care must be taken to avoid an intraneural injection with the unlikely possibility of causing local nerve sclerosis. Hind foot valgus deformities may benefit from orthoses.

When nonoperative measures fail in TTS, surgical intervention may be considered. The results of surgical decompression are not always rewarding. Release of the flexor retinaculum and fibrous origin of the abductor hallucis muscle are required. Local flexor tenosynovitis can be resected with radical tenosynovectomy. Enlarged and varicose veins can be ligated and resected. Postoperatively, an open shoe is used with partial weight bearing for 2 weeks.

Medications such as amitriptyline, carbamazepine, gabapentin, and venlafaxine may diminish pain intensity in all mononeuropathies.

PRIMARY SENSORY NEUROPATHIES OF THE LOWER EXTREMITY

Figure 87-2

Tibial Nerve

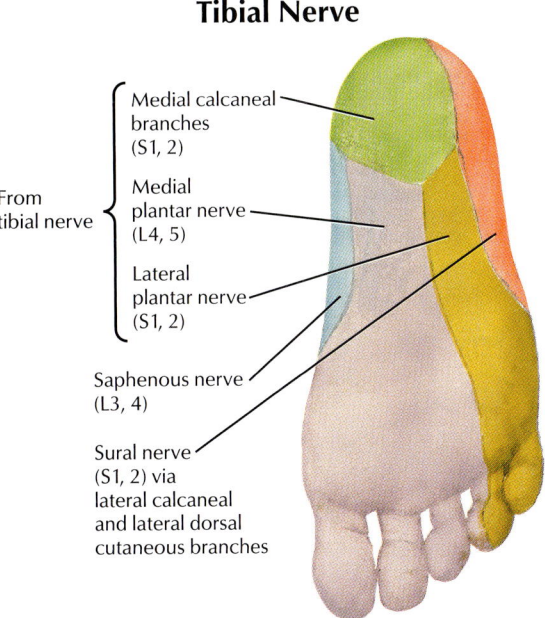

Cutaneous innervation of sole

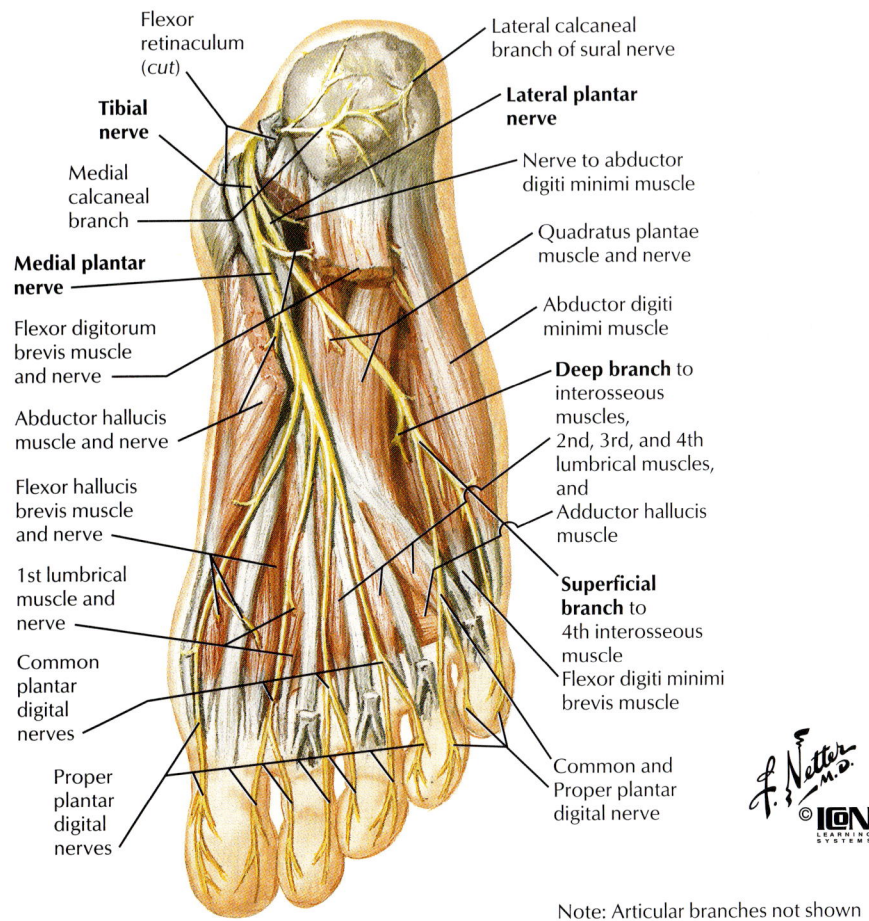

Note: Articular branches not shown

MONONEUROPATHIES

761

PROGNOSIS AND FUTURE DIRECTIONS

Prognosis of these mononeuropathies varies. Some respond to conservative treatment, whereas others resolve without intervention. A few relent after appropriate surgical intervention. Some progress to chronic conditions, apparently refractory to all interventions. Future directions will involve improved diagnosis through more sensitive neurophysiologic and neuroimaging techniques, and more specific and effective treatment of neuropathic pain syndromes.

REFERENCES

Kaplan PE, Kernahan WT. Tarsal tunnel syndrome. *J Bone Joint Surg Am.* 1981;63:96-99.

Mann RA, Plattner PF. Nerve entrapment syndromes of the foot and ankle. In: Szabo R, ed. *Nerve Compression Syndromes: Diagnosis and Treatment.* Thorofare, NJ: SLACK; 1989:273-291.

Stewart JD. *Focal Peripheral Neuropathies.* 3rd ed. Baltimore, Md: Lippincott Williams & Wilkins; 2000.

Section XXI
MOTOR NEURON DISORDERS

Chapter 88
Overview of Motor Neuron Disease 764

Chapter 89
Motor Neuron Disease Presenting in the Limbs With Lower Motor Neuron Features 777

Chapter 90
Primary Lateral Sclerosis: Motor Neuron Disease Presenting With Upper Motor Neuron Features in the Limbs 783

Chapter 91
Motor Neuron Disease: Bulbar, Head Drop, and Ventilatory Presentations 789

Chapter 92
Stiff Person Syndrome 794

Chapter 88
Overview of Motor Neuron Disease

James A. Russell and H. Royden Jones, Jr

Motor neuron diseases (MNDs) are characterized by degeneration of anterior horn cells and selective motor cranial nerve nuclei (Figures 88-1 through and 88-3). Sometimes these are multisystem disorders wherein the motor system is the first or most dramatically affected. Within the general population, they are relatively uncommon. The incidence of **amyotrophic lateral sclerosis** (ALS), Lou Gehrig disease, the most notorious MND, is 1 to 2 in 100,000. ALS is one of the most devastating neurologic disorders, physically and emotionally. Because the incidence of ALS seems to be increasing, its societal impact assumes even greater significance.

CLASSIFICATION

The absence of a satisfactory, universally agreed on classification scheme is common to all disorders of unknown cause. **Progressive muscular atrophy** (PMA) was initially considered a myelopathic disorder because of the associated ventral root atrophy; anterior horn cell degeneration was previously thought to be a secondary finding. **Progressive bulbar palsy** (PBP) was distinguished by its progressive dysphagia and dysarthria. Reports of PBP with concomitant degeneration of corticospinal tracts and anterior horn cells represented the first descriptions of **ALS**. **Primary lateral sclerosis** (PLS) was first described as a progressive disorder of upper motor neurons (UMNs), ie, the corticospinal tracts, without muscle atrophy, fasciculations, or weakness.

Despite their initial descriptions, ALS, PMA, PBP, and (equivocally) PLS are now recognized as related entities (Figure 88-4A). PMA and PBP are clinical syndromes that usually progress to ALS. At presentation, it is difficult to predict individuals' eventual temporal profile. Some patients have rapid progression to ALS with its poor prognosis; others continue with a more protracted form of limited MND. Therefore, it is appropriate to encourage the patient presenting early in the disease course to maintain hope. Although classification using these 4 acronyms is cumbersome and somewhat artificial, these definitions continue to be clinically preferred and descriptively useful. The PMA, PBP, ALS, and PLS continuum forms the basis of the World Federation of Neurology diagnostic criteria for ALS (the El Escorial criteria [EEC]).

Because of the shortcomings inherent in the ALS classification system of PMA, PBP, and PLS, the less specific and more encompassing term *MND* was proposed. Whether MND has a singular etiology with variable phenotypic expressions, ie, ALS, PMA, or PBP, is unclear. Each of these may be influenced by genetic variance or other confounding variables, including environmental contributions. Alternatively, the disorders now lumped under the acronym *MND* with similar but heterogeneous phenotypes may result from several primary insults operating through a unitary pathophysiologic cascade. To promote a predominantly clinically oriented approach, a practical classification of MND is suggested (Table 88-1).

The most common and recognizable phenotype of MND is ALS; the acronym *MND/ALS* is used throughout this section of the book. Where the initial clinical presentation is one of PMA, PBP, or PLS, the acronyms *MND/PMA*, *MND/PBP*, and *MND/PLS* are used.

Figure 88-1   **The Motor Neuron Pathway**

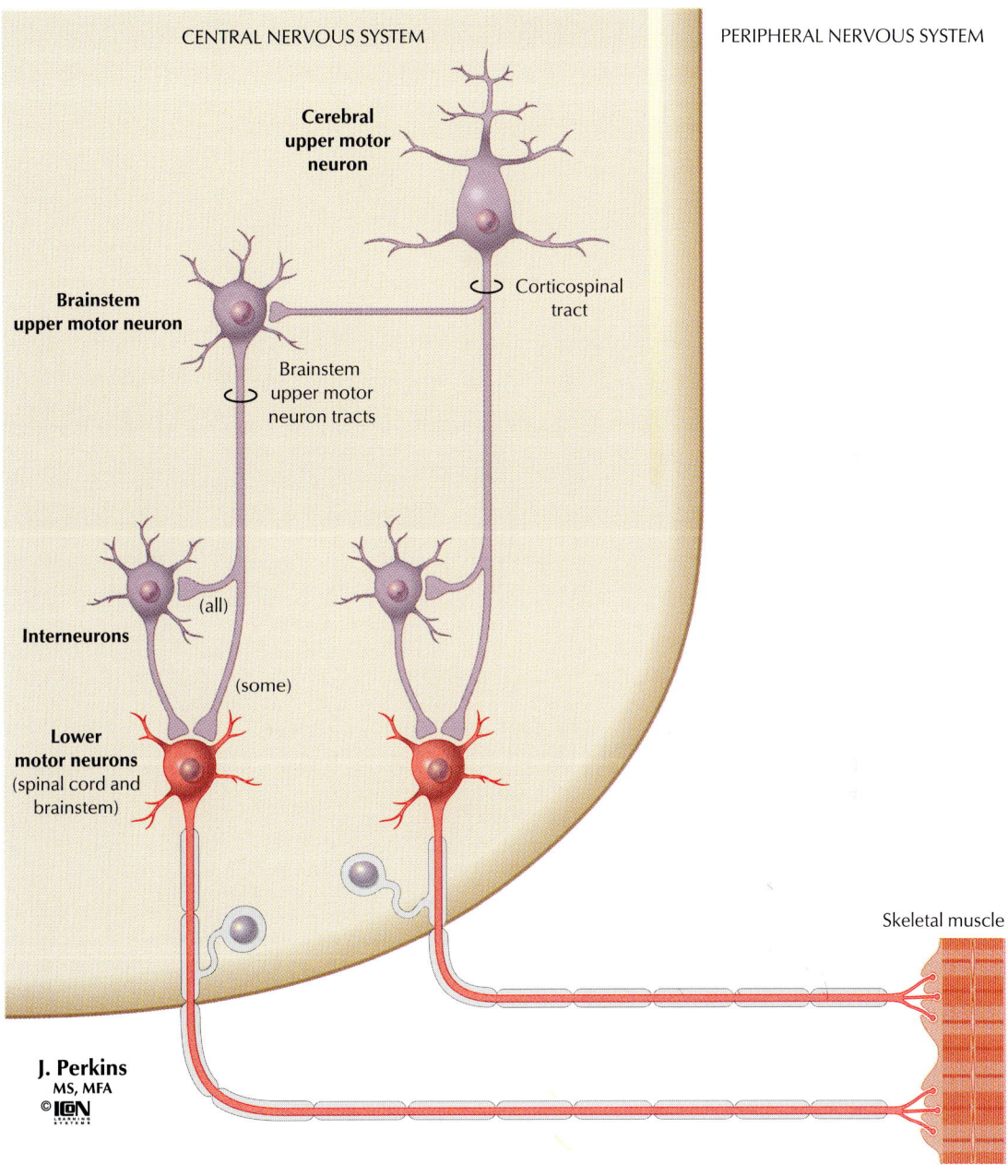

Multifocal motor neuropathies (MMNs) are not true motor neuron disorders. However, they typically mimic MND/PMA (Table 88-2). Because MMNs are eminently treatable disorders, consideration of them in the differential diagnosis is important (chapter 91). Diagnosis of MMN rests primarily on EMG findings and assays of anti-GM1 antibodies. Where MMN cannot be definitively excluded, therapeutic trials of immunomodulation may be warranted.

OVERVIEW OF MOTOR NEURON DISEASE

Figure 88-2 — Cerebral Cortex: Efferent Pathways

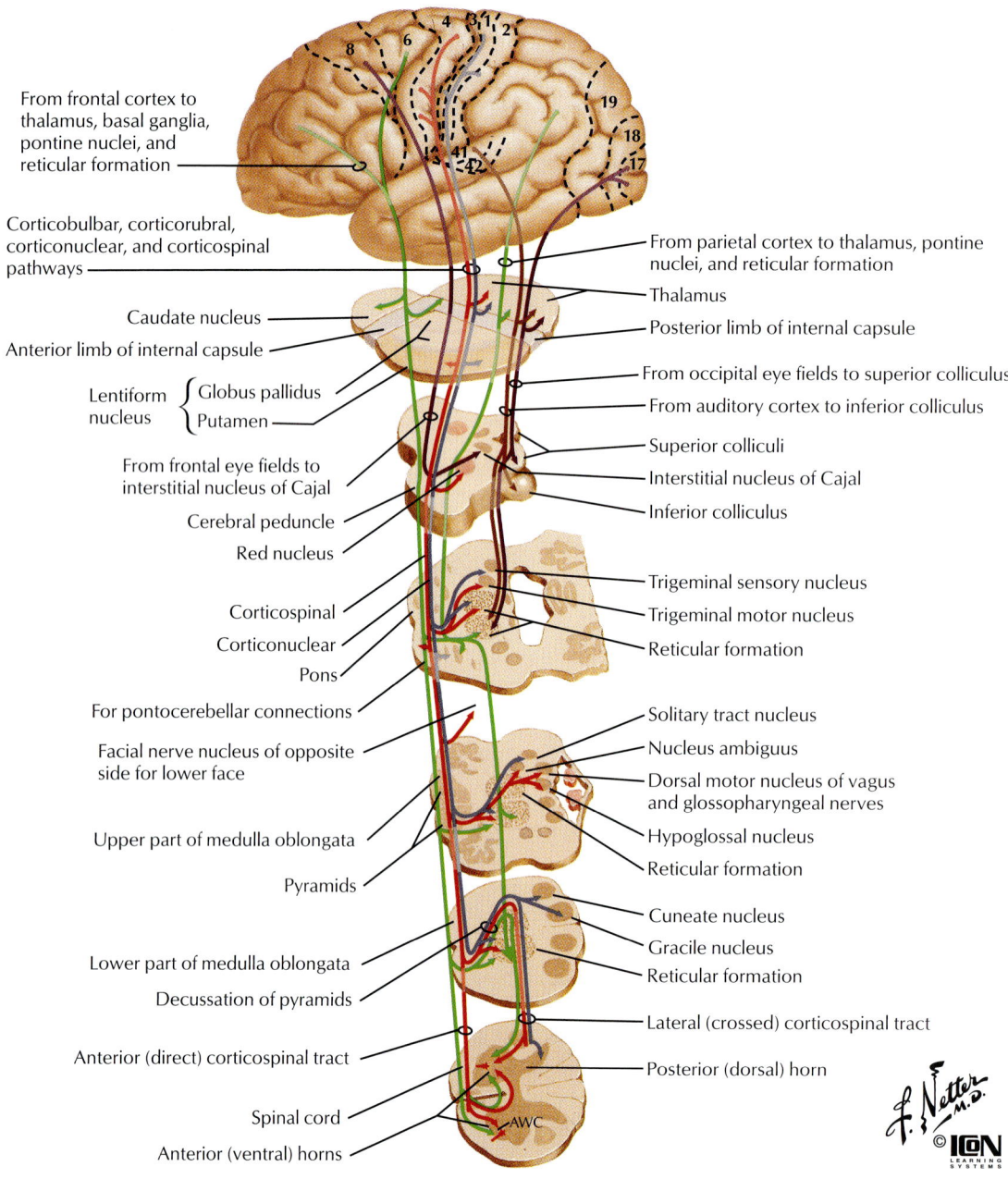

MOTOR NEURON DISORDERS

OVERVIEW OF MOTOR NEURON DISEASE

Figure 88-3 — Corticobulbar Fibers

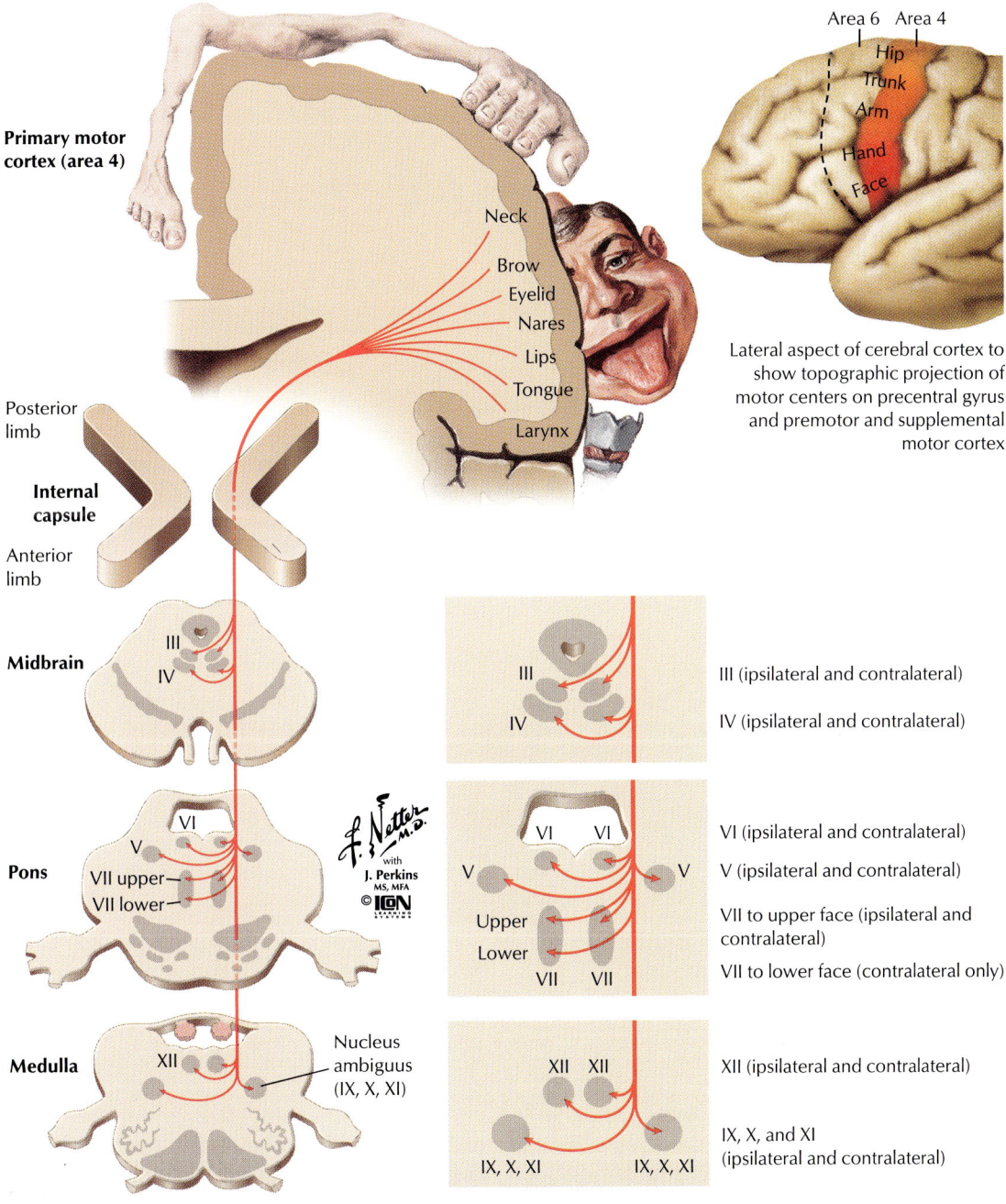

MOTOR NEURON DISORDERS

767

OVERVIEW OF MOTOR NEURON DISEASE

Figure 88-4A

Classification of Motor Neuron Disease

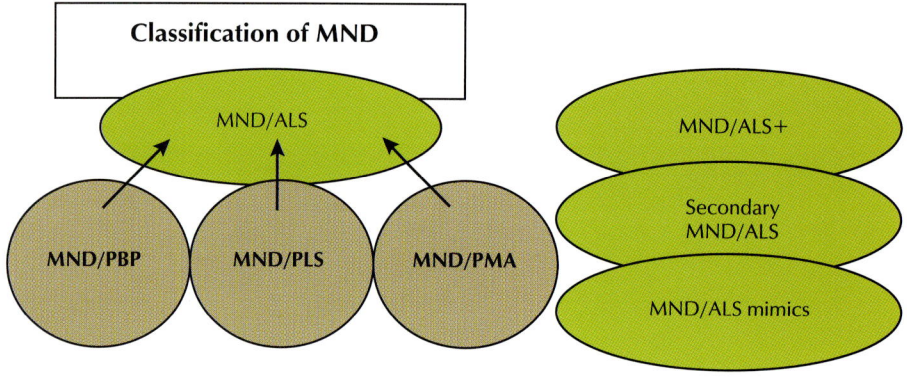

Figure 88-4B

Proposed Motor Neuron Disease Etiology and Pathophysiology

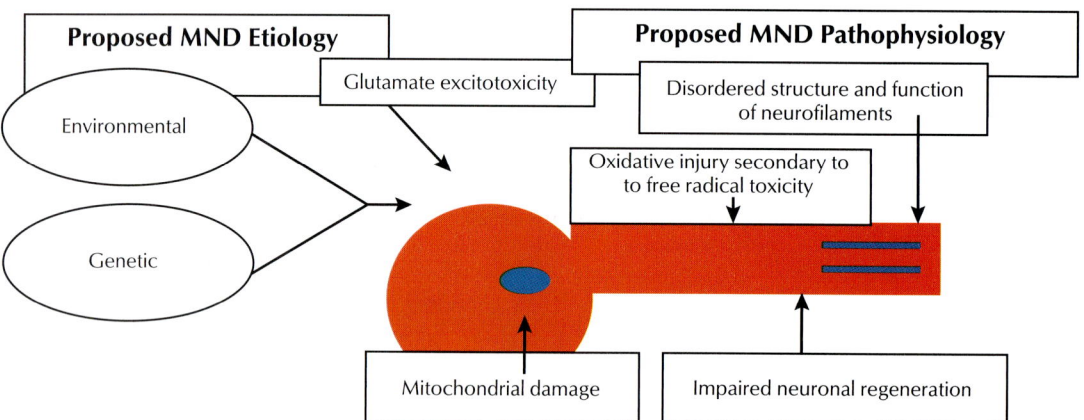

ETIOLOGY

The causes of MND remain unknown. In view of the strong phenotypic overlap between the familial and sporadic forms of ALS, many adhere to the hypothesis that MND/ALS results from an adverse environmental exposure in genetically susceptible individuals.

Our understanding of MND heredity and pathophysiology has advanced considerably, subsequent to the identification of mutations within the superoxide dismutase gene (SOD1) in 15% of familial ALS families. Some evidence supports each of the following mechanisms as potential contributors to the pathophysiology of MND/ALS: disordered structure and function of motor neuron neurofilaments, mitochondrial damage and dysfunction, glutamate excitotoxicity, oxidative injury secondary to free radical toxicity, and impaired neuronal regeneration secondary to microglial activation (Figure 88-4B). However, there is no evidence to support any of these mechanisms as the major cause of motor neuron injury in MND. It is unknown what triggers these different (although not necessarily mutually exclusive) mechanisms of cell injury or how they interact, if at all.

The cause of motor neuron death may differ from that promoting spread of disease from one group of anterior horn cells to another, which may be different from the initiating injury. Valid

MOTOR NEURON DISORDERS

Table 88-1
Clinical Classification of MND/ALS*

Phenotype	Subcategory	Comments
A: UMN and LMN presentations	sMND/ALS	Progressive diffuse UMN and LMN involvement
	fMND/ALS	Most mutations produce UMN and LMN involvement
	MND/ALS+	Association with frontotemporal dementia or other neurologic disorders
	Secondary MND/ALS	Guamanian MND Multisystem atrophy Prion disease (CJD)
B: UMN presentations	MND/PLS	May remain as UMN only or progress to MND/ALS
	HSP	Numerous mutations
	Secondary MND/PLS	HTLV-I, HIV Paraneoplastic (breast cancer)
C1: LMN, focal[†]—primary	MND/PMA	May remain as LMN only or progress to MND/ALS
	Juvenile segmental SMA (Hirayama disease)	Typically begins in one extremity in juveniles
	Motor neuropathies	See below
C2: LMN, focal[†]—secondary	Enterovirus, poliomyelitis, West Nile disease	Acute aseptic meningitis
	Paraneoplastic	Lymphoma, small cell lung cancer (anti-Hu+)
C3: LMN, regional[†] (weakness and atrophy occurring in discernable patterns)	X-linked bulbospinal muscular atrophy (Kennedy disease)	Male >>> female Proximal weakness Gynecomastia Sensory neuropathy
	Distal SMA	Mimics Charcot-Marie-Tooth disease
	Scapuloperoneal SMA	Mimics facioscapulohumeral and scapuloperoneal dystrophies
C4: LMN, generalized[†]	Types I-IV SMA Survival motor neuron gene at 5q1-13	Proximally predominant weakness Onset: • Infancy (I), ages 0-6 months • Childhood (II), ages 6-18 months • Juvenile (III), ages 2-16 years
D: Bulbar presentations	MND/PBP	UMN ± LMN signs—usually progresses to MND/ALS
	Fazio-Londe form of SMA	Rapidly progressive bulbar paralysis—onset <12 years
	Vialetto-van Laere	Bulbospinal atrophy and sensorineural hearing loss—onset <20 years

*ALS indicates amyotrophic lateral sclerosis; CJD, Creutzfeldt-Jakob disease; fMND, familial motor neuron disease; HSP, hereditary spastic paraparesis; LMN, lower motor neuron; MND, motor neuron disease; PBP, progressive bulbar palsy; PLS, primary lateral sclerosis; PMA, progressive muscular atrophy; SMA, spinal muscular atrophy; sMND, sporadic motor neuron disease; UMN; upper motor neuron.
[†]Focal, regional, and generalized presentations are relative in nature and may overlap on a case-by-case basis.

OVERVIEW OF MOTOR NEURON DISEASE

Table 88-2
Motor Neuropathies*

Type	Characteristics
MMN	Typically slowly progressive, asymmetric weakness of a hand or foot EMG/NCS: conduction block ± antiglycolipid antibodies (anti-GM1b)
Multifocal asymmetric motor axonopathy (MAMA) 17	Similar, perhaps identical to MMN without conduction block or antibodies
Proximal motor neuropathy	Similar to DMN with proximal onset of weakness
Inflammatory neuropathies (CIDP)	Variants of chronic inflammatory demyelinating neuropathy with limited involvement of sensory fibers
Paraneoplastic motor neuropathy	Rare—typically associated with lymphoma

*CIDP indicates chronic inflammatory demyelinating polyneuropathy; DMN, distal motor neuropathy; MMN, multifocal motor neuropathy; NCS, nerve condution studies.

explanations for MND must account for the semiselective vulnerability of anterior horn cells and corticospinal tracts.

PROBLEMS INHERENT IN ALS DIAGNOSIS

The diagnosis of MND/ALS is based on the typical clinical picture supplemented by ancillary studies. At presentation, it may be difficult to specifically determine whether the patient has a MND and, if so, what type of MND it is. It is appropriate to suspect this diagnosis in patients with asymmetric painless weakness, even when they do not have enough findings to meet the EEC for a diagnosis of ALS. Because of this uncertainty, neurologists are frequently conflicted about when to share diagnostic suspicions with patients and their families. It is always important to assure patients that the most careful differential consideration has been given before discussing a diagnosis of this magnitude.

Patients' need for answers and the potential for an early introduction of therapy are balanced against this conservative approach. A perceived "foot dragging" with consequent diagnostic uncertainty, as rare alternative diagnoses are excluded, may have equally deleterious effects on patients' trust in their physicians. It usually seems reasonable to disclose the diagnosis of suspected ALS as early as possible, after clear disease progression makes it more probable. The clinical diagnosis of MND/ALS becomes more certain with evidence of concomitant progressive UMN and LMN dysfunction within and beyond the originally affected anatomically defined region, provided potential secondary causes are excluded.

The **EEC** have attempted to achieve a balance between diagnostic sensitivity and specificity. Although imperfect, they remain important as they provide a diagnostic standard and basis for enrollment in clinical therapeutic trials. A major drawback to the EEC is their tendency to preclude individuals from enrollment in clinical trials at an early stage where therapeutic intervention may be the most effective. Some patients who die with pathologically confirmed ALS never fulfill the EEC. Also hampering use of these criteria is the problem of determining a reliable clinical (or paraclinical) sign of UMN or LMN pathology.

Particularly problematic is the difficulty of achieving an early, accurate diagnosis in patients who present with signs and symptoms affecting limited regions of the body or with restricted UMN or LMN features. Muscle atrophy, weakness in absence of UMN signs, diminished muscle stretch reflexes, widespread fasciculations, and reliable EMG parameters of active and chronic denervation are acceptable indicators of LMN disease. These findings are sometimes equivocal. For example, it is essential not to overcall atrophy and weakness in the arthritic hands of a 75-year-old woman. Fasciculations may be obscured by excessive subcutaneous tissue. The muscle stretch reflexes are often preserved because of concomitant UMN disease.

Demonstration of conclusive UMN signs, ie, spasticity, pathologically enhanced reflexes with clonus, and extensor plantar responses may be elusive particularly early in the illness. Some patients never have UMN signs. For example, a Babinski sign may never occur or may vanish when the extensor hallucis longus becomes too weak to support it. Absent abdominal reflexes, the presence of Hoffman sign, hyperactive jaw jerk, pseudobulbar affect, and preservation of reflexes from wasted weak muscles are often subtle signs that generally indicate UMN involvement.

The timing of discussions of the diagnosis and its implications is made on an individual basis, based on the physician's perception of what the patient wants and needs to know. In essence, the physician waits for the patient to ask. This approach must be tempered by the realization that some patients may be unwilling or unable to confront certain issues when they must be addressed. Under ideal circumstances, initial discussions regarding living wills, tracheostomy, and long-term mechanical ventilation would occur after the initial visit but before symptoms of ventilatory failure. All information needs to be presented with considerable tact and sensitivity as outlined in the ALS Practice Parameters.

Unfortunately, the clinical phenotype at presentation does not predict the natural history of individual ALS cases. Patients presenting with LMN features confined to the distal aspect of 1 extremity may have a relatively benign disorder with a long life expectancy or may rapidly progress to death with or without development of concomitant UMN features. Although age and sex (men younger than 45 years have the longest average life expectancy) and site of presentation (patients with bulbar palsy on average have a shorter life expectancy) have prognostic importance in large populations, they are not applicable to individual patients. The rate of clinical decline determines the disease course in individual patients. Although commonly linear during the early stages of MND/ALS, it varies 30-fold in speed. Serial evaluations, including measurements of strength and vital capacity, provide the best prediction of prognosis in individual patients.

DNA testing for familial MND/ALS provides a diagnostic conundrum; 90% of ALS cases are sporadic. Most familial MND/ALS cases seem to be dominantly inherited with high penetrance. ALS patients commonly ask about the genetic implications of their illness. Armed with the aforementioned information and a detailed family history, it is usually possible to state that progeny or siblings are at minimal risk. Unfortunately, recessively inherited forms of this disorder, the possibility of spontaneous mutation, false paternity, susceptibility genes, and lack of knowledge regarding the medical history of the patient's biologic relatives mean that this risk is never zero.

It seems reasonable to dissuade patients with no apparent risk of familial ALS from obtaining DNA mutational analysis. Because commercial testing is positive in only 15% of patients with familial MND/ALS, ie, 1.5% of patients with MND/ALS overall, a negative test result may give a false sense of security. Although false-positive results are uncommon in DNA mutational analysis, these chances are enhanced whenever a test is performed for dubious clinical indications. It is imperative that patients and families understand the myriad potential psychosocial consequences of both positive and negative results, especially in ALS, a disease wherein the natural history cannot be significantly altered, before testing is undertaken.

Another diagnostic problem are patients who seem to have MND but have additional clinical or laboratory evidence of disease in other neurologic systems, termed *MND+*, or in association with other neurologic or systemic disorders (secondary MND). Both MND+ and secondary MND may present as ALS, PBP, PMA, or rarely PLS. MND+ and secondary MND may result from multiple causes (Table 88-1).

DIAGNOSTIC APPROACH

The role of ancillary diagnostic studies in MND/ALS is 2-fold: to demonstrate with EMG that LMN disease is more widespread than it clinically appears, and to exclude ALS mimics, particularly MMN and secondary causes of MND (EMG, brain and spinal cord imaging, muscle biopsy, blood tests, etc). Other specific tests primarily depend on the clinical presentation. Although transcranial magnetic stimulation, PET, and magnetic resonance spectroscopy show promise in the ability to categorize UMN changes, their sensitivity, specificity, and availability remain suboptimal.

MANAGEMENT

The optimal treatment of patients with MND/ALS requires extensive effort and resources and exceeds the capacities of any single health care worker. Although potentially emotionally and physically overwhelming to the patient, the multidisciplinary clinic is the preferred model in the provision of MND/ALS care.

Information provided to patients by physicians (eg, regarding their disease, identification of resource support organizations) and from patients (identification of patient values and wishes, advanced directives) is the first priority.

No **specific therapies** have had any major prognostic impact. Although riluzole, available in the United States since 1994, may be of benefit, its effect is difficult to define in individual patients. Unfortunately, although it prolongs disease duration by approximately 10%, it does so without any noticeable improvement in patient strength or well-being. Long-term population-based studies are somewhat more optimistic, with treated patients having an increased survival over controls. It is reasonable to offer riluzole to patients despite its costs and limitations. Every effort must be made to ensure that patients and their families have reasonable expectations of its effect. If the patient cannot afford the medication and support for its cost cannot be obtained, it is unreasonable to expect a family to jeopardize their long-term financial stability to provide it.

Although **symptomatic treatments** do not provide the response desired by patients or physicians, they can provide substantial improvements in patient comfort, function, and safety. In addition, they promote assertive rather than passive patient and physician responses to the disease (Table 88-3 and Figure 88-5).

Supportive management includes involvement of other health care providers, services, medications and durable medical equipment to improve patient comfort, function and safety. Two aspects of management should be considered in each patient with MND/ALS. Deep vein thrombosis and pulmonary embolism are important potential complications of MND/ALS, for which prophylaxis may be warranted in immobilized patients. Weak ventilatory muscles can be readily attributed to dyspnea. Another concern is nocturnal and to a lesser extent diurnal oxygen desaturation. The frequency and severity of desaturation is greater in MND/ALS than in similarly disabling neurologic disorders, a phenomenon that is not explicable on the basis of reduced vital capacity or degree of handicap but that warrants consideration of nocturnal oximetry and treatment with noninvasive ventilation even before vital capacity measurements decline.

Support organizations within the Untied States, the Muscular Dystrophy Association and the ALS Association, have dedicated themselves to supporting ALS research and the well-being of individual patients. They also support the development and distribution of reliable disease-related information, development of local support groups, maintenance of "equipment closets" for durable medical equipment, provision of transportation and respite services, and, in some cases, financial support for individual patients.

An **"ALS-savvy" social worker** is an invaluable asset to afflicted families and physicians caring for patients with MND/ALS. Patients with MND/ALS require more services for longer periods of time than most medical insurers are willing to provide. A knowledgeable, willing, and assertive advocate can maximize patient support and act as a liaison with visiting nursing and hospice associations. Terminal care of MND/ALS patients at home would be woefully inadequate in most cases without the services provided by such agencies.

Many **allied health care workers** can benefit MND/ALS patients and their families. Occupational therapists, speech and swallowing therapists, and nutritionists are all essential to care of patients with ALS.

After the patient has accepted their diagnosis and developed a trusting relationship with the physician, meaningful discussions must occur about the potential goals, benefits, and limitations of various interventions, including percuta-

OVERVIEW OF MOTOR NEURON DISEASE

Figure 88-5   Motor Neuron Disease: Habilitation Devices and Procedures

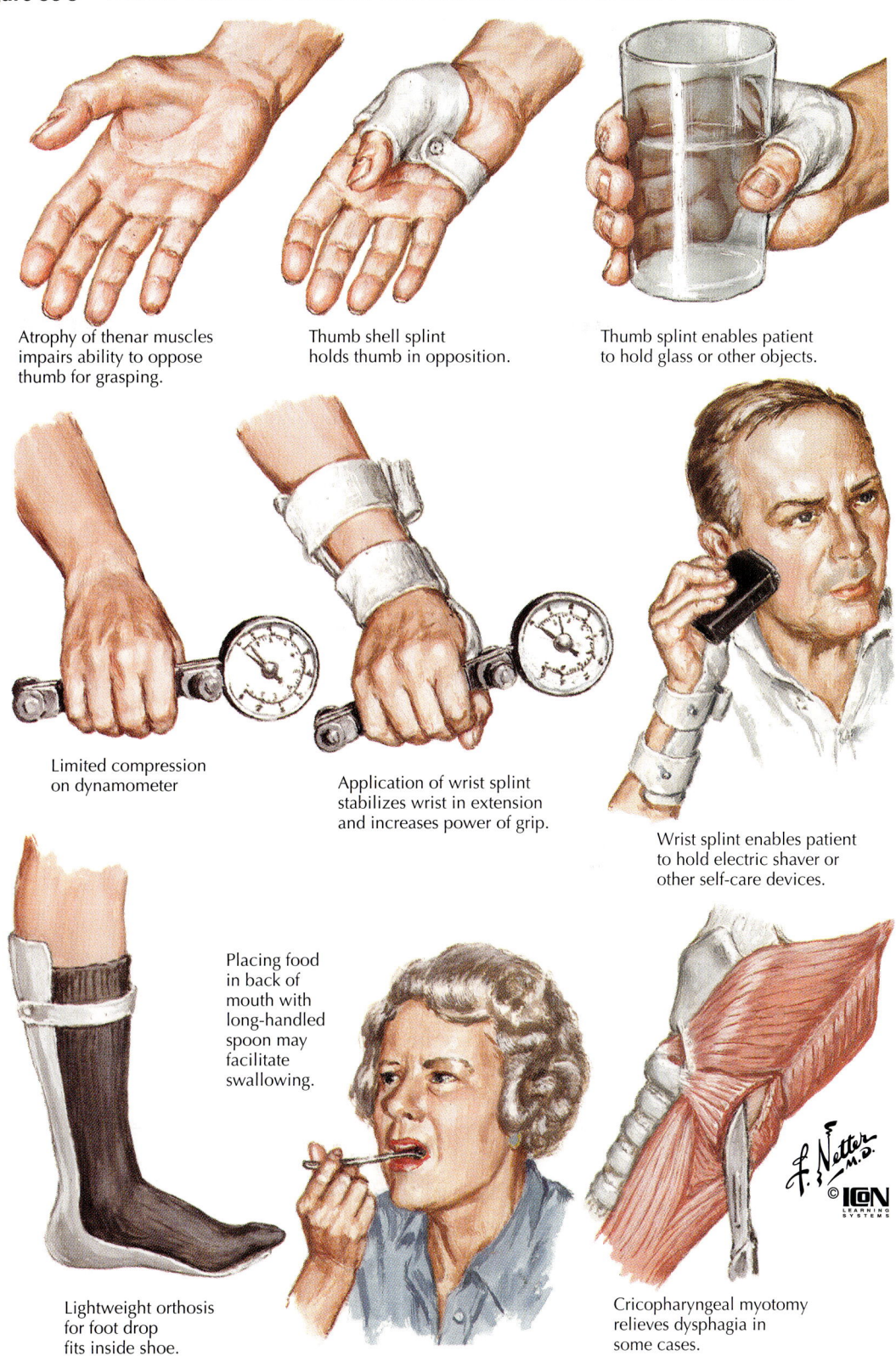

MOTOR NEURON DISORDERS

773

OVERVIEW OF MOTOR NEURON DISEASE

Table 88-3
Symptomatic Management of MND/ALS*

Symptom, Management Issue	Potential Treatments
Sialorrhea	Glycopyrrolate Tricyclic antidepressants Robinul Botulinum toxin Atropine Salivary gland radiation Scopolamine Chorda tympani section
Difficulty with secretion clearance	Tracheostomy Home suction In-exsufflator Guaifenesin β Blockers Nebulized saline and n-acetylcysteine
Pseudobulbar affect	Tricyclics Selective serotonin reuptake inhibitors
Laryngospasm	Antihistamines H_2 receptor blockers Antacids Proton pump inhibitors Sublingual lorazepam drops
Neck drop	Cervical collar High-back wheelchair with supports
Communication	Pad and pencil Erasable slates "Lite writers" Personal laptop computers
Breathing difficulties, morning headaches	BiPAP Cuirass Tracheostomy Morphine sulfate Benzodiazepines
Sleeping difficulties, morning headaches	Nocturnal oximetry BiPAP
Contractures	Night splints Range of motion exercises
Tripping from foot drop	Ankle-foot orthoses
Falling secondary to quadriceps weakness	Canes Crutches Walker Wheelchair
Bed mobility	Hospital bed with side rails, trapeze, or both
Bathroom safety and functionality	Stall shower Shower chair Transfer bench Toilet seat extension Shower and toilet bars

(continued)

Table 88-3
Symptomatic Management of MND/ALS* (continued)

Symptom, Management Issue	Potential Treatments
House accessibility	Stair lift or chair lift Hoyer lift elevators Ramps
Improved ADLs	Velcro for buttons and shoelaces Elastic shoelaces Long-handled grippers Foam collars for pens and utensils
Dysphagia, malnutrition	Neck positioning Feeding tube Change in food consistency Percutaneous gastrostomy
Constipation	Bulk Mobility Fiber Stool softeners/cathartics
Urinary urgency	Tolterodine
Cramps	Quinine sulfate Gabapentin Tizanidine Baclofen Benzodiazepines Phenytoin Carbamazepine Mexiletine Primrose oil Brewers' yeast
Safety	Lifeline Home safety evaluation

*ADL indicates Activities of Daily Living; ALS, amyotrophic lateral sclerosis; BiPAP, bilevel positive airway pressure; MND, motor neuron disease.

neous gastrostomy, tracheostomy, and long-term mechanical ventilation, and the location where the patient wishes to receive terminal care. It is important for patients to provide an advanced directive, identify a health care proxy agent, or both.

Experimental therapies such as numerous growth factors, riluzole, antiglutamatergic agents, and antioxidants have been studied without demonstrable success. Celecoxib, minocycline, and creatine are being studied in clinical trials based on theoretical benefit and positive results from in vitro MND models. Stem cell transplantation has been identified as a potential treatment for numerous disorders including MND/ALS. Unfortunately, realistic appraisals of its efficacy are not available.

Many patients with ALS ask physicians about **alternative therapies** for their disorder. A dogmatic opposing response by the physician risks losing the patient, particularly when the physician can offer no dramatically effective options. Conversely, physicians have a responsibility to dispel the perception that "natural" is synonymous with safe. Any substance biologically active enough to be beneficial is also biologically active enough to be harmful. "Natural" substances do not benefit from the same scrutiny and quality control as do pharmaceuticals and hence potentially pose risk.

FUTURE DIRECTIONS

Motor neuron disease/ALS has historically promoted nihilism from patients and their physicians, some of which is misplaced. Although current treatments are inadequate, they are still potentially helpful in improving patient comfort, function, and safety. With further basic research into this field, it is optimistic but not irrational to expect that MND/ALS, like cancer and AIDS, will no longer represent a universally lethal disorder ineffectively treated with a single drug. If not cured, MND/ALS may become controllable with a multidrug regimen successfully aimed at different components of its complex disease pathophysiology.

REFERENCES

Alblom M. *Tuesdays With Morrie*. New York, NY: Doubleday; 1997.

Brooks BR. El Escorial World Federation of Neurology criteria for the diagnosis of amyotrophic lateral sclerosis. *J Neurol Sci*. 1994;124(suppl):96-107.

Hand C, Rouleau GA. Familial amyotrophic lateral sclerosis. *Muscle Nerve*. 2002;25:135-159.

Miller RG, Rosenberg JA, Gelinas DR, et al. Practice parameter: the care of the patient with amyotrophic lateral sclerosis (an evidence-base review): report of the Quality Standards Subcommittee of the American Academy of Neurology: ALS Practice Parameters Task Force. *Neurology*. 1999;52:1311-1323.

Norris F, Shepherd R, Denys E, et al. Onset, natural history and outcome in idiopathic adult motor neuron disease. *J Neurol Sci*. 1993;118:48-55.

Ross MA, Miller RG, Berchert L, et al. Toward earlier diagnosis of amyotrophic lateral sclerosis. *Neurology*. 1998;50:768-772.

Rowland LP, Shneider NA: Amyotrophic lateral sclerosis. *N Engl J Med*. 2001;344:1688-1700.

Siddique T, Figlewicz DA, Pericak-Vance MA, et al. Linkage of a gene causing familial amyotrophic lateral sclerosis to chromosome 21 and evidence of genetic-locus heterogeneity. *N Engl J Med*. 1991;324:1381-1384.

Chapter 89

Motor Neuron Disease Presenting in the Limbs With Lower Motor Neuron Features

James A. Russell and H. Royden Jones, Jr

Clinical Vignette

Three years previously, a 75-year-old man noticed that he could no longer turn a key with his left hand. Weakness progressed to his right hand and then to his legs. Within a year, he could not raise his arms against gravity. After 2 years, he required a banister to climb steps. No pain or symptoms were referable to ventilation, sensation, or bulbar function.

Neurologic examination demonstrated weakness, atrophy, and fasciculations in all 4 extremities. The patient was areflexic. Although he could ambulate, he required both arms to get out of a chair. His mental status, cranial nerve, and sensory examination function were normal.

EMG revealed widespread active and chronic partial denervation and reinnervation consistent with a motor neuron disorder. A therapeutic trial of IV immunoglobulin was discontinued without benefit after the development of a rash.

Few neurologic disorders cause greater consternation to patients and physicians than motor neuron disease (MND). Its most common presentation is one of painless, asymmetric progressive weakness. Before confirming this diagnosis, critical consideration of the differential diagnosis and exclusion of alternative diagnoses—no matter how rare—is essential. There is no greater reward than to confirm a less serious and even potentially treatable illness when MND was initially suspected.

Isolated lower motor neuron (LMN) weakness in patients with the various forms of MND occurs in a varying percentage of patients (4-33%). Most patients eventually experience upper motor neuron (UMN) features and ultimately progress to "typical" MND/amyotrophic lateral sclerosis (ALS). Individuals with persisting isolated LMN signs for protracted periods may fare better. One study identified the duration of this form of MND as averaging 4 years (occasional cases remain stable for more than a decade).

The preceding vignette exemplifies a patient with insidiously progressive, asymmetric, painless weakness, beginning in one extremity and gradually generalizing, without development of concomitant symptoms in other neurologic systems or signs of a systemic disorder suggestive of an alternative diagnosis. This clinical profile fits that of MND/progressive muscular atrophy (PMA). The more common alternative diagnosis, MND/ALS, is inappropriate given this patient's absence of UMN signs. Most patients with MND/PMA, however, eventually have corticospinal tract signs compatible with MND/ALS.

CLINICAL PRESENTATION

Motor neuron diseases are the most common causes of painless asymmetric, multifocal weakness. Typically, these begin focally and segmentally progress to gradually affect multiple contiguous myotomes. Most patients demonstrate muscle atrophy, cramps, and fasciculations. In MND/ALS, upper extremity onset is approximately twice as common as lower limb onset. Distal weakness is more common than proximal. Impaired finger spread, thumb abduction, and wrist and finger extension are typically more severe than wrist and finger flexion (Figure 89-1). In

MOTOR NEURON DISEASE: PROGRESSIVE MUSCULAR ATROPHY

Figure 89-1 **Motor Neuron Disease: Early Clinical Manifestations**

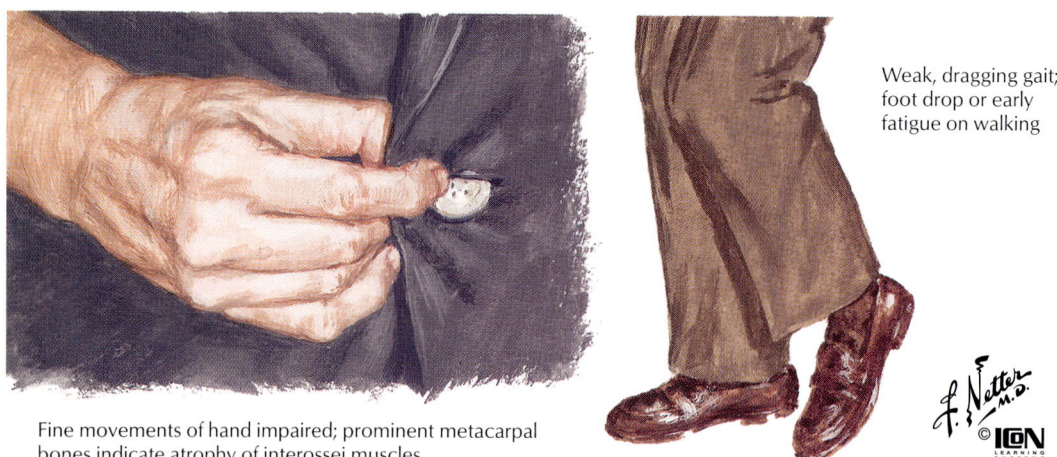

Fine movements of hand impaired; prominent metacarpal bones indicate atrophy of interossei muscles

Weak, dragging gait; foot drop or early fatigue on walking

the legs, foot dorsiflexion is usually more affected than plantar flexion.

Some MNDs are not classified as part of the MND/ALS complex; several do not present with focal patterns of weakness. Spinal muscular atrophies are genetically determined disorders of the anterior horn that are distinct from MND/ALS. The more common varieties, linked to the survival motor neuron gene on chromosome 5, usually present with generalized or proximally predominant weakness. These are primarily disorders of infancy and childhood.

DIFFERENTIAL DIAGNOSIS

The primary considerations in the evaluation of patients with progressive and isolated LMN weakness, unassociated with any concomitant sensory symptoms or signs, include typical and atypical MNDs, particularly distal forms of spinal muscular atrophy that present in a manner similar to that of Charcot-Marie-Tooth disease with bilateral foot drop but without sensory loss. However, their pattern of involvement and chronic course make these uncommon disorders an unlikely consideration.

Multifocal Motor Neuropathy

Multifocal motor neuropathy (MMN) necessitates special differential consideration. A presumed immune mediated disorder, MMN may clinically mimic MND but is exquisitely sensitive to immune modulatory therapy. This is a relatively uncommon disorder of middle-aged individuals. In MMN, the motor axon or its myelin sheath, rather than its anterior horn cell, is preferentially damaged.

Multifocal motor neuropathy often begins focally and is suspected when an individual nerve pattern of weakness develops rather than segmental distribution, eg, median C8-T1 innervated muscles may be affected to a significantly disproportionate degree to those of ulnar C8-T1 innervated muscles. This contrasts with segmental radicular denervation of MND, where all muscles innervated by a similar myotome are equally affected, regardless of nerve supply. There is often limited evidence of atrophy or fasciculations.

The diagnosis of MMN is verified when a patient with a focal LMN disorder has 1 or more of the following features: conduction block or other electrodiagnostic evidence of acquired demyelination, high anti-GM1 ganglioside antibody titers, and therapeutic response to immunosuppressive therapy. The diagnostic index of suspicion is further amplified when weakness occurs without a proportionate degree of atrophy, when weakness is confined to the distribution of a peripheral nerve, and when weakness begins distally in the upper extremity of a middle-aged man. This precise diagnosis remains difficult. Many patients present with a clinical picture similar to that of MMN but lack one of these

MOTOR NEURON DISEASE: PROGRESSIVE MUSCULAR ATROPHY

defining features; nevertheless, a therapeutic trial of IV immunoglobulin leads to gratifying clinical improvement. To further confuse the issue, some individuals thought to have MMN during life have spinal cord pathology identical to MND/ALS on postmortem examination. Unfortunately, there is no readily available, reliable, and universally acceptable paraclinical means by which to confirm concomitant corticospinal tract involvement in patients with an MND/PMA presentation. Therefore, a proactive therapeutic stance is advised, and a trial of IV immunoglobulin should be administered when any question exists about the presence of MMN. If patients are going to respond, they usually do so early in the course.

Spinal Muscular Atrophy Type III

Clinical Vignette

A 13-year-old boy had successfully played hockey for a few seasons; however, in the past year he had grown considerably. For the first time, he found it necessary to assume a squatting posture while defending the goal. This became more difficult. He attempted to compensate by bending from the waist into a pseudosquatting posture; otherwise, he could not properly provide goal cover. He was referred for neuromuscular evaluation. In retrospect, during the preceding year, his parents recalled his difficulty arising from low chairs, but there was no history of problems climbing stairs or using his arms over his head.

Neurologic examination demonstrated an inability to squat or rise and profound weakness of the iliopsoas and quadriceps muscles; muscle stretch reflexes were barely evocable.

Motor and sensory nerve conduction study results were entirely normal. Needle EMG demonstrated large motor unit potentials, markedly diminished in number, that fired at an increased frequency. No fasciculations or abnormal insertion activity was noted.

This vignette represents the typical presentation of spinal muscular atrophy type III (Kugelberg-Welander disease). The most benign of childhood spinal muscular atrophies, its presentation mimics that of a limb girdle muscular atrophy. EMG results prompt DNA testing for the survival motor neuron gene, enabling confirmation of the clinical diagnosis.

This genetic motor neuron disorder has an incidence of 1:10,000. Although usually presenting in infancy, it can present in adolescence or occasionally early adulthood. Its EMG findings can lead to confusion with PMA/MND. DNA testing is critical and can suggest a better long-term prognosis.

Juvenile Segmental Cervical Spinal Muscular Atrophy

A focal segmental disorder of motor neurons, juvenile segmental cervical spinal muscular atrophy, also called *benign focal amyotrophy* or *Hirayama disease*, occurs primarily in young men in their second and early third decades of life. It typically causes unilateral wasting and weakness of the hand and forearm, sometimes affecting the opposite extremity to a lesser degree. Rarely, weakness develops primarily in the leg rather than in the arm.

This uncommon disorder usually evolves relatively rapidly, reaching peak disability within a few years. Age of onset, clinical course, the tendency for serum creatine kinase determinations to remain normal, and the relative sparing of proximal arms and legs provide support for what may be a difficult distinction from early-onset MND/PMA. Fortunately, ALS/PMA is rare before the age of 18 years, and it is still atypical before the age of 40 years.

Bulbospinal Neuronopathy

An X-linked hereditary MND, bulbospinal neuronopathy (Kennedy disease) is primarily seen in middle-aged men. It may be confused with MND/PMA because of the patient's age at presentation; the progressive nature; the prominence of cramps and fasciculations; the presence of dysarthria, dysphagia, and tongue weakness; and the modest increase of serum creatine kinase. Features that help to distinguish it from classic MND/PMA include the absence of UMN features; a very slowly progressive course; a proximal, symmetric pattern of limb weakness; and prominent weakness of facial muscles. Kennedy disease is also characterized by androgen insufficiency, primarily gynecomastia, testicular atrophy, and impotence.

Diagnostically bulbospinal neuronopathy differs from PMA in the presence of associated sensory neuropathy on nerve conduction studies. Needle EMG demonstrates changes compatible

MOTOR NEURON DISEASE: PROGRESSIVE MUSCULAR ATROPHY

with primarily chronic partial denervation and reinnervation, with little if any concomitant changes of active denervation, in contrast to MND/ALS or PMA. DNA mutational analysis is commercially available. In the vignette at the beginning of this chapter, the asymmetric presentation, lack of bulbar findings and sensory neuropathy, and widespread active denervation rendered Kennedy disease unlikely.

Postpolio Syndrome

All patients presenting with focal weakness and atrophy must be questioned as to a history of poliomyelitis. The late evolution of seemingly healed old polio may mimic PMA but does not have its significantly progressive course.

Spinal Radiation Injury

Spinal radiation injury manifests with LMN weakness. Taking a careful history is important.

Neuromuscular Transmission Disorders

Neuromuscular transmission disorders present with focal, regional, or generalized weakness that is rarely confined to the limbs. Typically, they are confused with MND with "bulbar" presentations in which swallowing and speaking difficulties predominate. The absence of a history of fluctuating weakness and the presence of fasciculations and atrophy favor MND.

Myopathies

Myopathies are typically characterized by symmetric muscle weakness. Two myopathies are noted for their asymmetric tendencies. **Inclusion body myositis** (IBM) is most likely to be confused with MND/PMA. Fortunately, the pattern of weakness is diagnostically useful. IBM has a particular predilection for the quadriceps, finger and wrist flexors, foot dorsiflexors, and neck flexors. Other contiguous muscles may be involved but usually to a lesser extent. In MND, weakness spreads segmentally and regionally. Intervening muscles are not typically spared as in IBM.

Creatine kinase increases in IBM are similar to that in MND. Electrodiagnosis in IBM can be dominated by a combination of "neurogenic" and "myopathic" features; the former are readily confused with those of MND. Muscle biopsy is often necessary for specific diagnosis.

Facioscapulohumeral muscular dystrophy is also an asymmetric myopathy but is rarely confused with MND because the history is usually consistent with autosomal dominant inheritance. Facial and scapular weaknesses predominate in facioscapulohumeral muscular dystrophy, unusual for most MNDs.

Benign Fasciculations

Because many individuals are aware of the relation between fasciculations and MND, neurologists often evaluate patients who have observed fasciculations in themselves and become concerned about their significance.

Patients with MND/PMA are not specifically cognizant of their fasciculations until they are pointed out to them. Conversely, patients presenting with fasciculations without weakness rarely have MND. Patients in whom fasciculations are the chief symptom and who have otherwise normal neurologic examinations virtually never have MND. Patients presenting in this manner are usually reassured by expedient, carefully and thoroughly performed clinical neurologic and EMG evaluations, the results of which are almost invariably normal.

Neuromyotonia

Several rare disorders manifest with spontaneous fasciculations, sometimes with weakness, muscle cramps, or both. One of these, neuromyotonia, or Isaac syndrome, may mimic MND (chapter 92). EMG may provide a useful clue to this entity because it reveals continuous uninterrupted firing of normal motor unit potentials with no signs of denervation. The diagnosis is confirmed by testing for antibodies to voltage-gated potassium channels. These antibodies suppress outward potassium currents, inducing nerve hypersensitivity.

DIAGNOSTIC APPROACH

EMG is the definitive study for diagnosis of MND (Table 89-1). The 4 Ds, determinants, of EMG diagnosis are denervation, demyelination, differentiate, and distinguish: **Denervation** must be present in a widespread multisegmental dis-

Table 89-1
Evaluation of Patients With Suspected MND/PMA*

Major Studies: Recommended in Every Suspected Case	Selective Studies: Used Only With Certain Individuals
1. EMG and NCS: crucial to MND/PMA diagnosis	1. Muscle biopsy (query IBM)

2. CPK: generally should not be >1500 mg/dL in MND/ALS	2. Antibodies:
	   a. Anti–acetylcholine receptor binding (query MG)
	   b. Anti–voltage-gated calcium channel (query LEMS)

3. Anti-GM1 antibodies: with consideration of MMN after demyelination found on EMG	3. MRI of cervical spine, possibly brain
4. Serum protein immunofixation: rarely abnormal, but if so, bone marrow biopsy should be considered for lymphoma (query)	4. CSF, including IgG index and oligoclonal bands (query MS)

5. TSH	5. DNA mutational analysis
	   a. Androgen receptor gene (query Kennedy disease)
	   b. Superoxide dismutase gene (query familial ALS)
	   c. Survival motor neuron gene (query SMA I-III)

6. Forced vital capacity: baseline study	6. HTLV-I antibodies—blood and CSF
	7. Lyme serology—blood and CSF
	8. Hexosaminidase A levels (age <40 years)

	9. Generally not useful:
	   a. Bone survey
	   b. Heavy metal screen
	   c. Paraneoplastic antibodies
	   d. Single fiber electromyography

*ALS indicates amyotrophic lateral sclerosis; CPK, creatine phosphokinase; IBM, inclusion body myositis; LEMS, Lambert-Eaton myasthenic syndrome; MG, myasthenia gravis; MMN, multifocal motor neuropathy; MND, motor neuron disease; MS, multiple sclerosis; NCS, nerve conduction studies; PMA, progressive muscular atrophy; SMA, spinal muscular atrophy.

tribution, with preserved sensation, consistent with MND. **Demyelination** should **not be present**, particularly conduction block, which would be compatible with the treatable disorder multifocal motor neuropathy, rather than MND. The physician should **differentiate** MND from classic radiation neuropathy/plexopathy, myasthenia, or IBM. The physician should **distinguish** predominantly chronic denervation (eg, Kennedy disease) from MND where active denervation is prevalent (MND/ALS). Concomitant signs of a sensory neuropathy compatible with Kennedy disease should be sought.

Muscle biopsy is rarely indicated in suspected MND/PMA, except to exclude IBM in patients where the possibility exists based on clinical and EMG findings including prominent finger flexor weakness and myopathy abnormalities on EMG. Muscle biopsy cannot distinguish MND disease from other denervating disorders.

TREATMENT AND PROGNOSIS

General management principles of any patient with MND are described in chapter 88. Information must always be shared; potentially beneficial symptomatic intervention should be identified and instituted. Disease specific treatments such as riluzole are commonly used even if diagnostic criteria for MND/ALS are not met. Unfortunately, MND/PMA patients without UMN signs are not acceptable candidates for most clinical trials in MND/ALS.

Many neurologists offer a therapeutic trial of IV immunoglobulin to patients with atypical LMN syndromes without evidence of conduction block or anti-GM1, although cost and potential adverse effects must be borne in mind. This strategy stems from an inability to definitively exclude MMN on clinical or electrodiagnostic grounds. There is no consensus as to how long treatment should continue before deciding the patient is nonresponsive. Even more difficult are patients who wish to continue expensive and even potentially harmful treatments for subjectively perceived benefits that are unsupported by meaningful objective findings.

Prognosis varies for patients with an **MND/PMA phenotype** from those few with potentially treatable MMN to MND/ALS with its poor prognosis. No two patients follow a uniform natural history. Careful serial follow-up visits with quantitative clinical assessment remain the most useful and accurate diagnostic and prognostic tool.

REFERENCES

Blexrud MD, Windebank AJ, Daube JR. Long-term follow-up of 121 patients with benign fasciculations. *Ann Neurol.* 1993;34:622-625.

Dabby R, Lange DJ, Trojaborg W, et al. Inclusion body myositis mimicking motor neuron disease. *Arch Neurol.* 2001;58:1253-1256.

Gordon PH, Rowland LP, Younger DS, et al. Lymphoproliferative disorders and motor neuron disease: an update. *Neurology.* 1997;48:1671-1678.

Hirayama K, Tomonaga M, Kitano K, et al. Focal cervical poliopathy causing juvenile muscular atrophy of distal upper extremity: a pathological study. *J Neurol Neurosurg Psychiatry.* 1987;50:285-290.

Katz JS, Barohn RJ, Kojan S, et al. Axonal multifocal motor neuropathy without conduction block or other features of demyelination. *Neurology.* 2002;58:615-620.

Katz JS, Wolfe GI, Andersson PB, Saperstein DS, et al. Brachial amyotrophic diplegia. *Neurology.* 1999;53:1071-1076.

Kennedy WR, Alter M, Sung JH. Progressive proximal spinal and bulbar muscular atrophy of late onset: a sex-linked recessive trait. *Neurology.* 1968;18:671-680.

Mitsumoto H, Cwik VA, Neville HE, et al. Motor neuron diseases. *Continuum.* 1997;3(1).

Pestronk A, Chaudry V, Feldman EL, et al. Lower motor neuron syndromes defined by patterns of weakness, nerve conduction abnormalities, and high titres of antiglycolipid antibodies. *Ann Neurol.* 1990;27:316-326.

Traynor BJ, Codd MB, Corr B, et al. Clinical features of amyotrophic lateral sclerosis according to the El Escorial and Airlie House diagnostic criteria: a population based study. *Arch Neurol.* 2000;57:1171-1176.

Chapter 90

Primary Lateral Sclerosis: Motor Neuron Disease Presenting With Upper Motor Neuron Features in the Limbs

James A. Russell

Clinical Vignette

A previously healthy 47-year-old postal worker was evaluated for 1 year of progressive leg weakness. He felt that both legs were stiff, the right more so than left. He fatigued readily and could no longer run. He was unaware of any disturbances in his behavior, cognition, bulbar function, upper extremity, or genitourinary function. There was no family history of neurologic disease.

Examination disclosed a spastic quadriparesis. Tone and muscle stretch reflexes were increased in the extremities. The patient had slow and irregular repetitive movements. His legs were markedly spastic. He could not perform repetitive foot tapping. There was sustained clonus of both ankles with bilateral Babinski signs. His gait was stiff-legged with circumduction. He had no amyotrophy or fasciculations. Muscle strength, cranial nerves, mental status, and sensory examination results were normal. There was no pseudobulbar affect.

Ancillary testing was performed to exclude definable causes of progressive upper motor neuron (UMN) disease. His only abnormal test result was an increase CSF protein level: 76 mg%. MRI of the brain, cervical spine, and thoracic spine yielded normal results.

EMG disclosed no lower motor neuron (LMN) involvement. Test results for multiple sclerosis, Lyme disease, adrenoleukodystrophy, syphilis, vitamin B_{12} deficiency, anticardiolipin antibodies, and HTLV-I virus infection were normal.

A few years after the patient's initial evaluation, dysarthria with slowed tongue movements and a pseudobulbar affect developed. Three years later, he needed a cane to avoid falls. He still worked with some job modifications. Nine years after onset, he remained ambulatory, using a walker, and still had no LMN signs.

Primary lateral sclerosis (PLS) is a rare and poorly understood disorder without specific confirmatory tests. PLS therefore remains a diagnosis of exclusion in patients presenting with a slowly progressive UMN disorder. Motor neuron disease (MND) is rarely the underlying etiology in these patients. MND/amyotrophic lateral sclerosis (ALS) manifests predominantly as a LMN condition in the majority of cases; therefore, MND/PLS may not be initially considered in this differential diagnosis.

The findings in the preceding vignette are typical of a primary process affecting the corticospinal tracts (Figures 1-12 and 59-6); the patient is presumed to have MND/PLS. When a primary myelopathy is excluded, hereditary spastic paraparesis (HSP) is the other major diagnostic consideration.

CLINICAL PRESENTATION

In MND/PLS, the legs and, to a lesser extent, corticobulbar functions (speech and swallowing) are usually affected more than arms. The neurologic findings are often asymmetric, with prominent spasticity and a tendency to circumduct affected legs. Babinski signs and asymmetrically enhanced muscle stretch reflexes are common. Weakness is not even present in approximately 50% of cases. When present, it is usually mild and of UMN character, affecting primarily arm extensors and leg flexors rather than a LMN (segmental) distribution. The sensory examination is crucial and must be normal on repetitive examinations to exclude a myelopathic process, particularly cord compression.

DIAGNOSIS

Motor neuron disease/PLS is the working diagnosis usually made when a progressive UMN disorder occurs in the absence of LMN findings; sensory, extrapyramidal, cerebellar, or cognitive system involvement; similar family history; electrodiagnostic evidence of denervation or abnormal sensory potentials; or imaging, CSF, and serum test results supportive of other disease processes within the differential diagnosis. In essence, MND/PLS implies a lesion at any point along the corticospinal (pyramidal) tract (Figure 90-1).

Like other forms of MND, the PLS phenotype has a heterogeneous natural history. Diagnosis is based on progressive neurologic signs confined to pathology of the corticobulbar and corticospinal tracts. When MND/PLS remains a clinical UMN syndrome, life expectancy greatly exceeds that of MND/ALS. In one study, 10% of 383 patients with MND/ALS had exclusively UMN features at diagnosis, whereas only 4% remained devoid of LMN signs at the time of their last follow-up visit. No unequivocal criteria, at the time of presentation, distinguish patients with persisting MND/PLS and those who in whom MND/ALS eventually develops.

Confusing the MND classification further, in a manner similar to MND/progressive muscular atrophy, are those patients who die with seemingly exclusive UMN disease but at postmortem examination have evidence of anterior horn cell loss. Some patients with seemingly restricted UMN presentations and slow courses have clinical (cramps, fasciculations, atrophy), electrodiagnostic, or muscle biopsy evidence of restricted LMN involvement. Additionally, there are reports of individuals with otherwise typical **MND/PLS phenotypes** who have pathology of other neurologic systems. In a manner analogous to that of **MND/ALS plus**, it seems logical to recognize an even more uncommon **MND/PLS plus** category. As molecular biologic technology develops, some or all of these PLS phenotypes may eventually be classified within the HSP genotype.

Differential Diagnosis

Structural spinal cord (and occasionally brain) diseases with primary UMN signs are a common and often potentially treatable group of disorders that are within the differential diagnosis of PMD/ALS. Usually, their clinical features allow distinction from MND/PLS. Disorders such as multiple sclerosis, cervical spondylitic myelopathy, spinal cord or brain compression from benign tumors, spinal cord dural vascular malformations, and progressive multifocal leukoencephalopathy are also differentiated by characteristic abnormalities on neuroimaging. Vitamin B_{12} deficiency, HTLV-I, and adrenomyeloneuropathy are identified primarily by blood tests. The time course of many of these disorders and their frequent involvement of sensory and other systems represent notable differences helping to distinguish them from PLS.

Multiple sclerosis is a common and important differential diagnosis (chapter 62). Devic disease, an immune-mediated disorder with a specific IgG antibody that is distinct from multiple sclerosis, classically presents as an acute myelopathy with optic neuropathy.

Vitamin B_{12} deficiency is the most notable acquired metabolic derangement presenting with a myelopathy. Its usual presentation also includes paresthesias or a sensory ataxia that is often exacerbated in the dark. In contrast, **adrenomyeloneuropathy** is an untreatable inborn error of metabolism that primarily affects the corticospinal tracts.

Spinal cord or **frontal lobe tumors** and **cervical spondylosis** lead to cord or brain compression affecting the corticospinal tracts and presenting with a spastic gait.

Infectious/inflammatory diseases necessitate differential consideration, particularly those with a predilection for the spinal cord, including HTLV-I, HIV, to a lesser extent Lyme disease, and rarely syphilis in association with HIV. With the possible exception of HTLV1, most of these disorders are not likely to produce an isolated, chronic UMN phenotype. Sarcoidosis is uncommon but should always be considered.

A myelopathy may occur with the anticardiolipin antibody syndrome with or without **systemic lupus erythematosus**. There have been uncommon reports of a paraneoplastic myelopathy associated with breast cancer.

Hereditary spastic paraparesis is one of the primary clinical differential diagnostic considerations when uncommon but treatable disorders have been excluded. HSP also presents with UMN features affecting the legs more than the arms. It typically has more symmetric involvement than MND/PLS. This observation is useful, albeit somewhat limited, in its application to individual patients. Like MND/PLS, HSP can manifest at any time after childhood, but it most often presents in early adulthood. HSP has both "complicated" and "pure" forms, designated by the involvement or lack thereof of other non-UMN neurologic systems.

Unlike PLS, some patients with HSP have both clinical and lower extremity somatosensory evoked potential evidence of large fiber sensory dysfunction, correlating with the posterior column pathology commonly seen in HSP. Positive family history is a key distinction between MND/PLS and HSP. However, lack of knowledge regarding an individual's family history and the possibility of false paternity, spontaneous mutation, or recessive inheritance pattern preclude exclusion of HSP based on a negative family history. At least 16 different gene loci are identified for the various HSP phenotypes. These mutations can be dominant, recessive, or X-linked. Although the gene products for several different forms of HSP are identified, commercial DNA mutational analysis is costly and limited.

A number of **other hereditary/degenerative CNS disorders** also have prominent UMN features, including the hereditary leukodystrophies, spinocerebellar atrophies, and multisystem atrophy. In particular, **adrenomyeloneuropathy**, identifiable by an abnormal long-chain fatty acid ratio of C26:C22 lipids, is an X-linked disorder that affects young men, who present with a spastic paraparesis in early adulthood. It is sometimes mildly symptomatic in female carriers, ie, their mothers. Most affected individuals have only subtle cognitive and sensory involvement. Two clinical features usually distinguish MND/PLS from these disorders: neurologic signs and symptoms extending outside the motor system and, in certain cases, a positive family history.

Diagnostic Approach

Multiple options exist for evaluation of patients with a progressive UMN disorder in which MND/PLS is a consideration (Table 90-1). The primary tests routinely used are separated from those used in more specific clinical contexts, particularly those where the diagnosis may be defined but is untreatable. EMG is the primary modality for identifying rare patients with occult neurodiagnostic LMN findings.

TREATMENT AND PROGNOSIS

Treatment options for patients with MND/PLS are primarily supportive ones. One of the most important is reassurance that they do not have Lou Gehrig disease (MND/ALS). The peace of mind this counseling generates cannot be quantified but is of the utmost importance particularly among individuals in the health care profession.

Spasticity in this disorder may lead to significant patient morbidity. Its therapy in MND/PLS does not differ substantially from that of patients with MND/ALS. Baclofen, tizanidine, and, to a lesser extent, benzodiazepines and dantrolene may improve patient comfort and function. Unfortunately, both baclofen and tizanidine produce sedation at relatively low doses, often precluding dose escalation to a potentially effective level.

Additionally, spasticity may paradoxically improve patient mobility. At times, successful treatment of spasticity uncovers subclinical leg weakness, leading to the loss of ability to weight bear and transfer. Implantation of subcutaneous pumps enabling intrathecal delivery of baclofen to patients with spasticity can be effective for individuals who have inadequate control by oral medications. Although intramuscular botulinum toxin may be used to improve ambulation, it is most realistically beneficial in treating chair or bed bound patients with refractory painful spasms.

PRIMARY LATERAL SCLEROSIS

Figure 90-1

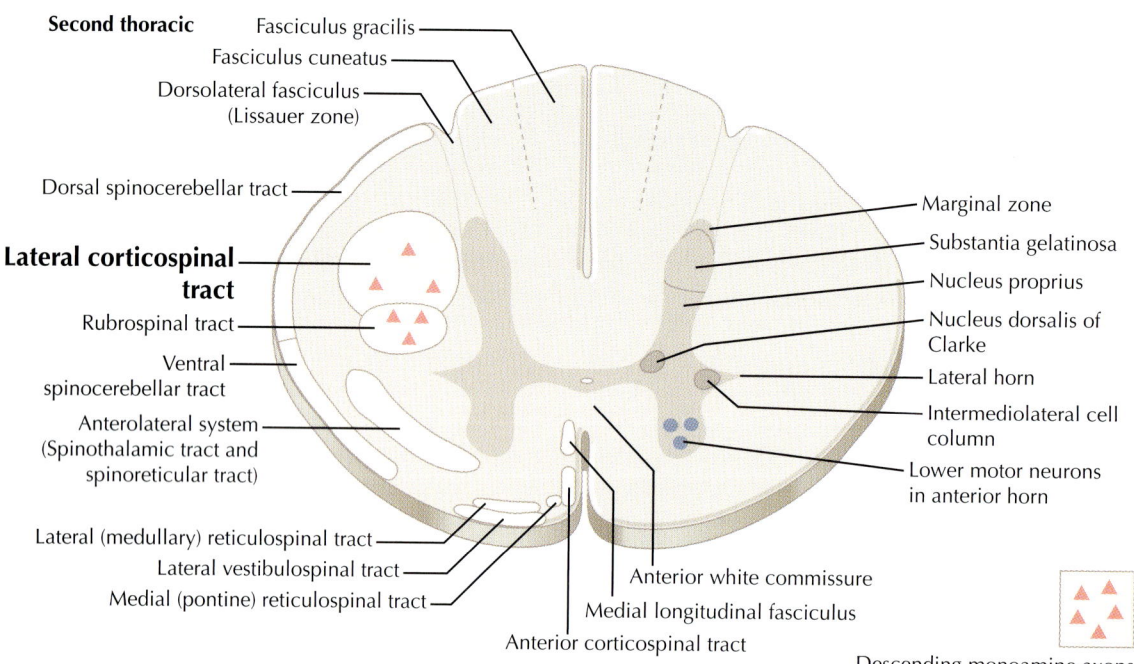

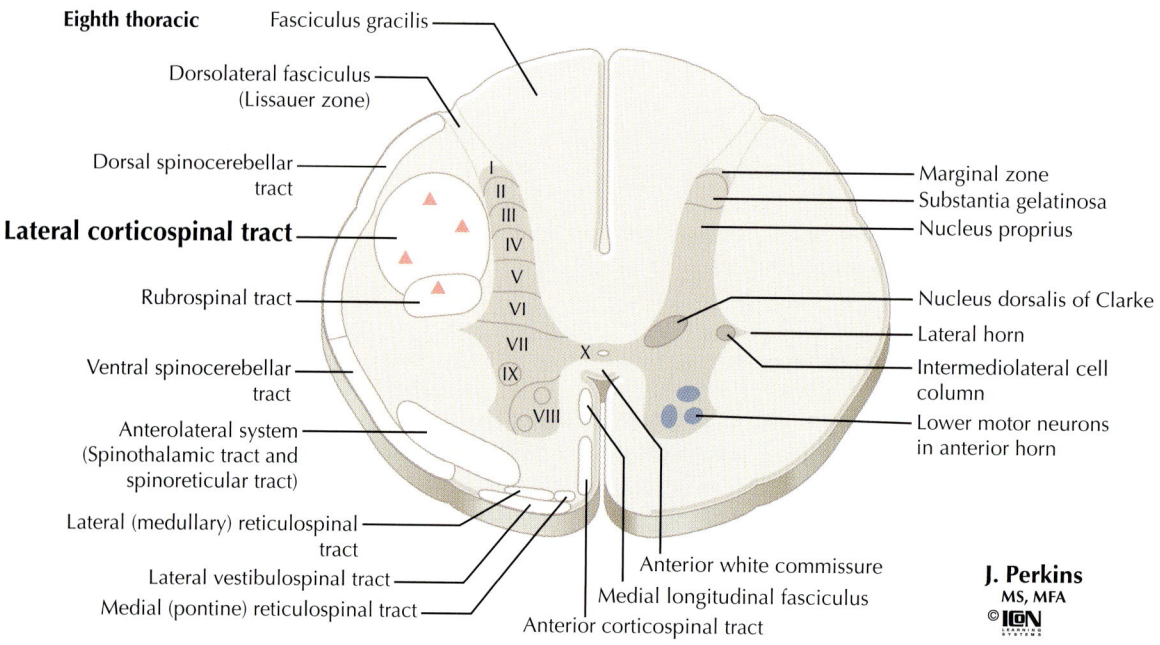

MOTOR NEURON DISORDERS

PRIMARY LATERAL SCLEROSIS

Figure 90-1

Corticospinal Tract Within the Thoracic Spinal Cord (continued)

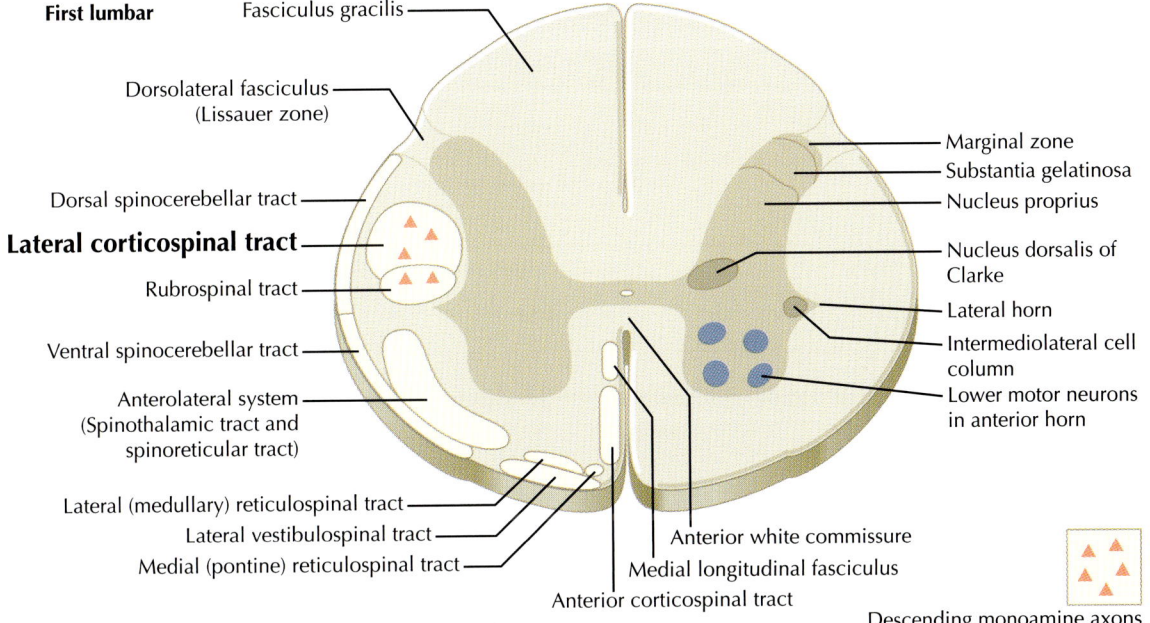

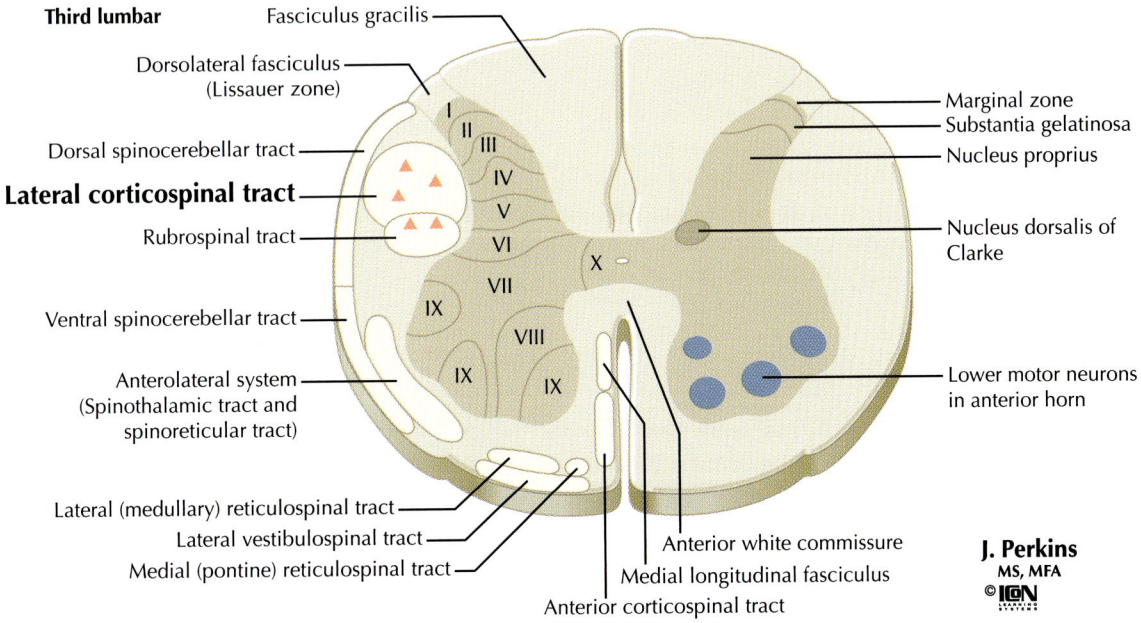

Table 90-1
Evaluation of Patients With Suspected MND/PLS*

Tests That Must Be Considered in Any Patient With Suspected MND/PLS	Tests That Should Be Considered in the Context of the Individual Patient
EMG and NCS	CSF evaluation, including IgG indexing and oligoclonal bands
MRI of brain	C26:C22 long-chain fatty acid ratio
MRI of cervical and thoracic spine	DNA mutational analysis for SCA
Vitamin B_{12} level	Neuromyelitis optica IgG antibodies
ACE level (serum and possibly CSF)	HTLV-I, HIV serologies
ESR, ANA, lupus anticoagulant, and anticardiolipin antibodies	Paraneoplastic antibodies, mammography
Lyme serology—blood and CSF	
RPR for syphilis	

*ACE indicates angiotensin-converting enzyme; MND, motor neuron disease; NCS, nerve conduction studies; PLS, primary lateral sclerosis; SCA, spinocerebellar atrophy.

Occasionally, surgical release of tendons may aid patient comfort, positioning, and hygiene. Fortunately, none of these invasive therapies are required frequently in the MND/PLS population.

Patients with MND/PLS may have symptoms of urinary urgency and incontinence. Tolterodine, oxybutynin, or the various antispasticity drugs may provide significant symptomatic relief.

Prognosis depends mainly on whether denervation and LMN signs develop. Although they are significantly handicapped, patients who have UMN disease only tend to have relatively full life expectancies. In one study, only 1 of 15 patients died after 15 years, far exceeding the median 3-year survival of patients with MND/ALS. Fifty percent of patients required a wheelchair after 4 years, although an additional 25% of individuals continued to ambulate unaided after 6 years. If and when LMN signs develop, prognosis becomes equated substantially with the MND/ALS, with prolonged life expectancy (>5 years) seen in less than 10% of patients.

FUTURE DIRECTIONS

Improved prognosis will occur with more rapid and exact means of differentiation between MNS/PLS and MND/ALS. Currently, no curative treatments for progressive motor neuronopathies exist. Development of such therapies depends on a better understanding of the molecular mechanisms of these disorders.

REFERENCES

Le Forestier N, Maisonobe T, Piquard A, et al. Does primary lateral sclerosis exist? A study of 20 patients and a review of the literature. *Brain.* 2001;124:1989-1999.

Mitsumoto H, Cwik VA, Neville HE, et al. Motor neuron diseases. *Continuum.* 1997;3(1).

Mitsumoto H, Norris FH Jr, eds. *Amyotrophic Lateral Sclerosis: A Comprehensive Guide to Management.* New York, NY: Demos Publications; 1994:4.

Pringle CE, Hudson AJ, Munoz DG, et al. Primary lateral sclerosis: clinical features, neuropathology and diagnostic criteria. *Brain.* 1992;115:495-520.

Traynor BJ, Codd MB, Corr B, et al. Clinical features of amyotrophic lateral sclerosis according to the El Escorial and Ailie House diagnostic criteria: a population based study. *Arch Neurol.* 2000;57:1171-1176.

Chapter 91
Motor Neuron Disease: Bulbar, Head Drop, and Ventilatory Presentations

James A. Russell

BULBAR PRESENTATIONS

Clinical Vignette

Five months before consulting a neurologist, a 77-year-old woman noted constant and progressive slurring of speech that had no diurnal variability. She had no diplopia or ptosis. Subsequent intermittent nasal regurgitation of liquids with drooling required her to change the consistency of her foods. No symptoms were referable to her limbs.

Neurologic examination demonstrated dysarthria and intermittently intelligible speech. The patient's tongue was weak and moved slowly, but there were no fasciculations or atrophy. Her jaw jerk and gag reflex were hyperactive, as were muscle stretch reflexes in her limbs.

The results of anti–acetylcholine receptor antibody determination, repetitive motor nerve stimulation, Tensilon testing, and a therapeutic trial of pyridostigmine were negative, excluding myasthenia. Brain MRI was unremarkable. EMG demonstrated no signs of denervation in limb or paraspinal muscles.

Left hand weakness was first noted 9 months later. During the next 5 years, generalized weakness gradually developed in the patient. A percutaneous gastrostomy was required because of progressive dysphagia with associated weight loss.

This vignette typifies the presentation of the progressive bulbar palsy (PBP) variant of motor neuron disease (MND), which occurs more frequently in women than in men. At presentation, patients with PBP commonly demonstrate predominant upper motor neuron (UMN) features; they lack clinical or electrodiagnostic evidence of bulbar and extremity denervation. When normal MRI excludes brainstem or clivus lesions, definitive diagnosis is often difficult. Usually, lower motor neuron (LMN) features do not develop for a few years; once tongue atrophy and fasciculations occur, myasthenia gravis and inflammatory myopathies are excluded. Such diagnoses should always be sought initially because both disorders are eminently treatable.

Dysarthria, dysphagia, or both are presenting symptoms in approximately 25% to 40% of patients with MND/amyotrophic lateral sclerosis (ALS) (Figure 91-1). Bulbar symptoms ultimately develop in almost 75% of patients with MND. Dysarthria is a more common presenting symptom than dysphagia. Unfortunately, MND/PBP is the most common neuromuscular mechanism for these "bulbar" symptoms.

Muscles innervated by cranial nerves IX through XII are more commonly involved than muscles innervated by the facial (CN-VII) or trigeminal nerves. Ptosis and ophthalmoparesis are rare in MND/progressive muscular atrophy; their presence is not compatible with a diagnosis of MND.

Motor neuron disease/PBP can present as a true bulbar palsy (LMN features only), a pseudobulbar palsy (UMN features only) or a combination of the two. Distinguishing between UMN and LMN bulbar presentations may be difficult but has pragmatic significance. The differential diagnosis of LMN bulbar disorders is limited. Disorders with both UMN and LMN features are fewer still. Tongue atrophy with fasciculation is the most reliable indicator of LMN disease. UMN involvement is suspected when patients' ability to blink or move the tongue rapidly is impaired in the absence of weakness or atrophy or when gag, snout, or jaw reflexes are exaggerated. Evidence of a pseudobulbar affect, ie, a tendency to

BULBAR, HEAD DROP, AND VENTILATORY PRESENTATIONS OF MND

Figure 91-1   Progressive Bulbar Palsy: Clinical Findings

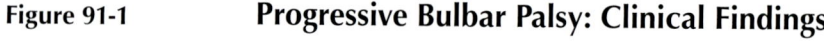

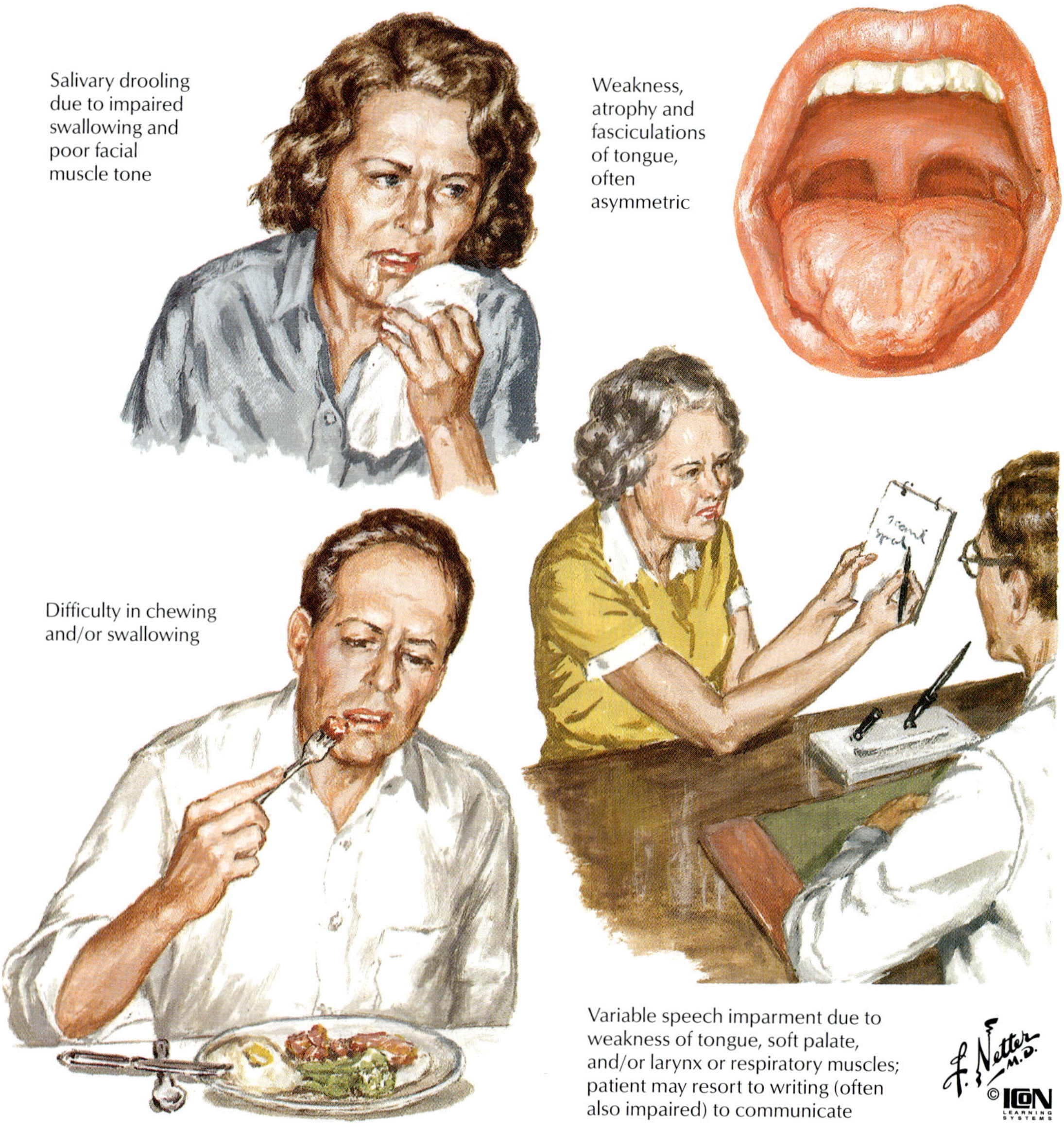

Salivary drooling due to impaired swallowing and poor facial muscle tone

Weakness, atrophy and fasciculations of tongue, often asymmetric

Difficulty in chewing and/or swallowing

Variable speech imparment due to weakness of tongue, soft palate, and/or larynx or respiratory muscles; patient may resort to writing (often also impaired) to communicate

laugh or cry without a typical associated emotional precipitant, suggests bilateral UMN pathology of the brain or upper brainstem.

Differential Diagnosis

Intramedullary brainstem disorders can sometimes be confused with MND/PBP or MND/ALS because both can affect cranial nerve motor nuclei and descending corticospinal tracts. Evidence of eye movement abnormalities, sensory signs, or both provide important clinical distinction from ALS.

A **stroke** is recognizable by its abrupt onset contrasting with the ingravescent course typical of PBP/MND. Occasionally, patients with small vessel strokes present with dysarthria, dysphagia, or both; however, vascular lesions rarely produce lower bulbar symptoms in isolation. MRI generally distinguishes between MND and a single or multiinfarct state.

MOTOR NEURON DISORDERS

Other cerebral disorders, particularly those involving white matter, such as multiple sclerosis or rarely either progressive multifocal leukoencephalopathy or a hereditary leukodystrophy, may produce a pseudobulbar state as a presenting sign.

Intrinsic brainstem tumors (ie, pontine gliomas or ependymomas) may present with slowly progressive dysphagia and dysarthria but are uncommon in adulthood.

Syringobulbia, an intramedullary lesion of the medulla, may affect multiple cranial nerve nuclei and requires consideration in patients presenting with swallowing or speech difficulties.

Multiple cranial neuropathies typically occur secondary to chronic meningitis, fungal or tuberculous infections, Lyme disease, parameningeal inflammations such as sarcoidosis, or leptomeningeal seeding of metastatic tumors at the skull base. More rare pathologies include benign tumors such as en plaque meningiomas, Paget disease, or an ectatic vascular structure.

Myasthenia gravis may be the most difficult disorder to distinguish from MND/PBP because of the absence of pain and sensory symptoms. However, fluctuating weakness, ptosis, or diplopia favor the diagnosis of myasthenia. Tongue atrophy or fasciculation and UMN findings are consistent with the MND/PBP diagnosis. Ancillary testing may be required in difficult cases. Diagnostic uncertainty sometimes remains, and sequential observation may be required for definitive diagnosis.

Some muscle disorders primarily affect speech and swallowing, especially **polymyositis**. Although approximately one third of patients with polymyositis report significant dysarthria or dysphagia, these are rarely isolated presenting symptoms. **Myotonic muscular dystrophy** often produces prominent bulbar and ventilatory weakness, usually relatively late in the disease course. **Oculopharyngeal muscular dystrophy** may present as dysphagia and ptosis in older individuals, usually in the context of a positive family history.

HEAD DROP AND VENTILATORY FAILURE PRESENTATIONS

Head drop and ventilatory failure are rarely the presenting symptoms of MND; both are more commonly associated with established disease. Ventilatory failure presents as dyspnea on exertion, orthopnea, fatigue, failure to wean from a ventilator, disordered sleep, or with symptoms of CO_2 narcosis, including early morning headache or encephalopathy. Head drop is commonly associated with posterior nuchal discomfort and is relieved with support.

Differential Diagnosis

The differential diagnosis is similar to that of PBP/MND. Both presentations result predominantly from LMN involvement. Head drop as an initial symptom is usually myopathic and relates to predominant involvement of the paraspinal muscles in conditions such as polymyositis and adult-onset congenital myopathies. Head drop can also develop after local radiation injury.

Orthopnea may suggest diaphragmatic paralysis due to involvement of the phrenic nerve. Ventilatory failure is sometimes the first symptom in MND/PBP and rarely in myasthenia gravis. Early-onset ventilatory compromise may occur in a few myopathies, namely acid maltase deficiency, myotonic muscular dystrophy, polymyositis, and the rigid spine syndrome.

Studies recommended in patients presenting with dysphagia, dysarthria, dysphonia, ventilatory muscle weakness, or head drop are listed in Table 91-1.

Muscles innervated by cranial nerves V, VII, IX, and XII are readily evaluated by needle electromyography. However, neurogenic abnormalities confined to these muscle groups cannot confirm a diagnosis of PBP, which remains uncertain until a more generalized picture of MND/ALS evolves. This evolution may be protracted. Limb or paraspinal muscle involvement or both may take months or even 4 to 5 years to manifest. Patients with PBP typically have normal electrodiagnostic examination results below the neck at presentation and do not fulfill the El Escorial criteria (chapter 88). This inability to make a definitive diagnosis often produces uncertainty and frustration for patients and physicians.

Repetitive motor nerve stimulation of CN-VII is often helpful to support a diagnosis of myasthenia, particularly when signs and symptoms

BULBAR, HEAD DROP, AND VENTILATORY PRESENTATIONS OF MND

Table 91-1
Evaluation of Patients With Suspected MND/PBP*

Primary Studies	Ancillary Studies
EMG with repetitive stimulation of facial nerve	CSF evaluation, including cytology, acid-fast and fungal cultures, RPR, Lyme serology, ACE
MRI of brain	Muscle biopsy
Serum CK	ESR
Anti–acetylcholine receptor binding antibodies	Anti–acetylcholine receptor modulating antibodies
Forced vital capacity	Single-fiber electromyography

*ACE indicates angiotensin-converting enzyme; CK, creatine kinase; MND, motor neuron disease; PBP, progressive bulbar palsy.

are restricted to the cranial musculature, but can be fraught with technical difficulties.

Normal brain MRI excludes structural brainstem lesions. CSF analysis can uncover leptomeningeal processes. When these are excluded, the differential diagnosis focuses on MND, myasthenia gravis, and polymyositis, all usually differentiated by EMG.

TREATMENT AND PROGNOSIS

General treatment principles address symptomatic control and emotional support (Figure 91-2 and Table 88-3).

Head drop is a frequent and troublesome symptom of MND and is often associated with posterior cervical discomfort. Head drop can also interfere with efficient swallowing, breathing, and secretion clearance. Probably no device provides adequate comfort, support, mobility, and ease of use in all patients. Finding the right cervical collar may necessitate trial and error and sometimes is not possible.

Percutaneous esophagogastrostomy (PEG) is eventually recommended in most patients with MND. PEG improves patients' quality of life by improving energy, improving nutrition, and lessening the time and effort associated with eating while minimizing the risk of choking and aspiration. It is unclear whether PEG tube placement significantly prolongs life expectancy. Patients opting for long-term mechanical ventilation require PEG or a suitable alternative. To minimize anesthetic risks, PEG placement should occur before the forced vital capacity decreases below 50% of the predicted value. Because most patients resist the concept of PEG, it should be discussed early and repeatedly, emphasizing the goal of improved quality rather than duration of life. Malnutrition, often insidious, may ensue in MND without PEG, impairing patients' strength and mood while increasing the risk of skin breakdown. PEG may reduce the risk of aspiration while minimizing concerns about choking episodes. PEG precludes neither oral intake nor showering.

Bilevel positive pressure is important in patients with dyspnea, orthopnea, or symptoms of CO_2 retention. Patient tolerance varies and is often a challenge; detailed attention to mask fit and machine settings is often rewarding.

Screening oximetry is essential in all patients with symptoms of restless sleep, excessive fatigue, morning headache, or irritability. Significant oxygen desaturation can occur in patients with MND, particularly nocturnally, even in individuals with seemingly adequate vital capacities.

Particularly onerous in MND/PBP is the inability to clear thick, viscous secretions. Expectorants have limited utility. Anticholinergic medications, when used for sialorrhea, usually have a paradoxical effect. Botulinum toxin injection into the parotid gland is a promising intervention. Providing a home suction device may be useful, although it is limited by the depth to which it can be inserted and by a hyperactive gag reflex in certain patients.

Pneumococcal and **yearly influenza vaccination** are recommended for MND patients with impaired ventilatory, swallowing or secretion clearance capabilities.

Regarding supplemental O_2 for the management of MND, many patients, families, hospice workers, and physicians are tempted to introduce O_2 when dyspnea develops. This practice should be avoided or initiated with great care because O_2 may depress ventilatory drive and aggravate rather than ameliorate the problem.

The percentage of patients with MND and their families that choose **long-term mechanical ventilation** varies considerably based on cultural and financial reasons. Estimated costs of maintaining a patient at home on mechanical ventilation exceed $150,000 per year. Patients with MND and their family members need to understand the logistical and financial implications of long-term mechanical ventilation. It is also important to anticipate that dementia may eventually occur, potentially robbing patients of whatever quality of life they might currently have.

Progressive bulbar palsy reduces life expectancy in the overall population of patients with MND, although the longevity of individual patients varies. The course of PBP/MND may be more protracted in older women. With adequate nutritional support, life expectancy can be doubled with bilevel positive pressure and quadrupled with tracheostomy-assisted mechanical ventilation.

REFERENCES

Chen R, Grand'Maison F, Strong MJ, Ramsay DA, Bolton CF. Motor neuron disease presenting as acute respiratory failure: a clinical and pathological study. *J Neurol Neurosurg Psychiatry.* 1996;60:455-458.

Chiò A, Finocchiaro E, Meineri P, et al. Safety and factors related to survival after percutaneous endoscopic gastrostomy in ALS. *Neurology.* 1999;53:1123-1125.

Miller RG, Rosenberg JA, Gelinas DF, Mitsumoto H, ALS Practice Parameters Task Force. Practice parameter: the care of the patient with amyotrophic lateral sclerosis (an evidence-based review). *Neurology.* 1999;52:1311-1323.

Oppenheimer EA. The critical role of respiratory care for quality of life and survival. *Amyotrophic Lateral Sclerosis.* 2001;2(suppl 2):7.

Sivak ED, Gipson WT, Manson MR. Long-term management of respiratory failure in amyotrophic lateral sclerosis. *Ann Neurol.* 1982;12:18-23.

Chapter 92
Stiff Person Syndrome

Ted M. Burns and H. Royden Jones, Jr

Clinical Vignette

A 53-year-old man reported episodic stiffness with variably severe muscle spasms and discomfort in his right leg. Episodes were brief (usually <1 minute), provoked by anxiety, and had occurred over 15 months. On 2 occasions while driving, he had transient, involuntary extension of his right leg that necessitated removing, by hand, his foot from the accelerator. One of these contributed to a minor motor vehicle accident. He had a history of pernicious anemia and thyroiditis. Family history included type 1 diabetes, thyroiditis, and pernicious anemia.

Neurologic examination demonstrated episodic right leg stiffening with knee extension and ankle dorsiflexion. The right patellar muscle stretch reflex was disproportionately brisk; its elicitation was followed immediately by prolonged spasm of the quadriceps femoris reproducing the patient's clinical symptoms.

Head and cervicothoracic spine MRI and CSF study findings were normal, as was the serum B_{12} level. EMG revealed prolonged motor unit activity in contracting muscles during episodes of stiffness and spasm but was otherwise normal.

Double-antibody radioimmunoassay demonstrated a high level of serum glutamic acid decarboxylase (GAD) 65 antibodies (199 nmol/L; reference range, ≤0.02 nmol/L). The patient was diagnosed with the appendicular variant of stiff person syndrome (SPS). Clonazepam alleviated symptoms but caused excessive drowsiness.

The patient was treated with 2 g/kg IV immunoglobulin, divided over 5 days, followed by prednisone (80 mg daily) in combination with diazepam and baclofen. He experienced gradual symptomatic improvement over the following 8 months but later developed similar problems with his other leg, necessitating increased medication dosages. Eventually, over 4 years, he was successfully weaned from corticosteroids.

Subsequently, his daughter developed a spinal axial variant with intermittent opisthotonic events that previously had been thought to represent hysteria. She was also anti-GAD65 positive.

Stiff person syndrome is a sporadic autoimmune disorder clinically characterized by severe stiffness and episodic painful muscle spasms. As is true of many autoimmune diseases, SPS is often accompanied by or historically associated with other organ-specific autoimmune disorders, including thyroiditis, type 1 diabetes mellitus, pernicious anemia, and vitiligo. SPS can be diagnosed on the basis of significantly increased levels of anti-GAD antibodies. Although uncommon, SPS is probably underrecognized, because its presenting symptoms (stiffness and pain) differ from those of most other neuromuscular disorders. Some affected individuals are initially thought to be hysterical or malingering.

The preceding vignette emphasizes that most SPS patients presenting with a focal stiff-limb form of SPS eventually have generalized, axially predominant, and painful muscular spasms. The anti-GAD65 antibody test allows early diagnosis, before patients become incapacitated by this potentially lethal disorder.

ETIOLOGY

Although SPS's designation as an autoimmune disorder has focused research initiatives, its precise pathogenesis remains unknown. GAD is the cellular enzyme that converts glutamic acid to GABA, a major inhibitory neurotransmitter. Consequently, one attractive theory of SPS pathogenesis is that GAD antibodies interfere with GABA production, leading to decreased spinal and supraspinal inhibition with development of rigidity and muscle spasms. Subsequently, Renshaw cell inhibitory input to the motor neurons diminishes, causing increased, less inhibited firing of anterior horn cells, similar to the pathophysiology of the lessening of Renshaw inhibitory input on the motor neuron cell seen in tetanus (Figure 92-1). Nosologically, SPS is not truly a motor neuron illness but rather a disorder of inhibition of normal motor neurons.

Intrathecal GAD65 antibody production in SPS supports an antibody-mediated pathogenesis. However, location of the antigen within neuronal cytoplasm may argue that the immunoglobulin is a biomarker of disease rather than a pathogenic antibody. GAD65Ab may also be accompanied by an unidentified effector autoantibody directed at a neuronal plasma membrane component.

CLINICAL PRESENTATION

Stiff person syndrome presents in middle-aged adults. Onset is usually insidious, with progression over months to years. However, 30% of affected individuals become significantly symptomatic in less than 1 month. Typical patients have intermittent axial or limb muscular rigidity with superimposed painful spasms. Spasms may be precipitated by simple sensory stimuli in a manner similar to that seen in tetanus. Pain occurs in all SPS patients and is often a major clinical concern.

Clinical Vignette

A 53-year-old woman was referred for "nonorganic" back pain of 1 month's duration. She had become increasingly disabled by severe spasmodic pains in her legs, abdomen, and back. Attempts to sit up, stand, or walk induced the spasms, which were associated with gait difficulty, episodic stiffening of her entire body, and sometimes incontinence. Her condition was so severe that she had been admitted to the hospital, where she promptly became a ward disturbance because of her distress during episodes of pain. Her medical history included a myeloproliferative disorder.

On neurologic examination, the patient was screaming "like a bellowing cow" according to the nurse, who stated, "She needs a psychiatric consult." However, the patient was alert, anxious, rational, and appropriately concerned about the illness. Initially, her body displayed total extensor spasm when touched for examination. The slightest sensory stimulus—touching her leg or trying to sit her up—produced severe pain and spasms. Except for marked, paravertebral spasm at times radiating to her abdomen and a right Babinski sign, her basic neurologic examination results were normal. When the neurosurgeon asked her to get out of bed, he went to hold her hand as she attempted to take a step. She developed a whole-body extensor spasm, became totally rigid, and bounced off the wall "like a telephone pole being cut."

A clinical diagnosis of an axial form of SPS was made in this vignette because the presentation resembled tetanus except that the patient had no trismus and no risk factors for tetanus. Antibody studies were not yet available. Soon thereafter, the patient experienced spells of thoracic wall spasm or brief "seizures" wherein she seemed unresponsive. EMG demonstrated continuous and conjoint firing of motor unit potentials in agonist and antagonist muscles. Treatment with benzodiazepines and immunosuppressants led to total remission in 4 to 5 years.

Falling, as in the preceding vignette, is common in SPS. Some SPS patients have also had their legs intermittently stiffen in "hiccupslike"

Figure 92-1

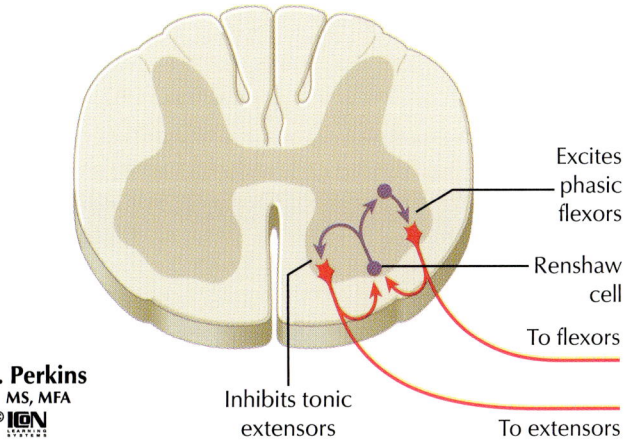

Renshaw Cell Bias

STIFF PERSON SYNDROME

spasms, throwing them to the ground. Another patient was reported to have fallen "like a wooden man, a wax dummy." At its extreme, simple parts of the examination, such as eliciting the quadriceps muscle stretch reflex, may put the patient into opisthotonic posture (Figure 92-2), sometimes confused with hysteria. Gait problems also occur but tend to be linked to precipitous spasms.

In patients in whom the diagnosis is unrecognized, insidious progression of the disorder causes development of chronic axial rigidity, leading to secondary spinal deformities such as lumbar hyperlordosis (Figure 92-3). The grandson of one patient with severe chronic hyperlordosis secondary to SPS used his grandfather as a tunnel to crawl through while playing.

Although initial muscle involvement is often confined to the trunk, the first symptoms may occur in the neck or shoulder or in one limb, usually a lower extremity (sometimes called **stiff leg syndrome**—see the first Clinical Vignette in this chapter). Such cases eventually progress to more widespread involvement, including the trunk, particularly if diagnosis is delayed. The proximal muscles are typically more prominently involved. When the back and abdomen become significantly affected, their muscles sometimes become hard and boardlike. Breathing may be compromised when the chest wall is affected by thoracic muscular spasms.

The neurologic examination is characterized by stimulus sensitive muscle spasms mimicking tetanus. These may be precipitated by sudden jarring, movement, or fright. The degree of muscular rigidity and spasm fluctuates. Stiffness is more likely to be extraordinarily severe versus moderate in the later stages. Despite this dramatic picture, patients with SPS have normal strength and sensation. Muscle stretch reflexes are so disinhibited that their elicitation, particularly the knee jerk, can recapitulate the clinical picture even early in the illness when no obvious rigidity or spasms are present.

DIFFERENTIAL DIAGNOSIS

Various previous diagnoses are reported, including functional hysteria, chronic tetany, dystonia, stroke, and arthritis. The possibility of a spinal cord disorder, ie, a myelopathy with spondylosis or disc herniation, versus a basal ganglia disorder, also requires consideration.

In any relatively acute setting, the possibility of tetanus must be considered because of the boardlike stiffening of the abdomen and the severity of muscle spasms. Sparing of the jaw muscles and absence of trismus make this diagnosis unlikely. Spasms are generally less violent and of less acute onset in SPS than in tetanus, but this is not invariable. Chronic tetanus is rare and typically presents with trismus and risus sardonicus.

Figure 92-2 **End-Stage Stiff Person Syndrome**

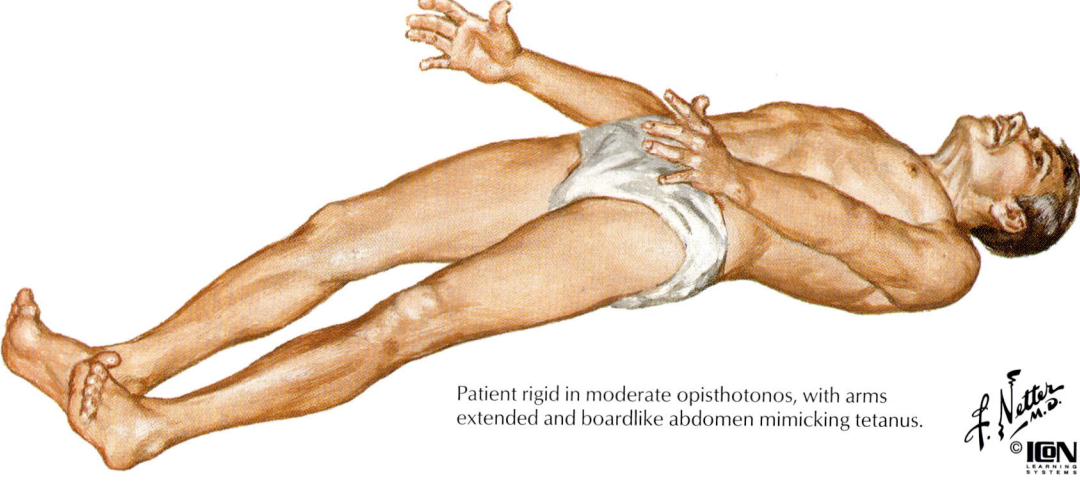

Patient rigid in moderate opisthotonos, with arms extended and boardlike abdomen mimicking tetanus.

STIFF PERSON SYNDROME

Figure 92-3
Stiff Person Syndrome

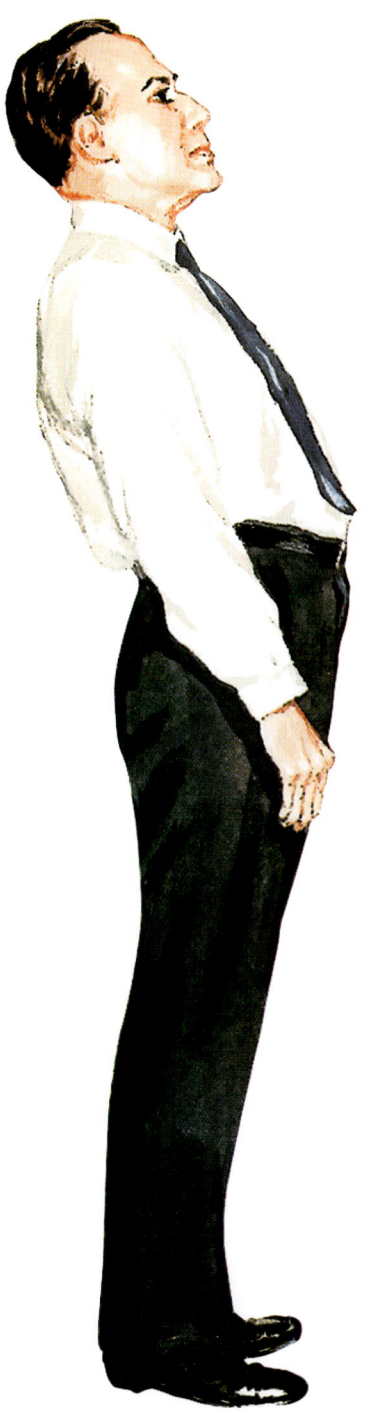

Occasional patient with stiff person syndrome assumes hyperextended posture with increased lordosis.

Startle-induced spasms occur in **hereditary hyperekplexia** or **startle disease**, a rare disorder caused by mutations in the glycine receptor, a receptor for a major inhibitory CNS neurotransmitter. Startle-induced spasms may also be seen in focal spinal cord lesions such as tumors or syringomyelia. Psychogenic muscle contraction or spasm is usually more variable but warrants consideration.

Other causes of muscular rigidity include disorders of muscle or neuronal membrane hyperexcitability. Two channelopathies with muscle rigidity, myotonia congenita and Isaac syndrome, deserve intellectual consideration in the differential diagnosis, but neither of these is associated with pain. Multiple sclerosis, poliomyelitis, Lyme disease, encephalomyelitis with rigidity, spinal myoclonus, tumors, and even strychnine poisoning are also in the differential.

There is a **paraneoplastic variant** of SPS associated with breast cancer. A 66-year-old woman with progressive rigidity leading to opisthotonus with physically and emotionally precipitated spasms was reported. Each woman with this variant had positive antineuronal antibody, leading to ultrasound identification of breast cancer. Treatment with tamoxifen, diazepam, and prednisone led to a cure.

DIAGNOSTIC APPROACH

A high level of antibody directed at the 65-kd isoform of GAD is a valuable serologic marker of SPS. This test has provided a means of early, accurate, reliable diagnosis in individuals who previously might have been thought to have a psychogenic disorder. Marked increased values support the clinical diagnosis of the stiff limb variety of SPS. Mild increases of this antibody are also seen in patients with diabetes mellitus, so caution is advised.

EMG usually reveals a characteristic abnormality with concomitant and continuous firing of motor unit potentials in agonist and antagonist muscles in those who are severely affected, but the findings of the study are often initially normal. The myotonic discharges of myotonia congenita and neuromyotonic discharges or nonpainful continual firing of motor units in Isaac syndrome are not easily confused with SPS.

MOTOR NEURON DISORDERS

TREATMENT AND PROGNOSIS

Treatment of SPS can be symptomatic or more specifically directed at the presumed underlying autoimmune process. Symptomatic treatment is dominated by agents that increase GABAergic transmission, including benzodiazepines (such as diazepam), baclofen, tizanidine, and anticonvulsants. Corticosteroids, azathioprine, IV immunoglobulin, and plasma exchange are commonly prescribed immunosuppressive or immunomodulating agents.

Of 14 cases at the Mayo Clinic between 1928 and 1956, 4 of the 11 patients with long-term follow-up died of the illness. Mortality is lower with specific treatment. In at least 1 case, a patient has died after inappropriate weaning of medication in an attempt to precipitate a diagnostic event.

REFERENCES

Burns TM, Jones HR, Phillips LH, Bugawan TL, Erlich HA, Lennon VA. Clinically disparate stiff-person syndrome with GAD65 autoantibodies in a father and daughter. *Neurology.* 2003;61:1291-1293.

Dalakas MC, Fujii M, McElroy B. The clinical spectrum of anti-GAD antibody-positive patients with stiff-person syndrome. *Neurology.* 2000;55;1531-1535.

Moersch FP, Woltman HW. Progressive fluctuating muscular rigidity and spasm ("stiff-man" syndrome): report of a case and some observations in 13 other cases. *Mayo Clin Proc.* 1956;31:421-427.

Saiz A, Graus F, Valldeoriola F, et al. Stiff-leg syndrome: a focal form of stiff-man syndrome. *Ann Neurol.* 1998;43:400-403.

Walikonis JE, Lennon VA. Radioimmunoassay for glutamic acid decarboxylase (GAD65) autoantibodies as a diagnostic aid for stiff-man syndrome and a correlate of susceptibility to type 1 diabetes mellitus. *Mayo Clin Proc.* 1998;73:1161-1166.

Section XXII
POLYNEUROPATHIES AND AUTONOMIC DISORDERS

Chapter 93
Overview of Peripheral Nerve Disease 800

Chapter 94
Length-Dependent Polyneuropathy 808

Chapter 95
Acquired Demyelinating Polyradiculoneuropathies: Guillain-Barré Syndrome and Chronic Inflammatory Demyelinating Polyradiculoneuropathy 818

Chapter 96
Multifocal Neuropathies 827

Chapter 97
Sensory Neuropathy and Neuronopathy 834

Chapter 98
Leprosy (Hansen Disease) 839

Chapter 99
Disorders of the Autonomic Nervous System 843

Chapter 93
Overview of Peripheral Nerve Disease

Ted M. Burns and James A. Russell

Clinical Vignette

A vigorous 42-year-old woman with a 26-year history of type 1 diabetes mellitus underwent a lumpectomy for breast carcinoma. She woke from anesthesia with severe burning pain prominent distally in all extremities, which was presumed to be related to her diabetes. She underwent chemotherapy with 5-fluorouracil, cyclophosphamide, and methotrexate, and the symptoms worsened. The pain became incapacitating; she could no longer work.

Neurologic examination demonstrated severe hyperpathia, interfering with the patient's ability to ambulate and with the examination because she could not tolerate any pressure against her skin. Absent muscle stretch reflexes and stocking-glove hypesthesias to touch, pain, temperature, and vibration sensory modalities were also found.

Previous neurologic evaluations suggested a small fiber sensory neuropathy related to the patient's diabetes, exacerbated by her malignancy and chemotherapeutic agents. Evaluation at Lahey demonstrated a very low serum vitamin B_{12} level. Replacement therapy led to complete symptom resolution.

Evaluating patients who have peripheral neuropathies is challenging. Myriad causes and disorders within the differential diagnosis must be addressed. Following a structured approach is essential, modifying the specific features of each case, including the nature, distribution, and evolution of symptoms and the context in which the disorder is occurring. The most rewarding approach to evaluating patients who have a polyneuropathy is a painstakingly thorough one. To interpret the patient's clinical picture, an understanding of peripheral nervous system anatomy and its varied capacity to respond to different pathologic injuries is required.

Frequently, a neurologist is requested to render an opinion in cases of severe painful incapacitating polyneuropathies. Each individual deserves a thorough investigation. In the preceding vignette, the history was key, as often occurs. Why did this woman who had no previous symptoms of a diabetic polyneuropathy awaken from her surgery with such a severe problem? Certainly it was not the temporal profile of a small fiber sensory neuropathy. The answer related to discovering that her anesthesia induction included nitrous oxide, known for its ability to precipitate a previously subclinical cobalamin deficiency leading to acute polyneuropathy and signs of subacute combined degeneration.

A 5-part strategy to acquire and organize information about peripheral neuropathies includes evaluation of symptoms and signs, definition of specific neuropathic patterns, differential diagnosis, the value and limitations of ancillary investigations, and treatment options.

CLINICAL PRESENTATION

Most neuropathies concomitantly affect sensory and motor function (Figure 93-1). When patients primarily present with weakness, disorders of the motor neuron, the neuromuscular junction, the skeletal muscle, and occasionally the spinal cord are considered. If symptoms are mainly sensory, predominant early sensory involvement of a mixed nerve, primary sensory neuronopathies, a radiculopathy, and occasionally myelopathies are the major diagnostic considerations.

Motor function is evaluated to define the pattern of weakness, ie, symmetric length-dependent, generalized non–length-dependent, or asymmetric, multifocal patterns. When the weakness is focal or multifocal, determination of

OVERVIEW OF PERIPHERAL NERVE DISEASE

Figure 93-1 Peripheral Neuropathies: Clinical Manifestations

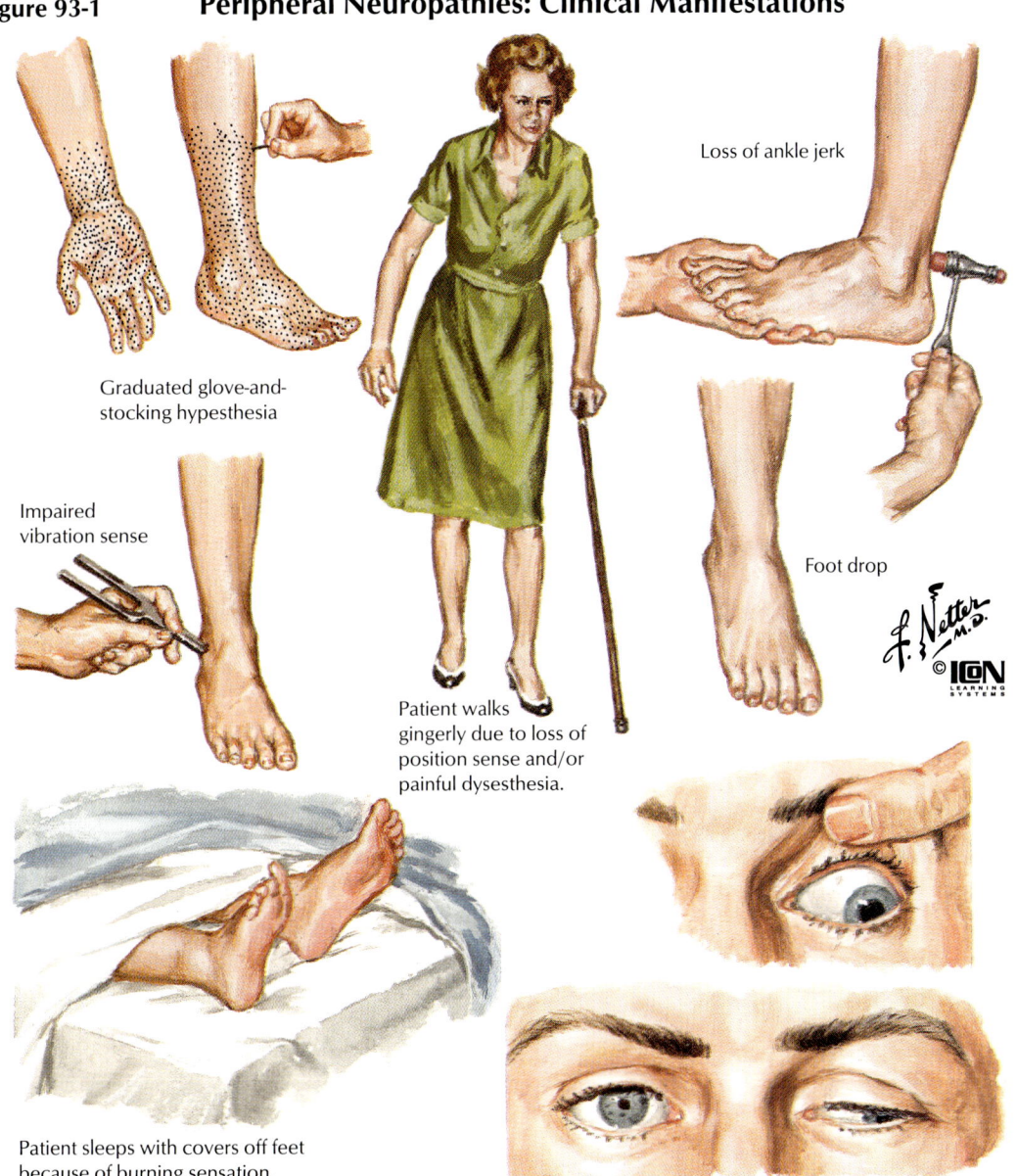

Graduated glove-and-stocking hypesthesia

Impaired vibration sense

Loss of ankle jerk

Foot drop

Patient walks gingerly due to loss of position sense and/or painful dysesthesia.

Patient sleeps with covers off feet because of burning sensation.

Oculomotor nerve palsy: ptosis, eye turns laterally and inferiorly, pupil dilated. Common finding with cerebral aneurysms, especially carotid-posterior communicating aneurysms.

whether it is primarily a nerve (eg, peroneal) or segmental (eg, L5) distribution is the next step (Table 93-1).

Sensory symptom characterization is important for patients with generalized polyneuropathies. Some disorders primarily affect certain fiber sizes, leading to specific symptoms. **Large fiber** sensory dysfunction is characterized by **negative** symptomatology with loss of sensation, numbness, a wooden stump–like or band sensation. Individuals with loss of proprioception frequently experience associated imbalance, particularly in the dark. In contrast, **small fiber** involvement is typified by **positive** sensory symptoms. These symptoms occur spontaneously, varying from painless, although sometimes uncomfortable, to unpleasant or definitely painful. **Painless positive** experiences include

POLYNEUROPATHIES AND AUTONOMIC DISORDERS

801

OVERVIEW OF PERIPHERAL NERVE DISEASE

Table 93-1
Pure Motor or Predominantly Motor Polyneuropathies*

Polyradiculoneuropathy Pattern

- Guillain-Barré syndrome
- Chronic inflammatory demyelinating Polyradiculoneuropathy (CIDP)
- Organophosphate toxicity
- Buckthorn wild cherry poisoning
- AIDS
- Porphyria
- Lyme disease?

Multifocal Neuropathy Pattern

- MMN with conduction block
- Motor neuropathies not meeting MMN criteria

Length-Dependent Polyneuropathy Pattern

- Charcot-Marie-Tooth disease
- Critical illness polyneuropathy
- Ara-C
- Buckthorn toxicity
- Dapsone
- Lead

Motor Neuron Disease Pattern

- ALS and progressive muscular atrophy (section XV)
- Spinal muscular atrophy
- Enterovirus

*ALS indicates amyotrophic lateral sclerosis; CIDP, chronic inflammatory demyelinating polyradiculoneuropathy; MMN, multifocal motor neuropathy.

perceptions such as asleep, prickling, tingling, swollen, and "bunched-up socks" under the toes. **Painful positive** symptoms include electriclike shock, burning, freezing, aching, tightness, and throbbing perceptions (Table 93-2). A paradigm for sensory testing is described in chapter 100. Patterns sought for patients with numb feet include those that can be localized to spinal cord (sensory level, suspended or dissociated) or peripheral nerve (length dependent, multiple nerve, multiple dermatome).

Only a few disorders affect both **autonomic** and **somatic nerves**; therefore, detection of clinical dysautonomia aids the differential diagnosis (Table 93-3). Autonomic symptoms include orthostatic intolerance or overt syncope, diarrhea, constipation, postprandial bloating, urinary symptoms, erectile dysfunction, abnormal or absent sweating, and dry mouth or eyes. Such symptoms in isolation, eg, constipation, do not implicate autonomic nervous system pathology. Judgment is required to assess relevance based on the distribution, comorbidities, and use of medications with potential autonomic side effects. Autonomic testing may clarify such cases.

Muscle stretch reflex diminution or absence is typical of many polyneuropathies. Because their presence relies on the viability of large myelinated fibers, these are sometimes spared in small fiber neuropathies. Typically, such reflexes are lost maximally in a distal distribution, particularly with axonal length-dependent neuropathies, ie, ankle jerks are lost first. Because active muscle stretch reflexes depend on the synchrony of impulse transmission, they tend to be characteristically suppressed with demyelinating neuropathies or polyradiculoneuropathies (multiple nerves and nerve roots).

Table 93-2
Painful Polyneuropathies*

Length-Dependent Polyneuropathy Pattern

- Diabetes and impaired glucose tolerance
- Alcohol
- Other toxins (certain) (with or without associated hypersensitivity vasculitis)
- B-vitamin deficiencies; B_{12}, B_6, thiamine
- Sjögren syndrome (often SN pattern)
- Amyloidosis—primary systemic and inherited
- Hepatitis C and cryoglobulinemia
- HIV neuropathy
- Hereditary sensory neuropathy
- Fabry disease
- Tangier disease

Multifocal Neuropathy or Length-Dependent Polyneuropathy Pattern

- Vasculitis (MM more typical; 25-30% of cases present as LDPN)
- Diabetes mellitus
- Hansen disease (leprosy)
- Lyme disease

Polyradiculoneuropathy Pattern

- Guillain-Barré syndrome
- Chronic inflammatory demyelinating polyradiculoneuropathy

*LDPN indicates length-dependent polyneuropathy; MM, mononeuritis multiplex; SN, sensory neuronopathy.

Table 93-3
Polyneuropathies With Autonomic Nervous System Involvement

Length-Dependent Polyneuropathy Pattern

- Diabetes mellitus
- Vincristine
- Sjögren syndrome (LDPN or SN)
- Amyloidosis (hereditary or primary systemic)
- Paraneoplastic polyneuropathy
- Hereditary sensory and autonomic neuropathies
- HIV-related polyneuropathy
- Pandysautonomia (idiopathic or autoimmune)

Polyradiculoneuropathy Pattern

- Guillain-Barré syndrome
- Porphyria

*LDPN indicates length-dependent polyneuropathy; SN, sensory neuronopathy.

Gait assessment is an important aspect of the suspected neuropathy evaluation. Ataxia, a major associated morbidity of neuropathy, commonly results from impaired large myelinated sensory fiber function. Wavering or loss of balance while standing with the eyes closed, disproportionate to the same stance with the eyes opened (positive Romberg sign), suggests significant proprioceptive loss.

Cranial nerve testing may identify trigeminal or greater occipital sensory disturbances as a clue to a non–length-dependent sensory neuropathy. Conversely, facial weakness is common in non–length-dependent demyelinating polyneuropathies, including Guillain-Barré syndrome or chronic inflammatory demyelinating polyradiculoneuropathies.

Definition of the Neuropathic Pattern

Initially, the history and examination are interpreted to determine whether a disorder affecting the peripheral neuromuscular system is likely to exist. This process facilitates the ultimate goal, identification of underlying etiology. The following clinical factors particularly implicate a peripheral nerve disorder.

The **history** focuses on the modalities affected (eg, motor, small fiber sensory, large fiber sensory, autonomic), geographic distribution of signs and symptoms (particularly at onset), temporal profile of symptom development, risk factor profile, the **quality** of symptoms (eg, a foreign skin, wooden, or burning sensation), and the **distribution** of symptoms (eg, a stocking-glove or multiple-nerve pattern that is unlikely to occur within a solitary CNS lesion).

The **examination** may afford confirmation of peripheral neuromuscular system involvement, reinforce the pattern of involvement, and exclude localizations that may mimic peripheral neuromuscular system disease (eg, spinal cord processes). **Peripheral neuromuscular system** pathology features include muscle wasting, absent muscle stretch reflexes, and stocking-glove sensory loss. **Absence of CNS involvement** is also a feature. Rarely, but more commonly in children, combined peripheral and CNS findings are present, eg, with inherited leukodystrophies.

DIFFERENTIAL DIAGNOSIS

Clinical presentation data is used to define polyneuropathy patterns that can focus the differential diagnosis into 1 of 5 recognized categories: length-dependent polyneuropathy, sensory neuropathy, polyradiculoneuropathy, multifocal neuropathy, and motor neuron disease. (Mononeuropathies and motor neuron disorders and mononeuropathies are discussed in sections XX and XXI.)

Length-dependent polyneuropathy is the predominant clinical type. Most forms are secondary to toxic, metabolic, or hereditary etiologies. The pathophysiology seems related to disordered peripheral nerve metabolism, resulting in a "dying back" process affecting the most distal aspects of the longest nerves first and shorter-length nerves later.

Length-dependent polyneuropathy is predominately an axon loss disorder affecting sensory more than motor fibers. Two basic differences in motor and sensory nerve anatomy in part explain this phenomenon. Sensory nerves are longer, having more distal distribution than motor axons, ie, there are no muscles in the toes. The motor system is essentially duplicated. For example, when the intrinsic toe flexor and extensor muscles are affected, clinical detection of weakness is masked because the long toe flexors and extensors located in the calf are not affected until later in the dying back process. Therefore, clinical but not EMG evidence of motor involvement may remain hidden until the process ascends to the calf.

In **sensory neuropathy**, the sensory cell bodies within the dorsal root ganglia are primarily affected. Autoimmune, toxic, or infectious etiologies are most commonly responsible. Primary abnormal sensory function is present clinically and electrodiagnostically. There is no motor involvement. The clinical pattern initially may seem length dependent, but careful evaluation often reveals patchy distribution with some proximal involvement.

Multifocal neuropathy is typically an axonal sensory-motor neuropathy. Motor or sensory signs and symptoms may predominate in variants. Multifocal neuropathy is often the result of disorders that infarct or infiltrate peripheral nerves or make them more susceptible to compressive injury. A careful history may identify that symptoms developed sequentially in a stepwise fashion, in the distribution of individual peripheral nerves. Deficits may become confluent in time, and only careful reconstruction of the history indicates the multifocal and asymmetric nature of the disease.

Polyradiculoneuropathy is typically a primary demyelinating disorder in contrast to the predominantly axonal process of length-dependent polyneuropathy, multifocal neuropathy, and sensory neuropathy. Usually, it is immune mediated. Although sensory involvement may begin distally with polyradiculoneuropathy, it often affects the hands, face, or other proximal areas sooner than in a length-dependent axonal disorder. Even though initial symptoms are often sensory in nature, many of these disorders are predominantly characterized by generalized, but asymmetric, and frequently severe motor neuropathies.

Ultimately, the differential diagnosis is generated by defining neuropathy patterns and comparing other illness features to those found in neuropathies known to produce such a clinical pattern. The differential diagnosis is then weighted by consideration of the patient's individual risks from family history, known systemic illnesses (Table 93-4), toxic exposures, and personal habits. A carefully elicited family history is the most important point in differential diagnosis of any nonacute polyneuropathy.

Table 93-4
Neuropathies Associated With Systemic Diseases

Diabetes mellitus
Toxins
Critical illness polyneuropathy
Vasculitis
Amyloidosis
HIV
Lyme
Uremia
Paraneoplastic
Sarcoidosis
Mitochondrial disorders
Fabry disease

DIAGNOSTIC APPROACH

Although many ancillary tests are available, a tailored evaluation is appropriate, in which the clinical phenotype, temporal profile, clinical context, and EMG results are considered in conjunction with various tests.

Familial predisposition is the most common cause of all polyneuropathies. Family histories and examinations of other family members at risk are some of the most time- and cost-effective means of evaluating patients with peripheral neuropathies.

EMG testing of a suspected polyneuropathy provides reasonably high specificity and sensitivity confirming its presence and facilitating its classification. EMG complements the clinical examination and may reveal evidence of motor nerve involvement that is not clinically apparent. Conversely, in hereditary neuropathies, such as Charcot-Marie-Tooth disease (CMT), where clinical sensory involvement may be inconclusive, sensory nerve conduction abnormalities provide confirmation of peripheral nerve disease, helping to distinguish CMT from distal forms of spinal muscular atrophy (Figure 94-2). EMG is critical to the evaluation of every suspected neuropathy.

EMG helps to determine classification of polyneuropathies into preferentially axonal or demyelinating processes. In particular, the definition of a primary demyelinating process, characterized by significant slowing (<70% of normal), greatly focuses the evaluation (Table 93-5). Next, differentiation of an acquired versus a hereditary process is accomplished by evaluating other EMG features. Acquired demyelinating polyneuropathies typically have nonuniform conduction slowing, temporal dispersion, conduction block, and "sural sparing."

The skill of the technicians and physicians who perform and interpret EMG is its foremost limitation. An EMG performed in isolation of other studies does not precisely identify the primary pathophysiologic cause of the neuropathy. Another limitation occurs as a consequence of aging. For example, lower extremity sensory nerve action potentials may diminish with age. Absent sensory nerve action potentials in the legs of an individual older than 70 years does not confirm a pathologic neuropathy. Therefore, distinguishing between a peripheral neuropathy and a chronic polyradiculopathy (eg, spinal stenosis), dependent on the presence or absence of sensory nerve action potentials, may be difficult in this age group.

Routine EMG, preferentially if not exclusively, tests large myelinated nerve fiber functions. Small fiber neuropathies typically present with painful, often burning feet without motor or reflex abnormalities. Conventional EMG studies are unfortunately insensitive for detection of these most common polyneuropathies. In this setting, other potentially supportive modalities are used, such as autonomic nervous system testing, quantitative sensory testing, and skin biopsy.

Laboratory blood tests are often valuable when used judiciously. There is no agreement on what a menu of screening tests must include, and none have had sensitivity, specificity, or cost effectiveness validated. Screening tests are rarely helpful. Tests should be ordered based on the differential diagnosis generated by clinical and electrodiagnostic evaluations. Tests performed under these circumstances have far greater likelihood of representing a true positive than those performed indiscriminately.

The low diagnostic yield that may accompany peripheral neuropathy evaluations is frustrating for physicians and patients. This undoubtedly promotes the practice of ordering commercially available "neuropathy panels" to increase the likelihood of a precise diagnosis; however, many panels consist of bundled tests with no relevance to the patient's clinical profile. Individual tests based on the specific patient context are a rational and economic approach. There is no substitute for careful evaluation by a knowledgeable and thoughtful physician. Judicious, general recommendations for use of commercially available serologic and DNA mutation analyses in peripheral neuropathy evaluation follow.

Testing options for the axonal form of CMT (type 2) are limited. The tests that are commercially available do not apply to most patients with CMT. DNA mutational analyses may be of use with demyelinating forms of type 1 CMT.

Anti-Hu (ANNA-1) antibody testing is indicated in an acute or subacute neuropathy patient with a significant smoking history or some-

Table 93-5
Primary Demyelinating Polyneuropathies*

Length-Dependent Polyneuropathy Pattern

Charcot-Marie-Tooth disease (types 1, 3, 4)
IgM monoclonal protein
Metachromatic leukodystrophy
Globoid cell leukodystrophy

Polyradiculoneuropathy Pattern

Guillain-Barré syndrome
CIDP
CIDP associated concurrent disease (eg, monoclonal protein [POEMS syndrome], diabetes, lupus)

Multifocal Neuropathy Pattern

Multifocal motor neuropathy with conduction block
Multifocal CIDP (Lewis-Sumner syndrome, MADSAM)
Hereditary neuropathy with liability to pressure palsy

*CIDP indicates chronic inflammatory demyelinating polyradiculoneuropathy; MADSAM, multifocal acquired demyelinating sensory and motor; POEMS, polyneuropathy, organomegaly, endocrinopathy, monoclonal gammopathy, and skin changes.

times with an ataxic sensory neuronopathy (Table 93-6).

GM-1 antibody testing is useful for patients with a motor neuropathy, without upper motor neuron signs, in whom unequivocal evidence of acquired demyelination, particularly conduction block, is not detected on EMG.

Myelin-associated glycoprotein antibodies are sometimes ordered in patients with sensory predominant, ataxic, demyelinating neuropathies who do not have circulating IgM monoclonal antibodies. Unfortunately the presence or absence of anti–myelin-associated glycoprotein activity does not define a different natural history or a potential therapeutic response.

Tests for potentially treatable disorders, even if fairly uncommon, are always indicated when possibly relevant to the patient's symptoms. Vitamin B_{12} deficiency mimicking a peripheral neuropathy and hypothyroid neuropathy are 2 notable examples. A peripheral neuropathy may occur with impaired glucose tolerance without overt diabetes. Because the natural history of this disorder is beneficially impacted by dietary modification and medication, 2-hour glucose tolerance testing should be performed in patients with burning feet and a small fiber sensory neuropathy phenotype.

CSF analysis is particularly helpful for implicating proximal involvement at the nerve root level, ie, suspected Guillain-Barré syndrome/demyelinating polyradiculoneuropathy. In such instances, CSF protein is usually increased. If an associated CSF pleocytosis (ie, increased WBCs in the CSF) exists, concerns about HIV, Lyme disease, sarcoidosis, or neoplastic meningoradiculitis prompt further serologic, cytologic, or histologic testing.

Of the more than 150 causes of peripheral neuropathy, fewer than 15 are associated with diagnostic sensory nerve biopsies. They tend to be relatively uncommon.

Sensory nerve biopsy (typically sural or superficial peroneal nerve) is primarily used when vasculitis, amyloidosis, or nerve tumor is strongly suspected. A concomitant muscle biopsy (gastrocnemius or peroneus brevis) may increase the diagnostic yield if vasculitis is suspected. Unfortunately, the biopsy yield in the most common pattern of length-dependent polyneuropathy is poor. Diabetes and most hereditary neuropathies may have suggestive but not diagnostic pathologic features. There are few other indications for biopsy. Clinicians should not biopsy simply because less invasive testing results are normal.

TREATMENT AND PROGNOSIS

Therapeutic options are ideally determined by the cause of the polyneuropathy. In general, treatment can be categorized into specific therapy, supportive treatment, and counseling.

The therapeutic goal is that identifying the precise cause of the neuropathy will lead to specific treatment. However, there are a limited number of treatable neuropathies, commonly those with an acute or subacute temporal profile such as Guillain-Barré syndrome/demyelinating polyradiculoneuropathy, mononeuritis multiplex, POEMS syndrome (polyneuropathy, organomegaly, endocrinopathy, monoclonal gammopathy, and skin changes), certain vitamin deficiencies, and various toxins that, when identified and withdrawn, lead to relatively good resolution of symptoms and findings. Some primary nerve injuries, particularly those with a significant axonal component, heal slowly; however, certain compression neuropathies have excel-

Table 93-6
Large Fiber, Sensory Predominant, Ataxic Neuropathies

Length-Dependent Polyneuropathy Pattern
IgM monoclonal protein
a-β Lipoproteinemia

Sensory Neuronopathy Pattern
Paraneoplastic sensory neuropathy
Sjögren syndrome (LDPN or SN)
Vitamin B_{12} deficiency
Pyridoxine toxicity
Cisplatin toxicity
Idiopathic
Spinocerebellar degeneration (Friedreich ataxia)

Polyradiculoneuropathy Pattern
Miller Fisher
Other sensory Guillain-Barré syndrome variants

*LDPN indicates length-dependent polyneuropathy; SN, sensory neuronopathy.

lent functional resolution. It may take months or years after treatment initiation to be certain neuropathy progression has arrested or reversed.

Nonspecific supportive, symptomatic treatment essentially refers to pain control. Simple, nonpharmacologic measures include wearing comfortable footwear and supports, soaking feet in cold (not ice-cold) water for 15 to 20 minutes each night followed by application of moisturizing lotion, and modification of daytime routine to avoid aggravating activities.

The clinician and patient must determine whether the degree of discomfort or pain warrants analgesics. Nocturnal pain is the most important to consider because it has the greatest impact on quality of life. Analgesic use may be targeted primarily at nocturnal pain, thus improving the efficacy of the medication by intermittent use and perhaps minimizing chances for abuse. Topical agents are generally disappointing. Nonnarcotic agents such as the tricyclic antidepressants, anticonvulsants including carbamazepine, gabapentin, and venlafaxine are successful in many patients.

Although traditionally most neurologists have avoided narcotic analgesics in chronic conditions such as painful polyneuropathies, pain medicine research is reshaping these ideas. Nonescalating doses of narcotics are reasonable for appropriately motivated patients whose function and quality of life are impaired and in whom other forms of analgesia have failed.

The risk of patients losing balance and falling secondary to severe neuropathies should always be considered. If the patient has a foot drop and is tripping, an ankle-foot orthosis (AFO) can be helpful. Long leg braces are useful in some patients whose quadriceps are weak and whose knees tend to buckle.

It is important to recommend the use of night-lights to minimize fall risk (particularly in patients with sensory ataxia), daily foot inspection to prevent infection of unrecognized wounds, and reinforcement of the importance of blood sugar control in patients with diabetes. Individuals with hereditary neuropathies must be made aware that they are susceptible to cumulative effect of other neurotoxins, particularly chemotherapeutic agents. Because many patients with polyneuropathy harbor the unexpressed fear that the neuropathy will become paralyzing or lead to amputation, reassurance that these are rare occurrences is appropriate. Prognosis in peripheral nerve disease varies, dependent on the primary etiology and the availability and timely application of specific therapies.

REFERENCES

Apfel SC, Asbury AK, Bril V, et al. Positive neuropathic sensory symptoms as endpoints in diabetic neuropathy trials. *J Neurol Sci.* 2001;189:3-5.

Barohn RA. Approach to peripheral neuropathy and neuronopathy. *Semin Neurol.* 1998;18:7-18.

Boerkoel CF, Takashima H, Garcia CA, et al. Charcot-Marie-Tooth disease and related neuropathies: mutation distribution and genotype-phenotype correlation. *Ann Neurol.* 2002;51:190-201.

Bromberg MB, Smith AG. Toward an efficient method to evaluate peripheral neuropathies. *J Clin Neuromusc Dis.* 2002;3:172-182.

Gardner E, Bunge RP. Gross anatomy of the peripheral nervous system. In: Dyck PJ, Thomas PK, eds. *Peripheral Neuropathy.* 3rd ed. Philadelphia, Pa: WB Saunders; 1993:8-27.

Harati Y, Machkhas H. Spinal cord and peripheral nervous system. In: PA Low, ed. *Clinical Autonomic Disorders.* 2nd ed. Philadelphia, Pa: Lippincott-Raven Publishers; 1997:25-45.

Hughes RC. Peripheral neuropathy. *BMJ.* 2002;324:466-469.

Pourmand R. Evaluating patients with suspected peripheral neuropathy: do the right thing, not everything. *Muscle Nerve.* 2002;26:288-290.

Chapter 94
Length-Dependent Polyneuropathy

Jennifer A. Grillo, James A. Russell, and H. Royden Jones, Jr

Clinical Vignette

A 72-year-old man reported a 4-year history of numb feet characterized as a feeling of "cotton between the toes." Walking in bare feet gradually became uncomfortable. The numbness ascended circumferentially to his ankles. He no longer trusted his balance to put on his pants without support. Difficulty wiggling the toes was the only indication of weakness. He had no symptoms in his hands or face, indications of dysautonomia or systemic illness. His medications included a diuretic and a multivitamin. He had no toxic exposure or affected family members.

The patient appeared well and had bilateral hammertoe deformities. Neurologic findings included an inability to spread his toes and intrinsic foot muscle atrophy. Muscle stretch reflexes were normal in the arms, diminished at the knees, and absent at the ankles. There was a distal maximal graded stocking distribution sensory loss to light touch, pinprick, temperature, vibration, and proprioception to midcalf bilaterally. He wobbled slightly on Romberg testing but did not fall.

EMG demonstrated a length-dependent, primarily axonal, sensory motor polyneuropathy. An undefined hereditary sensory neuropathy could not be excluded, although his children were examined clinically and electrodiagnostically. Laboratory investigation did not demonstrate an etiologic mechanism. Nerve biopsy was not indicated.

The symmetric pattern of sensory and reflex loss and the subtle distal motor involvement supported the length-dependent nature of his neuropathy. Although his hammertoes were compatible with a hereditary neuropathy, positive sensory symptoms, the sensory predominance, his age, and the absence of affected family members made Charcot-Marie-Tooth disease (CMT) an unlikely consideration.

Distal sensory symptoms could occur with myelopathies; however, the characteristic distribution of clinical findings and absence of urinary sphincter problems was consistent with a length-dependent polyneuropathy (LDPN). Annual follow-up revealed minimal progression of his neuropathy.

Polyneuropathies are one of the most common neurologic disorders; the length-dependent pattern is the most prevalent. Although there are many recognized causes of polyneuropathy, specific mechanisms have not been identified in many patients (Table 94-1). Many have a genetic but unidentified pathophysiologic basis.

Peripheral nerve axons are fine-caliber distal portions of long individual cells, sometimes longer than one meter. They depend on their cell bodies for homeostasis, within dorsal root ganglia or anterior horns, and their axonal transport mechanisms. Length-dependent patterns of dysfunction are thought to relate to impaired cell body metabolism or axonal transport within the nerves' most vulnerable components. As the neuropathy progresses to involve shorter length nerves, the fingers typically become symptomatic when lower extremity symptoms have ascended to approximately the midshin to knee level. Very rarely in advanced cases, the chin, nose, and midline trunk are involved.

Toxic or metabolic etiologies (Figure 94-1) are common causes of sensory LDPN, whereas genetic mechanisms underlie most motor-predominant distal polyneuropathies. The preceding vignette illustrates the frequent difficulty in achieving a specific diagnosis while attaining a reasonable prognosis in this most common clinical scenario.

CLINICAL PRESENTATION

Acquired length-dependent neuropathies are characterized by sensory more than motor

Table 94-1
Length-Dependent Polyneuropathies*

Hereditary
Charcot-Marie-Tooth disease
Hereditary sensory neuropathy (HSN or HSAN)
Idiopathic
Amyloidosis
Mitochondrial disorders

Idiopathic
Cryptogenic sensory or sensorimotor polyneuropathy

Dysimmune/Inflammatory
Amyloidosis
Monoclonal gammopathy of unknown significance
Sjögren syndrome (LDPN most common phenotype, may associate with SN, trigeminal neuropathy)
Rheumatoid arthritis
Sarcoidosis (LDPN most common phenotype, may produce MM, cranial neuropathy, usually occurs in established disease)
Vasculitis (25-30% of neuropathy cases present as LDPN, may be presenting manifestation, MM more typical)

Infectious
HIV
Lyme disease

Malnutrition
B-vitamin deficiency (B_{12}; thiamine)

Metabolic
Critical illness polyneuropathy
Diabetes mellitus and impaired glucose tolerance
Gluten-sensitive enteropathy
Hypothyroidism
Uremia

Toxic
Alcohol abuse
Pyridoxine (B_6) toxicity (sensory neuronopathy mimicking LDPN)
Environmental or industrial exposure
  Arsenic
  Hexacarbons
  Lead
  Mercury
  Organophosphates
  Thallium
Prescription drugs
  Amphiphilic cationic drugs (amiodarone, chloroquine, perhexiline)
  Colchicine (neuromyopathy)
  Disulfiram
  Hydralazine
  Isoniazid
  Metronidazole
  Nitrofurantoin
  Nitrous oxide
  Nucleosides (ddC, ddI, d4T for AIDS)
  Paclitaxel
  Thalidomide
  Vincristine
  Statins, questionably

*LDPN indicates length-dependent polyneuropathy; MM, mononeuritis multiplex; SN, sensory neuropathy.

---

symptoms and signs, in contrast with hereditary LDPN such as CMT wherein motor findings predominate. Typical patients with primary sensory LDPN note tingling, numb, or burning sensations, often pronounced at rest, particularly at night. Occasionally, exercise exacerbates these unpleasant sensations.

When weakness is present, foot and toe extensors and foot evertors are more affected than plantar flexors, ie, peroneal nerve predominant. **Pes cavus** is often the presenting sign in motor lesions such as CMT type 1. Gait is compromised because of weakness, manifested by foot drop, or painful dysesthesias, often increased with walking. Muscle stretch reflexes are variably affected but commonly ankle jerks are diminished.

Charcot-Marie-Tooth disease is the most common genetically determined neuropathy (Figure 94-2). Mutations of various genes give rise to specific DNA abnormalities in demyelinating forms. To date, very few definite genetic mutations have been identified for the axonal forms. CMT is characterized by a slowly progressive, chronic course with variable severity. Presenting symptoms include weakness of foot and toe dorsiflexors and evertors with concomitant orthopedic problems, particularly pes cavus. Clinical recognition usually occurs in late childhood or early adulthood. Typically, sensory loss is subclinical and may not be recognized by the patient. There are both demyelinating and axonal forms of CMT.

Hereditary sensory neuropathy is less common than CMT. These patients present with sensory ataxia, painless foot ulcers, or foot pain. Foot deformities may occur without demonstrable weakness.

Acquired metabolic disorders are common causes of LDPN. Diabetes mellitus may produce a number of neuropathic phenotypes, most commonly an LDPN sensory-predominant painful phenotype. Typically, it occurs with long-standing diabetes, but a small-fiber neuropathy may be the presenting feature of impaired glucose tolerance.

Many potential peripheral **neurotoxins** exist, including alcohol and therapeutic drugs. In some pharmaceuticals, neurotoxicity limits the dose. Neuropathies resulting from cryptic sources such as heavy metals are uncommon or uncommonly recognized (Figure 94-3). However, in certain parts of North America arsenic poisoning is still seen. The role of nutritional and vitamin de-

LENGTH-DEPENDENT POLYNEUROPATHY

Figure 94-1 Peripheral Neuropathies: Metabolic, Toxic, and Nutritional

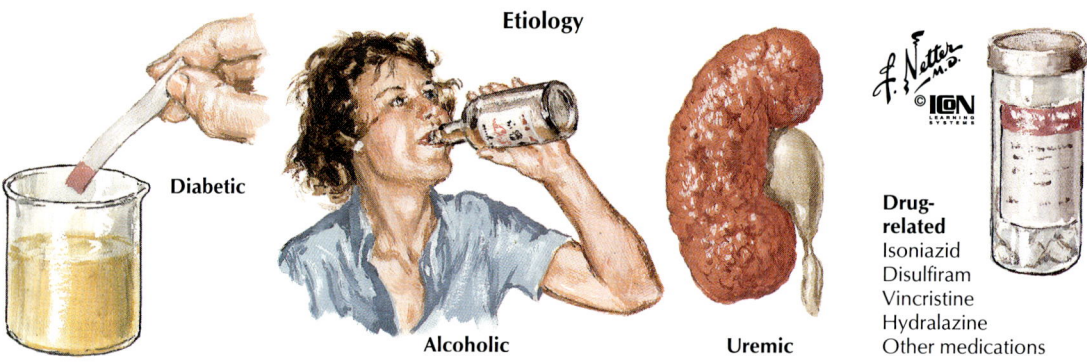

ficiency versus that of ethanol in the development of "alcoholic" neuropathy is uncertain.

Immune-mediated neuropathies are associated with monoclonal proteins, antibodies, or both directed against peripheral nerve constituents. Monoclonal proteins occur more commonly in patients with polyneuropathy than in age-matched controls without neuropathy. However, a precise cause and effect relationship is unproven. The strongest association occurs with IgM-κ monoclonal proteins, with or without presence of associated antimyelin associated glycoprotein antibodies.

In addition to severe polyneuropathy, patients with Sjögren syndrome (SS) have signs of dysautonomia with dry mouth and eyes. This immune-mediated neuropathy is associated with a length-dependent or sensory neuropathy pattern that can be incapacitating as a large-fiber ataxic neuropathy. A painful small fiber variety is less common. SS may be more common than is clinically appreciated; it is potentially treatable as described in the following vignette.

Clinical Vignette

A 62-year-old woman reported a 1-year history of progressive sensory symptoms with prominent ataxia causing marked gait difficulty, associated sicca symptoms, and 40-lb weight loss. Her examination results were remarkable for moderate to severe polyneuropathy, more sensory than motor, with marked positive Romberg sign and wide-based, ataxic gait.

The patient's 69-year-old brother reported a 5-year history of progressive stocking-glove distribution sensory symptoms. His examination revealed polyneuropathy, also more sensory than motor, with marked ataxia and positive Romberg sign.

Both siblings had significantly increased SSA and SSB antibodies. Electrodiagnostic testing demonstrated predominantly axonal sensorimotor polyneuropathy. The sister's lip biopsy, performed for evaluation of SS, revealed prominent lymphocytic infiltration supportive of SS. Her sural nerve biopsy demonstrated perivascular inflammation of small epineurial vessels and multifocal myelinated nerve fiber loss.

Both were treated with 2 g/kg IV immunoglobulin over 10 days followed by 0.4 g/kg every 3 weeks (sister) or every week (brother). After 3 months of treatment, sensory symptoms, gait, and functional status showed dramatic marked improvement.

Many symptomatic neuropathies associated with malignancy relate to treatment side effects. Subclinical forms may be related to impaired nutrition or end organ failure. **Paraneoplastic sensory neuropathies** are the notable exceptions that do not always conform to the LDPN pattern. They are most commonly associated with small cell lung cancer where the relation can be identified by finding the specific paraneoplastic antibody, anti-Hu. Other than obtaining a chest CT and anti-Hu in patients who smoke and have sensory polyneuropathies, an extensive search for occult malignancies is not warranted.

Infectious causes of LDPN are less common; **HIV** is an exception. Distal symmetric and often painful polyneuropathies are most commonly associated with HIV infection. Usually associated with low CD4 counts, in advanced disease, they may be complicated by neuropathies associated with antiretroviral drug treatments. **Lyme disease** may cause an LDPN pattern but this is uncom-

LENGTH-DEPENDENT POLYNEUROPATHY

Charcot-Marie-Tooth Disease

Figure 94-2A

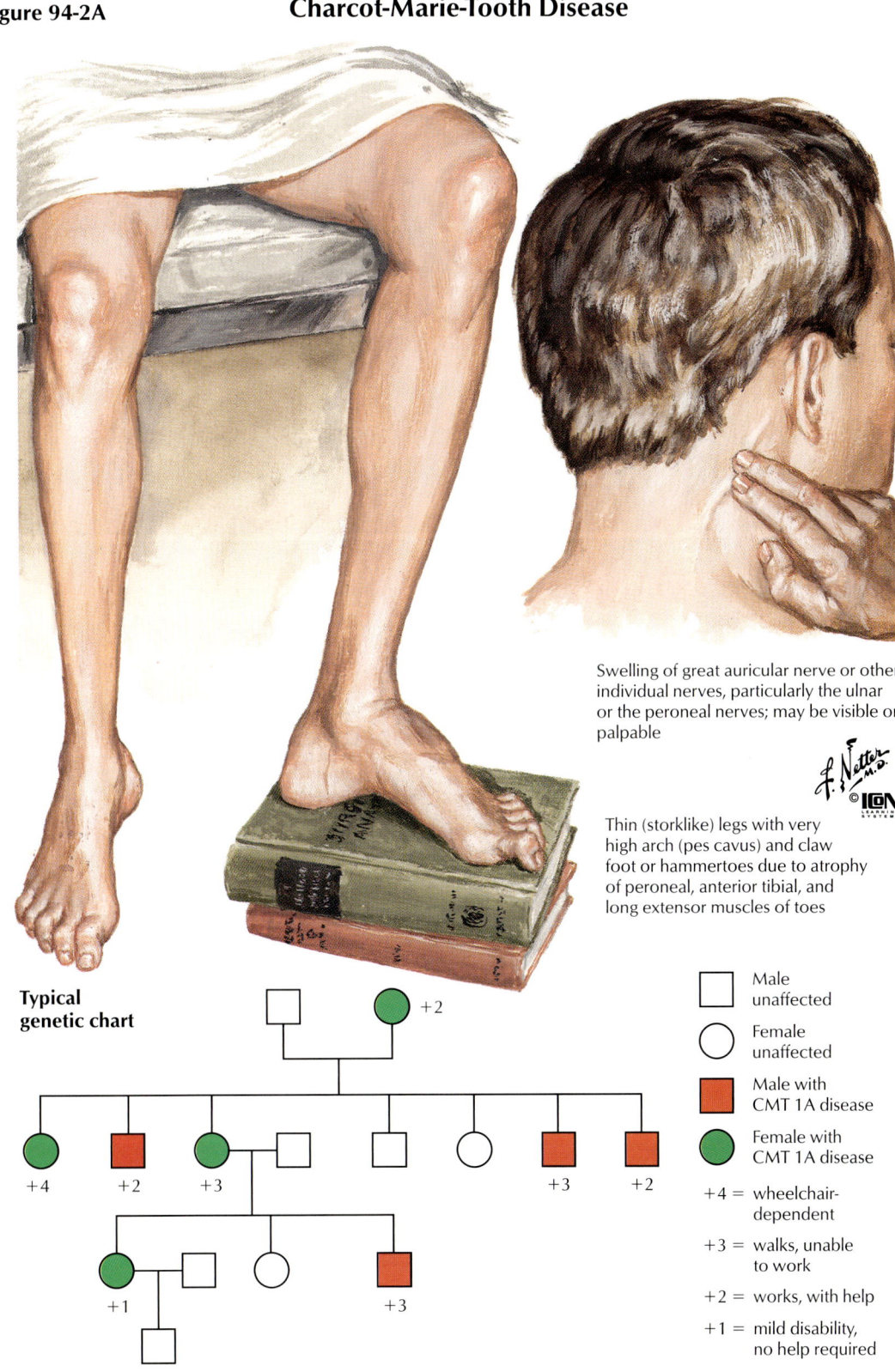

Swelling of great auricular nerve or other individual nerves, particularly the ulnar or the peroneal nerves; may be visible or palpable

Thin (storklike) legs with very high arch (pes cavus) and claw foot or hammertoes due to atrophy of peroneal, anterior tibial, and long extensor muscles of toes

Typical genetic chart

- ☐ Male unaffected
- ○ Female unaffected
- ■ Male with CMT 1A disease
- ● Female with CMT 1A disease

+4 = wheelchair-dependent
+3 = walks, unable to work
+2 = works, with help
+1 = mild disability, no help required

POLYNEUROPATHIES AND AUTONOMIC DISORDERS

LENGTH-DEPENDENT POLYNEUROPATHY

Figure 94-2B Charcot-Marie-Tooth 1A: Motor Nerve Conduction Velocity

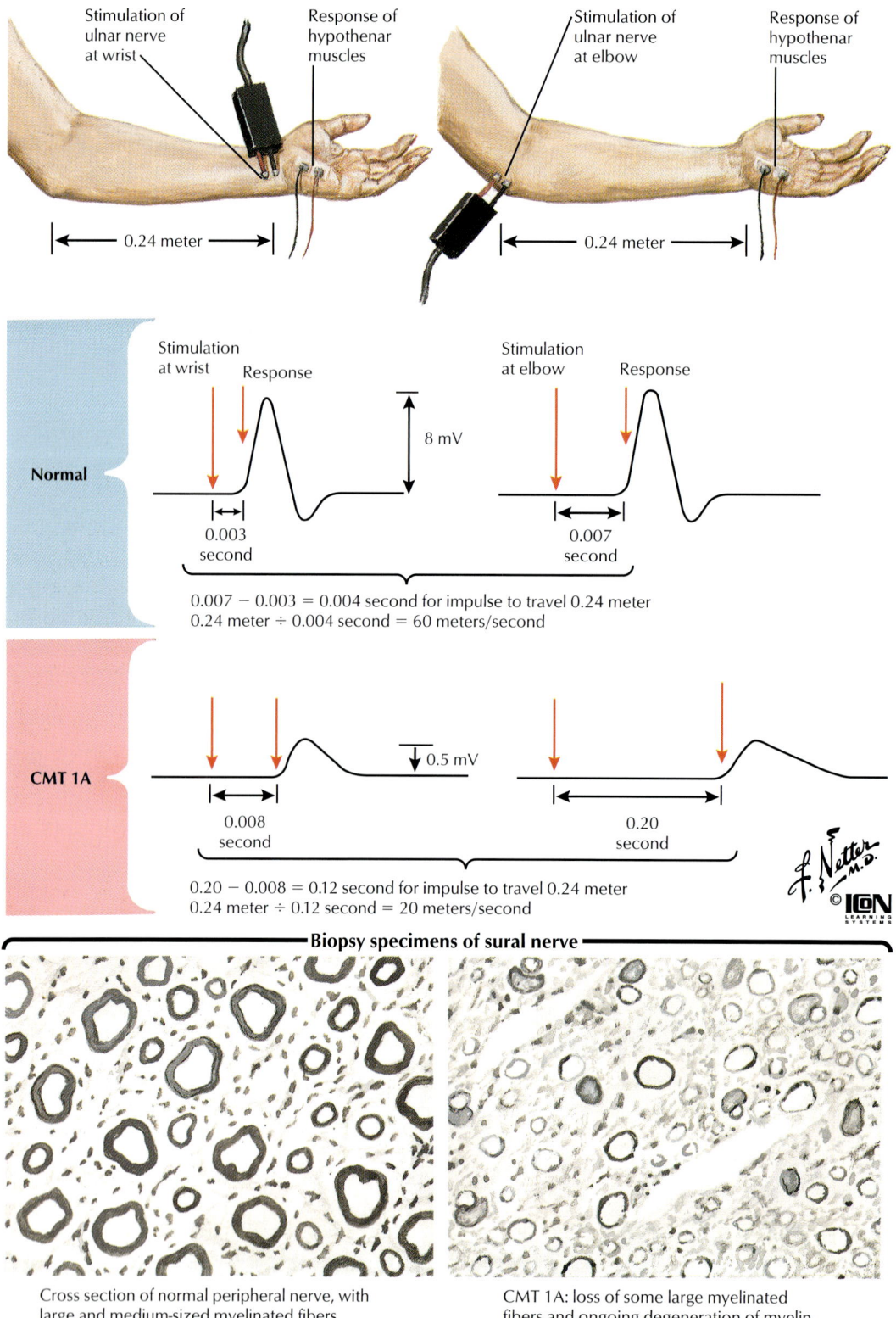

LENGTH-DEPENDENT POLYNEUROPATHY

Figure 94-3   **Peripheral Neuropathy Caused by Heavy Metal Poisoning**

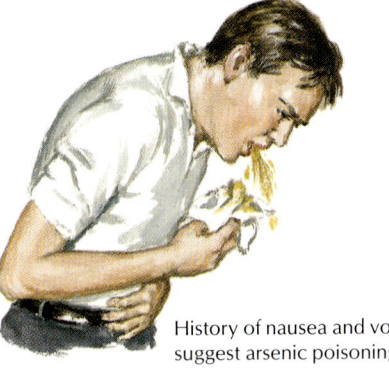

History of nausea and vomiting may suggest arsenic poisoning in patient with peripheral neuropathy.

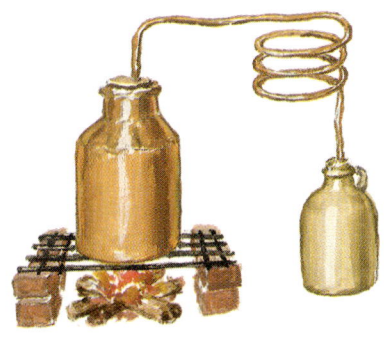

Antique copper utensils (eg, still for bootleg liquor) and runoff waste from copper smelting plant may be sources of arsenic poisoning.

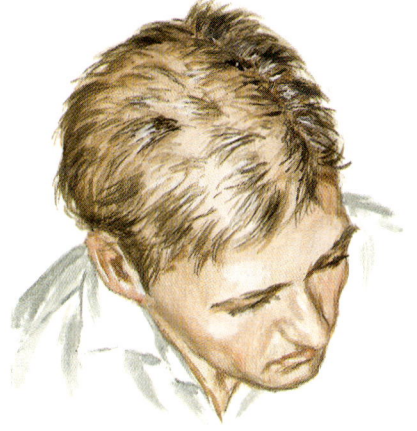

Spotty alopecia associated with peripheral neuropathy characterizes thallium poisoning.

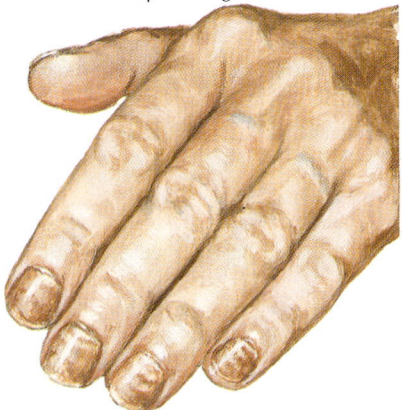

Mees lines on fingernails and hyperpigmentation of the soles are characteristic of arsenic poisoning.

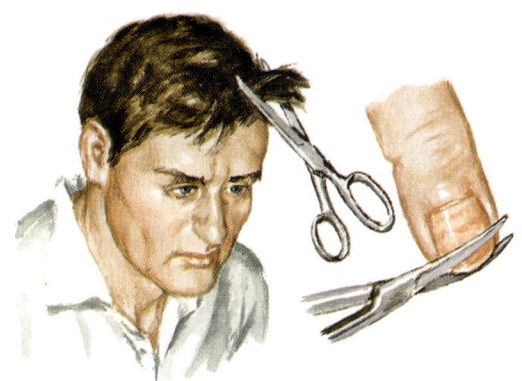

Although 24-hour urinalysis is best diagnostic test for arsenic, hair and nail analysis may also be helpful.

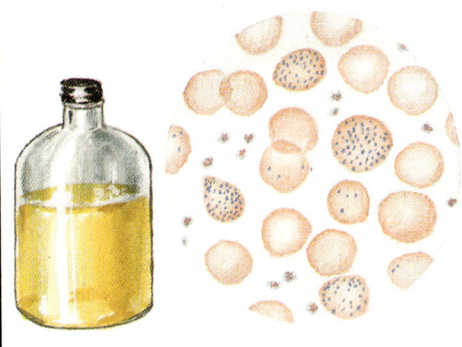

Lead poisoning, now exceedingly rare, causes basophilic stippling of red blood cells. 24-hour urinalysis is diagnostic test for this and other heavy metal poisons.

POLYNEUROPATHIES AND AUTONOMIC DISORDERS

mon compared with the **polyradiculoneuropathy** or **mononeuritis multiplex pattern**.

DIFFERENTIAL DIAGNOSIS

Identifying the LDPN per se is usually the easiest part of the evaluation. Determination of etiologic mechanism requires careful consideration and thorough investigation, although this does not always yield precisely identifiable mechanisms. For example, not all neuropathies in patients with diabetes mellitus are related to that disorder. Other mechanisms may be responsible and must be sought.

After determining that a neuropathy best fits an LDPN pattern, the clinician searches for additional clues to the differential diagnosis. These may come from determination of the relative contribution of motor and sensory involvement, presence or absence of dysautonomia, findings of sensory dissociation, and features favoring a predominantly demyelinating instead of axonal neuropathy.

Evaluation of a patient's risk factor profile from personal and family history, toxic exposures, and other symptoms such as pain or indications of a systemic disorder is important. A careful evaluation leads to specific diagnosis in 50% to 60% of patients. Diagnosis is often made on an associative basis without absolute proof of causation. Treatable neuropathies are more common among disorders presenting acutely or subacutely.

Motor-predominant LDPNs have a limited number of etiologies. These are primarily genetically determined (ie, CMT) or, less commonly, immunologically-acquired, multifocal motor neuropathies. More common motor disorders related to diseases affecting the motor neuron (anterior horn cell), neuromuscular junction, or skeletal muscle base usually have asymmetric or generalized patterns of involvement. There are few toxic or hereditary disorders that produce motor, probably length-dependent neuropathies, and the motor component may be clinically obscured (Table 93-1).

Pure sensory neuropathies fit into the LDPN pattern such as with diabetes mellitus, renal disease, vitamin deficiencies, various toxins, and amyloidosis (Figure 94-4), or represent a primary sensory ganglionopathy as discussed in chapter 97. The latter may be clinically suspected by its initially proximal, non–length-dependent pattern of involvement. EMG can aid confirmation.

Overt dysautonomia features accompanying a peripheral neuropathy are uncommon. When present, they suggest limited etiologies including diabetes mellitus, amyloidosis, and rare hereditary processes.

Dissociation of separate sensory modalities may lend valuable clues. A **small-fiber sensory neuropathy** is suggested by burning in the feet of patients with impaired pain and thermal sensation and sparing of vibration and proprioceptive sense. Many demonstrate marked distal hyperpathia to touch or stocking sensory loss. A number of small fiber neuropathies do not have identifiable etiologic mechanisms.

Sensory ataxia suggests predominantly **large fiber involvement.** The sensory neuronopathies, particularly paraneoplastic ganglionopathies, Sjögren syndrome, and pyridoxine or cisplatinum toxicity are associated with this syndrome.

Determining whether a neuropathy is predominantly **axonal or demyelinating is key** to differential diagnosis. Predominantly demyelinating neuropathies of an acquired nature usually adhere to a polyradiculoneuropathy pattern, ie, Guillain-Barré syndrome, and have non–length-dependent features. Weakness is more generalized than in typical LDPN. Generalized hypoflexia or areflexia is the norm.

Chronic predominantly demyelinating polyneuropathies most often have genetic bases ie, CMT. Their chronic nature and frequently associated foot deformities provide important clinical clues.

The neuropathy associated with IgM monoclonal neuropathy represents a relatively unique demyelinating LDPN. This acquired disorder may mimic the multitude of other sensory-predominant LDPN syndromes. Unlike most sensory predominant LDPN syndromes, generalized areflexia and EMG/NCS findings indicate a predominantly demyelinating pathophysiology.

Chronic neuropathies are usually identified by temporal course. The true duration of these disorders may go unrecognized by patients and their families for many years. A history of poor athletic performance or foot deformity in childhood lends support to an early onset. Pes cavus and hammertoes suggest disproportionate weakness of toe

LENGTH-DEPENDENT POLYNEUROPATHY

Figure 94-4 Dysproteinemia (Amyloid Neuropathy)

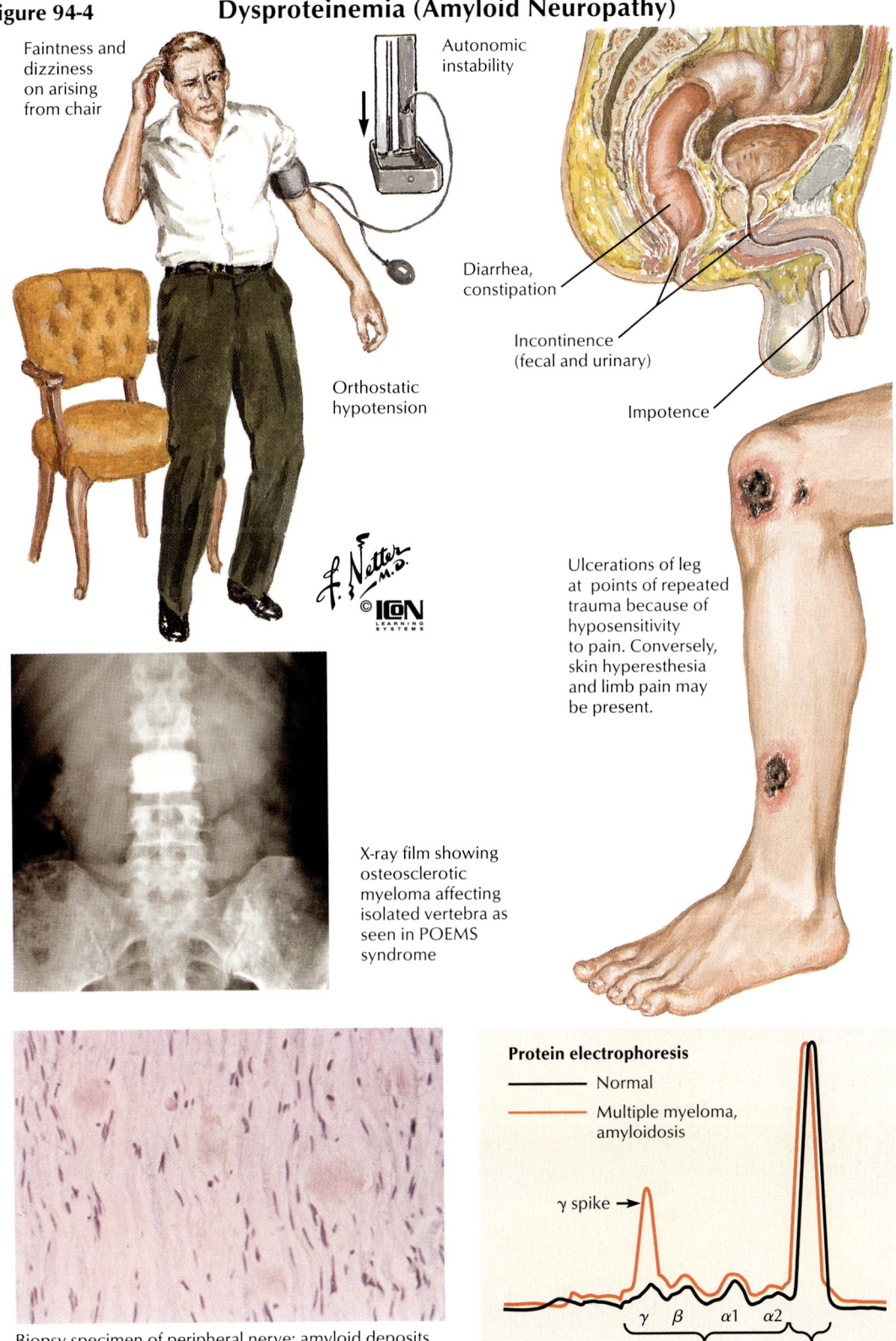

POLYNEUROPATHIES AND AUTONOMIC DISORDERS

flexor and extensor muscles when the bony architecture of the foot was not fully developed.

DIAGNOSTIC APPROACH

Etiologic identification is sometimes difficult in LDPN, providing incentive for significant usage of a myriad of diagnostic studies including sensory neuropathy profiles. Careful clinical evaluation is important, particularly with a history of familial disorder. A negative family history is insufficient to exclude a hereditary diagnosis. Clinical examination, brief electrodiagnostic testing, and DNA mutational analyses of first-degree family members commonly uncover unrecognized affected individuals. Forthright history taking in reference to medications, addictions (including alcohol and tobacco), intravenous drugs with predilection for hepatitis C and cryoglobulinemia, and occupational or environmental exposure such as glue sniffing or the classic bull's eye rash of Lyme disease can point to a specific LDPN diagnosis.

A thorough physical examination may suggest signs of CMT with pes cavus, Sjögren syndrome with dry eyes and mouth, arsenic poisoning with Mees lines, Raynaud phenomena and purpuric skin eruptions with cryoglobulinemia, pinch purpura with amyloidosis, angiokeratoma in the groin with Fabry disease, and enlarged yellow-orange tonsils of Tangier disease. Exploring these historic and physical findings can often prevent undirected selection of diagnostic tests. Individualized investigations for each clinical circumstance are encouraged to avoid the risk of providing a false conclusion, often at considerable expense.

Electrodiagnostic testing is indicated as outlined in chapter 93. Abnormal EMG findings are difficult to define with small fiber neuropathies because nerve conduction studies only test the larger proprioceptive fibers and not the small pain fibers affected in these disorders. Therefore, normal findings do not preclude the existence of small fiber neuropathies. Autonomic nervous system, quantitative sensory testing, and skin biopsy may be required for diagnostic support. Sural nerve or abdominal fat pad biopsy may be helpful for patients with LDPN with suspected amyloidosis, particularly those with orthostatic hypotension, where amyloidosis is more likely.

DNA mutational analyses are available only for some forms of CMT. Most apply to different forms of CMT type 1, the demyelinating forms. These is little need to utilize these for individuals with typical clinical, familial, and EMG features of CMT. Potential uses primarily include genetic counseling and helping individuals who know nothing of their family history.

Testing for the X-linked form of CMT is more relevant because the familial nature of the disorder is not often as clearly defined. Furthermore, in patients with CMT X, EMG features may sometimes mimic chronic inflammatory demyelinating polyradiculoneuropathy.

TREATMENT AND PROGNOSIS

Specific therapies are sometimes available when the etiology can be identified, but this is achieved in a frustratingly modest percentage of cases. Stabilization or reversal of neuropathy, or both can occur with successful treatment of uremia, nutritional deficiencies, and hypothyroidism. Removing neurotoxic drugs may completely reverse mild neuropathies or curtail further progression in more severe cases.

A therapeutic trial of prednisone, IV immunoglobulin, or plasmapheresis may have striking results for patients with an immune-mediated etiology. Unfortunately, some patients with LDPN respond poorly to treatment. In the absence of a definite diagnosis known to respond to immunomodulating agents, it is prudent to curtail treatment if no significant response occurs in a therapeutic trial of 3 to 4 months.

For patients with hereditary neuropathies, counseling should include likelihood of disease transmission to offspring and the extent of effect. Women with CMT of child-bearing age should be counseled that their neuropathy might worsen during pregnancy. All patients with CMT should be advised of their increased susceptibility to neurotoxic effects of drugs, eg, vincristine, which should be definitely avoided when possible. Patients, particularly those with decreased pain and thermal perception such as occurs in hereditary sensory neuropathies, need to understand the importance of diligent foot care to prevent secondary infectious complications of unrecognized wounds, particularly osteomyelitis.

The underlying causes of neuropathies determine the prognosis. Idiopathic neuropathies usually progress slowly over years and are infrequently disabling. In particular, most of these LDPNs rarely lead to need for ambulatory support, ie, a wheelchair. Often the physician needs to specifically discuss this with the patient and his or her family. Frequently, although the patient is concerned about such, he or she is too frightened to ask. This time taken for discussion is very reassuring to patients in whom no cause is found.

REFERENCES

Barohn RJ. Approach to peripheral neuropathy and neuronopathy. *Semin Neurol.* 1998;18:7-18.

Burns TM, Quijano-Roy S, Jones HR. Benefit of IVIg for long-standing ataxic sensory neuronopathy with Sjögren's syndrome [letter]. *Neurology.* 2003;61:873.

Katz JS, Saperstein DS, Gronseth GS, et al. Distal symmetric demyelinating symmetrical neuropathy. *Neurology.* 2000;54:615-620.

Lacomis DA. Small-fiber neuropathy. *Muscle Nerve.* 2002;26:173-188.

Rutkove SB, Nardin RA, Raynor EM, Levy ML, Landrio MA. Lumbosacral polyradiculopathy mimicking distal polyneuropathy. *J Clin Neuromusc Dis.* 2000;2:65-69.

Sumner CJ, Sheth S, Griffin JW, Cornblath DR, Polydefkis M. The spectrum of neuropathy in diabetes and impaired glucose tolerance. *Neurology.* 2003;60:108-111.

Wolfe GI, Barohn RJ. Cryptogenic sensory and sensorimotor polyneuropathies. *Semin Neurol.* 1998;18:105-111.

Chapter 95
Acquired Demyelinating Polyradiculoneuropathies: Guillain-Barré Syndrome and Chronic Inflammatory Demyelinating Polyradiculoneuropathy

Ted M. Burns, James A. Russell, and H. Royden Jones, Jr

Clinical Vignette

A 47-year-old man reported a 10-day history of progressive distal and proximal weakness and paresthesias in his arms and legs. He did not report bowel or bladder dysfunction, dysarthria, dysphagia or dyspnea. He remembered a mild and transient upper respiratory infection 2 weeks before onset of his neuropathic symptoms but otherwise had been well. His medical, family, and social history were unremarkable. He was not taking medications.

The patient's general examination was normal. Vital signs were normal without orthostatic hypotension or tachycardia. Forced vital capacity and negative inspiratory force were normal.

Neurologic examination demonstrated mild facial and symmetric primarily distal weakness in the lower and upper extremities. The patient was areflexic, and his toes were flexor to plantar stimulation. Vibration and joint position sensation were abnormal at the toes and ankles but normal at the fingers. Pinprick, temperature, and light touch sensation were normal, with no spinal cord "sensory level." The patient displayed mild dysmetria with heel-to-shin testing but performed well on finger-to-nose testing. His gait was characterized by weakness, with bilateral foot drop, and he was unsteady. The Romberg test was abnormal.

CSF examination results demonstrated increased protein of 107 mg/dL and only 3 WBCs. EMG disclosed multifocal signs of demyelination.

The degree of weakness made him a good candidate for immunomodulatory therapy. Plasmapheresis (PE) was begun on the second hospital day with intravenous immunoglobulin (IVIG) held in reserve. Autonomic and respiratory status were monitored closely. Except for mild intermittent tachycardia, the patient remained free of dysautonomia or respiratory compromise. By day 9 of hospitalization, the patient was walking without assistance. He was transferred to a rehabilitation unit after completing the PE. At follow-up 4 weeks later, he was asymptomatic.

The patient's rapidly evolving polyneuropathy affected motor and sensory function in a non–length-dependent fashion. Presentation with generalized areflexia, concomitant with antecedent respiratory infection was typical of Guillain-Barré syndrome (GBS). Subsequent electrodiagnostic and CSF examination results confirmed this diagnosis.

Guillain-Barré syndrome is a classic acute autoimmune polyneuropathy. Characteristically, it presents in a previously healthy person with the rapid onset of symmetric weakness, areflexia, and generally minimal sensory symptoms with the exception of severe pain in some individuals.

Typical CSF findings are albuminocytologic dissociation with increased protein and less than 50 WBCs. Additional findings include cranial nerve, gait ataxia, and autonomic involvement. Although GBS is the most common cause of acute flaccid paralysis, a primary spinal cord lesion must always be considered early in the clinical course.

Guillain-Barré syndrome, sometimes known as **acute inflammatory demyelinating polyradiculoneuropathy**, and **chronic inflammatory demyelinating polyradiculoneuropathy** (CIDP) are common acquired polyradiculopathies. Both are autoimmune processes that share the unusual feature of significant widespread peripheral, often including nerve root, and sometimes cranial nerve, involvement. Consequently, these disorders are categorized as **polyradiculoneuropathies** rather than polyneuropathies.

ETIOLOGY

The immune attack in GBS and CIDP is widespread and occurs proximally at the nerve roots and distally at the motor axon terminal. These 2 sites are theoretically more vulnerable because of their less complete blood-nerve barriers. Both cellular and humoral immune mechanisms seem to be involved. Lymphocytes and macrophages are the effector cells involved in damaging myelin and the adjacent axons (Figure 95-1). Motor, sensory, and autonomic nerves are affected. The weakness and sensory disturbances are due to nerve fiber action potential conduction block (secondary to demyelination) or conduction failure (due to axon damage).

In cases of GBS, and perhaps CIDP, the immune system probably is first primed as it responds to foreign molecules, such as a virus or bacteria. Later, the immune system inappropriately attacks host tissue that shares homologous epitopes, for example gangliosides found on the cell wall of certain bacteria and the peripheral nerve myelin of the host. This pathologic process has been termed molecular mimicry.

CLINICAL PRESENTATION
History

In keeping with molecular mimicry, approximately two thirds of patients with GBS give a history of antecedent infection. Campylobacter jejuni and **cytomegalovirus** are the most frequent antecedent infections in GBS, usually as gastroenteritis or respiratory infection 1 to 4 weeks before the appearance of GBS symptoms. Antecedent infection is observed less commonly in CIDP. Although antibody testing has improved understanding of the mechanisms of GBS and CIDP, it is not routinely performed because it is costly and does not influence management.

The cardinal features of GBS and CIDP are predominantly symmetric motor symptoms with less consistent sensory symptoms affecting all limbs, often with distal proximal gradient, particularly with GBS. The added proximal involvement in GBS and CIDP, rather than the classic distal weakness of a polyneuropathy, aids the distinction of a polyradiculoneuropathy. This typifies the patient with an autoimmune etiology rather than, for example, a toxic or metabolic etiology as seen with LDPN (chapter 94).

Typically, in GBS and CIDP, motor symptoms overshadow sensory paresthesias such as "tingling" or "pins and needles." These symptoms are more pronounced distally in a stocking-glove distribution. Back pain is common in GBS, particularly in children, but is not found in CIDP. At times, pure motor or pure sensory variants of GBS or CIDP occur but remain recognizable because of the frequently associated prodrome; the acute, symmetric, and generalized pattern of weakness; the areflexia; and the supportive information gained by electrodiagnostic and CSF examinations.

Gait difficulty often occurs early in polyradiculoneuropathies. It may manifest as trouble climbing stairs, arising from chairs, unsteadiness, falls, or difficulty with arm use. Facial weakness occurs in more than half of patients with GBS but is much less common in CIDP. Ophthalmoplegia, dysarthria, and dysphagia may occur in both disorders, more frequently in GBS.

Neurologic Examination

Neurologic examination demonstrates prominent proximal and distal weakness; rarely is this slightly asymmetric. More subtle proximal and distal strength should be sought by having the patient rise from a chair, step up on a step, kneel on one knee and stand, walk on the heels, and walk on the toes. Reduced or absent muscle stretch reflexes are important clues that the symptoms are likely from a peripheral nerve disorder rather than myopathies, a disorder of neuromuscular transmission, or a CNS process. However, retention of reflexes may occur in early GBS and occasionally in CIDP with rela-

ACQUIRED DEMYELINATING POLYRADICULONEUROPATHIES

Figure 95-1 — Guillain-Barré Syndrome

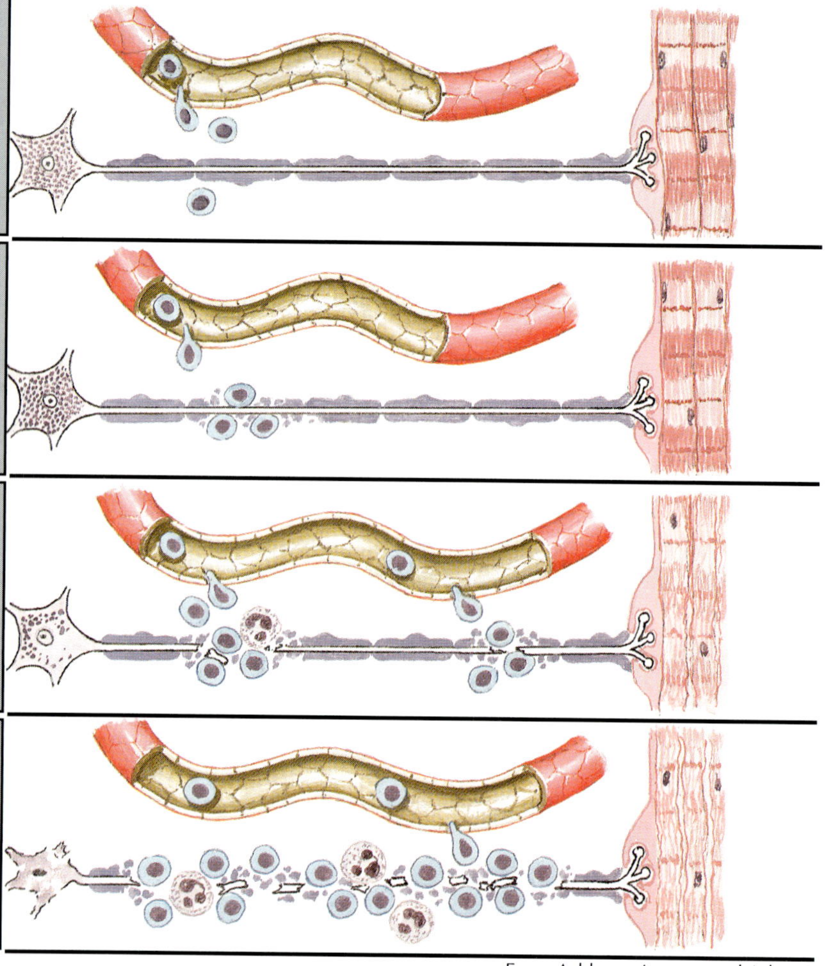

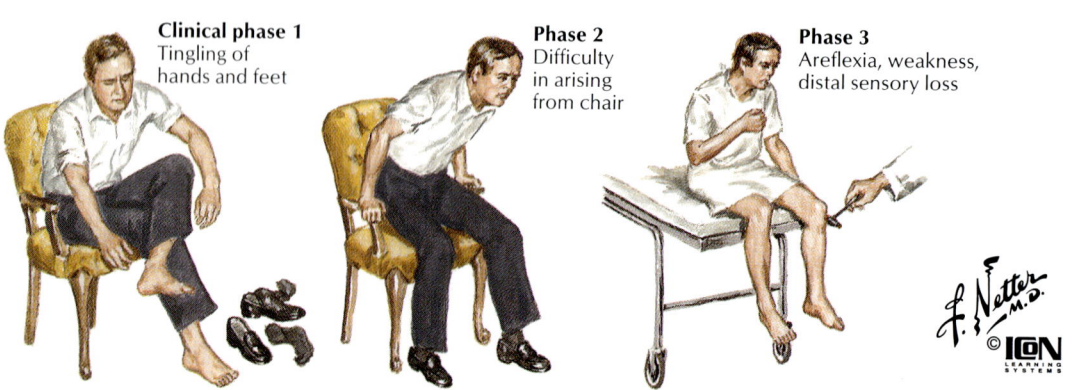

From Ashbury, Arnson, and Adams

ACQUIRED DEMYELINATING POLYRADICULONEUROPATHIES

Figure 95-1   Guillain-Barré Syndrome (continued)

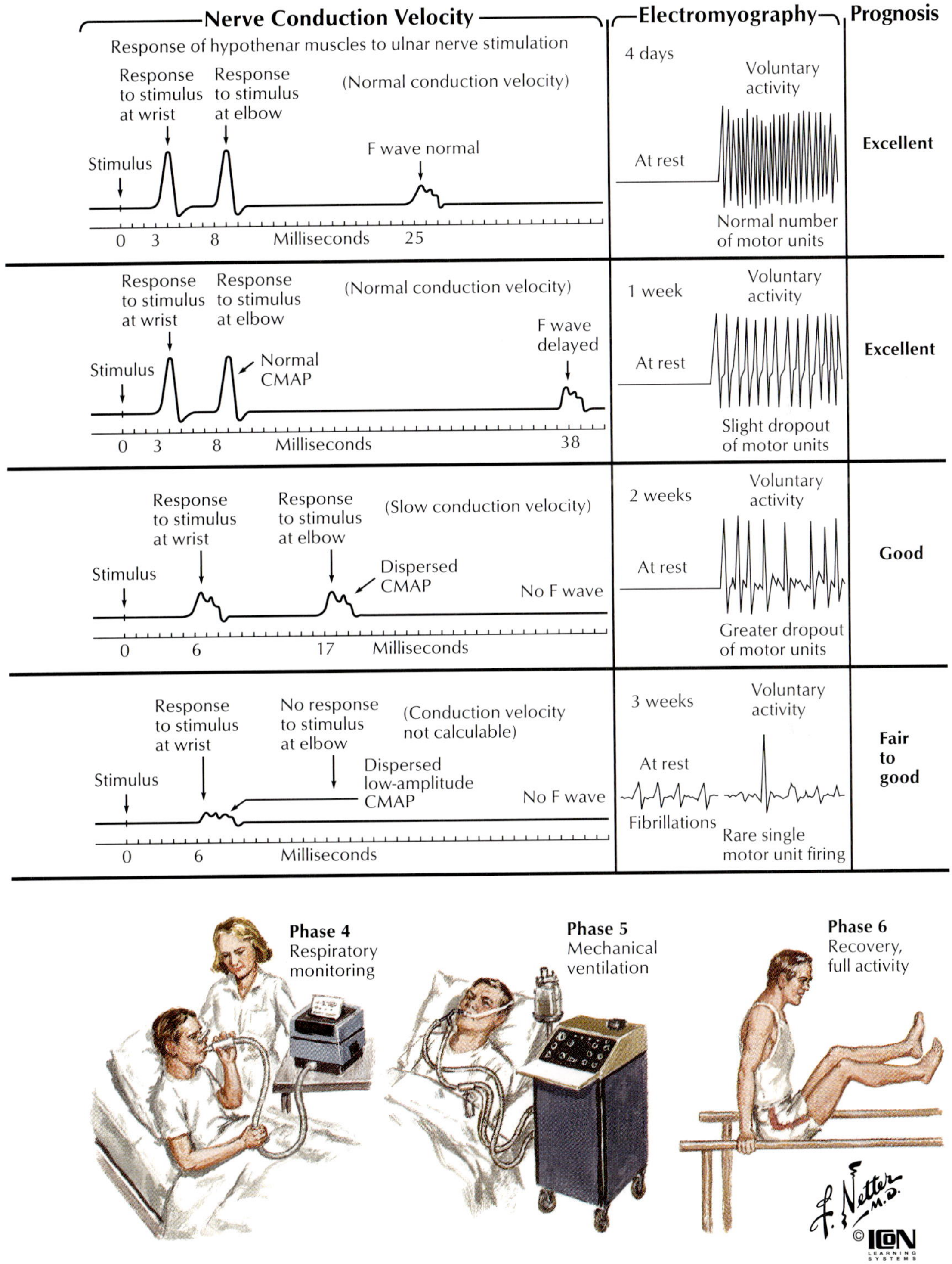

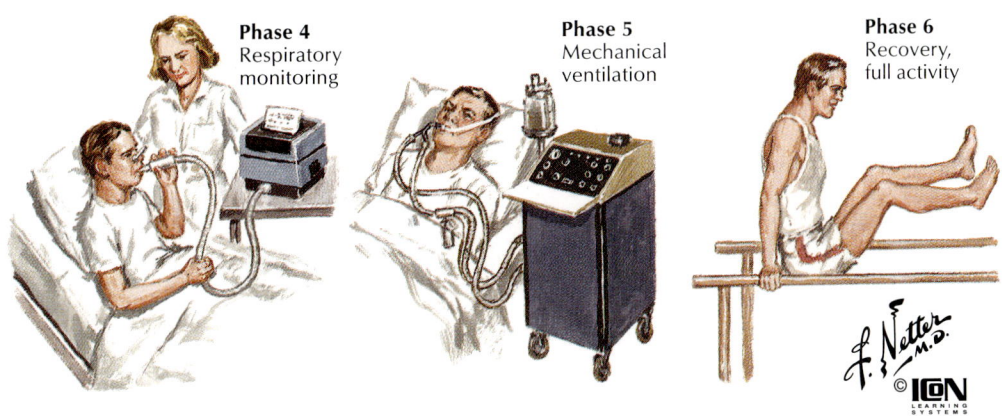

POLYNEUROPATHIES AND AUTONOMIC DISORDERS

ACQUIRED DEMYELINATING POLYRADICULONEUROPATHIES

tively mild sensory impairment distally in the feet. Despite the symptoms, the sensory examination results often seem normal.

Respiratory compromise occurs in 15% to 30% of patients with GBS. Endotracheal intubation for airway protection and mechanical ventilation for diaphragmatic weakness are necessary. Airway and respiratory compromise are rare in CIDP.

The autonomic nervous system is frequently involved in GBS, especially in severe cases. Dysautonomia in GBS commonly manifests as sinus tachycardia but may result in other cardiac arrhythmias or labile blood pressures that may be life threatening and warrant close observation. Urinary retention, adynamic ileus, and constipation sometimes occur. Overt dysautonomia in CIDP is rare.

Temporal Profile

The major clinical difference between GBS and CIDP is the temporal course. GBS is a monophasic illness of acute onset that usually reaches a nadir within 1 to 4 weeks and then gradually improves (Figure 95-1). CIDP has a slower onset and more prolonged course that is progressive, monophasic, or relapsing. Most cases of childhood or adult CIDP present within 6 months of symptom onset. Sometimes CIDP can present acutely, mimicking GBS, only later to be diagnosed correctly when a clinical relapse occurs.

DIFFERENTIAL DIAGNOSIS

Subjective sensory symptoms have differential diagnostic importance favoring GBS or CIDP over other motor unit disorders, including myopathies, neuromuscular transmission disorders, or motor neuron disorders. However, the possibility of acute spinal cord lesion or other fulminating forms of polyneuropathy should always be considered.

Myelopathies

Because sensory symptoms also occur with **myelopathies**, the possibility of an acute or subacute myelopathy with evolving spinal cord compression that may necessitate emergent intervention must always be considered, especially early in the patient's clinical course. Important clues to the possibility of a myelopathy include the preservation or hyperactivity of muscle stretch reflexes, Babinski signs, and a cord level on careful sensory testing. Patients presenting with a polyradiculoneuropathy do not have a spinal cord sensory level, and preservation of muscle stretch reflexes is unusual in GBS and CIDP, although such may occasionally occur for 48± hours.

Transverse myelitis (TM) is the most common acute spinal cord lesion leading to confusion in the differential diagnosis of GBS. Criteria for diagnosis of TM include paraparesis, a well-defined sensory level, severe bladder dysfunction, and myelitic findings on MRI. Often motor and sensory symptoms present equally but motor findings may predominate; only occasionally are sensory symptoms the presenting feature. Sphincter control is lost in most patients with TM. It may be difficult to make a clinical differential between GBS and TM in some individuals without spinal cord MRI.

Although urinary retention and constipation occasionally occur in GBS for the first day, these symptoms are very suggestive of a myelopathy, a conus medullaris and/or cauda equina disorders. Bowel and bladder symptoms are not typical of GBS or CIDP.

Back pain is common in GBS but not in CIDP. However, when it has a radicular quality, particularly in the thoracic distribution, a thoracic **spinal mass lesion**, **dural AVM**, or TM should be considered.

Often, these differential findings may not be precisely defined initially; therefore, fastidious reevaluation for clinical differentiation is essential. Because MRI is noninvasive, an initial spinal cord MRI to determine a potentially treatable lesion is advised.

Polyneuropathies

The temporal course is of primary importance for differentiating GBS and CIDP from many other peripheral neuropathies. Patients with GBS and CIDP can usually give a specific date of symptom onset. This contrasts with many other acquired or inherited polyneuropathies wherein the onset is so insidious that the patient has no recall as to its precise timing.

Patients with **mononeuritis multiplex** usually have an associated systemic or primary peripheral nervous system vasculitis. The clinical symptomatology's precise temporal profile, ie, stepwise and asymmetric, is the primary diagnostic clue, in direct contrast to CIDP, which has a symmetric evolution. Patients have sudden acute mononeuropathies, often affecting 4 to 6 specific nerves, particularly the peroneal, median, and ulnar, within a 2- to 6-week time period. If many nerves become involved, the subsequent clinical picture can mimic a symmetric generalized polyneuropathy. An increased erythrocyte sedimentation rate and a peripheral nerve biopsy demonstrating vasculitis provide important diagnostic information. High-dose immunosuppressive therapy, such as 60 to 100 mg prednisone daily, is indicated.

In **tick paralysis**, an unidentified tick saliva toxin most likely interacts with nerve ion channels producing an acute paralytic illness mimicking GBS. This is most common in girls and young women, in whom ticks can become hidden in their scalps' prominent quantity of hair. Examiners should search for ticks in any patient with an acute flaccid paralysis. Early pupillary involvement is helpful in differentiating tick paralysis from GBS. In North America, the recovery is rapid and complete after the tick is dislodged. In Australia, the course may be prolonged.

A number of **toxins**, including marine origin (red tide, ciguatoxin), metals (arsenic), solvents (hexacarbons), insecticides (organophosphates), and native plants such as Buckthorn, may produce acute generalized neuropathy. Most patients present with sensory motor syndromes associated with elements of systemic (often gastrointestinal) toxicity.

Guillain-Barré syndrome may be the presenting sign of **HIV** before AIDS is definitively diagnosed. The findings of a disparate CSF examination with an inordinate pleocytosis are clues to search for CD4 cell count deficiencies and other clinical and laboratory signs of AIDS.

Diphtheria is no longer of concern in industrialized nations with the exception of parents who withhold immunization from their children. However, it still occurs in less fortunate economic settings.

Acute intermittent and variegate **porphyria** may produce an acute generalized sensory motor neuropathy mimicking GBS. Previous attacks, a family history of similar disorders, concomitant abdominal pain, and mental status changes are clinical clues that typify this rare biochemical disorder. An axonal character defined by EMG, rather than the typical demyelinating neuropathy of GBS, raises the possibility of porphyria.

Leigh disease is an inborn metabolic disorder that may be precipitated or enhanced by certain medications, particularly barbiturates.

Patients with Charcot-Marie-Tooth type 1A have such gradual symptom onset that they are unable to identify when they became aware of clinical problems. Therefore, they rarely come into the differential diagnosis of GBS or CIDP. An exception is the patient with Charcot-Marie-Tooth type 1A who requires chemotherapy, particularly including vincristine, because the otherwise clinically manageable polyneuropathy may suddenly decompensate.

Neuromuscular Transmission Disorders

Botulism and **myasthenia gravis** may produce an acute generalized weakness. Botulism is typically acute in onset and myasthenia is usually more indolent, although myasthenia gravis can have a relatively rapid presentation with cranial nerve and peripheral distribution weakness. Neither produces sensory system involvement. Both have a predilection for oculobulbar musculature. Botulism may also have prominent manifestations of cholinergic dysautonomia. EMG may be required for distinction from GBS.

Lambert-Eaton myasthenic syndrome (LEMS) may mimic CIDP with a subacute onset of proximal weakness and areflexia. History of tobacco addiction and a dry mouth suggest LEMS (chapter 101).

Poliomyelitis

Paralytic polio is preceded by a prodrome that includes back pain similar to GBS. Its multifocal and asymmetric pattern, the absence of sensory signs or symptoms, and CSF pleocytosis are distinguishing features. EMG demonstrates axon loss confined to motor nerves, consistent with anterior horn cell localization.

Electrolyte Disorders

Severe **hypokalemia** and **hypophosphatemia** may produce weakness on an acute, generalized basis. Weakness severe enough to mimic GBS does not usually occur until potassium decreases to less than 2 mEq/mL and phosphate decreases to less than 1 mg/mL. Both typically occur in clinical contexts where severe hypokalemia or hypophosphatemia could be anticipated.

Hypokalemia weakness is thought to be myopathic and is unassociated with sensory changes. Manifestation of proximal renal tubular acidosis has rarely mimicked GBS. **Hyperkalemia** with acute severe generalized weakness may also mimic GBS. Addison disease becomes an important diagnostic consideration. Barium carbonate poisoning, severe vomiting and diarrhea, and clay ingestions have also presented with similar clinical pictures.

Sensory symptoms and signs in **hypophosphatemia** resemble GBS more closely than hypokalemic and hyperkalemic states.

Chronic Inflammatory Demyelinating Polyradiculoneuropathy

Chronic inflammatory demyelinating polyradiculoneuropathy associated with an IgG or IgA monoclonal gammopathy of undetermined significance usually presents clinically like CIDP, without a monoclonal protein, and treatment response is similar. However, an IgG-λ monoclonal gammopathy always suggests the possibility of **POEMS syndrome** (polyneuropathy, organomegaly, endocrinopathy, monoclonal gammopathy, and skin changes, particularly hyperpigmentation). Whether an osteosclerotic or osteolytic bony lesion is identified, focused beam radiation therapy to these tumors can dramatically improve all POEMS syndrome aspects.

In contrast, an acquired demyelinating polyneuropathy associated with an IgM monoclonal protein frequently presents with more predominant sensory symptoms and signs, including sensory ataxia. It is less responsive to standard CIDP treatments. Many patients with a demyelinating polyneuropathy with an IgM monoclonal protein have high titers of antibodies to myelin-associated glycoprotein. It is thought that the IgMs are directed at myelin-associated glycoprotein epitopes on peripheral nerve constituents, and thereby are possibly pathogenic. GBS is not associated with monoclonal gammopathies.

DIAGNOSTIC APPROACH

Although the confirmation of GBS or CIDP primarily rests on clinical features, CSF analysis, EMG (Figure 95-1), serum immunophoresis, and treatment response provide the best means to make a precise diagnosis.

Spinal Fluid

An increased level of CSF protein (>50 mg/dL) without pleocytosis (<10 cells/mm^3) is common in GBS and CIDP. CSF examination is often normal within the first week of GBS; however, approximately 90% of patients with CIDP and patients with late GBS have an increased level of CSF protein. Although 10 to 50 cells/mm^3 in the CSF may occur in GBS, more than 50 cells/mm^3 should arouse suspicion of an alternate diagnosis, including **Lyme neuroborreliosis**, **HIV-associated polyradiculoneuropathy**, **poliomyelitis**, or **lymphomatous meningoradiculitis**.

Electromyography

EMG definitively defines whether the clinical picture is the result of a peripheral neuropathic process, ruling out other causes of weakness, such as disorders of neuromuscular transmission or myopathy. EMG can demonstrate widespread involvement of spinal roots and peripheral nerves, usually defining the process as demyelinating, although well-recognized axonal variants exist with GBS.

In GBS or CIDP, the motor and sensory conduction velocities are abnormally slow, with prolonged distal motor and F-wave latencies and often absent H reflexes. However, these parameters do not distinguish acquired from inherited demyelinating polyneuropathies, such as CMT type 1A.

Nonuniform slowing, conduction block at sites not prone to entrapment and abnormal temporal dispersion are commonly found in GBS and CIDP but not in most inherited demyelinating polyneuropathies. Conduction block is present with significant reductions in compound motor nerve action potential amplitude and area, and with proximal versus distal stimulation. Temporal dispersion is characterized by abnormal prolongation of compound motor nerve action potential duration with proximal but not distal stimulation. Conduction velocities on routine nerve conduction studies may be normal when inflammatory lesions are more proximal, for example in nerve roots or early in the disease course. Documentation of absent F waves, conduction block, temporal dispersion, or both is helpful for diagnosis of early GBS wherein more widespread slowing of conduction is not yet present.

Caution is important when the only nerve conduction studies abnormality is absent F waves in the legs or arms but they are preserved in the unaffected extremities. This finding is also seen with TM when the primary spinal damage is at the L4-S1 or C6-8 cord levels, where the anterior horn cells innervating the fibers responsible for F waves originate.

Usually, blood laboratory study results are unremarkable in GBS and CIDP. The most important exception is the occasional occurrence of a monoclonal protein in patients with CIDP. Usually representing a monoclonal gammopathy of undetermined significance. When this is a λ monoclonal antibody, it may signify a malignancy, such as **osteosclerotic** or **osteolytic myeloma**, **multiple myeloma**, or **Waldenstrom macroglobulinemia**.

TREATMENT
Guillain-Barré Syndrome

Care of patients with GBS varies from watchful waiting to emergency intervention, but initially always in a hospital because of the potential for rapid respiratory compromise. Patients with mild GBS who are able to ambulate are often cared for without specific treatment. These individuals who are unable to walk, who develop respiratory compromise, or who exhibit rapid progression require treatment with PE or IVIG. Both treatments are effective, but only if given within 1 to 2 weeks of onset, when the autoimmune attack is still active.

Concomitant or sequential use of these therapies usually has no value, although rarely one seems to work when the other has been ineffective. IVIG is given as a 2.0 g/kg over 2 to 5 days. PE is given as 5 plasma exchanges of 1 plasma volume over 9 to 10 days. Oral steroids are not effective for GBS.

Patients are observed closely (Figure 95-1). Respiratory failure is common in GBS; one third of patients require mechanical ventilation. Negative inspiratory force and vital capacity must be monitored closely in all patients with GBS.

Autonomic dysfunction is also seen frequently. Labile hypertension and arrhythmias occur frequently, often prompting observation and management in the ICU. Either pulmonary or autonomic complications are the primary causes of the rare GBS fatality.

Chronic Inflammatory Demyelinating Polyradiculoneuropathy

Treatment of patients with CIDP having significant disability with oral corticosteroids, IVIG, and PE is useful. Predetermined neurologic end points, such as strength, gait, and reflexes, must be monitored closely. In CIDP, clinical improvement usually occurs within a few weeks.

Intravenous immunoglobulin is the primary treatment for CIDP because of its superior adverse effect profile and excellent efficacy and because it can be given at home. Drawbacks include cost and availability. IVIG may be dosed initially at 2.0 g/kg over 2 to 5 days and subsequently once every 10 to 21 days at 0.4 g/kg. When clinically significant improvement occurs, the frequency of IVIG treatment is gradually tapered and later completely withdrawn.

Oral steroids, usually prednisone, are also efficacious in CIDP. The initial dose is usually 40 to 60 mg/d, transitioned to every-other-day dosing, then tapered and discontinued. The potential acute and chronic risks must be considered when deciding on steroid treatment and its duration. PE is not used as frequently as oral steroids or IVIG for CIDP because it is more invasive and not any more efficacious. In addition, the response to PE may be more transient. Nonetheless, PE remains an option, especially for patients who do not respond to IVIG or steroids.

PROGNOSIS

Most patients with GBS have a good prognosis, particularly those who primarily have the disorder limited to demyelination without significant axonal involvement where the course may be more prolonged. Most recover within a few months, although recovery is not always complete. A small percentage are left with some disability, and rarely, permanent disability primarily involving distal weakness in the feet.

Occasional (approximately 1-2%) mortalities do occur in GBS. Most deaths are from preventable respiratory complications or autonomic derangement. Supportive care, including emotional and nutritional support, judicious pain management, and prophylaxis for common complications of hospitalized, immobile patients (deep venous thrombosis and decubitus ulcers) is important.

The long-term outcome varies for patients with CIDP who are treated with conventional therapy. Most return to normal strength although some require intermittent IVIG to maintain improvement. Unfortunately, a rare patient progresses despite aggressive immunotherapy.

REFERENCES

Asbury AK, Arnason BG, Adams RD. The inflammatory lesion in idiopathic polyneuritis: its role in pathogenesis. *Medicine*. 1969;48:173-215.

Barohn RJ, Kissel JT, Warmolts JR, Mendell JR. Chronic inflammatory demyelinating polyradiculoneuropathy: clinical characteristics, course, and recommendations for diagnostic criteria. *Arch Neurol*. 1989;46:878-884.

Dutch Guillain-Barré Syndrome Trial Group. Plasmapheresis and acute Guillain-Barré syndrome. The Guillain-Barré Syndrome Study Group. *Neurology*. 1985;35:1096-1104.

Dyck PJ, Lais AC, Ohta M, Bastron JA, Groover RV. Chronic inflammatory polyradiculoneuropathy. *Mayo Clin Proc*. 1975;50:621-637.

French Cooperative on Plasma Exchange in Guillain-Barré syndrome. Efficiency of plasma exchange in Guillain-Barré syndrome: role of replacement fluids. *Ann Neurol*. 1987;22:753-761.

Jones HR. Guillain-Barre syndrome: perspectives with infants and children. *Semin Pediatr Neurol*. 2000;7:91-102.

Plasma Exchange/Sandoglobulin Guillain-Barré Syndrome Trial Group. Randomized trial of plasma exchange, intravenous immunoglobulin, and combined treatments in Guillain-Barré syndrome. *Lancet*. 1997;347:225-230.

Ropper AH. The Guillain-Barré Syndrome. *N Engl J Med*. 1992;326:1130-1136.

van der Marché FG, Schmitz PI. A randomized trial comparing intravenous immune globulin and plasma exchange in Guillain-Barré syndrome. Dutch Guillain-Barré Syndrome Trial Group. *N Engl J Med*. 1992;326:1123-1129.

Chapter 96
Multifocal Neuropathies
Monique M. Ryan, Ted M. Burns, James A. Russell, and H. Royden Jones, Jr

Clinical Vignette

A 53-year-old man experienced a left hand tremor. Within 6 months, he noted bilateral weakness and paresthesias of his hands. Three years later, he noted a tendency to trip over his right foot while walking.

Examination demonstrated weakness of both arms, greater on the left as well as the right leg. This was most marked in radial, median, and right peroneal innervated musculature. No sensory level was documented. Bilateral asymmetric muscle stretch reflex loss was limited to the triceps, brachioradialis, and right gastrocnemius.

Nerve conduction studies revealed low-amplitude compound motor action potentials from 5 nerves. Conduction block was identified at the median and peroneal nerves. Other motor and all sensory nerve conduction studies parameters were normal. Serologic assay for anti-GM1 antibody was markedly abnormal at 1:40,000 (reference range, <1:800). Other blood and CSF study results were normal.

The patient was treated with high-dose IV immunoglobulin (IVIG) and experienced a marked improvement in symptoms within 3 months. An attempt at withdrawal of immunosuppressive therapy resulted in clinical relapse, but sustained improvement occurred after resumption of IVIG therapy.

The patient had weakness in multiple nerve distributions over a 3-year period. Although paresthesias were present, no clinical or EMG evidence of sensory involvement was defined, characteristic of a multifocal motor neuropathy (MMN) diagnosis. Conduction block on motor conduction studies and anti-GM1 antibodies in high titer confirmed this eminently treatable multifocal motor neuropathy.

An important subgroup of neuropathies is characterized by a unique temporal profile, having stepwise involvement of individual peripheral nerves. Despite a broad range of primary pathophysiologic mechanisms, from hereditary to those associated with systemic disorders, most commonly diabetes mellitus, a number of these conditions are eminently treatable. Their early recognition, with subsequent initiation of specific therapy, is an important consideration in patients presenting with peripheral neuropathy.

ETIOLOGY AND CLINICAL PRESENTATION

Multifocal neuropathies are caused by disorders that infarct, infiltrate, inflame, or render peripheral nerves more vulnerable to compression. Many are vasculitides, particularly diabetes mellitus. These conditions have affinities for small blood vessels the size of those that perfuse peripheral nerves, ie, the vaso nervorum. In **MMN** and the **Lewis-Sumner variant** of **chronic inflammatory demyelinating polyneuropathy**, an immune-mediated attack on peripheral nerve myelin occurs. It is unclear why these disorders present with multifocal clinical distribution as opposed to the symmetric manifestations of more common acquired demyelinating neuropathies. The precise pathophysiologic mechanism leading to genetically determined alteration in peripheral nerve myelin, ie, **hereditary tendency to pressure palsies**, is not understood but somehow predisposes the peripheral nerve to increased susceptibility to compression.

Patients may have an acute, potentially devastating temporal profile, as in an acute vasculitis, or one that evolves over months, as in an immunologically mediated or hereditary conditions. In the acute setting, patients' symptoms may develop so rapidly that presentation may be easily confused with generalized polyneuropathy. The basic mechanism is best appreciated by carefully recording each step in the history outlining the precise temporal profile of the illness.

Patients with classic **mononeuritis multiplex** suddenly develop foot drop or numbness and weakness within a single nerve's distribution in the arm or hand (Figure 96-1). This then repeats

MULTIFOCAL NEUROPATHIES

Figure 96-1

Mononeuritis Multiplex
With Polyarteritis Nodosa

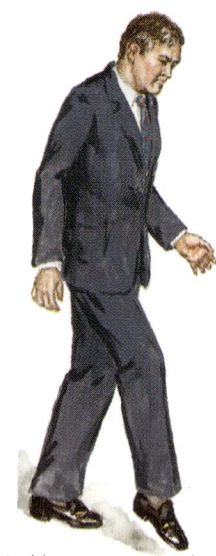

Sudden occurrence of foot drop while walking (peroneal nerve)

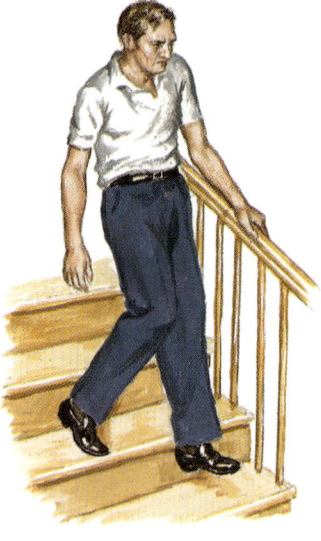

Sudden buckling of knee while going downstairs (femoral nerve)

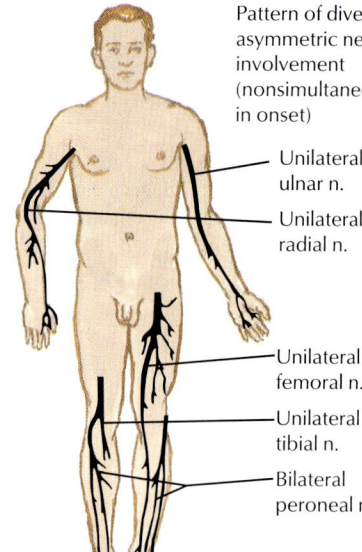

Pattern of diverse, asymmetric nerve involvement (nonsimultaneous in onset)

- Unilateral ulnar n.
- Unilateral radial n.
- Unilateral femoral n.
- Unilateral tibial n.
- Bilateral peroneal nn.

(Lower limb more commonly affected)

Polyarteritis nodosa with characteristic multisystem involvement

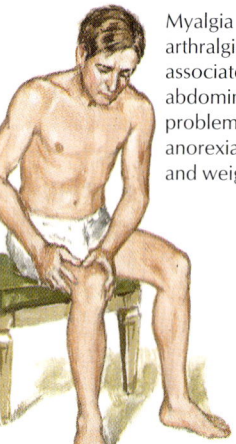

Myalgia and/or arthralgia often associated with abdominal problems, anorexia, fever, and weight loss

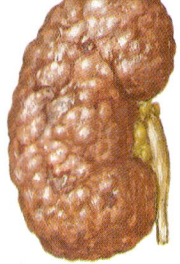

Nephropathy, a most serious effect; RBCs, WBCs, and casts in urine; eventual renal failure

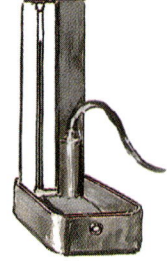

Hypertension common

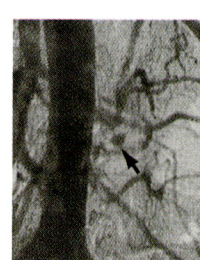

Angiogram showing microaneurysm of small mesenteric artery

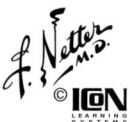

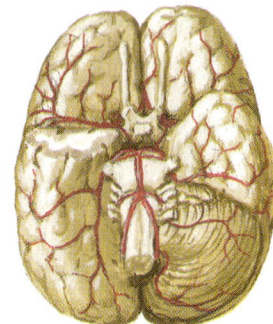

CNS involvement may cause headache, ocular disorders, convulsions, aphasia, hemiplegia, and cerebellar signs.

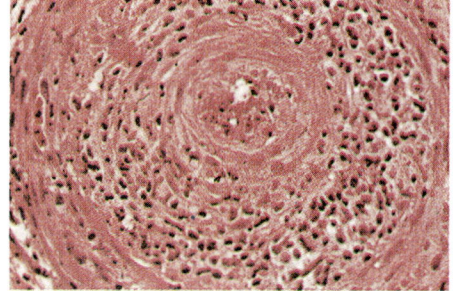

Inflammatory cell infiltration and fibrinoid necrosis of walls of small arteries lead to infarction in various organs or tissues.

POLYNEUROPATHIES AND AUTONOMIC DISORDERS

in another nerve as described in the preceding vignette.

DIFFERENTIAL DIAGNOSIS

The temporal profile of **mononeuritis multiplex** is so characteristic that the primary clinical issue is recognition of the process and identification of the etiologic mechanism. Multiple nerve root involvement also should be excluded. It is then necessary to differentiate various primary multiple mononeuropathies, the most prominent being mononeuritis multiplex.

Multifocal Polyradiculopathy

Various **multifocal polyradiculopathies** are the other motor unit processes that require consideration in differential diagnosis because they also produce multifocal neuropathic signs and symptoms in a staccato fashion, affecting multiple nerve roots and cranial nerves. These multifocal nerve root disorders have entirely different sets of predisposing pathologic processes, particularly metastatic malignancies or granulomatous conditions, including tuberculosis or sarcoidosis. This contrasts with the predominance of underlying vasculitis in mononeuritis multiplex with a predilection for specific peripheral nerve damage.

Often painful and usually accompanied by sensory symptoms, polyradiculopathies can be distinguished from mononeuritis multiplex in most instances by the sensory involvement distribution, segmental rather than peripheral nerve distribution of clinical findings, results of EMG and CSF abnormalities. Both groups of patients often have serious systemic complications with malaise, anorexia, weight loss, and low-grade fever.

Vasculitic Neuropathy

Mononeuritis multiplex is a frequent manifestation of **systemic necrotizing vasculitis**. Systemic illness signs and symptoms in the setting of a multifocal neuropathy strongly suggest vasculitis as the diagnosis (Table 96-1). Mononeuritis multiplex may occur in a more indolent form as a **nonsystemic necrotizing vasculitis** wherein peripheral nerves are selectively vulnerable. Ischemic neuropathies are commonly painful at onset, typically affecting sensory and motor function.

Clinical Vignette

A 12-year-old girl presented with fever, arthritis, and nephritis. She was diagnosed with systemic lupus erythematosus. Cerebritis, seizures, and chronic renal failure complicated her disease course.

At the age of 16 years, left hand numbness developed, and soon thereafter, an acute left foot drop occurred. Three weeks later, the patient reported right hand and foot paresthesias and weakness. Neurologic examination results demonstrated right median and ulnar and bilateral peroneal neuropathies. The patient was uremic, anemic, and thrombocytopenic. EMG revealed damage to these nerves in an asymmetric distribution appropriate to her clinical examination results. These EMG findings were consistent with a clinical diagnosis of mononeuritis multiplex.

Sural nerve biopsy revealed small-vessel vasculitis with thrombosed vessels, focal fibrinoid necrosis of vessel walls, and transmural infiltration by neutrophils. The internal elastic lamina was focally destroyed in several vessels, with destruction of the media and concentric perivascular fibrosis (Figure 96-1).

Several days after initiation of treatment with high-dose IV methylprednisolone, the patient had recurrent hematemesis. Gastroscopy revealed diffuse gastric ulceration, biopsy of which demonstrated necrotising vasculitis similar to the nerve biopsy. She was treated with prednisolone and cyclophosphamide, with full recovery other than a persistent left foot drop. She subsequently underwent renal transplantation and remained free of further neurologic symptoms. She recovered all function except for some residual loss in her peroneal nerve.

This vignette depicts the classic presentation of an acute mononeuritis multiplex. The rapidity with which the patient developed multiple mononeuropathies is typical for patients with a necrotizing vasculitis. It is important to recognize this clinical scenario and proceed with definitive diagnosis and high immunosuppressive therapy to avoid significant residual damage.

Diabetic Mononeuritis

Acute diabetic mononeuropathies also result from focal nerve ischemia. Clinically, some seem to be **femoral neuropathies**; however, EMG often discloses these as regional polyradiculoneuropathies, ie, **diabetic radiculoplexus neuropathy (diabetic amyotrophy)**. True mononeuritis multiplexes occur occasion-

MULTIFOCAL NEUROPATHIES

Table 96-1
Differential Diagnosis—Multifocal Neuropathies*

Mechanism	Category	Disease
Immune mediated	Demyelinating	MMN
		MADSAM
	Axonal	Multifocal acquired motor axonopathy and other non-MMN motor neuropathies
Ischemic	Vasculitis	Polyarteritis nodosa
		Nonsystemic vasculitis
		Systemic lupus erythematosus
		Churg-Strauss syndrome
		Wegener granulomatosis
		Essential mixed cryoglobulinemia
		Rheumatoid arthritis
	Hypersensitivity vasculitis	Henoch-Schönlein purpura
		Amphetamines, cocaine
		Antibiotics (sulfonamides, penicillin, isoniazid, etc)
	Diabetes	
Infectious	Spirochete	Lyme disease
	Hansen bacillus	Leprosy
	Viral	HIV infection
		CMV
Infiltration	Lymphoproliferative	Neurolymphomatosis
		Lymphomatoid granulomatosis
	Granulomatous	Sarcoidosis
	Protein	Amyloidosis
Susceptibility to compression	Genetic	HNPP
	Metabolic	Diabetes

*CMV indicates cytomegalovirus; HNPP, hereditary tendency to pressure palsies; MADSAM, multifocal acquired demyelinating sensory and motor neuropathy; MMN, multifocal motor neuropathy.

ally as the presenting manifestation in patients with diabetes. They are less common than the prototypic diabetic length-dependent polyneuropathies.

Diabetic nerves are more susceptible to compression injury. Multifocal neuropathy in patients with diabetes from median neuropathies at the wrist, ulnar neuropathies at the elbow, and peroneal neuropathies at the knee are fairly common.

Multifocal Motor Neuropathy

Multifocal motor neuropathy, a pure-motor syndrome, commonly evolves in an indolent fashion leading to gradually increasing weakness, mimicking patients with lower motor neuron presentation of motor neuron disease. Symptoms may evolve more acutely. Although typically affecting the distal upper extremity asymmetrically in middle-aged men, it may present in the legs.

Careful examination demonstrates neurologic findings in MMN that reflect involvement of multiple motor nerves rather than segmental root distribution more typical of motor neuron disease. For example, patients with MMN often have weakness with distal median motor distribution, sparing the ulnar muscles. However, it is unusual for patients with motor neuron disease or progressive muscular atrophy to have median without ulnar involvement because the involvement of the motor neurons is at C8 for both. Cramps, fasciculations, and atrophy also occur in MMN. MMN must be a major differential diagnostic consideration in every patient thought to have the primary muscular atrophy form of **amyotrophic lateral sclerosis.**

The diagnostic criteria and boundary limitations of MMNs are still being defined. However, major diagnostic features help to indicate the MMN diagnosis. These include high titers of antibodies directed against the GM1 ganglioside, demonstration of conduction block on motor nerve conduction studies (typically at sites not prone to external compression), and positive response to IVIG therapy. Individual patients commonly lack 1 or more of these features. The axonal variant of this disorder, called *multifocal acquired motor axonopathy*, may also exist.

Multifocal Acquired Demyelinating Sensory and Motor Neuropathy

Multifocal acquired demyelinating sensory and motor neuropathy is an acquired, multifocal demyelinating neuropathy affecting motor and sensory fibers. It is probably another variant of chronic inflammatory demyelinating polyneuropathy, with similar responsiveness to treatment.

Hereditary Liability to Pressure Palsy

Multifocal neuropathy resulting from apparently trivial external compression typically occurs related to a genetically determined hereditary tendency to pressure palsies. Patients usually present with multiple painless compressive neuropathies developing over time. Lesions occur at typical sites where peripheral nerves are vulnerable to compression, such as the peroneal nerve at the fibula head or the radial nerve in the upper arm. A family history may or may not be apparent. EMG demonstrates focal slowing and amplitude loss in sensory and motor nerves at compression points in combination with more generalized neuropathy manifested by mild slowing of peripheral nerve conduction.

Infiltrative Disorders

Nerves may be infiltrated by hematologic malignancies (particularly lymphoma), infectious agents, sarcoidosis, and byproducts of abnormal metabolism. **Neurolymphomatosis** is an uncommon manifestation of non-Hodgkin lymphoma characterized by development of typically painful, subacute peripheral nerve deficits and sensorimotor involvement in a focal or multifocal distribution. **Lymphomatoid granulomatosis** is another lymphoproliferative disorder that may affect peripheral nerves and lungs. Uncommonly, neurofibromas infiltrate nerves, producing **neurofibromatous neuropathy**. **Amyloidosis** typically presents as a length-dependent sensory predominant neuropathy but may rarely have a distinct multifocal presentation because of its infiltrative and angiocentric tendencies.

Infectious Disorders

Leprosy, HIV, Lyme disease, and cytomegalovirus are infectious disorders affecting the peripheral nervous system in a multifocal fashion by infiltrative and other mechanisms. Most are rare in North America. Each necessitates a high index of suspicion and specific tissue acquisition for diagnosis.

DIAGNOSTIC APPROACH

Because these disorders are associated with systemic illness, tests directed at other organ systems are frequently helpful. Nerve biopsy in multifocal neuropathy is useful in many patients in contrast to the individual with length-dependent polyneuropathy. Biopsy of nerve or other clinically affected tissue should be considered if diagnosis cannot be obtained by less invasive means, particularly in patients with rapidly evolving illness and associated systemic illness.

EMG is performed in all patients with an apparent multifocal neuropathy. A comprehensive

MULTIFOCAL NEUROPATHIES

study is necessary to define the pattern as multifocal. Side-to-side amplitude asymmetries of 50% or more on conduction studies are required to conclude that pathologic asymmetry exists. A careful search for conduction block or other acquired demyelination manifestation, such as focal conduction slowing, is necessary. If either conduction block or conduction slowing is documented, diagnostic considerations include hereditary tendency to pressure palsies, diabetes, mononeuritis multiplex, MMN, and multifocal acquired demyelinating sensory and motor neuropathy.

Of various additional laboratory studies, anti-GM1 antibodies are the most specific and useful (Table 96-2). An increased ESR is a nonspecific but important finding indicating a possible vasculitis and need for sural nerve biopsy. Serologic markers are usually abnormal in systemic vasculitis and normal or mildly abnormal in nonsystemic primary neurologic vasculitis. No other serologic tests have proven specific diagnostic roles in these syndromes. However, changes in antinuclear antibody, extractable nuclear antigens, rheumatoid factor, perinuclear and cytoplasmic antineutrophil cytoplasmic antibody, cryoglobulins, hepatitis C serology, serum and urine monoclonal proteins, angiotensin-converting enzyme level, and HIV serology sometimes provide support for more aggressive evaluation and therapeutic trials with various immunosuppressive therapies.

DNA mutational analysis for hereditary tendency to pressure palsies is indicated in patients with indolent multifocal neuropathy and a family history suggestive of a similar disorder, or clinical or electrodiagnostic evidence of an underlying multifocal neuropathy. Although nerve biopsy may be supportive, it is indicated only in individuals with a strongly suggestive phenotype in whom DNA mutational analysis is normal. Nerve biopsy is particularly valuable in suspected amyloidosis, sarcoidosis, and leprosy.

TREATMENT AND PROGNOSIS

Mononeuritis multiplex has an excellent response to immunosuppressive therapies; prednisone is the primary initial treatment modality. The multifocal variant of chronic inflammatory

Table 96-2
Evaluation of Patients With Multifocal Neuropathies

Tests Standards in Patients With Suspected Multifocal Neuropathy	Other Tests That Are Often Useful
Electrodiagnostic studies (EMG and NCS)	CSF evaluation including cytology, Lyme serology, and CMV serology
Fasting blood sugar	Ace level (serum and possibly CSF)
ESR	HIV serology
Urinalysis	Anti-GM1 antibodies
CBC, including eosinophil count	DNA mutational analysis for HNPP
	Lyme serology—blood and CSF
	Chest and abdominal imaging
	Antineutrophilic cytoplasmic antibodies
	Lymph node biopsy
	Serum and urine immunoelectrophoresis
	DNA mutational analysis for familial amyloidosis
	Serum cryoglobulins
	Nerve biopsy
	Biopsy of kidney, rectum, abdominal fat

*CMV indicates cytomegalovirus; HNPP, hereditary tendency to pressure palsies; NCS, nerve conduction studies.

demyelinating polyneuropathy and MMN usually responds to immunosuppressive therapies. Long-term treatment is often required; some patients have significant permanent motor and sensory deficits.

Multifocal motor neuropathy is treated with IVIG or cyclophosphamide, a cytotoxic agent. Corticosteroid therapy is not effective for MMN but may be beneficial in multifocal acquired demyelinating sensory and motor neuropathy.

Time is essential in treatment of systemic necrotizing vasculitis, with or without multifocal neuropathy. Before the introduction of immunomodulating therapy, death was virtually universal in these disorders. Treatment involves prednisone and a cytotoxic agent. Cyclophosphamide is typically required for months to a year or more, with gradual tapering titrated to response.

Nonsystemic vasculitic neuropathies are typically more indolent disorders with better prognoses than systemic vasculitis. Treatment is usually less aggressive and may be unnecessary in some cases. Neurologic deficits often have spontaneous recovery over time, and nonsystemic vasculitic neuropathy does not seem to alter survival.

Sarcoidosis is typically treated with prednisone and other immunosuppressive agents. Lymphoproliferative disorders typically require chemotherapy. Infectious causes of multifocal neuropathy are treated with appropriate antimicrobial regimens. Genetic counseling is important for patients with hereditary tendency to pressure palsies, which is typically inherited in an autosomal dominant fashion with variable penetrance.

The chance for excellent recovery of a vasculitic neuropathy is good if it is promptly recognized and appropriately treated. Substantial morbidity and mortality result if treatment is delayed or neglected. Diabetic multifocal neuropathies are associated with a good recovery, depending somewhat on blood sugar control. Up to 80% of patients with MMN respond rapidly to therapy with IVIG. Unfortunately, the durability of treatment may wane in some patients.

REFERENCES

Brown WF. Acute and chronic inflammatory demyelinating neuropathies. In: Brown WF, Bolton CF, eds. *Clinical Electromyography*. 2nd ed. Boston, Mass: Butterworth Heinemann; 1993:553-560.

Burns TM, Dyck PJB. Treatment of vasculitic neuropathy. In: Johnson RT, Griffin JW, McArthur JC, eds. *Current Therapy in Neurologic Disease*. 6th ed. St. Louis, Mo; 2002:390-394.

Chaudhry V, Corse AM, Cornblath DR, et al. Multifocal motor neuropathy: response to human immune globulin. *Ann Neurol*. 1993;33:237-242.

Dyck PJ, Benstead TJ, Conn DL, Stevens JC, Windebank AJ, Low PA. Nonsystemic vasculitic neuropathy. *Brain*. 1987;110:843-854.

Kissel JT, Collins MP, Mendell JR. Vasculitic neuropathy. In: Mendell JR, Kissel JT, Cornblath DR. *Diagnosis and Management of Peripheral Nerve Disorders. Contemporary Neurology Series*. New York, NY: Oxford University Press; 2001:202-232.

Lewis RA, Sumner AJ, Brown MJ, Asbury AK. Multifocal demyelinating neuropathy with persistent conduction block. *Neurology*. 1982;32:958-964.

Olney RK, Lewis RA, Putnam TD, Campellone JV. Consensus criteria for the diagnosis of multifocal motor neuropathy. *Muscle Nerve*. 2003;27:117-121.

Parry GJ, Clarke S. Multifocal acquired demyelinating neuropathy masquerading as motor neuron disease. *Muscle Nerve*. 1988;11:103-107.

Tyson J, Malcolm S, Thomas PK, Harding AE. Deletions of chromosome 17p11.2 in multifocal neuropathies. *Ann Neurol*. 1996;39:180-186.

Chapter 97

Sensory Neuropathy and Neuronopathy

Jennifer A. Grillo, James A. Russell, and H. Royden Jones, Jr

Clinical Vignette

A 64-year-old lifelong smoker woke with unexplained, poorly described pain in her left groin unrelated to position or movement. Within 2 weeks, pains developed in a multifocal distribution. Her feet, her hands, and the right posterior part of her scalp became numb. She experienced increasing difficulty maintaining balance and walking, particularly in the dark or with her eyes closed.

Examination revealed a chronically ill woman who initially seemed to give incomplete effort during manual muscle testing. This was corrected by having her directly visualize tested body parts. Muscle stretch reflexes were absent in the ankles and knees and diminished but present in the arms. Vibration, position, and, to a lesser extent, pain and temperature sensations were absent in the feet and variously diminished more proximally. Pinprick was less well perceived in the right posterior part of the scalp than in the left.

Within 2 months of onset, the patient could not open her mouth and reported blurred vision. Examination disclosed apparent trismus and a direction-changing nystagmus. EMG revealed absent sensory nerve action potentials in the lower extremities and reduced sensory nerve action potentials in the hands. Motor conduction and needle electrode examination results were normal.

An acute-onset sensory polyneuropathy developed in this patient. Her clinical profile suggested a non–length-dependent process typical of a dorsal root ganglion cell sensory neuronopathy.

This rapid temporal evolution in a smoker was a particularly ominous sign suggestive of a paraneoplastic sensory neuronopathy. Her subsequent development of trismus and nystagmus suggested concomitant brainstem encephalitis, another paraneoplastic syndrome that occurs in patients with small cell lung cancer.

Chest imaging and subsequent biopsy of an anterior mediastinal mass confirmed the suspected small cell lung cancer. Anti-Hu antibodies confirmed the paraneoplastic relation between the sensory neuronopathy and lung tumor.

Most patients with peripheral neuropathies present with sensory symptoms and signs typical of a **length-dependent polyneuropathy** (LDPN). In most patients with sensory LDPN, the condition is slowly ingravescent. Their symptomatology follows a course of gradually evolving, distal-predominate numbness. Various toxic, metabolic, and genetic mechanisms cause the primary neuropathology within sensory axons.

However, in many patients no identifiable cause can be found.

Another, smaller population of sensory-impaired individuals has pathophysiology primarily affecting the sensory neuron cells within the dorsal root ganglion (in contrast to neuropathies, affecting the distal nerve axon) (Figure 97-1). They are described as having **sensory neuronopathy**. The acute onset is often typified by a painful, noxious clinical picture with a generalized distribution.

Because the basic pathophysiologic mechanism is frequently idiopathic or assumed to be related to underlying type 2 diabetes mellitus, there may be some tendency to disregard these patients, particularly because of the mistaken belief that specific therapy is unavailable. However, a thorough and in-depth analysis occasionally identifies an esoteric but eminently treatable pathophysiologic mechanism.

ETIOLOGY AND CLINICAL PRESENTATION

Most peripheral sensory polyneuropathies are immune mediated or toxic. With sensory neuronopathies, the dorsal root ganglia (DRG) sen-

SENSORY NEUROPATHY AND NEURONOPATHY

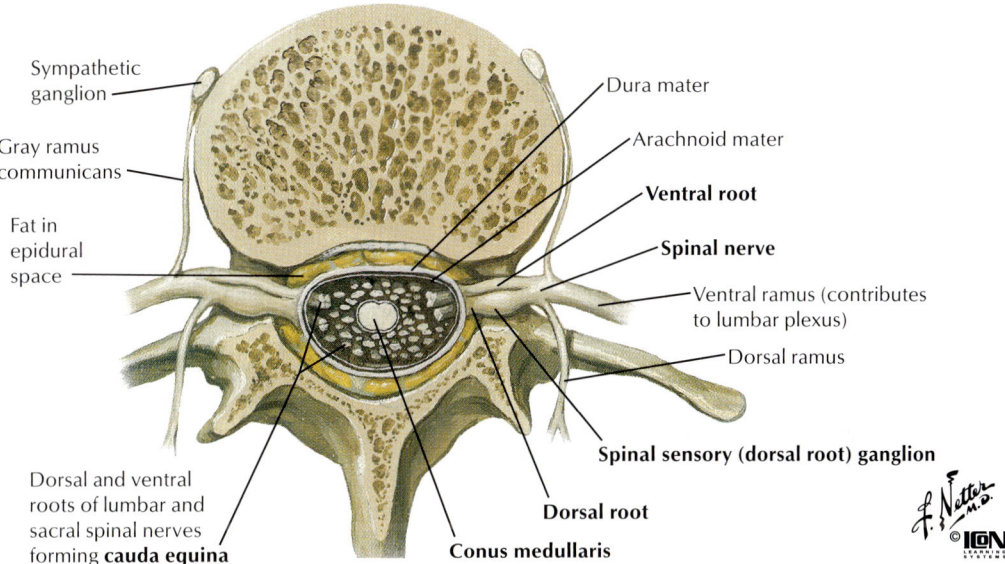

Figure 97-1 **Spinal Nerve Origin: Sensory Components**

sory peripheral nerve cell bodies are the primary target of the disease process, explaining why these disorders present with a non–length-dependent clinical pattern.

In **paraneoplastic sensory neuronopathy**, it is proposed that similar molecular and antigenic components in DRG and small cell lung carcinoma cells set the stage for molecular mimicry. A similar mechanism has not been determined for Sjögren syndrome and other presumed immune-mediated processes to explain the DRG-selective vulnerability that occurs with various toxins.

Characterized by damage to primary sensory axons, **LDPNs** are the most common pathologic entities with peripheral sensory system involvement. These patients have a small-fiber axonal sensory polyneuropathy with stocking-glove or pain and temperature sensory loss. Touch and vibration are affected to a lesser degree. The entities leading to this presentation are discussed in chapter 94.

A sensory neuronopathy secondary to inflammation or other damage to the DRG occurs less commonly. Both types of peripheral sensory lesions are often painful. However, severely affected individuals typically have primary DRG cell damage. Disproportionate loss of position and other discriminatory modalities occur when large sensory fibers are affected. Severe sensory ataxia frequently presents.

Distinguishing between sensory LDPN and sensory neuronopathy is important because their differential diagnoses vary considerably. Often, a clinically suspected diagnosis can be confirmed with EMG.

DIFFERENTIAL DIAGNOSIS

Sjögren syndrome is an immunologically mediated process associated with several neuropathy phenotypes that may evolve acutely or chronically. The classic sensory neuronopathy form is not the most common. It is clinically indistinguishable from other DRG lesions, particularly paraneoplastic sensory neuronopathy. Women are more commonly affected. Diagnostic findings include the sicca complex with dry eyes and mouth, antibodies directed against SSA and SSB, inflammatory involvement of salivary glands on lip biopsy, or a combination of these.

Sensory neuronopathy is a well-recognized dose-related and dose-limiting **toxicity of cisplatin and carboplatin**.

Paraneoplastic sensory neuronopathy typically has an acute to subacute painful presentation. It occurs in approximately 1% of patients with small cell lung cancer, rarely with other malignancies. The paraneoplastic syndrome may precede malignancy recognition by years. One or more additional paraneoplastic neurologic syndromes eventually develop in approximately 75% of these patients.

Pyridoxine in large doses (1-2 g daily) may cause irreversible sensory neuronopathy syndromes. Doses as small as 200 mg/d over extended periods may have similar toxic potential.

Vitamin B$_{12}$ deficiency and **tabes dorsalis** have strong predispositions to affect the posterior columns. They present with sensory ataxia. Patients with B$_{12}$ deficiency frequently experience paresthesias, first in the hand in a non–length-dependent manner, but may also have generalized painful neuropathies (see chapter 93; Clinical Vignette). **Tabes dorsalis** is rarely seen today. This complication of tertiary syphilis is typified by its unusual clinical manifestations, including paroxysms of severely uncomfortable lightning pains and ataxia.

Many sensory neuronopathy patients with ataxic neuropathies do not have definable pathophysiologic mechanisms. As with idiopathic or cryptogenic disease categories, this remains a diagnosis of exclusion. Often clinically indistinguishable from paraneoplastic sensory neuronopathy presenting with a sensory ataxia, these disorders may evolve acutely or chronically and occur predominantly in women. In contrast to many DRG disorders, they are often painless.

DIAGNOSTIC APPROACH

EMG is the initial study because it provides a means to differentiate between LDPN and sensory neuronopathy. Almost all patients with LDPNs, even those without clinical weakness, have EMG evidence of motor involvement. These are recognized by motor nerve conduction study changes, needle electrode examination abnormalities, or both (Figure 97-2). Patients with a primary DRG lesion, ie, sensory neuronopathy, have only sensory nerve conduction study abnormalities.

When sensory neuronopathies are confirmed, subsequent ancillary testing is limited to disorders known to cause such patterns (Table 97-1). The various causes of sensory LDPN may also require consideration (Table 97-2).

Testing for serum anti-Hu antibodies is indicated in sensory neuronopathy evaluation, particularly for patients with a smoking or asbestos-exposure history. They are sensitive and specific for paraneoplastic neurologic disorders, particularly those with occult malignancies such as small cell lung cancer. Chest CT is indicated because the neuropathy may precede malignancy recognition by several years.

Patients with suspected Sjögren syndrome require serologic tests, particularly SSA and SSB antibodies. Other potentially beneficial studies include the Shirmer test of lacrimation and slit lamp examination of the conjunctiva after Rose-Bengal staining. Minor salivary gland (usually lip) biopsy is performed if the diagnosis remains unconfirmed with less invasive means.

Vitamin B$_{12}$ levels and a serologic test for syphilis are important for evaluation of patients with large-fiber sensory dysfunction. If the vitamin B$_{12}$ level is borderline, the more sensitive blood or urine tests for homocysteine, methylmalonic acid, or both are helpful. No common causes of sensory neuronopathies are likely to produce diagnostic findings in a peripheral nerve biopsy specimen in contrast to amyloid with LDPN.

TREATMENT AND PROGNOSIS

Symptomatic treatments for discomfort associated with sensory neuronopathy and other sensory predominant neuropathies are discussed in chapter 93.

Potential neurotoxins require identification and subsequent elimination. An empiric approach may include carefully considering discontinuation of medication begun at illness inception. The degree of recovery depends on the nature, intensity, and duration of the exposure. Successful recovery may occur rapidly or be protracted, in keeping with known limitations of nerve regeneration.

Patients with severe sensory ataxia may require canes, crutches, walkers, or wheelchairs. Although frequently considered cosmetically unappealing and undignified, these allow safe, independent mobility. An empathetic discussion about the potential risks of falling with subse-

SENSORY NEUROPATHY AND NEURONOPATHY

Figure 97-2 Hereditary Sensory Neuropathy

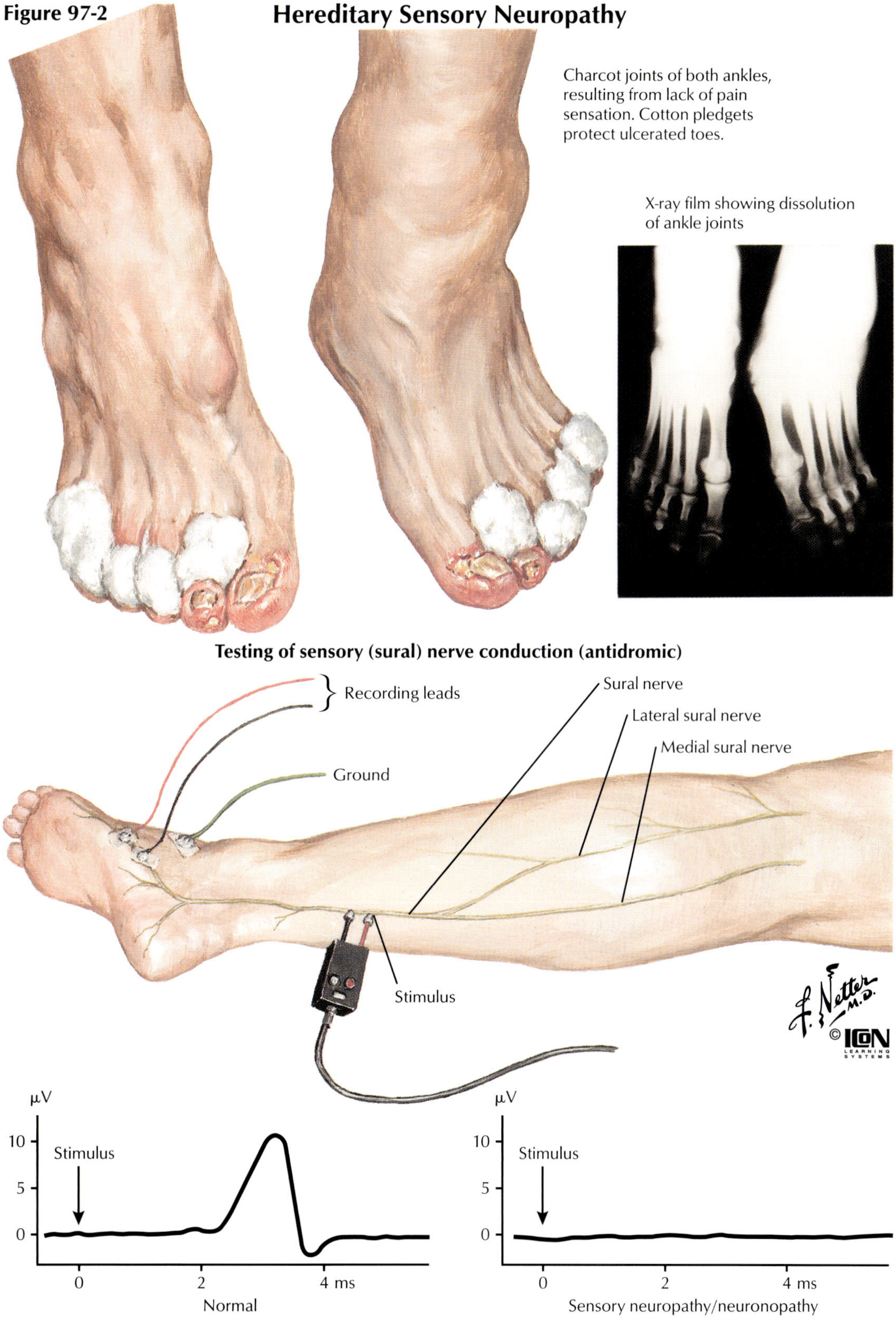

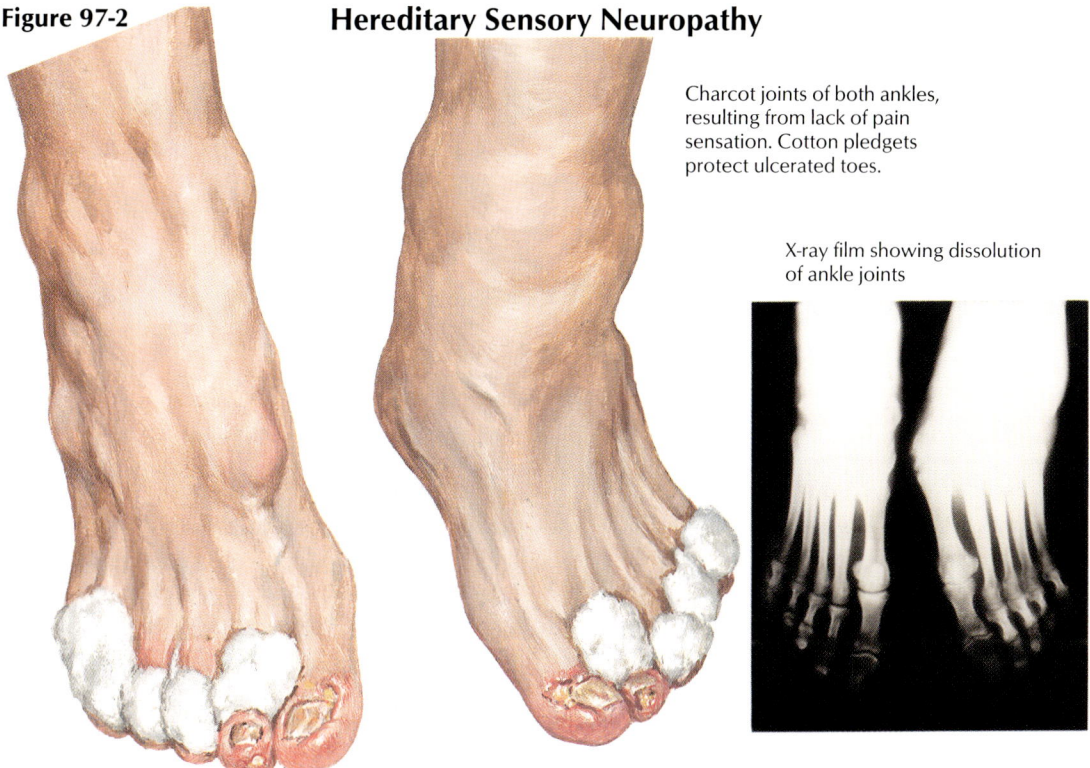

POLYNEUROPATHIES AND AUTONOMIC DISORDERS

Table 97-1
Sensory Neuronopathy Pattern Dorsal Root Ganglion

Sjögren syndrome

Cancer
  Paraneoplastic
    Small cell lung
    Non-Hodgkin lymphoma
  Cisplatin toxicity

Other medications
  Pyridoxine
  Thalidomide

Idiopathic

Table 97-2
Causes of Length-Dependent Sensory Polyneuropathy (LDPN)*

Axonal Sensory Neuropathy (by order of frequency)

- Idiopathic or chronic benign sensory polyneuropathy of the elderly
- Diabetes mellitus
- Small-fiber neuropathy
- Toxins
- B-vitamin deficiency
- Sjögren syndrome
- Amyloidosis (primary systemic or hereditary)
- HIV
- Hereditary sensory neuropathies
- Fabry disease?
- Spinocerebellar ataxias

Demyelinating Sensory Neuropathy

- Sensory polyneuropathy associated with IgM monoclonal protein with or without anti-MAG activity
- Guillain-Barré syndrome (sensory variant)

*MAG indicates myelin-associated glycoprotein.

---

quent hip fracture or head or neck injury is an important aspect of guidance for patients with moderately severe polyneuropathies. Ankle-foot orthoses (AFOs) or walkers are alternatives for those with milder disabilities. A home safety evaluation by a physical therapist may prove beneficial.

Meticulous foot hygiene should be emphasized when patients have prominent loss of pain perception. This includes monitoring for unnoticed painless injuries with the predisposition to become easily infected.

Pain is a prominent component and necessitates empathetic management and appropriate use of analgesics, including narcotics.

In Sjögren syndrome, reports of successful responses to various immunomodulating therapies are gaining recognition. IV immunoglobulin was effective in a patient who had been ill for 5 years before treatment.

Paraneoplastic sensory neuropathies are generally resistant to therapies, including a variety of immunomodulating agents. This seems paradoxical to the excellent evidence supporting an underlying autoimmune mechanism. Specific treatment of the underlying neoplasm, when identified, may be successful, but seems to have little or no impact on the neuropathy. These patients usually have an inexorable downhill course.

Prognosis varies depending on the underlying cause of the neuropathy and the extent of axonal damage before treatment initiation. Specific treatments for sensory neuropathies are lacking, disappointing most patients. Sometimes sensory neuronopathies are debilitating with loss of independence. Severe cases may prevent independent ambulation, even with gait aids.

REFERENCES

Burns TM, Quijano-Roy S, Jones HR. Benefit of IVIg for long-standing ataxic sensory neuronopathy with Sjogren's syndrome [letter]. *Neurology.* 2003;61:873.

Jones HR. Case presentation and discussion March 24, 1983. Case records of the Massachusetts General Hospital. Scully RE, Mark EJ, McNeeley BU, eds. *N Engl J Med.* 1984;310:445-455.

Chapter 98
Leprosy (Hansen Disease)

Jayashri Srinivasan and Winnie Ooi

Clinical Vignette

A 56-year-old woman from Southern India was examined because she had been tripping on her left foot for 6 months. For the past month, she had noticed difficulty gripping objects with the right hand and had experienced associated elbow and median forearm pain.

Neurologic examination of the right hand demonstrated weakness of finger abduction and adduction, mild clawing of the fourth and fifth digits, and sensory loss of the medial 1½ fingers, consistent with a right ulnar neuropathy. Examination results of the left leg revealed focal weakness of foot dorsiflexion and eversion with sensory loss on the lateral aspect of the left calf and the foot dorsum indicating a left common peroneal neuropathy. Both ulnar and peroneal nerves were thickened and palpable. Two subtle hypopigmented, anesthetic macules were found on the upper arm and trunk. Sensation was diminished on the ear pinna and tip of the nose.

EMG confirmed moderately severe right ulnar and left peroneal axonal neuropathies. Sural nerve biopsy revealed a noncaseating granuloma with lymphocytic infiltration and Langhans giant cells; a few acid-fast bacilli were seen on the modified Fite-Faraco stain. The diagnosis was tuberculoid leprosy, and dapsone, clofazimine, and rifampin were administered.

Leprosy is a chronic infectious granulomatous disease of skin and peripheral nerves. Worldwide, it is one of the most common causes of neuropathy. Any patient from an area endemic for leprosy who has multiple mononeuropathies, particularly ulnar and peroneal, and skin lesions in superficial sensory areas that have colder ambient temperatures is suspect for this disorder. The etiologic agent is *Mycobacterium leprae*, an acid-fast bacillus identified by Hansen in 1873. Today, leprosy is seen primarily in Asia, Africa, and Latin America. The incidence of new cases is approximately 750,000 per year, with a prevalence of 1.3 million patients; approximately 70% of registered patients live in India.

BACTERIOLOGY

The leprosy bacillus' genome demonstrates reductive evolution with extensive deletion and inactivation of genes and abundant pseudogenes; less than 50% of the genome contains functional genes. That may explain the unusually long generation time and the inability to culture *M leprae* in artificial media.

Leprosy is transmitted by respiratory droplets and direct skin contact during close and frequent exposure to untreated patients. Other routes of infection include contact with armadillos (a reservoir in Texas), infected soil, and rarely direct dermal implantation during procedures such as tattooing. The incubation period is usually 2 to 7 years. Because of an affinity for peripheral nerves, *M leprae*/laminin-$\alpha 2$ complexes bind to α/β dystroglycan complexes expressed on Schwann cells. Clinical development of leprosy depends on host immune responses and genetic factors. The disease spectrum varies widely from limited tuberculoid forms to an extensive **lepromatous** form.

CLINICAL PRESENTATION AND DIAGNOSIS

The 3 cardinal diagnostic criteria are anesthetic skin patches, thickened nerves, and acid-fast bacilli in skin smears (Figure 98-1). The World Health Organization recommends classification based on clinical criteria: **paucibacillary** if fewer than 5 skin lesions and/or 1 nerve is involved, or **multibacillary** if there are more than 5 skin lesions, more than 2 nerves involved, or both. This system determines the therapy type and duration for patients evaluated in the field where laboratory help is not available. The commonly used classification is based on the clinical

LEPROSY (HANSEN DISEASE)

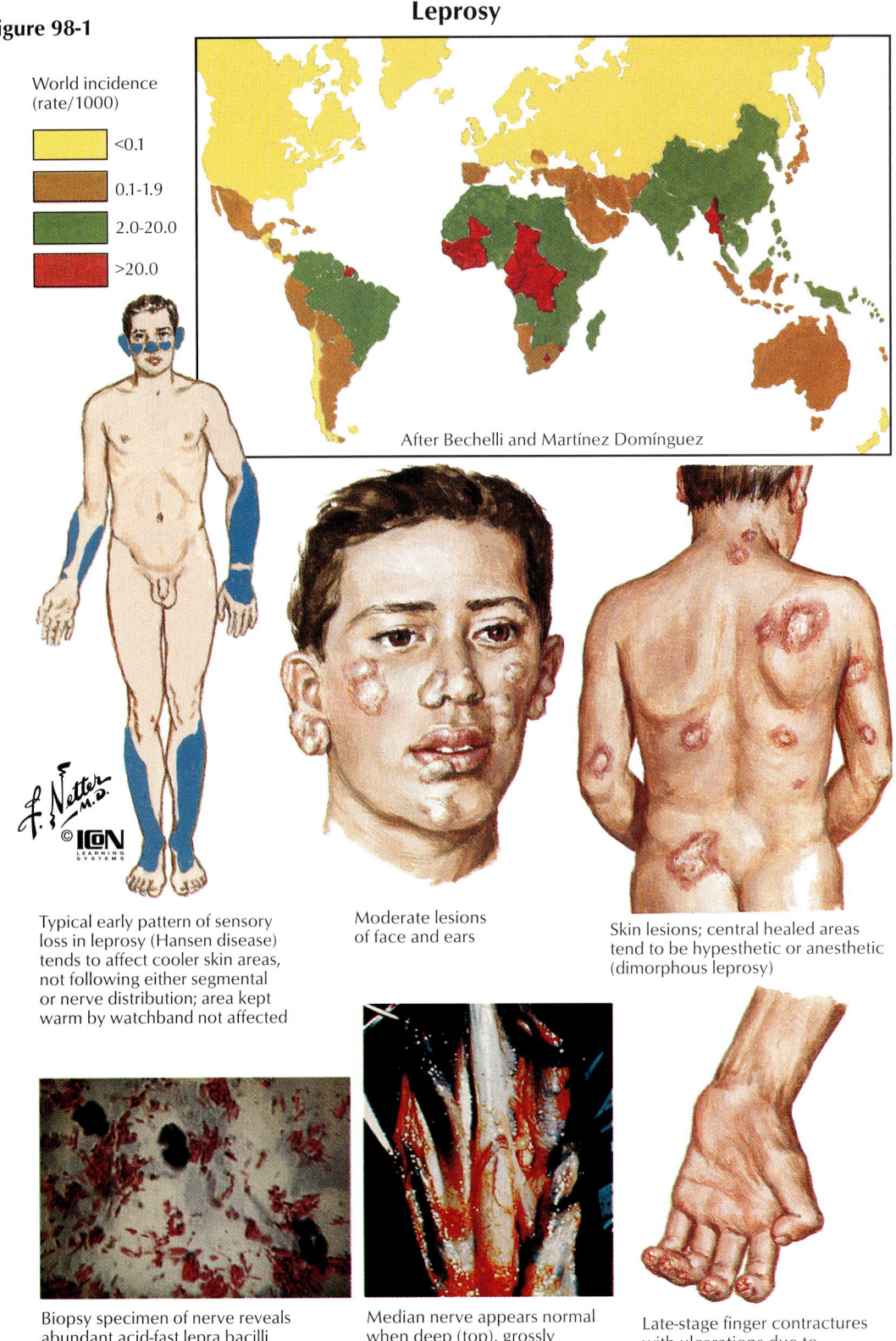

Figure 98-1

POLYNEUROPATHIES AND AUTONOMIC DISORDERS

840

spectrum of leprosy, extending from **tuberculoid** to **borderline tuberculoid**, **borderline**, **borderline lepromatous**, and **lepromatous**. Indeterminate leprosy, seen early in the infection, is diagnosed by the presence of a single or a few skin macules having variable sensory loss.

In **tuberculoid** (tuberculoid and borderline tuberculoid) **leprosy**, the preserved cell-mediated immunity prevents significant dissemination of the bacillus, precluding more severe disease. Patients usually have asymmetrically distributed hypopigmented anesthetic lesions with erythematous margins and an associated asymmetric multifocal neuropathy (mononeuritis multiplex). Involved nerves are concomitantly enlarged, particularly the ulnar, posterior auricular, peroneal, and posterior tibial nerves. Skin or nerve biopsies demonstrate well-demarcated, noncaseating granulomas with many lymphocytes, Langhans giant cells, and few bacilli.

Borderline leprosy stands between lepromatous and tuberculoid leprosy in severity and disease manifestation. After patients receive treatment, they usually move toward the tuberculoid pole of the spectrum.

Lepromatous and borderline lepromatous leprosy are the most severe forms with unrestricted bacterial multiplication and hematogenous dissemination. They particularly multiply in cooler body areas, such as the superficial nerves, nose, earlobe, skin, testes, and eyes. Nerve involvement is symmetric and more extensive than in tuberculoid leprosy. Cutaneous lesions are skin-colored nodules or papules that coalesce to form extensive symmetric raised plaques. On the face, they result in leonine facies. Skin biopsies demonstrate vacuolated foam cells within the dermis containing large numbers of *M leprae*, with few inflammatory cells, and no granulomas.

The ulnar is the most commonly involved peripheral nerve; when associated with median nerve involvement, the combination leads to clawing of the hand. Peroneal neuropathies are most common in the leg. At its extreme, patients with leprosy neuropathies develop autoamputation of digits, recurrent nonhealing ulcers that often result in osteomyelitis, and nasal bridge collapse.

Erythema Nodosum Leprosum and Reversal Reactions

Leprosy can be complicated by different reactional states, namely **erythema nodosum leprosum** and reversal reactions. Erythema nodosum leprosum is characterized by the development of crops of new, small, tender subcutaneous nodules accompanied by fever, arthralgias, adenopathy, and neuritis. Reversal reactions present as inflamed, indurated skin plaques with neuritis and represent a change in the patient's immune response to the infection. Tumor necrosis factor a is considered a key mediator in Hansen disease and reactional states.

DIAGNOSTIC APPROACH AND TREATMENT

Other disorders that may present with similar skin lesions include **sarcoidosis**, **leishmaniasis**, **lupus vulgaris**, **syphilis**, **yaws,** and **granuloma annulare**. However, no other disease has hypopigmented anesthetic skin lesions. Leprosy diagnosis depends on clinical findings and the results of skin biopsy, a less invasive procedure than nerve biopsy.

Multidrug treatment with the antibiotic combination of rifampin, dapsone, and clofazimine is highly effective. Recurrence occurs with high bacterial loads and after 5 years of initial treatment. Severe neural damage is the major complication of reactional states and responds to oral prednisone. Thalidomide, the preferred medication for severe erythema nodosum leprosum, has significant teratogenic potential. Management also includes injury prevention to anesthetized areas, hygiene maintenance, and reconstructive plastic surgery such as nasal reconstruction.

FUTURE DIRECTIONS

Multidrug treatment has resulted in a 90% reduction in disease prevalence. The global leprosy elimination campaigns aim toward early disease detection and completion of predefined treatment regimens. The World Health Organization hoped that leprosy would be eliminated (<1 case per 10,000 persons) as a public health problem by the year 2000; however, this was not achieved. Although specific preventive vaccines are not available, bacille Calmette-Guerin is variably effective. The mapping of the genome for the *M leprae* bacterium and better understanding of disease pathogenesis may result in more effective prevention and therapies.

The main drawback to treating this eminently curable disease is the limited resource availability in countries where leprosy is endemic. Greater provision of funds and medical expertise by the international community would help to overcome this.

REFERENCES

Ooi WW, Moschella SL. Update on leprosy in immigrants in the United States: status in the year 2000. *Clin Infect Dis*. 2001;32:930-937.

Ooi WW, Srinivasan J. Leprosy and the peripheral nervous system: basic and clinical aspects. *Muscle Nerve*. 2004;30:393-409.

Sabin TD, Swift TR, Jacobson RR. Leprosy. In: Dyck PJ and Thomas PK, eds. *Peripheral Neuropathy*. Philadelphia, Pa: WB Saunders; 1993:1354-1379.

Chapter 99
Disorders of the Autonomic Nervous System

Ted M. Burns, Jayashri Srinivasan, and James A. Russell

Clinical Vignette

A 56-year-old man presented with subacute onset of severe unexplained constipation. Over the next 2 weeks, he developed dry mouth, dry eyes, decreased sweating, urinary hesitancy, and orthostatic intolerance resulting in syncope. His previous medical history was unremarkable. His only medication was aspirin. He smoked 1 pack per day and drank sparingly. His family history was noncontributory.

The patient's blood pressure was 124/76 mm Hg supine and 66/40 mm Hg standing at 1 minute, with bradycardia while supine and standing, impaired pupillary responses to light and accommodation, and dry mucous membranes. His remaining general and neurologic examination results were normal.

Tilt table testing results confirmed bradycardia with orthostatic hypotension. Sweat testing demonstrated profound anhidrosis.

Paraneoplastic autoantibody studies revealed increased antibodies to ganglionic nicotinic acetylcholine receptors. Chest CT demonstrated left hilar adenopathy. Small cell lung carcinoma was diagnosed at bronchoscopic biopsy. The patient's orthostatic intolerance and constipation resolved after the third course of chemotherapy. Remission has persisted. Development of signs and symptoms related to parasympathetic and sympathetic dysfunction in the absence of central or other peripheral nervous system abnormalities was compatible with an autonomic neuropathy.

Primary autonomic polyneuropathies represent an uncommon subgroup of disorders. However, many length-dependent polyneuropathies have various degrees of autonomic fiber involvement, occasionally with important implications. An associated dysautonomia is the major pathophysiologic mechanism leading to rare deaths in **Guillain-Barré syndrome**. More commonly, patients' daily living activities are impacted by dysautonomic complications of common polyneuropathies. Impotence is a prime example in young patients with diabetic polyneuropathies.

CLINICAL PRESENTATION

Typically, patients have combinations of parasympathetic and sympathetic dysfunction (Figure 99-1). The former is characterized by dry mucous membranes, particularly noticeable in the eyes and mouth, with varying gastrointestinal involvement manifested as early satiety, nausea, vomiting, constipation, diarrhea, urinary bladder dysmotility, and erectile dysfunction.

Disorders of sweating and sudden feelings of severe light-headedness or syncope when assuming an upright posture are usual symptoms of impaired sympathetic function. Combinations of parasympathetic and sympathetic disorders affect sexual function. Signs of autonomic dysfunction include fixed heart rates, tonic pupils, and orthostatic hypotension, with normal strength and sensory examination (ie, sparing the somatic nerves).

Acute or subacute autonomic neuropathies are usually related to toxic, metabolic, or autoimmune disorders. In the absence of toxic or metabolic influences, **autoimmune paraneoplastic disorders** should be considered the primary mechanism.

DIFFERENTIAL DIAGNOSIS
Acute Disorders

Antecedent viral infections occur in more than half of patients with autoimmune autonomic neuropathy, suggesting that it may be a Guillain-Barré syndrome variant. Patients with **acute**

DISORDERS OF THE AUTONOMIC NERVOUS SYSTEM

Figure 99-1A

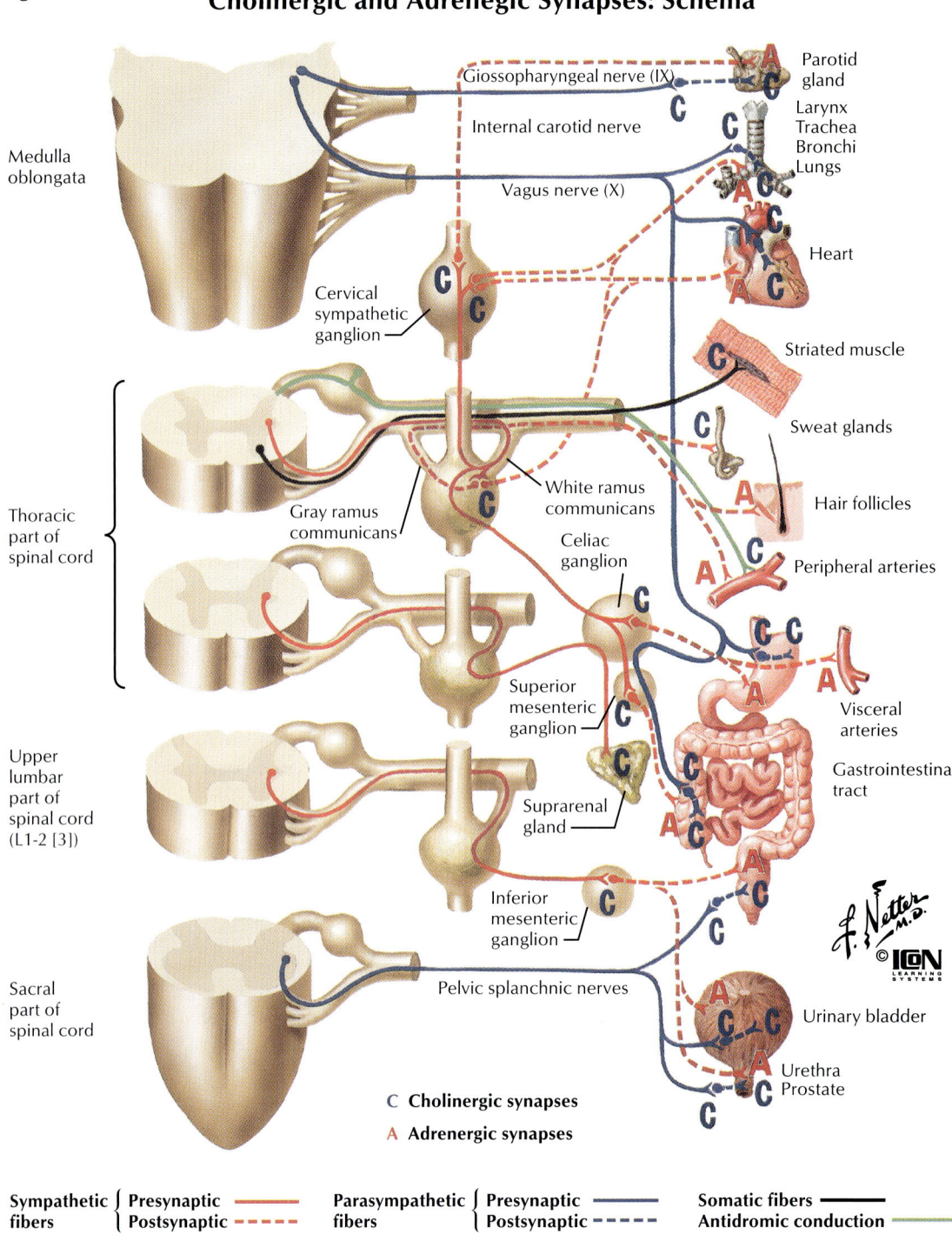

POLYNEUROPATHIES AND AUTONOMIC DISORDERS

DISORDERS OF THE AUTONOMIC NERVOUS SYSTEM

Figure 99-1B **Symptoms of Dysautonomia With Polyneuropathies**

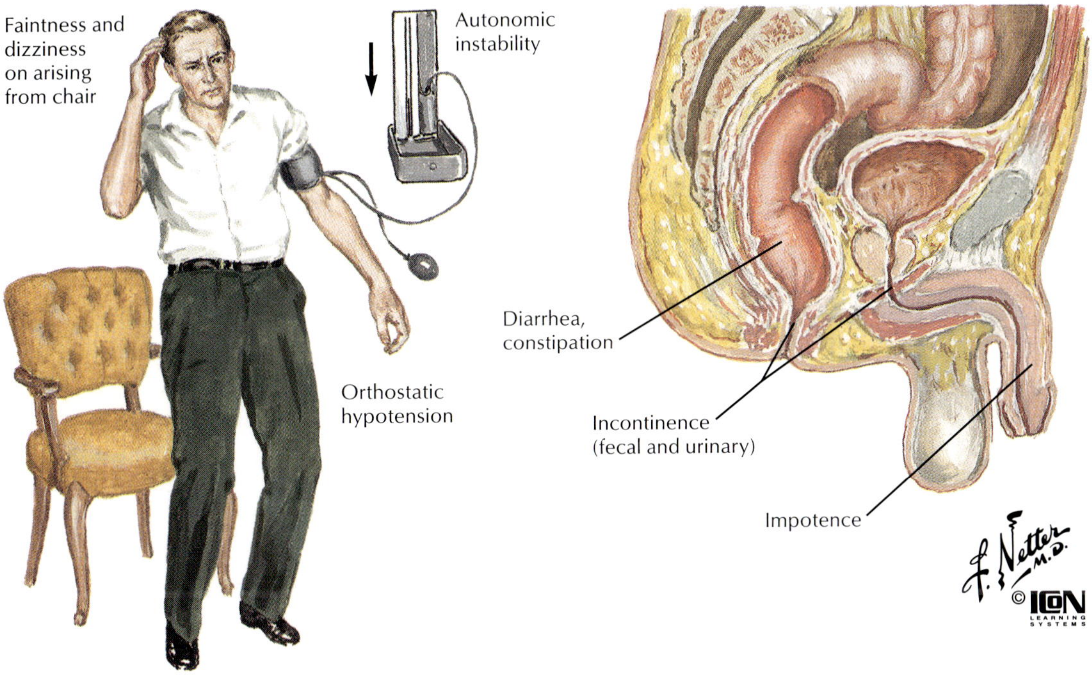

- Faintness and dizziness on arising from chair
- Autonomic instability
- Orthostatic hypotension
- Diarrhea, constipation
- Incontinence (fecal and urinary)
- Impotence

pandysautonomic neuropathy present with rapid onset of sympathetic and parasympathetic dysfunction. They may have generalized and severe disorders, but restricted milder forms also occur. Orthostatic intolerance and gastrointestinal dysmotility are common presentations.

Autonomic tests are almost always abnormal. Nerve biopsies demonstrate inflammatory infiltrates supporting an immune-mediated hypothesis. Recovery is slow and often incomplete. High titers of ganglionic acetylcholine receptor antibodies are reported in approximately half of these patients, supporting the presumed autoimmune basis.

Guillain-Barré syndrome preferentially involves somatic motor fibers but also causes dysautonomia in two thirds of cases, especially affecting the cardiovascular and gastrointestinal systems. Bladder dysfunction is less common. Autonomic complications may be life threatening; patients often must be monitored in the ICU.

Paraneoplastic autonomic neuropathy is often indistinguishable from primary autoimmune autonomic neuropathy. Gastrointestinal dysmotility is a common presenting manifestation. Antineuronal nuclear antibody type 1 is associated with small cell lung cancer. It is the most frequently demonstrated abnormal paraneoplastic neurologic antibody, including paraneoplastic autonomic neuropathy.

Hereditary **porphyria** presents with acute attacks of dysautonomic symptoms (abdominal pain, vomiting, constipation, hypertension, and tachycardia) in addition to predominantly motor polyneuropathies. Diagnosis requires demonstration of increased urinary excretion of porphobilinogen.

Certain chemicals, including various **medications**, particularly cisplatinum and vinca alkaloids, cause peripheral neuropathies, sometimes including autonomic features. Other specific **nerve toxins** such as organophosphates, heavy metals (ie, thallium and arsenic), hexacarbons, and acrylamide may produce autonomic peripheral neuropathies.

Chronic Disorders

Diabetic autonomic neuropathies are common complications of diabetic (somatic) neuropathies and often correlate with the duration of diabetes. Early clinical autonomic testing often reveals evidence of cardiovagal dysfunc-

POLYNEUROPATHIES AND AUTONOMIC DISORDERS

DISORDERS OF THE AUTONOMIC NERVOUS SYSTEM

tion manifested by impairment of heart rate response to Valsalva maneuver or to deep breathing.

Postural orthostatic tachycardia syndrome is seen predominantly in young women. It is characterized by orthostatic symptoms associated with significant rise in heart rate on standing without orthostatic hypotension or other clinical or laboratory evidence of autonomic neuropathy, except for distal sweat loss. The pathophysiology of postural orthostatic tachycardia syndrome is heterogeneous. It may include limited autonomic neuropathies, hypovolemia, and deconditioning.

Amyloidosis is a multisystem disorder that may be sporadic or familial. Autonomic neuropathy may occur and may present with symptoms of somatic small fiber dysfunction, orthostatic intolerance, and constipation alternating with diarrhea.

Pure autonomic failure is also known as ***idiopathic autonomic hypotension***. It is an insidious process with typical signs of disordered autonomic function. The absence of parkinsonian features helps differentiate this disorder from multiple systems atrophy. It results from postganglionic sympathetic neuron degeneration.

Hereditary autonomic neuropathies are rare disorders. **Hereditary sensory and autonomic neuropathy type III**, also known as ***Riley Day syndrome***, is an autosomal recessive disorder presenting with defective control of blood pressure, sweating, temperature, and lacrimation in children. Dysautonomic manifestations are less pronounced in the other hereditary sensory and autonomic neuropathies.

Central Disorders

Parkinson disease results in loss of pigmented substantia nigra dopaminergic cells and other pigmented nuclei, including the locus ceruleus and the dorsal vagal nucleus, at least partially explaining the associated autonomic dysfunction. Peripheral sympathetic heart denervation is common, resulting in orthostatic hypotension in severe cases.

Multiple systems atrophy is a degenerative disorder characterized by parkinsonian features with autonomic, cerebellar, and corticospinal involvement. When autonomic symptoms predominate, the disorder is called ***Shy-Drager syndrome***. Depletion of catecholaminergic neurons in the brainstem contributes to development of orthostatic hypotension. Other autonomic symptoms include bladder dysfunction, constipation, sexual dysfunction, orthostatic intolerance, and stridor.

Autonomic symptoms are also seen with spinal cord disorders such as **trauma**, **syringomyelia**, and **multiple sclerosis**. They usually consist of arrhythmias, blood pressure lability, and bladder atony.

DIAGNOSTIC APPROACH

Patients with dysautonomic symptoms require careful, complete neurologic examinations to find concomitant features of CNS involvement. EMG is necessary to search for somatic neuropathy findings.

Heart rate responses to Valsalva maneuvers and deep breathing are used to assess cardiovagal parasympathetic function. Commonly used parameters to assess sympathetic competency include blood pressure responses to standing and to Valsalva maneuvers and quantitative measurements of sweat production in response to cholinergic stimuli. The latter is typically done at 4 standardized locations to detect the abnormality pattern.

Quantitative sensory testing comparing thresholds for vibration to cold- and heat-pain thresholds is helpful for detecting small myelinated and unmyelinated somatic peripheral nerve dysfunction. Quantitation of intraepidermal nerve fiber density by **skin punch biopsy** and subsequent immunostaining directed at axons is performed at some centers to assess the severity of small-fiber loss.

Comprehensive screening for all recognized paraneoplastic antibodies is recommended in acute to subacute cases where **paraneoplastic autonomic neuropathy** is possible.

TREATMENT AND PROGNOSIS

Primary treatment consists of specific therapies for underlying diseases and, when possible, symptomatic relief. **Nonpharmacologic treatments** of orthostatic hypotension include increasing intake of dietary salt and water, eating smaller and more frequent meals, avoiding alcohol, and wearing elastic stockings or abdominal binders. **Medications** include sympathetic agents such as midodrine and fluid- and salt-conserving agents such as fludrocortisone. Orthostatic symptoms in postural tachycardia syndrome may respond to low-dose β blockers or low-dose midodrine.

Bladder dysfunction in most dysautonomic conditions is characterized by failure to empty. Treatments include timed voiding, intermittent catheterizations and, rarely, indwelling catheters. Pharmacologic agents that promote bladder emptying, such as bethanechol, have limited efficacy. Bladder pacemakers may benefit select patients.

Treatment of erectile dysfunction includes agents such as sildenafil, yohimbine, topical nitroglycerin or minoxidil, injections of prostaglandins, or penile implants.

Gastrointestinal dysfunction is best aided by strategies to maintain hydration and nutrition. Gastroparesis is treated with prokinetic agents such as metoclopramide; constipation is treated with increased fiber and laxatives.

Plasma exchange and IV immunoglobulin are used for the treatment of suspected immune-mediated autonomic neuropathy with variable success.

Prognosis depends on the etiology, severity, and overall degree of autonomic dysfunction. Autoimmune autonomic neuropathies often have a limited, unsatisfactory improvement. Patients with Guillain-Barré syndrome usually experience complete resolution of autonomic dysfunction in parallel with clinical recovery of strength. Prognosis for chronic peripheral and central autonomic disorders is less favorable.

REFERENCES

Benarroch EE, Smithson IL, Low PA, Parisi JE. Depletion of catacholaminergic neurons in the rostral ventrolateral medulla in multiple system atrophy with autonomic failure. *Ann Neurol.* 1998;43:56-163.

Cohen J, Low P, Fealey R, Sheps S, Jiang N-S. Somatic and autonomic function in progressive autonomic failure and multiple system atrophy. *Ann Neurol.* 1987;22:692-699.

Low PA, Vernino S, Suarez G. Autonomic dysfunction in peripheral nerve disease. *Muscle Nerve.* 2003;27:646-661.

Vernino S, Low PA, Fealey RD, Stewart JD, Farrugia G, Lennon VA. Autoantibodies to ganglionic acetylcholine receptors in autoimmune autonomic neuropathies. *N Engl J Med.* 2000;343:847-855.

Section XXIII
NEUROMUSCULAR TRANSMISSION DISORDERS

Chapter 100
Neuromuscular Junction Anatomy and Physiology . .850

Chapter 101
Lambert-Eaton Myasthenic Syndrome 858

Chapter 102
Myasthenia Gravis 864

Chapter 100
Neuromuscular Junction Anatomy and Physiology

Monique M. Ryan

NORMAL NEUROMUSCULAR TRANSMISSION

As motor nerves approach the endplate, they branch repeatedly and lose their myelin sheaths. Single nerve fibers ultimately divide into smaller branches, ending in swollen tips (terminal boutons) just before reaching the muscle endplate (Figure 100-1). Individual nerve terminals contain thousands of vesicles aligned near the presynaptic membrane. Each vesicle holds 5000 to 12,000 acetylcholine (ACh) molecules. Neuronal depolarization triggers an increase in free calcium within the nerve terminal, causing the opening of voltage-gated calcium channels and mobilization of synaptic vesicles. The synaptic vesicles then fuse with the terminal membrane (Figure 100-2). Vesicular packets, or quanta, of ACh are released into and diffuse across the synaptic cleft (Figure 100-3). Some ACh binds to postsynaptic nicotinic receptors; the rest is hydrolyzed by acetylcholinesterase within the basement membrane of the synaptic cleft. Choline thus released is absorbed back into the presynaptic terminal and recycled.

The **postsynaptic endplate** is a specialized region of the muscle membrane with involuted crests and valleys. **ACh receptors** (AChRs) are concentrated on the shoulders of each crest. The nicotinic AChR is assembled from 5 subunits: two a and single β, δ, and ε subunits. Fetal AChRs contain γ rather than epsilon subunits. Adult nicotinic AChRs include a transmembrane pore and binding sites for ACh and other agonists and antagonists. Binding of ACh molecules to the a subunit of AChR initiates conformational changes that result in opening of ligand-binding cation channels, causing local sodium entry. Each quanta of ACh thus results in a small local postsynaptic depolarization called a *miniature endplate potential*.

When summation of the endplate potentials is sufficient (usually requiring 20-200 quanta) to reach the depolarization threshold of the muscle fiber, activation of voltage-gated sodium channels causes an electrical propagation wave and generalized depolarization of the muscle cell membrane, ie, the muscle fiber action potential. This depolarization then triggers activation of dihydropyridine and ryanodine receptors within the transverse tubules and sarcoplasmic reticulum. A subsequent release of large amounts of calcium results in muscle contraction. Repolarization of nerve and muscle cells occurs by closure of sodium channels, slower opening of chloride channels, and return of the membrane potential to its resting level (-70 to -90 mV).

ALTERATION OF NEUROMUSCULAR TRANSMISSION

Pharmacologic agents can influence neuromuscular transmission by altering ACh release, ACh degradation, or the response of the neuromuscular junction to ACh (Tables 100-1 and 100-2).

Presynaptic ACh release is inhibited by botulinum toxin, which blocks exocytosis of synaptic vesicles and hence decreases ACh release after neuronal depolarization. Hypocalcemia and hypermagnesemia also decrease ACh release; quantal size is normal, but fewer quanta are released. Muscle weakness results from failure to release sufficient ACh quanta to trigger muscle endplate action potentials and contraction.

Acetylcholine synthesis and release is also diminished by pharmacologic agents, such as

NEUROMUSCULAR JUNCTION ANATOMY AND PHYSIOLOGY

Figure 100-1   Somatic Neuromuscular Transmission

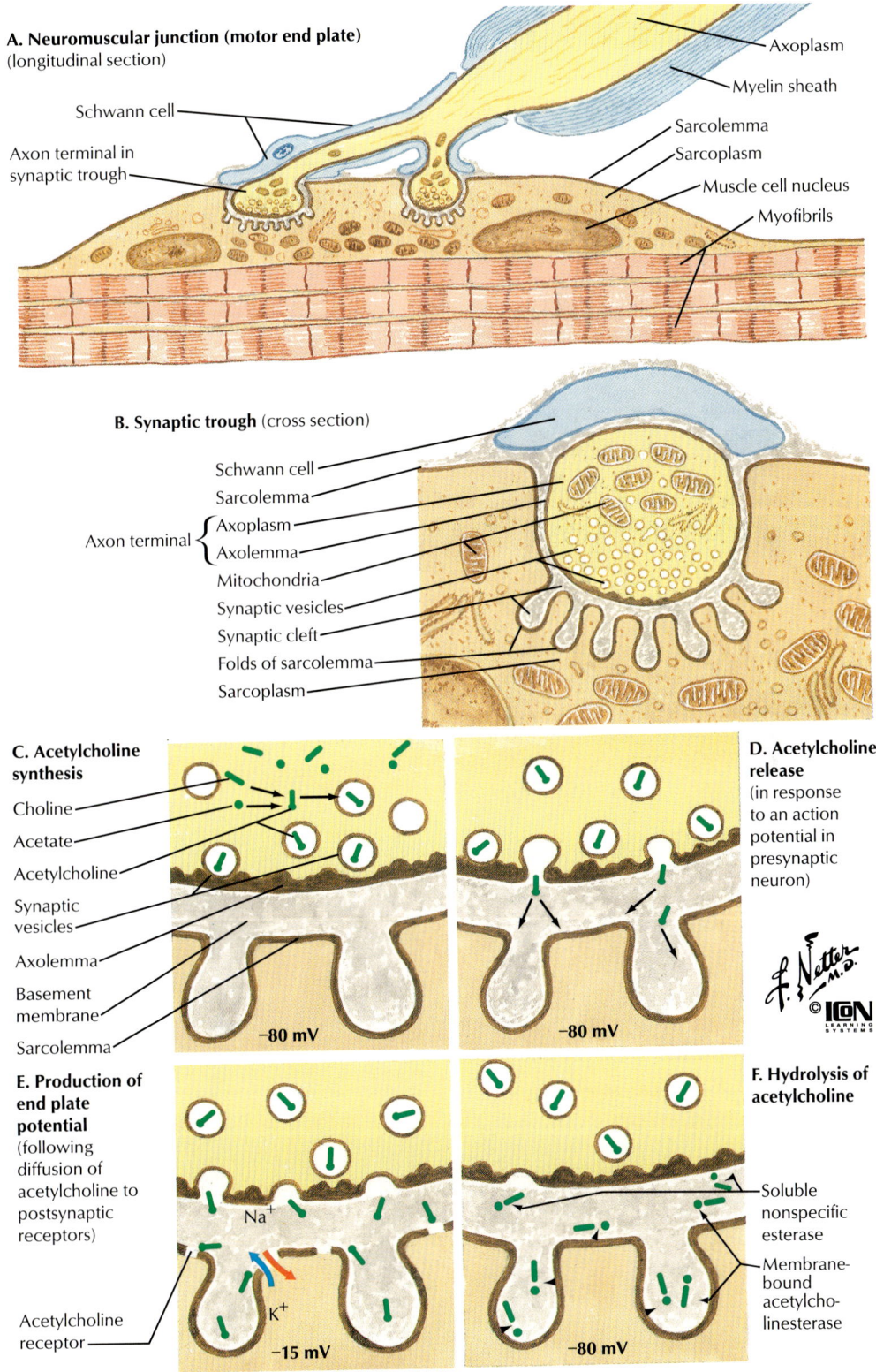

NEUROMUSCULAR TRANSMISSION DISORDERS

NEUROMUSCULAR JUNCTION ANATOMY AND PHYSIOLOGY

Figure 100-2

Neuromuscular Transmission

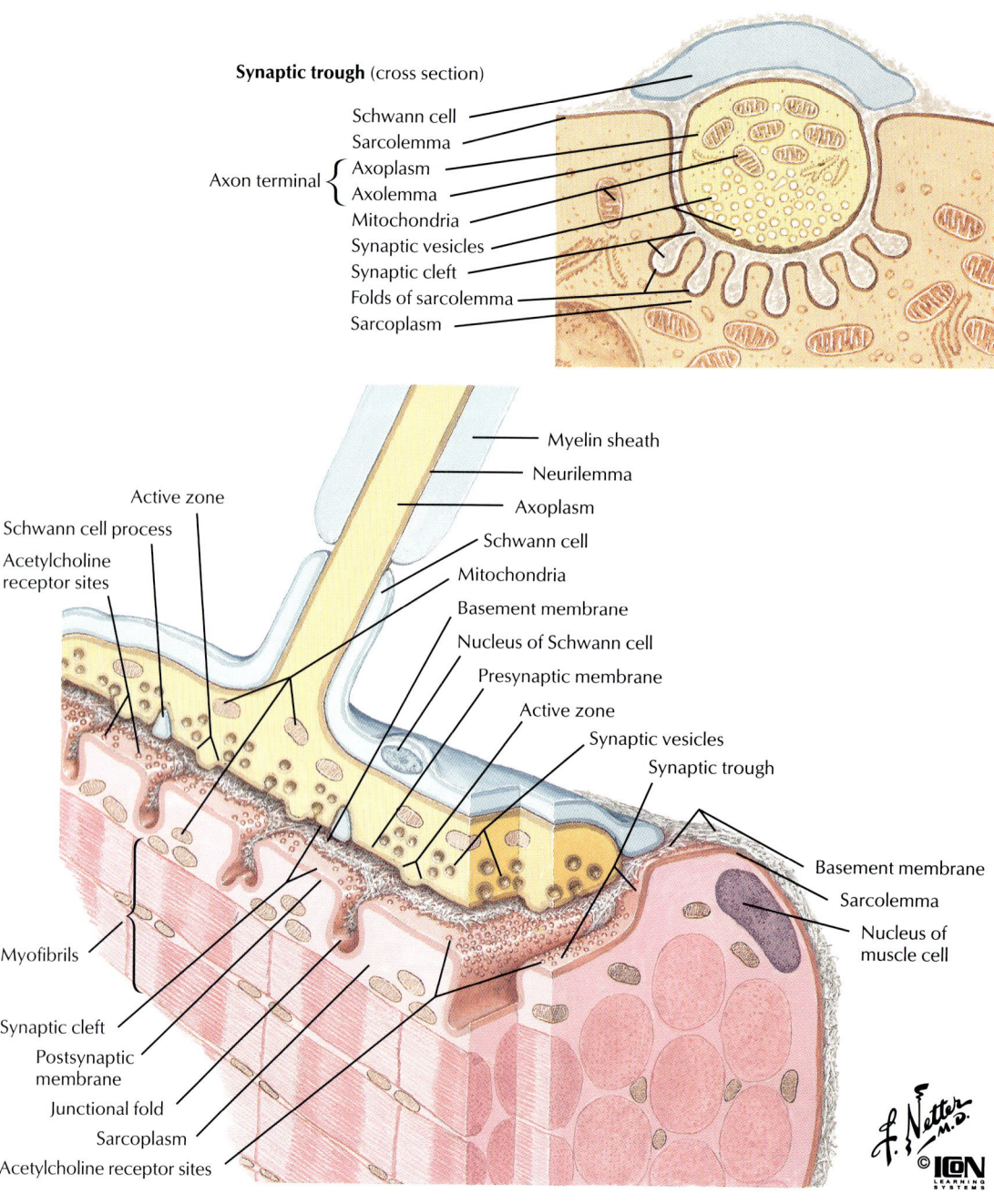

NEUROMUSCULAR TRANSMISSION DISORDERS

NEUROMUSCULAR JUNCTION ANATOMY AND PHYSIOLOGY

Figure 100-3

Neuromuscular Junction

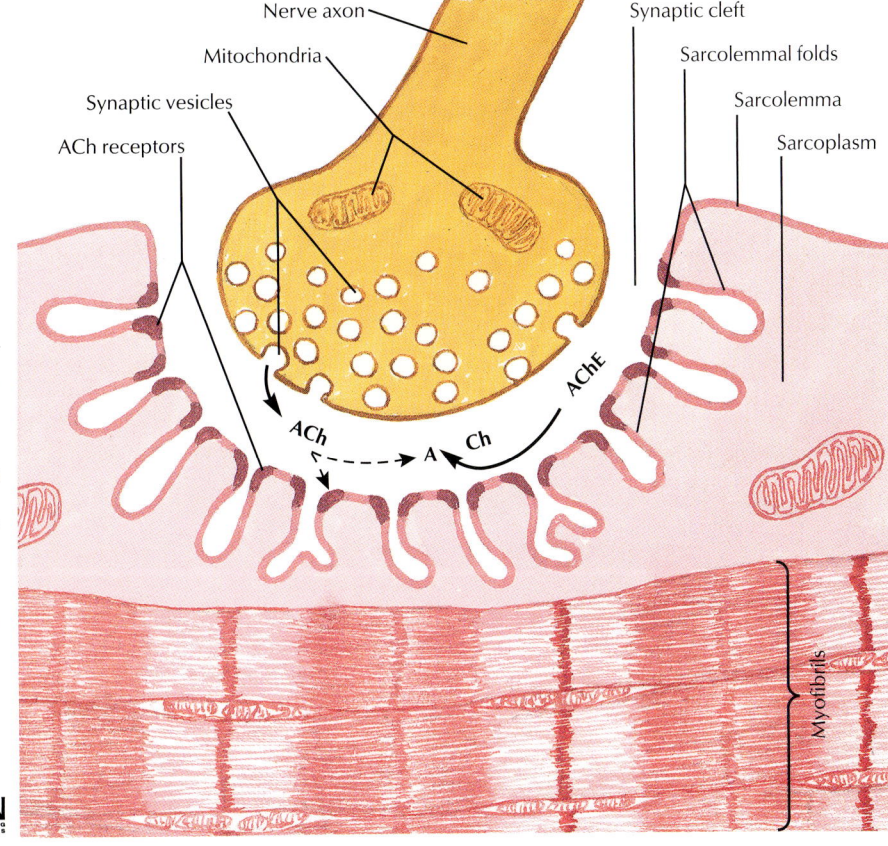

Normal neuromuscular junction
Synaptic vesicles containing acetylcholine (ACh) form in nerve terminal. In response to nerve impulse, vesicles discharge ACh into synaptic cleft. ACh binds to receptor sites on muscle sarcolemma to initiate muscle contraction. Acetylcholinesterase (AChE) hydrolyzes ACh, thus limiting effect and duration of its action.

hemicholinium, which decrease choline reuptake at the presynaptic membrane. The resultant ACh depletion results in release of smaller quanta and a decreased likelihood of endplate action potential generation after neuronal depolarization.

Acetylcholinesterase inhibitors increase ACh availability at the postsynaptic membrane and produce larger endplate potentials, thereby inhibiting ACh degradation. Some of these compounds are structurally similar to ACh and may have some direct depolarizing effect at the postsynaptic AChR. Compounds such as physostigmine, neostigmine, and edrophonium are used therapeutically to increase ACh availability in conditions of impaired neuromuscular transmission, such as myasthenia gravis, and to reverse competitive neuromuscular blockade, used with anesthesia, after surgical procedures.

In contrast, the organophosphorous compounds, such as malathion and parathion, irreversibly bind to acetylcholinesterase. The return of cholinesterase activity therefore depends on synthesis of new receptors. Organophosphorous compounds are used as agricultural insecticides and in chemical warfare.

The depolarizing action of ACh at the neuromuscular junction is inhibited by the ACh antagonists, or nondepolarizing neuromuscular blockers, such as tubocurarine and pancuronium. Chemically related to ACh, they compete with it for binding sites within the AChR. By occupying AChR sites but not causing local membrane depolarization, they decrease the size of endplate potentials in response to ACh release. These agents are used clinically as adjuncts to anesthesia to relax skeletal muscle and facilitate intubation.

NEUROMUSCULAR TRANSMISSION DISORDERS

853

NEUROMUSCULAR JUNCTION ANATOMY AND PHYSIOLOGY

Table 100-1
Action of Drugs on Nerve Excitability

Drug	Action on Membrane	Changes in Membrane Potential and Action Potential	Clinical Effects
Tetrodotoxin (puffer fish toxin) Saxitoxin (shellfish toxin)	Blocks voltage-sensitive Na^+ channels	Blocks action potential	Nerve block, paralysis, death
Tetraethylammonium (TEA)	Blocks K^+ permeability channels	Decreases resting potential (partial depolarization); prolongs action potential	?
Increased external potassium concentration	Makes K^+ equilibrium potential (E_{K^+}) less negative	Decreases resting potential (partial depolarization), thereby causing accommodation that decreases action potential size and increases threshold for action potential	Nerve block, plus action on many systems causing varied clinical picture
Metabolic inhibitors (cyanide) Cardiac glycosides (ouabain)	Block active transport, allowing Na^+ to accumulate in axoplasm, K^+ to leak out		
Low external calcium concentration	Destabilizes membrane: A. Ionic permeability increased B. Increases change in Na^+ permeability produced by depolarization	A. Resting potential shifts in depolarized direction (partial depolarization) B. Threshold level shifts in hyperpolarized direction A. and B. may induce repetitive firing	Hyperexcitability, tetany
Local anesthetics (procaine)	Stabilizes membrane: A. Ionic permeability produced by depolarization B. Decreases change in Na^+ permeability produced by depolarization	A. Resting potential constant B. Threshold level shifts in depolarized direction until approaching impulse can no longer trigger action potential	Nerve block

Such agents as nicotine and succinylcholine, the cholinomimetics, chemically resemble ACh and cause endplate depolarization. Their effect is more prolonged than that of ACh, causing an initial brief period of repetitive excitation, which may appear clinically as muscle fasciculations. Ultimately, however, the prolonged depolarization of the muscle endplate causes a conformational change in the adjacent sodium channels, rendering them inactive. The neuromuscular junction becomes refractory to ACh, causing a complete block of neuromuscular transmission and a flaccid paralysis. The only depolarizing neuromuscular blocker in common clinical usage is succinylcholine (suxamethonium).

Neuromuscular junction physiology is also affected by a range of pharmacologic interactions and diseases (Figure 100-4). Many antibiotics, including aminoglycosides and tetracycline, may reduce quantal release from the presynaptic terminals. Anesthetic agents, antiarrhythmics, and phenytoin stabilize the postjunctional membrane and render it less likely to depolarize.

Table 100-2
Pharmacology of Neuromuscular Junction*

	Effect on Supply of ACh in Terminal	Effect on Amount of ACh Released in Terminal by Action Potential	Effect on Amplitude of Endplate Potential	Effect of Muscle Response to Application of ACh	Direct Effect on Muscle Membrane Resting Potential	Clinical Effect
AChR blockers Botulinum toxin Low Ca^{2+} or high Mg^{2+} concentration	—	Decreased (fewer quanta)	Decreased	—	—	Paralysis (low Ca^{2+} concentration may also produce tetany by direct action on nerves)
Choline uptake inhibitors Hemicholinium Triethylcholine	Decreased	Decreased (smaller quanta)	Decreased	—	—	Paresis
Cholinesterase inhibitors Physostigmine Neostigmine Edrophonium	—	—	Increased; prolonged	Increased; prolonged	Depolarized slightly in high doses	Muscle power and duration of contraction increased
Organophosphorous compounds (nerve gases)	—	—	Increased; prolonged	Increased; prolonged	No change	Convulsions
ACh (nicotinic) antagonists D-Tubocurarine Pancuronium triethiodide Vecuronium	—	—	Decreased	Decreased	Depolarized (in high dosage)	Paralysis
Cholinomimetics Nicotine Decamethonium Succinylcholine	—	—	Decreased (by desensitization)	Decreased (by desensitization)	Strongly depolarized	Paralysis

*ACh indicates acetylcholine; AChR, acetylcholine receptor.

NEUROMUSCULAR JUNCTION ANATOMY AND PHYSIOLOGY

Figure 100-4A

Physiology of Neuromuscular Junction

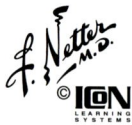

Labels (left side):
- Sarcolemma
- Basement membrane
- Synaptic cleft
- Schwann cell
- Axon terminal
- Axolemma
- Axon
- Myelin sheath
- Electric impulse propagated along axon by inflow of Na$^+$ and outflow of K$^+$
- Electric impulse
- Acetylcholine (ACh) formed in nerve terminal from acetate derived from acetyl CoA of mitochondria plus choline, catalyzed by choline acetyltransferase. ACh enters synaptic vesicles.
- Electric impulse traverses sarcolemma to transverse tubules where it causes release of Ca^{2+} from sarcoplasmic reticulum, thus initiating muscle contraction.

Labels (right side):
- Sarcoplasm
- Electric impulse causes channels to open in presynaptic membrane, permitting Ca^{2+} to enter nerve terminal.
- Postsynaptic membrane
- Ca^{2+} binds to sites at active zone of presynaptic membrane, causing release of ACh from vesicles.
- Junctional fold
- ACh receptors
- ACh attaches to receptors of postsynaptic membrane at apex of junctional folds, causing channels to open for inflow of Na$^+$ and outflow of K$^+$, which results in depolarization and initiation of electric impulse (action potential).
- Acetylcholinesterase (AChE) promptly degrades ACh into acetate and choline, thus terminating its activity.
- Choline reenters nerve terminal to be recycled.

NEUROMUSCULAR TRANSMISSION DISORDERS

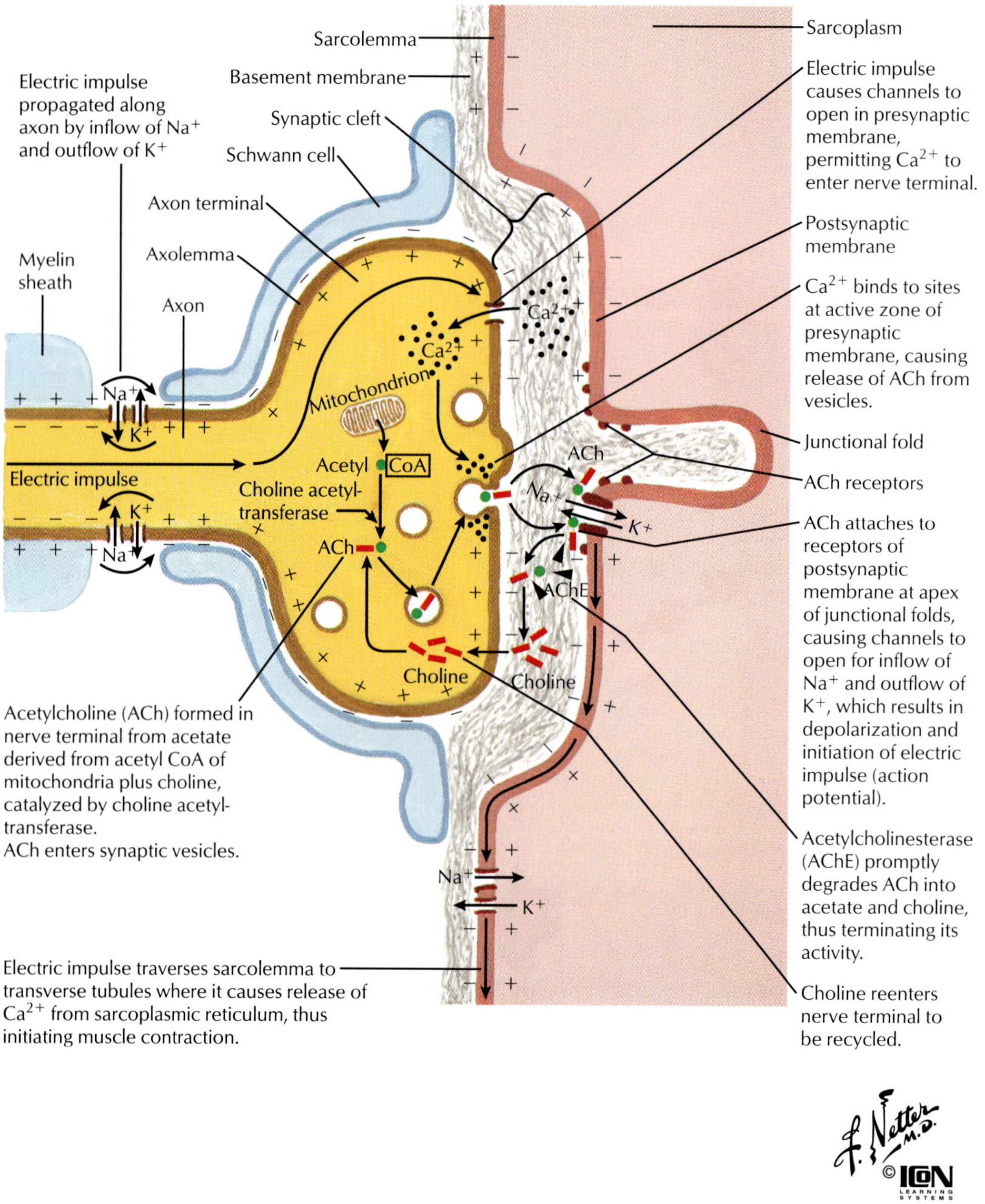

NEUROMUSCULAR JUNCTION ANATOMY AND PHYSIOLOGY

Figure 100-4B   Pharmacology of Neuromuscular Transmission

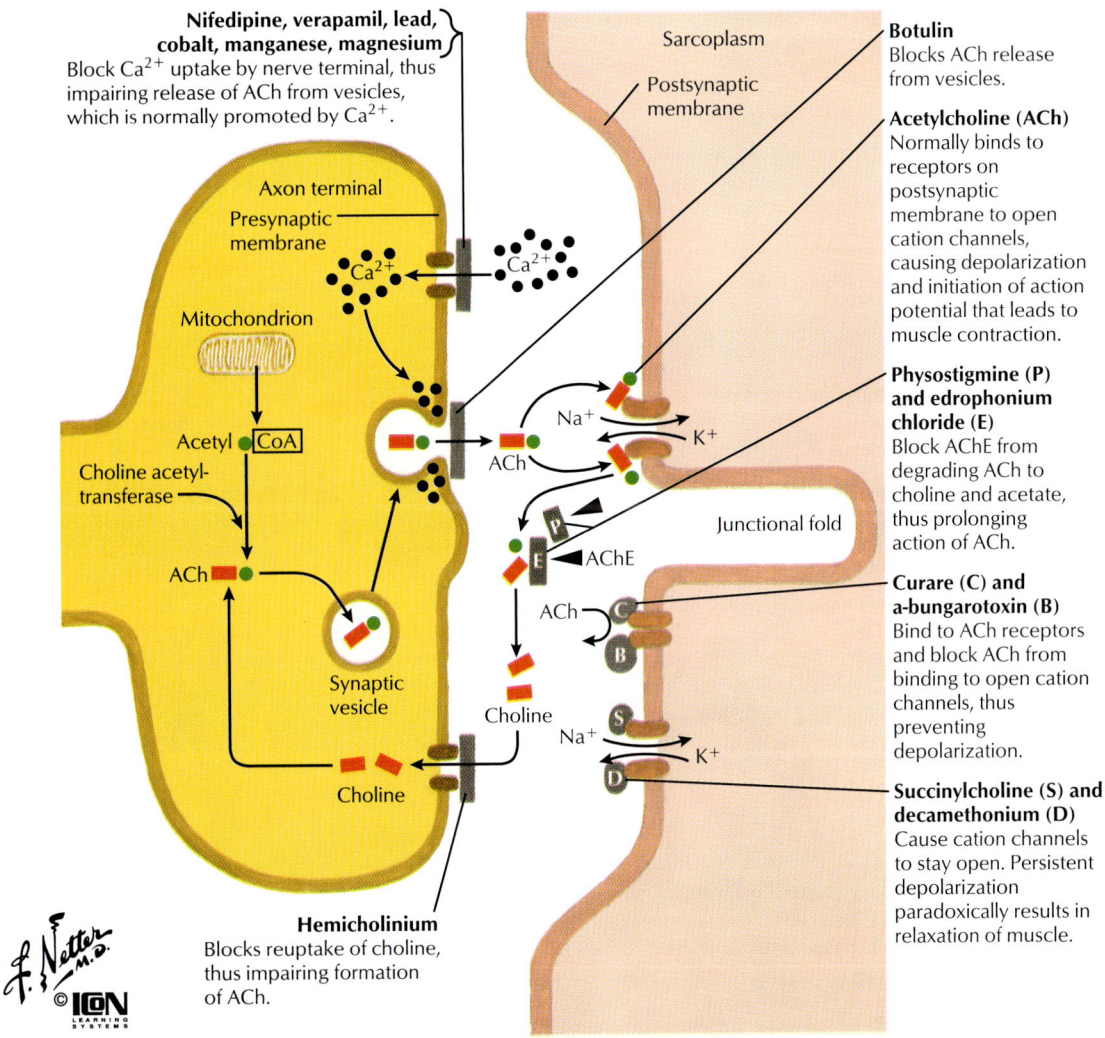

REFERENCES

Jennekens FG, Veldman H, Wokke JH. Histology and pathology of the human neuromuscular junction with a description of the clinical features of the myasthenic syndromes. In: DeBaets MH, Oosterhuis HJ, eds. *Myasthenia Gravis.* Boca Raton, Fla: CRC Press, 1993:99-145.

Kim YI, Lomo T, Lupa MT, Thesleff S. Miniature end-plate potentials in rat skeletal muscle poisoned with botulinum toxin. *J Physiol.* 1984;356:587-599.

Simpson LL. Kinetic studies on the interaction between botulinum toxin type A and the cholinergic neuromuscular junction. *J Pharmacol Exp Ther.* 1980;212:16-21.

Whittaker VP. The nature of acetylcholine pools in brain tissue. *Prog Brain Res.* 1969;31:211-222.

Chapter 101
Lambert-Eaton Myasthenic Syndrome

Ted M. Burns and H. Royden Jones, Jr

Clinical Vignette

A 64-year-old woman presented with a 1-year history of progressive fatigue, particularly trouble walking up and down stairs and difficulty arising from a chair. Lately she had noted slightly slurred speech, transient horizontal diplopia with ptosis, dry mouth, and tingling in the feet and legs. She had a 40-pack-year history of cigarette smoking.

Examination abnormalities included mild weakness of orbicularis oculi, neck flexors, deltoids, triceps, and iliopsoas muscles with difficulty arising from a chair. Her speech was slightly dysarthric. Muscle stretch reflexes were absent but displayed postexercise enhancement.

Serum creatine kinase and acetylcholine (ACh) receptor antibody study results were normal. The results of a previous quadriceps muscle biopsy were unremarkable.

EMG revealed low compound muscle action potentials (CMAPs). A 15% decrement of CMAP amplitude was observed with 2-Hz repetitive motor nerve stimulation of the ulnar nerve. After 10 seconds of exercise, the ulnar CMAP facilitated 226%, typical of a presynaptic neuromuscular transmission disorder compatible with Lambert-Eaton myasthenic syndrome (LEMS). Serum voltage-gated calcium channel (VGCC) antibodies were increased.

A chest radiograph showed a right hilar mass; its biopsy revealed small cell lung cancer (SCLC). The patient received chemotherapy and 3,4-diaminopyridine for symptomatic treatment of LEMS, resulting in some improvement in strength. She died 16 months later.

Although rare, LEMS is the most frequently occurring presynaptic neuromuscular transmission disorder in adults. In approximately 50% of cases, LEMS is associated with cancer, especially SCLC. When LEMS is not associated with cancer, a primary autoimmune etiology is suspected. The paraneoplastic and nonparaneoplastic forms of LEMS share an autoimmune pathophysiologic mechanism. LEMS associated with lung cancer usually presents in past or present smokers, and clinical manifestations often begin months to years before diagnosis of the malignancy. Therefore, a timely LEMS diagnosis may expedite the lung cancer diagnosis and influence treatment and prognosis.

The vignette in this chapter illustrates cardinal LEMS symptoms: proximal extremity weakness, reduced muscle stretch reflexes, fatigue, and dry mouth, with milder symptoms of cranial nerve–innervated muscle weakness. Because of the patient's history of cigarette smoking with its increased lung cancer risk, LEMS was a prime consideration. The muscle stretch reflexes and weakness demonstrated postexercise improvement after 10 seconds of exercise, corresponding with the EMG findings.

Lambert-Eaton myasthenic syndrome often provides an early diagnosis of SCLC because the immune response producing LEMS is believed to begin early in tumor evolution. However, by the time LEMS was diagnosed in the preceding vignette, the SCLC had metastasized.

ETIOLOGY AND PATHOPHYSIOLOGY

Under normal conditions, neuronal depolarization opens VGCCs on the presynaptic axon terminal membrane, resulting in calcium influx within the nerve terminal. Intracellular calcium binds to calmodulin and mobilizes ACh synaptic vesicles that are released into the synaptic cleft (see chapter 100).

The VGCCs are the primary site of immunopathology in LEMS. Divalent IgG autoantibodies cross-link the calcium channels, disrupting their function, resulting in inadequate release of presynaptic ACh vesicles from motor and autonomic cholinergic nerve terminals. The release of fewer ACh quanta at the neuromuscular junction decreases the probability of reaching the depolarization threshold of a muscle fiber and thus the likelihood of the muscle fiber action potential generation.

The VGCCs present in SCLC cells and other neoplasms provides the presumed antigenic stimulus for antibody production in the paraneoplastic form of LEMS. The precise antigenic stimulus in the nonparaneoplastic varieties of LEMS remains to be identified. Muscle weakness, fatigue, and autonomic symptoms result because the VGCC autoantibodies reduce the ACh release at motor and autonomic nerve terminals, impairing synaptic transmission.

CLINICAL PRESENTATION

Fatigue is a prominent muscular symptom; it is often the initial LEMS manifestation as well as proximal weakness mimicking a myopathy. Complaints of patients with LEMS typically seem disproportionate to objective examination findings. Some individuals even have a characteristic inconsistency or "give way" finding on examination, suggesting nonorganic weakness. The combination of vague weakness, dry mouth, and paresthesias sometimes mimics the hyperventilation syndrome, hysteria, malingering, or depression, errors the unwary clinician must avoid. When patients with suspected LEMS do not have objective detectable weakness, it may be better appreciated by watching individuals rise from a chair or climb stairs (Figure 101-1).

Oculobulbar weakness in the form of diplopia, ptosis, dysphagia, and dysarthria are frequently reported and are usually relatively mild. Additional symptoms include fatigue, dry mouth, impotence in men, and sometimes vague thigh paresthesias. Presentation is similar in primary autoimmune and secondary paraneoplastic LEMS.

Autonomic symptoms, including dry mouth or erectile dysfunction in men, often prompt clinicians to consider LEMS. Muscle stretch reflexes are typically depressed or absent. Postexercise potentiation of depressed or absent muscle stretch reflexes and of muscle strength is often demonstrable.

DIAGNOSTIC APPROACH

EMG is crucial in the diagnosis of LEMS (Figure 101-2). Most patients with LEMS have low-amplitude CMAPs on routine nerve conduction studies. Rare in patients with myasthenia gravis (MG), low baseline CMAPs should lead to postexercise facilitation testing. Subsequently, repetitive motor nerve stimulation can help to differentiate presynaptic (eg, LEMS) from a postsynaptic (eg, MG) neuromuscular transmission disorder. The crucial differentiation between a presynaptic and a postsynaptic neuromuscular transmission disorder is that brief (10-15 seconds) voluntary exercise or rarely, if necessary, high-frequency (20-50 Hz) repetitive motor nerve stimulation leads to marked (>100%) facilitation that is at least twice the baseline of the CMAP in patients with LEMS but not those with MG.

Voltage-gated calcium channel antibody testing provides the definitive means to confirm the clinical and EMG impressions of LEMS, in both paraneoplastic and primary autoimmune forms. Abnormally high titers of VGCC antibodies are found in approximately 90% of patients with LEMS but also in 20% to 40% of patients with SCLC who do not have LEMS. Therefore, a positive VGCC antibody test result does not diagnose LEMS. The typical clinical and EMG findings are needed to support the diagnosis.

Because approximately 50% to 75% of patients with LEMS have an associated cancer, a search for malignancy, primarily SCLC, must be initiated in each patient diagnosed with LEMS.

A **lung CT** is indicated even if the initial chest radiograph is normal. If the CT is negative, pulmonary cytologic studies, including sputum analysis and bronchial washings, may be valuable to diagnose occult lung tumors. Repeat chest CT or other chest imaging is needed for up to 4 years in all patients with LEMS, particularly those with significant tobacco addiction.

LAMBERT-EATON MYASTHENIC SYNDROME

Figure 101-1

Lambert-Eaton Syndrome

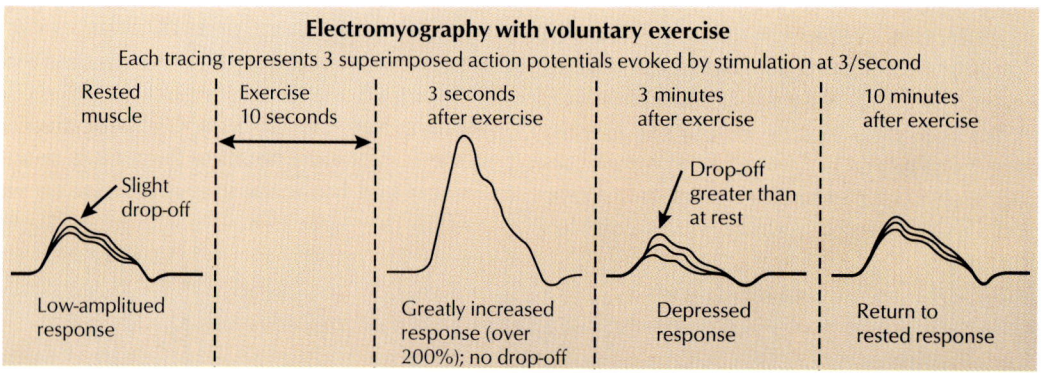

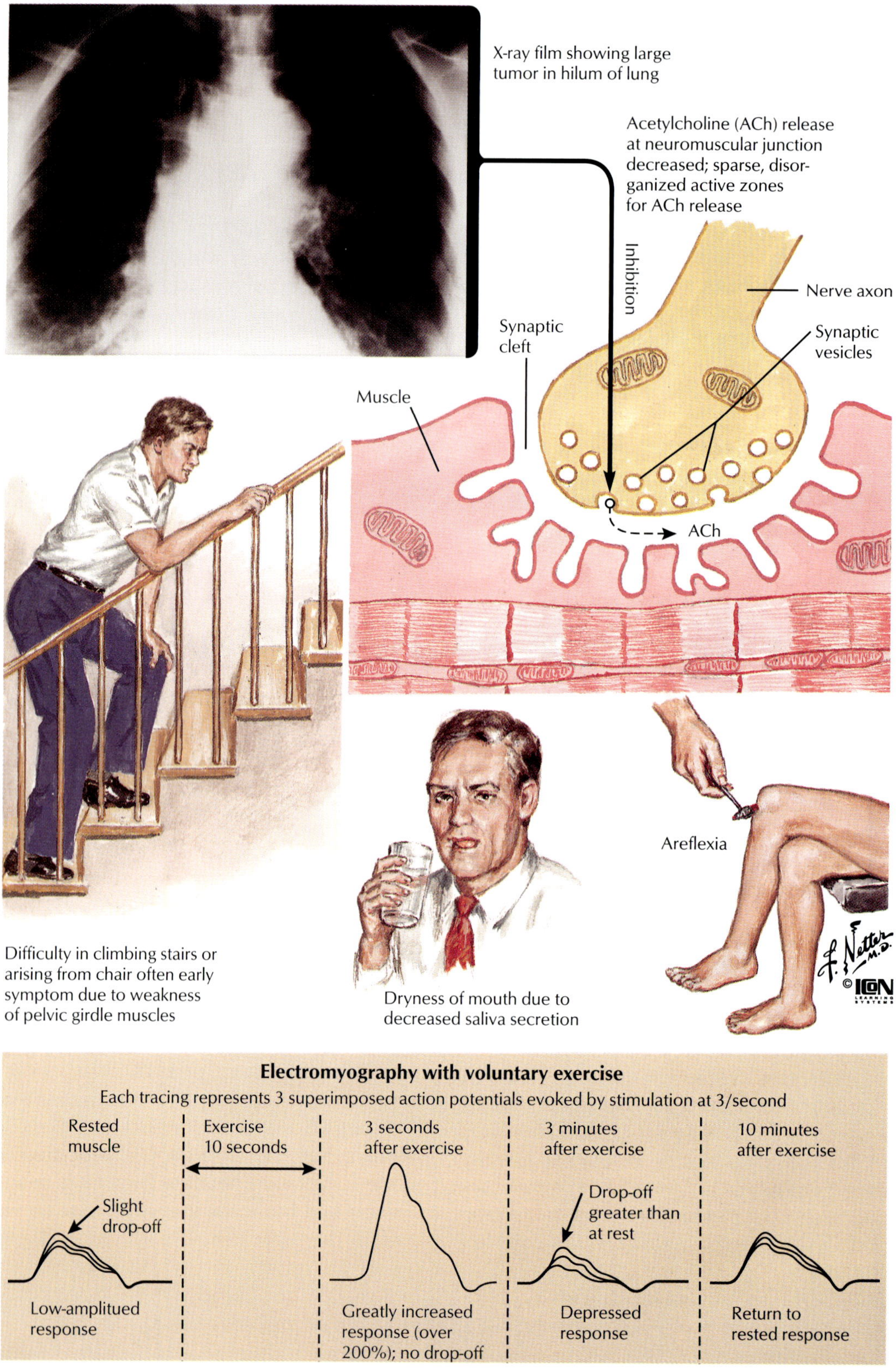

NEUROMUSCULAR TRANSMISSION DISORDERS

LAMBERT-EATON MYASTHENIC SYNDROME

Figure 101-2
Neuromuscular Manifestations of Bronchogenic (Small Cell) Carcinoma

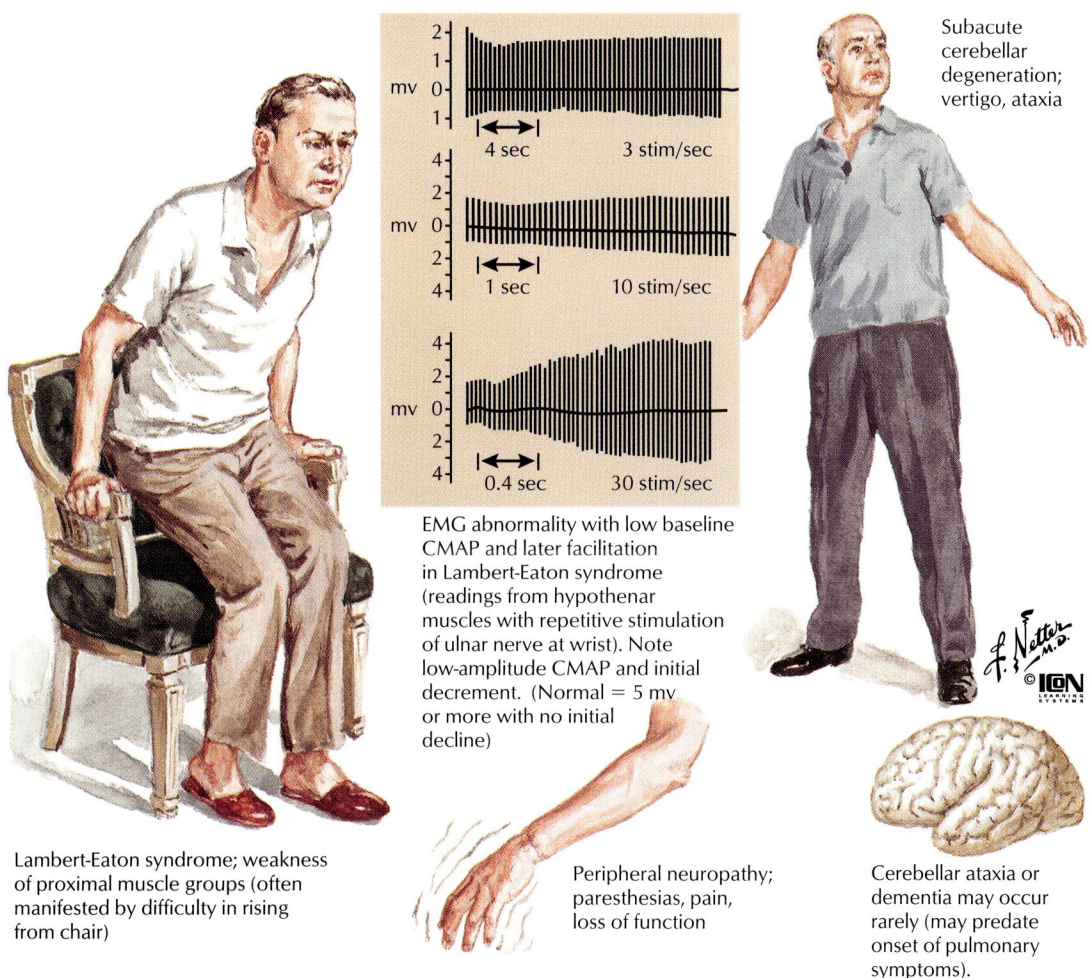

DIFFERENTIAL DIAGNOSIS

A variety of neurologic disorders, particularly **MG**, are included in the differential. Unlike LEMS, MG typically has a preponderance of ocular or bulbar symptoms—diplopia, ptosis, dysarthria, and dysphagia—early in its course, whereas in LEMS, oculobulbar symptoms are less commonly the presenting symptom and are usually mild. Occasionally, patients with LEMS who have prominent oculobulbar symptoms are misdiagnosed with MG. Prominent autonomic symptoms, such as dry mouth and erectile dysfunction, are characteristic of patients with LEMS but are often overlooked by patients or clinicians.

Other rare presynaptic neuromuscular transmission disorders (eg, botulism and magnesium intoxication) present acutely. In contrast, patients with LEMS rarely have a sudden clinical onset.

Inflammatory myopathies, namely polymyositis and dermatomyositis, typically also have predominant proximal limb and neck weakness and are occasionally associated with an underlying malignancy. However, they do not have the relatively subtle facilitation of strength immediately subsequent to testing of each muscle. The muscle stretch reflexes are usually preserved in patients with polymyositis and dermatomyositis, who also lack the typical autonomic and vague sensory symptoms classically seen with LEMS. Inflammatory and some metabolic myopathies are associated with increased levels of serum creatine kinase.

Chronic inflammatory demyelinating polyradiculoneuropathy (CIDP), with its insidious onset of proximal weakness and areflexia, also enters the LEMS differential diagnosis. Nerve conduction studies in chronic inflammatory demyelinating polyradiculoneuropathy demonstrate features of acquired demyelination (eg, slowed conduction velocities, conduction block, temporal dispersion), findings never seen with LEMS.

It is important to consider a LEMS diagnosis in patients with **fatigue** whose referring physician suspects **depression**, **hysteria**, or **malingering**. Psychiatric misdiagnoses occur because of the vague, nonspecific nature of the complaints. Furthermore, the "weakness" reported is usually disproportional to that observed. However, hyporeflexia or areflexia, with potentiation (enhancement) of muscle stretch reflexes and muscle strength, after 10 seconds of sustained exercise may provoke astute clinicians to include EMG testing.

TREATMENT AND PROGNOSIS

Chemotherapy, radiation therapy, surgery, or a combination are the primary treatment modalities for LEMS-associated lung malignancy. Cancer treatment often leads to symptomatic improvement in LEMS, presumably by removing the antigenic stimulus. Symptomatic treatment of LEMS aims to improve neuromuscular transmission. By prolonging the VGCC open time, **3,4-diaminopyridine** promotes ACh release from the presynaptic portion of the neuromuscular junction. It is available for LEMS primarily in Europe but in the United States requires local institutional review board approval and a concomitant submission to the FDA for compassionate use. The initial dose is 5 mg 3 times daily, with a typical maintenance dose of 20 mg 3 times daily. Caution is advised because central nervous system irritability, manifested by seizures, is a major adverse effect. The anticholinesterase medication **pyridostigmine (Mestinon)** also improves neuromuscular transmission. In contrast to MG, pyridostigmine alone is not very effective for LEMS. However, anticholinesterases potentiate the effects of 3,4-diaminopyridine, and pyridostigmine may be particularly beneficial when combined with 3,4-diaminopyridine.

Despite its disadvantages, immunomodulation therapy is also sometimes used. Although **prednisone** lessens the autoimmune response of patients with LEMS and therefore may improve the muscle weakness, it also inhibits the inherent attempt of the body to suppress the malignancy and thus may counteract the effects of cancer treatment. Therefore, in patients with SCLC or older LEMS patients at high risk for SCLC in whom a tumor has not been identified, initiation of immunosuppressive therapy may theoretically lessen the immunoresponsiveness of the body to patients' tumors and thus enhance the SCLC. **Plasmapheresis, IV immunoglobulin** therapy, or both are other immunotherapies useful for some significantly weak patients with LEMS. Unfortunately, these effects are transient, often ineffective after a few weeks.

Certain common **medications sometimes exacerbate LEMS** symptoms and should be used cautiously in LEMS: cardiac drugs, ie, adrenergic and calcium channel blocking agents, and antiarrhythmic agents, such as procainamide and quinidine. The aminoglycoside antibiotics, magnesium citrate cathartics, quinine, and lithium may also exacerbate the neuromuscular transmission defect, increasing weakness. Anesthesiologists must be aware of a LEMS diagnosis so they select medications that will not prolong postoperative respiratory depression. On rare occasions, this is the initial manifestation of LEMS.

Prognosis depends on whether LEMS is associated with malignancy and, if so, on the type and stage of malignancy. Most patients with LEMS have SCLC, with a median survival of a few years. However, early detection improves prognosis. In contrast, the prognosis in patients with primary autoimmune LEMS without SCLC is good; some patients live for more than 20 years after diagnosis. These patients with nonparaneoplastic LEMS often respond positively to immunomodulation and symptomatic therapy.

REFERENCES

Burns TM, Russell JA. Lachance DH, Jones HR. Oculobulbar involvement is typical with Lambert-Eaton myasthenic syndrome. *Ann Neurol.* 2003;53:270-273.

Gutmann L, Phillips LH, Gutmann L. Trends in the association of Lambert-Eaton myasthenic syndrome with carcinoma. *Neurology.* 1992;42:848-850.

Howard JF, Sanders DB, Massey JM. The electrodiagnosis of myasthenia gravis and the Lambert-Eaton syndrome. *Neurol Clin North Am.* 1994;12:305-330.

Lambert EH, Eaton LM, Rooke ED. Defect of neuromuscular conduction associated with malignant neoplasms. *Am J Physiol.* 1956;187:612-613.

Lambert EH, Rooke ED. Myasthenic state and lung cancer. In: Brain WR, Norris FH, eds. *The Remote Effects of Cancer on the Nervous System.* New York, NY: Grune and Stratton; 1965:67-80.

Lennon VA, Kryzer TJ, Griesmann GE, et al. Calcium-channel antibodies in the Lambert-Eaton syndrome and other paraneoplastic syndromes. *N Engl J Med.* 1995;332:1467-1474.

McEvoy KM, Windebank AJ, Daube JR, Low PA. 3,4-diaminopyridine in the treatment of Lambert-Eaton myasthenic syndrome. *N Engl J Med.* 1989;321:1567-1571.

O'Neil JH, Murray NMF, Newsom-Davis J. The Lambert Eaton myasthenic syndrome: a review of 50 cases. *Brain.* 1988;111:577-596.

Sanders DB. Lambert-Eaton myasthenic syndrome: clinical diagnosis, immune-mediated mechanisms, and update on therapies. *Ann Neurol.* 1995;37(suppl 1):S63-S73.

Tim RW, Sanders DB. Repetitive nerve stimulation studies in the Lambert-Eaton myasthenic syndrome. *Muscle Nerve.* 1994;17:995-1001.

Chapter 102
Myasthenia Gravis

Ted M. Burns, Monique M. Ryan, and H. Royden Jones, Jr

Clinical Vignette

During a period of several weeks, blurred vision and "droopy eyes" developed in a previously healthy 38-year-old woman. Her symptoms worsened toward the end of each day and often cleared overnight. Friends commented that her speech had become more difficult to understand and softer in volume. She also described increased tiredness on climbing stairs; sometimes she had to stop and rest while cleaning her teeth or brushing her hair. Neurologic examination revealed bilateral ptosis and dysconjugate eye movements in several directions of gaze. There was weakness of eye closure and neck flexion and mild proximal limb weakness.

An edrophonium (Tensilon) test resulted in marked improvement for 3 to 4 minutes. EMG showed normal motor and sensory action potentials. Repetitive motor nerve stimulation testing demonstrated a 15% decrease in the ulnar compound muscle action potential amplitude between the first and fifth stimuli. Anti–acetylcholine receptor (AChR) antibodies were present in significantly abnormal titers. Results of CT scanning of the mediastinum were unremarkable. Immunosuppressive and pyridostigmine bromide (Mestinon) treatments were initiated, with plans for the patient to undergo thymectomy when her symptoms were under control.

This vignette is typical of myasthenia gravis (MG), primarily presenting in a young woman with ocular signs. Generally, these individuals respond well to therapy, although they require careful long-term care with a neurologist who is comfortable using needed medications with numerous potential adverse effects over many years.

Myasthenia gravis is an uncommon disorder of neuromuscular transmission manifested by abnormal muscle fatigability and weakness, which commonly fluctuate. An autoimmune basis for MG has been recognized since 1960. Women are more commonly affected. Peaks of onset are seen in women in the second and third decades and in men in the fifth and sixth decades.

The overall prevalence, estimated at 1 per 10,000, has increased markedly during the past 40 years because of improved recognition, treatment, and survival. Other autoimmune disorders, including hyperthyroidism, Hashimoto thyroiditis, pernicious anemia, vitiligo, rheumatoid arthritis, and systemic lupus erythematosus, are seen in up to 10% of patients.

ETIOLOGY AND PATHOGENESIS

Autoimmune MG is caused by the development of autoantibodies to immunogenic regions (epitopes) on or around the nicotinic AChR of the postsynaptic endplate region at the neuromuscular junction (NMJ). These antiacetylcholine antibodies may block the binding of acetylcholine (ACh) molecules to their receptors or may trigger immune-mediated degradation of the acetylcholine receptors and their adjacent postsynaptic membrane (Figure 102-1).

Loss of large numbers of functional AChRs within muscles limits the number of fibers depolarized during motor nerve terminal activation, resulting in a decreased generation of muscle action potentials and subsequent muscle fiber contraction. Blocking of neuromuscular transmission causes clinical weakness when it affects large numbers of fibers.

The nicotinic AChR contains 5 subunits arranged radially around a transmembrane ion channel. The autoantibodies generated in MG are usually directed against the α subunit of the AChR. These antibodies may bind at or near the ACh binding site, directly preventing ACh binding, or may alter receptor function through other mechanisms, such as increased receptor degradation or complement-mediated receptor lysis. The autoimmune response of MG is primarily mediated by T lymphocytes derived from the thymus.

MYASTHENIA GRAVIS

Figure 102-1
Myasthenia Gravis: Pathophysiologic Concepts

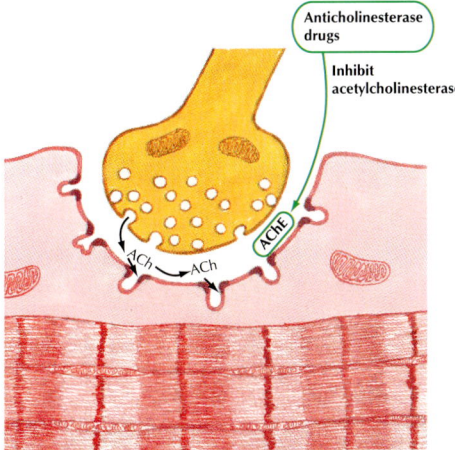

Myasthenia gravis: Marked reduction in number and length of subneural sarcolemmal folds indicates that underlying defect lies in neuromuscular junction. Anticholinesterase drugs increase effectiveness and duration of ACh action by slowing its destruction by AChE.

CLINICAL PRESENTATION

Myasthenia gravis is typically classified as ocular, generalized, neonatal, congenital, or drug-induced. At presentation, weakness is confined to the extraocular muscles in 50% to 60% of patients. Within 2 years, more generalized weakness develops in 85% to 90% of these individuals with primary ocular MG (Figure 102-2). In those few patients with primary ocular MG in whom bulbar or generalized weakness does not develop within this period, further progression is unlikely. However, such muscle involvement of wider distribution may occasionally develop even 8 to 10 years later.

The generalized form of MG is the most common. **Cardinal symptoms** include **fluctuating or fatigable weakness**, variably affecting the extraocular, bulbar, and extremity musculature. Most patients initially report diplopia and ptosis. Involvement of the extraocular muscles is commonly intermittent and asymmetric. Pupillary reactions are spared. Lower cranial nerve dysfunction, ie, bulbar weakness, may occasionally be the presenting symptomatology. Typically, the speech becomes soft with a nasal "twang" to the voice, chewing is difficult, and nasal regurgitation occurs with the potential for aspiration. Characteristically, these patients have no problem when they begin to eat their meal, but increasing difficulties develop within the same sitting, particularly as they attempt to chew foods such as meats. Facial weakness is typified by an expressionless facies with a transverse smile (the "myasthenic snarl") and weakness of eye and mouth closure.

Respiratory muscle involvement is potentially life threatening because of the risk of respiratory failure from hypoventilation. Neck extension weakness leads to patients' having difficulty holding up their heads. Increasing proximal muscle weakness results in problems with raising the arms overhead and with climbing stairs.

Fatigability is characteristic of MG. Patients commonly describe worsening of their symptoms late in the day or with exercise. Transient improvement occurs with rest. Symptoms often progress during the day. On examination, fatigability can be demonstrated on sustained upward gaze, which may exacerbate ptosis and diplopia.

Untreated MG has a variable course. Weakness may progress during weeks or months, or fluctuate; long-lasting spontaneous remission rarely occurs. On some occasions, after a brief period of symptoms, patients with new-onset MG may have a precipitous crisislike presentation, as in the second vignette in this chapter. Exacerbations may be precipitated by hot weather (which affects the kinetics of the ACh esterase enzyme), intercurrent illness, menstruation, pregnancy, or concurrent thyrotoxicosis. Certain medications that affect NMJ function, ie, some antibiotics (such as aminoglycosides), antihypertensives, and particularly β blocker or calcium channel blocker classes, may exacerbate and even precipitate incipient MG. Myasthenic crises may cause respiratory failure, requiring assisted ventilation and treatment with plasmapheresis, intravenous immunoglobulin, and corticosteroids.

Clinical Vignette

A 16-year-old girl presented with a 6-week history of difficulty speaking and swallowing, which initially led

MYASTHENIA GRAVIS

Figure 102-2

Myasthenia Gravis: Clinical Manifestations

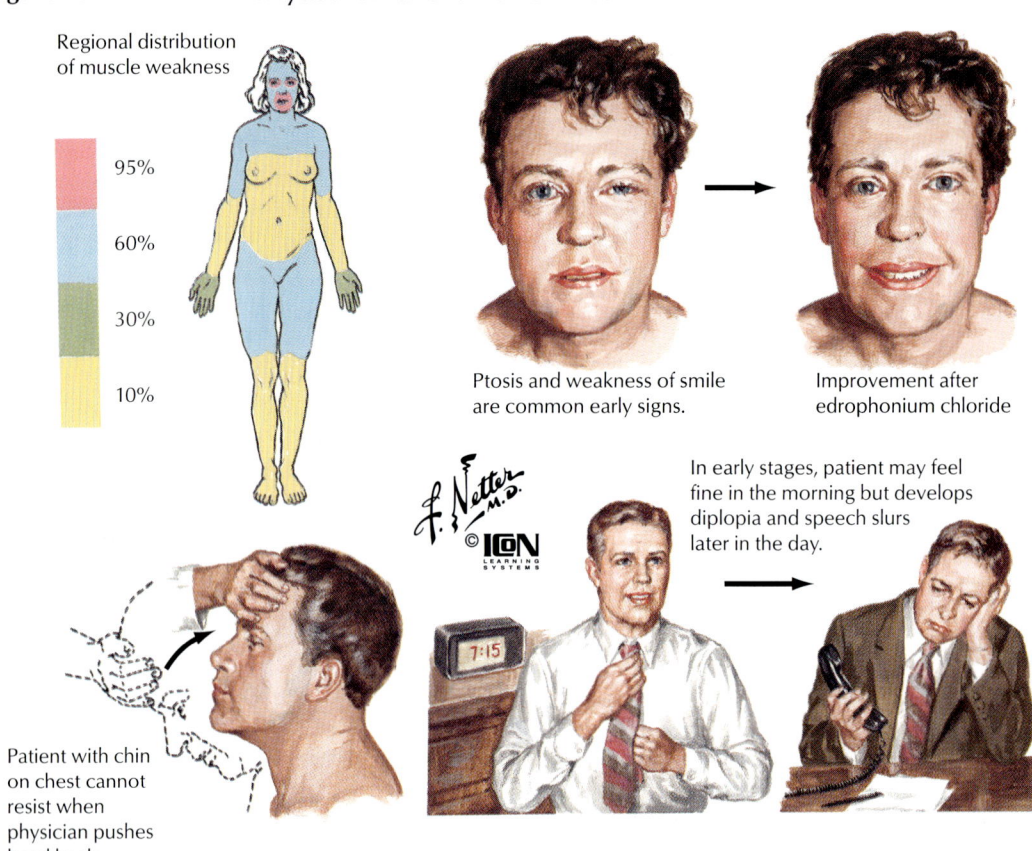

to a nondiagnostic otolaryngologic evaluation. During the next 2 weeks, generalized weakness, weight loss, ptosis, and diplopia developed. Within a few weeks, the illness had progressed to severe respiratory distress, and the patient presented to the ED. Her neurologic examination demonstrated bilateral ptosis, marked limitation of gaze, diminished gag, nasal voice, and proximal weakness with associated fatigability. She was in respiratory distress.

Results of Tensilon testing were positive; there was improvement in most abnormal clinical parameters. EMG demonstrated normal routine motor and sensory nerve conduction studies. Repetitive motor nerve stimulation of the ulnar nerve was normal at 2 Hz before and after 60 seconds of full exercise. In contrast, repetitive motor nerve stimulation of the facial nerve demonstrated a 50% decrement at rest, which was significantly repaired with 10 mg IV Tensilon. A needle examination demonstrated an increased percentage of low-amplitude, short-duration MUPs. The AChR antibody level was increased. Plasmapheresis was initiated, and after 4 exchanges, the patient was almost fully recovered. Subsequently, a thymectomy was per-

formed. Later, prednisone therapy was initiated when a modest relapse occurred.

The teenager in this vignette had a rapid onset of MG, which was not initially appreciated when she presented with atypical lower bulbar dysfunction. A diagnosis of a postsynaptic defect in neuromuscular transmission was confirmed by repetitive motor nerve stimulation of the facial nerve, illustrating the diagnostic importance of EMG. Sometimes, EMG of multiple nerves is needed, particularly proximal ones such as the spinal accessory or the facial nerve, to achieve a positive diagnosis. EMG can be diagnostic in the acute care setting, while the patients awaits the more specific anti-AChR antibody testing results.

Women with MG have a 15% to 20% chance of having a child who is affected by transient weakness, poor suck, and respiratory depression related to transplacental transfer of anti-AChR antibodies. Usually, the infant is affected for only a few months, and management with anticholinesterase medication, such as neostigmine, is sufficient. Transient neonatal myasthenia should be differentiated from the uncommon congenital myasthenia, which is a genetic condition arising from altered NMJ structure or function.

DIFFERENTIAL DIAGNOSIS

Myasthenia gravis presenting with ophthalmoplegia may mimic **isolated cranial nerve palsies**. Some patients with myasthenia have a pseudointernuclear ophthalmoplegia mimicking multiple sclerosis. In patients with initial oculomotor and bulbar weakness, **multiple sclerosis** is also suspected, but is less likely because of the absence of optic nerve pallor and cerebellar, corticospinal tract, and sensory signs. **Brainstem tumors** may present similarly but are sometimes associated with symptoms of increased intracranial pressure, peripheral weakness, and hyperreflexia with Babinski signs. The sudden development of diplopia, dysarthria, and weakness may suggest **vertebrobasilar emboli** or small-vessel cerebrovascular disease affecting the brainstem. Rarely, **multiple cranial neuropathies** are the presenting sign of **leptomeningeal inflammatory disorders**, such as sarcoidosis, tuberculosis, or fungal infections. Similarly, metastatic cancer can invade the leptomeninges, sometimes as the presenting sign, and mimic MG. A brain MRI is particularly useful for differentiating these conditions.

When bulbar dysfunction is prominent, and diplopia and ptosis are absent, the bulbar presentation of **amyotrophic lateral sclerosis** always requires consideration. **The Miller Fisher variant** of Guillain-Barré syndrome presents with extraocular muscle paresis, mimicking MG, but is usually associated with ataxia and areflexia. The **Lambert-Eaton syndrome** occasionally involves the bulbar musculature, but peripheral weakness and systemic symptoms are more prominent. Rarely, **polymyositis** presents with lower bulbar weakness. Prominent proximal weakness may suggest an acquired myopathy or muscular dystrophy. These conditions usually spare the extraocular muscles, and fatigability is uncommon. EMG can differentiate among myopathies, neuropathies, and disorders of neuromuscular transmission.

Disorders uncommon in countries with modern public health measures need consideration; **poliomyelitis**, **diphtheria**, and **botulism** may present with an acute-onset bulbar weakness. Although uncommon, they are still encountered in the United States. They can best be differentiated from myasthenia by their variable pupillary involvement and prominent peripheral weakness and by EMG.

DIAGNOSTIC APPROACH

Intravenous administration of edrophonium chloride (**Tensilon**) is usually the initial test for suspected MG. Tensilon is an acetylcholinesterase inhibitor that rapidly improves muscle strength for up to 3 to 5 minutes in most patients. The Tensilon test is more likely to be diagnostic in patients with obvious ptosis, diplopia, slurred speech, or peripheral weakness related to generalized myasthenia. Typically, Tensilon is packaged in a 1-mL vial containing 10 mg, enough for an adequate test of 1 suspected case of MG. Because some patients are hypersensitive to Tensilon, a test dose of 2 mg is usually given first, followed by gradual administration of the remaining 8 mg over a 1-minute period. The test result is deemed negative if no improvement occurs after the second dose.

Tensilon may cause muscarinic adverse effects, such as asystole, bradycardia, syncope, nausea, excessive lacrimation, and salivation. *Caution is advised when administering it to patients with cardiac disorders; its use is avoided in older patients unless performed in the presence of a physician intensivist.* Nicotinic adverse effects of anticholinesterases include muscle cramping and fasciculation. **False-positive results** on Tensilon tests may occur with the Lambert-Eaton syndrome, amyotrophic lateral sclerosis, neuropathies, and intracranial tumors.

Assays for **AChR binding**, **modulating**, and **blocking antibodies** are positive in up to 90% of patients with generalized MG. Individuals with purely ocular MG have an approximately 50% incidence of positive striated muscle antibodies. Such patients, usually men older than 50 years, have a higher incidence of associated thymomas. Muscle-specific kinase (MUSK) is another

MYASTHENIA GRAVIS

antibody that sometimes tests positive in patients with suspected MG who have otherwise negative immunologic studies. In seronegative instances, the diagnosis becomes more clinical, but may be confirmed by electrophysiologic testing.

The **electrodiagnostic EMG hallmark** finding of MG is the presence of an **electrodecremental response** with repetitive motor nerve stimulation. Inherent functional reserve in neuromuscular transmission (the safety factor) usually enables preservation of compound muscle action potential amplitude on repetitive stimulation in clinically unaffected individuals. However, in MG, the loss of functional AChRs results in a decrement of 10% to 15% or more in action potential size on repeated stimulation, a decrease that is apparent by the third to fifth stimulus. This decrement may be reversed by exercise or Tensilon. Repetitive stimulation of peripheral nerves may be normal in those with ocular myasthenia or mild generalized disease, whereby testing of the facial or spinal accessory nerves or both is often diagnostic. Although antibody testing is the first choice in patients with mild symptoms, EMG is useful in seriously ill individuals who require an immediate diagnosis before commencing specific therapies.

Single-fiber EMG, a more technically demanding test of NMJ function, records single muscle fiber discharges. In MG, the firing interval of individual muscle fibers, or jitter, is increased, and there may be intermittent blocking of neuromuscular transmission. Single-fiber EMG has a sensitivity of more than 90% in ocular and generalized MG, when appropriate muscles are tested.

CT or MRI imaging of the mediastinum is important in suspected MG, because 10% to 15% of patients with myasthenia have benign or malignant thymic tumors. Of those without tumors, 70% have thymic lymphoid follicular hyperplasia. Anti–striatal muscle antibodies are present in 90% of patients with myasthenia and thymoma. Thymectomy is indicated whenever a thymoma is identified.

MANAGEMENT AND PROGNOSIS

Acetylcholinesterase inhibitors are the primary means to achieve early symptomatic remissions in patients with MG. Pyridostigmine bromide (Mestinon) is the most commonly used agent. Treatment is generally started at 30 to 60 mg orally every 4 to 6 hours. The dosage is titrated relevant to the clinical response of the patient.

Doses of more than 120 mg every 3 to 4 hours may cause **cholinergic crisis**, with paradoxically increased weakness (sometimes to a marked degree), increased salivation, abdominal cramping, and muscle fasciculations. This is a rare event because other medications offer therapeutic options. Withdrawal of the anticholinesterase therapy is the treatment of choice. These medications do not affect the basic pathophysiologic process. Therefore, most patients with moderate or severe myasthenia commonly require some form of immunosuppressive therapy.

Corticosteroids are the initial treatment of choice to induce remission of this autoimmune disorder. Oral prednisone is generally effective for bringing patients with MG into remission, especially when anticholinesterase medications have not. Prednisone in large, eventually remission-achieving dosages of 60 to 100 mg/d has the potential to transiently, but significantly, exacerbate weakness, which is a particular concern for patients with significant respiratory compromise. Hence, outpatient induction of steroid therapy is usually performed with initial low dosages of 10 to 20 mg/d, gradually increasing every 5 to 15 days by 10 mg, until remission is achieved. Another option for the more seriously ill patient is to initiate corticosteroid therapy in the hospital, where prednisone dose can be increased every few days as tolerated, achieving a maximum dose within 7 to 10 days. Alternatively, prednisone can be given on an every other day basis, starting with approximately 20 mg and increasing to 120 mg one day, the "on day," with no medication on the "off day" or "low day."

Steroid treatment induces remission in up to 80% of patients. With high-dose therapy, most patients achieve sustained improvement within 4 to 12 weeks. After individuals have been stable for 1 to 2 months, prednisone is gradually withdrawn. If they have been on a daily dosage schedule, for example, 60 mg at remission, they can be switched to alternate-day therapy, initially decreasing the off- or low-day dose by 10-mg increments every 2 to 4 weeks. After a low-day dose of 10 to 20 mg (ie, 60/10-20 mg) is reached by this slow reduction schedule, the high-day dose is gradually diminished. Patients must be taught that they may have an exacerbation at any time during this reduction therapy. This often occurs from overly eager attempts by physicians unfamiliar with MG patient management to totally withdraw steroids in a relatively short time.

Myasthenia gravis is a chronic illness requiring fastidious attention to therapeutic detail and especially an understanding that most individuals will continue to take some prednisone for a number of years. Some patients may continue on prednisone therapy for more than 25 years, when each attempt to totally withdraw leads to exacerbations. The concomitant use of azathioprine enhances the potential to totally discontinue corticosteroids.

The well-known precautions to avoid the adverse effects of indefinite, maintenance, low-dose prednisone therapy must be followed with each patient. Some steroid therapy complications are significant, including aseptic necrosis of the femoral head, osteoporosis, the enhanced likelihood of infections developing in an immunocompromised host, and serious psychomotor depression. Nevertheless, patients must also be made aware that until a dosage schedule was developed to prevent the initial MG exacerbation associated with corticosteroid therapy, morbidity and mortality were significant when anticholinesterase medications were the only available therapies.

Azathioprine is excellent for the treatment of MG, although the timing of its introduction into the care of each patient varies. It is typically used as the first autoimmune therapy by some, but a response to this medication may not be seen for 6 to 12 months after its initiation. It is effective as a secondary autoimmune therapeutic modality, particularly when decreasing corticosteroid dosage in patients is thwarted because of recurrent exacerbations. Azathioprine is begun relatively early in older adults, because they are more likely to experience some significant corticosteroid adverse effects. The usual dosage is 100 to 150 mg/day. Rarely, patients experience significant hepatic toxicity, and therefore, frequent liver function monitoring is appropriate.

Plasma exchange removes acetylcholine receptor antibodies from the blood and produces rapid but transient clinical improvement. Plasmapheresis is particularly useful during myasthenic crises or steroid-related exacerbations, in preparation for thymectomy and other surgical procedures, and occasionally as maintenance therapy in patients refractory to other therapies.

Intravenous immunoglobulin has an effect similar to plasmapheresis and is easier to administer. It is also used for temporary control of myasthenic weakness. The usual dosage is 2.0 g/kg, in 5 daily aliquots of 0.4 mg/kg.

Thymectomy is a standard treatment modality for all patients younger than 60 years with generalized MG. It induces remission in up to 60% of patients with MG. Clinical improvement after thymectomy is usually delayed at least 6 to 12 months, but in some cases not for several years. The maximal benefit is seen in those who undergo thymectomy within 2 years of disease onset. However, thymectomy may not be as beneficial in patients who are antibody negative.

Approximately 10% to 15% of patients with MG have an associated thymoma. Ten percent of these thymomas are malignant. Both the benign and malignant entities are associated with a significant elevation of the anti–skeletal muscle antibody level. The significance of increased antibody in patients who have no signs of thymoma on CT imaging but have significantly increased titers of anti–skeletal muscle antibodies is unknown. All patients with a thymoma, regardless of their age, must undergo a thymectomy.

Because the thymus gradually involutes with aging, thymectomy is not generally recommended for adult patients older than 60 years. Its role in the treatment of patients with isolated ocular myasthenia is still under investigation.

Cyclosporine A is the only immunosuppressive therapy for MG that is proven effective by prospective, double-blind, placebo-controlled trials. However, both corticosteroids and azathioprine were used before such trials became commonplace. Their effectiveness is so very well documented that no one would participate in a "blinded" trial because it would be unethical. Clinical improvement with cyclosporine typically begins within 2 weeks of treatment and is maximal by 3 to 4 months, but relapse after discontinuation is common. The major drawback to cyclosporine is its potential for significant renal toxicity. **Cyclophosphamide** and **mycophenolate mofetil** have also been used in refractory MG. Although they may have an increased role in early MG treatment, both are considered second-level therapies.

Respiratory failure, secondary to intercostal and diaphragmatic muscle weakness, is the most serious potential complication with MG. Pulmonary function should be carefully monitored in newly diagnosed patients and those experiencing disease relapses. Should myasthenic patients require anesthesia, their clinical status must be optimized preoperatively.

Many medications affect NMJ function and **should be avoided in MG**. These include some antibiotics (aminoglycosides, macrolides, and ampicillin), antiarrhythmics (quinidine, procainamide, lidocaine, and β blockers), depolarizing neuromuscular blocking agents, chloroquine, trimethadione, and phenytoin. Some medications and therapies reportedly cause MG. These include penicillamine, interferon alfa, and bone marrow transplantation.

Long-term outcome in MG has improved markedly. In previous decades, up to 25% of patients died of respiratory failure within 3 years after diagnosis. However, with the widespread availability of multiple immunomodulatory therapies and the improved treatment of respiratory failure, more than 90% of patients, even those with severe generalized myasthenia, can achieve a status that is compatible with most activities of daily living within 1 year. A few patients continue to be more resistant to treatment, particularly those with the antibody-negative forms of the disease, for which therapeutic concepts are being reevaluated.

REFERENCES

Drachman DB. Myasthenia gravis. *N Engl J Med.* 1994;330:1797-1810.

Grob D, Arsura EL, Brunner NG, Namba T. The course of myasthenia gravis and therapies affecting outcome. *Ann N Y Acad Sci.* 1987;505:472-499.

Howard JF, Sanders DB, Massey JM. The electrodiagnosis of myasthenia gravis and the Lambert-Eaton myasthenic syndrome. *Neurol Clin North Am.* 1994;12:305-330.

Oosterhuis HJ. Observations of the natural history of myasthenia gravis and the effect of thymectomy. *Ann N Y Acad Sci.* 1981;377:678-689.

Oosterhuis HJ. The natural course of myasthenia gravis: a long term follow up study. *J Neurol Neurosurg Psychiatry.* 1989;52:1121-1127.

Pascuzzi RM, Coslett HB, Johns TR. Long-term corticosteroid treatment of myasthenia gravis: report of 116 patients. *Ann Neurol.* 1984;15:291-298.

Sanders DB, Howard JF Jr, Johns TR, et al. High dose daily prednisone in the treatment of myasthenia gravis: report of 116 patients. In: Dau PC, ed. *Plasmapheresis and the Immunobiology of Myasthenia Gravis.* Boston, Mass: Houghton Mifflin; 1979:289-306.

Section XXIV
MYOPATHIES

Chapter 103
Overview of Muscle Disease 872

Chapter 104
Acute or Subacute Proximally Predominant or Generalized Myopathies Presenting With Weakness 884

Chapter 105
Myopathies: Chronic Proximally Predominant or Generalized Weakness 892

Chapter 106
Distal Predominant Myopathies 906

Chapter 107
The Channelopathies: Myopathies Presenting With Episodic Weakness 909

Chapter 108
Myopathies Presenting With Exercise Intolerance ..914

Chapter 103
Overview of Muscle Disease

James A. Russell and H. Royden Jones, Jr

Myopathies are disorders that adversely affect muscle function. Although there is usually a demonstrable alteration in myofiber histology, this is not always the rule.

Insights from molecular biology are changing the traditional classification of muscle disorders and opening new areas of investigation. For example, certain clinically similar myopathic phenotypes may result from different gene mutations. Conversely, mutations of the same gene may result in disparate myopathic or nonmyopathic manifestations, even within the same family.

CLASSIFICATION

Current classifications of the myopathies remain suboptimal because of incomplete knowledge of the precise pathogenesis of many disorders and the complexity of genotypic-phenotypic correlations. Historic classifications begin by distinguishing between acquired and inherited myopathies, not always an easy clinical task. For the clinical setting, a useful classification system can be based on presentation: proximal acute and subacute (Table 103-1), proximal chronic (Table 103-2), distal (Table 103-3), exercise induced (Table 103-4), and periodic (Table 103-5).

DIFFERENTIAL DIAGNOSIS

Myopathies typically present with symmetric signs and symptoms of fixed skeletal muscle weakness affecting the proximal limbs and paraspinal musculature (Table 103-6). Asymmetric, distal, generalized, or regional patterns of weakness also occur in myopathies (Table 103-7). Less commonly, smooth, ventilatory, or cardiac muscle are concomitantly affected. Myopathies occasionally present with exercise-induced muscle pain or stiffness or periodic paralysis. Strikingly asymmetric or focal myopathies are uncommon.

Myopathies are typically considered in the same differential diagnosis as neuromuscular transmission disorders and motor neuron disease. Muscle stretch reflexes are often spared, and sensation is usually unaffected. Certain findings narrow the differential diagnosis when the patient is suspected of having a myopathy. These include an evaluation of the pattern of weakness (eg, presence of ptosis, ophthalmoparesis, ventilatory muscle weakness, scapular winging, and head drop) and other clinical features predominant in certain myopathies (eg, contractures, skeletal dysmorphisms, calf hypertrophy, myotonia, or cardiac involvement) (Table 103-6). Additionally, it is important to assess the temporal profile (eg, the rate of progression), any relapsing (periodic) weakness, and symptoms that occur only with exertion. Assess the patient for other risk factors, including genetic predisposition, medication and toxic exposure, and other organ system involvement. Acquiring a family history deserves emphasis; a simple inquiry as to whether any relatives are affected is insufficient. A detailed medical history of first-degree family members is always indicated, with reference to deformities and orthopedic problems, handicaps, early cataracts, and sudden death. A brief neurologic examination of potentially affected family members should always be considered.

DIAGNOSTIC APPROACH

Patients who present with myalgia and muscle weakness without objective signs and with or without concomitant increases in serum creatine kinase (CK) levels are common in clinical practice. Such patients are diagnostically and therapeutically challenging. Definable myopathic and neuropathic disorders are uncommon in patients who present with muscle pain, stiffness, fatigue, or exercise intolerance in the absence of objective clinical or laboratory ab-

OVERVIEW OF MUSCLE DISEASE

Table 103-1
Proximal Predominant Acute/Subacute Myopathies

Acquired
- Inflammatory/immune-mediated myopathies
  - Polymyositis
  - Dermatomyositis
  - Granulomatous myositis
  - Sarcoid myopathy
  - Eosinophilic myositis
- Endocrine
  - Adrenal: Cushing syndrome/disease, Addison disease
  - Thyroid: hypothyroidism, hyperthyroidism
  - Parathyroid: hyperparathyroidism
- Metabolic
  - Hypokalemia
  - Osteomalacia
- Systemic illness
  - Critical illness myopathy
  - Paraneoplastic
- Infectious
  - Viral—influenza, coxsackie, HIV
  - Bacterial—pyomyositis, *Staphylococcus*, *Legionella*, typhoid, *Clostridia*, *Aeromonas*, *Vibrio*
  - Parasitic—trichinosis, toxoplasmosis, cysticercosis
- Toxic
  - Alcohol
  - Aminocaproic acid
  - Amiodarone
  - Chloroquine/hydroxychloroquine
  - Cholesterol-lowering agents, statins
  - Cimetidine
  - Colchicine
  - Corticosteroids
  - Cyclosporine
  - Emetine (Ipecac)
  - Illicit drugs (IM injections)
  - Labetalol
  - Lamotrigine
  - Leuprolide
  - Lithium
  - Neuromuscular blocking agents
  - Omeprazole
  - Penicillamine
  - Propofol
  - Rifampin
  - Tacrolimus
  - Toluene (inhalation)
  - L-Tryptophan
  - Vincristine
  - Vitamin E
  - Zidovudine

Inherited
- Channelopathies
  - Periodic paralysis

Table 103-2
Proximal Predominant Chronic Myopathies*

Acquired
- Idiopathic-inflammatory myopathies
  - Inclusion body myositis
  - Sarcoidosis
- Infectious
  - HTLV-I
- Metabolic
  - Osteomalacia
  - Amyloidosis

Inherited
- Dystrophic
  - Dystrophinopathy (Duchenne/Becker)
  - Limb-girdle muscular dystrophy types 1A-E, 2A-I
  - Facioscapulohumeral muscular dystrophy
  - Myotonic muscular dystrophy types I and II (PROMM)
  - Oculopharyngeal muscular dystrophy
  - Congenital muscular dystrophy
  - Emery-Dreifuss muscular dystrophy
  - Ullrich/Bethlem myopathy
- Congenital
  - Nemaline myopathy
  - Centronuclear/myotubular myopathy
  - Central core myopathy
  - Myofibrillary (desmin) myopathy
  - Others
- Glycogen (GSD) and lipid storage
  - Acid maltase deficiency (GSD II)
  - Primary carnitine myopathy
  - Acyl-coenzyme A dehydrogenase deficiencies
- Channelopathies
  - Myotonia congenita (recessive)
  - Periodic paralysis (hypokalemic, hyperkalemic)
- Mitochondrial
  - Numerous mutations

*GSD indicates glycogen storage disease; PROMM, proximal myotonic myopathy.

MYOPATHIES

OVERVIEW OF MUSCLE DISEASE

Table 103-3
Distal Predominant Myopathies*

Acquired
Idiopathic-inflammatory myopathies
Inclusion body myositis
Inherited
Dystrophic
Late-onset type I (Welander)
Late-onset type II (Markesbery-Griggs-Udd)
Early-onset type I (Nonaka)
Early-onset type II (Miyoshi)
Early-onset type III (Laing)
Distal dystrophy with vocal cord paralysis and pharyngeal weakness
Myotonic muscular dystrophy
Scapuloperoneal muscular dystrophy
Facioscapulohumeral muscular dystrophy
Emery-Dreifuss muscular dystrophy
Hereditary inclusion body myopathy
Congenital
Myofibrillar (desmin storage) myopathy
Nemaline myopathy
Central core myopathy
Centronuclear myopathy
Congenital fiber type disproportion
Glycogen and lipid storage
Acid maltase deficiency (GSD II)
Debrancher deficiency (GSD III)
Phosphorylase b kinase deficiency (GSD VIII)

*GSD indicates glycogen storage disease.

Table 103-4
Exercise Intolerance Myopathies*

Acquired
Metabolic
Hypokalemia
Hypothyroidism
Inherited
Glycogen storage
Phosphorylase deficiency (GSD V)
Phosphofructokinase deficiency (GSD VII)
Other possibilities
Phosphoglycerate kinase deficiency (GSD IX)
Phosphoglycerate mutase deficiency (GSD X)
Lactate dehydrogenase deficiency (GSD XI)
Lipid storage
Carnitine palmitoyltransferase II deficiency
Very-long-chain acyl-coenzyme A dehydrogenase deficiency
Trifunctional protein deficiency
Short-chain 3-hydroxyacyl CoA dehydrogenase deficiency
Mitochondrial disorders (respiratory chain)
Complex I, III, or IV deficiency
Coenzyme deficiency Q_{10}

*GSD indicates glycogen storage disease.

gain an objective temporal profile of the clinical findings of the patient. An exact diagnosis also may prove elusive in patients who present with myoglobinuria, for whom a number of additional studies may be diagnostically helpful (Table 103-8).

Table 103-5
Periodic Weakness Myopathies

Inherited
Channelopathies
Hypokalemic periodic paralysis
Hyperkalemic periodic paralysis
Paramyotonia congenita
Others

normalities. Such individuals may have (as yet) undefined disorders of mitochondrial or other muscle metabolism. Some of them are inappropriately diagnosed with chronic fatigue syndrome, fibromyalgia, or even psychosomatic illness. Diagnostic judgment should be made cautiously. Patients with Lambert-Eaton syndrome, presenting with symptoms of proximal but "give way" weakness, have been incorrectly diagnosed with psychologic disorders. It is appropriate to recheck patients in 4 to 6 months to

OVERVIEW OF MUSCLE DISEASE

Table 103-6
Myopathies Associated With Distinctive Clinical Features and Patterns of Weakness*

Calf hypertrophy
- Dystrophinopathy
- Hypothyroidism
- Amyloidosis
- Sarcoidosis
- Glycogen storage disorders
- Limb-girdle muscular dystrophy types 1C, 2B, 2C-F

Contractures
- Emery-Dreifuss muscular dystrophy
- Congenital muscular dystrophy
- Ullrich/Bethlem myopathy
- Limb-girdle muscular dystrophy types 1A, 1B, 2A

Cardiac conduction abnormalities
- Anderson syndrome (periodic paralysis)
- Dermatomyositis/polymyositis (rare)
- Emery-Dreifuss muscular dystrophy
- Mitochondrial (Kearns-Sayres)
- Myotonic muscular dystrophy

Cardiomyopathy
- Carnitine deficiency
- Dermatomyositis/polymyositis
- Dystrophinopathy
- Emery-Dreifuss muscular dystrophy
- Glycogen storage disease types II, III, and IV
- Limb-girdle muscular dystrophy types 1B, 1D, 2C-F, 2G, 2I
- Myofibrillar myopathy
- Nemaline myopathy

Dysphonia
- Limb-girdle muscular dystrophy type 1A

Ptosis and ophthalmoparesis
- Ptosis only
  - Central core disease
  - Centronuclear myopathy
  - Myotonic muscular dystrophy

(continued)

Table 103-6
Myopathies Associated With Distinctive Clinical Features and Patterns of Weakness* (continued)

- Nemaline myopathy
- Oculopharyngeal muscular dystrophy

Ptosis and ophthalmoparesis
- Oculopharyngeal muscular dystrophy
- Oculopharyngeal distal muscular dystrophy
- Mitochondrial myopathy
- Myotubular myopathy

Gastrointestinal motility problems
- Dystrophinopathy
- Mitochondrial myopathy (MNGIE)
- Myotonic dystrophy

Head drop
- Carnitine deficiency
- Congenital myopathies
- Dermatomyositis/polymyositis/IBM
- FSH dystrophy
- Hyperparathyroidism
- Isolated paraspinal myopathy
- Myotonic muscular dystrophy

Myotonia (clinical)
- Myotonia congenita
- Myotonic muscular dystrophy
- Paramyotonia congenita
- (Hyperkalemic periodic paralysis; EMG primarily)

*FSH indicates facioscapulohumeral; IBM, inclusion body myositis; MNGIE, mitochondrial neurogastrointestinal encephalopathy syndrome.

Creatine Kinase

Increased CK level, or hyperCKemia, is a nonspecific finding vis-à-vis the existence of myopathies. Other motor unit disorders (such as motor neuron disease/amyotrophic lateral sclerosis or spinal muscular atrophy) and systemic processes (particularly myxedema) are commonly associated with CK increases 2 to 5 times higher than normal levels. Conversely, CK determinations are normal in several of the congenital myopathies that typically lack myofiber necrosis. Patients with persistently increased CK levels, sometimes associated with mus-

OVERVIEW OF MUSCLE DISEASE

Table 103-7
Regional Patterns of Weakness*

Asymmetric
IBM
FSH
Scapuloperoneal dystrophy
Miyoshi
Distal
Foot dorsiflexors
Myotonic muscular dystrophy
Acid maltase
Caveolin-3
Central core disease
Centronuclear myopathy
Debrancher deficiency
Dysferlinopathies
Laing
Markesbery-Udd
Nemaline myopathy
Nonaka
Oculopharyngeal distal muscular dystrophy
Foot plantar flexors
Dysferlin (Miyoshi)
Wrist and finger extensors
Welander
Wrist and finger flexors
IBM
Facioscapulohumeral
FSH
Scapuloperoneal
Scapuloperoneal
Emery-Dreifuss
Acid maltase
Nemaline myopathy
Central core disease
Humeroperoneal
Emery-Dreifuss
Biceps and hamstrings greater than triceps and quadriceps
Limb-girdle muscular dystrophy type 2C-F

(continued)

Table 103-7
Regional Patterns of Weakness*
(continued)

Adductor much greater than abductor weakness
Limb-girdle muscular dystrophy type 2A (calpain)
Ventilatory muscle weakness
Acid maltase deficiency
Carnitine deficiency
Centronuclear myopathy
Congenital muscular dystrophy
Dystrophinopathy
Emery-Dreifuss muscular dystrophy
Limb-girdle muscular dystrophy
Mitochondrial myopathy (rare)
Myotonic muscular dystrophy
Nemaline myopathy
Polymyositis (rare)

*FSH indicates facioscapulohumeral; IBM, inclusion body myositis.

cle pain but without clinically demonstrable weakness, contributory family histories, or exposure to potentially myotoxic substances, are classified as having **hyperCKemia**. Despite thorough clinical and laboratory examination, the cause for hyperCKemia is often elusive (Figure 103-1).

Electromyography

EMG evaluation of patients with suspected myopathies is important, with several caveats. Results of routine nerve conduction studies are normal in myopathies, with the exception of diminished compound muscle action potential amplitudes in more severe disorders. EMG abnormalities in the myopathies are often limited to the needle examination.

Destruction of myofibrils or muscle membrane results in the classic myopathic EMG abnormalities of low amplitude, short duration, and polyphasic motor unit potentials sometimes associated with abnormal insertional activity, particularly fibrillation potentials and complex repetitive discharges. Inflammatory myopathies, several dystrophies, and various muscle disorders associated with myotonic discharges are well defined by EMG.

OVERVIEW OF MUSCLE DISEASE

Table 103-8
Evaluation of a Patient With Suspected Muscle Disease*

Primary Studies	Studies That May Be Indicated in Some Patients
EMG	Muscle biopsy
CK	Potassium (serum)
Aldolase	Lactate (serum)
	Thyroid function tests, electrolytes
	Anti–acetylcholine receptor antibodies
	Ischemic forearm exercise testing (lactate, ammonia)
	Ischemic forearm exercise testing (venous O_2)
	Total eosinophil count
	Immunofixation (serum)
	DNA mutational analysis for dystrophinopathy
	DNA mutational analysis for FSH muscular dystrophy
	DNA mutational analysis for oculopharyngeal muscular dystrophy
	DNA mutational analysis for specific mitochondrial disorders
	DNA mutational analysis for myotonic muscular dystrophy types I and II
	Myositis-specific antibodies
	Forced vital capacity
	Electrocardiogram, echocardiogram
	Slit lamp examination

*CK indicates creatine kinase; FSH, indicates facioscapulohumeral; IBM, inclusion body myositis.

Concomitantly, EMG helps to exclude disorders that affect other anatomical sites within the peripheral motor unit, particularly those presenting with symmetric proximal weakness mimicking a myopathy. These include chronic inflammatory demyelinating polyneuropathies, neuromuscular transmission disorders (particularly Lambert-Eaton myasthenic syndrome), and myasthenia gravis.

Results of EMG are often normal in the endocrine, mitochondrial, and congenital myopathies. Disorders of energy metabolism do not affect the muscle fibers. The morphologic abnormalities characteristic of the congenital myopathies (nemaline rods, central cores, and fiber-type disproportion) do not lead to myofibril destruction or to sarcolemma membrane damage, ie, phenomena that cause "myopathic" abnormalities on an EMG.

Forearm Exercise Testing

Forearm exercise testing screens for certain glycogen storage disorders and myoadenylate deaminase deficiency. Its role is somewhat controversial because it is painful, has at least a theoretical potential to trigger rhabdomyolysis, and has perhaps been superceded by newer means of diagnosis. In the ischemic forearm test, patients with glycogen storage disease type V or VII do not develop a meaningful (>3 times baseline) increase in serum lactate levels after periods of repeated contraction in relatively ischemic conditions. Simultaneous serum ammonia measurements are performed,

MYOPATHIES

OVERVIEW OF MUSCLE DISEASE

Figure 103-1 **Laboratory Studies in Neuromuscular Diseases: Electromyography and Serum Enzymes**

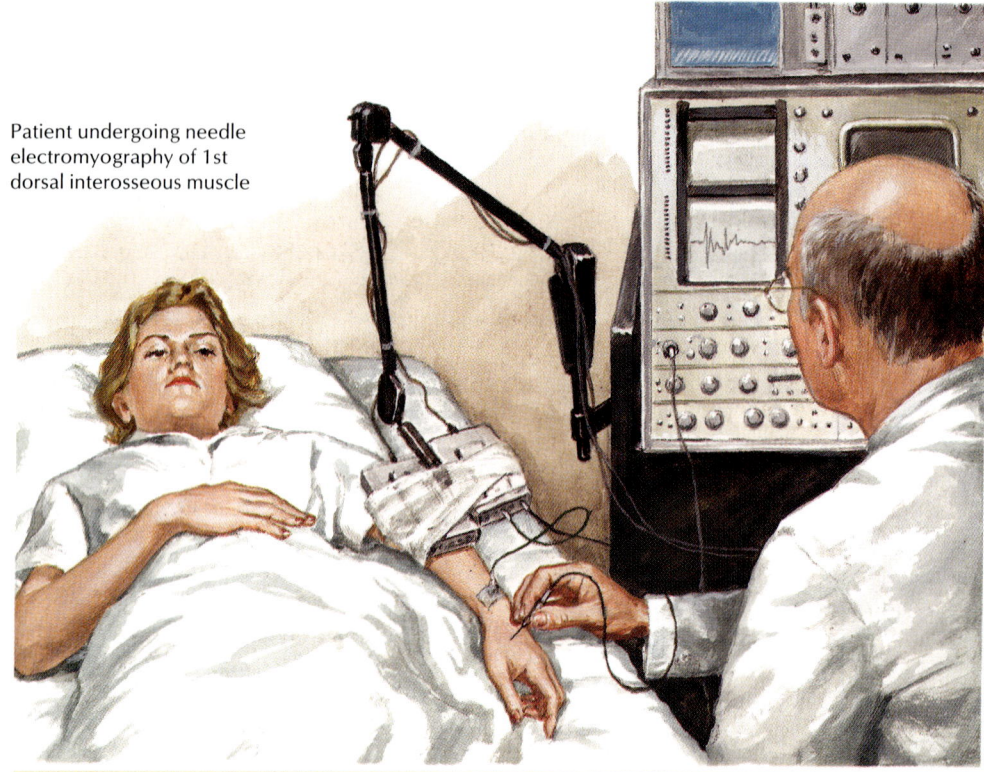
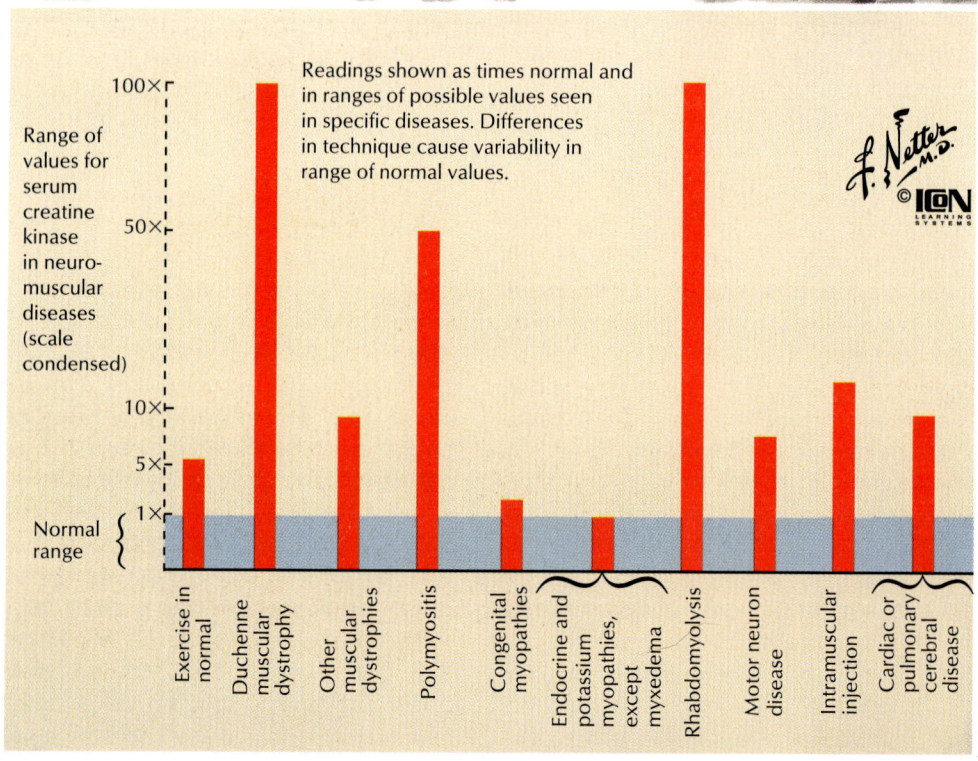

MYOPATHIES

providing a means to determine adequate effort. With myoadenylate deaminase deficiency, lactate levels increase, but ammonia levels do not.

Mitochondria Evaluations

Diagnosing mitochondrial myopathies is often difficult. Confirmatory testing has significant limitations. Serum and CSF lactate and pyruvate levels may be increased at rest but are not adequately sensitive or specific. Muscle biopsy is too invasive to be routinely used as a screening tool for vague and nonspecific symptoms. In addition, the histologic hallmark of mitochondrial disease, the "ragged red fiber," as well as succinate dehydrogenase and cytochrome C oxidase evaluations, lack sensitivity and specificity.

Commercially available tests for mutations in mitochondrial or nuclear DNA are few and costly. Forearm exercise testing, analogous to that used in suspected glycogen storage disorders, may prove useful in screening for mitochondrial disorders. Venous O_2 levels decrease when obtained from the exercised forearm in healthy individuals. However, in patients with mitochondrial disorders, the partial pressure of venous O_2 increases during exercise.

Muscle Biopsy

Muscle biopsy is the definitive diagnostic tool for many myopathies (Figure 103-2). The selection of the biopsy site is important; muscles that are unaffected, are at end stage, or have been recently subjected to EMG evaluation need to be avoided. Muscle should be divided into separate aliquots for formalin fixation, paraffin embedding, and immediate freezing. The formalin-fixed piece reacts with a limited number of stains; hematoxylin and eosin staining is most commonly used because it is rapid and especially useful for identifying inflammatory myopathies with potential for therapeutic intervention. Frozen specimens are particularly suited to extensive batteries of stains, including NADH, modified Gomori trichrome, adenosine triphosphatase, and lipid and glycogen stains (Figure 103-3).

Muscle biopsy specimens are also commonly subjected to biochemical analysis, mutational analysis, and electron microscopy, when these techniques are available. Immunohistochemical stains, immunoblotting, or both are available for calpain, caveolin, dysferlin, the dystroglycans, dystrophin, laminin-2 (formerly merosin), and the sarcoglycans.

DNA Mutational Analysis

DNA mutational analysis is an increasingly valuable diagnostic tool in heritable myopathies. False-positive results are rare. False-negative results occur for at least two reasons. Most clinical phenotypes occur from mutations on more than one chromosome. A commercially available test may exist for one genotypic form of a disorder but not another. False-negative results may also occur if technology allows for the detection of one type of mutation, eg, duplication or deletion, but not another, eg, point mutation.

Mutational analysis may also be useful for prenatal evaluation, in carriers, and in presymptomatic individuals. Before testing, patients and their families should have a thorough understanding of potential test benefits and risks. A listing of commercially available mutational analyses for heritable muscle diseases can be found at www.genetests.org.

Malignant Hyperthermia Evaluation

In vitro testing is available at a few laboratories for the potentially fatal trait leading to malignant hyperthermia. This is significant in congenital myopathies and in individuals with hyperCKemia.

Antibodies

Fewer than half of all patients with polymyositis and dermatomyositis have serum myositis-specific and myositis-associated antibodies. Serologic testing for these antibodies has a limited but sometimes useful role. Anti-Jo-1 antibodies suggest potential end organ comorbidity, eg, interstitial lung disease. Anti–signal recognition particle antibodies confer the probability of poor treatment response. The presence of these antibodies can aid in the diagnosis of the occasional patient for whom the history is not definitive and there is confusion between the possibility of an acquired inflammatory myopathy and a genetically determined dystrophy in which these antibodies are not present.

OVERVIEW OF MUSCLE DISEASE

Figure 103-2 Muscle Biopsy: Technique

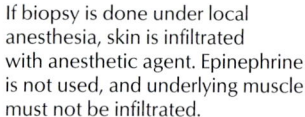

If biopsy is done under local anesthesia, skin is infiltrated with anesthetic agent. Epinephrine is not used, and underlying muscle must not be infiltrated.

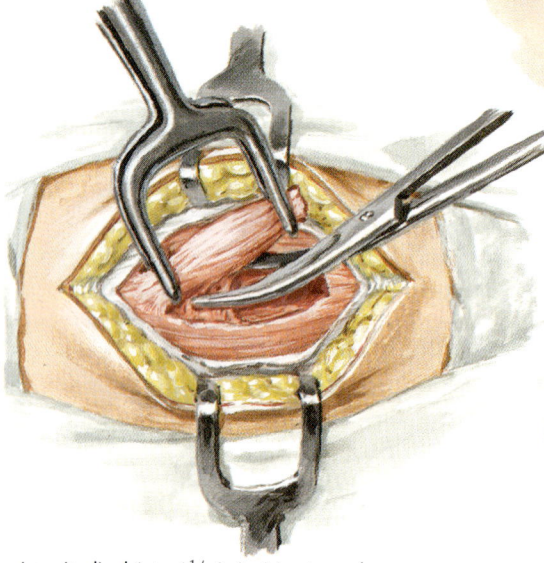

Longitudinal 1- to 1½-in incision is made and fascia incised, exposing muscle belly. Thin cylinder of muscle for ultrastructural study is excised in clamp and promptly immersed in glutaraldehyde.

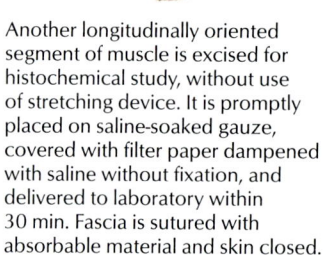

Another longitudinally oriented segment of muscle is excised for histochemical study, without use of stretching device. It is promptly placed on saline-soaked gauze, covered with filter paper dampened with saline without fixation, and delivered to laboratory within 30 min. Fascia is sutured with absorbable material and skin closed.

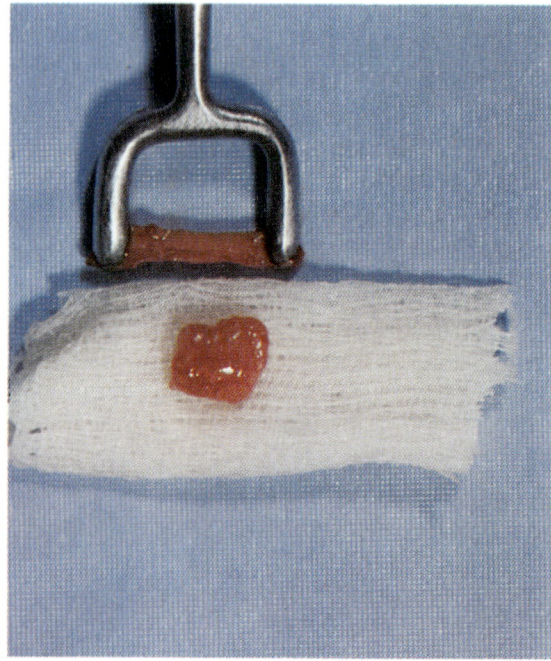

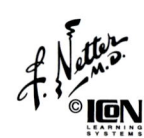

Clamped portion of biopsy specimen must be promptly fixed in glutaraldehyde and processed for electron microscopy. Free portion on saline-soaked gauze must be frozen within 30 min, cryostat-sectioned and stained for histochemical study.

MYOPATHIES

OVERVIEW OF MUSCLE DISEASE

Figure 103-3   Sections From Muscle Biopsy Specimens

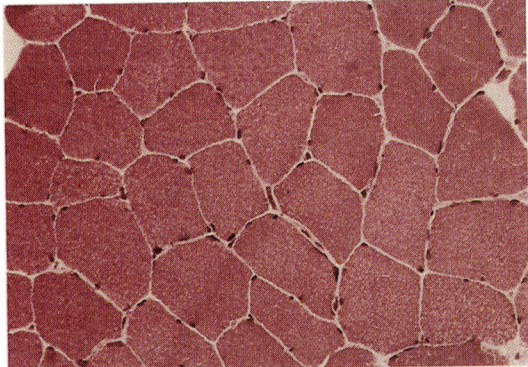

Cryostat section of normal adult muscle stained with hematoxylin and eosin. Muscle fibers are uniform in size and stain pink with eosin; their sarcolemmal nuclei are peripherally located and stain blue with hematoxylin.

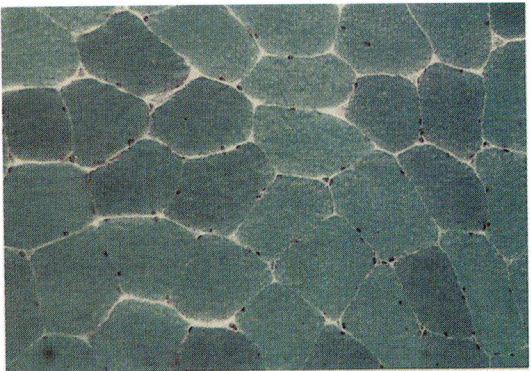

Cryostat section of normal adult muscle treated with modified Gomori trichrome stain, which stains muscle fibers greenish blue and sarcolemmal nuclei dark red.

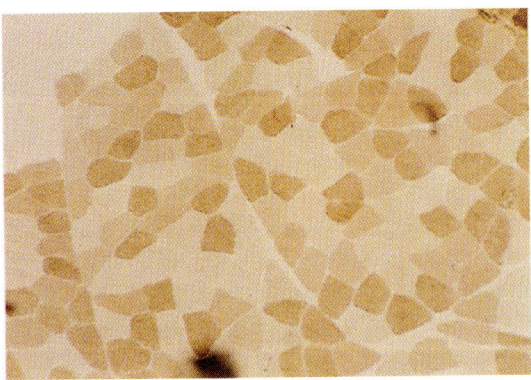

Cryostat section of normal muscle from adult male (ATPase stain, pH 4.6). Type II fibers, which contain low amounts of acid-stable ATPase, are subtyped into IIA (lightest) and IIB (intermediate) fibers. Type I (darkest) fibers contain largest amount of acid-stable ATPase. Each of these 3 fiber types amount to about 1/3 of total number.

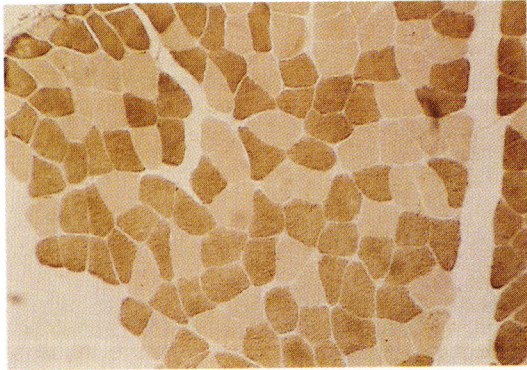

Cryostat section of norma muscle from adult male (ATPase stain, pH 9.4), showing typical checkerboard pattern with about twice as many type II fibers, which are high in alkali-stable ATPase and hence stain darkly.

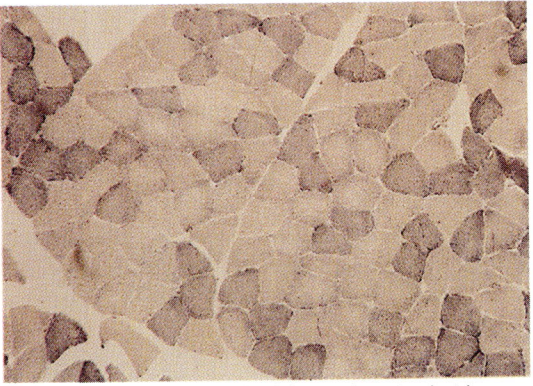

Cryostat section of normal adult muscle stained with NADH, an oxidative enzyme that reacts with mitochondria, sarcoplasmic reticulum, and T tubules. Type I fibers stain more darkly.

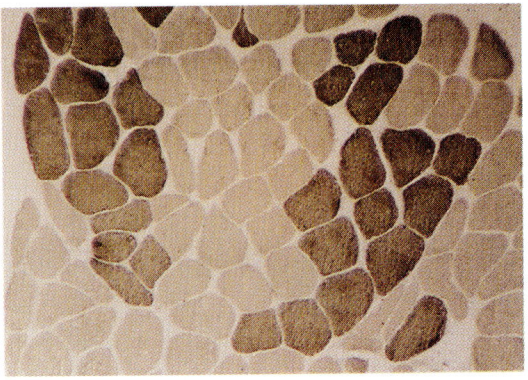

Cryostat section of reinnervated skeletal muscle stained with ATPase (pH 9.4), showing grouping of 2 fiber types: type I (lighter), type II (darker). Compare with normal section stained with ATPase (pH 9.4) above.

MYOPATHIES

OVERVIEW OF MUSCLE DISEASE

In summary, many laboratory studies are available for evaluating patients with suspected myopathies. Testing is case based and should be interpreted in the context of clinical phenotype.

TREATMENT

Muscle disorders are best managed by considering disease-specific therapies, genetic counseling, and various forms of supportive care. Unfortunately, few specific pharmacologic therapies are currently available for the myopathies. Directed therapies are anticipated for a number of genetic disorders.

Specific Pharmacologic Therapies

Polymyositis, dermatomyositis, and idiopathic, inflammatory, granulomatous, and sarcoid myopathies are often somewhat responsive to immunomodulating treatments. Prednisone is considered the gold standard, although its effect has never been confirmed in a well-designed prospective study. Other immunomodulating therapies are used, but none is the clear best second-line therapy. Immunomodulating treatments have no significant benefit in inclusion body myositis.

Steroids may benefit boys with Duchenne dystrophy by slowing disease progression and prolonging independent ambulation. This may occur at the expense of normal growth. There is no place for steroids in other dystrophies with potential inflammatory components, such as fascioscapulohumeral muscular dystrophy.

Replacement and suppression therapies for endocrine and other metabolic myopathies are important modalities for these eminently treatable disorders. Carbonic anhydrase inhibitors often effectively prevent attacks of periodic paralysis, but they do not prevent the fixed weakness that commonly develops in older patients. Mexiletine can suppress symptomatic myotonia. Carnitine replacement may benefit patients with lipid storage myopathies resulting from primary carnitine deficiency. Other disease-specific therapies include withdrawal of myotoxic agents.

Genetic Counseling

Patients need to understand the significance of the diagnosis, its anticipated natural history and response to treatment, and the pertinent genetic implications. Many patients perceive that a myopathic diagnosis is synonymous with Duchenne muscular dystrophy and its dismal prognosis. This should be clarified when relevant. Some patients want to understand as completely as they can what the future may hold. Patients often harbor fears, expressed or unexpressed, about eventually requiring a wheelchair. This concern should be anticipated and discussed when appropriate. If ventilatory failure is a future possibility, it is important to engage the patient in long-range treatment considerations.

The **Muscular Dystrophy Association** and its local support groups provide excellent sources of genetic information and support. Social workers knowledgeable in the resources available to patients and the means by which to access them are a most important resource for many patients with myopathy. Involvement of dedicated genetics services may provide further scientific detail and the means for psychologic support.

In conditions in which disease progression may cause ventilatory failure, patients must be engaged in consideration of long-range treatment options, including the possibility of long-term respiratory support. Tracheostomy may also be necessary for adequate secretion control.

Supportive Therapies

The goal of all treatments is maximization of patient function. Most patients with significant myopathies benefit from the involvement of a physiatrist early in the course of their illness. Rehabilitation specialists are best able to decide what form of support aids, including braces, canes, crutches, walkers, wheelchairs, lift chairs, stair lifts, elevators, bed rails, and lifting devices, are best suited for the individual patient. Lift chairs are beneficial to ambulatory patients with proximal weakness that precludes them from independently rising from a chair. Elevators and stair lifts are valuable when accessing more than 1 floor. Newer lift systems allow patient transfers with the help of a single individual. Crutches are of limited value for patients with myopathy because of concomitant arm weakness.

REFERENCES

Dabby R, Lange DJ, Trojaborg W, et al. Inclusion body myositis mimicking motor neuron disease. *Arch Neurol.* 2001;58:1253-1256.

Ferrante MA, Wilbourn AJ. Myopathies. In: Levin KH, Luders HO, eds. *Comprehensive Clinical Neurophysiology.* Philadelphia, Pa: WB Saunders; 2000:268-281.

Griggs RC, Mendell JR, Miller RG. *Evaluation and Treatment of Myopathy.* Philadelphia, Pa: FA Davis Co; 1995.

Kissel JT, Amato AA, Barohn RJ, et al. Muscle disease. In: American Academy of Neurology. *Continuum.* Philadelphia, Pa: Lippincott Williams & Wilkins; 2000;6:No 2.

Lacomis D, Oddis CV. Myositis-specific and -associated autoantibodies: a review from the clinical perspective. *J Clin Neuromusc Dis.* 2000;2:34-40.

Taivassalo T, Abbott A, Wyrick P, Haller RG. Venous oxygen levels during aerobic forearm exercise: an index of impaired oxidative metabolism in mitochondrial myopathy. *Ann Neurol.* 2002;52:38-44.

Wagner KR. Genetic diseases of muscle. *Neurol Clin.* 2002;20:645-678.

Chapter 104

Acute or Subacute Proximally Predominant or Generalized Myopathies Presenting With Weakness

Jayashri Srinivasan, James A. Russell, and H. Royden Jones, Jr

Clinical Vignette

A 40-year-old woman experienced 4 weeks of progressive difficulty climbing stairs and lifting heavy objects. For the previous 2 weeks, she had noted difficulty swallowing.

Examination disclosed an erythematous rash over the malar region of her face, eyelids, and dorsum of her hands. She had difficulty getting out of her chair when meeting her physician, in addition to weakness of neck flexors, shoulder abduction, knee extension, and hip flexors and extensors. Muscle stretch reflexes were hypoactive, and results of the sensory examination were normal.

The patient's serum creatine kinase (CK) level was increased to 20 times the upper limit of normal, and antinuclear antibodies at a titer of 1:160 were present in her serum. EMG demonstrated low-amplitude, short-duration, polyphasic motor unit potentials recruited in large numbers with relatively modest effort. On insertion of the needle electrode, there were many fibrillation potentials and complex repetitive discharges in multiple proximal muscles including the paraspinals.

The subacute onset of proximal symmetric weakness suggested an acquired myopathy. The time course and distribution of weakness, rash presence and distribution, CK values, increased ANA, and EMG results were strongly suggestive of dermatomyositis (DM). Muscle biopsy demonstrated myofiber necrosis and regeneration, typical findings in DM. Absent was the characteristic inflammatory response and perifascicular atrophy, the latter a highly specific although insensitive feature of this disorder in adults. Immunohistochemical staining for the membrane attack complex was required for confirmation of the clinical impression and demonstrated widespread uptake in the walls of capillaries and small arterioles.

Patients who begin to experience symmetric difficulty using the large muscles of the hip girdle and, less commonly, the proximal muscles of the shoulders and neck present the clinician with an interesting, important diagnostic challenge. When patients experience problems climbing stairs, getting out of low chairs, or holding objects (such as hair dryers) overhead, primary myopathic lesions are suggested (Figure 104-1). However, if the entire peripheral motor unit is always considered in differential diagnosis of this clinical presentation, important and often treatable lesions will also be recognized, particularly at the peripheral nerve level and the neuromuscular junction.

DIFFERENTIAL DIAGNOSIS

Other motor unit abnormalities may present with proximal weakness mimicking primary myopathic processes. These deserve careful consideration in the acute and subacute settings. The most familiar acute entities include acquired demyelinating peripheral nerve lesions such as Guillain-Barré syndrome and, less commonly, myasthenia gravis (MG). The latter is usually recognized by concomitant ocular and bulbar find-

ACUTE PROXIMAL MYOPATHIES

Polymyositis/Dermatomyositis

Figure 104-1

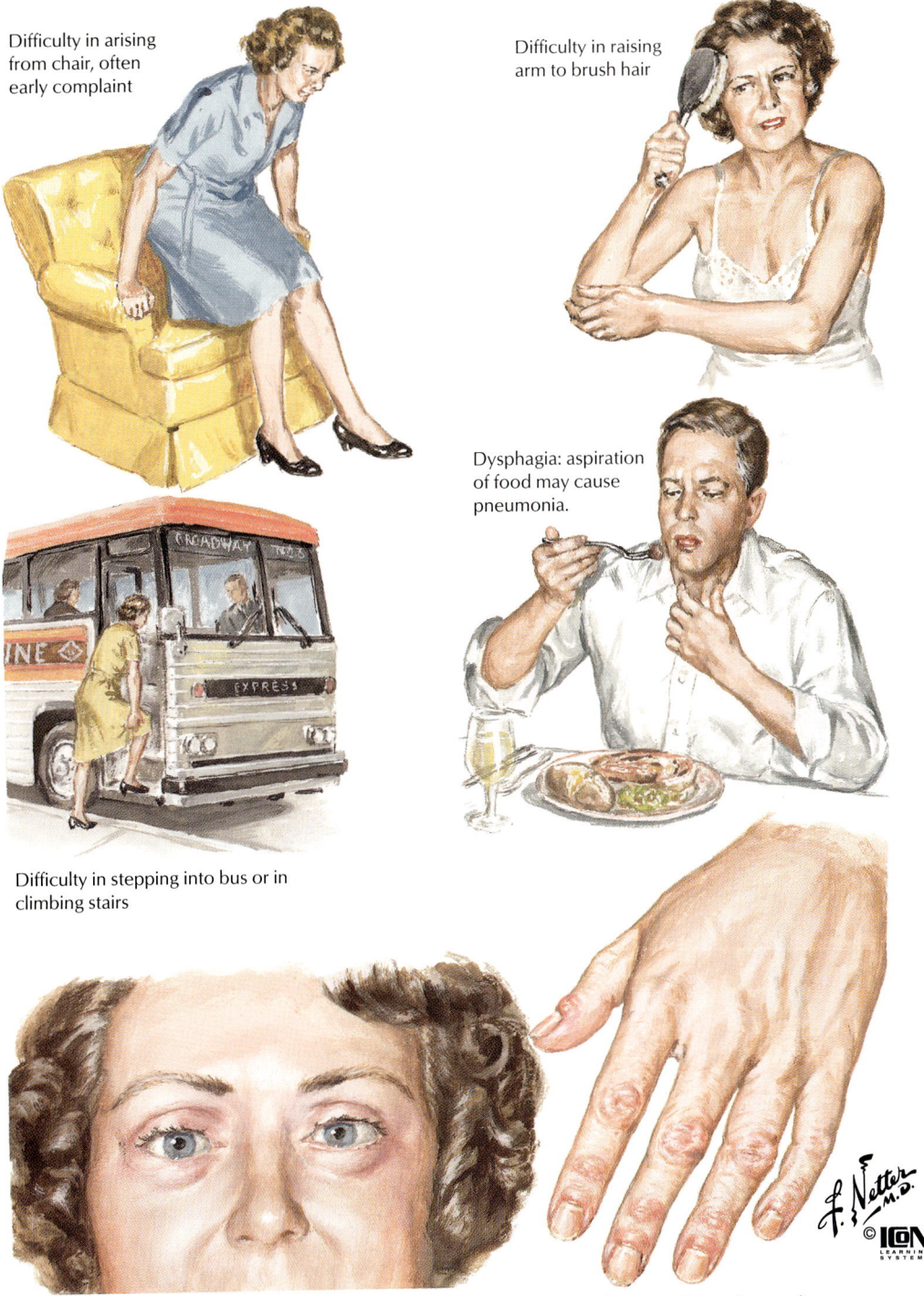

Difficulty in arising from chair, often early complaint

Difficulty in raising arm to brush hair

Dysphagia: aspiration of food may cause pneumonia.

Difficulty in stepping into bus or in climbing stairs

Edema and heliotrope discoloration around eyes a classic sign. More wisespread erythematous rash may also be present.

Erythema and/or scaly, papular eruption around fingernails and on dorsum of interphalangeal joints

MYOPATHIES

885

ACUTE PROXIMAL MYOPATHIES

ings. Subacute considerations include chronic inflammatory demyelinating polyneuropathy and Lambert-Eaton myasthenic syndrome. Hypoactive or absent muscle stretch reflexes are important initial clues to Guillain-Barré syndrome, chronic inflammatory demyelinating polyneuropathy, and Lambert-Eaton myasthenic syndrome. Guillain-Barré syndrome and chronic inflammatory demyelinating polyneuropathy usually have some sensory component. Autonomic symptomatology such as xerostomia and impotence in men point toward Lambert-Eaton myasthenic syndrome.

Immunologically Mediated Myopathies

Patients with DM present subacutely, with symptoms developing over several weeks. Rarely, the onset is precipitous. DM differs from polymyositis (PM) in its specific rash, tendency to involve multiple systems, greater frequency in children, histology, and possibly greater risk of underlying malignancy in adults.

Dermatomyositis occurs with a bimodal age distribution with peaks at 5 to 20 years and 40 to 60 years. Proximal muscles are affected primarily. Weakness of wrist extension, foot dorsiflexion, and swallowing occur in approximately one third of patients with DM. Dysphagia and other bulbar symptoms rarely occur. Significant muscle pain and tenderness are uncommon and are usually not predominant symptoms.

Characteristic cutaneous changes include an erythematous rash on the face, trunk, and limbs; heliotrope discoloration of upper eyelids; papular erythema over the knuckles (Gottron sign) (Figure 104-1); and, in adolescents, subcutaneous calcification over pressure points. The rash may precede or occasionally occur without a clinical myopathy. In contrast to children, systemic involvement is uncommon in adults but may include cardiomyopathy, enteric infarction, and interstitial lung disease.

Polymyositis is the least common idiopathic inflammatory myopathy. PM in most adults is clinically indistinguishable from DM. The pattern of weakness is identical. The arms are often affected to an equal or greater degree than the legs. Facial weakness is occasionally identified. Systemic manifestations are less prevalent than in DM, and rash is not present in PM.

Inclusion body myositis, the most common autoimmune myopathy, has a chronic presentation as described in chapter 105.

Toxic Myopathies

Many chemicals cause myopathies (Table 104-1). **Statin class lipid-lowering agents** lead to necrotizing myopathies in a small percentage of patients using them. A slightly larger percentage of individuals have asymptomatic increases of

Table 104-1
Toxic Myopathies

Alcohol
Aminocaproic acid
Amiodarone
Chloroquine/hydroxychloroquine
Cholesterol-lowering agents
Cimetidine
Colchicine
Corticosteroids
Cyclosporine
Emetine
Illicit drugs (IM injections)
Ipecac
Labetalol
Lamotrigine
Leuprolide
Lithium
L-Tryptophan
Neuromuscular blocking agents
Omeprazole
Penicillamine
Procainamide
Propofol
Rifampin
Tacrolimus
Toluene (inhalation)
Vincristine
Vitamin E
Zidovudine

ACUTE PROXIMAL MYOPATHIES

the serum CK, presumably related to subclinical muscle inflammation. The risk increases in patients simultaneously exposed to more than 1 drug.

HMG-CoA-reductase inhibitors (statins), fibric acid derivatives, and niacin all have myotoxic properties. Patients present with myalgias, proximal weakness, or both but rarely with rhabdomyolysis. Muscle biopsies in severely affected patients demonstrate necrosis and mitochondrial changes.

Chloroquine may cause amphiphilic neuromyopathies. CK is often increased. Muscle biopsy characteristically reveals autophagic vacuolation, with markedly increased staining for acid phosphatase.

Colchicine may also cause myopathy or neuropathy, which relate to colchicine-induced alteration of microtubular function. CK is usually increased, and muscle biopsies demonstrate autophagic vacuoles. Symptoms improve with drug discontinuation.

Zidovudine (AZT), a primary therapy for HIV infection, can induce a myopathy related to mitochondrial dysfunction. The myopathies caused by zidovudine and by HIV infection are clinically indistinguishable. CK values are usually increased. EMG does not distinguish between toxic AZT and HIV myopathies. Muscle biopsies demonstrate endomysial inflammation. Prominent ragged red fibers suggest AZT-induced mitochondrial abnormalities. AZT myopathies usually improve on drug cessation.

Critical Illness Myopathy

Critical illness myopathy, also referred to as *acute quadriplegic myopathy* or *myopathy associated with thick filament (myosin) loss*, is probably the most common cause of generalized weakness in the ICU. Critical illness myopathy is commonly seen in patients treated with high doses of corticosteroids or neuromuscular blocking drugs or who have sepsis with multiorgan failure. Weakness develops over several days and may be first detected when ventilator weaning is attempted. Clinical examination reveals profound, possibly asymmetric, weakness, reduced muscle stretch reflexes, and a normal sensory examination. Serum CK is increased in less than half of these patients. Muscle biopsies may show muscle fiber necrosis, atrophy of type 1 and 2 fibers, and patchy loss of uptake with adenosine triphosphatase stains. The latter correlates with electron microscopic demonstration of thick filament (ie, myosin) loss. The pathogenesis is not understood.

Hypokalemic Myopathies

Hypokalemia is a rare metabolic cause of acute myopathy (Figure 104-2). The presentation may mimic Guillain-Barré syndrome. ICU observation is recommended because of potential serious arrhythmias that may result from severe hypokalemia. Important etiologies include adrenal insufficiency (Addison disease), renal disease, and various potassium-losing diuretics and corticosteroids.

Endocrine Myopathies

Disorders of the adrenal, thyroid, and parathyroid glands can result in a number of subacute or, less commonly, acute myopathies. Interestingly, muscle involvement in such conditions may be apparent before patients have more typical clinical findings of their primary endocrinopathy.

Endogenous (Cushing disease) or exogenous (Cushing syndrome) corticosteroid excess is the most common cause of endocrine myopathy. Patients with Cushing syndrome, irrespective of etiology, experience proximal muscle weakness with atrophy usually starting in the hip girdles. Distal, bulbar, and ocular muscles are usually unaffected. Women seem to be more susceptible than men.

Alternate-day corticosteroid dosing schedules and enriched protein diets may reduce susceptibility. The serum CK level is usually normal. EMG is usually normal in iatrogenic steroid myopathy but is occasionally "myopathic" in patients with true Cushing syndrome. Type II fiber atrophy is apparent on muscle biopsy. The pathogenesis is poorly understood but may be related to increased protein catabolism.

Clinical Vignette

A 38-year-old woman had typical myopathic symptoms. Her husband noted that her emotions were more labile. Neurologic examination demonstrated moderate proximal weakness.

ACUTE PROXIMAL MYOPATHIES

Figure 104-2

Myopathies Related to Disorders of Potassium Metabolism

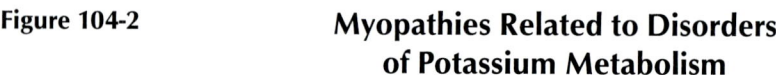

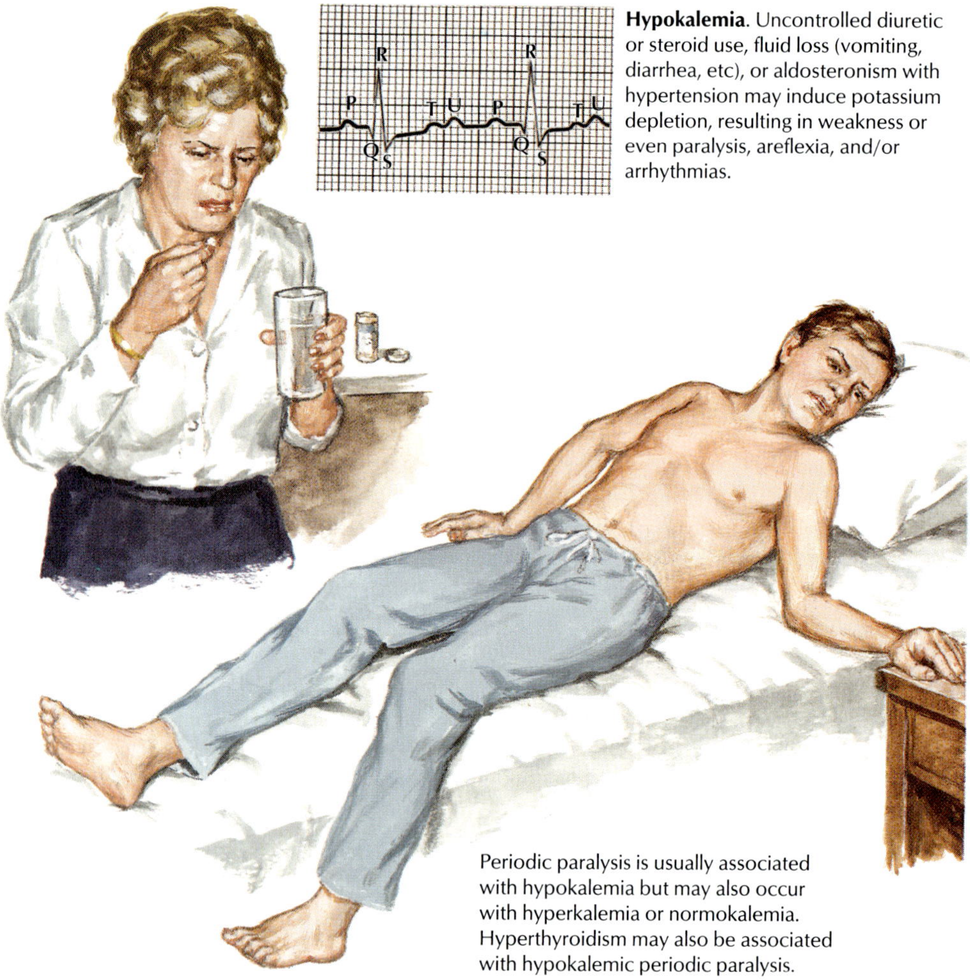

Hypokalemia. Uncontrolled diuretic or steroid use, fluid loss (vomiting, diarrhea, etc), or aldosteronism with hypertension may induce potassium depletion, resulting in weakness or even paralysis, areflexia, and/or arrhythmias.

Periodic paralysis is usually associated with hypokalemia but may also occur with hyperkalemia or normokalemia. Hyperthyroidism may also be associated with hypokalemic periodic paralysis.

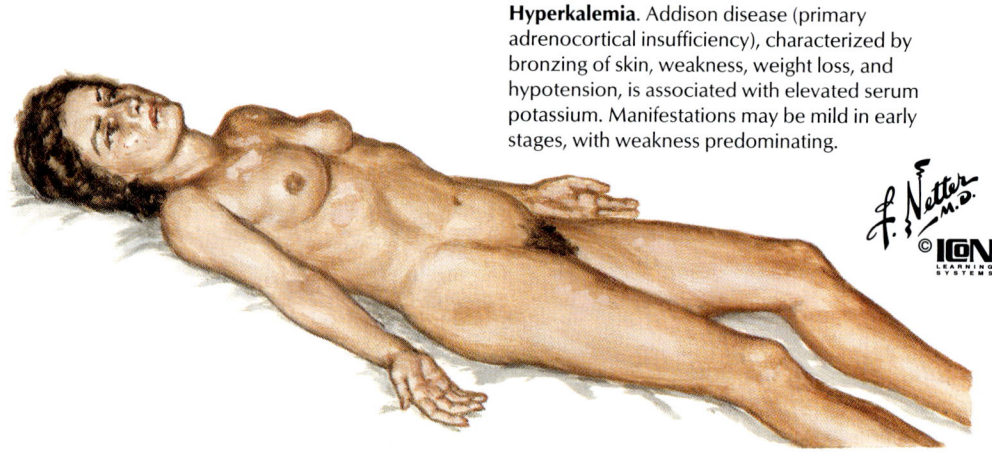

Hyperkalemia. Addison disease (primary adrenocortical insufficiency), characterized by bronzing of skin, weakness, weight loss, and hypotension, is associated with elevated serum potassium. Manifestations may be mild in early stages, with weakness predominating.

ACUTE PROXIMAL MYOPATHIES

When she returned for her EMG, the neurologist noted generalized bruising that resembled that of patients taking corticosteroids. Although she did not have other common stigmata of Cushing syndrome, it seemed that the bruising was similar to that of patients with hypercortisolism. The muscle strength testing thus led to the bruising.

The patient's EMG demonstrated myopathic motor unit potentials with fibrillation potentials. The EMG findings were surprising because most endocrine myopathies, including corticosteroid-induced myopathies, are not associated with abnormal insertional activity. Despite such, Cushing syndrome was considered in the differential of this slowly evolving myopathy when there were no abdominal striae, truncal obesity, or buffalo hump present. Serum cortisol levels were increased, and a corticotropin-producing pituitary tumor was found on neuroimaging.

Hyperthyroidism and Hypothyroidism

In addition to typical myopathic features, hyperthyroid patients have brisk muscle stretch reflexes, dysthyroid orbitopathy with proptosis, and impairment of extraocular muscle function. Thyrotoxicosis is associated with myasthenia gravis in approximately 5% of cases. Asian males also have a propensity to hypokalemic periodic paralysis with hyperthyroidism. Serum CK and routine electrodiagnostic study results are usually normal.

Hypothyroid patients present with proximal weakness, fatigue, myalgia, and cramps. Needle EMG is usually normal. Serum CK is usually increased 10 to 100 times and may lead to searching for primary myopathies such as PM. The differential diagnosis should include hypothyroidism in any patient presenting with an adult-onset myopathy.

Granulomatous Myopathies

Patients with **sarcoid myopathy** have granulomas in muscle tissue, often without symptoms. Focal pain, atrophy, or generalized proximal weakness may be seen. Diagnosis usually requires involvement of other end organs typically involved by sarcoidosis, particularly the liver or lungs.

Nonspecific inflammatory granulomatous myopathies are rare, although they may be seen with underlying myasthenia gravis and thymoma. Ocular and bulbar symptoms attributable to myasthenia may accompany proximal weakness.

Eosinophilic Myositis

Eosinophilic myositis is usually a component of hypereosinophilic syndrome. The pattern of weakness is indistinguishable from that of DM/PM. Systemic features of hypereosinophilic syndrome involving the heart, lungs, skin, kidneys, and gastrointestinal tract are usually present.

Infectious Myopathies

HIV infection may produce a primary inflammatory myopathy with subacute or chronic proximal weakness and myalgia. Typically seen in patients with CD4 counts of less than 200/mm^3, HIV myopathy may be difficult to distinguish from PM.

Viral syndromes cause significant myalgia, particularly in their prodromal phases. Acute myositis is occasionally seen in children and presents with prominent calf pain and toe walking. The CK level is usually increased; muscle biopsy reveals scattered necrotic and regenerating fibers. The course is self-limiting. Rarely, there may be severe muscle rhabdomyolysis with significant increase of CK, myoglobinuria, and consequent metabolic derangement.

Trichinosis, typically caused by the ingestion of inadequately cooked pork, is the most common parasitic infection of muscle. Some patients have a prodrome of nausea, vomiting, and periorbital edema within days after exposure. Severe myalgia, weakness, fever, and sometimes encephalopathy then develop. Occasionally, trichinosis causes a chronic myopathy.

In eosinophilic leukocytosis, the serum CK level may be increased. Muscle biopsy sometimes demonstrates organisms and eosinophilic infiltration.

Pyomyositis is a rare primary bacterial infection of muscle primarily seen in the tropics that is more common in immunodeficient individuals and can be caused by a number of gram-positive and -negative organisms. Muscle pain, tenderness, and fever are prominent. Neutrophilic leukocytosis and bacteremia also occur. CT and MRI of muscle may demonstrate muscle abscesses.

Paraneoplastic Necrotizing Myopathy

Paraneoplastic necrotizing myopathies are rare and are typically associated with lung, gas-

ACUTE PROXIMAL MYOPATHIES

Figure 104-3 Polymyositis/Dermatomyositis

A. Electromyography

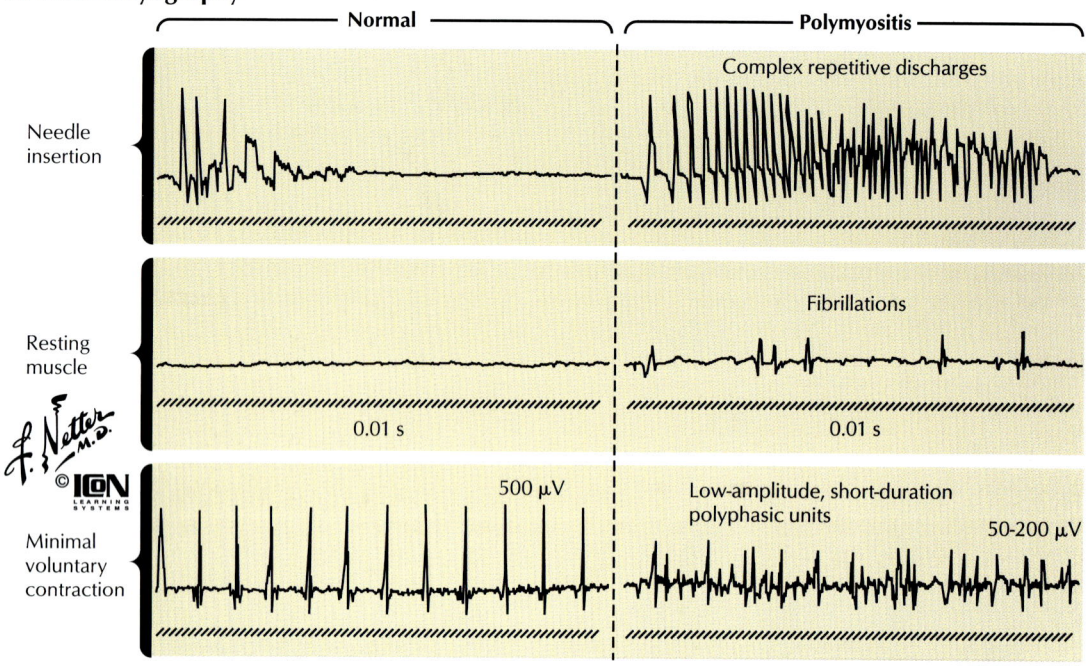

B. Muscle Biopsy

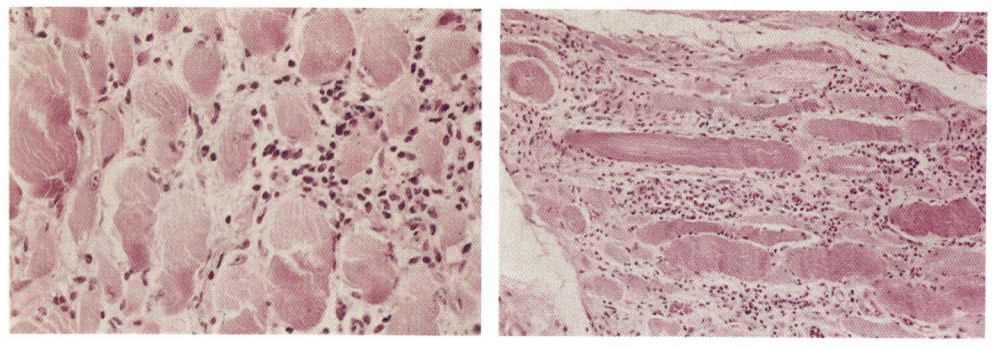

Transverse section ← Muscle biopsy specimens → Longitudinal section
Inflammatory reaction: muscle fiber necrosis and regeneration

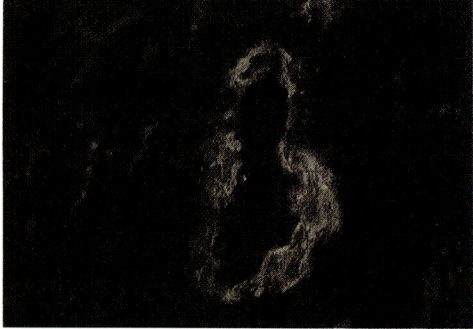

Anti-IgG immunofluorescence of frozen muscle section with positive staining within blood vessel wall, indicating immunologic basis of dermatomyositis

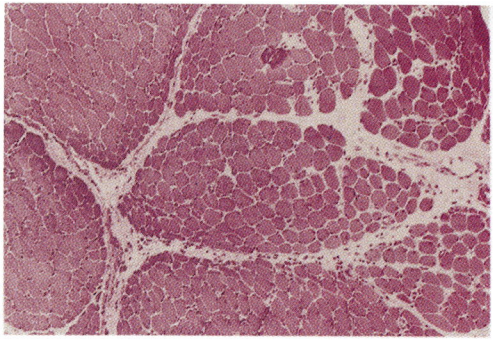

Perifascicular muscle atrophy in child with dermatomyositis

trointestinal, or adenocarcinoma. They typically present with gradually progressive proximal weakness with or without myalgias. The serum CK level may be increased. Necrotic muscle fibers with "pipestem" arterioles and capillaries with perivascular inflammation are notable histologic findings.

DIAGNOSTIC APPROACH

The diagnostic approach must be tailored to the index of clinical suspicion and impact of potential diagnoses. Serum CK determinations and EMG are routine screening procedures (Figure 104-3). Muscle biopsy is performed in many patients with suspected muscle disease and is especially valuable when histologically documenting an indication for treatment with immunosuppressive agents. Myositis-specific antibodies have limited utility.

Dermatomyositis may convey an increased, albeit very small, risk of occult malignancy. The intensity of diagnostic evaluation for a potential occult cancer is determined individually. A general physical examination, a thorough review of systems, a chest radiograph or CT, a mammogram (in women), a CBC, urinalysis, and stool guaiac are considered a reasonable screening protocol.

TREATMENT AND PROGNOSIS
Immunomodulating Therapies

Immunomodulating therapies are preferred treatments for DM and PM. Corticosteroids are the first-line drugs, typically prednisone equivalents of 1 to 1.5 mg/kg. Alternate-day dosing and appropriate dose tapers should be considered as soon as symptoms are adequately controlled. Sequential CK measurements may be useful in following disease activity.

Previous tuberculosis exposure should be excluded before initiation of steroid treatment. Vitamin D and calcium are regularly supplemented in patients on prednisone, particularly in women. Bone densitometry is indicated for patients at risk of osteopenia.

Other immunosuppressants are sometimes indicated for treatment of DM or PM when steroid response is inadequate or as steroid-sparing agents. IV immunoglobulin and plasma exchange may be useful for rapidly improving patient strength during myopathic crises.

Other Treatments

Toxic myopathies and critical illness myopathy most commonly resolve within weeks to months of withdrawal of the offending agent. Treatment is supportive, and most patients fully recover muscle strength.

The myotoxicity of cholesterol-lowering agents creates a common and vexing clinical problem. In some patients, CK increases and myalgia persist long after cholesterol-lowering agents are withdrawn. The basis for this phenomenon is unknown.

Endocrine myopathies are responsive to treatment of hormonal excess or inadequacy. Corticosteroid-induced endocrine myopathies usually respond to cessation of steroid therapy or treatment of primary pituitary or adrenal lesions. Some infectious myopathies, such as trichinosis, may respond to antimicrobial agents, corticosteroids, or both. Treatment of pyomyositis consists of appropriate antibiotics and surgical drainage of abscesses.

Prognosis

Control rather than immediate cure is often the most realistic initial management goal. DM and PM eventually stabilize or achieve remission, but drug therapy may be required for months or years.

Patients with infectious, toxic, and metabolic or endocrine myopathies that are amenable to treatment generally have excellent prognoses. The prognosis of paraneoplastic necrotizing myopathies is dependent on that of the underlying malignancy.

REFERENCES

Dalakas MC, Hohlfeld R. Polymyositis and dermatomyositis. *Lancet*. 2003;362:971-982.

Srinivasan J, Amato AA. Myopathies. *Phys Med Rehabil Clin North Am*. 2003;14:403-434.

Chapter 105
Myopathies: Chronic Proximally Predominant or Generalized Weakness

Jayashri Srinivasan, James A. Russell, and H. Royden Jones, Jr

Clinical Vignette

A 60-year-old man reported a 5-year history of slowly progressive diminished exercise tolerance and difficulty climbing stairs. Within the last 2 years, he had begun to have difficulty opening jars or car doors with his right hand and had begun to choke on food.

His examination revealed atrophy and significant weakness of the right wrist and finger flexors, bilateral knee extensors, ankle dorsiflexors, and neck flexors. Ankle jerks were diminished but present. The remainder of his muscle stretch reflexes and sensory examination results were normal.

Serum creatine kinase (CK) was increased 4 times normal. EMG revealed normal nerve conduction studies with abnormal results of a needle examination consisting of a mixture of short-duration, low-amplitude motor unit potentials and a second population of enlarged individual motor unit potentials, suggesting denervation and reinnervation compatible with a diminished number of functioning muscle fibers. Scattered fibrillation potentials and complex repetitive discharges were also present. A muscle biopsy specimen revealed endomysial inflammation, myofiber degeneration and regeneration, variation in myofiber size with atrophic and hypertrophic fibers, and rimmed vacuoles.

The myopathies have in common predominantly proximal muscle weakness with variable involvement of the facial and bulbar musculature. Most are lifelong conditions with a slowly progressive or essentially static course. Most muscle disorders of childhood and adolescence—the congenital myopathies and muscular dystrophies—are genetic in origin, whereas causation is more varied in adult patients. Several gradually evolving adult-onset myopathies are secondary to inflammatory, endocrine, metabolic, or toxic disorders. The man in the preceding clinical vignette exhibited virtually all of the clinical, electrodiagnostic and histologic aspects of the most common of these, inclusion body myositis (IBM). Its distinctive pattern of weakness usually allows accurate clinical diagnosis. CK values are typically 2 to 10 times normal. EMG demonstrates active myopathy in many cases, but chronic neurogenic features are also common and sometimes the dominant feature.

ETIOLOGY AND CLINICAL PRESENTATION

The recognized primary inciting mechanisms of the chronic myopathies of adulthood include immunologically mediated, endocrine, toxic, infectious, and, rarely, metabolic acquired disorders such as osteomalacia. The causative gene mutations in several of the congenital myopathies and muscular dystrophies have now been identified.

The pathophysiology of structural muscle changes and nature of changes engendered by mutated genes and abnormal protein products is now defined in some chronic myopathies. Many result from a deficiency of protein constituents of an extensive subsarcolemmal, transsarcolemmal, and suprasarcolemmal complex that provides myofibers with structural integrity.

The predominant involvement of the shoulder and limb-girdle musculature in all chronic myopathies, regardless of etiology, is not understood. Protein loss and abnormal structure may promote sarcolemmal instability, rendering these muscles more susceptible to injury.

Clinical presentation is similar in most chronic myopathies. Symmetrically distributed, proximal weakness insidiously develops in patients. Symptoms include problems arising from low chairs or toilet seats, climbing stairs, reaching things from overhead shelves, or holding the arms above the head for sustained amounts of time, as when blow-drying one's hair.

Patchy and selective patterns of weakness (ie, involvement of muscle groups with limited or nonexistent involvement of contiguous muscle groups) as described in the Clinical Vignette, suggest IBM or one of several muscular dystrophies. Such patterns often allow for specific clinical identification; for example, facioscapulohumeral muscular dystrophy presents with predominant facial musculature involvement. Notable asymmetry is characteristic of a few myopathies, IBM, facioscapulohumeral muscular dystrophy, and, to a lesser extent, dysferlinopathies.

DIFFERENTIAL DIAGNOSIS AND DIAGNOSTIC APPROACH

The differential diagnosis of the chronic myopathies includes a broad range of acquired and genetic conditions (see below). Other motor unit disorders, including those with multifocal, regional, or diffuse weakness without sensory involvement and/or myalgia, must also be considered. These include motor neuron diseases, uncommon motor neuropathies including chronic inflammatory demyelinating polyneuropathies, and disorders of neuromuscular transmission.

Acquired Chronic Myopathies (Table 105-1)

Sporadic IBM is characterized by slowly progressive weakness affecting older individuals, particularly men. The weakness is most pronounced in the wrist and finger flexors, neck flexors, quadriceps, and foot dorsiflexors. This presentation is rarely mimicked by other disorders. Dysphagia and facial weakness develop in approximately one third of patients. IBM rarely has any associated systemic involvement and is not associated with malignancy.

Polymyositis and **dermatomyositis** occasionally have a slowly ingravescent onset followed by the very gradual evolution of chronic proximal weakness without prominent myalgia (chapter 104).

Toxic myopathies are uncommon but occasionally cause slowly progressive painless myopathies affecting the extremities and tending to spare the facial and bulbar musculature (Table 104-1).

Endocrinopathies, including disorders of adrenal, thyroid, and parathyroid function, are particularly prone to affect skeletal muscle. These typically present in a subacute fashion but also require consideration in any patient with chronic proximal weakness.

Osteomalacic myopathy is associated with bone pain, loss of appendicular height, and kyphoscoliosis. Although usually considered in chronic renal failure, osteomalacic myopathy may also relate to long-term treatment with phenytoin. Serum CK and electrodiagnostic studies are normal. Muscle biopsy, if performed, demonstrates type II fiber atrophy.

Occasionally, acquired chronic myopathies accompany inflammatory or infectious processes. **Trichinosis** classically presents acutely, although rarely, it has a chronic or subacute temporal profile. **Sarcoidosis** and **amyloidosis are** usually associated with other features indicative of systemic involvement. The myopathy of **human T-cell lymphotropic virus** (HTLV-I) infection is usually overshadowed by concomitant myelopathy.

Genetically Determined Chronic Myopathies (Table 105-2)

Muscular Dystrophies

Muscular dystrophies are genetically determined myopathies distinguished from congenital myopathies by their generally progressive clinical course and characteristic dystrophic histology profile, ie, myofiber degeneration, regeneration, and fibrosis (Figure 105-1). The milder dystrophies, eg, oculopharyngeal and facioscapulohumeral muscular dystrophy, may lack some of these histologic features. Although Bethlem myopathy and hereditary inclusion body myopathies are not always classified as dystrophies, they have a hereditary predisposition and are somewhat progressive (Table 105-2).

CHRONIC PROXIMAL MYOPATHIES

Table 105-1
Acquired Myopathies*

Myopathy	Diagnosis	Pathology	Treatment

Immunologic mediated
  Dermatomyositis
  Polymyositis
  Inclusion body
	CK
	EMG/biopsy
	MRI
		Primary inflammation	Corticosteroids, IVIG

Endocrine
  Adrenal
    Addison
    Cushing
  Thyroid
  Myxedema
  Hyperthyroidism
  Hyperparathyroidism
	
	Serum cortisol
	
	TSH
	T4
	Ca^{2+}/parathormone
		
		Type 2 atrophy
			
			Cortisol replacement
			Determine primary cause
			
			Thyroid

Toxic
  Ethanol
  Prednisone
  Statins
  Chloroquine
  Zidovudine
	
	History
	Medication list
			
			Gradually withdraw
			  toxin/Rx as tolerated

Infectious/inflammatory
  Sarcoidosis
  Trichinosis
	
	Biopsy
		
		Granulomas
			
			Corticosteroids

Osteomalacia	Phenytoin Rx		

*CK indicates creatine kinase; IVIG, intravenous immunoglobulin; Rx, treatment; TSH, thyroid-stimulating hormone.

Chloride channelopathies are the most common adult forms of muscular dystrophy. They are genotypically heterogeneous. The classic autosomal dominant form, **myotonic muscular dystrophy** (DM1), usually presents in early adulthood but may be recognized from the neonatal period (Figure 105-2) presenting as a floppy infant similar to some of the congenital myopathies and congenital dystrophies.

Myotonia is a channelopathy dominated by muscle stiffness, not weakness. DM1 is clinically defined by delayed skeletal muscle relaxation. It is best demonstrated with a forceful handgrip or by thenar muscle eminence percussion. Temporalis, masseter, and sternocleidomastoid wasting, frontal balding, and ptosis contribute to the characteristic myotonic facies (Figure 105-3). Facial, pharynx, tongue, and neck muscles are also weak. Limb weakness predominantly affects distal extensor muscle groups and then progresses proximally.

Various systemic problems occur concomitantly with DM1: impaired gastrointestinal dysmotility, alveolar hypoventilation, cardiac conduction defects, and cardiomyopathy. The last three often shorten life expectancy. Neurobehavioral manifestations include hypersomnolence, apathy, depression, personality disorders, and cognitive impairment. Premature posterior subcapsular cataracts are common and may lead to initial diagnosis of DM1. Testicular atrophy and impotence occur in men. Pregnant women have a high fetal loss.

Proximal myotonic myopathy (DM2), is another autosomal dominant myotonic disorder that develops in adults or, rarely, children. Patients present with myotonia, myalgia, and proximal weakness. Weakness begins in the legs and is slowly progressive. Patients may describe episodic fluctuation in their weakness and may experience severe muscle pain. Ptosis, facial weakness, and weakness of the respiratory mus-

CHRONIC PROXIMAL MYOPATHIES

Figure 105-1

Other Types of Muscular Dystrophy

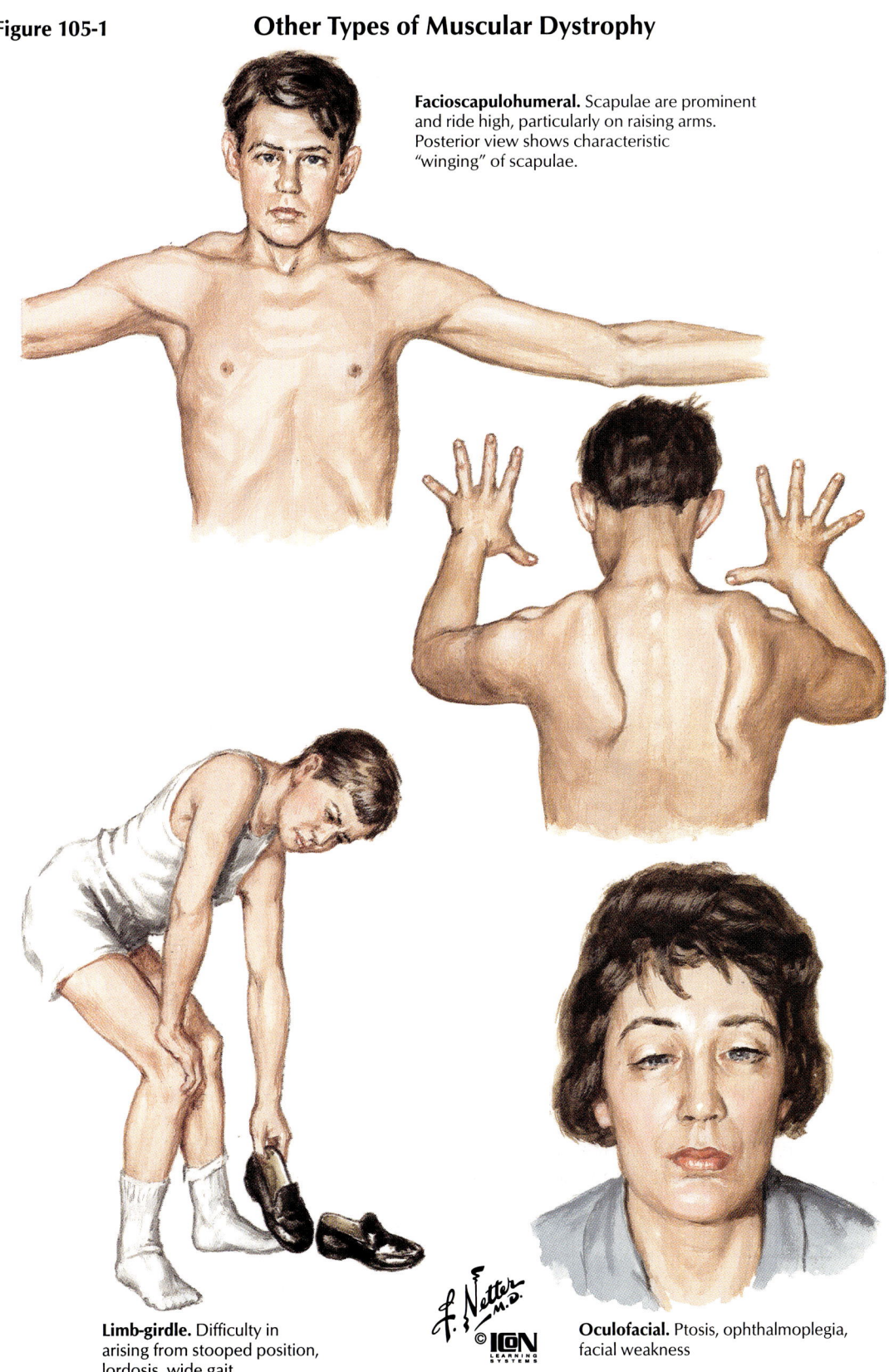

Facioscapulohumeral. Scapulae are prominent and ride high, particularly on raising arms. Posterior view shows characteristic "winging" of scapulae.

Limb-girdle. Difficulty in arising from stooped position, lordosis, wide gait

Oculofacial. Ptosis, ophthalmoplegia, facial weakness

CHRONIC PROXIMAL MYOPATHIES

Table 105-2
Chronic Genetically Determined Myopathies*

Myopathy	Type	Locus	Gene Product
Dystrophies			
Myotonic			
Classic distal	1†	AD 19q13	Myotonin protein kinase
Proximal (PROMM)	2†	AD 3q21	ZNF9 (zinc finger protein)
Limb-girdle	1A	AD 5q22-34	Myotilin
	1B	AD 1q11-21	Lamin A/C
	1C	AD 3p25	Caveolin-3
	1D	AD 6q23	FDC-CDM
	1E	AD 7	?
	2A	AR 15q15	Calpain-3
	2B‡	AR 2p13	Dysferlin
	2C‡	AR 13q12	γ Sarcoglycan+
	2D‡	AR 17q12	α Sarcoglycan+ (adhalin)
	2E‡	AR 4q12	β Sarcoglycan+
	2F‡	AR 5q33	δ Sarcoglycan+
	2G	AR 17q11	Telethonin
	2H	AR 9q31-33	E3 ubiquitin ligase
	2I	AR 19q13.3	Fukutin-related protein
	2J	AR 2q31	Titin
Dystrophinopathies			
	Duchenne		
	Becker		
Facioscapulohumeral	‡	AD 4q35	?
Scapuloperoneal		AD 12	?
Emery-Dreifuss	1‡	X Xq28	Emerin
	2	AD 1q11-q21	Lamin A/C
Oculopharyngeal	‡	AD 14q11.2-q13	Poly (A) binding protein 2
Bethlem		AD 21q22, 2q37	Collagen type VI
			Subunit α1 or α2
		AD 2q37	Collagen type VI
			Subunit α3
Congenital muscular dystrophy			
	Classic CMD‡	AR 6q22-23	Laminin-α2 chain of merosin
	α7 Integrin CMD	AR 12q13	Integrin α7
	Fukuyama	AR 9q31-33	Fukutin
	Walker-Warburg	AR ?	?
	Muscle-eye-brain	AR 1p32-34	O mannose β-1,2 N-acetylglucosaminyl transferase
	Rigid spine	AR 1p35-36	Selenoprotein N1

(continued)

Table 105-2
Chronic Genetically Determined Myopathies* (continued)

Myopathy	Type	Locus	Gene Product
Congenital myopathies			
	Central core	AD 19q13.1	Ryanodine receptor
	Nemaline	AD 1q21-23	α Tropomysin
	Nemaline	AR 2q21.2-22	Nebulin
	Nemaline	AR 1q42	a Actin
	Nemaline	AD 9p13	β Tropomysin
	Nemaline	AR 19q13	Troponin T
	Centronuclear	AR?	?
	Myotubular	X Xq28	Myotubularin
	Myotubular	AR?	?
	CFTD	?	?
	Myofibrillar	AD 11q22	α, β Crystallin
	Myofibrillar	AD 2q35	Desmin
	Myofibrillar	AR?	?
Metabolic			
Glycogen storage			
	II—acid maltase deficiency§	AR 17q21-23	α 1,4 Glucosidase
	III—debrancher deficiency§	AR 1p21	Amylo-1,6 glucosidase
	IV—branching enzyme deficiency§	AR 3	Branching amylo-1,4-1,6 transglucosidase
	V—myophosphorylase deficiency		
	VII—phosphofructokinase		
Lipid storage	Carnitine deficiency	AR/AD	

*AD indicates autosomal dominant; AR, autosomal recessive; CFTD, cogenital fiber–type disproportion; CMD, congenital muscular dystrophy; PROMM, proximal myotonic myopathy.
†DNA mutational analysis commercially available.
‡Immunostain commercially available.
§Biochemical analysis available.

cles are uncommon in DM2. Associated systemic abnormalities include cataracts, cardiac arrhythmias, and testicular atrophy. The proximal weakness and absence of signature features make DM2 a more difficult clinical diagnosis than DM1.

Serum CK may be mildly increased. EMG demonstrates myotonia, which may provide an important diagnostic clue when evaluating patients with typical clinical pictures of proximal myopathies. DNA studies are diagnostic in some kinds.

The **limb-girdle muscular dystrophies** (LGMDs) are a genetically heterogeneous group of disorders in which classification is rendered more complicated by the frequency of variable

CHRONIC PROXIMAL MYOPATHIES

Figure 105-2

Congenital Myopathies: Floppy Infant

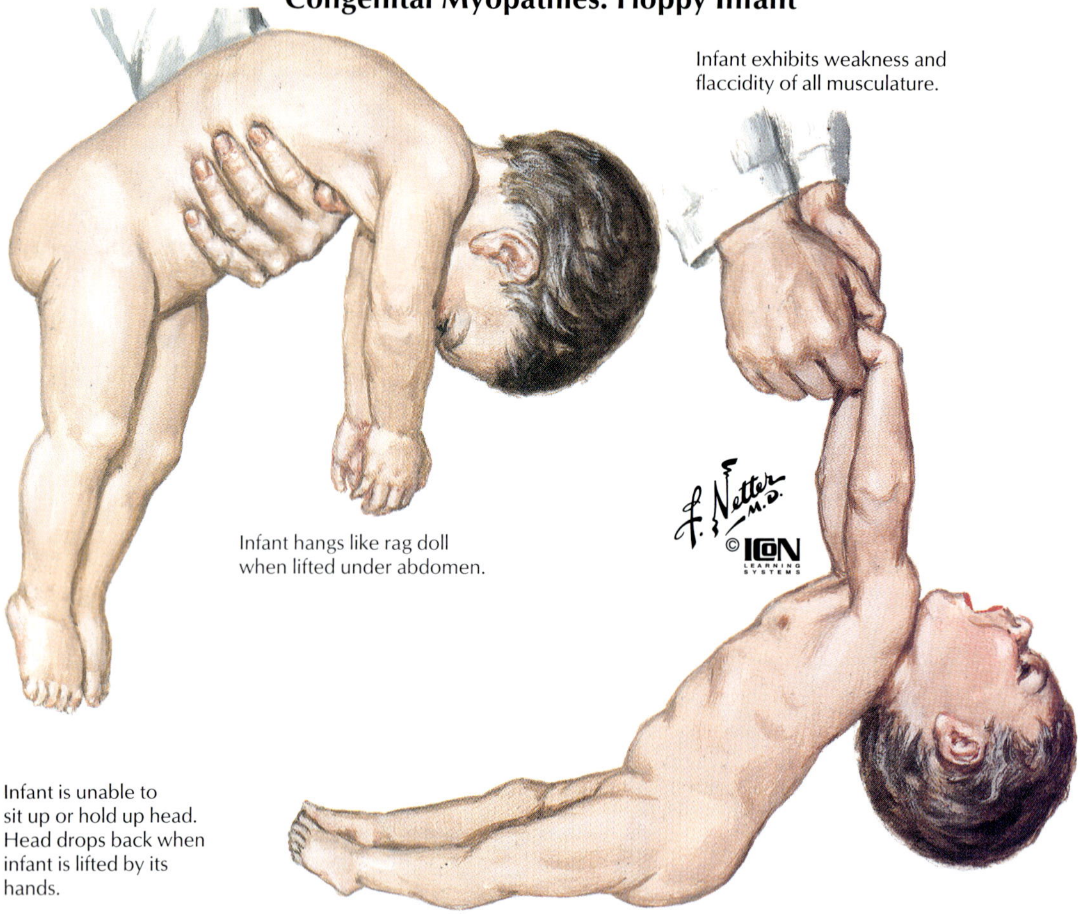

Infant exhibits weakness and flaccidity of all musculature.

Infant hangs like rag doll when lifted under abdomen.

Infant is unable to sit up or hold up head. Head drops back when infant is lifted by its hands.

Muscle biopsy specimens in different cases

Nemaline Rod

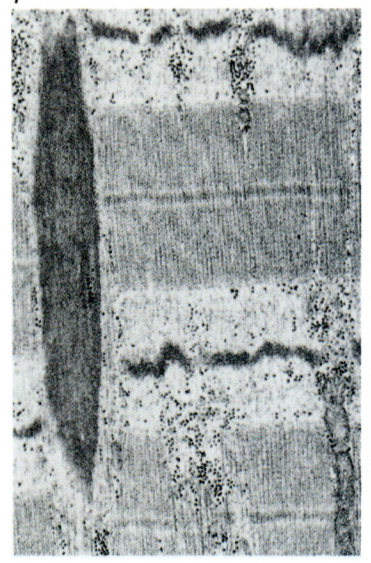

Electron micrograph showing nemaline body continuous with Z band (×30,000)

Central Core

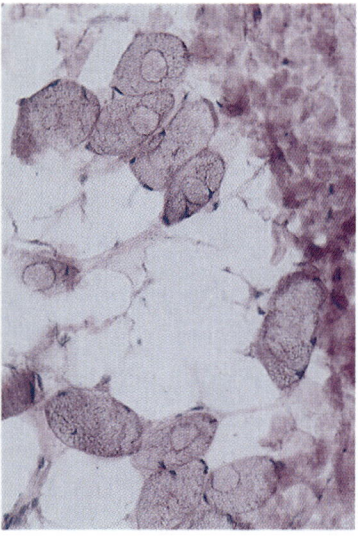

Muscle fibers with well-defined "cores." Muscle is largely replaced by adipose tissue (PAS stain).

Centronuclear

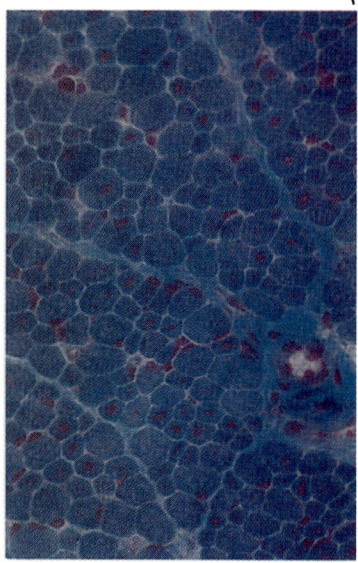

Large number of small fibers with abnormally located central nuclei (trichrome stain)

MYOPATHIES

CHRONIC PROXIMAL MYOPATHIES

Figure 105-3

Myotonic Dystrophy

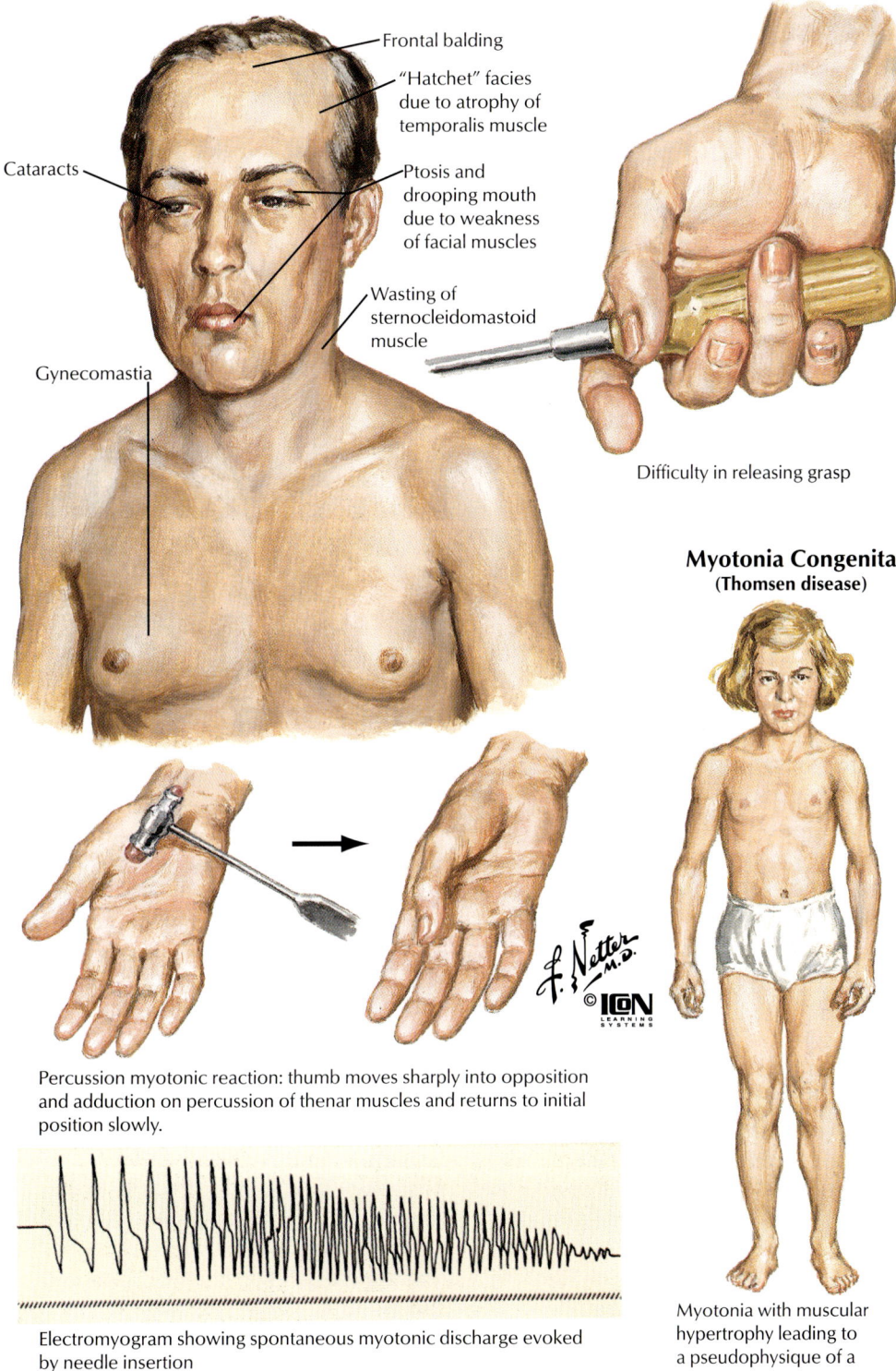

Myotonia Congenita
(Thomsen disease)

Difficulty in releasing grasp

Percussion myotonic reaction: thumb moves sharply into opposition and adduction on percussion of thenar muscles and returns to initial position slowly.

Electromyogram showing spontaneous myotonic discharge evoked by needle insertion

Myotonia with muscular hypertrophy leading to a pseudophysique of a highly trained athlete.

MYOPATHIES

899

myopathic and nonmyopathic phenotypes resulting from mutations of the same gene. It is difficult to clinically distinguish the various subtypes of LGMD, although patterns of weakness or other clinical features may suggest various genotypes. The LGMDs are classified by number (1 for dominant inheritance, 2 for recessive) and letter (order in which the chromosomal locus was discovered).

Weakness is characterized by a symmetric limb-girdle pattern, usually affecting the proximal leg muscles before the shoulder girdle. Facial, oculomotor, pharyngeal, and neck muscles are relatively spared. Onset is usually before the age of 20 years, although LGMD is frequently not recognized until early middle life. Systemic involvement is uncommon. CK increases range from normal to 20 times normal.

Duchenne muscular dystrophy (DMD) is an X-linked recessive dystrophinopathy presenting in early childhood with proximal weakness and difficulty walking (Figure 105-4). Untreated patients become wheelchair dependent by mid adolescence. Calf hypertrophy, heel cord shortening, and blunted intellect help to differentiate this disorder from other myopathies. Common initial signs are a clumsy gait, frequent falls, and proximal lower extremity weakness. An associated cardiomyopathy is common and can cause arrhythmias or congestive heart failure. Smooth muscle involvement may occur, manifesting as ileus or gastric atony. Most patients die of respiratory complications in the third decade of life unless they choose long-term mechanical ventilation. Long-term corticosteroid therapy may help somewhat to ameliorate the course of DMD. Female carriers often have asymptomatic CK increases but rarely may present with symptomatic myopathies as adults.

Diagnosis is primarily based on abnormal serum levels of dystrophin. EMG and muscle biopsy, once mainstays of diagnosis, are no longer necessary in most cases. Serum DNA mutational analysis is positive in approximately two thirds of patients. When DNA analysis is negative, a muscle biopsy is indicated for dystrophin immunostaining, immunoblotting, or Western blot analysis. Immunostaining demonstrates that most fibers are devoid of dystrophin in DMD.

Becker muscular dystrophy (BMD) is another dystrophinopathy and is allelic to DMD. The phenotype is similar but has delayed expression, with patients experiencing difficulty walking in the late first or early second decade of life. BMD can also manifest with exertional myalgias, cardiomyopathy, and asymptomatic increased serum CK levels. Increased CK may not manifest early on; some patients have normal values before increased serum CK levels develop later in their 20s. Life expectancy is still somewhat reduced but usually significantly longer than in DMD.

Diagnosis is similar to that of DMD. In BMD or female DMD, muscle biopsy shows a mix of staining and nonstaining fibers. Both immunoblotting and immunostaining results for dystrophin are quantitatively and qualitatively abnormal in BMD. The identified mutation may allow prediction of phenotype (DMD or BMD).

Facioscapulohumeral (FSH) muscular dystrophy is a dominantly inherited disorder with variable penetrance. Patients present with facial weakness and scapular winging in the second decade of life. Atrophy and weakness of biceps and triceps are accompanied by relative sparing of deltoid and forearm strength. Ankle dorsiflexors are usually first affected in the lower extremity. Variations include absence of facial weakness. An infantile form is rapidly progressive with wheelchair dependency by the age of 10 years.

Scapuloperoneal syndromes enter into the differential diagnosis of FSH. These may be autosomal dominant or recessive, sometimes X-linked or sporadic. Usually, these children present with arm weakness before foot drop. Most patients have normal longevity with relatively mild disability.

Emery-Dreifuss muscular dystrophy can be inherited in an X-linked or autosomal dominant manner. Distinctive features include a humeroperoneal (elbow flexion and extension, foot dorsiflexion) pattern of weakness and contractures (especially of the Achilles tendons, elbows, and posterior cervical muscles). Most patients present with contractures causing difficulty extending the elbows and dorsiflexing the ankles. Cardiac conduction defects are common causes of stroke and life-threatening arrhythmias.

Bethlem myopathy is an autosomal disorder similar to Emery-Dreifuss muscular dystrophy with early childhood onset. It is an indolent myopathy also having prominent elbow flexion contractures but without cardiac complications.

Oculopharyngeal muscular dystrophy is an autosomal dominant myopathy that is more prevalent in those of French Canadian ancestry. Most patients present in mid to late adulthood with ptosis and dysphagia. Mild proximal weakness and ophthalmoparesis may develop.

The ***congenital muscular dystrophies*** are a heterogeneous group of recessively inherited neonatal disorders commonly confused with congenital myopathies, particularly when infants are hypotonic. Children with congenital muscular dystrophy often have joint contractures or arthrogryposis. Some forms are associated with associated brain or ocular abnormalities. These clinical features coupled with increased CK values and dystrophic muscle histology distinguish congenital muscular dystrophies from congenital myopathies and other infantile neuromuscular diseases.

Congenital Myopathies

Congenital myopathies are usually evident at birth or in infancy. They may be severe but often tend to be only minimally progressive if the child survives infancy. Affected children are often limited in their physical capacities, but many live to adulthood. These myopathies are typically named for key histological features, eg, nemaline (threadlike) rods.

The most common congenital myopathies are **centronuclear (myotubular) myopathy**, **central core disease**, and **nemaline myopathy**. These are well-defined clinically and genetically heterogeneous disorders. Concomitant congenital skeletal changes such as high arched palates and kyphoscoliosis are commonplace and are suggestive of these genetically determined disorders. Although the presentation is usually that of a floppy infant, some individuals are mildly affected and may not present until early to mid adulthood. Babies surviving infancy tend to have minimal progression and reasonable life expectancy.

Myotubular myopathy is an X-linked recessive neonatal disorder frequently causing death from respiratory insufficiency in infancy. Ptosis and ophthalmoparesis help distinguish this from other congenital myopathies. **Centronuclear myopathy** is a more indolent disorder, having similar histopathology to myotubular myopathy. It manifests later in life with slowly progressive generalized weakness. **Myofibrillar myopathy** is clinically heterogeneous and can present at any age with proximal or distal weakness. Surveillance for associated cardiomyopathy, ventilatory insufficiency, or both is required. **Central core myopathy** is associated with an increased risk for malignant hyperthermia. When exposed to volatile anesthetics or depolarizing neuromuscular blockers, one fourth of central core patients develop this dreaded complication. **Nemaline myopathy** can present at any age from infancy to adulthood. Affected children have delayed motor milestones, but those surviving past infancy eventually achieve some degree of functional independence.

The diagnosis of congenital myopathies is usually confirmed with routine histochemical staining of muscle in concert with the appropriate phenotype. A few metabolic myopathies can be diagnosed by histochemical staining, but many require biochemical analysis of the muscle biopsy specimen or other tissue.

The **hereditary IBMs** are difficult to classify. They manifest in the second or third decades of life and are histologically identical to sporadic IBMs but without inflammation. Two forms are allelic to distal myopathies (chapter 106).

Disorders of Energy Metabolism

Acid maltase deficiency is an autosomal recessive metabolic disorder that presents as a severe infantile form (Pompe disease) or as a less virulent juvenile or adult type. Cardiomegaly, hepatomegaly, macroglossia, hypotonia, feeding difficulties, and respiratory weakness in the infantile form leads to death by the age of 2 years. The juvenile and adult forms present with progressive, primarily proximal weakness. Ventilatory muscles may be preferentially and severely involved early on. Serum CK is usually increased.

The **myopathic form of primary carnitine deficiency** presents in childhood or early adulthood with progressive proximal weakness. Secondary carnitine deficiency may be triggered by malnutrition, sepsis, hepatic failure, renal failure, and therapeutic interventions such as valproate, zidovudine, and total parenteral nutrition. In the

CHRONIC PROXIMAL MYOPATHIES

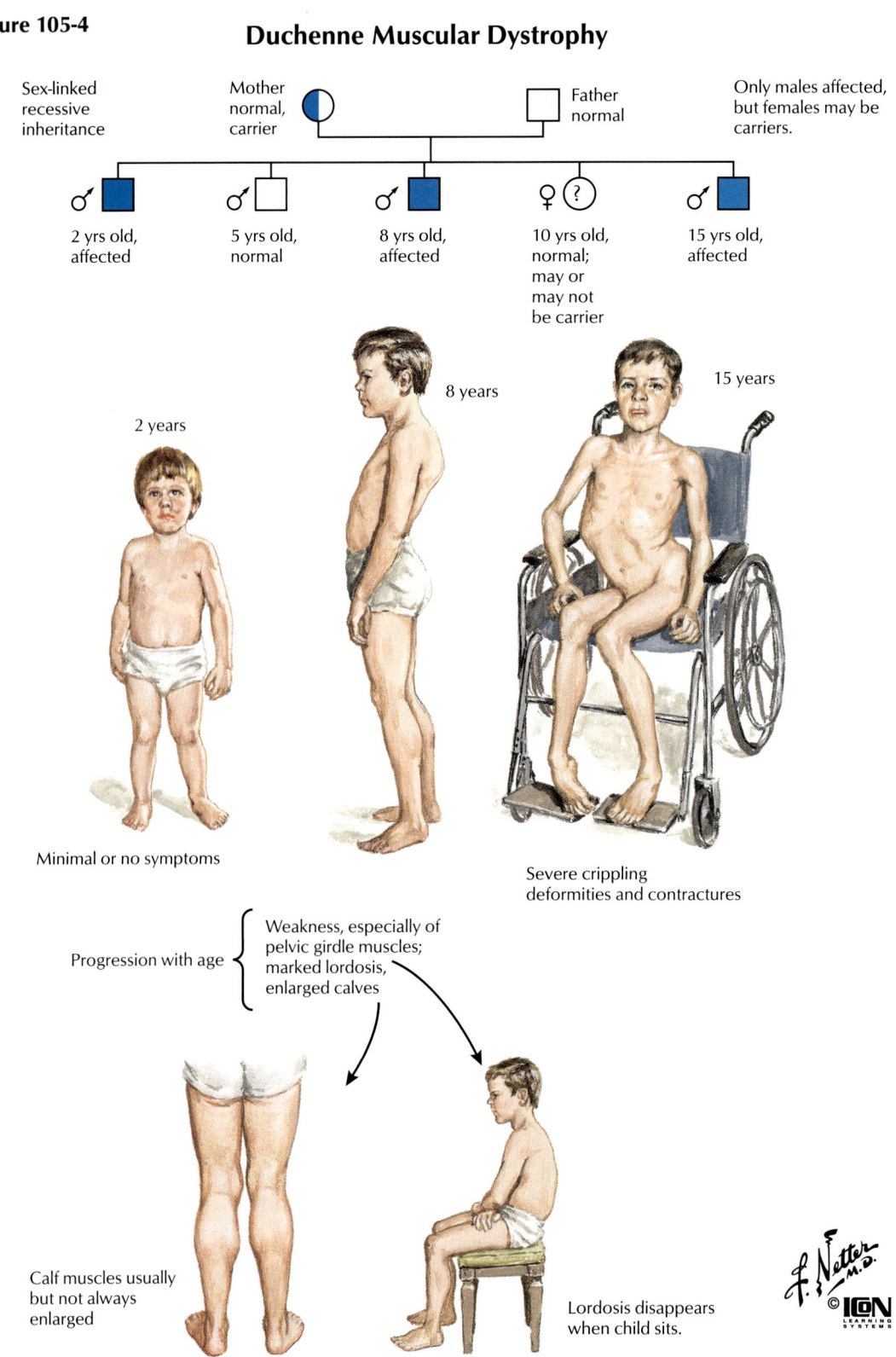

Figure 105-4 Duchenne Muscular Dystrophy

MYOPATHIES

CHRONIC PROXIMAL MYOPATHIES

Figure 105-4

Duchenne Muscular Dystrophy (continued)
Gowers maneuver

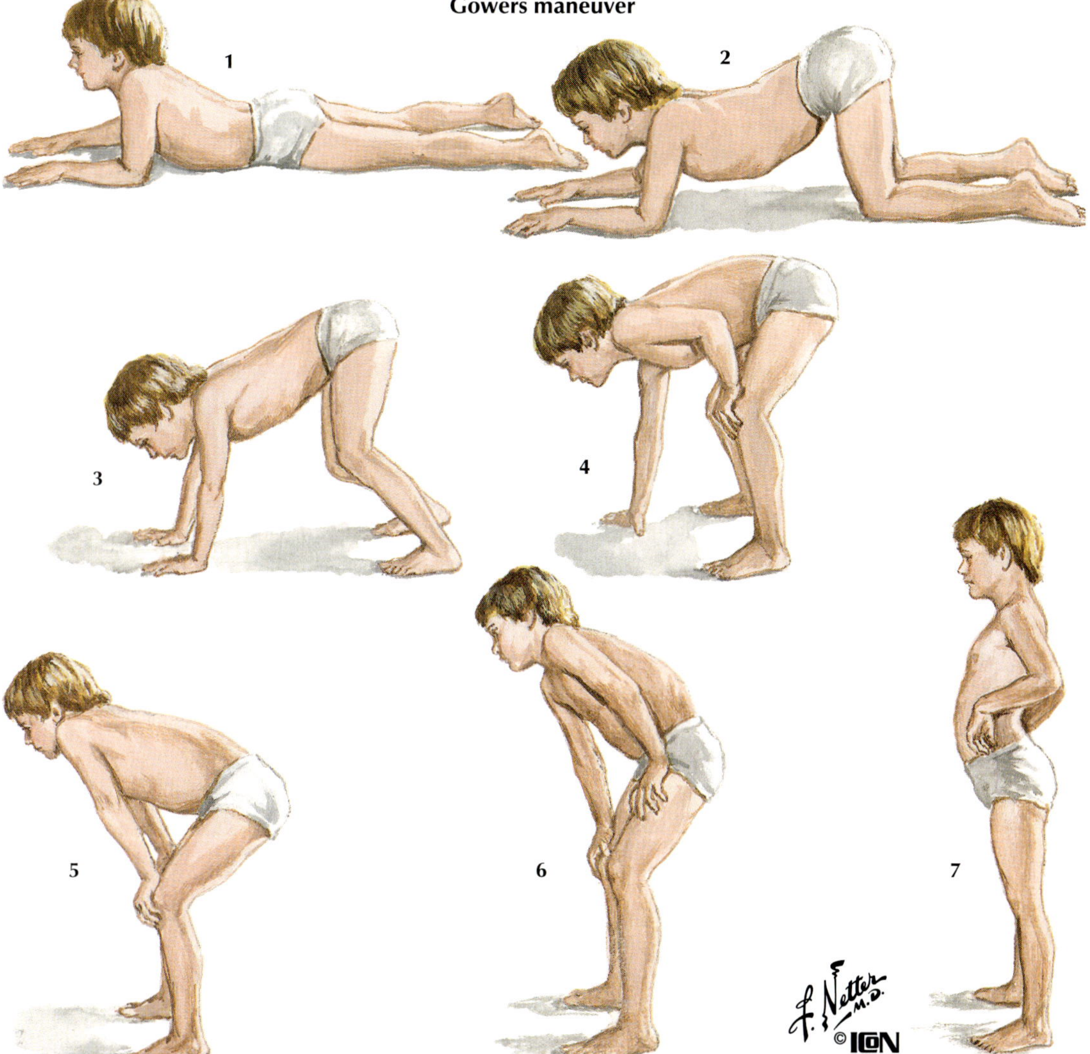

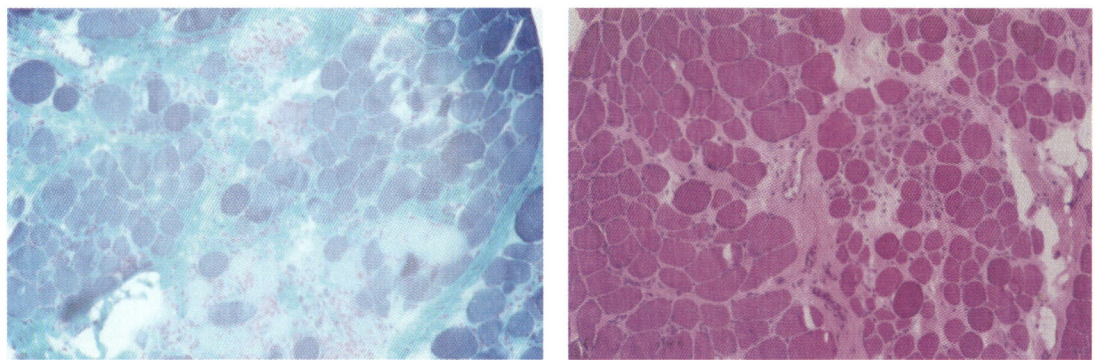

Characteristically, child arises from prone position by pushing himself up with hands successively on floor, knees, and thighs because of weakness in gluteal and spinal muscles. He stands in lordotic posture.

Muscle biopsy specimens showing necrotic muscle fibers being removed by groups of small, round phagocytic cells (left, trichrome stain) and replaced by fibrous and fatty tissue (right, H and E stain)

MYOPATHIES

903

myopathic form, low carnitine levels are found only in muscle and not in serum. Serum CK levels may be normal or increased.

Primary **systemic carnitine deficiency** is the prototypic lipid-storage disorder. In the systemic form, infants or children present with features of Reye syndrome, ie, vomiting, hepatomegaly, and encephalopathy. Plasma levels of carnitine are decreased, and histopathology demonstrates small fibers with abnormal lipid accumulation in the subsarcolemmal and intermyofibrillar region, demonstrable with oil red O or other fat stains.

Periodic paralysis patients (chapter 106) sometimes have fixed weakness late in their disease course.

Diagnostic Approach

The diagnostic testing required in patients with generalized or proximally predominant chronic myopathies varies depending on clinical presentation. Table 103-8 provides guidelines for routinely and selectively ordered tests. Many diagnostic tools are available for evaluating a patient with an apparent myopathy. Extensive analyses of muscle should be undertaken only when warranted by a reasonable index of clinical suspicion.

TREATMENT

General goals for the management of chronic myopathies are largely supportive rather than disease specific and do not usually impact the natural disease course (Table 105-3).

The chronic forms of polymyositis and dermatomyositis are treated in a fashion similar to their acute forms (chapter 104).

Despite its inflammatory characteristics, sporadic IBM does not respond to immunomodulating therapy. A 3-month therapeutic trial of steroids or IV immunoglobulin may be used in hope of identifying a rare responder, but evidence suggests that the risk of this practice exceeds the benefit when there is unequivocal clinical and histologic evidence of sporadic IBM.

Corticosteroids are often used in ambulatory patients with DMD or BMD. There is evidence suggesting that these drugs may delay wheelchair dependency by years in afflicted males. This benefit occurs despite the potential drawbacks of steroids in individuals who have not grown to full stature and who are prone to complications of immobility.

Table 105-3
Management Goals in the Chronic Myopathies Presenting With Proximally Predominant or Generalized Weakness

- Maintenance of optimal, independent neuromuscular function for as long as possible, with particular attention to ambulation, via durable medical equipment and occupational therapy evaluation and intervention
- Reduction in the risk of falls and injury through home modification, durable medical equipment, or physical therapy instruction
- Maintenance of patient comfort
- Prevention or correction of joint contractures, particularly spine deformities and kyphoscoliotic cardiopulmonary disease
- Maintenance of appropriate nutrition (adequate calories in those with feeding difficulties; caloric restrictions in those with a propensity to obesity)
- Provision of genetic counseling where needed
- Prevention or prompt treatment of aspiration and other forms of pneumonia (when appropriate)
- Recognition and treatment of associated congestive heart failure, symptomatic cardiac conduction defects, and pulmonary hypertension
- Avoidance of malignant hyperthermia
- Identification of patient (or parental) goals in situations in which the severity of the illness may be anticipated to significantly shorten the patient's life expectancy (with provision of adequate counseling)

Myoblast transfer in the dystrophinopathies and gene transfer in LGMD have been attempted without notable success.

Carnitine supplementation in lipid-storage myopathies is effective in few patients, presumably those with primary rather than secondary causes of carnitine deficiency.

Symptomatic myotonia is uncommon in DM1 and DM2. Mexiletine is probably the most effective treatment but requires caution in light of the risk of aggravating possible cardiac conduction problems.

Cardiomyopathies, with or without cardiac conduction abnormalities, occur in several of these disorders. Serial ECG surveillance and echocardiographic screening is important if the natural disease history or the patient's symptoms raise the possibility of accompanying cardiac dysfunction. Cardiac transplantation is rarely considered in BMD or other myopathies wherein congestive heart failure is the dominant symptom.

PROGNOSIS

Despite the paucity of disease-specific therapies, accurate diagnosis remains important for prognostic and counseling purposes. Precise definition of inheritance patterns is particularly important in myopathic disorders wherein the activities of daily living and life expectancy are diminished, especially where prenatal testing may be available. Affected patients, and sometimes their families, need to be made aware of all implications of their diagnoses as tactfully and honestly as possible. The issues are even more compelling when dealing with an affected child.

Many patients and their families have the misconception that all muscle diseases have a natural course similar to DMD. Those with more indolent disorders including certain congenital myopathies and milder forms of muscular dystrophy can often be reassured that the expected natural history is one of mild progression and normal life expectancy.

REFERENCES

Jones HR. Case presentation and discussion. June 5, 1997. Case records of the Massachusetts General Hospital. *N Engl J Med.* 1998;339:182-191.

Moxley R. Channelopathies affecting skeletal muscle in childhood. In: Jones HR, De Vivo D, Darras. *Neuromuscular Disorders of Infancy, Childhood, and Adolescence.* Philadelphia, Pa: Butterworth-Heinemann; 2003:783-812.

North K, Goebel HH. Congenital myopathies. In Jones HR, De Vivo D, Darras BT. *Neuromuscular Disorders of Infancy, Childhood, and Adolescence.* Philadelphia, Pa: Butterworth-Heinemann; 2003:601-632.

North K, Jones K. Congenital muscular dystrophies. In Jones HR, De Vivo D, Darras BT. *Neuromuscular Disorders of Infancy, Childhood, and Adolescence.* Philadelphia, Pa: Butterworth-Heinemann; 2003:633-648.

Olafsson E, Jones HR, Guay AT, Thomas CB. Myopathy of endogenous Cushing's syndrome: a review of the clinical and electromyographic features in eight patients. *Muscle Nerve.* 1994;17:692-93.

Snyder R. Bioethical issues. In: Jones HR, De Vivo D, Darras. *Neuromuscular Disorders of Infancy, Childhood, and Adolescence.* Philadelphia, Pa: Butterworth-Heinemann; 2003:1279-1286.

Wicklund MP, Mendell JR: The limb girdle muscular dystrophies: our ever expanding knowledge. *J Clin Neuromusc Dis.* 2003;5:12-28.

Chapter 106
Distal Predominant Myopathies

Monique M. Ryan and James A. Russell

Clinical Vignette

A 22-year-old woman reported fatigability and difficulty climbing stairs. Her calves had become noticeably thinner over the preceding 3 years. She had no family history of weakness, pes cavus, or gait handicap.

Examination demonstrated weak plantar flexion bilaterally. She was unable to rise on her toes. The gastrocnemius muscles were atrophied. All muscle stretch reflexes were preserved, and the results of a sensory examination were normal.

The serum creatine kinase level was increased 50 to 75 times. A muscle biopsy specimen revealed nonspecific myopathic changes. No rimmed vacuoles were present. There was no dysferlin on immunohistochemical testing and immunoblotting.

Patients presenting with predominantly distal symmetric weakness are usually found to have peripheral neuropathies. In contrast, patients in whom proximal distribution weakness develops are usually found to have myopathies. However, there are myopathies whose presentation mimics that of polyneuropathies and vice versa.

This clinical vignette illustrates one of these uncommon distal myopathies. Whenever there is symmetric distal weakness without sensory involvement, myopathies are a possibility. Initial involvement of the calves in a young adult with high creatine kinase values is strongly suggestive of the Miyoshi phenotype.

ETIOLOGY AND CLINICAL PRESENTATION

Mutations of a single gene can lead to multiple phenotypes, even within the same family. For example, individuals with absent dysferlin may have 3 different clinical manifestations, including the classic Miyoshi phenotype with posterior compartment weakness, a limb girdle (type 2B) phenotype, or, rarely, a distal myopathy with preferential anterior compartment weakness. Caveolin-3 deficiency rarely presents as a distal myopathy, but it may be associated with a limb girdle muscular dystrophy (type 1C), rippling muscle disease, or asymptomatic increased levels of serum creatine kinase. Nonaka distal myopathy and hereditary inclusion body myopathy also seem to be allelic.

Primary distal myopathies were originally characterized by muscle weakness and hand or foot atrophy with cranial nerve sparing and no sensory involvement. A number of specific phenotypes have been defined (Table 106-1). Distinguishing clinical variables include inheritance pattern, age, onset in an upper or lower extremity, and preferential involvement of the anterior or posterior leg compartment.

Distal predominant myopathies with underlying generalized mild weakness also occur, including myotonic dystrophy, sporadic inclusion body myositis, myofibrillar myopathy, acid maltase deficiency, nemaline myopathy, and dystrophies including scapuloperoneal, facioscapulohumeral, and oculopharyngeal distal dystrophy.

DIFFERENTIAL DIAGNOSIS

Peripheral neuropathy is the first consideration in patients presenting with symmetric distal weakness. Well-defined sensory symptoms and signs are the primary distinguishing findings with most polyneuropathies. Because most distal myopathies share with Charcot-Marie-Tooth disease a tendency to primarily weaken ankle dorsiflexion, Charcot-Marie-Tooth disease is the peripheral neuropathy most likely to be confused with them. High arched feet (pes cavus) and sensory loss, particularly for large-fiber modalities such as vibration sense, are typical in patients with Charcot-Marie-Tooth disease.

Table 106-1
The Distal Myopathies*

	Age at Onset	Initial Muscle Group Involved	Serum CK	Muscle Biopsy	Inheritance	Chromosome Linkage	Gene
Nonaka	Early adulthood	AC legs	N or sl ↑	Rimmed vacuoles	AR	9p1-q1	
Miyoshi	Early adulthood	PC legs	↑ × 10-150	Myopathic changes	AR	2p12-14	Dysferlin
Laing	Early adulthood	AC legs, neck flexors	↑ × 1-3	Myopathic changes	AD	14q11	
Desmin (myofibrillar) myopathy	Childhood to adulthood	Hands or AC legs	N or sl ↑	Myopathic changes with vacuoles or cytoplasmic inclusions	AD, sporadic, ? AR, ? X-linked	2q35, 11q21-23, 12q, 10q22.3	
Welander	Late adulthood	Finger and wrist extensors	N or sl ↑	Myopathic changes, rarely vacuoles	AD	2p13	
Markesbery-Griggs/Udd	Late adulthood	AC legs	N or sl ↑	Vacuolar myopathy, occasional rimmed vacuoles	AD	2q31-33	? Titin
Distal myopathy with vocal cord and pharyngeal weakness	Late adulthood	AC legs, finger extensors, late vocal cord and pharyngeal weakness	N or ↑ × 3-6	Vacuolar myopathy	AD	5q31	

*AC indicates anterior compartment; AD, autosomal dominant; AR, autosomal recessive; CK, creatine kinase; N, normal; PC, posterior compartment; sl, slight; ↑, increased.

Distal spinal muscular atrophy has a phenotype similar to that of Charcot-Marie-Tooth disease. It is considered a motor neuron disease, not a polyneuropathy. Distal spinal muscular atrophy has preserved sensory function clinically and electrodiagnostically.

Intraspinal processes affecting the cauda equina or conus medullaris are rare possibilities. However, it is unlikely for them to affect the calves symmetrically without some associated pain, sensory involvement, or bowel and bladder dysfunction.

DIAGNOSTIC APPROACH

Serum creatine kinase is useful for acquired myopathies. Markedly increased levels characterize Miyoshi myopathy, whereas moderate increases occur with Laing, Nonaka, and desmin myopathies. Normal or mildly increased levels typify the late adult-onset distal myopathies.

Nerve conduction studies are normal, but EMG examination demonstrates myopathic changes in all distal myopathies. MRI shows characteristic patterns of involvement in several conditions.

Muscle biopsy shows typical myopathic changes with degrees of dystrophic change in all distal myopathies but one. Because routine muscle biopsy histochemical staining in Miyoshi has nonspecific myopathic features, special immunologic studies are required to identify the absence of dysferlin. Moderately weak muscles are the best sites for biopsy. The hamstrings are better alternatives to the gastrocnemius, which may already be at end stage.

Rimmed vacuoles are nonspecific findings found in a number of distal myopathies including oculopharyngeal and oculopharyngodistal dystrophies and the sporadic and familial forms of inclusion body myositis or myopathy.

Immunohistochemical stains for dysferlin, caveolin-3 (absence), and desmin (presence in myofibrillar myopathy) provide strong diagnostic support for their respective disorders. Their utility is lessened by limited availability and the understanding that secondary rather than primary factors may contribute to their presence or absence.

TREATMENT AND PROGNOSIS

No specific treatments are available for distal myopathies. Symptomatic treatment includes physical and occupational therapy and various orthotic devices.

Early adult-onset distal myopathies may progress rapidly, with some patients becoming nonambulant as soon as 10 years after development of symptoms. Myofibrillar (desmin) myopathy may cause rapid evolution of distal and proximal weakness with subsequent development of bulbar, respiratory, and cardiac involvement. In contrast, late adult-onset distal myopathies are slowly progressive conditions that uncommonly cause loss of ambulation.

Genetic counseling requires specific inheritance pattern identification. Antenatal diagnosis is not generally available.

REFERENCES

Argov Z, Tiram E, Eisenberg I, et al. Various types of hereditary inclusion-body myopathies map to chromosome 9p1-q1. *Ann Neurol.* 1997;41:548-551.

Barohn RJ, Amato AA, Griggs RC. Overview of distal myopathies: from the clinical to the molecular. *Neuromuscul Disord.* 1998;8:309-316.

Barohn RJ, Miller RG, Griggs RC. Autosomal recessive distal dystrophy. *Neurology.* 1991;41:1365-1370.

Horowitz ST, Schmalbruch H. Autosomal dominant distal myopathy with desmin storage: a clinicopathologic and electrophysiologic study of a large kinship. *Muscle Nerve.* 1994;17:151-160.

Illarioshkin SN, Ivanova-Smolenskaya IA, Greenberg CR, et al. Identical dysferlin mutation in limb-girdle muscular dystrophy type 2B and distal myopathy. *Neurology.* 2000;55:1931-1933.

Saperstein DS, Amato AA, Barohn RJ. Clinical and genetic aspects of the distal myopathies. *Muscle Nerve.* 2001;24:1440-1450.

Chapter 107
The Channelopathies: Myopathies Presenting With Episodic Weakness

Monique M. Ryan and James A. Russell

Clinical Vignette

A 7-year-old boy presented with recurrent episodes of generalized weakness, usually after hockey games. Each event resolved within 30 minutes after onset, without associated respiratory distress, dysarthria, or dysphagia. At his worst, the boy could not stand or raise his hands over his head. During the winter months, he noted stiffness in his hands and found it difficult to open his eyes quickly after blinking. His mother recalled having several similar episodes but none since late adolescence. Physical examination results were normal.

The stiffness of the hands and problems with eyelid opening suggested myotonia as later confirmed by EMG. Myotonia is a nonspecific finding of the periodic paralyses and myotonic syndromes. During another episode, the patient had an increased serum potassium level of 6.4 mmol/L, confirming the diagnosis of hyperkalemic periodic paralysis. His symptoms responded to carbohydrate loading before exercise and administration of albuterol at the onset of muscle weakness.

The channelopathies are genetically determined, phenotypically similar disorders of muscle membrane ion channels, often having associated hypokalemia or hyperkalemia. Symptoms usually occur during childhood or adolescence. Typically, patients present with intermittent episodes of generalized, relatively short-lived weakness lasting 1 or 2 hours to a few days. Although relatively severe extremity paralysis may occur, respiratory-related musculature and muscles innervated by cranial nerves are spared. If there is associated hyperkalemia and no relevant family history, adrenal insufficiency must be considered with the patient's initial presentation.

ETIOLOGY

Periodic paralyses and myotonic disorders are caused by mutations in genes encoding muscle membrane ion channels (Table 107-1). During episodes of periodic paralysis, muscle membrane excitability is transiently lost, which is a poorly understood phenomenon.

Most conditions are inherited in an autosomal dominant fashion. A family history is usually present, although intrafamilial symptom severity may vary considerably. The condition is typically more symptomatic in men than in women.

Patients with **hypokalemic periodic paralysis** have mutations in the gene for a dihydropyridine-sensitive voltage-gated **calcium** channel. Few cases are due to sodium channel gene mutations. **Hyperkalemic periodic paralysis** and **paramyotonia** are **sodium** channel disorders. **Congenital myotonias** are **chloride** channel disorders inherited in a dominant (Thomsen disease) or recessive (Becker disease) manner.

CLINICAL PRESENTATION

Significant clinical and genetic overlap occurs in periodic paralyses and myotonic syndromes. Recurrent attacks of usually generalized (but occasionally focal or asymmetric) weakness are the hallmark of periodic paralyses (Figure 107-1). Typically, bulbar and respiratory muscles are spared. Muscle stiffness and pain, without sensory symptoms, are the most common associated symptoms occurring with or without periodic paralysis.

THE CHANNELOPATHIES

Table 107-1
Channelopathies Affecting Skeletal Muscle*

	Age at Onset	Duration of Episodes	Weakness	Myotonia	Precipitants	Alleviating Factors	Gene Mutation/Inheritance and Cation
Hyperkalemic periodic paralysis	Infancy-early childhood	Minutes-hours	Episodic, possibly permanent later in life	Possibly (between episodes of weakness) EMG (+)	Potassium loading, cold, fasting, rest after exercise	Carbohydrate loading, exercise	CN4A 17q23: AD Sodium channel
Paramyotonia congenita	Infancy	Minutes	Very uncommon	Present EMG (+)	Repeated exercise, cold, fasting	Warming	SCN4A 17q23: AD Sodium channel
Sodium channel myotonia	Childhood-adolescence	Variable	Very uncommon	Present (often painful)	Rest after exercise, potassium loading, fasting	—	SCN4A 17q23: AD Sodium channel
Hypokalemic periodic paralysis	Puberty	Hours-days	Episodic, possibly permanent later in life	Absent	Cold, rest after exercise, carbohydrate loading	Potassium loading, exercise	CACNLA3, SCN4A 17q23: AD Calcium channel
Myotonia congenita	Infancy-early childhood	Minutes	Uncommon	Present EMG (+)	Exercise after rest, cold	Repeated exercise	CLC-1 7q: AD (Thomsen), AR (Becker) Chloride channel

*AD indicates autosomal dominant; AR, autosomal recessive.

THE CHANNELOPATHIES

Figure 107-1   **Periodic Paralysis**

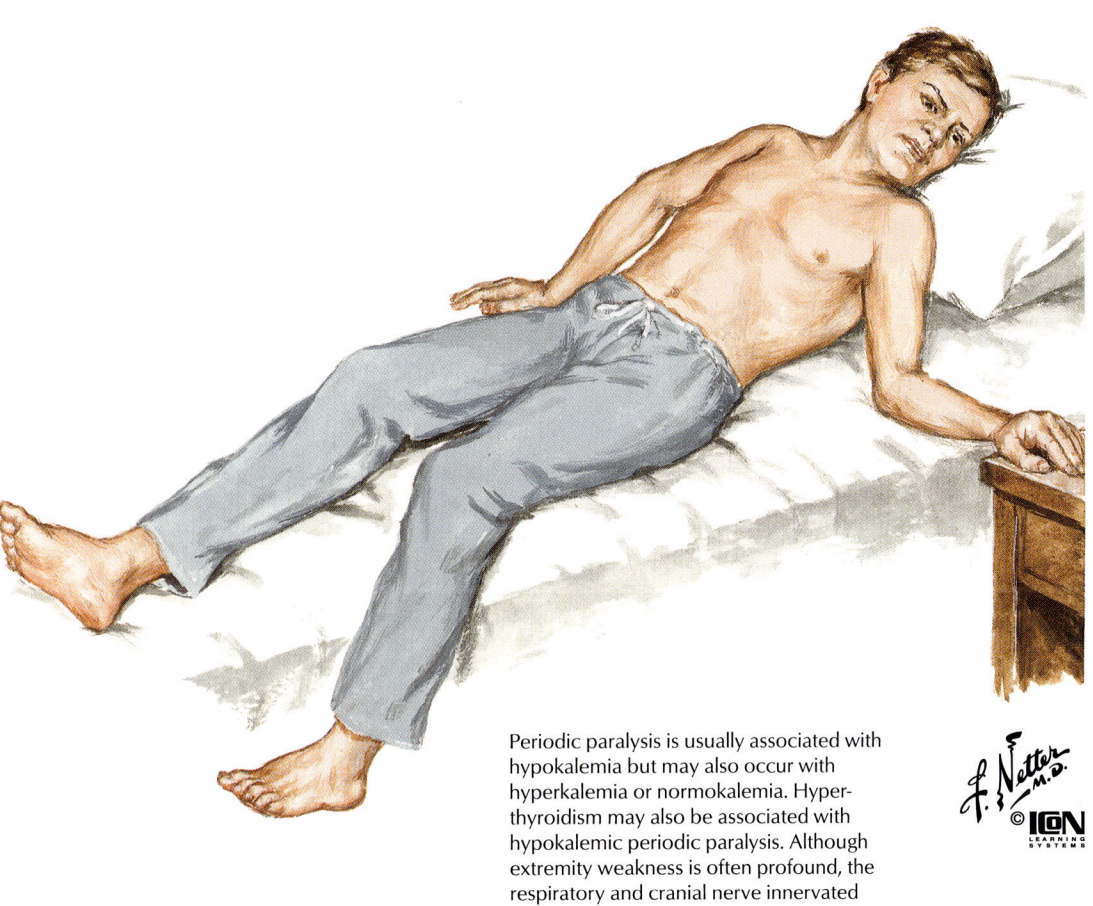

Periodic paralysis is usually associated with hypokalemia but may also occur with hyperkalemia or normokalemia. Hyperthyroidism may also be associated with hypokalemic periodic paralysis. Although extremity weakness is often profound, the respiratory and cranial nerve innervated muscles are spared.

Hyperkalemic periodic paralysis usually presents in early childhood with episodic weakness lasting minutes to hours. Events are triggered by immobility, rest after exercise, and fasting. Serum potassium is increased during episodes. Cold-induced and EMG-defined myotonia occurs between episodes. With age, periodic spells of weakness become less frequent, but fixed weakness may develop and impose its limitations.

Hypokalemic periodic paralysis is associated with a decrease in serum potassium levels during episodes, which are precipitated by rest after exercise, carbohydrate-rich meals and alcohol, and cold. Weakness usually persists for hours or days. Affected patients often have permanent weakness late in life.

Myotonia congenita is aggravated by immobility and ameliorated by exercise and warming; it is usually easily elicited on physical examination. Though weakness is rarely a feature of dominant myotonia congenita; patients with the recessive form may have mild progressive weakness and transient episodes of true weakness precipitated by sudden movements after rest and relieved by exercise. Interesting examples of brief weakness after a short "rest" include a baseball player who cannot run after hitting the ball or a subway rider who is frozen in place when the train stops and he wishes to get off.

Paramyotonia congenita is allelic with hyperkalemic periodic paralysis. Similar to myotonia congenita, muscle stiffness in paramyotonia is

MYOPATHIES

THE CHANNELOPATHIES

exacerbated by cold. In contrast to myotonia congenita, exercise exacerbates stiffness.

DIFFERENTIAL DIAGNOSIS

Episodes of transient, sometimes recurrent generalized hypotonia or weakness occur in brainstem ischemia, cataplexy, and seizures. These are best diagnosed through discriminating aspects of the history, EEG, and MRI with MRA.

Myasthenia gravis is typically characterized by fluctuating, rarely acute weakness. Myasthenia gravis preferentially affects oculobulbar muscles (chapter 102). Episodic muscle symptoms are the hallmark of many of the channelopathies, but typically myotonia and stiffness, rather than weakness, dominate.

Patients with nonorganic weakness often report episodic muscle pain. In such instances, there is usually no family history of neuromuscular disease. Importantly there is a "consistent inconsistency" or "giveaway component" in the distribution, duration, and triggers of the muscle paresis and the nature of any associated clinical symptoms and signs.

Addison disease requires urgent consideration during the evaluation of any acute, generally weak patient with hyperkalemia. Patients with periodic paralyses (particularly young Asian men) must be screened for clinical signs and laboratory findings of thyrotoxicosis because of its symptomatic link with periodic paralysis.

DIAGNOSTIC APPROACH

Diagnosis of channelopathies is predicated on clinical history. This may be relatively simple in patients with a positive family history who are examined while symptomatic with an abnormal serum potassium level or who have demonstrable myotonia on EMG. In sporadic cases, diagnosis may prove elusive, especially when clinical examination results are normal and no biochemical or neurophysiologic abnormalities are detected with provocative testing.

Whenever possible, abnormalities of serum potassium should be sought during spontaneous episodes of periodic paralysis. If identified, other mechanisms of hypokalemia or hyperkalemia must be excluded.

Provocative testing is occasionally required in patients with highly suggestive clinical histories. This allows for documentation of abnormal serum potassium levels during episodes of weakness. A controlled clinical setting with appropriate monitoring equipment and facilities for emergent care must be available before initiating this testing.

As more DNA-specific studies become available, provocative studies will be required less often. Currently, however, there are only a few DNA studies available in the evaluation of a patient with question of periodic paralysis. These include for the skeletal muscle sodium channel hyperkalemic periodic paralysis and the skeletal muscle calcium channel for hypokalemic periodic paralysis.

Serum creatine kinase levels are usually normal or minimally increased in the periodic paralyses and myotonic disorders.

Nerve conduction studies may demonstrate decreased compound motor action potential amplitudes during episodes of periodic paralysis but are otherwise normal. Prolonged periods of exercise may cause progressive diminution in compound motor action potential amplitudes in patients with periodic paralyses.

During episodes of periodic paralysis, needle EMG demonstrates that affected muscles are depolarized and electrically inactive. Myotonic discharges may be seen on EMG in most of the channelopathies, particularly hyperkalemic and paramyotonic varieties.

Muscle biopsy is normal early in the course of periodic paralyses. However, after patients develop persistent weakness, biopsy may demonstrate vacuolar myopathies with tubular aggregates. Biopsy is rarely necessary for diagnosis.

TREATMENT AND PROGNOSIS

Acute attacks of periodic paralysis are best treated by correction of abnormal potassium levels. Severe hyperkalemia necessitates emergent treatment with IV glucose and insulin. Less severe episodes are treated with inhaled β-adrenergic agents or ingestion of carbohydrates. With an initial event of paralysis and hyperkalemia, Addison disease is always a possibility; a large dose of corticosteroids should be administered after a serum cortisol level is obtained.

Hypokalemic episodes are managed with oral or IV potassium supplementation and may be prevented by avoiding dietary carbohydrate loads.

Maintenance therapy with the carbonic anhydrase inhibitors acetazolamide and dichlorphenamide is usually indicated to prevent attacks. Both medications are effective in patients with hyperkalemic or hypokalemic periodic paralysis.

When treatment of myotonia is required, therapy with mexiletine or other membrane stabilizers is usually effective.

Generally a diminution in frequency and severity of periodic paralysis attacks occurs in middle age. However, in some patients with periodic paralysis, a permanent proximal weakness develops with increasing age. This is only minimally responsive to carbonic anhydrase inhibitors and awaits a better therapy.

REFERENCES

Davies NP, Hanna MG. The skeletal muscle channelopathies: distinct entities and overlapping syndromes. *Curr Opin Neurol.* 2003;16:559-568.

Griggs RC, Engel WK, Resnick JS. Acetazolamide treatment of periodic paralysis. *Ann Int Med.* 1970;73:39-48.

McManis PG, Lambert EH, Daube JR. The exercise test in periodic paralysis. *Muscle Nerve.* 1986;8:704-710.

Moxley RT III. Channelopathies affecting skeletal muscle in childhood: myotonic disorders including myotonic dystrophy and periodic paralysis. In: Jones HR, De Vivo DC, Darras BT, eds. *Neuromuscular Disorders of Infancy, Childhood, and Adolescence.* Philadelphia, Pa: Butterworth-Heinemann; 2003:1017-1035.

Rudel R, Lehmann-Horn F. Membrane changes in cells from myotonia patients. *Physiol Rev.* 1985;65:310-56.

Chapter 108
Myopathies Presenting With Exercise Intolerance

Monique M. Ryan and James A. Russell

Clinical Vignette

A 17-year-old boy presented with severe pain, stiffness, and "hardening" of his forearm muscles while moving the contents of his friend's house. In the immediate aftermath, he noticed that his urine was "Coca-Cola" colored.

Hours later, his physical examination results were normal with the exception of muscle tenderness to palpation. His serum creatine kinase (CK) level was increased 50 times normal. His BUN was increased, and myoglobin was in his urine. The patient was admitted to the hospital and treated with vigorous IV hydration. His symptoms resolved within several days.

A forearm exercise test demonstrated the expected increase in venous ammonia levels without the expected increase in lactate, implicating a glycogen storage disease. Subsarcolemmal blebs seen on a periodic acid-Schiff–stained muscle biopsy specimen were consistent with glycogen excess. Biochemical analysis demonstrated decreased levels of myophosphorylase, confirming the diagnosis of McArdle disease.

Rarely, one sees an individual who develops periodic, painful weakness with muscle cramps and myoglobinuria after a period of vigorous exercise. Such symptoms, particularly when associated with profound increases of CK and "pigmenturia," suggest a metabolic myopathy (Figure 108-1). Usually, they are related to inborn errors of glycogen or, less commonly, lipid, mitochondrial, or purine metabolisms (Table 108-1). Although these are usually generalized processes, on occasion, one can have focal involvement. Precise diagnosis requires histochemical analysis, biochemical analysis of muscle or other tissue, or both. Muscle phosphorylase deficiency, an inborn error of glycogen metabolism, is the most common of these myopathies.

ETIOLOGY

Muscle metabolism depends on varied energy sources derived from circulating glucose and free fatty acids (Figures 108-2 and 108-3). At rest, muscles use fatty acids for basal metabolic demands. Glucose is preferentially used as an energy source during periods of low-intensity exercise, and fatty acids are mobilized from lipid oxidation after prolonged periods of exercise. At higher-intensity levels of exercise, oxidative glycolysis of glycogen stored in muscles becomes more important. With vigorous exercise, there is a switch to anaerobic glycolysis. Disorders of these metabolic processes may lead to myopathies.

Myophosphorylase deficiency may be dominantly inherited. Phosphoglycerate kinase deficiency is usually X-linked. The other glycogenoses, the disorders of lipid metabolism, the respiratory chain defects, and muscle adenylate deaminase deficiency are usually recessively inherited.

DIFFERENTIAL DIAGNOSIS

Clinicians commonly encounter patients with myalgias and exercise intolerance, with or without increases of CK. The diagnostic clues that implicate metabolic myopathies are the precipitation of symptoms by exercise, the localization of symptoms to muscle (as opposed to joint or soft tissues), muscle stiffness, and a history of myoglobinuria. Although specific defects of muscle energy metabolism are sometimes recognized, more commonly, specific enzymatic defects cannot be identified.

MYOPATHIES PRESENTING WITH EXERCISE INTOLERANCE

Myoglobinuric Syndromes

Figure 108-1

Paroxysmal rhabdomyolysis

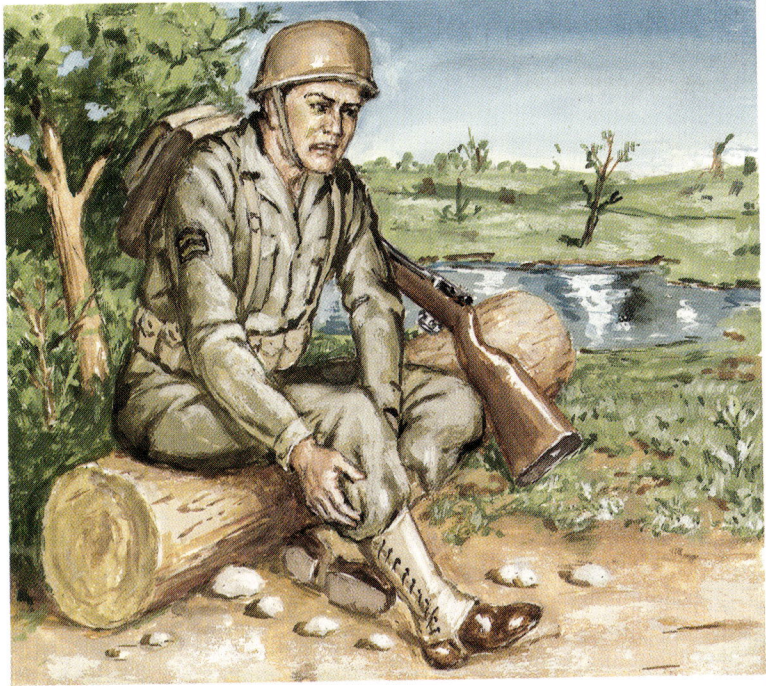

Severe muscle cramps and collapse on exertion (as in soldier on long march)

Malignant hyperthermia

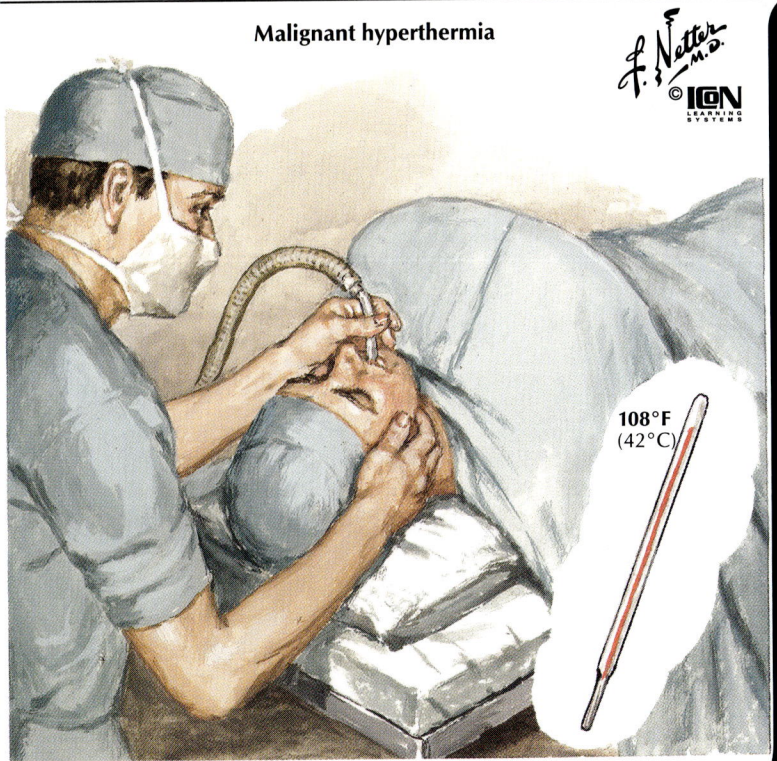

Extreme temperature elevation in anesthetized patient

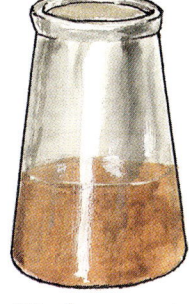

Urine brown, scanty (myoglobinuria)

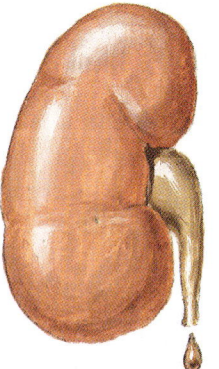

Renal shutdown

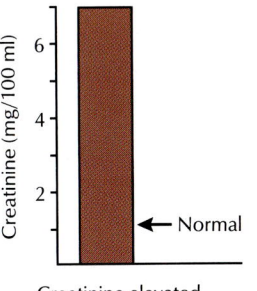

Serum CK elevated

Creatinine elevated

MYOPATHIES

MYOPATHIES PRESENTING WITH EXERCISE INTOLERANCE

Table 108-1
Myopathies Presenting With Exercise Intolerance

Glycogenoses	Respiratory Chain Defects	Lipid Metabolism Disorders
Phosphorylase deficiency (McArdle disease)	Complex 1 deficiency	Carnitine palmitoyltransferase II deficiency
Phosphorylase kinase deficiency	Coenzyme Q_{10} deficiency	Very long chain acyl CoA dehydrogenase deficiency
Phosphofructokinase deficiency	Complex III deficiency	Trifunctional protein deficiency
Phosphoglycerate kinase deficiency	Complex IV deficiency	Short chain 3-hydroxyacyl CoA dehydrogenase deficiency
Phosphoglycerate mutase deficiency		
Lactate dehydrogenase deficiency		

Muscle glycogenoses interfere with effective glycolysis, depriving muscle of glucose, an important energy source, while allowing the accumulation of underutilized glycogen within muscle. There are 12 different types (I-XII) based on the enzyme deficiency. **Type V, McArdle disease**, is the most common, presenting with dynamic symptoms: muscles that have been exercised are painful. Cramping and stiffness occur after strenuous exertion. There may be a characteristic "second wind" phenomenon, where brief periods of rest at the onset of myalgia alleviate symptoms and enable prolonged exercise. Symptomatic relief may come with rest. Recurrent myoglobinuria is common, and permanent weakness may develop in older patients. A few patients present with fixed, often progressive weakness with no clear history of episodic symptomatology. Similar phenotypes occur with types VII, IX, X, and XI (Figure 108-4).

Muscle adenylate deaminase deficiency is controversial because it is not clear that this is a discrete biochemical disorder. These patients experience exertional muscle cramping, stiffness, weakness, and pain and do not demonstrate an appropriate increase in serum ammonia levels after ischemic exercise. However, they have a normal increase in serum lactate, indicating normal glycogen metabolism. Myoglobinuria is rare in muscle adenylate deaminase deficiency, which may represent a disorder of defective purine metabolism.

Carnitine palmitoyltransferase II deficiency is the most common disorder of lipid metabolism. Dynamic symptoms include myalgia without muscle cramping. Most commonly, young men present with recurrent myoglobinuria after prolonged but not necessarily strenuous exercise. Brief periods of exercise are usually well tolerated. Episodes also may be triggered by fasting, cold, or stress. Unlike the glycogenoses, no "second wind" phenomenon is seen, fixed weakness does not develop, and serum CK values may normalize between episodes.

Mitochondrial myopathies are defined by alterations in mitochondrial structure and function. Other family members may or may be affected. There is marked clinical heterogeneity. Ptosis and ophthalmoparesis are clinical signatures of mitochondrial myopathies but are not present in every phenotype. Mitochondrial myopathy frequently occurs in apparent isolation, but involvement of other end organs, particularly those with high energy requirements such as the kidneys, liver, and brain, is typical.

DIAGNOSTIC APPROACH

Baseline CK levels are typically highest in black men and lowest in white women. Healthy individuals have mild postexercise CK increases. These are typically less than 5 times the upper limit of normal and return to normal standards within 3 to 8 days. The degree of increase is related to duration and intensity of exercise.

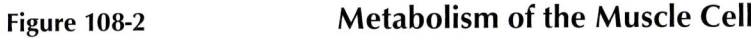

Figure 108-2 — Metabolism of the Muscle Cell

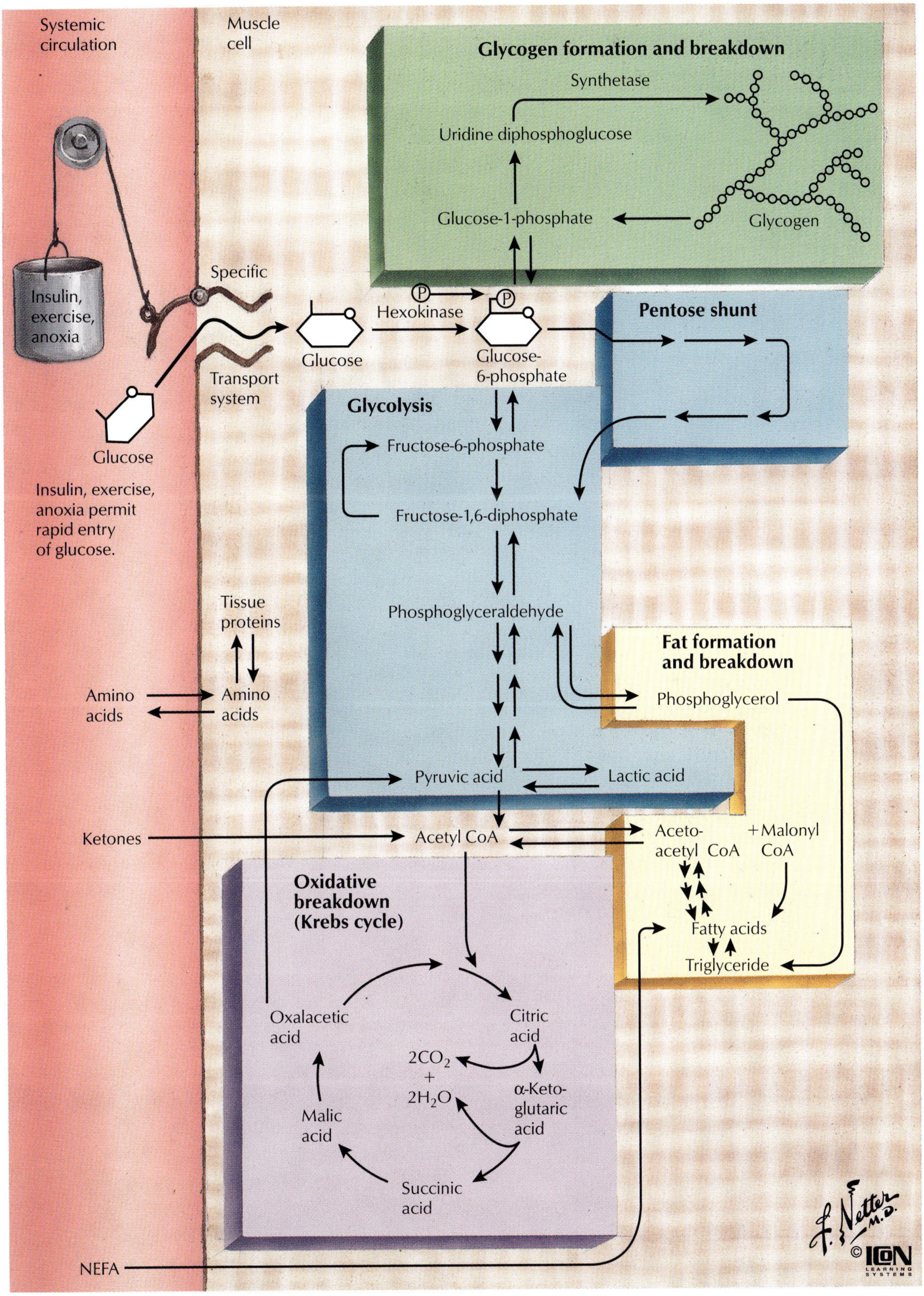

MYOPATHIES PRESENTING WITH EXERCISE INTOLERANCE

Figure 108-3
Regeneration of ATP for Source of Energy in Muscle Contraction

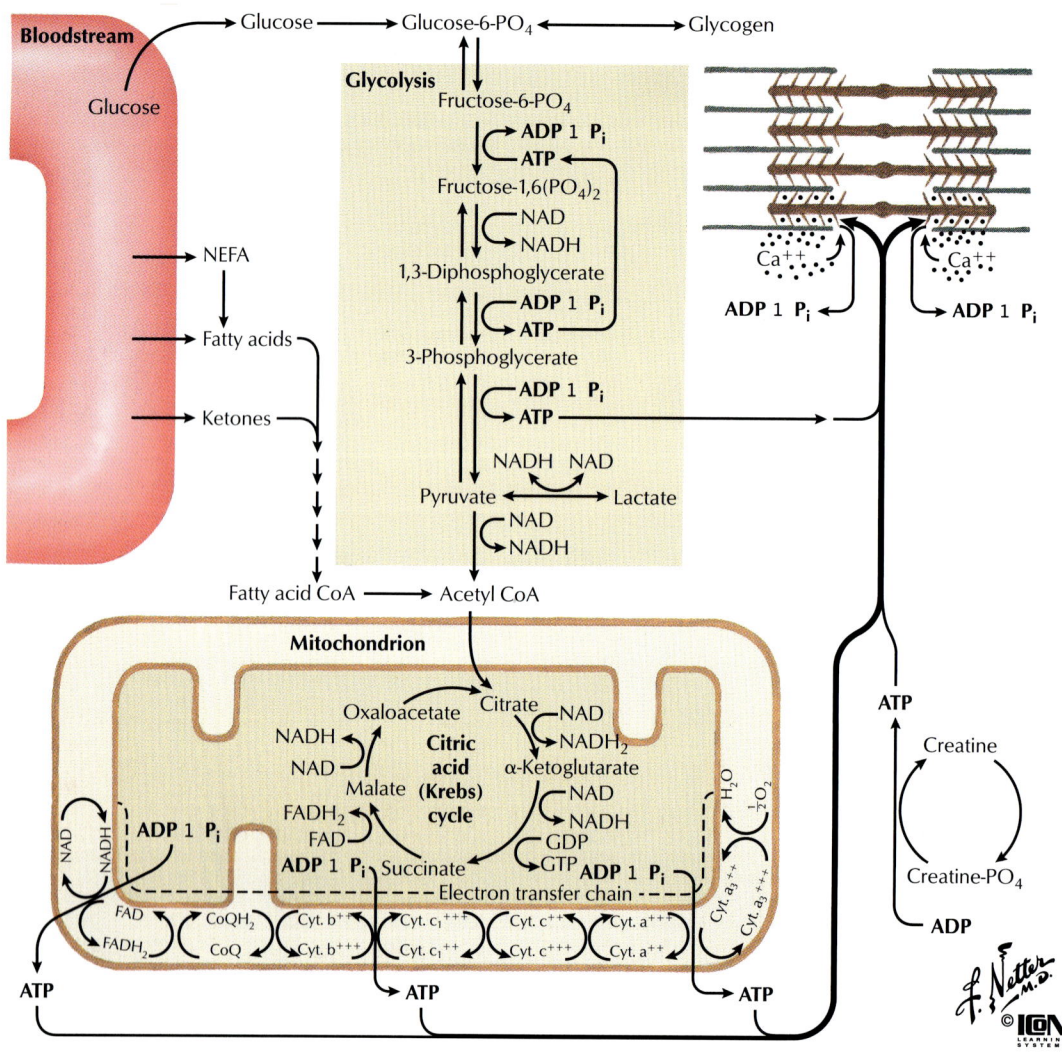

Evaluation of patients who have nonspecific symptoms or who are serendipitously found to have increased CK is often frustrating in the absence of clinically demonstrated weakness or specific EMG abnormalities. The yield of muscle biopsy in search of glycogen or lipid storage changes is relatively low, even with extensive histochemical staining and biochemical tests. Abnormalities found on routine analysis of muscle biopsy specimens do not accurately predict abnormalities on biochemical testing.

One crucial caveat is that patients with increased CK levels, regardless of cause, have an increased risk for development of malignant hyperthermia (Figure 108-1), the serious anesthetic complication of certain fluorinated hydrocarbon inhalation anesthetic agents such as halothane.

Some metabolic myopathies are muscle specific and necessitate tests of the involved muscles. Others are more systemically distributed and can be detected on enzymatic testing of fibroblasts or leukocytes.

MYOPATHIES

MYOPATHIES PRESENTING WITH EXERCISE INTOLERANCE

McArdle Disease

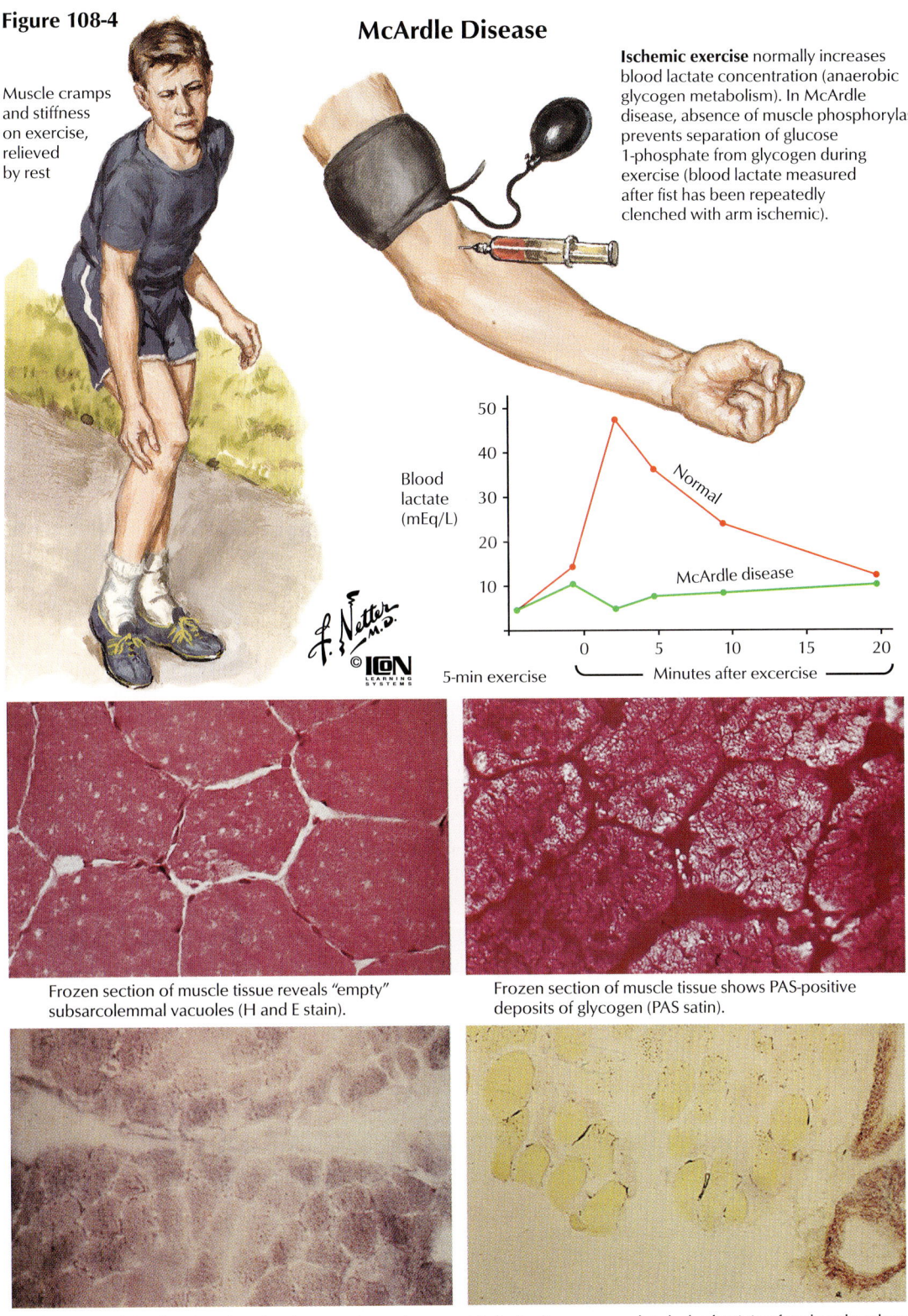

Figure 108-4

Muscle cramps and stiffness on exercise, relieved by rest

Ischemic exercise normally increases blood lactate concentration (anaerobic glycogen metabolism). In McArdle disease, absence of muscle phosphorylase prevents separation of glucose 1-phosphate from glycogen during exercise (blood lactate measured after fist has been repeatedly clenched with arm ischemic).

Frozen section of muscle tissue reveals "empty" subsarcolemmal vacuoles (H and E stain).

Frozen section of muscle tissue shows PAS-positive deposits of glycogen (PAS satin).

Positive staining for phosphorylase in normal muscle

McArdle disease: complete lack of staining for phosphorylase

MYOPATHIES

MYOPATHIES PRESENTING WITH EXERCISE INTOLERANCE

The **forearm ischemic exercise test** is useful for screening for metabolic myopathies. Baseline measurement of plasma lactate, pyruvate, and ammonia are obtained. The patient exercises an arm for 1 minute, and then a sphygmomanometer inflated significantly above systolic blood pressure is applied to make the arm ischemic. Serial lactate, pyruvate, and ammonia determinations are made immediately after exercise and 1, 3, 6, and 10 minutes thereafter.

Glycogen metabolism disorders are suspected where there is failure to achieve the normal transient 3- to 6-times increase of serum lactate from baseline. The forearm ischemic exercise test result is normal in defects of lipid metabolism. Muscle adenylate deaminase deficiency is defined by a lack of the expected increase in plasma ammonia after exercise.

The test sensitivity is dependent on patient effort. Permanent weakness after the ischemic forearm test is rarely reported. Rhabdomyolysis precipitated by testing may rarely cause renal impairment. Forearm ischemia sometimes causes painful muscle cramping in glycogenoses. These tests should therefore be performed in carefully controlled laboratory settings.

Respiratory chain disorders are suggested by marked increases in the serum lactate or pyruvate, metabolic acidosis, and dicarboxylic or aminoaciduria.

With one exception, EMG is not helpful because the results are normal or nonspecific to a myopathy. Its role is to exclude other motor unit processes before subjecting the patient to other studies. However, if an EMG can be performed while the patient is experiencing an active contracture, the electrical silence demonstrated is unique to glycogen storage disorders.

Lymphocyte or cultured skin fibroblast analysis supercedes the need for muscle biopsy in certain metabolic myopathies. Testing is available for many glycogenoses and disorders of lipid metabolism (Table 108-2). With the exception of complex IV deficiency, analysis for respiratory chain disorders is generally available only on a research basis.

Abnormal accumulation of glycogen or lipid may be detected in a muscle biopsy specimen using periodic acid-Schiff or oil red O staining, respectively. Muscle phosphorylase, phosphofructokinase, and myoadenylate deaminase deficiency are the only specific stains available for metabolic myopathies. Lipid stains may be normal or show mild lipid accumulation in carnitine palmitoyltransferase II deficiency. Biochemical testing of muscle is available for some myopathies.

A mitochondrial myopathy diagnosis is supported by ragged red fibers detected by the modified Gomori trichrome and succinic dehydrogenase stains or by myofibers that do not stain with cytochrome-c oxidase. Mitochondrial mutational analysis is available for a limited number of mutations.

TREATMENT AND PROGNOSIS

Most patients with metabolic myopathies learn to adapt to limited exercise tolerance. No

Table 108-2
Biochemical Analyses Available for Specific Metabolic Myopathies

Glycogen Storage	Lipid Storage	Mitochondrial	Purine
Acid maltase	Carnitine	NADH dehydrogenase	Myoadenylate deaminase
Neutral maltase	Carnitine palmitoyltransferase	NADH cytochrome-c reductase	Adenylate kinase
Phosphofructokinase		Succinate dehydrogenase	
Phosphorylase		Succinate cytochrome-c reductase	
Phosphorylase b kinase		Cytochrome-c oxidase	
Phosphoglycerate kinase		Citrate synthase?	
Phosphoglycerate mutase		Fumarase	

specific treatments are available for most of these conditions. Isolated reports attribute clinical benefit in the glycogenoses to aerobic training, high-protein diets, and creatine supplementation. However, none are proven reliable therapies. Patients with carnitine palmitoyltransferase II deficiency often can prevent attacks by increasing dietary carbohydrate intake before prolonged exercise.

Myoglobinuria with its risk of renal failure is always a significant concern with glycogenoses and lipid disorders of muscle metabolism. As many as 50% of patients with recurrent myoglobinuria experience episodes of acute renal insufficiency. Patients who are at risk for myoglobinuria are advised to seek prompt medical attention if such occurs. Treatment includes forced diuresis and alkalinization. A complete recovery is expected if the episodes are appropriately managed.

Metabolic myopathies are generally nonprogressive, although fixed weakness develops with increasing age in some patients with glycogenoses.

In few patients with carnitine palmitoyltransferase II deficiency, respiratory muscle involvement may require ventilatory support during episodes of severe weakness. Generally, these episodes are reversible with appropriate supportive care.

REFERENCES

DiMauro S, Lamperti C. Muscle glycogenoses. *Muscle Nerve*. 2001;24:984-999.

Felice KJ, Schneebaum AB, Jones HR. McArdle's disease with late onset symptoms. *J Neurol Neurosurg Psychiatry*. 1992;55:407-408.

Haller RG, Knochel JP. Metabolic myopathies. In: Johnson RT, Griffin JW, eds. *Current Therapy in Neurologic Disease*. St. Louis, Mo: Mosby-Year Book, 1993:397-402.

Katirji B, Al-Jaberi MM. Creatine kinase revisited. *J Clin Neuromusc Dis*. 2001;2:158-163.

Simmons A, Peterlin BL, Boyer PJ, Towfighi J. Muscle biopsy in the evaluation of patents with modestly elevated creatine kinase levels. *Muscle Nerve*. 2003;27:242-244.

Tonin P, Lewis P, Servidei S, DiMauro S. Metabolic causes of myoglobinuria. *Ann Neurol*. 1990;27:181-185.

Warren JD, Blumberg PC, Thompson PD. Rhabdomyolysis. *Muscle Nerve*. 2002;25:332-347.

INDEX

Note: Page numbers followed by *t* indicate tables.

A

α-bungarotoxin
A-α fibers, 34, 36
A-β fibers, 34, 36
　at neuromuscular junction, 857
A-δ fibers, rapidly conducting, 35–36
ABC assessment, 301
　for spinal cord injury, 658
　for traumatic head injury, 644, 645
Abdominal binders, 846–847
Abducens fasciculus, 89–92
Abducens internuncleus neuron, 12, 91
Abducens nerve (VI), 4, 83, 87, 90, 91, 224
　in cavernous sinus, 228, 229
　clinical vignette of, 89
　disorders of, 92–93
　distribution of, 5
　in nystagmus, 13
　schema of, 80, 86
　testing of, 11–14
Abducens nerve (VI) palsy, 78, 89, 92, 231
　with cerebral aneurysm, 251
　unilateral or bilateral, 93
Abducens nucleus, 6, 12, 80, 86, 89, 91, 105
　depressed, 13
Abductor digiti minimi muscle, 751, 761
Abductor hallucis muscle, 751, 761
Abductor hallucis nerve, 761
Abductor pollicis brevis muscle, 727
Abscess
　brain, 270, 567, 568, 609
　　magnetic resonance imaging for, 608
　cerebral and dural, 230
　dental and peritonsillar, 594–596
　epidural, 505
　multiple nocardial, 590
　paraspinous, 584
　spinal epidural, 566–567
　subdural, 567
　of tooth, 186
Absence seizures, 273
　atypical, 272
　clinical presentation of, 271–272
Absence status epilepticus, 275
Accessory nerve, 6, 105, 160, 224
　anatomy of, 157–158
　cranial root of, 151, 154, 158
　distribution of, 5
　spinal nucleus of, 6, 105
　spinal root of, 158
　testing of, 19
Accessory obturator nerve, 710
Accessory oculomotor (Edinger-Westphal) nucleus, 6, 8, 80, 81, 86, 105
Accessory optic tract nucleus, 68
Accommodation, 9
　oculomotor nerve in, 77
Acetaminophen, 174–175
Acetate, 851
Acetazolamide, 62
　for channelopathies, 913
Acetylcholine, 329, 853
　blocking of, 857
　formation of, 856
　hydrolysis of, 851

mobilization of, 858
presynaptic release of, 850
release of, 851, 860
synthesis of, 850–853
Acetylcholine antagonists, 855t
Acetylcholine receptor, 850, 851, 853
　blockers of, 855t
　nicotinic, 864
　sites of, 852
Acetylcholine receptor binding assays, 867–868
Acetylcholinesterase, 850, 856
　hydrolysis of, 853
　membrane-bound, 851
Acetylcholinesterase inhibitors, 853
　for myasthenia gravis, 868
Acetylsalicylic acid, 174–175
Achondroplasia, 692
Acid maltase deficiency, 901
Acoustic artery, internal. See *Labyrinthine artery*
Acoustic meatus
　external, 135
　internal, 16, 115, 114, 135
Acoustic neurinoma, 129
　filling cerebellopontine angle, 110
　in trigeminal neuralgia, 109
Acoustic neuroma, 113
　clinical presentation of, 624, 625
　diagnostic studies for, 624
　tinnitus with, 140
　treatment of, 626
　in trigeminal neuralgia, 106
Acoustic reflex testing, 125
Acoustic stria, 136
Acoustic tumor, 137
Acral paw lick syndrome, 377
Acromion, 704
Acrylamide, autonomic neurotoxicity of, 845
ACTH secreting tumors, 627
Acupuncture
　for cervical radiculopathy, 676
　for pain of multiple sclerosis, 554
Acute central disc, 506
Acute compartment syndrome, 754
Acute disseminated encephalomyelitis (ADEM), 544, 555
　clinical presentation of, 555
　diagnosis and treatment of, 555–557
Acute dystonic reactions, 432
　drugs causing, 433t
Acute pandysautonomic neuropathy, 843–845
Acute quadriplegic myopathy, 887
Acute respiratory distress syndrome, 257
Acute spinal cord syndromes
　evolution of symptoms in, 504
　pathology, etiology, and diagnosis of, 505, 636
　trauma in, 503–506
Acyclovir
　for facial palsy, 119
　for herpes simplex encephalitis, 574
　for herpes zoster encephalitis, 609
　for herpes zoster ophthalmicus, 108
　for herpes zoster virus, 581
Addison disease, 887, 888
　treatment of, 912
Adductor brevis muscle, 755
Adductor hallucis muscle, 751, 761
Adductor hiatus, 755
Adductor longus muscle, 755

NEUROLOGY

923

INDEX

Adductor magnus muscle, 750, 755
Adductor pollicis muscle, 727
Adenocarcinoma, parotid gland, 124–125
Adenohypophysis, 626
Adenylate deaminase deficiency, 916, 920
Adie tonic pupil, 84
Adrenergic synapses, 844
Adrenocortical insufficiency, 887, 888
Adrenoleukodystrophy, X-linked, screening for, 529
Adrenomyeloneuropathy, 784, 785
Advanced Trauma Life Support ABCs, 658
Affect concentration, 4
Affect consonant delusions, 366
Afferent ascending spinal connections, 499
Afferent auditory pathways, 136
Aging, pathological, 329
Agnosia
 evaluation for, 4
 visual, 51–52
Agoraphobia, 378
AIDS-associated vacuolar myelopathy, 531
Airway, poor protection of, 146
Akathisia, drug-induced, 433t, 435
Albendazole, 588
Albuminocytologic dissociation, 818–819
Alcohol
 cross-tolerances of, 390
 for essential tremor, 424
 fetal teratogenicity of, 390
 psychiatric illness and, 394
 toxic effects of, 394
 withdrawal from, 395, 398
  tremor in, 430t
Alcohol abuse
 clinical presentation of, 390–394
 diagnosis of, 394
 etiology of, 390
 signs of, 393
 treatment of, 394–398
Alcohol dependence, 390, 392
Alcoholic delirium, 322–324
Alcoholics Anonymous, 394
Alcoholism
 dopamine DR-2 receptor allele and, 390
 problem drinking patterns in, 391
Alexia, 49
Allied health care workers, 772
Alopecia, in heavy metal poisoning, 813
α-adrenergic agents, 465
α motor neurons, 34
α-synuclein, 402–405
 in parkinsonian syndromes, 414, 415t
ALS Association, 772
Altered consciousness, 206
Altitudinal scotomata, 57
Alveolar nerve
 anterior superior, 103
 inferior, 15, 102, 104, 107
 middle superior, 103
 posterior superior, 103
 superior, 107
Alzheimer disease
 amyloid cascade hypothesis in, 330
 clinical presentation of, 327, 339–341
 corticocortical and subcorticocortical projection circuits in, 337
 dementia with, 358

versus dementia with Lewy bodies, 349t
development and progression of, 333
diagnostic approach to, 341–343
differential diagnosis of, 341
epidemiology of, 327
family history of, 335
gross pathology in, 335
impaired smell in, 100
Lewy body variant of, 347, 348–349, 350
memory circuits and, 336
pathogenesis of, 327–329
pathology in, 331–335
presenile forms of, 335–339
progressive phases of, 340
risk factors for, 329–339
taupathies in, 352
treatment of, 343–346, 359
Amantadine
 for fatigue of multiple sclerosis, 554
 for Parkinson disease, 412
Amblyopia, 75
American Association of Neurological Surgeons "Think First" program, 658
Americans With Disabilities Act, 658
Amine precursors, 368
Aminoglycosans, 213
Aminoglycosides, 137
 in myasthenia gravis, 865
 in neuromuscular transmission, 854
Amitriptyline
 for herpes zoster virus, 581–582
 for lateral femoral nerve neuropathy, 759
 for progressive supranuclear palsy, 417
 for sensory neuropathies of lower extremity, 760
Ammonium tetrathiomolybdate, 470
Amnesic syndrome, 324
Amphetamine salts, 554
Amphetamines
 for narcolepsy, 291
 in thrombosis, 199
Amphotericin B, 592
Ampicillin
 for bacterial meningitis, 564
 for listeriosis, 592–593
Amygdala, 99
Amygdaloid complex, 96
Amyloid angiopathy, 244, 247
Amyloid cascade hypothesis, 330
Amyloid neuropathy, 815
Amyloid precursor protein (APP)
 altered metabolism of, 328
 in Alzheimer disease, 327–329
Amyloidogenesis, 328
Amyloidosis, 831, 846
 in chronic myopathy, 893
Amyotrophic lateral sclerosis (ALS), 121
 classification of, 764–768, 769t
 diagnostic approach to, 771–772
 diagnostic criteria for, 764
 diagnostic problems in, 770–771
 differential diagnosis of, 831, 867
 etiology of, 768–770
 future directions for, 776
 with lower motor neuron features, 777
 management of, 772–775
 in voice disorders, 155, 156
Analgesics

INDEX

for migraine, 175
   precipitating delirium, 399, 400
Anaplastic glioma, 611, 614
Anastomotic vein, inferior, 225
Anemia, megaloblastic, 532
Anesthetics, 854t
   complications of, 918
Angiography, 517
Angioplasty, 217
   for cerebral vasospasm, 256
   percutaneous, for carotid atherosclerosis, 222
Angiotensin-converting enzyme inhibitors, 314
Angular gyrus, 42
   lesions of, 46
Anhedonia, 366
Ankle clonus, 516
Ankle-foot orthosis, 754
   for neuropathies, 807
   for peripheral neuropathies, 807
   for sensory polyneuropathy, 838
Ankle jerk
   loss of, 801
   for mononeuropathies of lower extremity, 748
Ankle joints, dissolution of, 837
Ankylosing spondylitis, 694
ANNA-1 antibody testing, 805–806
Annulus fibrosus
   fissure in, 684
   nociceptors in, 684
Anococcygeal nerve, 711
Anosmia, 7, 97
Anosognosia, 50
Anoxia, diffuse, 52
Ansa cervicalis, 160, 163, 164
Ansa lenticularis, 403
Antebrachial nerve, 705
Anterior chamber, 56
Anterior commissure, 99, 226
Anterior compartment syndrome, 746
Anterior horn cell
   in generalized weakness, 25
   in motor disorders, 26
Anterior interosseous syndrome, 730, 731, 732
Anterior spinal artery syndrome, 191, 523
Anterior tarsal tunnel syndrome, 748
Anterograde amnesia, 324
Anterolateral central arteries, 193
Anti-GAD antibodies, 794
Anti-GM1 antibodies, 765
   for motor neuron disease, 781–782
Anti-Hu antibodies, 810
   in polyneuropathies, 805–806
   in sensory neuronopathy, 834
   testing of, 836
Anti-Jo-1 antibodies, 879
Anti-signal recognition particle antibodies, 879
Antiacetylcholine antibodies, 864
Antibiotics
   for bacterial meningitis, 564
   for childhood-onset obsessive-compulsive disorder, 377
   for comatose patient, 300
   for tetanus, 596
Antibodies, myopathic, 879
Anticholinergic drugs
   for dystonia, 446
   for Parkinson disease, 411–412
Anticholinesterase drugs, 865

Anticoagulant therapy
   for cerebral venous thrombosis, 232
   in intracerebral hemorrhage, 244
Anticonvulsants
   for bipolar disorder, 370–371
   for essential tremor, 426t
   for peripheral neuropathies, 807
   for stiff person syndrome, 798
   teratogenic effects of, 278
Antidepressants
   for Alzheimer disease, 344
   for bipolar disorder, 371
   for dysthymia, 383
   for major depression, 367
   for migraine, 175
   for obsessive-compulsive disorder, 375–377
   for panic disorder, 380
   for progressive supranuclear palsy, 417
Antidiuretic hormone, 628
Antidopaminergic drugs, 429–430
Antiemetics, 175
Antiepileptic therapy, 277
Antiglutamatergic agents, 775
Antihypertensives, 865
Antioxidants
   for chorea, 459
   for Friedreich ataxia, 535
   for motor neuron disease, 775
   for tardive dyskinesia, 437
Antiplatelets, 216
Antiprogesterone agents, 624
Antipsychotics
   for borderline personality disorder, 386
   for delirium, 326
   for tics, 465
Antiretroviral drugs, 531
Antispasmodics
   for AIDS-associated vacuolar myelopathy, 531
   for multiple system atrophy, 420
Antithrombin III deficiency, 199
Antithrombotics, 244
Antoni B pattern, 640
Anxiety, 407, 408
Aorta
   dissection aneurysms of, 512
   segmental arteries from, 501
Aortic arch, 155
Aortic valve endocarditis, 245
Apathetic states, 352, 354
Aphasia, 41–45
   characteristics of, 45t
   classification of, 41
   forebrain lesions in, 46
   primary progressive, 351, 353, 354
   sensory transcortical, 45
   thalamic, 239
Apnea test, positive, 318
Apneustic breathing, 311
ApoE genotype, 339
Apolipoprotein E genotyping, 342–343
Apraxia, 49
   evaluation for, 4
   of swallow mechanism, 152
Apraxic gait, 22
Aqua therapy, 554
Arachnoid, 116, 493
Arachnoid granulations, 191–194

INDEX

Arachnoid mater, 495, 496, 835
Arcuate ligament, 733
Areflexia, 32–35
    with complete transverse cord lesion, 501
    with Friedreich ataxia, 534
    in Lambert-Eaton myasthenic syndrome, 860
Argyll Robertson pupils, 570–571
Argyll Robertson syndrome, 10t
Arm, deep artery of, 704
Arnold-Chiari malformation, 167
    in multiple sclerosis, 541–542
    with syrinx, 528
Arnold-Chiari syndrome, 130
Arrhythmia, 195
    in cardioembolism, 207–209
Arterial dissection, 199, 211–212
Arterial pressure monitoring, 653
Arterial vascular syndromes, 92
Arteries, to brain and meninges, 188–194
Arteriography, 255
Arteriosclerotic heart disease, 208
Arteriosclerotic parkinsonism, 410
Arteriovenous fistulas, 517
Arteriovenous malformations, 270
    in brain abscess, 568
    differential diagnosis of, 609
    intradural, 517–519, 520
    in multiple sclerosis, 544–545
Articular nerve, recurrent, 747
Articularis genus muscle, 753, 758
Artificial synapse, 124
Aryepiglottic fold, 148
Arytenoid muscles, 153
Asomatognosia, 48–49
Aspergillus fumigatus meningitis, 588
Aspiration
    barium, 152
    clinical presentation of, 147
    silent, 146
Aspirin
    for migraine, 174–175
    for TIAs and stroke, 216
Astasia-abasia, 545
Asterixis, 429, 447
    drugs causing, 434t
Astrocytes, 611
Astrocytoma, 612, 613
    anaplastic, 614
    cerebellar, 618, 620
    intramedullary spinal cord, 642
    myelographic and CT characteristics of, 524
    of spinal cord, 638
Asymptomatic Carotid Atherosclerosis Study, 218–219
Ataxia
    with cerebrovascular disease, 483
    Friedreich, 488, 532–535
    frontal, 481
    in motor disorders, 26
    with neurodegenerative disorders, 487
    treatment of, 489
    with vertebrobasilar ischemia, 206
Ataxia telangiectasia, 485t
Ataxic cerebral palsy, 440
Ataxic hemiparesis, locations of, 211t
Ataxic intention tremor, 429
Ataxic neuropathy, 806t
Atherosclerosis, 196
    of basilar artery, 204
    carotid system, 195
    in hearing loss, 141
Atherosclerotic parkinsonism, 417
Atherosclerotic plaque, 198
Athetoid cerebral palsy, 440
Athetoid dystonia, 438
Athetoid movements, 469
Athetosis
    in cerebral palsy, 440
    versus chorea, 453
Atlas, 494
    Jefferson fracture of, 668
    posterior arch of, 184
Atlastin, 529
Atonic cerebral palsy, 440
ATP, regeneration of, 918
Atrial fibrillation, 208
    in cardioembolism, 207
Atrial myxoma, 199, 246
Atrial myxomatous tumor emboli, 215
Atrial septum
    aneurysm of, 199
    defects of, 209
Atrial vein
    lateral, 226
    medial, 226
Attention deficit disorder (ADD)
    clinical presentation of, 387
    diagnosis of, 387
    treatment of, 387–389
Attention deficit hyperactivity disorder (ADHD), 387–389
    with Tourette syndrome, 462, 464
Audiogram, 138
Audiometric testing, 141
Auditory artery, internal, 189
Auditory canal
    foreign bodies in, 137–138
    neoplasms of, 138
Auditory cortex, efferent pathway from, 500, 766
Auditory evoked responses, absence of, 318
Auditory hallucinations, 322
Auditory meatus, intracranial and internal, 118
Auditory neoplasms, 140
Auditory nerve, 128
    anatomy of, 134–136
    clinical vignette of, 134
    disorders of
        clinical presentation of, 137–138
        diagnostic approach to, 138
        differential diagnosis of, 138–141
        treatment of, 141
    testing of, 15–19
Auditory tube. See *Pharyngotympanic tube*
Auricle, 135
Auricular artery, posterior, 184, 189
Auricular muscles
    branches to, 115
    nerves to, 16
Auricular nerve, 15
    anterior, 102
    greater, 160, 183, 184
    posterior, 16, 104, 115, 122
Auriculotemporal nerve, 15, 102, 104, 107, 150, 183
Autoantibodies, 864
Autoimmune paraneoplastic disorders, 843
Autonomic fibers, facial nerve, 112

INDEX

Autonomic hypotension, 846
Autonomic nervous system
    disorders of
        clinical presentation of, 843
        diagnostic approach to, 846
        differential diagnosis of, 843–846
        in parkinsonism, 407, 408
        treatment and prognosis of, 846–847
    of eye, 8
    neuropathies of, 802
    polyneuropathies involving, 803t
Autonomic peripheral neuropathy, 845
Autonomic seizures, 51
AVMs. See *Arteriovenous malformations*
Axial cervical spine injury, 663
Axilla
    anterior view of, 704
    radial nerve compression in, 738
Axillary artery, 704
Axillary nerve, 703, 704, 705, 742
    lesions of, 706
    neuropathy of, 744
Axolemma, 851, 852, 856
Axon terminal, 851, 852, 856
Axonal multifocal neuropathies, 830t
Axonal transport, 717
Axonotmesis, 718
Axons, 717
    damage to, 721
    electric impulse propagated along, 856
Axoplasm, 717, 851, 852
Azathioprine
    for multiple sclerosis, 552
    for myasthenia gravis, 869
    for stiff person syndrome, 798
Azygous vein, 501

B

B_{12} vitamin deficiency, 545
    clinical presentation of, 531–532
    diagnosis of, 836
    differential diagnosis of, 784, 836
B vitamins
    deficiency of
        in alcoholism, 394
        gait disturbances in, 488
    for gait disorders, 488–489
    in vascular dementia treatment, 359
    for Wernicke encephalopathy, 324
Babinski response, 3
Babinski sign
    in amyotrophic lateral sclerosis, 771
    in brain hemorrhage, infections and tumors, 181
    in comatose patient, 301
    elicitation of, 35
    with head injury, 648
    in motor disorders, 26
    in primary lateral sclerosis, 783
    in pseudotumor cerebri, 606
    in spondylosis, 515, 516
Bacille Calmette-Guérin vaccine, 841–842
Back pain
    functional, 694–696
    lumbosacral, 708–714
    psychosomatic, 694–696
    rheumatologic, 694–696
Baclofen
    for primary lateral sclerosis, 785
    for stiff person syndrome, 798
    for tardive dyskinesia, 436–437
    for tics, 465
Bacterial infections
    audiometric testing in, 141
    in immunocompromised hosts, 586–593
Bacteroides
    in brain abscess, 568
    in subdural empyema, 568
BAER. See *Brainstem auditory evoked response*
Balance centers, testing of, 489
Balance training, 535
Balint syndrome, 52
Ballism, 453
Ballismus, 23–25
Balloon dilation, 221
Barany maneuver, 19
Barbiturates
    alcohol and, 390
    for increased intracranial pressure, 313
    overdose of, 300
Barium swallow, 147–152
Basal ganglia gait disorder, 483
Basal ganglion
    dopaminergic transmission in, 432
    efferent pathway to, 766
    in motor disorders, 26
    in motor tone, 30
    in Parkinson disease, 405
Basal skull
    fractures of, 646
    sinus thrombosis of, 229
Basal vein, 225, 227, 226
Base of skull sinus thrombosis, 229
Basement membrane, 98, 852, 856
    acetylcholine synthesis in, 850, 851
Basic pedunculi, 403
Basilar artery, 65, 78, 83, 189, 191, 193
    atherosclerosis of, 204
    embolus of, 204–207
Basilar artery migraine, 174
Basilar bifurcation aneurysm, 254
Basilar plexus, 224
Basilar skull fracture, 647
Basilic vein, 704
Bathroom safety, in motor neuron disease, 774t
Battle sign, 646, 647
    in comatose patient, 300
BCNU, 615
Becker muscular dystrophy, 900, 909
    treatment of, 904–905
Bed mobility, in motor neuron disease, 774t
Behavior, interpersonal, 44
Behavioral disorders
    clinical features of, 322–324
    diagnostic approach to, 325
    epidemiology of, 324
    treatment and counseling for, 325–326
Behavioral therapy
    for borderline personality disorder, 384–386
    for obsessive-compulsive disorder, 377
Behçet disease, 246
Bell palsy, 4
    clinical presentation of, 117
    differential diagnosis of, 117–119
    pathogenesis of, 117

INDEX

recurrence of, 123–124
  treatment and prognosis of, 119
Bell phenomenon, 14, 117
Bence Jones protein, 636
Benedict syndrome, 81
Benign childhood epilepsy, 274
Benign cough headache, 179
Benign exertional headache, 179
Benign febrile convulsions, 274
Benign focal amyotrophy, 779
Benign paroxysmal positional vertigo, 130, 133
Benzamide-induced parkinsonism, 432–433
Benzodiazepines
  for action tremor, 428
  alcohol and, 390
  for Alzheimer disease, 344
  in borderline personality disorder, 386
  for cervical radiculopathy, 676
  for chorea, 459
  for comatose patient, 300
  for delirium, 326
  for essential tremor, 426t
  for frontotemporal dementia, 355
  in increased intracranial pressure, 314
  for myoclonus, 452
  for night terrors, 294
  for panic disorder, 380
  for primary lateral sclerosis, 785
  for status epilepticus, 275
  for stiff person syndrome, 798
  for tardive dyskinesia, 436–437
  for vestibular disorders, 132
  withdrawal from, 397
Benztropine, 446
Bereitschaftspotential, 461
Berg Balance Scale, peripheral vestibulopathies, 132
Berry aneurysms, 234
  Hunt-Hess grading scale for, 252t
β-amyloid, 327–329
β-amyloid peptide deposition, 331
β-amyloid peptide plaques
  in Alzheimer disease, 334
  formation of, 333
β blockers
  for essential tremor, 426t
  for migraine, 175
  in myasthenia gravis, 865
  for orthostatic hypotension, 847
  for syncope, 280
β-receptor agonists, 423
β-sympathetic blockers, 314
Bethanechol, 847
Bethlem myopathy, 893, 896t, 900–901
Bezold-Jarisch reflex, 278
Biceps brachii muscle, 704, 742
Biceps femoris muscle
  long head of, 750
  tendon of, 747
Biceps tendon, rupture of, 744
Bilevel positive pressure, 792, 793
Binswanger disease, 357–358
Biochemical analysis, 920t
Biochemical pathways, 403
Bipolar affective disorder
  childhood-onset, versus attention deficit disorder, 387
  clinical presentation of, 369–370
  depression in, 366–367
  treatment of, 370–371
Bitemporal hemianopsia, 64, 66
Bladder dysfunction
  in multiple sclerosis, 554–555
  treatment of, 847
Bladder dysmotility, 843
Blepharoptosis, bilateral, 77
Blepharospasm, 441
  diagnosis of, 445
  treatment of, 446
Blind spots
  enlargement of, 11, 62
  with papilledema, 11
Blindness
  with cerebral artery occlusion, 205
  sudden unilateral, 61
Blocking tics, 461t
Blood-brain barrier, compromised, 235
Blood pressure control, intracranial, 313–314
Blood tests, 805
Blood volume expanders, 280
Blurred vision, 61, 541
  in myasthenia gravis, 864
Bone densitometry, 891
Bone marrow transplantation, 614
Bone spicules, 54
Bonnet syndrome, 51
Border zone ischemia, 319
Borderline personality disorder
  clinical presentation of, 384, 385
  treatment of, 384–386
Borderline schizophrenics. See *Borderline personality disorder*
Borrelia burgdorferi *antibodies,* 120
Botox. See *Botulinum toxin*
Botulin, at neuromuscular junction, 857
Botulinum toxin
  for corticobasal degeneration, 416
  for dystonia, 446
  for essential tremor, 426t
  for motor neuron disease, 792
  for progressive supranuclear palsy, 417
Botulism
  differential diagnosis of, 823
  primary sites of motor disorder in, 26
Bovine spongiform encephalopathy, 360
Bow tie atrophy, 69
Bowler's thumb, 720
Braces, cervical spine, 666, 669
Brachial artery, 704
Brachial nerve, medial, 705
Brachial plexitis, 676
Brachial plexopathy
  anatomical correlations of, 701–705
  clinical presentation of, 700–701, 706–707
  diagnostic approach to, 705
  differential diagnosis of, 705–707
  future research on, 707
  treatment and prognosis of, 707
Brachial plexus, 160, 494
  axillary anatomy and, 704
  embryonic limb organization compared to, 703
  etiologies of, 701t
  idiopathic neuropathy of, 705
    treatment of, 707
  neoplasms of, 674
  neuritis of, 745

INDEX

pathologic processes in, 700
Brachial veins, 704
   lateral, 227
Brachialis muscle, 704, 742
Brachiocephalic trunk, 189
Brachioradialis muscle tendon, 737
Bradykinesia
   in dementia with Lewy bodies, 349
   drug-induced, 433–435
   in parkinsonism, 405, 408
Brain
   abscesses of, 567, 568
      diagnosis of, 609
      magnetic resonance imaging for, 608
   arterial supply to, 188–194
   arteries of, 71
   compromised, rostrocaudal signs of, 307–312
   cysticercosis of, 588, 589
   deep and subpendymal veins of, 225
   hemorrhage of, 181
   injury of
      extraaxial traumatic, 646–654
      intraaxial traumatic, 655–657
      outcomes from, 657
      posterior fossa, 657
      signs suggesting need for operation for, 648
   magnetic resonance imaging of, 610
   malignant tumors of, 611–621
      epidemiology of, 611
   normal CT scan of, 651
   olfactory cortex of, 96
   superolateral surface of, 42
   traumatic injury to, 644–657
   tuberculosis of, 583–585
   tumors of, 609
      benign, 622–633
      in children, 619
      common manifestations of, 606–607
      future treatments for, 620–621
      headache in, 181
      intraventricular, 632
      metastatic, 615–616, 617
      primary intraaxial, 611–615
   venous drainage of, 223–229
   venous structures of, 191–194
   in weakness, 28
Brain biopsy
   for herpes simplex encephalitis, 576
   for nocardiosis, 588–589
   stereotactic, 612
   for transmissible spongiform encephalopathy, 363
Brain death
   clinical presentation of, 316
   criteria for, 316–318
   differential diagnosis of, 317
   mitigating factors in, 318–320
Brain imaging, gadolinium-enhanced, 615–616
Brainstem
   cranial nerve nuclei in, 105
   dysfunction of, 128, 303
   in gait disorders, 480
   glioma of, 113
   infarction of, 167
   intramedullary disorders of, 790
   intrinsic tumors of, 791
   in motor tone, 30
   trigeminal lesions of, 108t

tumors of, 867
ventral aspect of, 24
Brainstem auditory evoked response, 134, 138, 140
   in acoustic neurinoma, 625
   in multiple sclerosis, 548–549
   for severe head injury, 302
Brainstem reflexes, 296
   absence of, 318
Brainstem stroke, 506
Brainstem upper motor neuron, 765
Breast cancer
   metastatic, 110
   metastatic to brain, 617
   paraneoplastic myelopathy with, 785
Breathing, with increased intracranial pressure, 308–311
Broca aphasia, 41–45, 46, 47
Brodmann areas
   aphasia and, 45
   in eye movement control, 12, 91
   in visual cortex, 72
Brown-Séquard syndrome, 38–39, 492, 501, 522, 523
   clinical presentation of, 641, 642
Brudzinski maneuver, 249
Brudzinski neck sign, 560, 562, 563
Buccal nerve, 15, 102, 104, 107, 183
Buccinator muscle, 16, 104, 115
Budge-Waller, ciliospinal center of, 85
Bulbar palsy, primary, 792t. See also *Progressive bulbar palsy (PBP)*
Bulbopontine angle, 112
Bulbospinal muscular atrophy, 121
Bulbospinal neuronopathy, 779–780
Buprenorphine, 398
Burr hole trephine, 650
Burr holes
   exploratory, 656
   for subdural hematoma, 650, 652
Burst fracture
   in acute spinal cord syndrome, 505
   of vertebral body, 660
Buspirone, 355

C

C fibers, conducting, 35
C7 nerve root irritation, 672–674
C2 pars interarticularis fracture, 663
C5 radiculopathy, 743
C7 radiculopathy, 36–38
   differential diagnosis of, 736
C8 radiculopathy, 736
C-reactive protein, 181
CADASIL, 358
Caffeine, 175
CAGE questionnaire, 394
Cajal, interstitial nucleus of, 12, 91, 500
   efferent pathways to, 766
Calcarine artery, 69, 72, 193
Calcarine fissure, 9, 70, 73
Calcarine infarction, 205
Calcarine sulcus, 42
Calcium
   for acute proximal myopathies, 891
   intracellular, 858
   in nerve terminal, 850
   in neuromuscular junction, 856
Calcium channel, voltage gated, 862
Calcium channel blockers

INDEX

for essential tremor, 426t
for migraine, 175
in myasthenia gravis, 865
for tics, 465
in vascular dementia treatment, 359
Callosomarginal artery, 193
Callosotomy, 278, 284
Calmodulin, 858
Caloric testing
    with increased intracranial pressure, 309
    for severe head injury, 302
Campylobacter jejuni, 819
Canalith repositioning, 131
Carbamazepine
    for bipolar disorder, 370–371
    for epilepsy, 277
    for lateral femoral nerve neuropathy, 759
    in myoclonus, 452
    for peripheral neuropathies, 807
    for sensory neuropathies of lower extremity, 760
    for tics, 465
Carbon monoxide, 410
Carbonic anhydrase inhibitors
    for cerebral venous thrombosis, 233
    for channelopathies, 913
    for essential tremor, 426t
    for myopathies, 882
Carboplatin, 835
Carcinomatous meningitis, 121
Cardiac artery, dissection of, 199
Cardiac embolism, 195–199
Cardiac glycosides, 854t
Cardiac transplantation in
    for Becker muscular dystrophy, 905
Cardioembolic disease, 207–209
Cardioembolic stroke, 235
Cardiomyopathy, 886
    treatment of, 905
Cardiomyopathy, with Friedreich ataxia, 535
Caregiving
    for Alzheimer disease, 345–346
    for frontotemporal dementia, 354–355
Carnitine
    deficiency of
        myopathic, 901–904
        primary systemic, 904
    replacement of, 882
    supplementation of, 905
Carnitine palmitoyltransferase II deficiency, 916
    treatment of, 921
Caroticotympanic nerve, 16, 115, 150
Carotid angiograms, 226
Carotid angioplasty-stent, 217
Carotid artery, 65
    in cavernous sinus, 229
    common, 150, 160, 164, 188, 189
    dissection of, 4
        extracranial, 211–212
        Horner syndrome signs with, 163
        internal, 167
    external, 150, 160, 171, 188, 189
    extracranial atherosclerosis of, 218–222
    internal, 8, 80, 83, 86, 87, 90, 114, 150, 160, 164, 171, 188–191, 193, 224, 228
        cavernous segment of, 188–190
        cervical segment of, 188
        petrous segment of, 188

supraclinoid segment of, 190
intracranial occlusive disease of, 202
ischemia of, ocular signs of, 201
occlusion of, 199–201
thalamoperforate branches of, 190
Carotid artery trunks, 64
Carotid atherosclerosis, 195
Carotid body, 150, 189
Carotid-cavernous fistula, posteriorly draining, 88
Carotid endarterectomy, 159, 163
    for atherosclerosis, 219–222
    benefits of, 218–219
    introduction of, 218
    for stroke, 217
Carotid nerve, internal, 844
Carotid plexus, 80, 86, 87
    internal, 8, 16, 90, 115
Carotid-posterior communicating aneurysm, 78
Carotid sinus, 150, 189
Carotid siphon, 188–190
Carpal tunnel, 728
    compression at, 720
    compression neuropathy at, 722
    surgical decompression of, 729
Carpal tunnel syndrome
    clinical presentation of, 726–730
    diagnosis of, 532
    differential diagnosis of, 730
    epidemiology of, 716
    testing for, 726–730
Carpopedal spasms, 596
Cataplexy, 290
Cataract, 79
Catastrophic thinking, 378, 380
Catechol-O-methyl-transferase (COMT) inhibitors, 412
Catecholamine synthesis, 444
Cauda equina, 494, 497
    spinal nerves forming, 496
Cauda equina syndrome, 635–637
Caudal pons, 112
Caudate nucleus, 500, 766
    anterior vein of, 225
    degeneration and atrophy of, 456
    head of, 225
    hemorrhage of, 238
    posterior vein of, 225
    transverse veins of, 225
Caudate vein, 226
Caveolin-3, 908
    deficiency of, 906
Cavernous angioma, 519
    in intracerebral hemorrhage, 243
Cavernous distention, 88
Cavernous hemangioma, 242
Cavernous malformations, 519
Cavernous plexus, 80, 86
Cavernous sinus, 65, 81–82, 83, 189, 190, 194, 224, 228–229
    abducens nerve in, 89
    coronal section through, 90
    cranial nerves of, 228
    cross section of, 230
    thrombosis of, 83, 229–231, 230
Cavernous sinus syndrome, 83
C26:C22 long-chain fatty acid analysis, 529
CCNU regimen, 613
Cefotaxime, 564

INDEX

Ceftriaxone
    for bacterial meningitis, 564
    for herpes simplex encephalitis, 574
    for neurosyphilis, 571–573
Celecoxib, 775
Celiac ganglion, 144, 844
Central canal, 165
Central cord compression, 525
Central cord damage, 502
Central cord syndrome, 523, 661
    decompression for, 662
Central core disease, 901
Central nervous system
    disorders of, 128
    in gait control, 480
    lesions of, 749
    lymphoma of, 618
        mimicking multiple sclerosis, 544
    motor neuron pathway in, 765
    pathology of in multiple sclerosis, 539
    tumors of in voice disorders, 155
Central neurogenic hyperventilation, 311
Central pain pathway, 171
Central spinal canal, syrinx in, 526–528
Central sulcus, 42
Central vein, 501
Centronuclear myopathy, 901
Centrotemporal spikes, 274
Cephalic vein, 704
Cephalosporin
    for bacterial meningitis, 564
    for brain abscess, 568
Cerebellar artery, 78
    aneurysm of, 254
    anterior inferior, 189, 191, 193
        occlusion of, 92
    infarction of, 128
    lateral medullary, 191
    posterior, 189
    posterior inferior, 189, 191, 193
        occlusion of, 202–207
    superior, 189, 191
        ectatic loop of, 106
Cerebellar astrocytoma, 618
    cystic, 620
Cerebellar ataxia, 81
    primary sites of motor disorder in, 26
Cerebellar gait disorders, 483–488
Cerebellar hemispheric vein, inferior, 227
Cerebellar peduncle, 136, 227
    inferior, 165
    middle, 33
    superior, 33, 81
Cerebellar PICA syndrome, 204
Cerebellar syndrome, 420
Cerebellar vein, superior, 227
Cerebellitis, infectious or postinfectious, 486–488
Cerebellopontine angle
    acoustic neurinoma in, 110
    neoplasms of, 138
    tumors of, 109, 113
Cerebellum, 73, 226
    acquired processes affecting, 485t
    dysfunction of, 21
    in gait disorders, 480
    hemorrhage of, 230, 238, 240
    infarction of, 128–129
    lesions of in gait disorders, 481–483
    in motor disorders, 26
    in motor tone, 30
    parts of, 227
    trauma to, 129
    tumors of
        invasive, 483
        midline, 22
Cerebral afferent pathways, 33
Cerebral aneurysms, 234, 248–255
    congenital, 235
    diagnostic approach to, 252
    differential diagnosis of, 249–252
    distribution of, 235, 253
    frontotemporal approach to, 259
    management of, 255–261
    ophthalmologic manifestations of, 78, 251
    pathophysiology of, 252–255
    posterior approach to, 260
    ruptured, 248
        complications of, 255–257
        pathophysiology of, 255
        risk factors for, 255
    saccular, 257–258
    sizes of, 253
    unruptured, 257
    warning leak of, 248
Cerebral aqueduct, 226
Cerebral artery, 83, 171
    aneurysms of, 254
    anterior, 64, 65, 71, 74, 189, 190, 193
        A1 segment of, 190
        occlusion of, 203
    branches of, 193
    ischemia of, ocular signs in, 200, 201
    middle, 69, 71, 72, 74, 189, 190, 193, 203
    occlusion of, 75–76, 195, 203, 205
    posterior, 69, 71, 72, 74, 188, 193
        infarcts of, 207
        occlusion of, 205
    superior, 193
    terminal cortical branches of, 193
Cerebral artery stroke, 143
Cerebral autoregulation, 313, 314
Cerebral cortex
    abscess of, 230
    arterial supply of, 74
    arterial supply to, 191–194
    biopsy of for acute disseminated encephalomyelitis, 555
    contusions of, 655
    edema of
        in intracerebral hemorrhage, 246
        with subdural hematoma, 650–654
    efferent pathways of, 500, 766
    embolism of, 195–199
        cardiac sources of, 208
    fail-safe circulation systems of, 190
    function and association pathways of, 43
    functional organization of, 73
    ischemic damage of in brain death, 316
    lateral aspect of, 24
    mass lesions in mimicking multiple sclerosis, 544
    medial aspect of, 73
    in motor disorders, 26
    in motor tone, 30
    postcentral gyrus, 37
    superior margin of, 42

NEUROLOGY

931

INDEX

topographic projections of, 767
Cerebral crus, 71, 193, 225
Cerebral disorders, 790–791
Cerebral fissure, longitudinal, 225
Cerebral herniation, 307–312
Cerebral palsy, 440
Cerebral peduncle, 500, 766
    in parkinsonism, 406
Cerebral sinuses, 191–194
Cerebral tuberculomas, 585
Cerebral upper motor neuron, 765
Cerebral vasospasm, 256
Cerebral veins, 191–194
    anterior, 67, 225, 227, 226
    deep middle, 225, 227, 226
    deep thrombosis of, 229
    inferior, 224, 225
    internal, 225, 227, 226
    superficial middle, 224, 225
Cerebral venous system, 223–229
Cerebral venous thrombosis, 223–233
    causes of, 223t
Cerebrospinal fluid
    in congenital aneurysm rupture, 250
    drainage of, 194
    in increased intracranial pressure, 604–607
    for neurosyphilis, 571
    pressure of in cerebral venous thrombosis, 233
    shunting of for increased intracranial pressure, 607
Cerebrospinal fluid analysis
    for acquired demyelinating polyradiculoneuropathies, 824
    for acute disseminated encephalomyelitis, 555
    in Alzheimer disease, 343
    for bacterial meningitis, 560, 562–564
    for cerebral venous thrombosis, 232
    for cryptococcus, 592
    for demyelinating disorders, 610
    for headache, 181–182
    for hereditary spastic paraplegia, 529
    for herpes simplex encephalitis, 576
    of infiltrative processes, 167
    for lumbosacral plexopathies, 709
    for multiple sclerosis, 546–548
    in polyneuropathies, 806
    for progressive multifocal leukoencephalopathy, 588
    for rabies, 578
    for subarachnoid hemorrhage, 252
    for subdural empyema, 568
    for transmissible spongiform encephalopathy, 363
    for tuberculous meningitis, 583
Cerebrospinal fluid immunoassay, 548
Cerebrovascular disease, 483
Cerebrovascular embolus, 221
Cerulean, impaction of, 137–138
Ceruloplasmin, 467
    levels of in Wilson disease, 468
Ceruloplasmin gene, 468
Cervical artery
    deep, 189
    transverse, 704
Cervical disc
    herniation of
        clinical manifestations of, 675
        imaging of, 677
    ruptured, 677
Cervical lymph node biopsies, 157

Cervical lymphadenopathy, 589
Cervical nerve roots, 493
    compression of, 672, 674
        diagnosis of, 676
        with herniated disc, 675
    lesions of, 574t
        motor impairment related to, 673
Cervical nerves, 497
Cervical plexus, 494
    branches from, 183
    in situ, 160
Cervical radiculopathy, 706
    clinical presentation of, 672–674
    diagnostic approach to, 676
    differential diagnosis of, 674–676
    treatment and prognosis of, 676–677
Cervical spinal cord, tumors in, 637
Cervical spinal nerves, 183
Cervical spine injury
    compression, 660
    diagnosis of, 658–662
    flexion and flexion-rotation, 659
    hyperextension, 661
    on-site treatment of, 664–665
    rehabilitation for, 669
    traction and bracing for, 666
Cervical spine osteoarthritis, 178
Cervical spinous processes, wiring of, 667
Cervical spondylosis, 488, 502
    differential diagnosis of, 784
Cervical sympathetic ganglion, 844
    superior, 150, 164
Cervical vertebrae
    anterior dislocation of, 659
    fracture and dislocation of, 668
Channelopathies, 797
    chloride, 894
    clinical presentation of, 909–912
    diagnostic approach to, 912
    differential diagnosis of, 912
    with episodic weakness, 909–913
    etiology of, 909
    treatment and prognosis of, 912–913
Charcot joints, 837
Charcot-Marie-Tooth disease, 778
    characteristics of, 811
    clinical presentation of, 809
    diagnosis of, 804–805
    differential diagnosis of, 906
    motor nerve conduction velocity in, 812
    sensory loss in, 818
    type 1A, 124, 823
Charcot-Marie-Tooth syndrome, type 1, 816
Chelation therapy, 470
Chemoprophylaxis, meningitis, 565
Chemotherapy
    for anaplastic glioma, 614
    for glioblastoma multiforme, 615
    for gliomas, 621
    for intramedullary spinal cord tumors, 642
    for Lambert-Eaton myasthenic syndrome, 862
    for low-grade gliomas, 613–614
    for lymphoproliferative disorders, 833
    for meningioma, 624
    for nerve sheath tumors, 641
    for toxoplasmosis, 590
Cherry-red spots, near macula, 11

INDEX

Cheyne-Stokes respirations, 308–311
    in bacterial meningitis, 562
Chiari malformations, 126
Chiasmatic disorders, 64–67
Childhood neglect, 384
Children
    brain tumors in, 619
    gliomas in, 621
Chiropractic treatment, 676
Chloride channel disorders, 909
Chloride channelopathy, 894
Chloroquine, 54
    in toxic myopathies, 887
Cholesteatoma, 167
    in facial palsy, 121
Cholesterol-lowering agents, 891
Choline, 851
    blocked reuptake of, 857
    at nerve terminal, 856
Choline uptake inhibitors, 855t
Cholinergic crisis, 868
Cholinergic synapses, 844
Cholinesterase inhibitors, 855t
    for Alzheimer disease, 343, 344, 346
    for dementia with Lewy bodies, 350
    for frontotemporal dementia, 354–355
    for vascular dementia, 359
Cholinomimetics, 855t
Chondroma, trigeminal, 109–110
Chorda tympani nerve, 15, 16, 102, 104, 115, 114, 113
Chordoma, 167, 628, 630, 633
    intracranial, 628
Chorea
    causes of, 454t
    clinical presentation of, 453, 455–457
    diagnostic evaluation of, 458–459
    differential diagnosis of, 456, 457–458
    drug-induced, 434t, 435–437
    etiology of, 453
    evaluation of, 23–25
    future research on, 459
    pathophysiology of, 453–455
    versus tics, 460
    treatment of, 459
Choreiform movements, 436
    demonstration of, 458
    in Huntington disease, 456
Choriocarcinoma, pineal, 633
Choroid, 56
Choroid plexus, 71, 165, 225
    of lateral ventricle, 193
Choroid vein, superior, 225
Choroidal artery
    anterior, 69, 71, 190, 193
    lateral, 71
    medial, 71
    posterior lateral, 193
    posterior medial, 193
Choroidal vein, superior, 226
Chovstek sign, 596
Chromosome 17 gene mutation, 417–418
Chronic inflammatory demyelinating polyneuropathy, 886
    characteristics of, 770t
    Lewis-Sumner variant of, 827
    treatment of, 832–833
Chronic inflammatory demyelinating polyradiculoneuropathy
    differential diagnosis of, 824, 862
    versus Guillain-Barré syndrome, 822
    long-term prognosis for, 826
    treatment of, 825
Chronic multiple tic disorder, 462
Chronic wasting disease, 360
Cidofovir, 588
Ciguatoxin, 823
Cilia, olfactory cell, 98
Ciliary artery, 56, 190
Ciliary body, 56
Ciliary ganglion, 8, 15, 86, 87, 89, 90, 102, 103
    parasympathetic root of, 80, 86, 87, 90
    roots o f, 8
    sensory root of, 15, 80, 86, 87, 90, 102
    sympathetic root of, 80, 86, 87, 90
Ciliary muscle, 80, 86
    paralysis of, 77
Ciliary nerve
    long, 8, 15, 80, 86, 87, 90, 102, 103
    short, 9–10, 15, 80, 86, 87, 90, 102, 103
Ciliary vein, 56
Ciliospinal reflex, 9
Cingulate gyrus, 43
Circadian cycle, 288
Circadian rhythm disorder, 294
Circumferential arteries, long, 241
Circumflex humeral artery
    anterior, 704
    posterior, 704
Cirrhosis
    alcoholic, 391
    nodular, 467
    in Wilson disease, 469
Cisplatin, 835
Clarke column, 33
Claude syndrome, 81
Clavicle, 704
Clinical evaluation
    approach to, 3–4
    neurologic history in, 2–3
Clivus, chordoma of, 630
Clofazimine, 841
Clonazepam (Klonopin)
    for asterixis, 429
    for corticobasal degeneration, 416
    for essential tremor, 426t
    for REM sleep behavior disorder, 292
    for stiff person syndrome, 794
    for tics, 465
Clonidine, 465
Clonus, 32–35
Clopidogrel, 216
Clostridium perfringens, 568
Clostridium tetani, 594, 595, 596
Clozapine
    for bipolar disorder, 371
    for schizophrenia, 374
Cluneal nerve, inferior, 750
Cluster headache, 175–177, 176
    in subarachnoid hemorrhage, 249–252
CN-I fiber synapse, 96
Cobalt, uptake of, 857
Cocaine
    abuse of, 100
    addiction to, 398
    in thrombosis, 199

INDEX

Coccygeal nerves, 494, 497, 711
Coccygeal plexus, 711
Coccyx, 494
Cochlea, 135
Cochlear duct, 127, 135
Cochlear ganglion, 114
Cochlear nerve (VIII), 4, 114, 128, 135
    testing of, 14–19
Cochlear nucleus, 105, 134, 136
    ventral and dorsal, 6
Cognitive assessment, 3–4, 40–52
Cognitive-behavioral therapy, 383
Cognitive disorders
    clinical features of, 322–324
    diagnostic approach to, 325
    epidemiology of, 324
    in schizophrenia, 373
    treatment and counseling for, 325–326
Cognitive impairment
    in Alzheimer disease, 341–342
    in dementia with Lewy bodies, 349
    in frontotemporal dementia, 354
    in Huntington disease, 457
    in parkinsonism, 407, 408
    with transmissible spongiform encephalopathy, 361
    vascular, 356
Cognitive testing, 41
Cognitive therapy, 367
Cogwheeling, 26
Coital headache, 179
Colchicine, toxic, 887
Cold caloric test, 14
Cold stimulus headache, 177
Cold-water calorics, 11–14
Collar immobilization
    cervical, 662
        for cervical spine injury, 666
    for subaxial cervical spine injury, 663
Colliculus
    inferior, 134, 136, 227, 500, 766
    superior, 6, 12, 68, 91, 105, 227, 500–501, 766
Colloid cysts, 632, 633
Color perception, 73
Color vision loss, 54
Coma, 296–300
    with bacterial meningitis, 564–565
    with cerebral herniation, 307
    in cerebral venous thrombosis, 232–233
    in delirium, 323
    differential diagnosis of, 299, 317
    evaluation and treatment of, 300–303
    from metabolic disease, 311
    with pontine hemorrhage, 241
    prognosis of, 302, 303–304
    stages of, 297t
    toxic-metabolic induced, 296
Comatose patient
    evaluation and treatment of, 300–303
    eye movement in, 14
Communicating artery, 65, 83
    aneurysms of, 66, 82
    anterior, 71, 189, 190, 193
    lenticulostriate branches of, 190
    middle, 190–191
    posterior, 71, 78, 90, 189, 190, 193
        aneurysms of, 82

Communication disturbance, 774t
Compensation disorder, 696
Complex regional pain syndrome, 701
Compound muscle action potentials (CMAPs), 119, 858
Compression
    of peripheral nerve, 717
    severe acute, 718
    severe chronic, 718
Compression cervical injury, 660
Compression-induced venous ischemia, 719
Compression neuropathy, 716–719
    in athletes and musicians, 720
    clinical evaluation of, 722
    electrodiagnosis of, 723–724
    sites of, 722
    in workplace, 719
Compressive lumbosacral plexopathies, 712–713
Compulsive behavior, 375
Compulsive tics, 460, 461t
Computed tomography
    advantages and disadvantages of, 215t
    in Alzheimer disease, 343
    for aneurysmal subarachnoid hemorrhage, 248–249
    for brachial plexopathies, 705
    for brain abscess, 568
    for cerebral venous thrombosis, 232
    for cervical radiculopathy, 676
    for chorea, 458–459
    for compression neuropathy, 725
    for diffuse axonal or shear injury, 655
    for epidural hematoma, 650, 651
    in evaluation, 2
    for facial palsies, 124–125
    for herpes simplex encephalitis, 576
    for intracerebral hemorrhage, 243
    for ischemic stroke, 212
    for Lambert-Eaton myasthenic syndrome, 859
    for lumbar radiculopathy, 686
    for lumbar spinal stenosis, 693
    for lumbosacral plexopathies, 709
    for meningiomas, 622–624
    for myasthenia gravis, 868
    for neurosyphilis, 571
    for partial seizures, 268
    for progressive multifocal leukoencephalopathy, 588
    for pseudotumor cerebri, 606
    for spinal cord meningioma, 526
    of spinal cord tumors, 637
    of spinal tumors, 524
    for spine injury, 662
    for subdural hematomas, 650, 651, 654
    for syringomyelia, 528
    for vertebrobasilar occlusive disease, 202–203
    for vertebrobasilar stroke, 140
Computed tomography angiography, 252
    advantages and disadvantages of, 215t
    of circle of Willis, 213
Conduction aphasia, 46
Conduction block, 721
Conduction deafness, 19
Conductive olfactory disorders, 97
Confusion, 296
Confusional migraine, 174
Congenital aneurysm rupture, 250
Congestive heart failure, 208
Connective tissue disorder, trigeminal involvement of, 108
Connective tissue injury, 26

INDEX

Consciousness
    impaired, 322
    levels of, 296–298
        decreased, 648
        fluctuating, 322
Constipation
    in motor neuron disease, 775t
    treatment of, 847
Constructional dyspraxia, 50
Contractures, muscular, 774t
Conus medullaris, 494, 496, 497, 835
    tumors of, 637
Convergence, 92
Conversion disorder, back pain, 695, 696
Conversion hysteria, 157, 545
Coordination
    evaluation of, 4
    impaired, 21
Copper
    deposition of in tissues, 468
    hepatic metabolism of, 467
    renal excretion of, 468–470
Copper-transporting adenosine triphosphatase, 468
Coprolalia, 461t, 463
Coracobrachialis muscle, 704, 742
Coracoid process, 704
Cord capillary plexuses, 501
Cornea, 56
    hypesthesia of, 84
Corneal reflex, 14
    lost, 319
    unilateral loss of, 108
Coronal venous plexus, 501
Coronary artery aneurysm, 243
Corpectomy, 517
Corpus callosotomy, 284
Corpus callosum, 43, 73
    genu of, 226
    lesion in splenium of, 49
    rostrum of, 225
    splenium of, 225, 228, 227, 226
        clinical manifestations of infarction in, 205
Corpus striatum, 403
    in parkinsonism, 406
Corrugator supercilii muscle, 16, 115
Corti, spiral organ of, 135
Cortical cerebellar atrophy of Holmes, 485t
Cortical dysfunction, nondominant hemisphere higher, 50
Cortical dysplasia, 286
Cortical function, testing of, 44
Cortical magnification, 74–75
Cortical necrosis, diffuse, 319
Cortical neurons
    epileptic firing pattern of, 263
    normal, 332
    normal firing pattern of, 263
Cortical sensory abnormalities, 39
Cortical vein thrombosis, isolated, 229
Corticobasal degeneration, 415t
    clinical presentation of, 414, 416
    diagnosis of, 416
    in frontotemporal dementia, 351, 353
    pathophysiology of, 414
    treatment of, 416
Corticobulbar fibers, 767
Corticobulbar pathway, 500, 766
Corticocortical projection circuits, 337

Corticonuclear pathway, 500, 766
Corticoreticular fibers, 12, 91
Corticorubral pathway, 500, 766
Corticospinal pathway, 500, 766
Corticospinal tract, 493–500, 499, 765
    anterior, 24, 498, 500, 766, 786, 787
    bilateral damage to, 39
    degeneration of, 533
    dysfunction of, 521
    interruption of, 510
    lateral, 24, 498, 500, 766, 786–787
    lesions of, 502, 784
    in thoracic spinal cord, 786–787
Corticosteroid-releasing hormone inhibitors, 368
Corticosteroids
    for acute proximal myopathies, 891
    alternate-day dosing of, 887
    for bacterial meningitis, 564
    for chronic myopathies, 904
    for cluster headache, 175
    for facial palsy, 119
    for increased intracranial pressure, 607
    for lumbosacral plexopathies, 713–714
    for multifocal motor neuropathy, 833
    for myasthenia gravis, 865, 868
    for spinal injury, 663
    for stiff person syndrome, 798
    for temporal arteritis, 181
    for Tolosa-Hunt syndrome, 83
    for tuberculous meningitis, 585
Corti's basilar membrane, 134
Costocervical trunk, 189
Counseling
    for Alzheimer disease, 346
    for dysthymia, 383
CPAP, 289–291
Cramps, in motor neuron disease, 775t
Cranial fossa, posterior, veins of, 227
Cranial motor nerve nuclei, 26
Cranial nerve III palsy, 77
Cranial nerve palsy, 867
Cranial nerve VI palsy, 11
Cranial nerves, 4
    disorders of, 4
    distribution of motor and sensory fibers of, 5
    evaluation of, 4
    in lateral dissection, 6
    testing of, 4–17, 803
    viewed from behind, 6
Cranial neuralgia, 182–185
Cranial neuropathy, 4
    with bacterial meningitis, 564
    primary sites of motor disorder in, 26
    systemic disease and, 19–21
Craniectomy, posterior fossa, 657
Craniocervical traction, 662
Craniopharyngioma, 628, 629
Craniotomy
    for cerebral aneurysms, 258
    for cerebral contusions, 655
    for subdural hematomas, 654
Creatine, 775
Creatine kinase, 780
    in acid maltase deficiency, 901
    in channelopathies, 912
    in chronic proximal myopathies, 892
    in distal predominant myopathies, 908

INDEX

in myopathies, 872, 875–876, 884, 887
in myopathies with exercise intolerance, 914, 916, 918
in paraneoplastic necrotizing myopathy, 889–891
Crescendo-decrescendo respiratory pattern, 308–311
Creutzfeldt-Jakob disease
    clinical classification of, 769t
    diagnostic approach to, 363
    EEG in, 274
    epidemiology of, 360–361
    gait disorder in, 483–485
    in parkinsonism, 409
    pathogenesis of, 361–363
    prions in, 588
    variant, 360–363
Cribriform plate, 98, 99
Cricoarytenoid muscles, 153
Cricoid cartilage, 148
Cricopharyngeal muscle paralysis, 20
Cricopharyngeal myotomy, 773
Cricopharyngeal sphincter, 147
Cricopharyngeus muscle, 148, 149
Cricothyroid muscle, 151, 154
Crista, section of, 127
Crural interosseous nerve, 751
Crutchfield tongs, 666
Cryostat sections, muscle, 881
Cryptococcosis, 590–592
Cryptococcus, 590–592
Cryptococcus neoformans, 590–592
    in bacterial meningitis, 564
    in meningitis, 588
CT. See *Computed tomography*
Cubital tunnel, 733
    compression neuropathy at, 722
Cubital tunnel syndrome, 734
Cuneate fasciculus, 498
Cuneate nucleus, 37, 500, 766
    external, 165
Cuneocerebellar tract, 493
Curare, 857
Cushing disease, 626
    endogenous and exogenous, 887
    treatment of, 628
Cushing response, 313–314
Cushing syndrome
    with ACTH secreting tumors, 627
    iatrogenic, 521
    myopathy and, 889
Cutaneous nerves
    of arm, 703, 704
    dorsal, 747
    of forearm, 703, 704, 738
    of head and neck, 183
    lateral dorsal, 750
    of thigh
        lateral, 710, 753, 755
        posterior, 494, 711
Cyanide, 410
Cyanocobalamin deficiency, 502
Cyclophosphamide
    for multiple sclerosis, 552
    for myasthenia gravis, 870
    for systemic necrotizing vasculitis, 833
    for transverse myelitis, 511
Cyclosporine, 552
Cyclosporine A, 869–870
Cystic astrocytoma, 620

Cystic necrosis, 199
Cysticercosis, 588, 589
Cytarabine, 616
Cytochrome C oxidase, 879
Cytomegalovirus
    differential diagnosis of, 831
    in Guillain-Barré syndrome, 819
Cytotoxic drugs, 555

D

D-tubocurarine, 855t
Dacron velour patch, 220
Daily living assessment, 345
Dalteparin, 216
Danaparoid, 216
Dantrolene
    in neuroleptic malignant syndrome, 435
    for primary lateral sclerosis, 785
Dapsone, 841
Dawson fingers, vascular pathways of, 547
Deafness, 19
Decamethonium, 855t
    at neuromuscular junction, 857
Decerebrate rigidity, 31, 32
    with increased intracranial pressure, 308
Decompression
    after spinal injury, 663
    after spine injury, 662
    for spinal stenosis, 682
Decompressive laminectomy, 693
Decorticate posture, 308
Decussation, 24
Deep brain stimulation
    for dystonia, 446
    for movement disorders, 476, 477
Deep brain stimulator, 286
Deep tendon reflexes, 32
Deep venous thrombosis, 217
Defection energy metabolism, 23
Degenerative disorders, 485t. See also *Disc degeneration*
Deglutition
    mechanics of, 148–149
    neuroregulation of, 144–145
Deglutition center, 145
Deiters, ascending tract of, 91
Delayed sleep phase syndrome, 294
Delirium, 296–297, 322–323
    with alcohol withdrawal, 395
    clinical presentation of, 399–400
    versus dementia, 325
    treatment of, 325–326
Delirium tremens, 322–324, 398
Deltoid muscle, 704
Delusions
    affect consonant, 366
    in dementia with Lewy bodies, 349
    in neurosyphilis, 571
    in schizophrenia, 372–373
Dementia
    in Alzheimer disease, 330, 333, 341
    versus delirium, 325
    frontotemporal, 351–355, 357, 417–418
    lacking distinctive histology, 351
    in Lambert-Eaton myasthenic syndrome, 861
    with Lewy bodies, 347
        clinical presentation and differential diagnosis of, 348–350

INDEX

diagnostic approach to, 350
pathogenesis of, 347–348
treatment of, 350
progressive, with transmissible spongiform encephalopathy, 361–363
vascular, 356–359
Demyelinating disorders
differential diagnosis of, 609–610
of striate cortex, 75
in trigeminal neuralgia, 106
Demyelinating neuropathies, 814
multifocal, 830t
treatment of, 725
Demyelinating peripheral nerve lesions, 884
Demyelinating polyneuropathy
cranial nerve testing in, 803
primary, 805t
Demyelinating polyradiculoneuropathy
acquired
clinical presentation of, 818–822
diagnostic approach to, 824–825
differential diagnosis of, 822–824
etiology of, 819
pathogenesis of, 820–821
prognosis of, 825–826
treatment of, 825
differential diagnosis of, 862
Demyelination, 721, 781
in acute disseminated encephalomyelitis, 555–557
diagnosis of, 723
fatigue with, 553–554
in Guillain-Barré syndrome, 820
magnetic resonance imaging of, 550
monofocal acute inflammatory, 544
in multiple sclerosis, 538
with nerve compression, 718
optic radiation, 69
patchy, 539
in progressive multifocal leukoencephalopathy, 587
in upper extremity mononeuropathies, 739
Dendrites, olfactory cell, 98
Denervation, 780–781
Dens fractures, 663
Dental abscess, 594–596
Dental infections
in headache, 186
in spinal epidural abscess, 566
Dental plexus
inferior, 15, 102
superior, 103
Dentate gyrus, 99
Denticulate ligament, 495
Depolarization, 850
in neuromuscular junction, 853
Depression. See also *Dysthymia*
agitated, 369
alcoholism and, 394
in bipolar disorder, 369
double, 366, 381
major, 381
clinical presentation of, 366–367
epidemiology of, 366
treatment of, 367–368
in parkinsonism, 407, 408
spreading, 174
Depressor anguli oris muscle, 16, 115
Depressor labii inferioris muscle, 16, 115

Depressor septi nasi muscle, 16, 115
Dermal segmentation, 29
Dermatomes, upper limb, 673
Dermatomyositis
clinical presentation of, 884, 885
diagnosis of, 890
treatment of, 882, 891, 904
Dermoid tumor, intramedullary spinal cord, 642
Desmin, 908
Desmin myopathy, 907t, 908
Desmosomes, 98
Devic syndrome, 541
Dextroamphetamine (Dexedrine)
for fatigue of multiple sclerosis, 554
for tics, 465
Diabetes
auditory nerve disorders in, 134
femoral neuropathies in, 752
hearing loss in, 141
insipidus
pineal tumor with, 419
with pineal tumors, 631
mellitus, in epidural spinal abscess, 508
in nerve injury, 719
neuropathies of, 712, 725, 806
autonomic, 845–846
multifocal, 833
ocular complications of, 79
parameningeal infections in, 566
radiculopathies of, 713
third cranial nerve palsy in, 801
Diabetic amyotrophy, 712
future treatments for, 714
treatment of, 713–714
Diabetic mononeuritis, 829–830
Dialectical behavioral therapy, 384–386
3,4-Diaminopyridine, 862
Diaphragm, 710
Diaphragma sellae, 228
Diazepam (Valium), 426t
Dichlorphenamide, 913
Dieters, ascending tract of, 12
in nystagmus, 13
Diffuse axonal injury, 655–657
Diffuse Lewy body disease, 347–350
Diffuse plaques, 329
Digastric muscle, 16, 104, 115, 160
anterior, 106
nerve to, 122
Digestive enzymes, 146
Digit Span Backward test, 48
Digital arteries, palmar, 727
Digital compression test, 722, 729
Digital nerves, 728
compression at, 720
dorsal, 747
palmar, 727
to thumb, 727
Dihydropyridine receptors, 850
Diphtheria, neuropathology in, 823
Diplegia, 440
Diplopia
horizontal, 604
treatment of, 88
Dipyridamole, 216
Disability rating scale, 657
Disc degeneration, 689

INDEX

in cervical spondylosis, 514
Disc disease, 637t
Disc herniation
    in cervical spine injury, 525, 662
    clinical manifestations of, 675
    diagnosis of, 676
    interspinal, 30
Disc rupture, 662
Discectomy
    for lumbar radiculopathy, 688
    for spondylosis, 517
Discogenic nerve root compression, 689
Discogenic pain, 684
Disinhibited patients, 352
Distal spinal muscular atrophy, 908
Disulfiram, 398
Diuretics, 312–313, 607
Divalproex sodium, 277
Diving accident, 660
Dix-Hallpike test, 131
Dizziness, 126
DNA mutational analysis
    for amyotrophic lateral sclerosis, 771
    for channelopathies, 912
    for hereditary tendency to pressure palsies, 832
    for length-dependent polyneuropathy, 816
    for myopathies, 879
    for Wilson disease, 468, 470
Doll's eyes maneuver, 11–14, 319
    for increase intracranial pressure, 308
Doll's eyes phenomenon, 309
Donepezil
    for Alzheimer disease, 343
    for dementia with Lewy bodies, 350
Dopa, 406
Dopa-responsive dystonia, 443t
Dopamine. See also *Levodopa*
    brain receptors for, 412
    for dystonia, 445–446
    loss of in Parkinson disease, 405
    in parkinsonism, 406
    release of, with drug abuse, 398
    synthesis abnormalities of, 441
    transporters of, 412–413
Dopamine agonists
    advantages and disadvantages of, 412t
    in neuroleptic malignant syndrome, 435
    for Parkinson disease, 411
    for tardive dyskinesia, 436–437
Dopamine antagonists, 459
Dopamine D2-receptor antagonists, 441
Dopamine-depleting agents, 436–437
Dopamine DR-2 receptor allele, 390
Dopamine-producing cells, 413
Dopamine receptor-blockers, 409, 459
    excitotoxic mechanism of, 435–436
    inducing movement disorders, 432–437
    in secondary dystonia, 443
Dopaminergic agents, 411
Doppler ultrasonography, 256
Dorello canal, 89
Dorsal horn, 766
Dorsal ramus, 496, 703, 835
Dorsal root ganglion, 145, 835
    disorders of, 834–835
    sensory neuronopathy pattern of, 838t
Dorsal spinal roots, 495, 496

filaments of, 495
sensory, 493
Down syndrome, 339
Dressing apraxia, 49
Drug abuse/dependence, 398
    withdrawal signs and symptoms in, 396–397
Drug intoxication
    trigeminal involvement of, 108t
    wide-based gait of, 22–23
Duane syndrome, 82–83
Duchenne-Erbe palsy, 700
Duchenne muscular dystrophy
    clinical presentation of, 900
    diagnosis of, 900, 902–903
    prognosis for, 905
    treatment of, 882, 904
Dumbbell tumor, 638
Dura mater, 116, 493, 835
    layers of, 228
    spinal, 494, 495, 496
    venous sinuses of, 224
Dural abscess, 230
Dural arteriovenous malformation, 517, 518, 519–520
    differential diagnosis of, 822
Dural sac, termination of, 494
Dural sinus, 171
Duret hemorrhage, 247
Dynamic Gait Index, 132
Dynamic posturography, 132
Dynamometer, 773
Dysarthria, 163
    thalamic lesions in, 477
Dysarthria-clumsy hand, 211t
Dysautonomia
    focal, 721
    in Guillain-Barré syndrome, 822
    in hereditary autonomic neuropathies, 846
    with polyneuropathies, 845
    in primary autonomic polyneuropathies, 843
Dysdiadochokinesia, 21, 30
Dysembryoplastic neuroectodermal tumor, 286
Dysequilibrium
    in multiple sclerosis, 541–542
    nonpharmacologic therapy for, 132–133
Dysesthesia
    of lateral thigh, 758
    painful, 23
Dysferlin stain, 908
Dysgeusia, 163
Dyskinesia
    drugs causing, 434t
    evaluation of, 23–25
    tardive, 435–437, 457–458
Dysosmia, 7
Dysphagia, 19, 143
    clinical presentation of, 147
    cricopharyngeal myotomy for, 773
    in motor neuron disease, 775t
    in parkinsonism, 407, 408
    treatment of, 152
    with vertebrobasilar ischemia, 206
Dyspnea, 792
Dysphonia, 19, 156
    with vertebrobasilar ischemia, 206
Dysphoric mania, 369
Dyspraxia, constructional, 50
Dysproteinemia, 815

INDEX

Dysthymia
    clinical presentation of, 381, 382
    diagnosis of, 381
    treatment of, 381–383
Dysthymic state, 366
Dystonia
    classification of, 438t
    clinical presentation of, 438, 441–443
    deep brain stimulation for, 477
    diagnostic approach to, 445
    differential diagnosis of, 443–445
    drug-induced, 432, 434t
    focal, 438–441, 442
    generalized, 440, 441–442
    genetic primary, 441–443
        classification of, 442t
    heredodegenerative, 445
    kinesigenic, 443
    multifocal, 440–441
    paroxysmal, 443
    pathophysiology of, 441
    psychogenic, 443–445, 472–473
    restricted or fragmentary, 440
    secondary, 443
    segmental, 440
    sporadic primary, 441
    treatment of, 445–446
    types of, 438–441
    with Wilson disease, 466–467
Dystonia musculorum deformans. See *DYT1 dystonia*
Dystonia-plus disorders, 442–443
Dystonic postures, 436, 438
Dystonic reactions, 441
Dystonic spasms, 438
Dystonic tics, 460
Dystrophinopathy, 896t
    treatment of, 905
DYT7 adult-onset focal dystonia, 442
DYT5 dopa-responsive dystonia, 442–443
DYT1 dystonia, 441–442
    treatment of, 446
DYT1 gene, testing of, 445
DYT genetic defects, 441–443

E

E vitamin, 437
Ears
    anatomy of, 114
    hemorrhage of, 647
    middle, 8
Echocardiography
    for ischemic stroke, 212
    for syncope, 279
Echolalia, 45, 461t
    in Tourette syndrome, 463
Edinger-Westphal nucleus. See *Accessory oculomotor nucleus*
Edrophonium chloride, 855t
    for myasthenia gravis, 866
    at neuromuscular junction, 857
Edrophonium chloride (Tensilon) test, 864, 866, 867
EEG. See *Electroencephalography*
Efferent pathways, 500, 766
Ehlers-Danlos syndrome, 26
Elastic stockings, 846–847
Elbow
    compression at, 720
    extension of, 733
    flexion of, 733
    flexion testing of, 734
    ulnar neuropathies at, 739
Electrocardiography, 279
Electroconvulsive therapy
    for bipolar disorder, 371
    for major depression, 367–368
Electrodiagnosis
    for compression neuropathy, 724
    for length-dependent polyneuropathy, 816
    for mononeuropathies, 723
        with lower extremity weakness, 754
        of shoulder, 744–745
        of upper extremity, 738
Electroencephalography
    in absence seizures, 271–272
    for acute disseminated encephalomyelitis, 555
    in Alzheimer disease, 343
    in brain death, 318
    for coma, 303
    in delirium, 323
    for dementia with Lewy bodies, 350
    for demyelinating disorders, 610
    for epilepsy, 281
    ictal, 271
    in infantile spasms, 274–275
    for myoclonus, 451–452
    in normal versus epileptic person, 269
    for partial seizures, 268
    spikes in, 274
    in status epilepticus, 276
    in syncope, 278–279
    in tonic-clonic seizures, 271, 272
Electrolytes
    abnormalities of with subarachnoid hemorrhage, 257
    disorders of, 823–824
Electromyography
    for acquired demyelinating polyradiculoneuropathies, 824–825
    for atrophied tongue, 167
    for brachial plexopathies, 700, 705
    for carpal tunnel syndrome, 730
    for channelopathies, 912
    for compression neuropathy, 724
    for demyelination, 723
    for distal ulnar mononeuropathies, 732–736
    in Guillain-Barré syndrome, 821
    for Lambert-Eaton myasthenic syndrome, 859, 860
    for length-dependent polyneuropathy, 816
    for lumbosacral plexopathies, 709
    for mononeuropathies with lower extremity weakness, 754
    for motor neuron disease, 771–772
        with lower motor neuron features, 780–781
    for multifocal neuropathies, 831–832
    for myasthenia gravis, 866, 868
    for myoclonus, 451–452
    for myopathies, 876–877, 884
    for myopathies with exercise intolerance, 918
    normal versus polymyositis, 890
    for polyneuropathy, 804–805
    for primary lateral sclerosis, 783, 785
    for proximal median neuropathies, 732
    for sensory neuropathies of lower extremity, 760
    for sensory neuropathy and neuronopathy, 836
    for shoulder mononeuropathies, 744

INDEX

showing myelin loss, 721
spontaneous myotonic discharge in, 899
for stiff person syndrome, 797
for syringomyelia, 528
for upper extremity mononeuropathies, 738
Embolism
   intra-arterial, 195–199
   of lesser degree without infarction, 451
   pathology of, 196
   platelets in, 197
Embryonal carcinoma, pineal, 633
Embryonic limb organization, 703
Emery-Dreifuss muscular dystrophy, 896t, 900
EMG. See *Electromyography*
Encephalitis
   abscess in, 270
   clinical presentation and differential diagnosis of, 574–576
   diagnosis and treatment of, 576
   herpes, 608
   herpes simplex, 574–576
   herpes zoster, 609
   in immunocompromised hosts, 586–588
   rabies in, 576–578
   West Nile virus in, 578–579
Encephalitis lethargica, 409
Encephalomyelitis, postvaccinal, 510
Encephalopathy, 324
   transmissible spongiform, 360–363
End plate depolarization, 854
End plate potentials, 853
   miniature, 850
   production of, 850, 851
Endarterectomy, 218–222
Endocarditis
   infective, 209
   in intracerebral hemorrhage, 244–246
   septic emboli of, 234
   staphylococcal, 562
   subacute bacterial, 208
Endocrine myopathy, 887–889
   treatment of, 891
Endocrinopathy, 893
Endodermal sinus tumors, pineal, 633
Endoplasmic reticulum, 98
Endoscopic evaluation, swallowing, 147
Endovascular techniques, 217
Endovascular therapy, 258–261
Energy metabolism disorders, 901–904
Entacapone, 412
Enterobacteria, 568
Entorhinal cortex, 96, 99
   Alzheimer disease changes in, 336
Entrapment mononeuropathy, femoral cutaneous nerve, 757, 758
Entrapment neuropathy, 716–719
   fractures causing, 719
Eosinophilic myositis, 889
Ependymoma, 612, 616, 638
   diagnosis of, 522
   of fourth ventricle, 632
   intramedullary spinal cord, 642
   in lumbar radiculopathy, 686
   pontine, 791
   spinal cord, 635
Ephaptic transmission, 124
Epicranial aponeurosis, 184

Epidermoid
   spinal cord, 642
   trigeminal, 109–110
Epidural abscess, 506–508
   pathology, etiology and diagnosis of, 505
Epidural hematoma
   burr hole exposing, 656
   clinical presentation and diagnosis of, 646–650
   CT scan of, 651
   posterior fossa, 649, 657
   with skull fracture, 646
   subfrontal, 649
   temporal fossa, 649
   treatment and prognosis of, 650
Epidural infections, 686
Epidural lipomatosis
   clinical presentation of, 520–521
   diagnosis and treatment of, 521
   pathophysiology and etiology of, 521
Epidural space, fat in, 496, 835
Epidural venous plexus, 501
Epiglottis, 148, 149
Epilepsia partialis continua, 268
Epilepsy, 264. See also *Seizures*
   complex partial seizures in, 268–271
   ECG in, 269
   generalized seizures in, 271–274
   partial seizures in, 264–268
   preoperative assessment of, 281–284
   status epilepticus, 265–276
   surgical treatment for, 281–286
   syndromes of, 274–275
   therapy for, 277–278
Epineurium
   normal, 718
   of peripheral nerve, 717
   thickened, 718
Epiphora, 117
Episcleral artery, 56
Episcleral vein, 56
Epitympanic recess, 114, 135
Equilibrium, evaluation of, 4
Erb palsy, 702
Erectile dysfunction
   in autonomic nervous system disorders, 843
   treatment of, 847
Erythema nodosum leprosum, 841
Erythematous vesicular eruption, 580
Escherichia coli meningitis, 560
Esophagogastrostomy, percutaneous, 152
Esophagus, 147, 151
   stripping wave in, 149
Esterase, soluble nonspecific, 851
Ethambutol, 585
Ethmoid bone, cribriform plate of, 98, 99
Ethmoidal nerve, 107, 183
   anterior, 15, 80, 87, 90, 102, 103
   posterior, 15, 80, 86, 87, 90, 102, 103
Ethosuximide, 277
Evoked potentials, 548–550
Excitatory glutamate pathway, 453–455
Exercise-induced headache, 252
Exercise intolerance, myopathies presenting with, 872, 874t, 914–921
Extensor carpi radialis brevis muscle, 736–737
Extensor digitorum brevis muscle, 747
Extensor digitorum longus muscle, 747

INDEX

Extensor hallucis brevis muscle, 747
Extensor hallucis longus muscle, 747
Extensor response, 31
Extensor retinaculum muscle, inferior, 747
External beam radiation, 618
Extracranial occlusive disease, 198
Extraocular muscle palsy, 79
Extraocular muscle function, 11
Extrapyramidal system, 405
Eye movements
 central control of, 91
 control of, 12
 with increased intracranial pressure, 308, 309
Eyes
 autonomic innervation of, 8
 convergence of, 9
 optic chiasm and, 65
 trauma to, 647
 visual receptors of, 55

F

Facet disease, referred pain due to, 683
Facetectomy, 677
Facial anhidrosis, 701
Facial artery, 160, 189
Facial canal, 114
 lesions in, 118
Facial expression, 4
Facial muscles, 115
 innervation of, 16
Facial myokymia, 124
Facial nerve (VII), 4, 6, 102, 104, 135, 150, 224
 anatomy of, 112–113
 branches of, 15, 122
 cervicofacial division of, 122
 clinical correlations and entities of, 113–124
 course and distribution of, 118
 distribution of, 5
 fibers of, 16, 114
 geniculate ganglion of, 6, 16, 150
 geniculum of, 105, 114
 hyperactivity of, 124
 lesions of, 112
  diagnostic modalities for, 124–125
 main trunk of, 122
 mastoid segment of, 113
 motor nucleus of, 16, 115
 motor root of, 114
 motor trunk of, 113
 peripheral lesions of, 112
 schema of, 115–114
 temporofacial division of, 122
 testing of, 14
 topognostic testing of, 125
 in trigeminal nerve territories, 15
 tympanic segment of, 112–113
Facial neuroma, 138
 imaging studies for, 124–125
Facial nucleus, 6, 105, 500, 766
Facial numbness, 108
 unilateral, 113
Facial pain, 108
 abscessed tooth in, 186
 cranial nerve injury in, 4
Facial palsy, 113
 idiopathic
  clinical presentation of, 117
  differential diagnosis of, 117–119
  pathogenesis of, 117
  treatment and prognosis of, 119
 infectious, 119–120
 neuromuscular disorders with, 121–123
 recurrent, 123–124
 traumatic, 120–121
Facial paralysis, 26
Facial sensation
 cranial nerves in, 4
 trigeminal nerve in, 101
Facial vein, 160, 227
Facial weakness
 cranial nerve injury in, 4
 with facial nerve lesions, 112
 in Guillain-Barré syndrome, 819
Facioscapulohumeral muscular dystrophy, 123, 900
 differential diagnosis of, 780
Factitious disorder, 696
Factor V Leiden, 199
False localizing sign, 93
Falx, meningioma of, 623
Falx cerebri, 224, 227
Fascicles, peripheral nerve, 717
Fascicular injury, selective, 723
Fasciculations
 in amyotrophic lateral sclerosis, 770–771
 benign, 780
 in muscle weakness, 30
 in myasthenia gravis, 791
 tong atrophy with, 789–790
Fasciculus
 dorsolateral, 498, 499, 786, 787
 medial longitudinal, 11, 12, 91, 786, 787
  disruption of, 308
Fasciculus cuneatus, 37, 499, 786
Fasciculus gracilis, 37, 499, 786, 787
Fasciculus lenticularis, 403
Fasciculus thalamicus, 403
Fascioscapulohumeral muscular dystrophy, 895, 896t
Fat
 epidural accumulation of, 520–521
 formation and breakdown of, 917
Fatigue
 chronic, in dysthymia, 381, 382
 in Lambert-Eaton myasthenic syndrome, 859, 860, 862
 in multiple sclerosis, 553–554
 in myasthenia gravis, 865
 in myopathies, 872
Fatty acids, 918
Femoral nerve, 494, 709, 710, 752, 753, 755
 anterior cutaneous, 753
 knee buckling with injury to, 23
 lateral cutaneous
  anatomy of, 757
  sensory neuropathy of, 757–758
 posterior cutaneous, 750
Femoral neuropathy, 752–754
Femoral radiculopathy, diabetic, 713
Fetor hepaticus, 323
Fibrillary astrocytoma, 618
Fibrinoid necrosis, 199
Fibromuscular dysplasia, 199
Fibular nerves, 747
Fibularis brevis muscle, 747
Fibularis longus muscle, 747

NEUROLOGY

941

INDEX

Filum terminale tumor, 638
Finger-to-nose test, 21
    for chorea, 455
    for multiple sclerosis, 543
Fisher "one-and-a-half" syndrome, 92
Flaccid paralysis
    with complete transverse cord lesion, 501
    in paralytic polio, 598
Flaccid paraplegia, 510
Flaccidity, 30, 32
Flat affect, in schizophrenia, 373
Flexion-rotation spine injury, 659
Flexion spine injury, 659
Flexor aponeurosis, common, 733
Flexor carpi ulnaris aponeurosis, 733
Flexor digiti minimi brevis muscle, 751, 761
Flexor digitorum brevis muscle, 751, 761
Flexor digitorum brevis nerve, 761
Flexor digitorum longus muscle, 751
Flexor digitorum profundus muscle, 733
Flexor digitorum superficialis arch, compression at, 720, 722
Flexor digitorum superficialis muscle, 733
Flexor hallucis brevis muscle, 761
Flexor hallucis brevis nerve, 761
Flexor hallucis longus muscle, 751
Flexor pollicis brevis muscle, 727, 728
Flexor retinaculum, 751, 761
Flexor sheath, common, 727
Flexor tendons
    in carpal tunnel, 728
    of hand, 727
Flexor tenosynovitis, 760
Floor walking tests, 132
Floppy infant, 898
Fluconazole, 592
Flucytosine, 592
Fludrocortisone
    for multiple system atrophy, 420
    for orthostatic hypotension, 847
    for syncope, 280
Fluent aphasia, 239–240
Flumazenil, 300
Fluorine-18 deoxyglucose scanning, 282–284
Fluoxetine
    for narcolepsy, 291
    for progressive supranuclear palsy, 417
Focal encephalitis, 268
Focal resection, 284, 285
Focal slowing, EMG, 721
Focal weakness, 25
Folic acid, 359
Foot
    hygiene of in sensory neuropathy and neuronopathy, 838
    innervation of, 761
    sole of, cutaneous innervation of, 751, 761
Foot drop, 23, 25
    bilateral, 778
    lightweight orthosis for, 773
    management of, 754
    with motor neuron disease, 774t, 778
    in peripheral neuropathy, 801
    unilateral, 749
Foramen magnum, 158, 159
Foramen ovale, 103
Foramen ovale plexus, 81

Foramen rotundum, 103
Foramen spinosum, 104
    packing of, 656
Foraminal neurolemmoma, 638
Foraminotomy, 693
Forearm, unusual sensory neuropathies of, 738
Forearm ischemic exercise test, 920
    for myopathies, 877–879
Forebrain, functional regions of, 46
Fornix, columns of, 225
Fortification phenomena, 173, 174
Fortification spectra, 249
Forward flexion gait, 23
Fosphenytoin, 275
Foster-Kennedy syndrome, 100
Foville syndrome, 92
Fractures, skull, 646
Frataxin, 534
Free radical toxicity, 768
Friedreich ataxia, 488
    clinical presentation of, 532–533, 534–535
    diagnosis of, 535
    pathophysiology and etiology of, 534
    prognosis of, 535
    treatment of, 489, 535
Frohse, fibrous arcade of, 736–737
Frontal eye fields, 12, 91
    efferent pathways from, 766
    voluntary, 19
Frontal gyrus, 42
Frontal hematoma, 245
Frontal intracranial hemorrhage, 239
Frontal lobe, 73
    arterial supply to, 190–191
    connections of, 47
    dysfunction of, 45–47
        evaluation for, 4–7
    efferent pathways from, 500
    lesions of, 45
    lesions of in gait disorders, 481–483
    meningioma of, 481
    surface of, 42
    testing of, 47
    tumors of, 784
Frontal lobe syndrome, 357
Frontal nerve, 15, 80, 86, 87, 90, 102, 103, 107
Frontal opercula, 42
Frontal temporal atrophy, 41
Frontobasal artery
    lateral, 193
    median, 193
Frontocingulate pathway, 43
Frontoparietal opercula, 42
Frontopolar artery, 193
Frontopontine tract, 24
Frontopontocerebellar tracts, disruption of, 481
Frontotemporal atrophy, 40
Frontotemporal dementia, 357
    clinical presentation of, 351, 352–354
    diagnostic approach to, 354
    pathogenesis of, 351–352
    treatment of, 354–355
Frontotemporal dementia parkinsonism-chromosome 17 (FTPD-17), 415t, 416
    clinical presentation of, 417–418
    diagnosis and treatment of, 418
    pathophysiology of, 417

INDEX

Frontotemporal lobar degeneration, 354
Frontothalamic tract, 24
Functional back pain, 694
    diagnosis and treatment of, 694–696
    history of, 694–696
Functional hemispherectomy, 284
Funduscopy, 60
Furosemide, 313
Fusion
    of cervical spinous processes, 667
    for subaxial cervical spine injury, 663

G

γ motor neurons, 34
γ plate endings, 34
GABA inhibitory pathway, 455
GABA mimetics, 436–437
Gabapentin (Neurontin)
    for epilepsy, 277–278
    for essential tremor, 426t
    for herpes zoster virus, 581–582
    for lateral femoral nerve neuropathy, 759
    for pain of multiple sclerosis, 554
    for peripheral neuropathies, 807
    for sensory neuropathies of lower extremity, 760
    for trigeminal neuralgia, 106
GAD65 antibody production, 795
Gadolinium-enhanced magnetic resonance imaging, 138
Gag reflex, absence of, 146
Gait
    assessment of, 21–23
    CNS control of, 480
    disturbances in
        with dementia, 357–358
        in Guillain-Barré syndrome, 819
        in multiple sclerosis, 542
        in parkinsonism, 405, 407, 408
        in spondylosis, 515, 516
    evaluation of, 4
    in peripheral nerve disease, 803
    wide-based, 22
Gait ataxia, 480
Gait disorders, 21, 22–23
    cerebellar, 483–488
    clinical presentation of, 480
    evaluation of, 488
    frontal, 481–483
    Parkinson, 483, 484
    in parkinsonism, 484
    spinal cord, 488
    treatment of, 488–489
Galantamine
    for Alzheimer disease, 343
    for dementia with Lewy bodies, 350
Galen, great cerebral vein of, 194, 224, 225, 228, 227, 226
Gambling addiction, 375
Gangliocytoma, trigeminal, 109–110
Ganglionopathy, 108
Ganzfeld electroretinography, 62
Gardner-Wells tongs, 666
Gasserian ganglion, 89
Gastrocnemius muscle, 751
Gastrointestinal dysfunction, 847
Gastroparesis, 847
Gaze-dependent nystagmus, 126
Gaze deviation, 112
Gaze palsy, ipsilateral, 92

Gene therapy, 621
Gene transfer, 905
Genetic counseling, 833
    for distal myopathies, 908
    for myopathies, 882
Genetic linkage studies, 462–464
Genetic markers
    of optic nerve disorders, 62
    of Wilson disease, 467–468
Genetic screening
    for dystonia, 445
    for hereditary spastic paraplegia, 529
Geniculate body
    lateral, 6, 9, 38, 68, 70, 71, 105, 193, 225, 227
    medial, 38, 71, 136, 193, 225, 227
Geniculate ganglion, 105, 112, 115
    lesions in, 118
Geniculate nucleus
    dorsal lateral, 9
    lateral, 67–69
    projections on, 70
Geniculum, 104
Genioglossus muscles, 148, 164
Geniohyoid muscle, 164
Genitofemoral nerve, 710, 755
Genitofemoral neuropathy, 759–760
Gennari stripe, 72
Gentamicin, 592–593
Geode crystals, 54
Germ cell tumors, 633
Gerstmann-Sträussler-Scheinker syndrome, 360
    gait disorders in, 486–488
Gerstmann syndrome, 49
Giant cell arteritis, 59–62, 180
    headache in, 179–181
    ocular manifestations of, 61
Giant cell granuloma, 62
Giant congenital aneurysms, 254
Glasgow Coma Scale, 297, 298, 644
    in severe head injury, 302
    for traumatic brain injury, 657
Glatiramer acetate, 551
Glaucoma, 57, 59
    neovascular, 79
    optic disc and visual field changes in, 60
    treatment of, 62
Glial cells, 72
Glial cytoplasmic inclusions, 414
Glial tumors, 633
    supratentorial, 618
Glioblastoma, 611, 613t
    frontal lobe, 607
Glioblastoma multiforme, 611, 612, 614–615
    fulminating, 609
    treatment and prognosis of, 615
Glioma, 611
    anaplastic, 611, 613t, 614
    in children, 621
    of corpus callosum, 612
    future treatments for, 620–621
    in gait disorders, 481
    grades of, 613t
    low-grade, 286, 611–613
        treatment and prognosis of, 613–614
    mimicking multiple sclerosis, 544
    mixed, 613
    optic, 640

INDEX

of pineal region, 633
pontine, 620
spinal cord, 635
Gliosis
   with Friedreich ataxia, 534
   surrounded by syrinx, 527
Global aphasia, 46
Global Polio Eradication Program, 597
Globus pallidus, 500, 766
   parkinsonism toxins in, 410
   stimulation of, 446
      for movement disorders, 476, 477
Glomerulus, 99
Glomus jugular tumor, 167
Glossitis, 533
Glossodynia, 167
Glossopharyngeal nerve (IX), 4, 6, 16, 102, 105, 115, 151, 154, 224, 844
   disorders of, 147–152
      treatment of, 152
   distribution of, 5
   dorsal motor nucleus of, 500, 766
   function of, 143
   lesser petrosal nerve from, 15
   physiology of, 143–147
   schema of, 150
   in swallowing, 144
   testing of, 19
Glossopharyngeal neuralgia, 185
Glove-and-stocking hyperesthesia, 36, 801
Glucocorticoids, 530
Glucose
   in muscle cells, 914, 917
   in muscle contraction, 918
Glutamate excitotoxicity, 768
Gluteal artery
   inferior, 711
   superior, 711
Gluteal nerve, 494
   inferior, 711
   superior, 711
Glycogen
   formation and breakdown of, 917
   in muscle contraction, 918
Glycogen metabolism disorders, 920
Glycogen storage myopathy, 897t
   biochemical analysis for, 920t
Glycogenosis
   etiology of, 914
   treatment of, 921
   types of, 916t
GM1 antibodies
   in multifocal neuropathies, 831, 832
   in polyneuropathies, 806
Goldmann perimeter, 7
Golgi tendon organs, fibers from, 34
Gomori trichrome stain, 920
Gonioscopy, 79
Goodpasture syndrome, 470
Gottron sign, 886
Gouda frame, 612
Gowers maneuver, 903
Gracile fasciculus, 498
Gracile nucleus, 6, 37, 500, 766
Gracilis muscle, 755
Gradenigo syndrome, 92–93, 231
Graefe sign, 82

Gram-negative organisms, 686
Gram stain, 562–564
Grand mal seizures, 271–272
Grandmother cell, 75
Granule cell, 99
Granulomatous infections
   chronic, 4
   in cranial nerves, 4
   in facial paralysis, 120
Granulomatous multifocal neuropathies, 830t
Granulomatous myopathy, 882
Granulomatous skin disease, 839–842
Graphesthesia, 39
Graves orbitopathy, 82
Gray matter
   lateral horn of, 496, 498
   spinal, 495, 498
Gray ramus communicans, 8, 495, 496, 710, 711, 835, 844
"Green poultice" syndrome, 694–695, 696
Grip strength, 722
Growth factors, 775
Growth hormone-secreting tumors, 627
   treatment of, 628
GTP cyclohydrolase defect, 443
Guanfacine, 465
Guglielmi detachable coils, 258, 261
Guillain-Barré syndrome, 296, 884, 886
   areflexia in, 32
   clinical presentation of, 818–822
   diagnostic approach to, 824–825
   differential diagnosis of, 822–824, 843–845
   etiology of, 819
   with facial palsy, 117, 121
   Miller Fisher variant of, 867
   mortality in, 843
   pathogenesis of, 820–821
   peripheral neuropathy with, 545
   polyradiculoneuropathy pattern in, 814
   prognosis of, 825–826
   stages of, 820
   treatment of, 825
Gumma, neurosyphilitic, 571, 572
Guyon canal. See *Ulnar tunnel*

H

Habenula, 99
Habilitation devices, 773
Haemophilus influenzae
   in bacterial meningitis, 560–561
   vaccine for, 565
Hair cells, 136
   structure and innervation of, 127
Hallucinations
   with alcohol withdrawal, 395
   in delirium, 322
   in Huntington disease, 455–457
   in parkinsonism, 407, 408
   in schizophrenia, 372–373
   of smell, 100
   visual, 51
Halo traction brace
   for cervical spine injury, 666
   for spinal injury, 662
Halo vest immobilization, 663
Halogenated inhalation, 313
Haloperidol, 429
   for chorea, 459

INDEX

for tics, 465
Halter traction, 666
Hamate, hook of, 727
Hammertoe, 814–816
Hamstring, weakness of, 750
Hand muscle atrophy, 526, 527
Hands
   arteries and nerves of, 727
   impaired fine movement of, 778
   intrinsic muscles of, 733
   sensory distribution in, 722, 728, 733
Hangman's fracture, 663, 668
Hansen disease. See *Leprosy*
Head
   hyperflexion of, 659
   position of in increased intracranial pressure, 313
   trauma to
      in olfactory disorders, 97–99
      in parkinsonism, 410
Head and neck, cutaneous nerves of, 183
Head drop
   in motor neuron disease, 791–792
   treatment and prognosis of, 792
Head injury
   brain abscess with, 609
   closed, 4
      trochlear nerve damage in, 85
   from fall, 659
   general principles of care for, 644
   initial management of, 301, 645
   intensive medical management of, 653
   posterior communicating artery aneurysm and, 82
   prognosis of, 302
   respiratory exchange in, 310
   with vertical blow to head, 660
Head-on collision, 659
Head-up tilt-table test, 279
Headache. See also *Migraine*
   assessment of, 170
   chronic daily, 177
   contiguous structure, 186
   in dysthymia, 381, 382
   in increased intracranial pressure, 606
   low-CSF pressure, 607–608
   primary disorders of, 170–179
   with ruptured aneurysms, 255
   secondary disorders of, 179–186
   in subarachnoid hemorrhage, 249–252
   triggers for, 178
   with vertebrobasilar ischemia, 206
Hearing, 4
   loss of, 134
      conductive, 138
      history of, 137
      progressive, 140
      sensorineural, 138
      unilateral, 140
   normal, 19
   testing of, 138–140
Heart rate, 846
Heavy metal poisoning
   of autonomic nervous system, 845
   in peripheral neuropathy, 813
Heel-to-shin test, 21
Helicotrema, 135
Hemangioblastoma
   intramedullary spinal cord, 642

trigeminal, 109–110
Hemangioma, 636
   seventh nerve, 123
Hematologic disorders
   in hearing loss, 141
   in thrombosis, 199
Hematoma
   of dorsal-medial thalamic area, 239
   frontal, 245
   intracerebellar posterior fossa, 657
   intracerebral
      acute, 651
      headache in, 181
      temporal lobe, 652
   intraparenchymal, 655
   occipital, 239
   parietal, 239
   postauricular, 647
   surgical evacuation of, 247
   temporal, 239–240
Hemianesthesia, 648
Hemianopia
   complete, 70–71
   homonymous, 69, 70–71
Hemianopic visual field loss, 66, 67
Hemianopsia, 64, 205
   bitemporal, 606
   with vertebrobasilar ischemia, 206
Hemicholinium, 855t
   at nerve terminal, 857
Hemichorea, 453
Hemicord lesion, 501
Hemicraniectomy, 314
Hemifacial spasm, 124
Hemiparesis
   gait disorder in, 22
   with head injury, 648
Hemiplegia, 311, 440
   crossed, 92
   with head injury, 648
Hemiplegic migraine, 174
Hemispherectomy, 284, 285
Hemispheric dysfunction, nondominant, 49
Hemizygous vein, 501
Hemodilution, 256
Hemodynamic ischemia, 195
Hemodynamic strokes, 200
Hemorrhage
   intracerebral, 234–247
   intraventricular, 655
Hemorrhagic brain infarct, 235–237
Hemorrhagic tumors, 243, 244t
Heparin
   for cerebral venous thrombosis, 232
   in hemorrhagic brain infarct, 235–237
   for TIAs and stroke, 213–216
Heparinoids, 213, 216
Hepatic encephalopathy, 324
Hepatitis, alcoholic, 391
Hereditary autonomic neuropathy, 846
Hereditary brachial plexus neuropathy, 700–707
   differential diagnosis of, 705
Hereditary hyperekplexia, 797
Hereditary spastic paraparesis
   clinical classification of, 769t
   differential diagnosis of, 785
Herniated nucleus pulposus, 525, 688
   inflammation in, 684

INDEX

lumbar, 680t
Herniation, 307
Herniation syndromes, 654
Heroin-induced brachial plexopathy, 706
Herpes encephalitis, 608
Herpes simplex encephalitis, 574–576, 577
    clinical features of, 575
    routes of transmission of, 575
Herpes simplex virus, 117
Herpes zoster, 579
    in Bell palsy, 117
    clinical manifestations of, 579–581
    in facial pain, 108
    headache and, 185–186
    ophthalmicus, 109
    pathophysiology and diagnosis of, 579
    treatment of, 581–582
Herpes zoster encephalitis, 609
Herpes zoster oticus, 141
Heschl gyrus, 48, 134
Heubner, recurrent artery of, 71, 190, 193
Hexacarbons
    autonomic neurotoxicity of, 845
    neurotoxicity of, 823
High-frequency brain stimulation, 476, 477
Hippocampal commissure, 43
Hippocampal fimbria, 99
Hippocampal gyrus, 96
Hippocampal vein, 226
Hippocampus
    atrophy of, 286
    clinical manifestations of infarction in, 205
    resection of, 284
Hirano bodies, 329
    in Alzheimer disease, 334
Hirayama disease, 706–707, 779
HIV infection
    differential diagnosis of, 784–785, 831
    in length-dependent polyneuropathies, 810–814
    myopathies in, 889
    neuropathology in, 823
HIV-vacuolar myelopathy, 531
HLA-B27 test, 694
HMG-CoA reductase inhibitors, 887
Hoffman sign, 771
Holmes Adie syndrome, 10t
Holmes tremor, 429
Holter monitoring, 279, 280
Homocysteine levels
    in Alzheimer disease, 329, 342–343
    in vascular dementia, 359
Homonymous hemianopsia
    bilateral, 207
    in carotid occlusion, 200
    with cerebral aneurysm, 251
    with occipital hematomas, 239
    in posterior cerebral artery ischemia, 201
Homovanillic acid, 406
Horizontal conjugate gaze circuits, 11
Horizontal gaze paresis, 241
Horner syndrome, 10–11, 88, 701
    with carotid artery dissection, 163
    differential diagnosis of, 705–706
    ipsilateral, 92
    treatment of, 707
House accessibility, 775t
HTLV-1 antibodies, 530

HTLV-1 infection
    differential diagnosis of, 784–785
    gait disturbances in, 488
    treatment of, 489
HTLV-1 myelopathy
    clinical presentation of, 529, 530
    diagnosis of, 530
    pathophysiology and etiology of, 529–530
    treatment and prognosis of, 530–531
Humeral head, 733
Hunt-Hess grading scale, 252t
Huntington disease
    clinical presentation of, 455–457
    dystonia in, 445
    neurodegenerative changes in, 455
    treatment of, 459
Hutchinson syndrome, 10t
Hydrocephalus
    in bacterial meningitis, 563
    frontal lobe syndrome with, 357
    with infratentorial hemorrhage, 240
    in intracerebral hemorrhage, 246
    normal pressure, 481, 482
        apraxic gait of, 22
        FLAIR images in, 483
        treatment of, 489
    pineal tumor with, 419
    with subarachnoid hemorrhage, 256
5-Hydroxy-tryptophan
    for myoclonus, 452
Hydroxychloroquine, 54
Hyoid bone, 149, 155
Hyperactivity, 387, 388
Hyperacusis, 113, 118
Hypercapnia, chronic, 318
Hypercoagulable screen, 209
    for ischemic stroke, 212–213
Hypercortisolism, 521
Hyperexcitability, 854t
Hyperextended posture, 797
Hyperextension cervical injury, 661
Hyperkalemia, 824
    myopathy in, 888
Hyperkalemic periodic paralysis, 909, 911
    characteristics of, 910t
    diagnosis of, 912
    treatment of, 912–913
Hypernephromas, 243
Hypersensitivity vasculitis, 830t
Hypersomnolence, idiopathic, 291
Hypertension. See also *Intracranial hypertension*
    hearing loss in, 141
    in intracerebral hemorrhage, 241t, 243
    with polyarteritis nodosa, 828
    with subarachnoid hemorrhage, 257
Hyperthyroidism, 889
Hyperventilation
    central neurogenic, 311
    for increased intracranial pressure, 312
    in panic disorder, 378
    for syncope, 280
Hypervigilance, 322
Hypervitaminosis A, 604, 605
Hyphema, 79
Hypnic headache, 177
Hypocalcemic tetany, 596
Hypochondriasis, 696

INDEX

Hypoglossal muscle, 164
Hypoglossal nerve (XII), 4, 104, 160, 224
    anatomy of, 163–164
    disorders of
        clinical presentation of, 163–167
        diagnostic approach of, 167
        differential diagnosis of, 167
    distribution of, 5
    lesions of, 166
    paralysis of, 20
    testing of, 19
Hypoglossal nucleus, 6, 105, 164, 500, 766
    damage to, 19
Hypogonadotropic hypogonadism, 97
Hypokalemia, 823–824
    in channelopathies, 909
    in myopathy, 887, 888
Hypokalemic periodic paralysis, 911
    characteristics of, 910t
    treatment of, 912–913
Hypomania, 369
Hypoperfusion, 195
Hypopharynx, 147
Hypophosphatemia, 823–824
Hypophyseal portal system, 64
Hypophysis, 90
Hypopituitarism, 629
Hyposmia, 7
Hypotension, 658
Hypothalamus, 145, 403
Hypothenar muscles, arteries to, 727
Hypothyroidism
    myopathy and, 889
    in parkinsonism, 410
    in rapid mood cycling, 371
Hypotonia, 30
    in cerebellar dysfunction, 21
    primary sites of motor disorder in, 26
Hypotonic cerebellar tone, 30
Hypotonic fluids, 312–313
Hypoxia, 658
Hypoxic brain damage, 319
Hypsarrhythmia, 275
Hysterical gait, 481–483

I

Idebenone, 535
IgG synthesis, 548
IgM monoclonal neuropathy, 814
Iliacus muscle, 710, 711, 753
Iliohypogastric nerve, 494, 710, 755
Iliohypogastric neuropathies, 759
Ilioinguinal nerve, 494, 710, 755
    entrapment of, 759
Iliopsoas muscle weakness, 752
Imaging studies. See also specific techniques
    advantages and disadvantages of, 215t
    in Alzheimer disease, 343
    for attention deficit disorder, 387
    for dementia with Lewy bodies, 350
    in evaluation, 2
    for facial palsies, 124–125
    for visual cortex, 76
Imipramine, 417
Immobilization
    for spinal injury, 662
    for subaxial cervical spine injury, 663

Immune-mediated neuropathies, 810
Immunocompromised hosts
    demyelinating disorders of, 609
    infections in, 586–593
Immunoglobulin
    for acute disseminated encephalomyelitis, 555
    for chronic inflammatory demyelinating
        polyradiculoneuropathy, 825
    for chronic myopathies, 904
    for Lambert-Eaton myasthenic syndrome, 862
    for motor neuron disease, 781–782
    for multiple sclerosis, 553
    for myasthenia gravis, 865, 869
    for stiff person syndrome, 798
Immunohistochemical stains, 908
Immunomodulatory therapy
    for acute proximal myopathies, 891
    for Lambert-Eaton myasthenic syndrome, 862
    mechanisms of, 551
    for multiple sclerosis, 540, 550–551
    for myopathies, 882
    neutralizing antibodies in, 551–552
Immunosuppressive therapy
    in herpes zoster, 579
    for multifocal neuropathies, 832–833
Immunotherapy, 826
Impulse control disorders, 375
Inclusion body myopathy, hereditary, 893
Inclusion body myositis, 780, 892
Incomplete spinal cord syndromes, 523
Incus, 135
    lenticular process of, 114
    ligaments of, 114
    long limb of, 114
Indomethacin, 177
Infancy, benign myoclonus of, 448
Infantile spasms, 274–275
Infarct
    dementia with, 357
    with late petechial hemorrhage, 242
    pathology, etiology and diagnosis of, 505
Infectious disorders
    differential diagnosis of, 831
    in immunocompromised hosts, 586–593
    in length-dependent polyneuropathy, 810–814
    spinal, 784–785
Infectious myopathies, 889
Infiltrative disorders, 831
Inflammatory disease
    in Bell palsy, 117
    in lumbar pain, 684
    spinal, 784–785
Inflammatory myopathy, 861–862
    antibodies in, 879
    diagnosis of, 876
    treatment of, 882
Influenza vaccination, 792
Infraorbital canal, infraorbital nerve entering, 103
Infraorbital nerve, 15, 86, 102, 103, 107, 183
    alveolar branches of, 102
    branches of, 15
Infraspinatus muscle, 742
Infratentorial hemorrhages, 240–241
Infratrochlear nerve, 15, 87, 90, 102, 103, 183
Inguinal ligament, 710
Insomnia, 288
    in depression, 366

INDEX

Insula
　central sulcus of, 42
　circular sulcus of, 42
　gyri of, 42
Intact reflexive eye movement, 296
Interbody fusion, 667
Intercavernous sinus, 224
Intercostal nerves, 494, 496, 703
Intercostobrachial nerve, 704
Interfacet dislocation, 659
Interfascicular fasciculus, 498
Interferon beta-1a
　for multiple sclerosis, 550, 551
　neutralizing antibodies in, 552
Interferon beta-1b, 551, 552
Intermediate cranial nerve, 16, 115
　distribution of, 5
Intermediolateral cell column, 786, 787
Intermedullary tumors, 167
Internal capsule
　anterior limb of, 500, 766, 767
　posterior limb of, 500, 766, 767
　in pyramidal system, 24
Interneurons, 765
Interosseous muscles, 751, 761
Interosseous nerves
　anterior, 730
　posterior, 736, 737
Interspinal ligament tears, 659
Interthalamic adhesion, 226
Interventricular foramen, 225, 226
Intracardiac tumors, 195
Intracavernous carotid aneurysm, 92
　internal, 254
Intracavernous carotid dissection, 92
Intracerebral hemorrhage
　antithrombotic- and anticoagulant-induced, 244
　atypical locations of, 243-244
　causes of, 241t, 242-243
　clinical manifestations of by site, 486
　clinical presentation of, 234, 237-241
　differential diagnosis of, 241-246
　management and prognosis of, 246-247
　pathophysiology of, 234-237
　tumors causing, 243, 244t
Intracranial aneurysm, 252-255
Intracranial hypertension, idiopathic, 62, 181
　clinical presentation of, 604-607
　diagnostic studies of, 604-607
　treatment of, 607
Intracranial lesions, 230
　trigeminal, 108t
Intracranial metastases, 167
Intracranial pressure
　increased
　　in abducens palsy, 93
　　anatomical considerations in, 307
　　brain compromise in, 307-312
　　with diffuse axonal or shear injury, 655
　　eye movements with, 309
　　optic disk and visual fields effects of, 10-11
　　papilledema with, 78, 100
　　with subarachnoid hemorrhage, 256-257
　　with traumatic brain injury, 646
　　treatment of, 312-314
　monitoring of, 653
　　with intraparenchymal hematoma, 655

　triad of, 606
Intracranial surgical dissection, 258
Intraculminate vein, 227
Intrafusal muscle fiber, 34
Intraorbital nerve, 80
Intraparenchymal hemorrhage, 237
Intraparietal sulcus, 42
Intraspinal lesions, primary, 706-707
Intrinsic CN-VII topognostic testing studies, 125
Invasive electrode placement, 282, 283
Iris, 56
　incomplete reinnervation of, 84
Isaac syndrome, 797
Ischemic disease
　clinical manifestations of, 204t
　of visual cortex, 75-76
Ischemic optic neuropathy, anterior, 180
Ischemic stroke. See *Stroke, ischemic*
Ischio-coccygeus muscle, 711
Isoniazid, 585
Isopter, 7

J
Jackson-Pratt drain, 652
JC virus, 586-588
Jefferson fracture
　of atlas, 668
　surgery for, 663
Joint receptors, 34
Jugular foramen, 150, 151, 154, 158, 159, 194, 224
Jugular vein, 228
　cannulation of, 159
　internal, 160, 164, 226
Juvenile myoclonic epilepsy, 274, 448
　treatment of, 452
Juvenile segmental cervical spinal muscular atrophy, 779

K
Kallmann syndrome, 97
Kayser-Fleischer rings, 467, 468, 469
Kennedy disease, 121, 779-780
Keratitis, 109
Keratoacanthoma, 110
Kernig sign
　in bacterial meningitis, 560, 562, 563
　in epidural spinal abscess, 508
Kernohan notch phenomenon, 311
Ketamine, 313
Kidney tumor, 617
Kinetic perimetry, 7
Klebsiella *meningitis*, 561, 562
Knee
　innervation of, 755
　sudden buckling of, 23
Knee locking technique, 754
Kojewnikoff syndrome, 268
Korsakoff psychosis, 324, 394
Kraepelin, Emil, 372
Krebs cycle, 917, 918
Kuru, 360
Kyphoscoliosis, 893
Kyphotic deformity, postoperative, 677

L
L-dopa. See *Levodopa*
L5 radiculopathy, 748
Labyrinth

INDEX

membranous, 127
   tonic discharge of, 128
Labyrinthine artery, 193
Labyrinthine segment, 112
Labyrinthitis, 129
Lacrimal flow, 125
Lacrimal gland, 87, 90, 103
   postganglionic fibers to, 112
Lacrimal nerve, 15, 80, 86, 87, 90, 102, 103, 107
   cutaneous branch of, 103
   palpebral branch of, 183
Lacrimation, 112
Lactic acid infusion, 378
Lacunar infarction, 210
Lacunar small vessel disease, 209–211
Lacunes, 199
Lagophthalmos, 117
Laing myopathy, 907t
Lambert-Eaton myasthenic syndrome, 823, 858, 886
   cardinal symptoms of, 858
   clinical presentation of, 858, 859
   diagnosis of, 874
   diagnostic approach to, 859–860
   differential diagnosis of, 861–862, 867
   etiology and pathophysiology of, 858–859
   treatment and prognosis of, 862
Lamina cribrosa, 57, 58
Laminectomy
   for lumbar radiculopathy, 688
   for lumbar spinal stenosis, 693
Laminoplasty, 517
Lamotrigine
   for cortical myoclonus, 452
   for epilepsy, 277
Language
   assessment of, 2, 3–4, 40–52
   dysfunction of
      dominant hemisphere, 46
      evaluation of, 41–45
      frontal lobe, 45–47
   fluency, degree of, 41–45
Large artery occlusive disease, 195
   clinical presentation of, 199–201
   ocular signs of, 200, 201
Large fiber neuropathy, 806t, 814
Large fiber sensory dysfunction, 801
Large-vessel disease, dementia with, 357
Laryngeal artery, superior, 189
Laryngeal muscles
   innervation, action, and vocal function of, 153t
   intrinsic, 146, 153
   motor supply of, 153–154
Laryngeal nerve, 155
   recurrent, 4, 144, 151, 154–156
   superior, 151, 155, 156
Laryngeal tremor, 156
Laryngeal vestibule, 146
   in deglutition, 148
Laryngopharyngeal reflux, 147
Laryngopharyngeal sensation, 147
Laryngospasm, 774t
Larynx, 149
   anatomy of, 153–154
   innervation of, 155
   intrinsic muscle of, 154
   neurologic disorders of, 154–156
   ventricle of, 148

Lateral compartment syndrome, 746
Lateral gaze center, 91
Lateral sclerosis, gait disturbances in, 488
Latex agglutination, 592
Latissimus dorsi muscle, 704
Lead
   nerve terminal uptake of, 857
   toxicity of, 813
Leber hereditary optic atrophy, 62
Left ventricular aneurysm, 198
Leg. See also *Lower extremity*
   bracing in neuropathies, 807
   circumduction of in spondylosis, 516
   cutaneous innervation of, 750, 753, 755, 758
   muscles of, 753
   weakness of, 25
Leigh disease, 823
Leishmaniasis, 841
Lemniscus
   lateral, 136
   medial, 165
Lennox-Gastaut syndrome, 272, 274, 284
Lens, 56
Lenticular nucleus degeneration, 469
Lentiform nucleus, 500, 766
Leprosy
   bacteriology of, 839
   borderline, 841
   clinical presentation of, 839–841
   diagnosis of, 839–841
   differential diagnosis of, 831
   dimorphous, 840
   early sensory loss patterns in, 840
   facial palsy in, 120
   future research on, 841–842
   lepromatous, 839, 841
   reversal reactions in, 841
   treatment of, 841
   in trigeminal neuropathy, 108
   tuberculoid, 841
Leptomeningeal inflammatory disorders, 867
Leptomeningeal seeding, 4
Leptomeninges, 110, 496
   infiltrating lesions of, 167
   inflammation and suppurative process on, 563
   in subarachnoid space, 560–562
Leukemia, 141
Leukoencephalopathy
   acute hemorrhagic, 557
   progressive multifocal, 485, 589
      in immunocompromised hosts, 586–588
Levator anguli oris muscle, 16, 115
Levator ani muscle, 711
   nerve to, 711
Levator labii superioris muscle, 16, 115
Levator palpebrae muscle, 82
Levator palpebrae superioris muscle, 86, 87, 90
Levator scapulae muscle, 160
Levator veli palatini muscle, 151, 154
Levetiracetam
   for cortical myoclonus, 452
   for epilepsy, 277–278
Levodopa, 406
   for dystonia, 446
   for multiple system atrophy, 420
   in neuroleptic malignant syndrome, 435
   for Parkinson disease, 405–408, 411

NEUROLOGY

INDEX

in parkinsonism, 409–410
for progressive supranuclear palsy, 417
Lewy bodies
    in Alzheimer disease, 341
    dementia with, 347–350
    in Parkinson disease, 402
    in substantia nigra, 404
Lhermitte sign, 3
    in multiple sclerosis, 543
    in spondylosis, 515
Lidocaine patches, 582
Limb coordination, loss of, 21
Limb-girdle muscular dystrophy, 895, 896t, 897–900, 906
Limb-girdle musculature
    chronic myopathies involving, 892–893
    weakness of, 900
Limb paralysis
    total, 25
    unilateral, 25
Limb paresthesias, 515, 516
Limbic cingulate cortex, 73
Limbic region, 73
Linear skull fractures, 646
Lingual artery, 160, 189
Lingual nerve, 15, 16, 102, 104, 107, 115
Lioresal, 106
Lipid metabolism disorders, 916t
Lipid oxidation, 914
Lipid storage myopathy, 897t
    biochemical analysis for, 920t
Lipohyalinosis, 199
Lipoma
    intramedullary spinal cord, 642
    in lumbar radiculopathy, 686
Lisch nodules, iris, 640
Lissauer zone, 786, 787
Listening, in neurologic history, 2
Listeria monocytogenes, 592–593
    in bacterial meningitis, 560–561, 564
    in meningitis, 588
Listeriosis, 592–593
Lithium
    for bipolar disorder, 370–371
    for borderline personality disorder, 386
    for tics, 465
Lobar dementia, 353
Lobar hemorrhage, 239–240
Lobectomy, 284, 285
Locked-in syndrome, 296
    management of, 303
Long thoracic nerve
    compression of, 742
    damage to, 161
    palsy of, 159
Longissimus capitis muscle, 184
Loop diuretics, 137
Lorazepam, 322
Low back pain, 681. See also *Lumbar radiculopathy*
Low cerebrospinal fluid pressure headache, 181–182
Low-CSF-pressure headache syndrome, 607–608
Lower extremity
    cutaneous innervation of, 747
    mononeuropathies with weakness of, 746–756
    sensory neuropathies of
        primary, 757–759
        uncommon, 759–762
Lower motor neuron disease, bulbar, 789–790
Lower motor neuron weakness, 777

Lucid interval, in epidural hematoma, 646
Lumbar disc
    degeneration of, referred pain due to, 683
    extrusion of, 685
    herniation of, 22
        differential diagnosis of, 682
    neovascularization of, 684
    protrusion of, 497
    ruptured, 679–682
Lumbar nerve root compression, 680
Lumbar pain, inflammatory, 684
Lumbar plexus, 494, 710, 753, 755
Lumbar puncture
    for bacterial meningitis, 560–561
    for brain abscess, 568
    for multiple sclerosis, 546–548
    for subarachnoid hemorrhage, 252
    for transverse myelitis, 511
Lumbar radiculopathy, 709–712
    clinical presentation of, 679–682
    diagnostic approach to, 686
    differential diagnosis of, 682–686
    incidence of, 679
    nerve root signs of, 682t
    pain patterns in, 683
    treatment of, 686–689
Lumbar spinal nerves, 497
    dorsal and ventral roots of, 835
Lumbar spinal stenosis, 23
    clinical presentation of, 691
    diagnosis of, 691–693, 757
    with lumbar radiculopathy, 688
    treatment of, 693
Lumbar spinal tumors, 686
Lumbar vertebra, 496
Lumboperitoneal CSF shunt, 62
Lumbosacral plexopathy
    anatomical correlations of, 708–709
    clinical presentation of, 708, 712–713
    diagnostic approach to, 709
    differential diagnosis of, 709–712, 748
    future research on, 714
    treatment and prognosis of, 713–714
Lumbosacral plexus, 708
    disorders of, 759
    lesions of, 750
    tumors invading, 712
Lumbosacral plexus neuropathy, 712
Lumbosacral radiculoplexus neuropathy, diabetic, 712
Lumbosacral trunk, 710, 711, 753, 755
Lumbrical muscles, 727, 728, 761
Lunate sulcus, 42
Lung, 496
    metastatic cancer of, 616, 617
    tumors of in voice disorders, 155
Lupus erythematosus, 457
Lupus vulgaris, 841
Luschka, lateral aperture of, 226
Lyme disease
    cranial nerves in, 4
    in cranial neuropathies, 4
    differential diagnosis of, 784–785, 831
    in facial palsy, 117, 120
    in length-dependent polyneuropathy, 810–814
Lymphocyte analysis, 920
Lymphoma
    to cranial nerves, 4

INDEX

mimicking multiple sclerosis, 544
primary CNS, 618
spinal canal, myelographic and CT characteristics of, 524
trigeminal, 109–110
Lymphomatoid granulomatosis, 831
Lymphoproliferative malignancies, 110
Lymphoproliferative multifocal neuropathies, 830t
Lysosomal storage disorders, 445

M

Machado-Joseph-Azorean disease, 485t
Macroglobulinemia, 141
Macula, 56
    cherry-red spots near, 11
    degeneration of, 54
    section of, 127
Macular arteriole, 56
Macular sparing, 76
Macular venule, 56
Macular zone, 9, 70
Mad cow disease, 360, 361
Magendie, median aperture of, 226
Magnesium, uptake of, 857
Magnetic gait, 481
Magnetic resonance angiography, 214
Magnetic resonance imaging
    for acoustic neuroma, 140, 624
    for acute myelopathies, 512
    advantages and disadvantages of, 215t
    in Alzheimer disease, 343
    for brachial plexopathies, 705
    for cerebral venous thrombosis, 232
    for cervical radiculopathy, 676
    for chorea, 458–459
    classification of spinal abnormalities of, 637t
    for compression neuropathy, 725
    for demyelinating disorders, 610
    diffusion-weighted, for ischemic stroke, 212
    for epidural lipomatosis, 521
    for epilepsy, 264, 281
    in evaluation, 2
    for facial palsies, 124–125
    functional, for epilepsy, 284
    for hereditary spastic paraplegia, 529
    for hypoglossal disorders, 167
    for intracerebral hemorrhage, 243
    for low-CSF-pressure headache syndrome, 608
    for lumbar radiculopathy, 686
    for lumbar spinal stenosis, 693
    for lumbosacral plexopathies, 709
    for meningiomas, 622–624
    for mononeuropathies with lower extremity weakness, 754
    for multiple sclerosis, 539, 545–546, 547
    for myasthenia gravis, 868
    for neurosyphilis, 571
    of optic pathways, 71
    for partial seizures, 268
    for pituitary tumors, 628
    for progressive multifocal leukoencephalopathy, 588
    for proximal median neuropathies, 732
    for spinal cord meningioma, 522–526
    of spinal cord tumors, 637
    for spine injury, 662
    for syringomyelia, 528
    for transmissible spongiform encephalopathy, 362, 363
    for transverse myelitis, 511
    for upper extremity mononeuropathies, 738–739
    for vertebrobasilar occlusive disease, 202–203
Magnetic resonance venography
    for cerebral venous thrombosis, 232
    showing sagittal sinus thrombosis, 231
Magnetoencephalography, 452
Malathion, 853
Malignant hyperthermia, 915
    creatine kinase levels in, 918
    in myopathies, 879
Malignant myeloma, 636
Malignant tumors, 705–706
Mallear fold
    anterior, 114
    posterior, 114
Malleus, 135
    anterior process of, 114
    handle of, 114
    head of, 114
    ligaments of, 114
Malnutrition, 775t
Mandible, ramus of, 122
Mandibular foramen, 104
Mandibular nerve, 80, 86, 87, 90, 102, 103, 104, 150, 183
    innervation zone of, 107
    meningeal branch of, 87, 90
    in trigeminal nerve territories, 15
Manganese
    nerve terminal uptake of, 857
    toxicity of, 410
Mania
    in bipolar disorder, 369, 370
    childhood, versus attention deficit disorder, 387
    classic, 369
Mannitol, 312–313
Marantic emboli, 215
Marfan syndrome, 199
    primary sites of motor disorder in, 26
Markesbery-Griggs/Udd myopathy, 907t
Mass lesions, 588–593
Massage, cervical, 676
Masseter muscle, 122
    innervation of, 106
Masseteric nerve, 102, 104
    lateral, 15
Mastectomy, edema after, 702
Mastication
    cranial nerves in, 4, 106
    muscles of, 106
Mastoid process, 122
Maxillary artery, 104, 188, 189
Maxillary nerve, 80, 86, 87, 90, 102, 103, 104, 183
    branches of, 15
    in cavernous sinus, 228
    innervation zone of, 107
    meningeal branch of, 87, 90
Maxillary sinus, mucous membrane of, 103
McArdle disease, 23, 919
    type V, 916
Mechanical ventilation, 793
Mechanoreceptors, 35
Meckel cave, 89, 101
Meclizine, 132
Median mononeuropathy
    distal, 729–730

INDEX

proximal, 730–732
Median nerve, 703, 704, 727
    in carpal tunnel, 728, 729
    communicating branch of, 727
    distal entrapment of, 726–730
    proximal compression of, 730–732
    recurrent branch of, 727
    sensory distribution of, 728
Median neuropathy, at wrist, 739
Median sulcus, dorsal, 495
Medroxyprogesterone, 289–291
Medulla oblongata, 37, 73, 114, 136, 500, 767, 844
    infarction of, 129
    lower part of, 766
    upper part of, 766
Medullary arteries, 517–519
Medullary lamina, 403
    external, 38
    internal, 38
Medullary reticulospinal tract, 498
Medullary vein, 501
    anterior, 227
Medulloblastoma, 616–618
    in children, 619
Megaloblastic anemia, 532
Meige syndrome, 441
Melanoma
    hemorrhagic, 243
    metastatic to brain, 617
Melatonin secretion, 68
Melkersson-Rosenthal syndrome, 123–124
Memantine, 346
Memory
    in Alzheimer disease, 336
    examination of, 4
    loss of in cerebral artery infarction, 205
    short-term problems of, 48
    testing for, 44
    testing of, 48
    voluntary and involuntary, 48
Ménière disease, 129
    differential diagnosis of, 140
    hearing loss with, 137
    in multiple sclerosis, 541
Meningeal artery, middle, 104, 171, 189
Meningeal vein, middle, 224
Meninges
    arterial supply to, 188–194
    outer, 228
    signs of irritation of, 250
    of spinal cord, 493
Meningioma, 4, 167
    of auditory canal, 138
    clinical presentation of, 622, 623
    in facial palsy, 121
    of falx, 607
    histology of, 623
    hormonal receptors in, 633
    in lumbar radiculopathy, 686
    mimicking multiple sclerosis, 544
    myelographic and CT characteristics of, 524
    olfactory groove, 96, 99–100
    of spinal cord, 635, 638
        clinical presentation of, 521, 522
        diagnosis of, 522, 526
        pathophysiology and etiology of, 521–522

        treatment and prognosis of, 526
    subfrontal, 97
    of thoracic spine, 501
    treatment of, 622–624
    trigeminal, 109–110
    in trigeminal neuralgia, 106
Meningismus, 562
Meningitis, 120
    bacterial
        clinical presentation of, 560, 562
        complications of, 564–565
        diagnosis of, 562–564
        pathophysiology of, 560–562
        treatment of, 564
    carcinomatous, 616
    in facial palsy, 121
    in gait disorders, 481
    headache in, 181, 185
    in immunocompromised hosts, 588–593
    migraine with, 249
    nonparalytic aseptic, 598
    syphilitic, 570
    tuberculous, 583–585
Meningoencephalitis, 579
Meningovascular syphilis, 570–571
Menke syndrome, 468
Mental nerve, 15, 102, 104, 107, 183
Mental status
    in Alzheimer disease, 341–342
    assessment of, 2
    fluctuating, 348–349
Mentalis muscle, 16, 115
Mesencephalic nucleus, 102, 105
Mesencephalic reticular formation, 68
Mesencephalic subnucleus, 106
Mesencephalic vein
    lateral, 227
    posterior, 227, 226
Mesencephalon, 37
Mesenteric ganglion
    inferior, 844
    superior, 844
Mesial temporal sclerosis, 264
    in epilepsy, 286
    partial seizures in, 268
Mesothelial septum, 495
Metabolic coma, 297, 311
Metabolic disorders
    acquired, 809–810
    in peripheral neuropathies, 810
Metabolic-endocrine disorders, 297
Metabolic multifocal neuropathies, 830t
Metabolic myopathy, 897t
    biochemical analysis for, 920t
    treatment of, 921
Metacarpal arteries, palmar, 727
Metamorphopsia, 173
Metastatic disease
    in acute central disc, 506
    to intramedullary spinal cord, 638, 642
    pathology, etiology and diagnosis of, 505
    to spinal cord, 635, 636
Metastatic tumor
    brain, 615–616, 617
    extradural
        differential diagnosis of, 674

INDEX

in lumbar radiculopathy, 686
lumbosacral, 708
Methadone, 398
Methazolamide (Glauc Tabs, Neptazane), 426t
Methotrexate
    for carcinomatous meningitis, 616
    for CNS lymphoma, 618
    for multiple sclerosis, 552–553
Methylphenidate
    for fatigue of multiple sclerosis, 554
    for tics, 465
Methylprednisolone
    for acute disseminated encephalomyelitis, 555
    intravenous, 59
    for multiple sclerosis, 553
    for spinal injury, 663
    for transverse myelitis, 511
Methylsergide
    for cluster headache, 175
    for migraine, 175
Metoclopramide
    for gastroparesis, 847
    inducing parkinsonism, 432–433
Metoprolol (Lopressor, Toprol), 426t
Metronidazole
    for brain abscess, 568
    for subdural empyema, 568
Mexiletine, 905
Meyer loop, 9, 69, 70
Meynert cells, in striate cortex, 72
Microaneurysm rupture, 236
Microcatheter navigation, 261
Microcystic adnexal carcinoma, 109–110
Microhemagglutination test, 138
Microscopic analysis, 540
Microtubules, 717
    patent, 718
Microvascular disease, 141
Midbrain, 24, 136, 767
    clinical manifestations of infarction in, 205
    hemorrhage in, 240–241
    lesions of
        breathing patterns with, 311
        differential diagnosis of, 88
Middle ear fossa hematoma, 656
Midodrine, 847
Migraine, 170–174
    with aura, 170–174
    chronic or transformed, 177
    considerations in, 174
    mechanisms of, 172
    spreading depression in, 174
    in subarachnoid hemorrhage, 249
    treatment of, 174–175
Miliary aneurysm, 234
Milkmaid's grip, 455
Millard-Gubler syndrome, 92
Miller-Fisher syndrome, 121
Mineralocorticoids, 280
Minerva jacket brace, 666
Mini-Mental Status Examination (MMSE), 41
    in Alzheimer disease, 342
Minimally invasive techniques, 642
Minocycline, 775
Minoxidil, 847
Mitochondria, 851, 852, 853
    damaged to, 768

disorders of, 445
evaluation of in myopathies, 879
Mitochondrial mutational analysis, 920
Mitochondrial myopathy, 916
    biochemical analysis for, 920t
    diagnosis of, 920
Mitoxantrone, 552
Mitral cell, 99
Mitral valve
    defect of in intracerebral hemorrhage, 245
    prolapse of, 215
    stenosis of, 208
Miyoshi myopathy, 907t
    diagnosis of, 908
Miyoshi phenotype, 906
Mobilization, post-spine injury, 662
Modafinil
    for fatigue of multiple sclerosis, 554
    for narcolepsy, 291
Molecular mimicry, 819
Monoamine oxidase B inhibitors, 412
Monoamine oxidase inhibitors
    for major depression, 367
    for panic disorder, 380
Monoclonus tremor, 429
Monocular fields, 9, 70
Monocular homonymous defect, 75
Monocular occlusion, 75
Monocular visual blurring, 61
Monofocal acute inflammatory demyelination (MAID), 544
Mononeuritis multiplex
    clinical presentation of, 827–829
    differential diagnosis of, 822–823, 829
    pattern of, 810–814
    polyarteritis nodosa with, 828
    treatment and prognosis of, 832–833
Mononeuropathy, 706
    clinical presentation of, 721–723
    diagnostic approach to, 723–725
    differential diagnosis of, 723
    epidemiology of, 716
    future research on, 725
    individual, 36
    with lower extremity weakness, 746–756
    mechanisms of pathophysiology of, 716–721
    peripheral, 30
    with shoulder pain and weakness, 741–745
    therapy and prognosis of, 725
    ulnar, 732–736
    with upper extremity symptoms, 726–739
    weakness in, 25
Mononucleosis, infectious, 120
Monoparesis, 25
Monoradiculopathy, 723
Mood stabilizers
    for bipolar disorder, 370–371
    for borderline personality disorder, 386
    for frontotemporal dementia, 355
Mood states
    atypical, 369
    diurnal fluctuations of, 366
    rapid cycling of, 370, 371, 384
Motor aphasia, 112
Motor apraxia, 49
Motor cortex
    primary, 24, 73

NEUROLOGY

953

INDEX

supplemental, 73
Motor deficits/disorders
    in Huntington disease, 457
    primary sites of, 26
    with transmissible spongiform encephalopathy, 361–363
Motor end plate, 26
Motor fibers
    cranial, distribution of, 5
    of facial nerve, 112
Motor function
    evaluation of, 800–801
    impaired, 673
Motor impersistence, 50
Motor neuron disease, 159, 167, 908
    alternative therapies for, 775
    bulbar presentations of, 789–791
    classification of, 764–768, 769t, 784
    dementia of, 351
    diagnostic approach to, 771–772
    diagnostic problems in, 770–771
    etiology of, 768–770
    frontotemporal lobar degeneration with, 354
    future directions for, 776
    habilitation devices and procedures for, 773
    head drop and ventilatory failure presentations of, 791–792
    impaired smell in, 100
    in limbs with lower motor neuron features, 777–782
    with lower motor neuron features
        differential diagnosis of, 778–781
        treatment and prognosis of, 781–782
    management of, 772–775
    pathophysiology of, 768
    primary sites of motor disorder in, 26
    symptomatic management of, 774–775t
    treatment and prognosis of, 792–793
Motor neurons, 499
    lower, 765
    pathways of, 25, 765
    upper, 765
Motor neuropathy, distal, 770t
Motor nucleus, 102, 106
Motor-predominant polyneuropathy, 802t
    length-dependent, 814
Motor tics
    chronic, 462
    complex, 460, 461t
    simple, 460, 461t
Motor tone, 30
    abnormalities in, 30–32
Motor tracts, descending, 493–501
Motor unit abnormalities, 884–886
Motor weakness
    with cervical herniated disc, 675t
    focal, 723
    pure, 28
Movement disorders, 23–25
    differentiation of, 461t
    drug-induced, 432–437
    psychogenic, 472–474
    surgical treatments for, 475–477
    versus tics, 460
Moyamoya, 246
MPTP, 410
MRI. See *Magnetic resonance imaging*
Mucormycosis *meningitis*, 588

Multifocal acquired demyelinating sensory and motor neuropathy, 831
Multifocal acquired motor axonopathy, 831
Multifocal motor neuropathy (MMN), 765
    characteristics of, 770t
    clinical presentation of, 827
    differential diagnosis of, 778–779, 830–831
    treatment of, 832–833
Multifocal neuropathy, 805t
    clinical presentation of, 827–829
    diagnostic approach to, 831–832
    differential diagnosis of, 804, 829–831
    etiology of, 827–829
    treatment and prognosis of, 832–833
Multifocal polyradiculopathy, 829
Multi-infarct dementia, 358
Multiple cranial neuropathies, 791
    differential diagnosis of, 867
Multiple myeloma, 636
Multiple sclerosis
    adjuvant medical problems and treatments of, 553–555
    benign, 540
    clinical features of, 509
    diagnostic approach to, 545–550
    differential diagnosis of, 541–545, 784, 846, 867
    epidemiology of, 538
    facial myokymia in, 124
    gait disturbances in, 488
    genetic factors in, 538
    in hearing loss, 141
    during heat waves, 555
    management and therapy for, 550–555
    medulla oblongata infarction in, 129
    MRI for, 2
    MS plaques of, 539
        microscopic analysis of, 540
    optic neuritis in, 59
    pathology of, 538–540
    during pregnancy, 555
    primary progressive, 541
    primary sites of motor disorder in, 26
    relapsing-remitting, 540
    secondary progressive, 540–541
    spinal cord lesions in, 502
    subtypes of, 540–541
    treatment of swallowing problems in, 152
    vertigo in, 128
Multiple sleep latency test, 291
Multiple subpial transections, 286
Multiple system atrophy, 415t
    clinical presentation of, 418–420
    diagnosis of, 420
    differential diagnosis of, 846
    pathophysiology of, 420
    treatment of, 420
Mural thrombus, 198–199, 208
Muscarinic agonists, 344
Muscle adenylate deaminase deficiency, 916, 920
Muscle biopsy, 771–772, 781
    for channelopathies, 912
    for congenital myopathies, 901
    in congenital myopathies, 898
    in distal predominant myopathies, 908
    for Duchenne muscular dystrophy, 903
    for myopathies, 879–881, 884, 890
    for myopathies with exercise intolerance, 919
    technique in, 880

INDEX

Muscle cells
    cardiac metabolism of, 917
    membrane depolarization and repolarization of, 850
    nucleus of, 851
Muscle contraction headache, 178
Muscle cramps, 23
Muscle diseases
    classification of, 872
    diagnostic approach to, 872–882
    differential diagnosis of, 872
    evaluating patient with, 877t
    treatment of, 882
Muscle energy metabolism defects, 914–921
Muscle metabolism, 914
Muscle receptors, 34
Muscle relaxants
    for cervical radiculopathy, 676
    for tetanus, 596
Muscle rigidity, 797
Muscle-specific kinase (MUSK), 867–868
Muscle spindles, 34
Muscle strength assessment, 4, 25–30
Muscle stretch, passive, 32, 34
Muscle stretch reflex
    diminished or absent, 26, 802, 819–822
    evaluation of, 4, 32–35
    in lumbar radiculopathy, 682t
Muscle stretch reflexes
    hypoactive or absent, 886
    testing of in Lambert-Eaton myasthenic syndrome, 861–862
Muscle tests, 27t
Muscle wasting
    in myotonia, 894
Muscle weakness
    in myasthenia gravis, 866
Muscles
    asymmetry of, 30
    ATP in contraction of, 918
    diseases of, 872–883
    injury of in motor disorders, 26
    severe cramping and collapse of, 915
    spasms of in tetanus, 594–595
    weakness of, 25
        grading of, 27–30
Muscular dystrophy
    congenital, 898, 901
    differential diagnosis of, 893–901
    genetic counseling for, 882
    hereditary, 902–903
    limb-girdle, 906
    prognosis for, 905
    treatment of, 904
    types of, 895
Muscular Dystrophy Association, 772
Musculocutaneous nerve, 703, 704, 742
    compression of, 742
    damage to, 744
Musculoskeletal disorders, 480
Myalgia, with polyarteritis nodosa, 828
Myasthenia, 791–792
Myasthenia gravis, 864–870, 884
    autoimmune-mediated, 470
    clinical presentation of, 864, 865–867
    diagnostic approach to, 867–868
    differential diagnosis of, 791, 823, 867, 912
    etiology and pathogenesis of, 864
    management and prognosis of, 868–870
    pathophysiologic concepts in, 865
    primary sites of motor disorder in, 26
    in voice disorders, 155, 156
Myasthenic crises, 865
Mycobacterium leprae, *839*
    biopsy specimen of, 840
    genome mapping for, 841–842
Mycobacterium tuberculosis, *585*
    in spinal epidural abscess, 566
Mycophenolate mofetil, 870
Mycotic aneurysms, 234
    in intracerebral hemorrhage, 245–246
Mydriasis, 10
    with Adie tonic pupil, 84
Myectomy, 446
Myelin
    loss of, 721
        in multiple sclerosis, 538
    susceptibility of to compression, 721
    thinned, 718
Myelin-associated glycoprotein antibodies, 806
Myelin basic protein, 538–539
    in multiple sclerosis, 548
Myelin sheath, 717, 718, 851, 852, 856
    multifocal damage to in Guillain-Barré syndrome, 820
Myelinated fibers, 493
Myelination, 538–539
Myelitis
    in AIDS-associated vacuolar myelopathy, 531
    in multiple sclerosis, 544
    transverse, 509–511
Myelography
    for cervical radiculopathy, 676
    for epidural lipomatosis, 521
    for lumbar radiculopathy, 686
    for lumbar spinal stenosis, 693
    for spinal arteriovenous malformations, 520
    for spinal cord meningioma, 526
    of spinal tumors, 524
    for syringomyelia, 528
Myelopathy, 492
    acute
        clinical presentation of, 512
        diagnosis and treatment of, 512–513
        extradural spinal lesions in, 503–508
        intradural intramedullary spinal lesions in, 509–512
    AIDS-associated vacuolar, 531
    anatomical aspects of, 492–502
    chronic, 514–535
    chronic extradural, 514–521
        causes of, 514t
    chronic intradural extramedullary, 521–526
    chronic intradural intramedullary, 526–532
    differential diagnosis of, 822
    extradural extramedullary, 501
    extramedullary, 492
    HIV-associated vacuolar, 502
    HTLV-1, 529–531
    intradural extramedullary, 501
    intramedullary, 492, 501–502
    in multiple sclerosis, 543–544, 545
    spinal cord ischemic, 511–512
Mylohyoid muscle, 104, 160
    innervation of, 106
    nerve to, 104
Mylohyoid nerve, 15, 102, 104, 144
Myoblast transfer, 905

INDEX

Myocardial infarction, 198
   in brain death, 316
   with mural thrombus, 208
Myocardiopathy, 215
Myoclonic dystonia, 438
Myoclonic encephalopathy, 274
Myoclonic seizures, 272–274
Myoclonus, 274
   action or intention, 447
   additional forms of, 448
   classification of, 447, 448t
   clinical presentation of, 447, 448
   cortical, 447
   diagnostic evaluation for, 449–452
   differential diagnosis of, 448–449
   drugs causing, 434t
   essential, 448, 450
   etiologies of, 449t
   familial essential, 448
   generalized, 449–451
   multifocal, 449–451
   negative, 447
      testing for, 451
   pathologic, 447
   pathophysiology of, 448
   physiologic, 447
   physiologic sleep, 448
   positive, 447
   precipitating factors of, 449–451
   psychogenic, 473
   reflex, 447
   rhythmic forms of, 449
   spinal, 447
   spontaneous, 447
   subcortical, 447
   treatment and prognosis of, 452
Myofiber necrosis, 884
Myofibrillar myopathy, 907t
   treatment of, 908
Myofibrils, 851, 852
   destruction of, 876
Myoglobinuria, 889, 915
   history of, 914
   recurrent, 916
   treatment of, 921
Myoglobinuric syndromes, 915
Myopathy
   acquired chronic, 894t
      differential diagnosis of, 893
   antibodies in, 879
   Bethlem, 900–901
   chronic proximal
      differential diagnosis and diagnostic approach to, 893–904
      etiology and clinical presentation of, 892–893
      management goals for, 904t
      prognosis of, 905
      treatment of, 904–905
   chronic proximally predominant, 892–905
   classification of, 872
   congenital, 877, 896–897t, 898, 901
   critical illness, 887
   diagnostic approach to, 872–882, 908
   differential diagnosis of, 780, 872, 906–908
   distal predominant, 874t, 906–908
      etiology and clinical presentation of, 906
   with distinctive clinical features and weakness, 875t
   DNA mutational analysis for, 879
   endocrine, 887–889
   with episodic weakness, 909–913
   exercise intolerance, 874t
   with exercise intolerance, 914
      diagnostic approach to, 916–920
      differential diagnosis of, 914–916
      etiology of, 914
      treatment and prognosis of, 920–921
   forearm exercise testing for, 877–879
   gait disorder in, 23
   with generalized weakness, 892–905
   genetically determined chronic, 893–901
   hypokalemic, 887, 888
   immunologically mediated, 886
   infectious, 889
   inflammatory, 861–862
   malignant hyperthermia evaluation in, 879
   mitochondria evaluations in, 879
   in multiple sclerosis, 545
   muscle biopsy for, 879–881
   paraneoplastic necrotizing, 889–891
   periodic weakness, 874t
   presenting with weakness, 884–891
   primary sites of motor disorder in, 26
   proximal predominant acute/subacute, 873t
   proximal predominant chronic, 873t
   with regional patterns of weakness, 876t
   toxic, 886–887
   treatment and prognosis of, 908
   treatment of, 882
   weakness in, 28
Myophosphorylase deficiency, 914
Myosin loss, 887
Myositis, eosinophilic, 889
Myositis-associated antibodies, 879
Myositis-specific antibodies, 891
Myotomes, of upper limb, 673
Myotonia, 894
   in channelopathies, 909
   congenital, 909, 910t
   treatment of, 905, 913
Myotonia congenita, 797, 899, 911
Myotonic muscular dystrophy, 121–123, 899
   congenital, 123
   differential diagnosis of, 791
Myotubular myopathy, 901
Myxopapillary ependymoma, 616
   in lumbar radiculopathy, 686

N

Nadroparin, 216
Nalidixic acid, 604, 605
Naltrexone, 398
Narcolepsy, 290, 291
   clinical presentation of, 291
   diagnosis of, 291
   treatment of, 291
Nasal nerve
   external and internal, 107
   posterior, 107
Nasal regurgitation, 146
Nasal retina, 56
   fibers of, 64
Nasal sinus infection, 186
Nasal step, 57
Nasal wall, 98

INDEX

Nasalis muscle, 16, 115
Nasociliary nerve, 8, 15, 80, 86, 87, 90, 102, 103, 107
Nasopharyngeal carcinoma, 110
Nasopharynx, 90, 135, 146
National Prion Disease Pathology Surveillance Center, 363
Nausea and vomiting
    in increased intracranial pressure, 606
    in subarachnoid hemorrhage, 249
Neck
    pain in, 515
    range of motion of, 658–662
    trauma to, 167
    tumors of in voice disorders, 155
Neck drop, 774t
Necrotizing vasculitis
    differential diagnosis of, 829
    treatment of, 833
Neglect, left-sided stimuli, 50
Neglect syndrome, 48–49
Negri bodies, 578
Neisseria meningitidis, 560–561, 562
    vaccine for, 565
Nemaline myopathy, 901
Neoplasms
    of facial nerve, 119
    in facial palsy, 121
    with hypoglossal paralysis, 167
    trigeminal, 109–110
    of visual cortex, 75
Neostigmine, 855t
Neovascular glaucoma, 79
Nephrectomy, 512
Nephropathy, 828
Nerve axon, 853
Nerve block paralysis, 854t
Nerve cell axons, 717
Nerve cell transplantation, 413
Nerve conduction studies, 723
    for carpal tunnel syndrome, 730
    for channelopathies, 912
    for compression neuropathy, 724
    in distal predominant myopathies, 908
    for upper extremity mononeuropathies, 738
Nerve conduction velocity, 821
Nerve deafness, 19
Nerve fiber
    myelinated, 717
    unmyelinated, 717
Nerve root dermatomes, sensory territories of, 29, 30
Nerve root-dura interface inflammation, 684
Nerve roots
    compression of
        in lumbar radiculopathy, 688, 689
        radicular pain due to, 683
    in lumbar radiculopathy, 682t
Nerve sheath tumors, 641
Nerve terminal, 857
Nerves
    drugs in excitability of, 854t
    entrapment of
        management of, 754
        treatment of, 725
    injury to, Sunderland classification of, 718
    ischemia of, 719
    toxins of in autonomic neuropathy, 845
Nervous system, viral infections of, 574–582
Nervus intermedius, 112, 224

Neural grafting, 413, 745
Neuralgic amyotrophy, 705
Neurapraxia, 718
Neurilemma, 852
Neurinoma, 167
    acoustic, 625
    trigeminal, 109
Neuroacanthocytosis, 458
Neuroborreliosis, 120
Neurodegenerative disorders
    classification of, 485–486
    clinical manifestations of, 487
    impaired smell in, 100
Neurodegenerative processes, 48
    in gait disorder, 483–488
Neurofibrillary tangles, 329
    in Alzheimer disease, 330–331, 332, 333, 334
    in Parkinson disease, 404
    in parkinsonian syndromes, 414
Neurofibroma, intradural spinal cord, 640
Neurofibromatosis
    type I, 640
    type II, 625
Neurofibromatous neuropathy, 831
Neurogenic pulmonary edema, 257
Neurogenic thoracic outlet syndrome, 706
Neuroimaging studies
    advances in techniques of, 756
    advantages and disadvantages of, 215t
    for dystonia, 445
    for epilepsy, 264
    for myoclonus, 451–452
    for partial seizures, 268
Neurolemmoma, 638
Neuroleptic malignant syndrome, 350, 435
    drugs causing, 434t
Neuroleptics
    for dementia with Lewy bodies, 350
    for frontotemporal dementia, 355
    for schizophrenia, 373–374
    in secondary dystonia, 443
    for tics, 465
    tremor with, 429–430
Neurologic examination
    for back pain, 696
    basic tenets of, 3–4
    for gait disorders, 488
    in Guillain-Barré syndrome, 819–822
Neurologic history, 2–3
Neurolymphomatosis, 831
Neuroma, acoustic, 624–626
Neuromelanin, 405
Neuromuscular blockers, 853
    depolarizing, 854
Neuromuscular disorders
    with cerebral aneurysm, 78, 251
    with facial palsy, 121–123
    in voice disorders, 156
Neuromuscular junction
    acetylcholine release at, 860
    anatomy and physiology of, 849–857
    defects of in myasthenia gravis, 864, 865
    fold of, 852
    folds of, 856, 857
    motor end plate of, 851
    normal, 853
    pharmacology of, 854, 855t

INDEX

Neuromuscular transmission
    alteration of, 850–854
    mechanisms of, 852
    normal, 850
    pharmacology of, 857
    somatic, 851
Neuromuscular transmission disorders, 545
    differential diagnosis of, 780, 823, 872
Neuromyelitis optica, 510
    in multiple sclerosis, 541
Neuromyotonia, 780
Neuronopathy, sensory, 834–838
Neurons
    activation patterns of, 75
    depolarization of, 850
    impaired regeneration of, 768
    loss of in Alzheimer disease, 330, 333, 336
Neuro-oncology, 604–610
Neuropathy
    alcoholism and, 393
    anterior interosseous, 731, 732
    associated with systemic diseases, 804t
    chronic, 814–816
    multifocal, 827–833
    primary sites of motor disorder in, 26
    sensory, 834–838
        of lower extremity, 757–762
Neuropathy panels, 805
Neuroprotective agents, 359
Neuropsychological testing, 282
Neurosurgery, 506
Neurosyphilis
    clinical presentation of, 570–571
    diagnosis and treatment of, 571–573
    epidemiology of, 570
Neurotoxins
    elimination of, 836
    peripheral, 809–810
    in sensory neuropathy, 835–836
Neurotransmitters, 474
Neurotrophic growth factors, 459
Neutralizing antibodies
    in multiple sclerosis, 551–552
    for poliomyelitis, 600
Nicotine
    in endplate depolarization, 854
    neuromuscular effects of, 855t
Nicotine addiction, 398
Niemann-Pick type C disease, 410
Nifedipine, uptake of, 857
Night terrors, 293–294
Nigrostriatal projections, 403
Nimodipine (Nimotop), 426t
Nitroglycerin, 847
Nocardia
    branching hyphae of, 590
    in meningitis, 588–589
Nocardiosis, 588–589, 590
Nociceptors, 684
Nonaka distal myopathy, 906
    characteristics of, 907t
Nonlanguage cues, abnormal recognition of, 50
Nonsteroidal anti-inflammatory drugs (NSAIDs)
    for carpal tunnel syndrome, 729
    for cervical radiculopathy, 676
    for migraine, 174–175
    for pain of multiple sclerosis, 554

Norepinephrine reuptake inhibitors, 377
North American Symptomatic Carotid Endarterectomy Trial (NASCET), 218
Nuclear bag fiber, 34
Nuclear chain fiber, 34
Nucleoside analog, 588
Nucleus ambiguus, 6, 105, 145, 150, 151, 154, 158, 159, 165, 500, 766, 767
Nucleus cuneatus, 165
Nucleus dorsalis of Clarke, 786, 787
Nucleus gracilis, 165
Nucleus proprius, 786, 787
Nucleus solitarius, 165
Numb chin syndrome, 110
Numbness
    of lateral thigh, 758
    in multiple sclerosis, 540, 544, 545
    in spinal cord degeneration, 533
    transient, 540
    in ulnar mononeuropathy, 732
Nursing home placement, 346
Nutritional-related peripheral neuropathies, 810
Nutritional support, 152
Nystagmus, 14
    bilateral horizontal, 19
    cerebellar lesions in, 21
    downward gaze vertical, 126
    evaluation for, 19
    fast phase, 128
    fatiguing, 19
    with Friedreich ataxia, 534–535
    gaze-dependent, 126
    in multiple sclerosis, 542
    opticokinetic, 75
    palatal, 429
    in positional vertigo, 18
    rapid phase of, 13
    right beating, 19
    slow phase of, 13
    torsional, 19
    upward gaze vertical, 126

O

Obesity, in pseudotumor cerebri, 605
Obex, medulla-level of, 165
Oblique muscle, 80, 86, 87, 90, 91
Obliquus capitis inferior muscle, 184
Obliquus capitis superior muscle, 184
Obsessive-compulsive disorder
    clinical presentation of, 375
    with Tourette syndrome, 462, 464
    treatment of, 375–377
Obstructive sleep apnea syndrome, 289
Obtundation, 296
    in cerebral venous thrombosis, 232–233
Obturator externus muscle, 755
Obturator internus muscle, 711
Obturator nerve, 710, 711, 753, 755
Obturator neuropathies, 754
Occipital artery, 184, 189
    mastoid branch of, 189
Occipital condyle, 164
Occipital cortex, 7, 65
    pathways to, 9
Occipital eye fields, 12, 91
    efferent pathway from, 500, 766

INDEX

Occipital hematoma, 239
Occipital lobar white matter, hemorrhage of, 238
Occipital lobe, 42, 73
    arterial supply to, 191
    dysfunction of, 49–52
    infarcts of, 52
    projections on, 9, 70
Occipital nerves, 183, 184
    greater, 183
    lesser, 160, 183
Occipital neuralgia, 185
Occipital pole, 42
Occipital region, lesions of, 46
Occipital sinus, 194, 224, 227
Occipital sulcus, 42
Occipital vein, internal, 226
Occipitofrontalis muscle, 16, 115, 184
Occupational therapy, 908
Ocular dominance columns, 75
Ocular palsy, 648
Oculobulbar weakness, 859
Oculocephalic reflexes, 303–304
Oculofacial muscular dystrophy, 895
    myotonic, 894, 896t
Oculomotor fasciculus, 81
Oculomotor nerve (III), 4, 8, 83, 87, 91, 105, 224, 228
    aberrant regeneration of, 82
    anatomical correlations of, 77–82
    in cavernous sinus, 229
    clinical presentation of, 77
    clinical vignette of, 77
    course of, 77
    disorders of, 82–84
    distribution of, 5
    efferent and afferent fibers of, 6
    inferior division of, 80, 86, 90
    inferior division palsies of, 84
    in nystagmus, 13
    preservation of function of, 10
    schema of, 80, 86
    superior division of, 80, 86, 90
    testing of, 11–14
Oculomotor nerve (III) palsy, 78
    with cerebral aneurysm, 251
    differential diagnosis of, 82
Oculomotor nerve (III) root, 8
Oculomotor nucleus, 6, 12, 77–81, 86, 91, 105
Oculomotor paralysis, 77
Oculomotor paresis, 77
Oculopharyngeal muscular dystrophy, 791, 896t, 901
Odontoid process fracture, 668
Olanzapine, 465
Olecranon, 733
Olfaction, 4
Olfactory apparatus, mass compressing, 97
Olfactory axons, unmyelinated, 98
Olfactory bulb, 98
    fibers from, 99
Olfactory cells, 98
Olfactory cortex, 96
Olfactory discrimination, 100
Olfactory epithelium, 99
    distribution of, 98
Olfactory function, 7
Olfactory gland, 98
Olfactory groove meningioma, 99–100
Olfactory mucosa, 98

Olfactory nerve (I), 4, 99
    benign neoplasm of, 96
    clinical vignette of, 96
    congenital disorder of, 97
    damage to, 7
    disorders of
        acquired, 97–100
        differential diagnosis of, 97–100
    distribution of, 5
    functional testing of, 4–7
    testing of, 4–7
Olfactory pathways, 99
Olfactory receptor cells, 96
    life span of, 100
Olfactory receptors, 98
Olfactory rod, 98
Olfactory stria, 99
Olfactory tract, 99
Olfactory tract nucleus, 99
Olfactory trigone, 99
Olfactory tubercle, 99
Oligoastrocytoma, 613
Oligodendrocytes
    in brain myelin elaboration, 538–539
    in intraaxial brain tumors, 611
Oligodendroglial cytoplasmic inclusions, 420
Oligodendroglioma, 612, 613
Olivary complex, superior, 136
Olivary nucleus, 165
Olive, inferior, 68, 165
Olivopontocerebellar atrophy, 420
Olivopontocerebellar degeneration, 483
    gait disturbance in, 485t
Omega-3 fatty acids, 371
Omohyoid muscle, 160, 164, 704
Oncovirus, type C, 531
Ophthalmic artery, 8, 78, 188–190
Ophthalmic herpes zoster, 581
Ophthalmic nerve, 8, 80, 86, 87, 90, 102, 103, 104, 183
    in cavernous sinus, 228
    innervation zone of, 107
    meningeal branch of, 87, 90
    nasal branches of, 15
    tentorial branch of, 15
    in trigeminal nerve territories, 15
Ophthalmic vein, superior, 224
Ophthalmicus, herpes zoster, 108
Ophthalmoplegia, 84
    internuclear, 92
Ophthalmoplegic migraine, 174
Opiate abuse, 398
Opioids
    for herpes zoster virus, 581–582
    withdrawal from, 396
Opponens pollicis muscle, 727, 728
Optic atrophy, 251
Optic canal, 190
Optic chiasm, 7, 9, 70, 90, 225, 228, 226
    anatomy of, 64–67
    anterior lesions of, 66
    central lesions of, 66
    clinical vignette of, 64
    disorder of, 66, 67
    posterior lesions of, 66
    vascular supply of, 64
Optic cup, 58
Optic disc, 56

NEUROLOGY

INDEX

anatomy of, 57
atrophy of, 59
in glaucoma, 60
increased intracranial pressure on, 10–11
Optic fundus, 11
Optic nerve (II), 4, 8, 9, 56, 65, 70, 78, 87, 90, 224, 227
    anatomy of, 57, 58
    clinical appearance of, 58
    disorders of, 57–62
        genetic markers of, 62–63
    distribution of, 5
    elevation and swelling of, 62
    fenestration of for cerebral venous thrombosis, 233
    head of, 57
    layers of, 58
    pathoanatomical correlations of, 57–59
    testing of, 7–11
Optic nerve sheath
    fenestration of, 62
        for increased intracranial pressure, 607
    hemorrhage into, 78
        with ruptured cerebral aneurysm, 251
Optic neuritis, 59
    in benign multiple sclerosis, 540
    in multiple sclerosis, 544
Optic neuropathy, anterior ischemic, 59, 61
Optic radiations
    anatomy of, 69
    disorders of, 69–71
    vascular supply of, 69
Optic tract, 7, 9, 65, 67, 70, 71, 193, 227
    fibers in, 6
Optokinetic nystagmus, 126
Ora serrata, 56
Oral cavity, 146
Orbicularis oculi muscle, 16, 115
Orbicularis oris muscle, 16, 115
Orbit, 82
    nerves of, 87, 90
Orbital apex syndrome, 84
Orbital fissure, superior, 81–83
Orbital fissure syndrome, 83
Orbitofrontal artery
    lateral, 193
    medial, 193
Organophosphates
    autonomic neurotoxicity of, 845
    neurotoxicity of, 823
Organophosphorus compounds
    binding to acetylcholinesterase, 853
    neuromuscular effects of, 855t
Orgasmic postcoital headache, 252
Orientation, examination of, 4
Orofacial dyskinesia, 436
    drugs causing, 434t
Oropharyngeal cavity, 148
Oropharynx, 146
Orthopnea
    in motor neuron disease, 791
    treatment of, 792
Orthosis, for foot drop, 773
Orthostatic hypotension, 280
    treatment of, 846–847
Orthostatic tremor, 427–428
Orthotic devices, cervical spine, 669
Ortriptyline, 581–582
Oscillopsia, 130

Osmotic agents, 312–313
Osteoid osteoma, 636
Osteomalacic myopathy, 893
Osteomyelitis, 120
    of skull, 567
Otalgia, hearing loss with, 137
Otic ganglion, 15, 16, 102, 104, 115, 150
Otitis media, 120
Otorrhea, 647
    hearing loss with, 137
    persistent or recurrent, 648
Otosyphilis, 141
Ototoxic drugs, 137
Ouabain, 854t
Overgeneralization, in panic disorder, 378, 380
Overt dysautonomia, 814
Oxcarbazepine, 277
Oxidative breakdown, muscle cell, 917
Oximetry screening, 792
Oxybutynin
    for bladder dysfunction of multiple sclerosis, 554–555
    for multiple system atrophy, 420
Oxygen therapy, 793

P

P-com, 81, 190
    aneurysm of, 77
Pacemakers
    imaging guidelines with, 215t
    for syncope, 280
Paclitaxel (Taxol), 615
Pain
    capelike distribution of, 526, 527
    in lumbar disease, 683
    in multiple sclerosis, 554
    pathways of in migraine, 172
    poorly characterized or vague, 381, 382
    sciatic, 679
    sensation of, 493, 499
        central mechanisms of, 172
    in spinal arteriovenous malformations, 519
    with weakness, 28–30
Pain referral, 171
Pain-sensitive structures, 171
Painful polyneuropathies, 802t
Paired helical filaments, 332
    in Alzheimer disease, 333
Palatal monoclonus, 429
Palatal muscles, paralysis of, 156
Palatal tremor, 429
Palate, soft, 144, 146
    in deglutition, 148, 149
Palatine nerve, 107
    branches of, 15
    greater and lesser, 102, 103
Palatoglossus muscle, 151
Palatopharyngeus muscle, 151, 154
Pallia, 461t
Pallidotomy
    for dystonia, 446
    for movement disorders, 475–477
Palmar arch, superficial, 727
Palmar carpal ligament, 727
Palmaris brevis muscle, 735
Pancoast tumor, 705, 706
    differential diagnosis of, 528

INDEX

Pancreatitis, alcoholic, 391
Pancuronium triethiodide, 855t
Panda bear eyes, 646, 647
Panic attacks, 378
Panic disorders
    clinical presentation of, 378
    diagnosis of, 378
    somatic symptoms of, 379
    treatment of, 380
Papaverine, 256
Papilledema, 62, 100
    blurred vision from, 229
    with cerebral aneurysm, 251
    in cerebral venous thrombosis, 233
    in Horner syndrome, 10–11
    with increased intracranial pressure, 78, 606
    in pseudotumor cerebri, 605
Papillomacular bundle, 57–59
Papovavirus virions, 587
Paracentral artery, 193
Paracentral lobule, 73
Parahippocampal gyrus, 49, 99
Parakinesia, 453, 460
Paralysis, 504
    periodic, 911
        in channelopathies, 909
            diagnosis of, 912
            hyperkalemic and hypokalemic, 910t
    periodic, with carnitine deficiency, 904
Paralytic polio, 598
    differential diagnosis of, 823
Paralytic poliomyelitis, 599
Paramedian artery, 191
Paramedian basilar artery branch occlusion, 92
Paramedian penetrators, 240–241
Parameningeal granuloma, 583
Parameningeal infections, 566–568
Paramyotonia, 909
Paramyotonia congenita, 911–912
    characteristics of, 910t
Paranasal sinus disease, 97
Paraneoplastic autonomic neuropathy
    diagnosis of, 846
    differential diagnosis of, 845
Paraneoplastic cerebellar degenerations, 485
Paraneoplastic myelopathy, 785
Paraneoplastic necrotizing myopathy, 889–891
Paraneoplastic sensory neuronopathy, 835
    differential diagnosis of, 835–836
Paraneoplastic sensory neuropathy, 810
    treatment of, 838
Paraparesis, 25
    with epidural lipomatosis, 521
Paraphasia, with thalamic hemorrhage, 239
Paraplegia, 25
    with epidural spinal abscess, 508
    in multiple sclerosis, 543
    rehabilitation for, 669
Parapontine reticular formation, 91
    in nystagmus, 13
Parasomnias, 292–294
Paraspinous abscess, 584
Parasympathomimetic drugs, 10
Parathion, 853
Parent-child relationship disturbances, 384, 385
Paresis, neurosyphilic, 571, 572
Paresthesia
    with B_{12} vitamin deficiency, 532
    in cervical radiculopathy, 674
    in Guillain-Barré syndrome, 819
    in multiple sclerosis, 544–545
    pathophysiology of, 716
    with posterolateral column lesions, 502
    with shoulder girdle mononeuropathies, 741
    testing techniques for, 722
    in ulnar mononeuropathy, 732
Parietal hematoma, 239
Parietal lobe, 73
    arterial supply to, 190–191
    dysfunction of, 48–49
    efferent pathways from, 500
    surface of, 42
    testing of, 49
    visual pathway in, 51
Parietal lobule, 42
Parietocingulate pathway, 43
Parietooccipital artery, 72, 193
Parietooccipital sulcus, 42
Parietooccipital visual cortex, 76
Parinaud syndrome, 631
PARK1 gene, 402–405
Parkin (PARK2) gene, 402
Parkinson, James, 402
Parkinson disease
    biochemical pathways of, 403
    clinical presentation of, 402, 405–408
    deep brain stimulation for, 476
    degenerative causes of, 409t
    dementia of, 347–348
    diagnostic evaluation of, 410
    differential diagnosis of, 409–410, 846
    dystonia in, 445
    etiology of, 402–405
    exclusion criteria for, 408t
    future research on, 412–413
    gait dysfunction in, 21
    history of, 472
    impaired smell in, 100
    pathophysiology of, 405
    primary sites of motor disorder in, 26
    rating scales for, 410t
    rigidity in, 32
    surgical treatment for, 475
    treatment of, 411–412
    tremors of, 25, 427t
    voice disorder in, 155, 156
    with Wilson disease, 466
Parkinson gait, 483
Parkinson plus syndromes, 408
Parkinsonian syndromes, atypical, 414–420
Parkinsonism
    in Alzheimer disease, 341
    clinical stages of, 484
    with dementia, 358
    drug-induced, 432–435
    drugs causing, 433t
    psychogenic, 473
Parkinsonism toxins, 410
Parosmia, 7
Parotid duct, 122
Parotid gland, 122, 150, 160, 844
    adenocarcinoma of, 124–125
Paroxysmal atrial fibrillation, 195–198
Paroxysmal hemicrania, 177

INDEX

chronic, 176
  in subarachnoid hemorrhage, 252
Pars compacta degeneration, 405
Parsonage-Turner syndrome, 705, 712
Partial limb weakness, 25
Partial sensory seizures, 51
Past pointing, 21
Patellar muscle stretch reflex, diminished or absent, 752–754
Patent foramen ovale, 199, 209
Patient expectations, 2
Patient-physician relationship, positive, 2–3
Pectineus muscle, 753, 758
Pectoral nerve
  lateral, 703, 704
  medial, 703, 704
Pectoralis major muscle, 704
Pectoralis minor muscle, 704
Pectoralis minor tendon, 704
Peduncular hallucinosis, 241
Pemoline
  for fatigue of multiple sclerosis, 554
  for tics, 465
Penicillamine, 470
Penicillin
  for acute rheumatic fever, 459
  for brain abscess, 568
  for neurosyphilis, 573
Penicillin G, 564
Penile implants, 847
Pentobarbital, 275
Pentose shunt, 917
Percussion myotonic reaction, 899
Percutaneous esophagogastrostomy, 792
Perforating cutaneous nerve, 711
Pericallosal artery, 193
  posterior, 193
Pericallosal vein, posterior, 226
Perifascicular muscle atrophy, 890, 891
Periglomerular cell, 99
Perimesencephalic subarachnoid hemorrhage, 255
Perimetric devices, 7
Perimetry
  in glaucoma, 60
  retinal, 56
Periodic limb movements, 292
Peripheral facial paralysis, 120
Peripheral facial paresis, 113
Peripheral motor unit disorders, 748
Peripheral nerve cell body disorders, 835
Peripheral nerve disease
  clinical presentation of, 800–803
  defining neuropathic pattern in, 803
  diagnostic approach to, 804–806
  differential diagnosis of, 803–804
  treatment and prognosis of, 806–807
Peripheral nerves
  anatomy of, 717
  axons of, 818
  lesions of, 719
Peripheral nervous system
  disorders of, 128
  motor neuron pathway in, 765
  in muscle weakness, 30
  vasculitis of, 822–823
Peripheral neuropathy, 23
  autonomic and somatic nerves affected in, 802

heavy metal poisoning in, 813
  in Lambert-Eaton myasthenic syndrome, 861
  motor function in, 800–801
  in multiple sclerosis, 545
  sensory modalities in, 36
  sensory symptoms of, 801–802
Peripheral vestibulopathies, 129–130
Peripherin, gene mutation for, 54
Peristalsis, pharyngeal, 146
Peritonsillar abscess, 594–596
Pernicious anemia, 533
Peroneal nerve, 709
  common, 750, 751
  common fibular, 747
  compression of, 747
    management of, 754
  deep, 747
  iatrogenic injury of, 746
  injury of with foot drop, 23
  superficial fibular, 747
Peroneal neuropathy
  clinical presentation of, 746–748
  deep, 748
  differential diagnosis of, 748–749
  superficial, 748
Persistent asymmetric tonic reflex, 440
Personality disorder, obsessive-compulsive, 375–377
Pes cavus, 809
  in chronic neuropathies, 814–816
PET scan
  in Alzheimer disease, 343
  for chorea, 458
  for epilepsy, 264, 282–284
Petit mal seizures, 271–272
Petit pas gait, 26
Petrosal nerve
  deep, 16, 115, 150
  greater, 16, 87, 90, 112, 115, 114, 150
  lesser, 15, 87, 102, 104, 115, 150
Petrosal sinus
  inferior, 194, 224, 229
  superior, 194, 224, 229
  thrombosis of, 231
Petrosal vein, 224, 227
Petrous ridge, 116
Phalen maneuver, 726–730
Pharyngeal artery, ascending, 189
Pharyngeal constrictor muscles, 151, 154
Pharyngeal neurologic disorders, 156
Pharyngeal plexus, 144, 150, 151, 154
Pharyngeal swallow, 146
Pharyngeal wall, 144
Pharyngeal weakness, 907t
Pharyngopalatine muscle, 148
Pharyngotympanic tube, 114, 135, 150, 151, 154
Pharynx, structures in, 149
Phenobarbital, 277
Phenothiazines
  dystonic reactions to, 441
  in secondary dystonia, 443
  in tetanus, 596
  toxic retinopathy of, 54
Phenylalanine, 368
Phenylephrine hydrochloride (Neo-Synephrine), 256
Phenytoin
  in asterixis, 429

INDEX

for epilepsy, 277
for status epilepticus, 275
for trigeminal neuralgia, 106
Phlebitis, deep venous, 752
Phonemic tics, 460, 462
simple and complex, 461t
Phosphoglycerate kinase deficiency, 914
Photoreceptors, 54, 55
Phrenic nerve, 160, 703, 704
Physaliferous cells, 633
Physical therapy, 474
Physostigmine, 855t
at neuromuscular junction, 857
Pia, 493
Pia mater
overlying spinal cord, 495
spinal, 496
Pick bodies, cortical, 352
Pick cells, 352
Pick complex, 351
Pick disease, 351
clinical presentation of, 40, 352–354
treatment of, 354–355
Picornaviridae, 598
Pie in the sky defect, 69
Pigmenturia, 914
Pill-rolling tremor, 427
Pilocytic astrocytoma, 611, 618
Pimozide
for chorea, 459
for tics, 465
Pinch strength, 722
Pineal parenchyma tumors, 633
Pineal tumors, 419, 631, 633
Pineoblastoma, 631, 633
Pineocytoma, 633
Ping-pong ball skull depression, 648
Pinpoint pupils, 296
Piracetam, 452
Piriform lobe, 99
Piriformis muscle, 711, 751
nerve to, 711
Piriformis syndrome, 750–751
Pisiform, 727, 735
Pituitary apoplexy, 626
Pituitary gland, 73, 224, 228
adenoma of, 66
clinical presentation of, 626–627
diagnostic approach to, 628
nonsecreting, 626
treatment of, 628
macroadenoma of, 628
microadenoma of, 628
tumors of
anatomic classification of, 627
functional classification of, 627
suprasellar extension of, 627
Plantar digital nerves
common, 761
proper, 761
Plantar nerve
lateral, 750, 751, 761
medial, 750, 751, 761
neuropathies of, 760
Plantar stimulation, 4
Plantaris muscle, 750, 751
Plasma exchange

for autonomic nervous system disorders, 847
for multiple sclerosis, 553
for stiff person syndrome, 798
Plasmapheresis
for acquired demyelinating polyradiculoneuropathy, 818
for acute disseminated encephalomyelitis, 555
for childhood-onset obsessive-compulsive disorder, 377
for Lambert-Eaton myasthenic syndrome, 862
for multiple sclerosis, 553
for myasthenia gravis, 865, 866
Plate petechial hemorrhage, 242
Platelet-fibrin aggregation, 197
in arterial dissection, 211
Platelets
aggregation of, 196
in arterial thrombosis, 197
Platysma, 16, 115
Pleura, 496
Plexopathy, 36, 159
brachial, 700–707
differential diagnosis of, 723, 730
lumbosacral, 708–714
PMP22 gene mutations, 719
Pneumococcal meningitis, 560–562
vaccine for, 565
Pneumococcal vaccination, 792
Pneumonia, bacterial, 560–562
POEMS syndrome, 824
Polio vaccine, 597–598
oral, 599
Poliomyelitis, 159, 167
abortive, 598
clinical presentation of, 597, 598
diagnostic approach to, 600
differential diagnosis of, 823
etiology of, 598, 599
neuronal lesions in, 600
pathogenesis of, 598, 599
in peripheral facial paralysis, 120
transmission of, 597
vaccines for, 597–598
Polyarteritis nodosa
in intracerebral hemorrhage, 246
with mononeuritis multiplex, 828
Polycythemia, 141
Polymerase chain reaction (PCR) analysis
for cryptococcus, 592
for herpes simplex encephalitis, 576
for tuberculous meningitis, 583
Polymyalgia rheumatica, 180
Polymyositis, 791, 886
clinical presentation of, 885
diagnosis of, 890
differential diagnosis of, 867
treatment of, 882, 891, 904
Polyneuropathy
with autonomic nervous system involvement, 803t
differential diagnosis of, 730, 822–823
dysautonomia with, 845
generalized, 36
length-dependent, 805t
clinical presentation of, 808–814, 834, 835
diagnostic approach to, 816
differential diagnosis of, 803–804, 814–816
large fiber, sensory predominant, 806t
length-dependent sensory, 838t
painful, 802t

INDEX

primary autonomic, 843–847
pure motor or predominantly motor, 802t
treatment and prognosis of, 816–817
Polyomavirus, 586–588
Polyradiculoneuropathy, 805t, 810–814
    chronic inflammatory demyelinating, 818–826
    differential diagnosis of, 804
    inflammatory demyelinating, 803
    large fiber, sensory predominant, 806t
Pons, 24, 73, 500, 766, 767
    hemorrhage of, 238
Pontine
    efferent pathway to, 766
    gliomas of, 620
        differential diagnosis of, 791
        facial myokymia in, 124
    hemorrhage of, 240–241
    intramedullary lesions of, 113
Pontine artery, 193
Pontine reticular formation, 12
    projections of, 30
Pontine tegmentum
    arterial supply to, 191
    reticular nucleus of, 68
Pontocerebellar connections, 500, 766
Pontomedullary junction, 191
Pontomesencephalic veins, anterior, 227
Pontoreticulospinal tract, 498
Popliteus muscle, 751
    nerve to, 751
Porphyria, 823, 845
Portus acusticus, 116
Position sense loss
    with Friedreich ataxia, 534
    in multiple sclerosis, 543
Positional vertigo test, 18
Postcentral sulcus, 42
Postchiasmatic defects, 64
Postencephalitic parkinsonism, 409
Posterior column syndrome, 523
Posterior fossa
    hematoma of, 649
    lesions of, 657
Posterior interosseous syndrome, 736–737
Posterolateral column lesions, 502
Postictal stupor, 272
Postpolio syndrome, 598
    differential diagnosis of, 780
Postsynaptic membrane, 852, 856, 857
Postural instability, 407, 408
Postural orthostatic tachycardia syndrome, 846
Postural tremor, drug-induced, 433t
Posturography, 489
Potassium
    abnormalities of, 912
    for channelopathies, 912–913
Potassium metabolism disorders, 888
Pott disease, 584, 585
    in spinal epidural abscess, 566
Pott puffy tumor, 230
Praxis, constructional, 44
Praziquantel, 588
Precentral gyrus, 42
    motor centers on, 24
Precentral sulcus, 73
Precentral vein, 227
Prechiasmal plexus, 64

Prechiasmatic defects, 64
Preculminate vein, 227
Precuneal artery, 193
Prednisone
    for chronic inflammatory demyelinating polyradiculoneuropathy, 825
    for facial palsy, 119
    for length-dependent polyneuropathy, 816
    for multifocal neuropathies, 832–833
    for myasthenia gravis, 868
    for myopathies, 882
    for sarcoidosis, 833
Prefrontal artery, 193
Prefrontal circuit dysfunction, dorsolateral, 357
Prefrontal lobe, 45
Preganglionic parasympathetic fibers, 112
Pregnancy
    migraine in, 174
    multiple sclerosis during, 555
    pseudotumor cerebri during, 605
Prenatal abducens nerve dysgenesis, 83
Preoccipital notch, 42
Presbycusis, 141
Presenilins, 327–329
Pressure palsy, hereditary tendency to, 124, 827
    differential diagnosis of, 831
    DNA mutational analysis of, 832
    treatment and prognosis of, 833
Pressure sensation, 499
Presynaptic neuromuscular transmission disorders, 861–862
Pretectum, 68
Prevotella *brain abscess*, 568
Primary lateral sclerosis (PLS), 764
    clinical classification of, 769t
    clinical presentation of, 783–784
    diagnosis of, 784–785
    differential diagnosis of, 784–785
    future research on, 788
    patient evaluation for, 788t
    treatment and prognosis of, 785–788
Primary motor cortex, 767
Primary progressive aphasia, 351
Primidone (Mysoline)
    for epilepsy, 277
    for essential tremor, 426t
Primitive neuroectodermal tumors, 616–618
Princeps pollicis artery, 727
Prion diseases, gait disorders in, 486–488
Prion protein (PrP^c), 361
Prions, 588
Prismatic glasses, 88
Probe-patent foramen ovale transmitting venous clots, 215
Procaine, 854t
Procarbazine, 613
Procerus muscle, 16, 115
Progressive bulbar palsy (PBP)
    clinical classification of, 769t
    clinical presentation of, 789–790
    differential diagnosis of, 790–791
    treatment and prognosis of, 792–793
Progressive bulbar palsy (PBS), 764
Progressive multifocal leukoencephalopathy (PML), 362
Progressive muscular atrophy (PMA), 764, 765
    clinical classification of, 769t
    with lower motor neuron features, 777
    prognosis of, 782

INDEX

Progressive supranuclear palsy, 415t
    clinical presentation of, 416–417
    diagnosis of, 417
    etiology of, 416
    pathophysiology of, 416
    treatment of, 417
Prolactin secreting tumors, 627
    treatment of, 628
Prolactinoma, 626
Promontory, 135
Pronator syndrome, 730, 731
Pronator teres muscle, compression neuropathy at, 722
Pronator teres syndrome, 732
Propofol, 313
Propranolol, 426t
Proprioception, 499
    impaired, 502
    loss of, 23
Proprioceptive neurons, 106
Prostacyclin, secretion of, 197
Prostaglandins, 847
Protein C deficiency, 199
Protein electrophoresis, 815
Protein S deficiency, 199
Prothrombin gene mutation, 199
Protriptyline, 289–291
Proximal myotonic myopathy, 894–897
PrP gene mutation, 361
Pseudo-Graefe sign, 82
Pseudobulbar affect, 783
    in motor neuron disease, 774t
Pseudobulbar palsy, 789–790
Pseudoclaudication, 693
Pseudoptosis, 83
Pseudotumor cerebri, 62, 181, 604–607
Psoas major muscle, 710, 711, 753, 758
Psychiatric evaluation, 282
Psychic sensation, 460
Psychic tension, 460
Psychogenic movement disorders
    clinical presentation of, 472–473
    diagnostic evaluation of, 474
    differential diagnosis of, 473
    etiology of, 473
    future research on, 474
    treatment and prognosis of, 474
Psychophysiologic insomnia, 288
Psychosis, 366
Psychosomatic back pain
    clinical presentation of, 694
    diagnosis of, 696
    history of, 694–696
    treatment of, 696
Psychostimulants, abuse of, 398
Psychotherapy
    for dysthymia, 383
    for major depression, 367
    for panic disorder, 380
    for psychogenic movement disorders, 474
    for schizophrenia, 374
Pterygoid canal
    nerve of, 103
    vidian nerve of, 15, 16, 102, 115, 150
Pterygoid hamulus, 104
Pterygoid muscle
    lateral, 104, 106
    medial, 104, 106, 122
Pterygoid nerve
    lateral, 15, 102, 104
    medial, 15, 102
Pterygoid plexus, 81
Pterygopalatine ganglion, 15, 16, 80, 86, 102, 103, 112, 115, 150
    ganglionic branches to, 103
Ptosis
    in diabetes, 79
    in myasthenia gravis, 866
    in oculomotor palsy, 78
Pubic ramus, superior, 711
Pudendal artery, internal, 711
Pudendal nerve, 494, 711
Puffer fish toxin, 854t
Pulvinar, 38, 68, 71, 193, 225
Pulvinar vein, 227
Pupil
    in comatose patients, 81
    dilator muscle of, 80, 86
    dilator of, 8
    direct and consensual reactions of, 9
    examination of, 9
    parasympathetic, 82
    parasympathetic inputs to, 9–10
    sphincter muscle of, 80, 86
    sphincter of, 8
    unilateral dilatation of, 648
Pupillae sphincter paralysis, 77
Pupillary abnormalities, 10t
Pupillary dilatation. See *Mydriasis*
Pupillary light reflex, 302
Pupillary reactivity, 303–304
    in coma, 311
    with increase intracranial pressure, 308
Pupillary responses, 9
Purine myopathy, 920t
Putamen, 500, 766
Putaminal hemorrhage, 236, 237, 238
Pyomyositis, 889
Pyramidal cells, 72
Pyramidal system, 24
Pyramids, 165, 766
    decussation of, 24, 500, 766
Pyrazinamide, 585
Pyridostigmine bromide (Mestinon)
    for Lambert-Eaton myasthenic syndrome, 862
    for myasthenia gravis, 864, 868
Pyridoxine, 836
Pyrimethamine, 590

Q

Quadrantanopia, 251
Quadratus femoris muscle, nerve to, 711
Quadratus lumborum muscle, 710
Quadratus plantar muscle, 751, 761
Quadratus plantar nerve, 761
Quadriceps femoris muscle, 753, 758
Quadrilateral tunnel syndrome, 744
Quadriparesis, 241
Quadriplegia, 25
    with hyperextension injury, 661
    rehabilitation for, 669
Quantitative sensory testing, 846

INDEX

R

Rabies, 576–578
   encephalitis form of, 576–578
   paralytic form of, 578
Raccoon eyes, 646, 647
Radial artery, 727
   palmar branches of, 727
   recurrent, 736–737
Radial nerve, 703, 704, 705
   compression of, 716, 722, 736, 737–738
   entrapment of, 736
   superficial, 736–737
Radial neuropathy, 706, 723
   management of, 739
   predominant motor, 736
   predominant sensory, 736
Radial tunnel, compression neuropathy at, 722
Radial tunnel syndrome
   provocative tests for, 737
   sensory signs of, 736–737
Radialis indicis artery, 727
Radiation injury, spinal, 780
Radiation therapy
   for anaplastic glioma, 614
   for CNS lymphoma, 618
   for glioblastoma multiforme, 615
   in hypoglossal damage, 167
   for intramedullary spinal cord tumors, 642
   for low-grade gliomas, 613
   for lumbar radiculopathy, 689
   for malignant brain tumors, 620–621
   for meningioma, 624
   for metastatic brain tumors, 616
   for nerve sheath tumors, 641
   for spinal cord meningioma, 526
   for spinal cord tumors, 640
Radiculopathy, 36–37, 159
   cervical, 672–677
   lumbar, 679–689, 709–712
Radiography
   for lumbosacral plexopathies, 709
   for mononeuropathies with lower extremity weakness, 754
   for shoulder mononeuropathies, 745
Ragged red fibers, 879, 920
Ramsay-Hunt syndrome, 119, 581
   facial palsy in, 117
Ranvier, node of, 717
Rasmussen encephalitis, 268
Raymond syndrome, 92
Reanastomosis, 725
Rebleeding, cerebral aneurysm, 255–256
Recombinant tissue plasminogen activator
   contraindications for, 217t
   for ischemic stroke, 217
Rectus capitis posterior major muscle, 184
Rectus capitis posterior minor muscle, 184
Rectus femoris muscle, 753
Rectus motor neurons, 13
Rectus muscle, 86, 87, 90, 91
   in nystagmus, 13
   superior, 80, 82
Red nucleus, 6, 105, 403, 500, 766
Red thrombus, 197
Reflex signs, cervical herniated disc, 675t
Reflex sympathetic dystrophy, 701
Reflexive eye movements, 308

Reflexive vestibular-ocular movement, 19
Rehabilitation
   for cervical spine injury, 669
   for gait disorders, 489
   for spinal injury, 662
   vestibular, 132
Relaxation techniques, 288
REM sleep, 291
   deprivation of for depression, 368
REM sleep behavior disorder, 292–293
Renal failure, 300
Renshaw cell bias, 795
Renshaw cell inhibitory input, 794–795
Repetitive motion nerve injury, 720
Repolarization, 850
Reserpine
   for chorea, 459
   for tardive dyskinesia, 436–437
Respiratory alkalosis, hyperventilation-induced, 378
Respiratory arrest, 796
Respiratory chain disorders, 916t
   diagnosis of, 920
Respiratory chorea, 455
Respiratory compromise, 822
Respiratory disorders, with dysphagia, 152
Respiratory failure, 865
   with myasthenia gravis, 870
Respiratory infection, upper, 97
Respiratory muscle myotomy
   treatment of, 921
Respiratory muscle weakness, 864, 865
Respiratory stimulant medications, 289–291
Reticular formation, 37, 500
   efferent pathway to, 766
Reticulospinal tract, 499
   lateral and medial, 786, 787
Retina, 9
   anatomy and physiology of, 54
   architecture and perimetry of, 56
   changes in with cerebral aneurysm, 78, 251
   disease of, 54
      genetic markers of, 62–63
   layers of, 55
   neuroarchitecture of, 56
   photoreceptors and, 55
   projections on, 9, 70
   tomographic optical sectioning of, 62
Retinal artery, 54, 56
   central, 190
Retinal nerve
   fibers of, 58
   topography of, 56
Retinal vein, 56
Retinal vessels, 56
Retinitis pigmentosa, 54
Retrobulbar neuritis, 61
Retrocochlear lesions, 138
Retrograde amnesia, 324
Retroperitoneal hematoma, 712, 759
Retroperitoneal infections, 712–713
Retroperitoneal neoplasms, 759
Retrotonsillar vein
   inferior, 227
   superior, 227
Reverse counting, 44
Rhabdomyolysis, 920
Rheumatic chorea, 459

NEUROLOGY

INDEX

Rheumatic fever, 457
Rheumatic heart disease, 244–245
Rheumatic valvular disease, 198
Rheumatoid factor, 458
Rheumatologic back pain
    clinical presentation of, 694
    diagnosis of, 696
    history of, 694–696
    treatment of, 696
Rhinorrhea, 647
    persistent or recurrent, 648
Rhodopsin, gene mutation for, 54
Ribs, first, 494
Rifampin
    for leprosy, 841
    for tuberculous meningitis, 585
Rigid limbs, 31
Rigidity, 30, 32
    decerebrate, 31, 32
    in dementia with Lewy bodies, 349
    in Parkinson gait, 483
    in parkinsonism, 405, 407, 408
Riley Day syndrome, 846
Riluzole, 775, 781
Rinne test, 14–19, 17, 139
Risperidone, 465
Risus sardonicus, 594, 595
Ritualistic behaviors, 352–354
Rivastigmine
    for Alzheimer disease, 343
    for dementia with Lewy bodies, 350
Rocking bed, 662
Rod photoreceptor, 55
Rods, in light and dark, 55
Rolandic spikes, 274
Romberg sign
    with B_{12} vitamin deficiency, 532
    in neurosyphilis, 571
    in peripheral nerve disease, 803
    in peripheral vestibulopathies, 132
    in spinal cord degeneration, 533
Rosenthal, basal veins of, 67, 194
Rostrocaudal deterioration, 307–312
Rotating frame, 662
Rotator cuff tear, 743
Round window, 135
Rubeosis iridis, 79
Rubral tremor, 429
Rubrospinal tract, 498, 499, 786, 787
    origin of, 500–501
Ruffini terminals, 34
Ryanodine receptors, 850

S

Saccade, 126
Saccadic center, 13
Saccadic movement, 13
Saccular aneurysms, 255
    management of, 257–258
Saccule, 114, 127, 135
Sacral nerves, 497
    perineal branch of, 711
Sacral plexus, 494, 711
    compression of, 708
Sacral spinal nerves, dorsal and ventral roots of, 835
Sacral splanchnic nerves, 711

Sacrum, 494
    chordoma of, 630
Sagittal sinus
    inferior, 194, 224, 225, 227, 226
    meningioma invading, 623
    superior, 194, 224, 225, 228, 227, 226
Sagittal sinus thrombosis, 231
    superior, 229
Salicylates, ototoxicity of, 137
Saliva, 146
    secretion of, 860
Salivary gland
    adenocarcinoma of, 110
    biopsy of, 836
Salivation, 112
Salivatory nucleus, 6, 105
    inferior, 150
    superior, 16, 115
Salpingopharyngeus muscle, 151, 154
Saphenous nerve, 753, 758, 761
    infrapatellar branch of, 753, 758
    medial crural cutaneous branches of, 758
Sarcoid myopathy, 882
Sarcoidosis, 4
    in chronic myopathy, 893
    in cranial neuropathies, 4
    differential diagnosis of, 785, 841
    facial palsy in, 117
    in facial paralysis, 120
    in intracerebral hemorrhage, 246
    treatment of, 833
Sarcolemma, 851, 852, 853, 856
    folds of, 851, 852, 853
Sarcoma, trigeminal, 109–110
Sarcoplasm, 851, 852, 853, 856, 857
Sarcoplasmic reticulum, 856
Sartorius muscle, 753, 758
Satellite vessel rupture, 236
Saxitoxin, 854t
Scala vestibuli, 135
Scalene muscle, 703
    anterior, 160, 704
    middle, 160
Scalp injury, 644–646
Scapula, 161
    winging of, 159, 161, 742, 743, 895
Scapular artery, dorsal, 160, 704
Scapular nerve, dorsal, 703, 704
Scapuloperoneal muscular dystrophy, 896t, 900
Schirmer test, 125
Schistosoma mansoni infection, 510
Schizophrenia
    ambulatory or pseudoneurotic, 384
    clinical presentation of, 372–373
    forme fruste of, 384
    incidence and prevalence of, 372
    treatment of, 373–374
Schizophrenogenic mothers, 372
Schwann cell, 98, 717, 851, 852, 856
    nucleus of, 852
Schwannoma, 4
    in facial palsy, 121
    intradural spinal cord, 640
    in lumbar radiculopathy, 686
    spinal cord, 635
    trigeminal, 109
    vestibular, 140

INDEX

Sciatic nerve, 494, 709, 711, 749, 750
    common peroneal segment of, 750
    tibial segment of, 750
Sciatic neuropathy, 748
    clinical presentation of, 749
    differential diagnosis of, 750–751
Sciatica. See *Lumbar radiculopathy*
Scintillating scotoma, 173
Sclera, 56
Scleral venous sinus, 56
Sclerosis, sacroiliac joint, 694
Scoliosis
    with Friedreich ataxia, 535
    with spinal poliomyelitis, 600
Scopolamine, 132
Scotoma, 57, 59
    central, 61, 75–76
    junctional, 67
    posterior junctional, 66
    scintillating, 173
Scrapie, 360
Seborrheic dermatitis, 407, 408
Secretion clearance, 774t
Sedative-hypnotics, abuse of, 398
Sedative-precipitated delirium, 399, 400
Segawa syndrome, 442–443
Segmental cervical spinal muscular atrophy, 706–707
Seizures
    with alcohol withdrawal, 395
    alcoholism and, 393
    with arteriovenous malformations, 609
    with bacterial meningitis, 564–565
    in benign multiple sclerosis, 540
    causes of, 270
    in cerebral venous thrombosis, 232, 233
    chronic, in immunocompromised hosts, 588
    complex partial, 267, 268–271
    generalized, 271–274
    in immunocompromised hosts, 588
    intracranial hemorrhage and, 237
    with lobar hemorrhage, 239
    origin and spread of, 263
    partial, with secondary generalization, 271
    partial sensory and autonomic, 51
    simple partial, 264–271
    in subarachnoid hemorrhage, 249
    temporal lobe tumor in, 129
    treatment of in increased intracranial pressure, 314
Selective serotonin reuptake inhibitors (SSRIs)
    for frontotemporal dementia, 355
    for major depression, 367
    for narcolepsy, 291
    for obsessive-compulsive disorder, 375–377
    for syncope, 280
Selegiline, 412
Sella turcica, 64
    enlargement or erosion of, 627
Semantic dementia, 354
Semicircular canal, 127
    caloric testing of, 309
    in nystagmus, 13
Semicircular duct, 114, 135
Semimembranosus muscle, 750
Semispinalis capitis muscle, 184
Semispinalis cervicis muscle, 184
Semitendinosus muscle, 750
Senile plaques, 327–329, 331, 334

Senile tremor, 424
Senses, cranial nerves in, 4
Sensitivity value, 7
Sensorimotor stroke, 211t
Sensorineural hearing loss, 137
    etiologies of, 138
Sensory ataxia, 836–838
Sensory dissociation, 505
Sensory dysfunction syndromes, 36–39
Sensory examination, 35–39
Sensory fibers
    cranial, distribution of, 5
    of facial nerve, 112
    injury of, 721–723
Sensory loss
    with B_{12} vitamin deficiency, 532
    with cervical herniated disc, 675t
    dissociated, 38
    in leprosy, 840
    in motor disorders, 26
    in myelopathy, 492
    in spinal cord degeneration, 533
    with syringomyelia, 526, 528
    with weakness, 28–30
Sensory modalities
    evaluation of, 4
    in peripheral neuropathy, 36
Sensory nerve action potentials, 532
Sensory nerves
    biopsy of in polyneuropathies, 806
    conduction testing of, 837
Sensory neuronopathy, 834–838
Sensory neuropathy, 806t
    clinical presentation of, 834–835
    diagnostic approach to, 836
    differential diagnosis of, 804, 835–836
    etiology of, 834–835
    of forearm, 738
    hereditary, 837
    length-dependent, 814
    of lower extremity, 757–762
    treatment and prognosis of, 836–838
Sensory threshold testing, 722
Sensory tics, 461t
Sensory tracts, 24
    ascending, 493
Septal vein
    anterior, 226
    posterior, 226
Septomarginal fasciculus, 498
Septum pellucidum, 225
    anterior vein of, 225
Serologic tests, 836, 879
Serratus anterior muscle, 161, 704, 742
    weakness of, 743
Sex addiction, 375
Shape perception, 73
Shear injury, cerebral, 655–657
Shellfish toxin, 854t
Shiatsu massage, 554
Shingles, 579–582
    headache and, 185–186
Shirmer test, 836
Short ciliary nerve, 8
Shoulder
    chronic myopathies involving, 892–893

INDEX

mononeuropathies of
    future research on, 745
    management and prognosis of, 745
  pain and weakness of in mononeuropathies, 741–745
  proximal mononeuropathies of, 743–744
Shoulder girdle
  mononeuropathies of
    clinical presentation of, 741–743
    differential diagnosis of, 743
  weakness of, 706
Shunt placement, 219
Shy-Drager syndrome, 280, 420
  differential diagnosis of, 846
Sialorrhea, 774t
Sick sinus syndrome, 195
Sickle cell anemia, 141
Sigmoid sinus, 194, 224, 228
Sildenafil, 847
Sinus headache, 186
Sinus recanalization, 233
Sinuses, confluence of, 224, 225, 228, 227
Sinuvertebral nerve, 684
Situational syncope, 278
Sixth cranial nerve palsy, 79, 89
Sixth cranial nerve paresis, 89
Sjögren syndrome
  diagnosis of, 836
  differential diagnosis of, 835
  polyneuropathies in, 810
  treatment of, 838
  trigeminal involvement of, 108
Skeletal muscle, 765
  channelopathies affecting, 910t
Skill movement, spinal tracts for, 493–500
Skin punch biopsy, 846
Skin receptors, 35
Skull
  base of, 494, 497
    trigeminal lesions of, 108t
    tumors of, 110
  basilar fracture of, 647
  erosion of, 572
  fractures of, 646
  osteomyelitis of, 567
Sleep
  deprivation of for depression, 368
  disturbances in
    in dysthymia, 381, 382
    in motor neuron disease, 774t
    in muscle contraction headache, 178
    in parkinsonism, 407, 408
  periodic limb movements of, 448
Sleep apnea syndrome, 288–289
  clinical presentation of, 289
  diagnosis and treatment of, 289–291
Sleep disorders, 288–294
Sleep hygiene, 288
Sleep paralysis, 290
Sleep state misperception disorder, 288
Sleeping sickness, 409
Sleepwalking, 294
Slow virus infections, 362, 586–588
Small cell anaplastic carcinoma, metastatic, 617
Small cell lung carcinoma, 858
  neuromuscular manifestations of, 861
Small-fiber sensory dysfunction, 801
Small-fiber sensory neuropathy, 814

Small-vessel disease, 199
  dementia with, 357
Smell
  distortion of, 7
  evaluation of, 96
  impaired sense of, 100
Smile, asymmetric, 3
Smith craniotome drill, 656
Snellen vision chart, 7
Snoring, 289
Social workers, 772
Sodium amobarbital test, 283
Sodium amytal test, 281–282
Sodium channel blockers, 582
Sodium channel myotonia, 909, 910t
Sodium valproate
  for asterixis, 429
  for migraine, 175
Soft tissue injuries, 644–646
Soleus muscle, 750, 751
Solitary tract nucleus, 6, 16, 105, 115, 145, 150, 151, 154, 500, 766
Somatic nerve neuropathy, 802
Somatosensory association cortex, 73
Somatosensory evoked potentials
  in multiple sclerosis, 549, 550
  for myoclonus, 451–452
Somatostatin analog, 628
Somesthetic system, 37
Somnambulism, 294
Sound reception, pathway of, 135
Sound waves, 134
Spasmodic dysphonia, 156, 441
Spastic gait, 23
  in multiple sclerosis, 542
Spastic paraparesis tropical. See *HTLV-1 myelopathy*
Spastic paraplegia, hereditary
  clinical presentation of, 528, 529
  diagnosis and treatment of, 529
  pathophysiology and etiology of, 528–529
Spastic quadriparesis, 783
Spastic quadriplegia, 440
Spastic release, 32
Spasticity, 30, 32
  treatment of in primary lateral sclerosis, 785
  in Wilson disease, 469
Spatial disorientation, 50
Spatial visual pathway, 73
SPECT scanning
  in Alzheimer disease, 343
  for epilepsy, 264, 282–284
Speech
  assessment of, 3–4
  decreased discrimination of, 138
  impairment of, 163
    with progressive bulbar palsy, 790
  motor control of, 43
  nerves in, 4
  slurred, 4
Speech discrimination evaluation, 138
Speech prosody, 352
Speech therapy, 156
SPG3 gene, 529
SPG4 gene mutation, 528–529
Sphenoid sinus, 65, 81, 90
Sphenoparietal sinus, 194, 224, 225
Spinal abscess, epidural, 506–508

INDEX

Spinal accessory nerve, 157
   anatomy of, 157–159
   disorders of
      clinical findings in, 161
      clinical presentation and diagnostic approach to, 159
      differential diagnosis of, 159
      prognosis for, 160
   mononeuropathy of, 743–744
Spinal accessory nerve palsies, 159
Spinal artery
   anterior, 191, 193, 501
      damage to, 502
      infarction of, 38–39
   posterior, 191, 193, 501
Spinal artery syndrome
   anterior, 512
   posterior, 512
Spinal border cells, 33, 499
Spinal canal, 493
   narrowed, 514, 687, 692
Spinal cord, 766
   acute extradural lesions of, 503–508
   acute injury to, 503–506
   anatomy of, 494
   bulging of, 527
   compression of, 662
      with hyperextension injury, 661
      in spondylosis, 514–515, 516
   cross sections of, 498
   gait disturbances with disorders of, 488
   gross anatomy of, 493
   infarction of, 511–512
   internal structure of, 493
   intradural intramedullary lesions of, 509–512
   Intramedullary tumors of, 502
   lumbar, 844
   meningioma of, 521–526
   in motor disorders, 26
   in motor tone, 30
   normal segment of, 518
   in pyramidal system, 24
   sacral, 844
   spinal nerves and, 493
   thoracic, 8, 844
   tracts of, 493–501
   traumatic injury of, 658–670
   tumors of
      in acute central disc, 506
      classification of, 637t
      differential diagnosis of, 784
      evolution of symptoms of, 639
      extradural, 635–640
      future treatment of, 642
      intradural, 635
      intradural extramedullary, 638, 640–641
      intradural intramedullary, 641–642
      intramedullary, 638
   vascular supply of, 501
   in weakness, 28
Spinal cord arteriovenous malformations
   clinical presentation of, 517, 519–520
   diagnosis of, 520
   pathophysiology and etiology of, 517–519
   treatment and prognosis of, 520

Spinal cord injury
   chronic intradural extramedullary, 521–526
      myelographic and CT characteristics of, 524
      types of, 522t
   chronic intradural intramedullary, 526–532
      types of, 522t
   diagnostic approach to, 658–662
   myelographic and CT characteristics of, 524
   pathophysiology of, 658
   prognosis for, 663–670
   signs of, 28
   treatment of, 662–669
Spinal cord mass effect, 492–493
Spinal cord syndromes, 38–39
Spinal cord veins, superficial, 501
Spinal dura mater, 494
Spinal epidural abscess, 566–567
Spinal infections, 674
Spinal injury, primary sites of motor disorder in, 26
Spinal mass lesion, thoracic, 822
Spinal membranes, 495
Spinal muscular atrophy, 30, 778
Spinal muscular atrophy (SMA)
   clinical classification of, 769t
   type III, 779
Spinal nerve roots, 495
   filaments of, 494
   ventral, 495
   vertebrae and, 497
Spinal nerves, 158, 160, 493, 494
   anterior primary ramus of, 163
   dorsal ramus of, 495
   dorsal root of, 495
   in motor disorders, 26
   origin of, 496
   recurrent meningeal branches of, 496
   sensory components of, 835
   ventral ramus of, 495, 710
   ventral root of, 495
Spinal nucleus, 165
   of trigeminal nerve, 171
Spinal radiation injury, 780
Spinal radiography
   for cervical radiculopathy, 676
   for lumbar radiculopathy, 686
   for lumbar spinal stenosis, 693
Spinal segmental instability, 689
Spinal sensory ganglion, 495, 496
Spinal shock, 32, 492
   with complete transverse cord lesion, 501
   with spinal cord trauma, 503
Spinal stabilization, 503
   for cervical spine injury, 664
   with spine injury, 662
   for spondylosis, 517
Spinal stenosis, 30, 516
   differential diagnosis of, 682
   lumbar, 691–693
   in lumbar radiculopathy, 688
Spinal tap, 233
Spinal tract, 6, 102
Spinal tumors, 524
Spinal vein
   anterior, 227
   anterior median, 501
   posterior, 227

INDEX

Spine
    traumatic injury of, 658–670
    tuberculosis of, 583–585
Spinocerebellar tract, 165
    anterior, 498
    degeneration of, 533
    dorsal, 33, 493, 499, 787
    evaluation of, 32
    posterior, 498
    rostral, 33
    ventral, 33, 493, 499, 786, 787
Spinohypothalamic fibers, 498
Spinoolivary tract, 498
Spinoreticular tract, 165, 499, 786, 787
Spinothalamic tract, 37, 165, 499, 786, 787
    anterior, 493
    bilateral damage to, 39
    lateral, 493
Spiral ganglion, 136
Splanchnic nerves, 144
    pelvic, 711, 844
Splenius capitis muscle, 184
Splenius cervicis muscle, 184
Splinting
    for carpal tunnel syndrome, 729
    for cubital tunnel syndrome, 734
    for mononeuropathy, 725
    for motor neuron disease, 773
Spondylolisthesis
    of axis, 663
    differential diagnosis of, 682
    spinal stenosis with, 693
Spondylosis
    cervical
        clinical presentation of, 514, 515
        diagnosis of, 515
        pathophysiology and etiology of, 514–515
        treatment of, 515–517
    diagnosis of, 676
    with herniated lumbar disc, 682
    in spinal stenosis, 691–693
Spondylotic disease, degenerative, 686
Spondylotic subluxation, 687
Spongiform encephalopathy
    early cortical involvement of, 362
    gait disorder in, 483–485
    prions in, 588
    transmissible, 360–363
Sporadic motor neuron disease, 769t
Spurling maneuver, 675
Squamous cell carcinoma, trigeminal, 109–110
Stabilization traction board, 665
Stapedius muscle, 16, 115
Stapedius nerve, 16, 115, 113
Stapes, 135
Staphylococcus aureus
    in bacterial meningitis, 562
    in epidural spinal abscess, 508
    in intracerebral hemorrhage, 245
    in spinal epidural abscess, 566
Staphylococcus epidermidis
    in bacterial meningitis, 562
Staphylococcus *epidural infection*, 686
Staphylococcus *meningitis*, 300
Startle disease, 797
Startle-induced spasms, 797
Static perimetry, 7

Statins, toxic, 886–887
Status epilepticus, 265–276
    complex partial, 275
    generalized convulsive, 275
    nonconvulsive, 275
Stellate ganglion, 145
Stellate skull fractures, 646
Stem cell research, 670
Stem cell transplantation
    for motor neuron disease, 775
    for movement disorders, 477
Stents, for stroke, 217
Stereotactic needle guide, 476
Stereotactic radiosurgery
    for acoustic neuromas, 626
    future advances in, 642
    improvements in, 633
    for malignant brain tumors, 620–621
    for movement disorders, 475, 476
Stereotyped motor behavior, 460–461
Stereotypy, in frontotemporal dementia, 352–354
Sternocleidomastoid muscle, 158, 160, 184, 704
    innervation of, 157, 159
    tumors of, 439
    weakness of, 161
Sternohyoid muscle, 160, 164
Sternothyroid muscle, 160, 164
Steroids
    for acute hemorrhagic leukoencephalopathy, 557
    for carpal tunnel syndrome, 729
    for chronic inflammatory demyelinating
        polyradiculoneuropathy, 825
    for cysticercosis, 588
    for Guillain-Barré syndrome, 825
    inducing tremor, 430t
    for lateral femoral nerve neuropathy, 759
    for myasthenia gravis, 868–869
    for myopathies, 882
    for pituitary adenoma, 628
    in pseudotumor cerebri, 604, 605
    for sensory neuropathies of lower extremity, 760
Stiff leg syndrome, 796
Stiff person syndrome
    clinical presentation of, 794, 795–796
    diagnostic approach to, 797
    differential diagnosis of, 796–797
    etiology of, 794–795
    treatment and prognosis of, 798
Stimulants
    for attention deficit disorder, 389
    for fatigue of multiple sclerosis, 554
Straight leg raising, 695
Straight sinus, 194, 224, 225, 228, 227, 226
Strength testing, 25–30
Streptococcal M proteins, 455
Streptococcus *A infection*, 457
    in chorea, 458
Streptococcus aureus, 568
Streptococcus *infections, in obsessive-compulsive disorder*, 377
Streptococcus *meningitis*, 300
Streptococcus *milleri*, 568
Streptococcus pneumoniae
    in bacterial meningitis, 560–561
    vaccine for, 565
Striatal gait disorders, 483
Striate artery, medial, 71, 193

INDEX

Striate cortex, 72
   cells of, 75
   diseases of, 75–76
Striatonigral degeneration. See *Multiple system atrophy*
Striatum, 405
Striofugal system, 403
Striopetal system, 403
Stripping wave, 148–149
Stroke
   affecting optic radiation, 69
   border zone, 202t
   brainstem, 506
   in carotid occlusion, 200
   coma with, 297
   dementia with, 357, 358
   differential diagnosis of, 790
   dysphagia with, 143
   hemispheric, 112
   ischemic
      clinical presentation of, 199–212
      diagnostic approach to, 212–213
      etiology and pathophysiology of, 195–199
      future research on, 217
      treatment of, 213–217
   lacunar, 209–211
   mimicking brachial plexopathies, 707
   with multiple sclerosis, 544
   posterior cerebral artery, 207
   preventing recurrence of, 359
   primary sites of motor disorder in, 26
   pure motor, 211t
   pure sensory, 211t
   risk factors for, 199
   sensorimotor, 211t
   treatment of swallowing problems in, 152
   uncommon etiologic mechanisms of, 215
   vertebrobasilar, 140
Struthers ligament, 733
   compression neuropathy at, 722
Stupor, 296, 322
   in terminal TSE, 363
Stuttering, nonfluent, 47
Styloglossus muscle, 164
Stylohyoid muscle, 16, 104, 115, 160
   nerve to, 122
Stylomastoid foramen, 16, 115, 113, 122, 150
   lesions in, 118
Stylopharyngeus muscle, 146, 150, 154
Subarachnoid hemorrhage, 246, 248–255, 646
   aneurysmal, 248
   clinical presentation of, 249
   diagnostic approach to, 252
   differential diagnosis of, 249–252
   in gait disorders, 481
   headache in, 181
   management of, 255–261
   nonaneurysmal, 248
   pathophysiology of, 252–255
   in persistent vegetative state, 305
Subarachnoid oculomotor nerve, 81
Subarachnoid screw, 653
Subarachnoid space, 496
Subaxial cervical spine injury, 663
Subcallosal area, 99
Subclavian artery, 151, 160, 189, 704
   occlusion of, 198
   stenosis of, 203–204

Subclavian steal, 204
Subclavian vein, 160, 704
Subclavius muscle, 703, 704
Subcortical orbitofrontal circuit dysfunction, 357
Subcorticocortical projection circuits, 337
Subcostal nerve, 494, 710
Subdural abscess, 230, 567
Subdural empyema, 568
Subdural hematoma
   acute, 650, 651, 652, 654
   chronic, 651, 654
   differential diagnosis of, 609
   in gait disorders, 481
   headache in, 181
   in neurosyphilis, 572
   in normal pressure hydrocephalus, 482
   of posterior fossa, 657
   subacute, 651
   with traumatic head injury, 644
Subdural hemorrhage, 246
Subependymal veins, 226
Subependymoma, 632
Subfrontal hematoma, 649
Sublingual gland, 16, 104, 115
Sublingual nerve, 104
Submandibular ganglion, 15, 16, 102, 104, 112, 115
Submandibular gland, 16, 104, 115, 160
Suboccipital nerve, 184
Suboccipital triangle, 184
Subpendymal veins, 225
Subscapular artery, 704
Subscapular nerve, 705
   circumflex, 704
   lower, 703, 704
   upper, 703
Substance P inhibitors, 368
Substantia gelatinosa, 786, 787
Substantia nigra, 403
   depigmented, 404
   destruction of, 423
   in parkinsonism, 405, 406
   section of, 404
   stimulation of for movement disorders, 476
Subthalamic nucleus stimulation, 477
Succinate dehydrogenase evaluation, 879
Succinylcholine, 855t
   in endplate depolarization, 854
   at neuromuscular junction, 857
Suffocation alarm theory, 378
Suicidal ideation, 366
   alcoholism and, 393
   in bipolar disorder, 369
Sulcal vein, 501
Sulfadiazine, 590
Sulfonamides, 589
Sundowning, 399–400
Superoxide dismutase gene (SOD1) mutations, 768
Supinator muscle, 736–737
Suprachiasmatic nucleus, 68
Supraclavicular nerves, 183
Supraclinoid segment aneurysm, 254
Supraclinoid trunk, 64
Supramarginal gyrus, 42
Supraorbital nerve, 15, 87, 90, 102, 103, 107, 183
   branches of, 90
Suprarenal gland, 844
Suprascapular artery, 160, 704

INDEX

Suprascapular nerve, 703, 704, 706
   injury of, 741–743
Suprasellar craniopharyngioma, 628
   large cystic, 629
Supraspinatus muscle, 742
Supratentorial bleeds, 240
Supratentorial hemorrhage, 237–240
Supratrochlear nerve, 15, 87, 90, 102, 103, 183
Sural cutaneous nerve
   lateral, 751
   medial, 750, 751
Sural nerve, 747, 750, 751, 761
   sensory conduction testing of, 837
Surgery
   for brain abscess, 568
   for cervical radiculopathy, 676–677
   for dystonia, 446
   for epilepsy, 278, 281–286
   with lumbar radiculopathy, 689
   for movement disorders, 475–477
   for pituitary adenoma, 628
   for spinal arteriovenous malformations, 520
   for spinal injury, 663
   for subdural hematomas, 654
Surgical clipping, 258–261
Surgical decompression
   for carpal tunnel syndrome, 729
   for median neuropathy, 739
   for spinal cord tumors, 640
   for spondylosis, 517
   for ulnar neuropathy, 739
   for ulnar tunnel syndrome, 735
Surgical resection
   for acoustic neuromas, 626
   for chordoma, 633
   for colloid cysts, 633
   for epilepsy, 284–285
   for intramedullary spinal cord tumors, 642
   for intraparenchymal hematoma, 655
   for meningioma, 624
   pathologies found in, 286
Sustentacular cells, 98
Suxamethonium, 854
Swallowing
   difficulty in, 4
      with progressive bulbar palsy, 790
   endoscopic evaluation of, 147
   esophageal phase of, 147
   glossopharyngeal and vagus nerves in, 143–152
   oral phase of, 146
   oral preparatory phase of, 146
   pharyngeal phase of, 146
   physiology of, 143–147
Swallowing center, 146–147
Swallowing disorders
   clinical presentation of, 147
   diagnosis of, 147–152
   hypoglossal nerve in, 163–167
   treatment of, 152
Swallowing reflex testing, 19
Swan-Ganz balloon catheter, 653
Sweating, 843
Sydenham chorea, 453, 455
   choreiform movements in, 458
   clinical presentation of, 457
   diagnosis of, 458
   differential diagnosis of, 456
   treatment of, 459

Sylvian fissure, blood in, 243
Sylvius, sulcus of, 42
Sympathetic ganglion, 496, 835
Sympathetic trunk, 150, 710, 711
Sympathetic trunk ganglion
   first thoracic, 8
   superior cervical, 8
Sympathomimetics, 430t
Synaptic cleft, 850, 851, 852, 853, 856, 860
Synaptic trough
   axon terminal in, 851, 852
   cross section of, 851
Synaptic vesicles, 851, 852, 860
   acetylcholine in, 853
Syncope, 278–280
   management of, 279
   neurologic causes of, 280
   psychogenic, 280
Synkinesis, 124
Synovial cysts, 682–686
Syphilis
   diagnosis of, 836
   diagnostic tests for, 141
   differential diagnosis of, 841
   neurologic deficits of, 570–573
Syphilitic meningoencephalitis, 572
Syringobulbia, 167, 526
   differential diagnosis of, 791
Syringohydromyelia, Chiari I with, 527
Syringomyelia, 38, 159, 502, 706–707
   classification of, 637t
   clinical presentation of, 526, 528
   diagnosis of, 528
   differential diagnosis of, 674, 846
   pathophysiology and etiology of, 526–528
   treatment and prognosis of, 528
Syringotomy, 528
Systemic lupus erythematosus
   differential diagnosis of, 785
   in intracerebral hemorrhage, 246
   transverse myelitis in, 509–510
Systemic necrotizing vasculitis
   differential diagnosis of, 829
   treatment of, 833
Systemic sclerosis, trigeminal involvement of, 108
Systemic vasculitis, 713–714

T

T-wave abnormalities, 256–257
Tabes dorsalis, 571, 572
   differential diagnosis of, 836
Taenia solium, *588, 589*
Tarditive dystonia, 434t
Tardive dyskinesia syndromes
   differential diagnosis of, 457–458
   drug-induced, 435–437
Tardive tremor, 430
Tardy ulnar palsy, 739
Tarsal tunnel syndrome, 752, 760
   differential diagnosis of, 750–751
Taste, 4, 146, 150
Tau, 329
   bound to microtubule, 332
   dissociated, 332
Tau gene, 414, 415t
Tau protein, pathological, 352

INDEX

Tauopathy, 352, 417–418
    sporadic, 416
Tectospinal tract, 8, 165, 498
    origin of, 500–501
Tegmen tympani, 135
Tela choroidea, 225
Temozolomide
    for anaplastic glioma, 614
    for glioblastoma multiforme, 615
Temperature neurons, 493
Temperature sensation, 499
    loss of, 526, 527
Temporal arteritis, 180, 200
    headache in, 179–181
Temporal artery, 171, 193
    deep, 189
    posterior, 72
    superficial, 188, 189
Temporal cephalalgia, 180
Temporal crescent defects, 76
Temporal dispersion, 721
Temporal fascia, 104
Temporal fossa hematoma, 649
Temporal gyrus, 42
Temporal hematoma, 239–240
Temporal lobe, 73
    acoustic area of, 136
    arterial supply to, 190–191
    "burst," 652
    clinical manifestations of infarction in, 205
    contusions of, 655
    dysfunction of, 47–48
    herniation of, 311
    inferior, lesions of, 46
    middle, 73
    surface of, 42
    testing of, 48
    tumor of, 129
    visual pathway in, 51
Temporal lobe epilepsy, 264
Temporal lobectomy, 284, 285
Temporal nerve, deep, 15, 102, 104
Temporal opercula, 42
Temporal pallor, 57, 59
Temporal pole, 42
Temporal retina, 56
Temporal retinal arteriole, 56
Temporal tumor, 269
Temporalis muscle, 104
    innervation of, 106
Temporocingulate pathway, 43
Temporomandibular joint dysfunction, 178
Temporopontine tract, 24
Tendinous ring, common, 80, 86, 87, 90
Tension headache, 177
Tensor tympani muscle, 104, 114
Tensor tympani nerve, 15, 102, 104
Tensor veli palatini muscle, 104
Tensor veli palatini nerve, 15, 102, 104
Tentorial artery, 224
Tentorial nerve, 87, 90, 103
Tentorium, 116
Tentorium cerebelli, 87, 90, 171, 224, 227
Teratoma, pineal, 633
Teres major muscle, 704
Terminal filum
    external, 494
    internal, 494

Terminal vein, anterior, 226
Terson syndrome, 249
Tetanic spasm, 796
Tetanospasmin, 594
Tetanus, 794–795
    chronic, 796
    clinical presentation of, 594
    diagnosis of, 594–596
    focal, 594
    generalized, 594
    treatment and prognosis of, 596
Tetanus immunoglobulin, 596
Tetany, drugs causing, 854t
Tetrabenazine
    for asterixis, 429
    for chorea, 459
    for tardive dyskinesia, 436–437
    for tics, 465
Tetracycline, 604, 605
    in neuromuscular transmission, 854
Tetraethylammonium, 854t
Tetraplegia, 510
Tetrodotoxin, 854t
Thalamic aphasia, 41–45, 239
Thalamic hemorrhage, 237–239
    with AVM, 242
Thalamic pain syndrome, 39
Thalamic relay nucleus, 67–69
Thalamocortical motor pathway, disruption of, 453
Thalamostriate vein, 226
    superior, 225, 226
    inferior, 227, 226
Thalamotomy
    for dystonia, 446
    for movement disorders, 476, 477
Thalamus, 73, 145, 225, 227, 403, 500
    clinical manifestations of infarction in, 205
    efferent pathway to, 766
    multiple nuclei of, 38
    pulvinar of, 71, 193, 225
    schematic representation of, 38
Thalidomide, 841
Thenar muscle, atrophy of, 728, 773
Thermoanesthesia, 502
Thiamine
    deficiency of
        in alcoholism, 394
        in Wernicke disease, 488
    for Wernicke encephalopathy, 324
Thigh
    lateral cutaneous nerve of, 710, 753, 755
    numbness and dysesthesias in, 758
    posterior cutaneous nerve of, 494, 711
Third cranial nerve palsy, diabetic, 801
Thomsen disease, 899, 909
Thoracic artery
    internal, 189
    lateral, 704
    superior, 704
Thoracic nerves
    long, 703, 704
        mononeuropathy of, 743
    vertebrae and, 497
Thoracic outlet compression neuropathy, 720, 722
Thoracic outlet syndrome
    differential diagnosis of, 736, 750–751
    epidemiology of, 716

INDEX

Thoracic radiculopathy, diabetic, 713
Thoracic spinal cord
    corticospinal tract in, 786–787
    tumors in, 637
Thoracic sympathetic ganglionic chain, 145
Thoracic vertebra, 496
Thoracoacromial artery, 704
Thoracodorsal artery, 704
Thoracodorsal nerve, 703, 704, 705
Thoracolumbar spine injury, 663
    diagnosis of, 662
Thoracotomy, 512
Threshold, visual, 7
Thrombolytic agents, 232
Thrombophlebitis, 563
Thrombosis, 196
    cerebral venous, 223–233
    platelets in, 197
Thromboxane A_2, 197
Thumb, digital nerves and arteries to, 727
Thumb shell splint, 773
Thymectomy, 869
Thyrocervical trunk, 160, 189
Thyrohyoid membrane, 154, 155
Thyrohyoid muscle, 160, 164
Thyroid artery
    inferior, 160, 189
    superior, 160, 189
Thyroid cartilage, 148, 153, 155, 189
Thyroid disease, 341
Thyroid hormone, 371
Tiagabine, 277–278
Tibial nerve, 709, 750, 751, 761
Tibial neuropathy, 751–752
Tibialis anterior muscle, 747
Tibialis posterior muscle, 751
Tic disorders
    classification of, 460–461
    clinical presentation of, 460
    differential diagnosis of, 448
    drugs causing, 434t
    pathophysiology of, 461–462
    secondary, 461t, 464–465
    syndromes of, 462–465
    treatment of, 465
Tic douloureux, 4, 106
Tick paralysis, 823
Ticlopidine, 216
Timed Up and Go Test, 132
Tinel phenomenon, 674
Tinel sign, 36, 722
    in carpal tunnel syndrome, 726–730
    in cubital tunnel syndrome, 734
Tinnitus, 137
    with acoustic neuromas, 140
    pulsatile, 138
Titanic spasm, 595
Tizanidine
    for primary lateral sclerosis, 785
    for stiff person syndrome, 798
Tolcapone, 412
Tolosa-Hunt syndrome, 83, 84
Tongue
    atrophied, 167
        with fasciculation, 789–790
        in myasthenia gravis, 791
    burning pain in, 167
    in deglutition, 148
    deviation of, 163
    dysarthria of, 156
    fasciculations on, 19
    intrinsic muscles of, 164
    mobility of, 146
    sensory fibers of, 112
    in somatic sensation, 150
    in swallowing, 144
    in taste, 146, 150
    weakness of, 166, 167
Tonic-clonic seizures
    clinical presentation of, 271
    generalized, 272
Tonsil, 144
Top of the basilar syndrome, 191, 204–207
Topiramate (Topamax)
    for action tremor, 428
    for epilepsy, 277–278
    for essential tremor, 426t
Topographical disorientation, 49
Torcular herophili, 228
Torticollis, 439, 441
    diagnosis of, 445
    in DYT7 dystonia, 442
    with trochlear palsy, 85
Total parenteral nutrition, 901–904
Touch pressure sensation, 499
Touch sensation, light, 493
Tourette syndrome, 462
    clinical presentation of, 432
    criteria for, 464t
    genetics of, 462–464
Tourettism, 464–465
Toxic excitatory amines, 658
Toxic myopathy, 891
Toxic peripheral neuropathies, 810
Toxic retinopathies, 54
Toxic vestibular damage, 480–481
Toxin-induced neuropathy, 823
Toxoplasma gondii, *589–590, 591*
    in meningitis, 588
Toxoplasmosis, 589–590, 591
Trachea, 151, 154
Tracheoesophageal groove, 154
Tracheostomy, 882
Tracheostomy-assisted mechanical ventilation, 793
Traction
    for cervical radiculopathy, 676
    for cervical spine injury, 665, 666
    in peripheral nerve compression, 717
Traction birth injury, 702
Traction board, cervical spine, 664
Tractus solitarius, 165
Transcranial Doppler imaging, 215t
Transcranial magnetic stimulation, 368
Transesophageal echocardiography (TEE), 209
    for ischemic stroke, 212
Transient ischemic attack (TIA), 199–201
    in arterial dissection, 212
    infective endocarditis with, 209
    with multiple sclerosis, 544
    preceding stroke, 211
    prophylactic treatment of, 213–216
    in syncope, 280
    vertebrobasilar, 203–204

INDEX

Transient monocular blindness, 200
    in carotid artery ischemia, 201
Transient tic disorder of childhood, 462
Transmissible spongiform encephalopathy
    clinical presentation of, 360, 361-363
    diagnostic approach to, 363
    epidemiology of, 360-361
    hereditary, 360, 363
    pathogenesis of, 361
    sporadic, 360, 363
    treatment of, 363
Transport olfactory disorders, 97
Transverse carpal ligament, 727, 728, 735
Transverse cervical artery, 160
Transverse cord lesions, complete, 501-502
Transverse myelitis, 509-511
    differential diagnosis of, 822
Transverse pontine vein, 227
Transverse sinus, 116, 194, 224, 225, 227
Transversus abdominis muscle, 710
Trapezius muscle, 157, 158, 159, 161, 184, 704
Trapezoid body, 134, 136
Trauma
    brain, 644-657
    to lumbosacral plexus, 712
    of spine and spinal cord, 503-506, 658-670
Traumatic brain injury, 657
Traumatic facial palsy, 120-121
Trazodone, 355
Tremors
    action, 423, 425
        types of, 428t
    with alcohol withdrawal, 395
    ataxic intention, 429
    in cerebellar dysfunction, 21
    classification of, 424t
    clinical presentation of, 422
    differential diagnosis of, 449
    drug-induced, 429-430
    essential, 423-427
        drugs for, 426t
        versus Parkinson tremor, 427t
    evaluation of, 23-25
    exaggerated physiologic, 422-423
    familial or hereditary, 423-424
    frequency of, 423t
    intention, 543
    isometric, 423
    kinetic, 423
    in motor disorders, 26
    orthostatic and action, 427-428
    palatal, 429
    in parkinsonism, 405, 407, 408
    pathogenesis of, 422
    pathologic, 423-431
    pathophysiology of, 423
    physiologic, 422-423
    postural, 423, 424
    psychogenic, 430-431, 473
    rest, 423, 425
    resting, 427
    senile, 424
    with Wilson disease, 466
Treponema pallidum, *138, 570, 571*
Triceps brachii muscle, 704, 733
Trichinosis, 889
Trichotillomania, 375

Tricyclic antidepressants
    for herpes zoster virus, 581-582
    for major depression, 367
    for night terrors, 294
    for pain of multiple sclerosis, 554
    for peripheral neuropathies, 807
Triethylcholine, 855t
Trigeminal ganglion, 6, 8, 15, 87, 90, 101-105, 107
    cell bodies of, 108
    neuromas of, 109
Trigeminal motor nucleus, 500, 766
Trigeminal nerve (V), 4, 83, 116, 150, 151, 224, 227
    acoustic neurinoma compressing, 110
    anatomy of, 101-106
    branches of, 102, 103
    distribution of, 5
    divisions of, 101
    in headache, 171
    herpes zoster along course of, 580, 581
    lesions of, 106-110
    mandibular division of, 101, 183
    mandibular zone of, 107
    maxillary division of, 101, 183
    mesencephalic nucleus of, 6, 105
    motor component of, 106
    motor nucleus of, 6, 105
    neuropathy of, 108
    nuclei of, 15, 101, 102
    ophthalmic division of, 101, 183, 229
    ophthalmic zone of, 107
    pain pathway of in migraine, 172
    pontine, 101
    schema of, 102
    sensory component of, 101
    sensory distribution of, 107
    sensory divisions of, 101
    sensory nucleus of, 6
    spinal nucleus of, 6, 105
    testing of, 14
    trigger points of, 107
Trigeminal neuralgia, 106, 185
    sensory distribution in, 107
    treatment of, 106
    trigger points of, 107
Trigeminal sensory neuropathy, 108
Trigeminal sensory nucleus, 500, 766
Trigeminal sensory territory, 15
Trigeminal vascular reflex, 172
Triglycerides, 917
Trihexyphenidyl, 446
Triple flexion, 35
Triple-H therapy, 256
Trisomy 21, 339
Trochlear nerve (IV), 4, 6, 83, 87, 90, 91, 105, 224, 228
    in cavernous sinus, 229
    clinical vignette of, 85
    distribution of, 5
    lesions of, 88
    schema of, 80, 86
    testing of, 11-14
Trochlear nerve (IV) palsy
    clinical presentation of, 85
    diagnosis and treatment of, 88
    differential diagnosis of, 88
    treatment of, 88
Trochlear nucleus, 6, 12, 80, 86, 91, 105
Tropical spastic paraparesis. See *HTLV-1 myelopathy*

INDEX

Tryptophan, 368
Tuberculoma, 583
Tuberculosis
    of brain and spine, 583–585
    in cranial neuropathies, 4
    epidural infection of, 686
Tuberculous meningitis, 120
    basilar, 584
Tuberous sclerosis, 270
Tufted cell, 99
Tumor necrosis factor, mediating leprosy, 841
Tumors
    of abducens nerve, 92–93
    cerebellar, 483
    control of growth of, 621
    headache in, 181
    intracranial, 270
    invading lumbosacral plexus, 712
    in lumbar radiculopathy, 686
    of optic chiasm, 66, 67
    optic radiation, 69
    of pineal region, 419
    primary sites of motor disorder in, 26
    spinal cord, 635–642
    sternocleidomastoid, 439
    trigeminal, 109–110
Tuning fork, 138
    in cranial nerve testing, 14–19
    in sensory threshold testing, 722
Twist drill drainage, 654
Two-point discrimination, 722
Tympanic cavity, 104, 114, 135, 150
    lateral wall of, 114
Tympanic membrane, 14, 114, 134, 135
    decreased mobility of, 138
Tympanic nerve, 16, 115, 150
Tympanic plexus, 16, 115, 150
Tyrosine, 406

U

Ubiquitin-C-hyrdrolase-L2, 405
Ulnar artery, 727, 735
Ulnar canal, ulnar nerve in, 728
Ulnar head, 733
Ulnar mononeuropathies, 732
    differential diagnosis of, 736
    distal, 732–736
    proximal, 732
Ulnar nerve, 703, 704, 728, 735
    communicating branch of, 727
    compression of, 720, 733
        zones and clinical signs of, 735
    deep palmar branch of, 727
    lesions of, 706
    submuscular transposition of, 734
    superficial branch of, 727
Ulnar neuropathy, 739
Ulnar tunnel, 733
    compression neuropathy at, 722
Ulnar tunnel syndrome, 735
Ultrasonography
    advantages and disadvantages of, 215t
    for cerebral vasospasm, 256
    for ischemic stroke, 212
    for mononeuropathies with lower extremity weakness, 754
Uncal herniation, 311

Uncal vein, 225
Uncinate crises, 100
Uncus, 96, 99
Upper limb, dermatomes and myotomes of, 673
Upper motor neuron dysfunction, 113
Upper respiratory infections, 566
Urinary incontinence, 540–541, 543, 554–555
Urinary urgency, 775t
Utricle, 114, 127, 135
Uvular paralysis, 20

V

V1 area
    cells of, 76
    cortical magnification in, 74–75
    specialization of, 75
V2 area, 76
V3 area, 76
V4 area, 76
V6 area, 76
Vaccine, bacterial meningitis, 565
Vagal nucleus, 105
    dorsal, 6
Vagus nerve (X), 4, 6, 105, 158, 160, 224, 844
    auricular branch of, 183
    branches of, 151, 154
    caudal fibers of, 159
    distribution of, 5
    dorsal motor nucleus of, 500, 766
    inferior ganglion of, 158, 164
    in larynx, 155
    paralysis of, 20
    pharyngeal branch of, 150
    posterior nucleus of, 105
    schema of, 151, 154
    stimulation of for depression, 368
    stimulator of, 286
    superior ganglion of, 158
    in swallowing, 143–152, 144
    testing of, 19
    in voice disorders, 153–156
Vallecula, 148, 149
Valproate
    in carnitine deficiency, 901–904
    for cortical myoclonus, 452
    for tardive dyskinesia, 436–437
Valproic acid
    for action tremor, 428
    for bipolar disorder, 370–371
Valsalva maneuver, 846
Valsalva syncope, 278
Valsalva test, 182
Valve replacement, thrombus formation in, 208
Valvular thrombus, 208
Vancomycin, 564
Varicella vaccination, 579
Varicella-zoster virus
    in Bell palsy, 117
    in facial palsy, 119
    latent, 108, 579
    with probable keratitis, 109
    reactivation of, 579–581
Vascular cognitive impairment, 356
Vascular compromise, retinal, 54
Vascular dementia
    clinical presentation of, 356, 357–358
    differential diagnosis of, 357–358

INDEX

epidemiology of, 356-357
  prevention and treatment of, 358-359
Vascular headache, 249
Vascular malformations, 239
Vasculitic neuropathy
  differential diagnosis of, 829
  pathogenesis of, 719
Vasculitic plexopathy, 713-714
Vasculitis
  differential diagnosis of, 830t
  in intracerebral hemorrhage, 246
Vasculitis neuropathy, 833
Vasovagal cardiac reflex syncope, 278
Vasovagal edema, 246
Vasovagal syncope, 278
Vastus intermedius muscle, 753
Vastus lateralis muscle, 753
Vastus medialis muscle, 753
VDRL test, 571
Vecuronium, 855t
Vegetations, 208
Vegetative state, persistent, 32, 304-306, 319
  in brain death, 319
  with diffuse axonal or shear injury, 655-657
Vena cava, inferior, 501
Venlafaxine
  for lateral femoral nerve neuropathy, 759
  for peripheral neuropathies, 807
  for sensory neuropathies of lower extremity, 760
Venous hypertension, 517
Venous plexus, internal vertebral, 496
Venous sinuses
  draining into jugular vein, 228
  normal, 224
Venous thrombosis, 521
Ventilatory failure
  in motor neuron disease, 791-792
  treatment of, 793
Ventral horns, 766
Ventral motor roots, 493
Ventral nerve root, 835
Ventral parietal area (VP), 76
Ventral ramus, 496, 835
  in situ, 494
Ventral root, 496
  filaments of, 495
Ventricle
  fourth, 165, 227, 226
  lateral, 71, 193, 225, 226
  third, 225, 226
Ventricular aneurysm, 208
Ventricular fold, 148
Ventricular vein, inferior, 226
Ventriculoperitoneal shunt, 489
Ventromedial tegmentum lesions, 423
Verapamil, 175
  nerve terminal uptake of, 857
Vermian hemorrhage, 240
Vermian vein
  inferior, 227
  superior, 227
Vertebrae, 493, 494
  cross sections through, 496
  fracture and dislocation of, 668
  fractures of, 660
  lumbar, 835
  spinal nerve roots in relation to, 497

Vertebral angiograms, 227
Vertebral artery, 160, 189, 193
  anterior meningeal branch of, 189
  occlusion of, 198
Vertebral disc, extruded, 506
Vertebral tuberculosis, 585
Vertebrobasilar artery, 171
  extracranial, 191
  intracranial, 191
  occlusion of, 195
Vertebrobasilar cerebral artery, 188
Vertebrobasilar embolus, 867
Vertebrobasilar ischemia, 206, 486
Vertebrobasilar occlusion, 202-207
Vertebrobasilar stroke, 140
Vertebrobasilar system ischemia, 204t
Vertical conjugate gaze, center for, 14
Vertigo, 126
  causes of, 129
  in CNS disorders, 128
  evaluation for, 488
  hearing loss with, 137
  in multiple sclerosis, 541-542
  nonpharmacologic therapy for, 132-133
  peripheral nervous system disorders, 128
  positional test for, 18
  testing of, 131
  types of, 130
  with vertebrobasilar ischemia, 206
Vestibular damage, 480-481
Vestibular function, 4
Vestibular ganglion, 114, 127
Vestibular nerve (VIII), 4, 12, 91, 114, 116, 135
  anatomy of, 126-128
  in cerebral afferent pathway, 33
  clinical vignette of, 126
  CNS disorders of, 128
  disorders of
    diagnostic approach to, 130-132
    treatment of, 132-133
  peripheral nervous system disorders of, 128
  peripheral vestibulopathies of, 129-130
  testing of, 14-19
Vestibular neuritis, 130
Vestibular neuronitis, 541
Vestibular nucleus, 6, 12, 91, 105, 114
  lateral, 500-501
Vestibular-ocular reflex, 14, 130
Vestibular receptors, 127
Vestibular schwannoma, 140. See also *Acoustic neuroma*
Vestibular system, 127-128
  bilateral problems of, 130
  testing of, 11, 19
Vestibule, 135
Vestibulocochlear nerve, 6, 105, 114, 135, 224, 227
  anatomy of, 126-128, 134
  cochlear division of, 136
  distribution of, 5
  neuritis of, 129
Vestibulopathy, chronic, 130
Vestibulospinal tract, 498, 499
  lateral, 786, 787
  origin of, 500-501
Vibration sensation
  impaired, 36, 502
  loss of
    with B_{12} vitamin deficiency, 532

INDEX

with Friedreich ataxia, 534
in peripheral neuropathy, 801
in spinal cord degeneration, 533
in spondylosis, 516
Video electroencephalographic analysis, 281
Videofluoroscopy, 147–152
Videopharyngogram, 147–152
Vincristine
for length-dependent polyneuropathy, 816
for low-grade gliomas, 613
Violence, alcohol-related, 391
Viral infections
audiometric testing in, 141
of nervous system, 574–582
Vision, 4
blurred, 7
loss of, 7
monocular, 59
Visual acuity screening, 7
Visual agnosia, 51–52
Visual association cortex, 73
anatomy of, 72–75
clinical vignette of, 72
diseases of, 75–76
extrastriate association, 76
optic pathways of, 68
research on, 76
topographic organization of, 72–75
vascular supply of, 72
Visual disturbances, 541, 542
Visual evoked responses, 548–549
Visual field
central, 74
contralateral deficit of, 49
defects of, 64, 75–76
from anterior optic nerve disease, 57
in cerebral aneurysm, 251
macular sparing in, 76
evaluation of, 4, 7
in glaucoma, 60
information from, 72–74
loss of
progressive, 67
retinal pattern of, 54
overlapping, 9, 70
with papilledema, 11
temporal crescent of, 75
Visual hallucinations, 322
in dementia with Lewy bodies, 349
Visual information processing, hierarchy of, 75
Visual pathways, 9
in parietal and temporal lobes, 51
Visual receptors, 55
Visual/somatosensory interface, 76
Visual-spatial functions, 44
Vital signs, deterioration in, 648
Vitrectomy, 79
Vitreous chamber, 56
Vocal cord weakness
in distal myopathy, 907t
Vocal cords
dystonia of, 441
examination of, 19
Vocal fatigue, 156
Vocal folds, 148, 154, 155
paralysis of, 155
Vocal tics, 460

Voice disorders
causes of, 155–156
recurrent laryngeal nerve in, 154–156
superior laryngeal nerve in, 156
vagus nerve in, 153–156
Volar carpal ligament, 735
Voltage-gated calcium channel (VGCC) antibodies, 858–859
Voluntary movement, spinal tracts for, 493–500
Vomiting, with vertebrobasilar ischemia, 206
von Economo disease, 409
von Recklinghausen disease, 640
Vorticose vein, 56

W

Wada test, 284
for epilepsy, 278, 281–282, 283
Wakefulness, 554
Wallenberg syndrome, 191, 204
clinical manifestations of, 204t
Warfarin
for cardioembolism, 207
for cerebral venous thrombosis, 232
for TIAs and stroke, 216
Weakness
in acute or subacute myopathies, 884–891
clinical documentation of, 28t
episodic, 909–913
fluctuating, in myasthenia gravis, 865
generalized, 892–905
grading, 27–30
with Lambert-Eaton myasthenic syndrome, 874
with mononeuropathies, 723
muscle, 25–30
in myasthenia gravis, 866
in myopathies, 874t, 875t
regional patterns of, 876t
sudden onset of, 28
Weber syndrome, 81
Weber test, 17, 19, 134, 139
Wegener granulomatosis
in facial paralysis, 120
in intracerebral hemorrhage, 246
Weight loss, 521
Welander myopathy, 907t
Werdnig-Hoffmann disease, 30
Wernicke aphasia, 45, 46, 47–48
Wernicke encephalopathy, 324
coma in, 300
gait disorders in, 488
Wernicke syndrome, 394
West Nile virus, 578–579
West syndrome, 274–275
Wheelchairs, 669
Whiplash, 666
Whipple disease, 488
White commissure, anterior, 498, 786, 787
White matter, 493
spinal, 495, 498
White ramus communicans, 8, 495, 496, 710, 844
White thrombus, 197
Willis, circle of, 64, 190, 193
3-D reconstructed image of, 213
Wilson disease, 443
clinical presentation of, 466–467
diagnosis of, 468–470
dystonia in, 445

NEUROLOGY

979

INDEX

genetics of, 467–468
hepatic copper metabolism in, 467
treatment and prognosis of, 470–471
Wiring, of cervical spinous processes, 667
Withdrawal response, 35
Word list testing, 48
Wrisberg, intermediate nerve of, 112
Wrist
    compression neuropathy at, 722
    median neuropathies at, 739
    orthotic devices for in cervical spine rehabilitation, 669
    splinting of in motor neuron disease, 773
Wrist drop, 25, 723
    with radial nerve compression, 738
Writer's cramp, 442

X
Xerostomia, 886

Y
Yaws, 841
Yoga, 554
Yohimbine, 847

Z
Zidovudine (AZT)
    in carnitine deficiency, 901–904
    in toxic myopathies, 887
Zinc acetate, 470–471
Zinn-Haller, vascular circle of, 58
Zona incerta, 403
Zonisamide, 277–278
Zoster sin herpete, 581
Zygomatic nerve, 15, 80, 86, 102, 103
Zygomaticofacial nerve, 15, 102, 103, 107, 183
Zygomaticotemporal nerve, 15, 102, 103, 107, 183
Zygomaticus major muscle, 16, 115
Zygomaticus minor muscle, 16, 115